# DON'T GO TO THE COSMETICS COUNTER WITHOUT ME

Completely Revised and Updated **5**th EDITION

*A Unique Guide to Over 30,000 Products, plus the Latest Skin-Care Research*

# PAULA BEGOUN

Copy Editors: Sigrid Asmus, Kris Fulsaas, and Nicole Turgeon
Art Direction, Cover Design, and Typography: Erin Bloom, Beginning Press
Printing: Publishers Press
Research Assistants: Nicole Turgeon and Kathy Siegler
Contributing Editor and Writer: Bryan Barron

Copyright © 1991, 1992, 1993, 1994, 1995, 1996, 1997, 1998, 1999, 2001
by Paula Begoun

Publisher:        Beginning Press
                  13075 Gateway Drive, Suite 160
                  Seattle, Washington 98168

First Printing for this edition: January 2001

ISBN              1-877988-28-6
                  1 2 3 4 5 6 7 8 9 10

This book is distributed to the United States book trade by:
                  Publishers Group West
                  1700 Fourth Street
                  Berkeley, CA 94710
                  (800) 788-3123

and to the Canadian book trade by:
                  Raincoast Books
                  8680 Cambie Street
                  Vancouver, B.C. V6P 6M9
                  (800) 663-5714

# Also by Paula Begoun

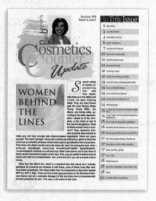

**Cosmetics Counter Update newsletter**

Keep up with the ever-changing cosmetics industry with Paula's bimonthly newsletter. Each issue includes the latest product reviews, full evaluations of new lines, clear explanations of new research and studies, and "Dear Paula" questions that cover a wide variety of skin, makeup, and hair-related topics.

1-Year Subscription (6 issues):
$25 US, $35 Canada, $45 Other Countries

**Don't Go Shopping for Hair Care Products Without Me, 2nd Edition**

Everything you always wanted to know about hair products but were afraid to ask your stylist! Over 4,000 product reviews to help you find which products work and which are a waste of your money!

$19.95, 642 pgs.

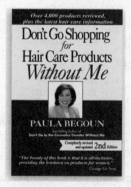

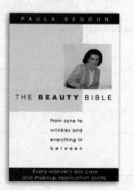

**The Beauty Bible: From Acne to Wrinkles and Everything in Between**

An in-depth guide to understanding what your skin needs and how to perfect your skin-care routine, as well as step-by-step instruction for flawless, easy makeup application.

$16.95, 382 pgs.

Visit www.CosmeticsCop.com for a complete product list, or call (800) 831-4088 to request a free catalog.
(Order form on next page.)

❏ 1 Year **Cosmetics Counter Update** (US)      $25.00 _____

❏ 1 Year **Cosmetics Counter Update** (Canada)      $35.00 _____

❏ 1 Year **Cosmetics Counter Update** (All Other Countries)      $45.00 _____

❏ e-mail Subscription to **Cosmetics Counter Update**      $12.50 _____

     **e-mail address** _____

❏ One-Time Introductory copy of **Cosmetics Counter Update**      $ 1.00 _____

❏ *The Beauty Bible*      $16.95 _____

❏ *Don't Go Shopping for Hair Care Products Without Me*, 2nd Edition      $19.95 _____

❏ *Don't Go to the Cosmetics Counter Without Me*, 5th Edition      $24.95 _____

❏ Paula's Choice/Paula's Select brochure      **FREE**

❏ Paula's e-mail Beauty Bulletin      **FREE**

     **e-mail address** _____

| | If your order totals | Add | |
|---|---|---|---|
| **Shipping Charges** | $ 0.00–$12.99 | $3.50 | **All Prices Are Listed in U.S. Funds** |
| | $13.00–$20.00 | $5.00 | |
| | $20.01–$40.00 | $6.00 | **Subtotal** _____ |
| | $40.01–$60.00 | $7.00 | |
| | $60.01–$80.00 | $8.00 | **WA State Residents Add 8.6% Sales Tax** _____ |
| | $80.01–$100.00 | $9.00 | **Shipping (for book orders only)** _____ |
| | $100.01 and up | $10.00 | **TOTAL** _____ |
| | **No shipping charges for newsletter** | | |

❏ My check or money order is enclosed. Make payable to Beginning Press and send your order to **Beginning Press, 13075 Gateway Drive, #160, Seattle, WA 98168.**

❏ Please charge my credit card (account number listed below)

**Printed Name** _____

**Address** _____

_____

**Phone #** _____

**Signature** _____

**Credit Card #** _____    **Expiration Date** _____

(Visa, MasterCard, American Express, and Discover Accepted)

# Call (800) 831-4088 to order now
## www.CosmeticsCop.com

DG5AI

# From the Publisher

Paula Begoun is the best-selling author of *Don't Go to the Cosmetics Counter Without Me, The Beauty Bible, Don't Go Shopping for Hair Care Products Without Me,* and *Blue Eyeshadow Should Be Illegal.* She has sold more than 2.5 million books, educating women about the facts and secrets the beauty industry doesn't want them to know.

Ms. Begoun is also a syndicated journalist with Knight-Ridder News Tribune Service, and her weekly "Dear Paula" column has been gaining popularity across the country in such newspapers as the *New York Daily News.*

Paula is nationally recognized as a consumer advocate for the cosmetics and hair-care industries. She is called upon regularly by reporters and producers from television, newspapers, magazines, and radio as a cosmetics industry expert. She has appeared on hundreds of talk shows over the years, including *DateLine NBC, Good Morning America, 20/20, Leeza,* the *Today* show, *Later Today, CBS Morning News, Hard Copy, Canada AM,* and *National Public Radio,* and has made more than 13 appearances on the *Oprah Winfrey* show. With the success of Paula's Web site, www.CosmeticsCop.com, women all over the world consider Paula the most reliable source for straightforward information about all their beauty questions.

In 1996 Ms. Begoun launched her own line of skin-care products called Paula's Choice and Paula's Select. This distinctive line of products is renowned for its effectiveness and affordability. While Paula is proud of her line, she realizes that there are vast numbers of product options for women to consider. As a result she continues to impart substantiated and documented studies and analysis about skin care and makeup products from other lines based on her extensive research and years of experience. There are as many "happy faces" as there are "unhappy" and "neutral" faces in this edition. It is clear that Paula maintains her evenhanded approach to her reviews and critiques offering readers an unprecedented assortment of choices for their cosmetic purchases.

# Publisher's Disclaimer

The intent of this book is to present the author's ideas and perceptions about the marketing, selling, and use of cosmetics. The author's sole purpose is to present consumer information and advice regarding the purchase of makeup and skin-care products. The information and recommendations presented strictly reflect the author's opinions, perceptions, and knowledge about the subject and products mentioned. Some women may find success with a particular product that is not recommended or even mentioned in this book, or they may be partial to a $250 skin-care routine. It is everyone's unalienable right to judge products by their own criteria and to disagree with the author.

More important, because everyone's skin can, and probably will, react to an external stimulus at some time, any product could cause a negative reaction on skin at one time or another. If you develop a skin sensitivity to a cosmetic, stop using it immediately and consult your physician. If you need medical advice about your skin, it is best to consult a dermatologist.

# Acknowledgments

I want to personally thank Nicole Turgeon, my research assistant, and Bryan Barron, a contributing editor and writer for this edition, for their dedication and loyalty to getting this book to print. Their skills and focus were truly a godsend. Without their feedback, patience, and contributions, this book would absolutely not have been possible.

# Contents

## Chapter Three— Product-by-Product Reviews

# Contents

# Contents

# Contents

## *Chapter Four—Baby's Skin-Care Products*

# Contents

# More questions?

# www.CosmeticsCop.com

13075 Gateway Drive, #160,   Seattle, WA  98168   (800) 831-4088

# Introduction

## From Paula

Those of you who are familiar with my books *Blue Eyeshadow Should Be Illegal, The Beauty Bible,* and previous editions of *Don't Go to the Cosmetics Counter Without Me;* subscribe to my newsletter *Cosmetics Counter Update;* read my syndicated newspaper column *Dear Paula;* or who have seen me on television know that I have strong feelings about the quality of information, marketing tactics, and types of products the cosmetics industry provides for women. From every corner of the industry, there are extensive research and documentation proving that the $45 billion-a-year cosmetics industry gives women misleading, deceptive, and often just plain false information. Whether it comes from cosmetics advertising, cosmetics salespeople, cosmetics companies' brochures, or so-called editorial pieces in fashion magazines, distorted, inaccurate, and specious explanations about skin-care and makeup products are continually being created and publicized. I have spent my career (over 20 years in the cosmetics industry) providing women with the information and substantiation to debunk all this, while showcasing the truly wonderful and helpful products that do exist. I hope this edition will help you travel wisely through the wide, ever more complicated world of cosmetics one more time.

## How I Got Started

I often marvel at how I happened into this unusual line of work. It's not as if you can answer an ad for this kind of job, and clearly the cosmetics industry and fashion magazines aren't interested in hiring someone to do what I do. Yet, as a result of interviews with and feedback from thousands and thousands of women over the years, it became clear to me that this kind of work needed to be done.

I started in 1977, when I took my first job at a department-store makeup counter to supplement my income as a freelance makeup artist. As a young makeup artist in Washington, D.C., I had built up a list of celebrity clients and was doing quite well, both financially and professionally. I found the artistry of creating beautiful makeup styles for women intriguing, and the world of fashion and glamour thoroughly exciting. At the age of 24, I was thrilled with my career. My clients wanted only me, and they were some of the most powerful and formidable women in Washington, D.C. But, as with any business, it had its ups and downs, and shoring up my income once in a while became necessary. A store at a mall in Silver Spring, Maryland, had an opening for a cosmetics salesperson. They hired me on the spot because, I was told, I looked the part, wearing nice makeup and dressing well. Amazingly, they weren't interested in my makeup experience.

Even back then I knew something was awry with a substantial number of cosmetics and the advertising for them, particularly in the skin-care area. Having struggled for years with oily skin and acne, I knew from personal experience that astringents didn't close pores, products claiming not to cause breakouts made me break out, and most products that promised to clear up acne only made my skin more red and irritated. I didn't yet know all the technical details of why this was so, but it was blatantly obvious that plenty of mascaras with claims of being flakeproof weren't, and that creams purporting to eliminate scarring and lighten "age spots" didn't. More often than not, the claims made about what the products would do rarely matched their performance. However, while it seemed unquestionable that much of the cosmetics industry was grossly misrepresenting its products, at the time I had no way to confirm my suspicions.

On my first day, I was assigned to work behind the counters for Calvin Klein (Klein had a makeup line then that lasted only a brief period; it was resurrected in 1999) and Elizabeth Arden. With no previous training or information about these lines, I was told to sell the products. I did the best I could. Unfortunately, my notion of how to help customers was completely different from that of the other salespeople and the line manager. My first mistake was telling several customers not to bother using an astringent because alcohol-based products could cause something called a "rebound effect." By irritating the skin, these products could actually stimulate oil production and make oily skin worse. Instead I recommended 3% hydrogen peroxide, available then for 50 cents at the drugstore. By the end of the second day, the woman working next to me was mortified. She called in the line representative, who made it clear that I should keep my personal opinions to myself and just sell the products. I said I would do my best. This was only my second day! Things had to get better, I thought. They didn't.

After I complained that the two lines I was assigned to didn't always have the best makeup colors or skin-care products for every woman I talked to, the cosmetics manager told me, "All the customer wants to know is what you tell her; the customers never ask questions, because they trust our products." Several disagreements later, I was out of a job.

Shortly after that incident, I read *The Great American Skin Game* by Toni Stabile. It changed my life. This landmark book conveyed in clear, concise terms the processes and techniques the cosmetics industry uses to sell hope to gullible and uninformed consumers. In fact, Ms. Stabile was largely responsible for proposing many present-day FDA regulations, including advertising guidelines, safety regulations, and mandatory ingredient lists. Her work confirmed what I had already reasoned must be true, and significantly changed the way I approached cosmetics.

Although it sounds a bit melodramatic, I couldn't continue selling something I knew to be a waste of money or bad for the skin. Consumers (including myself) deserved better. I wasn't anti-makeup—just the opposite—but I was (and am) anti-hype and against misleading information. As one newspaper reporter recently commented, "She's not Mother Teresa, but it does seem to be just Ms. Begoun against these huge cosmetics companies." Thus I took my first steps on a long career path—longer than I ever imagined—that went from owning my own cosmetics stores to working as a TV news reporter to owning my own publishing company, and back to owning my own skin-care company. With every step, my goal has been to do what it takes to find out and expose the truth behind the ads and the literally unbelievable claims thrown about by the cosmetics world. After all, one good sales pitch about an "exclusive patented secret" or a revolutionary new formula, and your pocketbook could easily be lighter—by $50 to $250 and up to $500—for a 1-ounce jar of standard cosmetic ingredients or ingredients that can't possibly live up to the claims made for them.

I know that I can't stop the cosmetics industry from force-feeding consumers an endless stream of products and misleading or erroneous claims and information, but I also know there are enough women who are interested in seeing the other side of the picture to motivate me to continue to do what I do. Knowing the "rest of the story" can help make you feel and look more beautiful in the long run.

"Inner beauty is priceless.

Outer beauty doesn't have to be."

Paula Begoun

# CHAPTER ONE

# Beauty in Conflict

What I do is controversial. I've known it almost since the beginning, when at my first cosmetics job I told a customer that "astringents can't close pores, and if they could, why would anyone still have pores—wouldn't they all be closed by now?" I knew I was in a precarious position. No doubt there were going to be salespeople who wouldn't be thrilled by my comments, and without question throngs of cosmetics company executives would be disturbed by someone challenging their claims.

Yet what I say or write is not unknown to those in the industry (at least not those involved in serious skin-care and makeup research and formulation). I draw my conclusions from many well-known cosmetics industry sources, which I encourage all of you to check out for yourselves. My primary references for the conclusions drawn and assessments used throughout this book are from *Drug and Cosmetics Industry* magazine, *Cosmetics & Toiletries* magazine, and *The Rose Sheet*. All of these are industry publications that report on or review ongoing cosmetics research, U.S. government's Food and Drug Administration (FDA) regulations, the creation and critique of formulations, and opinions from the people who make the products. I also constantly refer to medical journals such as *Cosmetic Dermatology, The Journal of the American Medical Association, The New England Journal of Medicine*, and *The Lancet* (a British medical research journal), as well as press releases from the American Academy of Dermatology, and published studies from the biochemistry world found in *The Blue Sheet* (a health and biomedical publication).

Two must-read sources for every cosmetics consumer are the FDA's Web site at www.FDA.gov and the medical research site www.Medscape.com. I also use several dermatology journal Web sites, including the *Dermatology Online Journal* at http://www.matrix.ucdavis.edu/DOJdesk/desk.html and the *American Academy of Dermatology* at www.AAD.org. Published, peer-reviewed* information is integral to my work, but I also spend a great deal of time interviewing cosmetics chemists, dermatologists, cosmetics ingredient manufacturers, biochemists, oncologists, and plastic surgeons. This accumulated research provides me with abundant sources of information that you may not get a chance to hear because the fashion magazines just leave out any information that their cosmetics advertisers don't agree with.

(*Note: Essentially, the peer-review process is a quality control mechanism for medical, academic, technical, research, and professional journals to assure that the articles they publish contain research and data that meet precise standards of objective and ethical scientific methodology.)

Despite the work I cite, I have been called everything from a charlatan to someone who has nothing more than a vendetta against the cosmetics industry, with no substantiation or proof backing up what I say (I guess ignoring credible sources is the only way to prove anyone wrong). Yet I truly feel that it only takes a quick perusal of this book's Appendix for someone to realize that I have extensive resources and data for my comments. The fundamental research I base my evaluations on is well documented and the specifics are detailed in my work.

I also receive complaints (particularly from cosmetics salespeople) saying I hate all cosmetics except my own products. Yet a quick flip through the pages of my book clearly reveals that I recommend hundreds and hundreds of products. Women who have written me often comment that they notice that people who sell cosmetics usually find my work both awful *and* wonderful. My book is considered insightful and helpful when I recommend the products they sell, but if I suggest that some of the products in their line are a waste of money or potentially damaging to skin, then their opinion is that I don't know what I'm talking about and that I should mind my own business.

While those in the cosmetics industry protest that I don't like anything, paradoxically I also get letters from readers objecting to my long lists of "best products." I am constantly asked to narrow the field to my absolute ten favorites in each category.

I've also received criticism for making my recommendations too complicated and convoluted. How ironic! The cosmetics industry has no problem with their hundreds of lines and thousands of products all claiming identical miracles of one sort or another. And I'm the one making it complicated? Sigh.

Do I hate the cosmetics industry? Hardly. I am in constant awe of the spectacular quality and performance in relation to a multitude of remarkable skin-care and makeup products. What I hate are the ludicrous claims, disproportionate prices, and the products that can hurt skin or mislead the consumer into taking poor care of the skin.

What is difficult for me to comprehend is why so many women give carte blanche belief to what the cosmetics industry tells them. It doesn't seem to cause any doubts or skepticism for women when cosmetics lines repeatedly have new miracle products every few months (but never tell us what was wrong with their previous products because they keep selling them). Lots of women can't wait to buy the products a celebrity claims to use or is selling, because it seems to be accepted as fact that being beautiful means you must know about product quality or what is best for skin care.

After the incessant hype and marketing distortion that accompany all of this, and despite the inevitable disappointment (if we weren't disappointed, the same lines wouldn't keep creating new antiwrinkle, acne, or myriad other skin-care items), we still buy whatever the next impressive ad or celebrity is selling—and repeat this pattern season after season, year after year.

There is a part of me that struggles with what I do. Not that I don't find the work rewarding, because I do. The wonderful feedback I get from thousands of readers touches me deeply in ways I can't even begin to describe. In spite of that, it still isn't easy being the pariah of the cosmetics industry. I am truly dedicated to providing accurate and complete information about skin care and makeup to help you, the consumer, make educated, wise decisions about your purchases. You may not agree with me, but at least you will have someone else's voice in your ear saying, "Here is research or data showing this product won't work or is bad for skin" or "Consider that this other far less expensive product is better than the expensive one you're looking at" or "It isn't worth the money but at least the product is good for your skin"—and then you can make up your own mind about what works best for you. I believe this is far better than basing a decision on the thousands of never-ending, incessant claims that "our product cures or gets rid of (whatever you don't like about your skin)."

## *Knowledge Is Beautiful*

*Have you ever purchased an antiwrinkle cream that didn't get rid of your wrinkles?*

*Did you every buy a product to get rid of puffy eyes but it didn't work?*

*Have you ever bought an all-day lipstick that didn't last all day?*

*Have you used oil-control products that didn't control oil?*

*Have you purchased more than five different products that claimed they would make you "look younger"?*

*Have you ever applied a foundation claiming to reflect light in such a way that your wrinkles wouldn't be so noticeable only to find that they still were completely noticeable?*

*Do you watch infomercials selling cosmetics and skin-care products and believe what they're saying is true, especially if it's from a celebrity?*

*Have you tried a product claiming to be hypoallergenic only to find you did have an allergic reaction?*

*Have you ever purchased a product claiming to be noncomedogenic and oil-free and found that you had breakouts after using it?*

If you answered yes to any of these questions, you definitely need the information in this book. I'd like to share with you the following letter from a reader that rather nicely sums up how I feel about my book and the overall work I do.

*Dear Paula,*

I just finished reading your book *Don't Go to the Cosmetics Counter Without Me*, and I have to admit that I'm a little depressed. You wouldn't believe what I (roughly) calculated that I have spent on ineffective, outrageously priced cosmetics purchased over the last two decades. (I guess you would believe it, given your experience, but it shocked the heck out of me!) The number of wasted dollars totals in the thousands (several of them), and makes my mild malaise more than understandable. I've regrouped only because I'm the kind of person who tends to look forward, not behind me, and now that I have you, I am bouncing back.

My quick recovery is due to the fact that I feel educated and armed to deal with the cosmetics companies in a manner that I did not think was possible. As a sales and marketing executive myself, in another industry, I always knew that I was being sold to by claims of questionable validity. However, cosmetics advertising is so damn slick and convincing that even I, seasoned professional that I am, just wasn't able to stop myself!

I have just ordered your book on hair-care products, and I am already beginning to brace myself for the ugly truth (though I know it will be beautiful and liberating in the long run). I know I'm going to start calculating the wasted money there, just like I did when I read your book on cosmetics, and, understandably, I'm getting a little nervous. Thank you, and keep up the great work. You are providing an invaluable consumer service. I only wish I had found you years ago!

**Depressed but Smarter**

This edition of *Don't Go to the Cosmetics Counter Without Me* presents product-by-product reviews of cosmetics from almost 250 of the most popular lines, which is 75 more lines (and thousands more products) than I covered in the last edition of the book.

If you've ever felt uncertain about a product, or too short of time or energy to figure out for yourself which foundations are too pink or too orange, which eyeshadows are too shiny or too difficult to use, which powders went on too chalky, which cleansers are too greasy, which toners are too harsh, what makes one moisturizer different from another, or how wrinkle creams differ, look no further. As you read the reviews in this book, you will start to get a better understanding of how the cosmetics industry really works. I've also included a summary chapter of best finds and best buys, but don't jump to that one first. It is important to read the individual product reviews so you understand *exactly* what you are buying. I might recommend 20 good mascaras, but each one might be good for a different reason.

In the reviews, each product is described in terms of its reliability, value, texture, application, and effect. Within every category of product—foundations, mascaras, blushes, eyeshadows, concealers, pressed powders, lipsticks, and pencils—I have established specific criteria, and I evaluate products using those standards. For example, a foundation meant for someone with oily skin, according to my criteria, should be matte, contain minimal to no greasy or emollient ingredients, blend easily, leave a smooth, even finish, and have no blatant ingredients known to cause breakouts. All foundations must match skin tones exactly; they cannot be any noticeable shade of orange, peach, rose, pink, or ash, because people are not orange, peach, rose, pink, or ash. I made similar determinations for mascaras, blushes, eyeshadows, concealers, pressed powders, lipsticks, and pencils. I relied on my more than 20 years as a professional makeup artist to help establish guidelines for the quality of a product and its application.

Skin-care products were evaluated almost entirely by analyzing the ingredient list and comparing it to the claims made about the product. If a toner asserts that it is designed for sensitive skin, it shouldn't contain ingredients that irritate the skin. If a moisturizer claims it can hydrate the skin, it should contain ingredients that can do just that. In addition, I have made a point of challenging the inflated claims made about such ingredients as yeast, herbal extracts, botanicals, seaweed extracts, placenta extracts, alpha hydroxy acids, vitamins, DNA, RNA, hyaluronic acid, liposomes, and other much-hyped ingredients. I also explain why some of these and other seemingly impressive-sounding ingredients might indeed benefit the skin, but more complete explanations for product claims and miracle ingredients are found in my book *The Beauty Bible*.

## *Due Diligence*

I can't stress enough how much time and effort my staff and I put into gathering our information. We are diligent about making sure we incorporate accurate and precise information or research for all of the products we review. To accomplish this, the first order of business with every edition is to contact every cosmetics company I'm including to ask them for their data or facts regarding any of their products or claims. We called every company, asking them to please send whatever they could regarding their products. It is always shocking to me how few companies are even willing to send their product list, let alone any research or studies substantiating their claims. And then there are those companies that actually say they don't provide information to Paula Begoun (a dubious distinction) and many that just never return our calls. Often we simply receive a press release without any other piece of information. Unbelievable!

Let me state clearly that I am more than open to presenting any documented research that substantiates information contradicting something I've stated. I am more than willing to alter previously stated opinions and positions as new research comes to light showing that earlier information is no longer correct. For example, over the years I have changed my opinion on sunscreens with regard to the new research on UVA protection. I have modified my attitude toward antioxidants, too, given the growing body of literature establishing the positives of these ingredients for skin care (not that they are miracles or will erase wrinkles, but they do have strong benefits that make them worthwhile for skin). I have been more open to layering products when different active ingredients are needed. I could go on, but I want to be explicit about my desire to present the most up-to-date, currently published research that exists when it comes to skin-care formulations and makeup products.

I want to thank the companies that did take the time to send me their information. While I may not agree on the quality of all their products or their advertising claims, their help was more than appreciated. The following companies are the only ones that provided me with full details and information regarding the products they sell:

Alpha Hydrox, Aqua Glycolic, Avon, Awake, bare escentuals, BeautiControl, Black Opal, CamoCare, Chanel, Clear LogiX, Color Me Beautiful, Dermablend, Dove, Dr. Mary Lupo, FACE Stockholm, Fancl, Flori Roberts, Guerlain, Iman, Jan Marini, Kiss My Face, Lip Ink, Models Prefer, Neostrata/Exuviance, Nivea Visage, Nu Skin USA, N.V. Perricone, M.D., Olay, Oxy Balance, philosophy, Pond's, Reflect.com, Renee Guinot Skincare, Sea Breeze, Shaklee, SkinCeuticals, Sothys, St. Ives, Suave, T. Le Clerc, Tony & Tina, Trish McEvoy, Youngblood, and Zia Natural Skin Care.

## *What You Aren't Told*

Cosmetics companies and cosmetics salespeople often attempt to defend their claims or products by spreading false information, particularly around the issue of ingredients. It is typical to hear the familiar refrain about how every product being sold is all natural and contains no chemicals or synthetic ingredients, which presupposes that chemicals and synthetic ingredients are inherently really bad for skin. For me to suggest that this is a completely bogus notion is an understatement: it is actually completely far-fetched. First, *everything* from water to herbal extracts to fragrance and minerals in a cosmetic is a "chemical." After a substance is extracted from a plant, preserved, and mixed with other "natural" and "unnatural" ingredients, the notion that it is still related to what came from the ground is ludicrous. How many skin-care or makeup products are you willing to sprinkle on your salad anyway? Second, there is plenty of research establishing that many synthetic ingredients are superior for the health of skin and preferred over botanical elements. Third—and this is a biggie—everything natural isn't good for the skin (think of poison ivy or ragweed), anymore than everything synthetic is bad.

While lots of cosmetics companies carry on at length about the glory of natural ingredients, the following research is something you won't be hearing from any of them. According to the November 9, 1998, issue of *The Rose Sheet* (an insider cosmetics industry newsletter), the National Toxicology Program Board of Scientific Counselors concluded that "methyleugenol, a component of a number of essential oils, has shown clear evidence of carcinogenic activity in male and female rats and mice." Methyleugenol is a natural constituent of such plant oils as rose, basil, blackberry, cinnamon, and anise. The FDA probably cannot set limits for the exact amount of methyleugenol as an ingredient because essential oils are not broken down into their components but are just listed as whole extracts. It is important to note that the study is an animal model (and so it may or may not relate to humans), but I assure you there isn't a cosmetics company with a prejudice for the natural that is going to tell you about this study even though they read about it in the same trade newsletter I did.

Here's another tidbit the "natural cosmetics" world won't tell you. An article in the September 1999 issue of *Cosmetics & Toiletries* (a professional cosmetics industry journal) states: "Bauman et al. have studied the effects of topical vitamin E on the cosmetic appearance of scars. ... Anecdotal reports claim that vitamin E speeds wound healing. ... " The study by Bauman to prove if any of this is true was a double-blind* one on 15 patients. "The results of the study show that topically applied vitamin E does not help in improving the cosmetic appearance of scars and, indeed, leads to a high incidence of contact dermatitis. . . . In 90 percent of the cases in this study, topical vitamin E either had no effect on, or actually worsened, the cosmetic appearance of scars."

(*In the double-blind process all information that identifies what is being tested, including the product, the researcher, and the results being sought, is not known either to the people who administer the test or to the test subjects, a procedure that ensures impartiality.)

One more particularly ominous omission from the world of fashion magazines and skin-care companies is the information about UVA-protecting ingredients. Despite the overwhelming evidence about the efficacy of titanium dioxide, zinc oxide, avobenzone (also called Parsol 1789 or butyl methoxydibenzoylmethane), and Mexoryl SX™ for complete UVA protection, fashion magazines and most all skin-care companies won't educate the consumer about this one. Why? Because a preponderance of the advertisers in fashion magazines don't reliably use those ingredients in their sunscreen products. Disagreeing with your advertisers is something fashion magazines never do.

Briefly, I would like to go over a few of the more salient points that you are never told regarding the marketing jargon, terms, and ingredients that get hyped and overhyped by the cosmetics industry:

**Hypoallergenic:** This term is not regulated by the FDA and has no legal meaning. A cosmetics company can slap the term "hypoallergenic" on a label with no requirement for what should or shouldn't be in the product. What is most absurd is how many products wear this word and yet contain everything from fragrance to alcohol, menthol, and a host of other irritating ingredients.

**Noncomedogenic:** This term is also not regulated by the FDA and has no legal meaning. The search for products that won't cause breakouts remains a struggle. Wouldn't it be nice if a product could live up to this claim? But given that most all cosmetic ingredients can trigger breakouts for some people, the term is not only bogus, it can never be true. Besides, all women have bought products labeled as noncomedogenic that made them break out.

**Dermatologist tested:** As impressive as this sounds, as long as there are no published data stating otherwise, all this can mean is that a doctor applied the product to his or her skin or watched someone else do that and said they liked the product. It doesn't tell you anything about efficacy or how it compares to an alternative product.

**Laboratory tested:** A laboratory sounds so scientific—but anyplace a study is done can be called a "laboratory" setting. Once you're past the scientific impression that term may give you, you realize that the testing issues are the same ones described in "Our Studies Show," below.

**Patented secrets:** There is no such thing as a patented secret. The very concept is an oxymoron. The only way to obtain a patent is to divulge the complete contents of the product and its intended use. Further, there are no patents regarding proof of efficacy. All a patent says is you can use this ingredient(s) for this purpose. That has nothing to do with whether or not those ingredients can do anything at all.

**All natural:** Please keep in mind the following facts about the notion of a product being "all natural":

1. According to the FDA, cosmetics companies do not have to prove their claims. That means that they get to say just about any little thing they want about their products, and these claims absolutely do not have to be true or have any proof.

2. The FDA also does not require safety documentation for cosmetics until after the product has been brought to market and the FDA starts receiving consumer complaints.

The only part of the cosmetics industry that is strictly regulated for the consumer is the ingredients label. Unfortunately, the vast majority of consumers don't know how to read a cosmetics label, or they just don't care about it and would rather rely on the unregulated claims and assertions the marketing copy boasts about.

I could go on, and I will over the next many pages as I explain and cite sources explaining what works and what doesn't when it comes to skin-care products. The information I provide is everything the cosmetics industry knows to be true (it's their information directly from their sources) but won't tell you: what you absolutely need to know to make rational decisions about what you put on your face.

## Our Studies Show

Ever wonder how so many companies can proclaim that their studies show a 154% improvement in skin firmness or an 87% increase in moisture content? If they would only show us their studies, we would know exactly why they are announcing those numbers, and, more importantly, whether or not those numbers have meaning or are contrived to sound impressive to the consumer. Of course, we won't ever see a company's actual study because either the study doesn't really exist, or, if it does, it is so completely unscientific and illogical that no reasonable person would accept the results.

Almost without exception, skin-care studies come up short on many counts. Either just a small group of women (usually less than 12) are studied, or the protocol (meaning how the study is handled) is just a joke. A typical skin-care study protocol in the cosmetics industry is to leave one side of the face without anything on it while the other gets the company's cream. Well of course there will be a dramatic improvement in the side with the cream, but that proves nothing. That would be true of most any product.

According to an article in the December 1999 issue of *Cosmetics & Toiletries* magazine, pages 52–53, "Skin moisturization studies using bioengineering methods are commonplace today. If data generated for a new test product demonstrate a statistically significant difference between the test product and untreated skin in favor of increased hydration, then claims indicating this to the consumer would be substantiated ... For example, [the claim] 'moisturizes your skin for up to 8 hours' would be substantiated by a study where a statistical difference was observed between the test product and untreated skin for up to 8 hours following application of the test product." In essence, what most if not all of those brochures, ads, product labels, and endorsements that celebrate what "our studies show" (and that actually do have studies, given that many companies don't, but bandy the phrase anyway) are basically telling you is this: when compared with plain, unmoisturized, washed skin, their moisturizer made skin moist. What a shock!

There is an entire industry of claim substantiation going on in the world of cosmetics, mostly in response to European claim standards that will go into effect in a year or two regarding proof of claims. That means the industry is fast and furiously establishing standards that basically meet regulatory standards but give you no information that is helpful for your skin. A test that looks at dry skin that is unmoisturized and dry skin that is moisturized, with the ensuing proclamation that "our product works great!" is like doing a test that measures how drunk you can get drinking orange juice and vodka versus just drinking orange juice, which provides no information at all because the result is already a given: of course you don't get drunk when you don't drink alcohol. Likewise, of course, moisturized skin looks better than skin that isn't moisturized.

Here is another example of how a skin-care study (this one from Estee Lauder) can be designed to look significant when it isn't. The following is a story that appeared in a London newspaper in July 1998: " 'Estee Lauder claims a daily application of the cream can counter the effects of aging, helping to prevent and reduce crow's-feet.' According to research promoted by Lauder, forehead wrinkles and crow's-feet around the eyes can be prevented and even reduced by daily application of a cream containing vitamins, green tea, and minerals. [The press release from Lauder stated:] 'The 18-month study involved 160 volunteer women, aged between 35 and 60, living in three climatically different regions of France. Half were given a cream containing antioxidant ingredients; the rest used an apparently identical cream with no antioxidants. Every six months, researchers from the universities in the three cities, led by Loic Vaillant, Professor of Dermatology at Tours University, measured their wrinkles. After 18 months the researchers carried out a series of tests to find out if there was any difference in the skin of those who had been given the antioxidant and those who had not. They discovered a significant improvement in many of those who had been using the special cream,' Daniel Maes, vice president of research and development at Estee Lauder laboratories, said. 'The study showed a 23 per cent reduction in the formation of new lines and wrinkles, and an 8 per cent reduction in existing lines and wrinkles among women who were using the antioxidant cream,' he said. Maes said 'that a suction test found that the cream gave a 4 percent protection against the loss of elasticity.' " If you don't know how to read between the lines, this could appear to be a very important study. But, as is true with any so-called research like this, it doesn't take much to see what an unscientific report this really is. All this study did was test a Lauder product against some unknown placebo cream. Without more controls, like applying pure antioxidants without the moisturizing ingredients, all you end up knowing is that the Lauder product made the skin look 23% better (whatever that means) than some unknown product. In other words, this would be like eating a piece of Godiva chocolate and saying it tasted 23% better than a ball of sugar and cocoa mixed together. Of course the Godiva chocolate tastes better, but what about compared with a piece of chocolate from a different company or some other chocolate decadence? Would the Godiva hold up? Without all the facts, there's no way to know if this study was comparing an apple to an orange or even to a horse.

(By the way, this story about Lauder's study appeared in that London newspaper in July 1998; what a shock that the Lauder cream used in the study went on sale in London the same month.)

I could go on and on about this kind of ludicrous claim-substantiation business taking place in the world of skin care and I do so numerous times throughout this book. What is important to note is that phrases like "our studies show" or "our research establishes" or "our test results demonstrate" aren't worth the paper they are written on unless you see the entire study and can judge exactly how the research was done and whether or not the results are significant or senseless.

## Crazy Things You See on the Web

Over the years I've debunked hundreds and hundreds of fictions and myths involving skin-care, makeup, and hair-care products. Some of the more notorious areas of fraudulent information have grown up around astringents and their promises to close pores, hair-care products claiming to repair damage, creams purporting to rid thighs of cellulite, natural ingredients being the best way to care for skin, and, of course, the notion that expensive products are better for skin. Now, with the accessibility of the Internet, some myths spread like wildfire and become twisted realities for lots of people. As is always true with hoaxes of this kind, you are just sent the story. Accurate sources or excerpts that document the information are never provided, but that rarely stops people from believing it's all true. The following are some of the more flagrant ones out there.

<u>Sodium Lauryl Sulfate and Sodium Laureth Sulfate:</u> I have received more e-mails and letters than I care to count about the concern over sodium lauryl sulfate (SLS) and sodium laureth sulfate (SLES) being serious problems in cosmetics. I believe that this entire mania was generated by several Neways Web sites, and has been carried over as fact into other so-called "all natural" cosmetics lines.

It seems that most of this entire issue is based on the incorrect reporting of a study done at the Medical College of Georgia. As a reminder, here is what is being quoted: "A study from the Medical College of Georgia indicates that SLS is a systemic, and can penetrate and be retained in the eye, brain, heart, liver, etc., with potentially harmful long-term effects. It could retard healing and cause cataracts in adults, and can keep children's eyes from developing properly. (Summary of report to Research to Prevent Blindness, Inc. Conference.)" The doctor who conducted the study and delivered the final report is Dr. Keith Green, Regents Professor of Opthalmology at the Medical College of Georgia, and received his doctorate of science from St. Andrews University in Scotland. Yes, Dr. Green is completely embarrassed by all this. He told me, "My work was completely misquoted. There is no part of my study that indicated any [eye] development or cataract problems from SLS or SLES and the body does not retain those ingredients at all. We did not even look at the issue of children so that conclusion is completely false because it never existed. The Neways people took my research completely out of context and probably never read the study at all." He continued in a completely perturbed voice, saying, "The statement like 'SLS is a systemic' has no meaning. No ingredient can be a systemic unless you drink the stuff and that's not what we did with it. Another incredible comment was that my study was 'clinical,' meaning I tested the substance on people, [but] these were strictly animal tests. Furthermore, the eyes showed no irritation with the 10 dilution substance used! If anything, the animal studies indicated no risk of irritation whatsoever!" Which is why as of 1987 Green no longer pursued this research. When I asked if anyone has done any follow-up studies looking at SLS and SLES in this regard, Dr. Green said, "No one has done this because the findings were so insignificant."

Resulting e-mails continued for some time, carrying on the SLS and SLES myth with a slightly different bent. Yet, according to Health Canada, they "looked into the matter and found no scientific evidence to suggest that SLS causes cancer … Upon further investigation, it was discovered that this e-mail warning is a hoax. The letter is signed by a person at the University of Pennsylvania Health System and includes a phone number. Health Canada contacted the University of Pennsylvania Health System and found that it is not the author of the sodium laureth sulphate warning and does not endorse any link between SLS and cancer."

Further, according to the American Cancer Society's Web site, "Contrary to popular rumors on the Internet, Sodium Lauryl Sulfate (SLS) and Sodium Laureth Sulfate (SLES) do not cause cancer. E-mails have been flying through cyberspace claiming SLS [and SLES] causes cancer … and is proven to cause cancer … [Yet] A search of recognized medical journals yielded no published articles relating this substance to cancer in humans."

That's not to say that SLS isn't a potent skin irritant, because it is. In amounts of 2% to 5% it can cause allergic or sensitizing reactions in lots of people. As a matter of fact, SLS is the standard sensitizing agent used in irritancy testing of other ingredients. In other words, when they want to establish whether or not an ingredient is problematic for skin, they compare the results to SLS. But irritancy is not the same as the other dire, erroneous warnings floating around the Web about this ingredient!

**Propylene Glycol:** Propylene glycol is a humectant and delivery ingredient used in cosmetics. There are Web sites and e-mails stating that propylene glycol is really industrial antifreeze, and the major ingredient in brake and hydraulic fluids. Tests show that it can be a strong skin irritant. Material Safety Data Sheets (MSDS) on propylene glycol warn users to avoid skin contact, as systemically (in the body) it can cause liver abnormalities and kidney damage. It is true that propylene glycol is anti-freeze, but—and this is a very big *but*—in cosmetics it is used in only the smallest amounts to keep products from melting in high heat or freezing when it is cold outside. It also helps active ingredients penetrate the skin. In the tiny amounts used in cosmetics, propylene glycol is not a concern. Women are not suffering from liver problems because of propylene glycol in cosmetics.

I have seen several studies indicating that propylene glycol is not a problem as it is used in cosmetics, while I have seen no studies indicating the opposite. The Material Safety Data Sheet warning concerned 100% concentrations of propylene glycol for industrial or manufacturing purposes only, not the extremely diluted form used in cosmetics. Furthermore, many other cosmetic or pharmaceutical ingredients, from alpha hydroxy acids to beta hydroxy acids, tretinoin (the active ingredient in Retin-A), preservatives (which show up in every cosmetic product), standard cleansing agents, and topical disinfectants, would make your skin melt if they were used in 100% concentrations.

And finally, according to the U.S. Department of Health and Human Services, within the Public Health Services Agency for Toxic Substances and Disease Registry, "studies have not shown these chemicals [propylene or the other glycols as used in cosmetics] to be carcinogens."

**Mineral Oil and Petrolatum:** The notion that mineral oil and petrolatum (Vaseline) are bad for skin has been around for some time, with Aveda being the most visible company to make a career of deriding these ingredients. According to many "natural" cosmetics companies, mineral oil (and petrolatum) comes from crude oil (petroleum), is used in industry as a metal-cutting fluid, and therefore can harm the skin by forming an oil film and suffocating it.

This foolish, recurring misinformation about mineral oil and petrolatum is maddening. After all, crude oil is as natural as any other earth-derived substance. Moreover, lots of ingredients are derived from awful-sounding sources but are nevertheless benign and totally safe. Salt is a perfect example. Common table salt is sodium chloride, composed of sodium and chlorine, but salt doesn't have either the poisonous gas-emitting properties of chlorine or the unstable explosiveness of sodium. In fact, it is a brand-new compound with properties of neither of its components.

Mineral oil and petrolatum are considered to be the safest, most nonirritating moisturizing ingredients ever found. Yes, they can keep air off the skin to some extent, but that's what a good antioxidant is supposed to do; it doesn't suffocate skin! In addition, in an article in *Cosmetics & Toiletries* magazine, Dr. Albert Kligman said, "Petrolatum is known to help in wound healing." Every cosmetics chemist I've ever interviewed is frustrated at the fact that consumers have become afraid of mineral oil and petrolatum.

**Lanolin:** Have you heard this one about lanolin? Supposedly lanolin has been found to be a common skin sensitizer causing allergic contact skin rashes because lanolin usually contains pesticides used on sheep and wool. First, lanolin isn't all that common a skin sensitizer. Many other cosmetic ingredients are far worse, including fragrance from natural, so-called essential oils, preservatives, plant extracts, vitamin E, and fruit extracts. Lanolin can cause problems for a percentage of the population, and if you have a tendency to break out, it can clog pores, but that leaves a lot of people risk-free. Further, cosmetic-grade lanolin is devoid of any pesticides or other impurities.

**Polyethylene Glycol (PEG):** Web sites gain a great deal of attention by attributing horror stories to PEG. For example, "Because of their effectiveness, PEGs are often used in caustic spray-on oven cleaners, yet are also found in many personal care products. Not only are they potentially carcinogenic, but they contribute to stripping the skin's Natural Moisture Factor, leaving the immune system vulnerable." There is no research substantiating any of this. Quite the contrary: PEGs have no known skin toxicity. The only negative research existing for this ingredient group indicates that large quantities given orally to rats can cause tumors. How that got related to skin-care products is a mystery to me.

**Deodorants:** According to some sources, deodorant is fine, but antiperspirant is not because it prevents you from sweating and blocks the lymph nodes, therefore causing a buildup of toxins in the breast area below the armpit.

This isn't true in the least because it is a physiological impossibility. The lymph nodes are deep beneath the skin, whereas sweat glands are on the surface. Antiperspirants may clog pores but they cannot absorb into skin and get anywhere near a lymph node. One of the great myth-busting Web sites is Urban Legends, which everyone should add to their bookmark page: http://urbanlegends.miningco.com. Here is a summary of their informed report on the rumor relating to whether or not antiperspirants have anything to do with breast cancer. "Antiperspirants have no known (or suspected) connection with breast cancer. In a May 25, 1999 article by Dawn MacKeen in *Salon* magazine, Dr. Mervyn Elgart of the department of dermatology at George Washington University eloquently characterized the rumor as (and I quote): 'a bunch of crap.' "

One important urging from Urban Legends is this: "before you believe or forward any supposed 'medical information' you receive by e-mail, check with your own doctor or another reliable source to find out if it's true." For more information about the issue of breast cancer and this rumor, check the following links on the Urban Legends Web site: American Cancer Society, "Email Rumor," Urban Legends Reference Pages, "Breast Defense," and *Salon* magazine, "No Sweat."

# Crazy Things Fashion Magazines Say

One of the recurring questions I get from women about many makeup and skin-care products is "I saw this product rated in a fashion magazine as a favorite of their readers" or "I read in a fashion magazine that [fill in the name of any celebrity] loved this product." Hasn't anyone noticed that fashion magazines only tell us about the products celebrities, models, readers, or editors liked? Yet all women have products they don't like. I get thousands of letters telling me about cosmetics mistakes and problems every month. If fashion magazines were truly being objective, why not tell us what products their readers, editors, or celebrities didn't like, or even hated? But NO-O-O-O, they'll never tell us that. They leave out a very significant part of the equation, and as a result I am entirely skeptical that any of what they declare they like is accurate.

The fact is that fashion magazines can't tell you the truth about cosmetics. Think about it; when was the last time you read an article in a fashion magazine that criticized a cosmetic of any kind? When was the last time a fashion magazine warned you that a particular product wasn't worth the money or was recalled by the FDA (which happens) or contained potentially harmful or risky ingredients? About as often as you see a model with acne or wrinkles. The only stories fashion magazines contain glorify the products their advertisers sell. If an article on cosmetics casts a critical eye on a product or topic involving beauty or fashion, or if it buries the cautionary words in the middle or end of the report with a summary that concludes this stuff works, be suspicious, very suspicious, because not every product works wonderfully.

Fashion reporters have their journalistic hands tied by the demands of the companies that advertise in the publications they write for. And there is little impetus to change things. If a magazine depends on advertisers, it is simply forbidden to tick them off. When cosmetics companies spend hundreds of thousands of dollars or millions of dollars a year advertising in a magazine, a fashion magazine cannot include information that incorporates contrary or unfavorable information and stay in business. This commingling of editorial and advertising control results in gushing "news" stories that are little more than cosmetics-company publicity pieces and biased product recommendations. *All the news that's fit to print—as long as it's what the cosmetics industry wants the consumer to know.*

# Crazy Things Dermatologists Say

Let me first say that I have the utmost respect for the field of dermatology and plastic or cosmetic surgery. For many different skin problems, from acne to rosacea, seborrhea, psoriasis, infections, and rashes of all kinds, or face-lifts, peels, laser resurfacing, and other options, dermatologists and plastic/cosmetic surgeons are an essential resource and are too often neglected in favor of cosmetics-counter advice. Yet I have encountered my own share of misinformation from dermatologists and plastic/cosmetic surgeons, and the letters I've received from women about their experiences make my heart sink.

Little more than ten years ago, most dermatologists and plastic/cosmetic surgeons eschewed cosmetics as being silly and a waste of time for women. Somewhere along the line, something changed and physicians stepped into the sphere of cosmetics sales. Over the past several years, dermatologists in search of better or more profitable patient care began selling skin-care products, often in tandem with makeup products. Fifteen years ago, when I first started my cosmetics research work, there were maybe four skin-care lines being wholesaled to dermatologists for retail sales; today there are more than a hundred.

What does this mean for the cosmetics consumer? While it is completely reasonable to expect your doctor to be an objective and impartial source for gathering information and options based on the most current, documented, and peer-reviewed published research, it is questionable whether that is truly happening when the only option being presented is the doctor's own products. In crossing the line from physician to cosmetics salesperson, doctors sidestep the issues of medical ethics and the use of impartial scientific modalities in treating or providing recommendations to patients. In doing so they sell standard cosmetic products and make claims about their being medically formulated when nothing could be further from the truth. Many so-called doctor lines sell products containing well-known skin irritants, poorly formulated sunscreens, and do-nothing wrinkle creams.

Highlighting just how prevalent and serious an issue this is, an article in the August 1999 issue of the *Tufts University Health & Nutrition Letter* stated that the "American Medical Association has issued guidelines advising physicians not to sell health-related products for profit. When a doctor stands to gain from something a patient buys, it creates a conflict of interest." The American College of Physicians–American Society of Internal Medicine issued ethical guidelines for physicians selling products, which were in turn reported in the *Annals of Internal Medicine*, December 7, 1999. The paper stated that sales of cosmetics and vitamins by physicians are "ethically suspect."

I am very concerned about the way many physicians portray their products as having special or unique formulations different from the rest of the cosmetics industry, which is rarely if ever the case. Rather, I find the same shortcomings in products sold by physicians that I find in the rest of the cosmetics industry: overpriced formulations promising miracles they can't live up to. And I've seen the same industry "trend hysteria" run amok among doctors. Much like other consumers, physicians will read a study from some researcher about an ingredient revelation and, without any further information or substantiation, begin selling products that contain the showcase ingredient. Of course, every skin-care revelation has to sell for at least $40 to $80 an ounce, even though the products contain standard cosmetic ingredients that show up in far less expensive versions.

It's clear from several surveys I've seen that lots of women buy products at their doctors' offices. It turns out (as you will see from many of the reviews for physician skin-care lines) that the hype and misleading information so pervasive in the world of skin-care products is no different at your doctor's office or from doctor-created lines than it is in infomercials, department stores, or in-home sales.

## *For Women of Color*

Many cosmetics lines are trying to make up for their past inequities by adding makeup products appropriate for women of color. Previously, the foundations of-fered in this area were too orange and greasy, the eyeshadows were strictly shiny, and the skin-care products were fairly drying. It seems unbelievable that it has taken so long for the major cosmetics companies to finally acknowledge and try to meet the needs of such a large group of women. Revlon, Prescriptives, M.A.C., Clinique, and Lancome are the leaders in this area, and they are to be commended. Not only are their color products appropriate, but they offer a large number of choices. Although some lines designed specifically for women of color, such as Flori Roberts and Fash-ion Fair, offer limited options and problematic colors, other lines, including Black Opal, Posner, and Iman, have incredible color selections and high-quality products.

One area in which these specialty lines often fail is in their approach to skin care. Although Black Opal or Flori Roberts would like to lead the consumer to believe that their products are specially formulated for African-American skin, there is noth-ing in their formulations supporting that claim. In fact, products for African-American women are often formulated to be either greasy, with heavy moisturizers and wipe-off cleansers, or drying, with alcohol-based toners. Both of these product types pose problems for darker skin tones. Alcohol can dry out the skin and increase ashiness, and greasy products can cause breakouts and make skin look dull.

A handful of cosmetics lines coming on the scene claim they are designed for Asian women. Their brochures say Asian skin is supposedly so different from Cauca-sian, Latin, and African-American skin that it requires a separate product line. Nothing could be further from the truth: the products in these lines are just like those in all the other lines on the market, and the formulations just as problematic. Creating a special marketing niche where none exists might be good business, but it isn't neces-sarily good for the consumer. As it turns out, according to marketing surveys, most

Asian and African-American women do not want a line directed specifically at them; they would rather just buy mainstream cosmetics that include them, too.

When it comes to skin-care routines, any differences having to do with your skin color are minimal to nonexistent. Product choices need to be based on skin type, not skin color. As surprising as this may sound, skin color does not affect skin type. If you have a blemish or dry skin, the treatment is the same regardless of your skin color. Darker skin tones may have more problems with keloidal scarring or ashy skin tones, but these problems are not addressed differently from those of scarring or freckling for Caucasian women. Many cosmetics lines aim their makeup and color products at Caucasian skin, but their skin-care routines can be suitable for any skin color. As long as a product line has gentle, effective cleansers, reliable sunscreens (SPF 15 or higher with UVA protection), nonirritating toners, effective blemish products, and lightweight moisturizers, there is little risk to any skin type or skin color.

# *International Readers*

For those of you who shop for cosmetics outside of the United States, let me give you a heads-up—that's American slang for advance warning—about how this book applies to where you live. For the most part, most cosmetic products sold here in the United States are similar or identical to those sold in Europe, Canada, and Australia. Occasionally there are differences in formulations, though they rarely affect a product's actual performance. However, I cannot guarantee that my reviews are the same for products sold outside of the United States.

Sunscreens are the one product for which there are a few significant differences between formulations found in the United States versus the rest of the world. Sunscreen formulations outside of the United States, for the exact same product, can be quite different. European, Canadian, and Australian formulators have been using the UVA-protecting ingredients avobenzone (also called Parsol 1789 or butyl methoxydibenzoylmethane), titanium dioxide, zinc oxide, and Mexoryl SX™ (a UVA-protecting ingredient not available in the United States) for years. Also, the international sunscreen formulations allow for very different combinations of active ingredients. Whether the products are from L'Oreal, Lancome, or Lubriderm, they may all have very different sunscreen formulations than their U.S. counterparts and, when there are differences, the international versions are preferable. Because of this discrepancy in sunscreen formulations, you cannot judge my SPF reviews as being applicable everywhere. You must always check the active ingredient list to be sure the UVA-protecting ingredients are included, and then be sure you are also buying an SPF 15, a sunscreen number that is universally important.

# CHAPTER TWO

# Face Facts

By now, your skepticism about cosmetics and the cosmetics industry should be firmly in place. However, you must be wondering, if the cosmetics industry's promises and claims aren't real—then what is real? What is and isn't possible when it comes to your skin? If you can accept the following premises, you are much less likely to waste money on overpriced or ineffective skin-care products, or to be swayed the next time you hear a sales pitch for a miraculous (or even semi-miraculous)-sounding skin-care product or routine. I base a great deal of my evaluation of skin-care products on the following facts:

**You can clean your skin, but you can't "deep-clean" it.** You can't get inside a pore and clean it out like a dentist with a drill. Scrubs work on the surface of skin regardless of the claim on the label. Even if you could get inside a pore and clean it out, the damage to the skin would negate any benefit of deep cleaning. (I know a blackhead looks like it's dirty, but dirt isn't what's making it look black!) Expensive water-soluble cleansers will not make your face any cleaner, nor are they necessarily any gentler than the less expensive water-soluble cleansers. In fact, the handful of standard cleansing agents used in cleansers is the same across the cosmetics spectrum. What is essential is to find a gentle, water-soluble cleanser that doesn't dry out the skin or leave it feeling greasy, and that can remove eye makeup without irritating the eyes. Many cleansers that claim to be water-soluble are really too greasy to rinse off completely and can cause clogged pores.

**Spending more money does not affect the status of your skin.** The amount of money you spend on skin care has nothing to do with how your skin looks. However, what products you use does. An expensive soap by Erno Laszlo is no better for your skin than an inexpensive bar soap such as Dove (though I would suggest that both are potentially too irritating and drying for all skin types). On the other hand, an irritant-free toner by Neutrogena can be just as good as, or maybe even better than, an irritant-free toner by Orlane or La Prairie (depending on the formulation), and any irritant-free toner is infinitely better than any toner that contains alcohol, peppermint, menthol, essential oils, eucalyptus, lemon, or other irritants, no matter how natural-sounding the ingredients are and regardless of the price. Spending less doesn't hurt your skin, and spending more doesn't necessarily help it.

**Even minimal sun exposure is damaging to the skin.** Women clamor for the latest skin-care products that contain antioxidants, vitamins, plants, and a host of other exotics, yet all of that is meaningless if you aren't using an effective sunscreen every day of your life or are getting any amount of a tan. If you are exposed to the sun, even for as little as a few minutes every day—and that includes walking to your car, walking to the bus, or sitting next to a window (the sun's damaging UVA rays come through windows)—at any time of the year, that cumulative exposure over the years will wrinkle your skin. No skin-care product except a sunscreen with a high SPF and appropriate UVA-protecting ingredients (see the section on "Sun Reflections," later in this chapter) can change that. If exposure that minimal can wrinkle the skin, imagine how much worse the impact of sunbathing is. In short, there is no such thing as careful, safe, or wrinkleproof tanning or sun exposure of any kind.

**A great number of skin-care problems are caused by the skin-care products used to prevent them.** Overly emollient moisturizers can clog pores, temporary face-lift products can cause wrinkles because of the irritation they generate on the skin, and products designed to control oily skin often contain ingredients that can make skin oilier (oil-free products often contain pore-clogging ingredients that don't sound like oils). Allergic reactions are often caused by products that contain plant substances, because plants are inherently potent sources of allergens. Lots of skin-care products from the most expensive lines contain irritating ingredients such as fragrance, alcohol, witch hazel, and on and on. All of those things can contribute to the very skin problems you want to eliminate from your life and face.

**Dry skin doesn't wrinkle any more or less than oily skin.** Oily skin may *look* less wrinkled, which means it can have a smoother, more fluid appearance, but wrinkles are caused by sun exposure, genetic inheritance, muscles sagging (not from lack of exercise but from gravity—they slip down on the face) or other facial trauma, and just plain growing older—but not because of dry skin. All the moisturizers in the world won't change a wrinkle on your face, or prevent one, regardless of the amount of vitamins or plants they contain. That's not to say moisturizers can't temporarily make dry skin look smoother, because they absolutely can. You can prove this to yourself: simply stop using the miracle lifting or firming product you've been using and in a day or two, very unmiraculously, your skin will be back the way it was.

**Your skin may become inflamed, dry, and blemished if you use too many scrubs, products that contain potentially irritating ingredients, or several AHA or BHA products, either at the same time or in combination with one another.** For example, the following combinations can hurt the skin: a granular cleanser used with a loofah, a washcloth used with an abrasive scrub, an AHA product used with a granular scrub, an astringent that contains alcohol (or other irritants) used with an AHA product, or more than one exfoliating product (more than one scrub, more than one

AHA, or BHA). If you use too many irritating products at the same time, you are likely to develop skin irritations, breakouts, dryness, and, possibly, wrinkles.

**Exfoliating the skin is helpful but it won't erase wrinkles.** It is good to exfoliate the skin, and it is very important for many skin types, but exfoliation doesn't create new skin or get rid of wrinkles. Exfoliation can smooth the skin and help moisturizers be better absorbed, and some amount of exfoliation can generate collagen production, but the amounts are so inconsequential that you will never notice it, not to mention that the effects are temporary. Even with Retin-A and Renova, the effects stop after you discontinue use.

**For the most part, the fewer products you use on your skin, the better.** The more you use, the greater your chances of allergic reactions, cosmetic acne (from product buildup in the pores), and/or irritation. Layering skin-care products to try to get as many "wrinkle" cures on your face as possible can cause more problems, and putting all this stuff on your skin doesn't give any added benefit anyway.

**Worry about skin-care products that "smell" nice or have pretty colors.** I know the pretty blue or pink shades of skin-care products are attractive, and a pretty wafting fragrance from a cream or lotion can be appealing, but these are problematic and completely unnecessary in skin-care products. Ingredients that add fragrance to a product, even natural fragrances, are notorious for causing allergic reactions or skin sensitivities. Coloring agents may be great in a lipstick or foundation, but a blue or pink moisturizer is not great when the purpose of the skin-care product is to be absorbed into the skin.

**Do not automatically buy skin-care products based on the notion of age.** Many products on the market are supposedly designed for women who are 30, 40, or more than 50. Before you buy into these arbitrary divisions, ask yourself why the over-50 group always gets lumped together. Isn't it odd that women between the ages of 20 and 49 have skin that requires three or four categories, but women over the age of 50 need only one? There are a lot of years between 50 and 90. According to this logic, someone who is 40 shouldn't be using the same products as someone who is 50, but someone who is 80 should be using the same products as someone who is 50. Categorizing products by decades is nothing more than a marketing device that sells products; it does not correlate with benefits to the skin. Skin has different needs based on how dry, sun-damaged, oily, sensitive, thin, blemished, or normal it is, all of which have little to do with age. Plenty of young women have severely dry skin, and plenty of older women have oily skin and breakouts (particularly those women experiencing perimenopausal hormone fluctuations). Turning 40 or 50 does not mean a woman should assume that her skin is drying up and that she should begin using overly emollient moisturizers or skin creams.

**Do not automatically buy skin-care products based on your skin type.** I know that sounds strange, but there are several reasons for this. It's not that skin type isn't important, but more often than not your skin type is not what you think it is. It's even possible that your skin type has been created by the products you are already using. Soap can severely dry the skin, wrinkle creams can clog pores and cause blemishes, and alcohol-based toners can irritate the skin and cause combination skin. The only way to know what your skin type really is, is to start from square one with the basics that won't alter or adversely affect your skin, such as a water-soluble cleanser, an irritant-free toner (or a disinfectant if you break out), an exfoliator (such as an AHA product if you have sun-damaged skin and a BHA product for breakouts), a sunscreen for the daytime (which can be included in your moisturizer or foundation), and a moisturizer at night (but only if you have dry skin). Please understand that the intense cosmetics hype that insists that everyone needs a moisturizer is absolutely not true. (I discuss this at length in *The Beauty Bible*.) If your skin is truly dry you can do the extra things, such as using a more-emollient moisturizer at night, a more-emollient foundation, or a moisturizer with sunscreen during the day. If you are really prone to breakouts, you can try varying topical disinfectants and oil-absorbing masks.

**Treat the skin you have today, not the skin you had last month, last week, or yesterday.** Skin type can fluctuate. Skin-care routines based on a specific skin type don't take into consideration the fact that your skin changes according to the season, your emotions, the climate (humidity, dryness, cold, and heat all affect your skin), and your menstrual cycle. Pay attention to what your skin tells you it needs at any given time. This month you might need an extra-moisturizing sunscreen during the day, and a more emollient nighttime moisturizer. Next month you may only need a lightweight sunscreen or a foundation with sunscreen during the day and no moisturizer at night. The same is true for oily skin and breakouts. Don't hold fast to the idea that your skin fits into only one group—it changes, and so should your skin-care routine. That doesn't mean you need new products every month, it just means you may need to use less of one item or more of another.

**Teenagers are not the only ones who have acne.** One of the biggest fallacies is that women over the age of 20 should not have blemishes. What a mistaken belief that is! Women in their 30s, 40s, and 50s can have acne just like teenagers. Not everyone who has acne as a teenager will grow out of it, and even if you had clear skin as a teenager, that's no guarantee that you won't get acne later in life.

**Oily skin types rarely, if ever, require a moisturizer.** Specialty products such as oil-free moisturizers are rarely if ever good for someone with oily skin, because even though they may truly not contain oil, they include plenty of ingredients that don't sound like oil but that can make the skin feel oily and clog pores. Furthermore, if you don't have dry skin you don't need a moisturizer. The notion that the skin needs to have a moisturizer even if it's oily may sound nice, but moisturizers contain a lot more than water, and any and all of those ingredients can clog pores and make skin look and feel like an oil slick. You only need moisturizer where you have dry skin. Lighter-weight or matte-finish moisturizers may be good for someone with oily skin over dry parts of the face, but they still should not be used over oily areas.

The basic rule of thumb for someone with oily skin is to always determine if the dryness you're experiencing is being caused by other skin-care products. If so, stop using those first before you decide to use a moisturizer.

**There are great skin-lightening products to be found that can have an impact on sun-damage spots.** You can expect about a 20% to 40% improvement if you use these products in association with an effective sunscreen. However, plants are not the best source of skin-lightening properties. Mulberry extract has one study showing it to have minimal effectiveness and almost none when compared to hydroquinone (Dong-II Jang et al. "Melanogenesis inhibitor from paper mulberry." *Cosmetics & Toiletries* 112 (1997) 59–62), and this was a pure concentration, not the minimal amounts used in cosmetics. Kojic acid, an extract from mushrooms, is another natural option though not as effective as hydroquinone, and kojic acid is considered to be more irritating and unstable. (Nakagawa, J. and K Kawai. "Contact allergy to kojic acid in skin-care products." *Contact Dermatitis* 32, no. 1 (1995) 9–13). Hydroquinone (1% to 2% concentrations are available over the counter, and 4% or higher concentrations are available from physicians) has the most established research showing it to inhibit melanin production.

There are other plant extracts claiming to lighten skin, and while I have seen studies for these demonstrating some amount of effectiveness in vitro (meaning in a petri dish), there are no studies showing they can do this on human skin.

AHAs and BHA can smooth skin but they can't stop wrinkling. A well-formulated AHA product (meaning one having a 4% to 10% concentration of AHA with a pH of 3 to 4—and possibly 4.5) can help encourage cell turnover; that is, help remove built-up surface skin cells. But it can't affect actual cell production.

**Tretinoin, the active ingredient in Retin-A and Renova, can change abnormal cell growth back to some level of normalcy.** In discussing antiwrinkling products or skin products designed to improve the appearance of sun-damaged skin, it is important to consider the use of a retinoid such as tretinoin. What retinoids deliver to the skin is significant because of the way they can positively affect cell production. But all retinoids need to be prescribed by a physician; the over-the-counter vitamin A products *cannot* perform like Retin-A or Renova.

**Antioxidants in theory are good skin-care ingredients but there is no evidence that they can change a wrinkle on your face or affect how your face ages.** More and more products are being formulated with antioxidants (in fact it's rare to find a line that doesn't include them, but the notion that they will get rid of or stop wrinkles is not substantiated. The antioxidant wars the cosmetics industry is waging these days as to which company has the best antioxidants are a fool's game. There is no "best," though there are a lot of good ones and research is discovering new ones every day.

## It Really Is Irritating

As I'll explain more in the section on antioxidants later in this chapter, preventing and reducing irritation is essential for all skin types. There are so many reasons why irritation is bad for skin, it is almost mind-boggling. Nearly the entire body of research regarding the effects of antioxidants on the skin has to do with reducing irritation, redness, and swelling as a result of sun exposure or other influences. The positive impact these substances have on the skin is impressive; however, it's all after the fact. It doesn't take into consideration what a woman can do if she simply avoids irritation and unprotected sun exposure from the get-go. Indeed, irritation is a bigger problem for the skin than even many researchers ever suspected. Irritation can dry up skin cells that need to retain water; it can cause increased dryness, which adds to cell debris that can clog pores; it can cause breakouts like a diaper rash over the skin; it can cause redness; it can bring out surface capillaries on the face; and it can diminish the skin's immune system. In short, irritation is hell on the skin.

While all that is problematic for the health of the skin, even more significant over time is that it seems clear from the research that irritation can destroy the skin's integrity by breaking down the skin's protective barrier, something that, long-term, damages the skin's structure and impairs the skin's natural immune functions and healing ability. Additionally, breaking down the skin's protective barrier can allow the introduction of bacteria, and therefore raise the risk of breakouts.

What's more startling is the histological evidence that even if your skin doesn't feel irritated when you apply a cosmetic or skin-care product containing irritants, it is still being irritated and the breakdown of the skin's protective barrier is nonetheless taking place. That means if a product contains potentially irritating or sensitizing ingredients, the irritating ingredients can still harm the skin, even if they don't sting or burn. Not paying attention to the irritation potential of ingredients can be damaging to the health of your skin. Ignoring the irritating effect many plant extracts have on skin, or of many other irritating ingredients that show up in skin-care products—of which the most popular are alcohol (SD alcohol, ethyl alcohol, benzyl alcohol, and grain alcohol), menthol, peppermint, eucalyptus, lemon, orange, and grapefruit—can cause problems in the short term as well as the long term.

I have long insisted that the issue of being gentle to skin is paramount for all skin types. Getting people to heed this warning has proven to be an uphill battle, particularly for those with oily skin who have a belief that they must dry up their skin to prevent breakouts. That's as far from the truth as you can get, and my position was substantiated in a recent study published in the *Proceedings of the Fourth International Symposium on Cosmetic Efficacy.* A paper entitled "The Effects of Cleansing in an Acne Treatment Regimen" concluded that 52% of the time, a hydrating face wash gave the best results in reducing comedones (both open and closed blackheads), papules, and pustules when used with benzoyl peroxide. By comparison, this type of gentle cleanser was more effective than either soap or a benzoyl peroxide cleanser. That means irritating and drying up skin isn't helpful and can make matters worse.

## *What Gets Rid of Wrinkles?*

Perhaps no other question keeps women more addicted to the hype served up by the cosmetics industry than "What gets rid of wrinkles?" According to the cosmetics industry, just about everything. But that leaves the consumer wondering what to choose. Is collagen the answer? What about gold, silver, algae, lotus seed, AHAs, proteins, amino acids, DNA, milk protein, yeast, elastin, mink oil, emu oil, kalaya oil, myriad plants ranging from ginseng to *Ginkgo biloba,* echinacea, green tea, bilberry, horsetail, or lavender? How many have jumped on the alpha lipoic acid, vitamin C, vitamin A, vitamin K, vitamin E, or coenzyme Q10 bandwagon? Did I forget to mention aloe, chamomile, Dead Sea water, beta-glucan, superoxide dismutase, selenium, or growth factors?

Sadly, most women buy into this insanity hoping one or a combination of these will finally be the answer. But how many secret, miraculous, antiwrinkle formulas can there be? Do we ever get tired of the onslaught? The answer seems to be "Never." Every few months there's another cosmetic product or company launched promising women perfect skin. And every month, women purchase another cache of products believing they've bought the answer to erase their wrinkles. Some doctor or renowned scientist will introduce a line, or some new natural, all-botanical line will be introduced, and I'll get a horde of letters asking, "What do you think of this? It sounds so good, surely this must be it." Usually there is some interesting research behind many popular skin-care ingredients, but I haven't seen any research indicating that "the answer" or the fountain of youth is finally out there. I truly do wish there were a miracle skin-care ingredient for wrinkles or blemish-prone skin because then this book would be one page thick and we would all look 20 again without a blemish in sight!

Promises of a new miracle ingredient for skin care have a long history. There was the lemon craze in the late 1970s, the vitamin E bandwagon from the early '80s, the collagen and elastin frenzy from the mid '80s, the retinol mania from the late '80s (yes, the retinol being touted in the new millennium is the same one that came and went in the late '80s), the AHA mania from the early '90s, and then the vitamin C hysteria. Women thought all of these at one point or another were the answers to their skin-care woes. Yet hundreds of these products were created and millions of units were sold—and women still had their wrinkles. It's not that vitamin E, vitamin C, retinol (vitamin A), collagen, elastin, and AHAs aren't good skin-care ingredients, because they are, but none of them are the fountain of youth we're being promised or that we're hoping for. For some desperate reason that social scientists may be better at ascertaining than I am, women need to believe there is a magic potion out there that will restore their youthful appearance or get rid of any and all skin flaws. To that end, women will accept most any sales pitch they're handed as long as the promise is for miraculous results.

Actually, the more unbelievable the claim, the more expensive the product, or the more well-known the celebrity endorsing it, the more likely it is to be bought by women. Vitamin E, collagen, elastin, and lemon are now merely memories, and vitamin C, vitamin A, and a host of plant extracts from weeds to flowers are now the big deal everyone is buying. But the next fad (such as growth factors and growth hormones) is on the horizon and it will have its swarms of devotees, and vitamin C and vitamin A, along with lots of other has-been skin-care miracles, will be hardly a memory.

## *The Signs of Aging*

One of the best ways to curb our appetite for wrinkle creams is to understand that the skin's aging process is more complicated than we can ever imagine. Researchers generally agree that the visible signs of aging on the surface of the skin—deep wrinkles, lines, and discolorations—are only one aspect of a multilevel composite of events. Surprisingly, furrowed, leathery skin and brown "liver" spots are directly caused by sun exposure and are not genetically predetermined. What do seem to be genetically predetermined are a vast range of occurrences in the skin that can cause it to look older.

Looking at the issue objectively can help us to better understand what is happening to our skin, and therefore gain some insight into why wrinkle products can only fractionally live up to any of their claims. For example, while we know that collagen and elastin are the support structures of the skin and that they break down and flatten as a result of exposure to the sun, they also become less pliant and more hardened with age, so the skin becomes less elastic. Even if a product could build more collagen or elastin in our skin, if our skin isn't pliant and flexible, what good is the product? Some products claim to build only collagen or only elastin. That is much like building a house with only crossbeams and no support beams: one without the other is useless, because the house won't stay erect. Additionally, the process that builds collagen isn't the same as the one that builds elastin. But for the sake of argument, let's say there are products that *can* selectively build more collagen or elastin. Simply rebuilding elastin or collagen or any other single part of the skin isn't enough to halt or reverse the intricate, convoluted aging process and its effect on our face, because collagen and elastin represent only a part of why the skin becomes wrinkled and sags.

One notable difference between older skin and younger skin is that younger skin has more fat cells in the dermis than older skin. That's one reason why older skin looks more transparent and thinner than younger skin. But of course no one is going to sell an antiwrinkle product by saying it increases fat content in the skin, despite the fact that if a product could do that, it would absolutely make the skin look younger.

Furthermore, for some unknown reason, the skin keeps growing and expanding as we age, despite the fact that the fat tissue in the lower layers of skin is decreasing. That is why the skin begins to sag. Too much skin is being produced, but there isn't enough bone (remember, bone also deteriorates with age) or fat to shore it up. Simultaneously, facial muscles begin to sag, moving down and in on the face, and giving the face a drooping appearance. All the facial exercises in the world can't stop that from happening; it isn't that the muscles of the face aren't toned or strong—facial muscles are the most used muscles of the body. Instead, with time, use, and sun damage, the facial muscles begin to stretch and sag away from their original position on the face. Sagging, stretched-out-of-place muscles (not untoned muscles) is what causes jowling and the deep folds that go from the nose to the mouth, called the "nasal-labial fold." One way that plastic surgeons deal with the issue of sagging jowls or improving the appearance of the nasal-labial folds is to anchor the muscles back to the position they had before they began to be pulled down by gravity. Exercise can't do that. Rather, if you tone up a muscle that is by the mouth (when it is supposed to be up by the cheek and temple area) you would only get more pooching in that area.

Furrowing the brow is also a major reason that part of the face gets horizontal or vertical lines. All the cosmetic lotions and potions can't change facial expressions. That's why a Botox treatment, a medical procedure involving injections that paralyze the facial muscles of the forehead, smoothes out the wrinkles in that area.

Certain components of the skin also become depleted with age. The water-retaining and texture-enhancing elements such as ceramides, hyaluronic acids, polysaccharides, vitamins, enzymes, coenzymes, and proteins are exhausted. Older skin is also more subject to allergic reactions and skin sensitivities than younger skin, which suggests that older skin is less capable of defending itself against irritants because of a weakening autoimmune system.

On a deeper molecular level, portions of the DNA codes within the skin cells can get lost or rearranged, either from sun damage or from aging itself. This change in the DNA (the fundamental cornerstone that controls aging throughout the entire body) prevents our skin cells from reproducing as they did when we were younger. Cells become abnormally shaped, which further changes the skin's texture and also prevents the cells from holding on to water. This inability to retain water is why older skin *tends* to be drier than younger skin. Companies that stick DNA and RNA in their products want you to believe they can help rectify this deterioration. They can't, and even if they could do something, do you really want to mess around with your genetic coding? If those ingredients really could change cell growth, it could put your skin at serious risk of cancer (cancer is about abnormal cell growth).

Cosmetics companies target many of these factors of aging (except the issue of fat depletion) by adding cosmetic ingredients that claim to counteract the effect of these specific depletions. Ceramide, hyaluronic acid, vitamins, proteins, and other components of skin are popular in wrinkle creams. The problem is that you can't put ceramide or hyaluronic acid back into the skin from the outside in (or even from the inside out); their molecular structure is too large to penetrate the skin. Moreover, even when these ingredients are chemically altered so they can penetrate skin, how much of the ingredient does skin need? A gram? A milligram? And what if it gets distributed unevenly? Plus, the quantity of skin substances being depleted numbers in the thousands.

Simply put, no product anywhere can handle all the multitudinous nuances of skin aging.

Like collagen and elastin, ceramide and hyaluronic acid are good water-binding agents and therefore are useful in moisturizers. Unfortunately, the cosmetics industry loves to use phrases such as "Replaces what skin has lost," leading you to believe that these ingredients can affect skin structure when all they are doing is working as a good moisturizer—which is great for skin; it's just not worth $25 to $325 an ounce.

Growing old cannot be reversed by the right skin-care routine, by jerking your face around with elaborate exercises, or by stimulating muscles with machines. As far as antiaging products are concerned, you are never going to get what you think you've paid for, unless you're buying a sunscreen, because sunscreens can truly prevent a great deal of sun damage, and that's what is primarily causing our skin to wrinkle.

Despite all these caveats, that doesn't mean there aren't great products out there that can have a profound impact on skin. However, your wrinkles will not be reversed, and with no permanent change in the inherent structure of skin, the results will be temporary.

## Stop the Moisturizing Madness

Not everyone needs or should be using a moisturizer, especially women with oily, combination, or acne-prone skin! And women with dry skin only need one moisturizer (not including sunscreen). That sums it up. I can't think of one skin-care product that is more misunderstood, misused, and abused than moisturizer. How did things get so out of hand? The only answer is that things tend to get out of hand in the world of cosmetics.

It's not that I don't think moisturizers can be vital for some skin types. I also find most moisturizers to be well formulated, which means I rate moisturizers favorably more often than not. And putting aside the nasty debate over cost versus performance, the main problem is that moisturizers are overused by most women, which can result in some pretty surprising skin problems. A lot of women (maybe most) still cling to the erroneous belief that moisturizers somehow prevent wrinkles. Not just moisturizers with a high sun-protection factor (SPF), which do stop further skin damage if they contain titanium dioxide, zinc oxide, or avobenzone (also called Parsol 1789 or butylmethoxydibenzoylmethane) for UVA protection, but all moisturizers. The mistaken notion that dry skin is more prone to wrinkles than oily skin remains firmly implanted in the mind of the consumer, and that's on top of all those claims about firming, toning, repairing, and lifting the skin with all sorts of creams, gels, and lotions. Or that these moisturizers contain some miracle ingredient like emu oil, mink oil, vitamins, copper, algae, or whatever, and if women don't get that on their skin, it will wrinkle away. It's just not true! Evidence alone tells us this is the way reality is. If these wrinkle potions worked, plastic surgeons would not be doing more face-lifts and resurfacing procedures than ever before. The statistics speak for themselves.

The only reason to use a moisturizer is if you have dry skin or wrinkled skin you want to look smoother (moisturizers can smooth over, not change, wrinkles). If you don't have dry skin, there is no reason to use a moisturizer. If you have oily skin or skin that breaks out, the worst thing you can do is use a moisturizer of any kind. At least not over the oily areas, that's for sure. It's that simple. What happens when you overuse a moisturizer? Pores get clogged and blackheads can develop; dead skin cells get trapped and have a harder time naturally sloughing off (which can leave the skin looking dull); and you run a higher risk of getting patches of dermatitis, increasing the number of breakouts, and creating your own combination-skin predicament. Additionally, oversaturating the skin can turn off the skin's own immune/healing response. Overdoing moisturizers can actually prevent the skin from repairing itself.

## What Makes a Good Moisturizer?

As you read my reviews for individual moisturizers, you may wonder why I state that one is a boring product while the other is a more interesting or state-of-the-art formulation. In essence the question is, are all moisturizers created equally? Or, to put it another way, do all moisturizers work the same?

Those are great questions with a complicated answer. Essentially, to one degree or another most all moisturizers (with very few exceptions) moisturize skin. However, there are differences, and what separates one moisturizer from another, what makes one potentially better than another, is what justifies the comments I make. Aside from active ingredients like AHAs, BHA (topical exfoliants), skin-lightening agents (hydroquinone-based products), sunscreen with UVA protection, and prescription medications such as Renova and Retin-A, there are a few definitive elements that go into establishing a state-of-the-art moisturizer that account for the difference in the content of my review versus the rating.

Just to be clear, we're not talking about products claiming to be firming, antiaging, or antiwrinkle creams, because they don't really exist, at least not in your moisturizer and not the way we want them to work (which is the way they are advertised). AHAs, BHA, Retin-A, and Renova do have a role in reducing the appearance of wrinkles (that I'll discuss later), but everything else, and I mean *everything* else, comes under the header of moisturizer. Regardless of the price tag, the name of the product, or the claim, moisturizers moisturize, and here's how they do that.

Essentially, a good moisturizer contains emollients, water-binding agents (sometimes called humectants, ingredients that attract water to the skin and help keep it there), soothing or anti-irritant substances (to reduce inflammation or irritation), and antioxidants (explained later in this chapter).

Emollients are lubricating ingredients that are essential for dry skin. They provide dry skin with the one thing it's missing—lubrication—in the form of ingredients that resemble the skin's own oil production. Emollients are ingredients like plant oils, mineral oil, shea butter, cocoa butter, petrolatum, cholesterol, and animal oils (including emu, mink, and lanolin, with the latter probably the one ingredient that is most like our own skin's oil). All of these are exceptionally beneficial for skin and easily recognizable. Far less easy to comprehend on the ingredient label are a wide range of ingredients like triglycerides, palmitates, myristates, and stearates, which I usually list as thickening agents. These substances are more waxy and less elegant than the other emollients I've listed, but they create the fundamental base and texture of the moisturizer and provide their own benefit when it comes to lubricating the skin. Silicones are another interesting group of lubricants for skin. These have the most exquisite silky texture and an incredible ability to prevent dehydration without suffocating skin.

All of these emollient ingredients, in endless variations, are spread over the skin to create a thin, imperceptible layer, re-creating the benefits of our own oil production, preventing evaporation, and giving the skin the lubrication it is missing. Without these ingredients, dry skin would remain parched and tight, and so as it turns out all moisturizers contain some combination of these.

Water-binding agents work great for dry skin and most are suitable for all skin types. "Water-binding agent" is a general term I use to refer to ingredients that keep water in the skin. Humectants attract water to skin, but what good is getting water in the skin if the structure isn't there to keep it from leaving? It turns out that skin cells usually have plenty of water if they don't become degraded or damaged. Once skin is irritated, overcleansed, exposed to the sun, dehydrated from air conditioning or heaters, and so on and so on, the integrity of the skin is compromised. That means the substances that keep the skin cells bound together to create the surface structure we see as skin are depleted. You may have heard this skin "glue" referred to as the intra-cellular structure or matrix of skin. This intracellular structure is made up of many different components, many of which can be included in a moisturizing formula-tion. Ingredients ranging from ceramide to lecithin, glycerin, polysaccharides, hyalur-onic acid, sodium hyaluronate, mucopolysaccharides, sodium PCA, collagen, elas-tin, proteins, amino acids (of which there are dozens), cholesterol, glucose, sucrose, fructose, glycogen, phospholipids, glycosphingolipids, and glycosaminogly-cans, to name just a few. All of these give the skin what it needs to keep skin cells intact, and they reinforce the skin's natural ability to retain water. When a skin-care product contains several forms of these water-binding agents, I consider that a more elegant formulation; that doesn't mean your skin will notice the difference, but that the research indicates that there is benefit for your skin when these are present.

Skin-care formulations are not as benign or harmless on skin as was once thought. First, the number of products a woman puts on her face can mean that an endless litany of ingredients get piled on the skin. Sometimes these ingredients are com-pletely useless and do nothing but irritate or injure the skin, or have no positive effect on skin—such as essential oils (fragrant components that can be sensitizing and irritating for most skin types), eucalyptus, peppermint, camphor, citruses, and menthol. Some of these ingredients are fairly innocuous, but others, like sunscreen agents, preservatives, AHAs, BHA, topical disinfectants and antibiotics, scrubs, and cleansing agents, though necessary, can still cause irritation. To that end, and to help skin handle the impact of all this stuff on the face, lots of cosmetics contain soothing agents and anti-irritants. These nifty little ingredients are secretly helpful in cosmetic products, and include substances with names like bisabolol, allantoin, burdock root, aloe, licorice root, glycyrrhetinic acid, green tea, and chamomile extract.

Antioxidants are a fascinating part of a moisturizing formula (I explain more about this below). What makes antioxidants so intriguing is that they seem to have the ability to keep air off the face and reduce some effects of sun exposure. All that is incredibly beneficial for cell turnover, healing, and reducing dehydration. I suspect that antioxidant research for skin will end up being even more fascinating over the next decade. Lots of antioxidants, such as selenium, superoxide dismutase, vitamin A (retinyl palmitate and retinol), vitamin C (ascorbyl palmitate and magnesium ascorbyl palmitate), beta-glucan, and vitamin E (tocopherol), to name the most popular ones, are showing up in skin care these days. All of these and many more are excellent additions to skin-care products and moisturizers of all sorts. Not that they will change one wrinkle on your face, and definitely not that one is better than another, but they all do help keep skin intact, soothed, and moisturized.

All of these, from emollients to water-binding agents, soothing or anti-irritating ingredients, and antioxidants, combined in more permutations than you can imagine, create the moisturizers I consider more interesting or state-of-the-art for skin. However, there's no point in searching for one single mixture or "best" ingredient. Vitamin C isn't the answer any more than collagen, elastin, or vitamin A is—or whatever hyped ingredient is being pushed on you as the absolute best there is. Just like there isn't one "best" chocolate cake recipe, there isn't one best anything in the world of moisturizers. I wish there were, but the brilliance of cosmetics chemists and ingredient manufactures lies in their ability to create and combine a profusion of ingredients, to produce lots and lots of wonderful products. There are just too many great options to sum it up in any one ingredient or product. But I assure you, when a product lacks these things, I will let you know!

## What Works? What Doesn't?

The endless parade of sensational ingredients being propagandized by the cosmetics industry is almost beyond comprehension. Throughout this book, depending on the line being reviewed, I will explain and often challenge the claims being made for a variety of ingredients. For now, I want to pinpoint a few of the more well-known gimmicks that are floating around on ingredient labels and being heralded in ads, to help establish some basic facts right from the start.

## Antioxidants

"Antioxidant" is a word freely bandied about in the cosmetics industry to explain the value of various skin-care ingredients used in myriad products. Basically, what we call antioxidants are any of the substances that inhibit oxygen. Inhibit oxygen? Don't we need oxygen? Absolutely. While humans unquestionably need oxygen for life, ironically oxygen can also be detrimental to life because it triggers free-radical damage in human and plant cells (as well as free-radical damage in *all* molecular systems). Free-radical damage can lead to cell destruction (just think about what happens to food when you leave it exposed to air as opposed to sealing it off in a Tupperware™ container or a tightly sealed plastic bag—keeping air off of the food prevents it from breaking down quite as fast as it would if you left it unprotected).

There is extensive, and I mean really extensive, evidence to implicate free radicals in the development of a number of degenerative diseases and health conditions including heart disease and arthritis.

What is free-radical damage? Free radicals are extremely busy chemical compounds that are naturally produced in the body during metabolism of foods, but that are also produced in connection with exposure to air pollution, smoke, and sunlight. Either way, oxygen is the major culprit. When a cell converts oxygen into energy, tiny molecules called free radicals are also made. When produced in normal amounts, free radicals work to rid the body of harmful toxins and also maintain many basic life functions, including the immune system, metabolism, and collagen production, keeping everything healthy. But when free radicals are produced in toxic amounts, they damage the body's cellular machinery, resulting in cell death and tissue damage.

So while free radicals are normal by-products of cells and have certain beneficial roles in the body and plants, increased levels in either body or plant tissue can be detrimental to the plant or our health. Regrettably, you just can't lock the body in Tupperware or a plastic bag to prevent free-radical damage. However, there is a vast body of research showing that the oral intake of antioxidants prevents air from interacting with other molecules and causing them to become unstable, and that can stop the free-radical chain reaction from spiraling out of control. Antioxidants range from vitamins A, C, and E to superoxide dismutase, flavonoids, beta-carotene, glutathione, zinc, green tea, and grape juice, among many, many others (and thousands of others yet to be identified).

While the mountain of evidence surrounding antioxidants for the body is extremely convincing, the question of what effect antioxidants have on skin hasn't been answered. The problem is that the skin is constantly exposed to oxygen and sunlight, so how could you ever use enough antioxidants to stop that? How much oxygen, sunlight, or air pollution can you really keep away from all skin cells, or even some skin cells? How fast do the antioxidants get used up? Do they last two minutes, ten minutes, one hour, two hours, five hours, or more on the skin? No one has the vaguest idea, and you can't block the skin and suffocate the body to find out.

Major investigation is being done in this fascinating area of human aging that most unquestionably influences wrinkling. Even though a lot of respected researchers are working on this issue, the research is in its infancy, at least in the arena of skin care, and suggesting anything else is sheer fantasy. According to Dr. Jeffrey Blumberg, Ph.D., Associate Director and Professor, Antioxidants Research Laboratory, Tufts University, "There isn't going to be a single compound or approach that is going to answer all of the questions about aging." When it comes to research regarding antioxidants, he said the "implication for cosmetics is just unknown [because] researchers are focused on the major serious diseases and conditions that kill people, and of the billions of dollars spent on this research there is little to none spent on skin care." He further explained that "If it was just a matter of replacing things [skin] lost with age … we would [apply those things] and be done with it. But that's not how it works, though most people wish it did. One myth I would like to dispel is that there isn't one [antioxidant] that is the magic bullet. Mother nature provided literally thousands of antioxidants and they work together in a synergistic capacity."

Almost every company these days makes moisturizers that contain antioxidants, each with varying claims and promises, so they aren't hard to find. You won't see any difference in your skin, but if free-radical damage, and thus the destruction of the skin's structure, can be slowed, or if sun damage can be reduced, then antioxidants should help. For now, it's all theoretical, and no one can give you any definitive amount or specific ingredients to look for, despite the cosmetics industry's attempts to do so.

It is also interesting to note that almost all antioxidants, ranging from retinol to green tea, vitamin C, grape juice, and on and on, are exceptionally unstable. That means these ingredients break down with exposure to sunlight and air. The likelihood that a product with these ingredients can maintain its content level after it's opened is highly doubtful.

## *Oxygen for Skin Care*

Many skin-care companies are touting the fact that their products can deliver oxygen to the skin, which is supposed to get rid of wrinkles and improve the overall health of the skin. It seems fitting to discuss this foolishness after the discussion of antioxidants. After all, if antioxidants are the be-all and end-all of skin care (since they keep oxygen off of the skin), how is it possible that giving the skin more oxygen is the right thing to do?

The irony about oxygen in skin-care products is that the skin doesn't like oxygen! According to an article by Dr. Peter Pugliese in the April 1999 issue of *Skin Inc.*, 90% of skin-cell activity takes place anaerobically, meaning without oxygen, or simply doesn't require oxygen. One of the reasons hydrogen peroxide works to disinfect is because it releases an extra oxygen molecule to skin. Because the bacteria causing acne (called propiobacterium) live in the pores where no air is present, this extra amount of oxygen can kill off the offending bacteria. Any claim that oxygen in skin-care products can penetrate the epidermis (the skin's surface) is simply not true.

Oxygen is perhaps the most confusing element among health concerns, both for the body and for the way it is built up in skin-care products. While we need oxygen to live, oxygen (as oxidation) also causes free-radical damage, as described above. To add to the confusion, there is strong evidence showing that seriously wounded skin can be helped by oxygen delivered in a hyperbaric chamber (like the ones divers use). But you can spend only so much time in a hyperbaric booth before it starts hurting you. Too much concentrated oxygen over time can actually cause damage to the body. Keep in mind that this research showing that oxygen in hyperbaric booths can be helpful is about ulcerated wounds that won't heal under any other conditions; it isn't related to how normal skin behaves. Ulcerated wounds and wrinkles are not related.

For the sake of argument, let's assume oxygen was good for normal, nonwounded skin: Could a skin-care product deliver oxygen to the skin? Separate from Pugliese's comment above, and given the nature of oxygen, once the product was put on the skin the release of oxygen would take place in about a hundredth of a second. That would give it no time to impact the skin in any way, shape, or form.

Even more to the point, what the companies selling products that supposedly give oxygen to the skin can't explain without a good deal of double-talk is how you can give the skin oxygen when oxygen causes free-radical damage. This oxygen paradox has no answer, although it's clear that putting oxygen in skin-care products isn't it.

## Vitamin C Wars

I don't know about you, but I'm really getting tired of this whole vitamin C skin-care craze. I thought for sure the vitamin A craze would take its place, but it hasn't seemed to dampen the fire; vitamin C products and claims keep on coming. You wouldn't think that one nebulous little ingredient would cause so much commotion—but then, we're talking about the cosmetics industry, where it only takes one ingredient to start a furor. Especially one ingredient that promises instant youth, and vitamin C is such an ingredient. This time the new angle with vitamin C appears to be more politically motivated than anything else, which in some ways does make it more intriguing, just not skin-worthy.

I've discussed at length the research surrounding vitamin C. It started with Dr. Sheldon Pinnell from Duke University, who looked at the effect of sun exposure in relation to applying L-ascorbic acid (a specific form of vitamin C) on hairless pigs. It seems the pigs with L-ascorbic acid applied to their skin did not get as badly sunburned as the pigs who didn't have L-ascorbic acid. From this study, and following theoretical models of vitamin C and its role as an antioxidant in healthy skin (discussed above), it was assumed by Pinnell that L-ascorbic acid was an exceptional antioxidant that could suppress sunburn. Pinnell also knew at the time that L-ascorbic acid was an exceptionally unstable ingredient. However, Pinnell didn't tell anyone that the L-ascorbic acid in the $70-an-ounce bottle of Cellex-C he was endorsing decomposed upon opening. Despite this known drawback, dermatologists and the cosmetics world became enthralled with Cellex-C, and the bottles flew off the shelf. Not to be left out, other cosmetics lines, from Lancome with its Vitabolic to Avon's Anew Formula C Treatment Capsules and La Prairie's Cellular Defense Shield with

SPF 15, to companies selling vitamin C patches, all launched products containing forms of this now famous vitamin.

The story has become more complicated since I originally wrote about the issues surrounding vitamin C. It turns out that in 1997, Pinnell stopped endorsing Cellex-C (he never endorsed the entire Cellex-C product line, by the way, which included more than 20 additional products). Yes, Pinnell has always recognized that the original L-ascorbic acid he researched was unstable. He now claims to have a stabilized version of L-ascorbic acid available only through his company, SkinCeuticals. Not surprisingly, this stabilized form of L-ascorbic acid is not available to the makers of Cellex-C. Of course, why we are supposed to believe Pinnell now is anyone's guess.

Vitamin C in the form used in Pinnell's new line will do well despite the lack of evidence, as Pinnell's brochure states "Each product contains a unique blend of botanical extracts that help restore a youthful, radiant experience." So much for his vitamin C being the ultimate for wrinkles, now you need plants, too. The original question I posed some time ago in regard to Cellex-C applies to SkinCeuticals: If L-ascorbic acid, stabilized or otherwise, is supposed to be so amazing for building collagen and repairing skin, why would you need to add botanical ingredients? Why do there have to be all these other products making more miraculous claims? Why would you need AHAs, toners, and other wrinkle creams if one product was doing all the work?

Furthering the confusion about vitamin C and creating more of a minefield is that some high-profile dermatologists are hawking the benefits of their versions of vitamin C. Pinnell has L-ascorbic acid, Dr. N.V. Perricone's line uses magnesium ascorbyl palmitate, and other so-called dermatologic lines use ascorbic palmitate or ascorbic acid. Dermatologists vying for consumer dollars with lines of cosmetics is a sad state of affairs. It's no longer about what the research confirms but how much product can be sold, regardless of consumer need or any basis in substantiated, peer-reviewed research.

What is true for any issue involving skin wrinkling is that aging is more complicated than just the loss or need of vitamin C—or any other vitamin, enzyme, protein, or fatty acid in the skin. It is the whole picture we should be concerned about, not one small aspect. Besides, there are many other antioxidants that are as good as or even more impressive than vitamin C, including beta-glucan, vitamin E, and vitamin A, to name a few; and, according to many researchers dedicated to the study of antioxidants, there are probably thousands of undiscovered antioxidants out there that may be even more significant.

The entire arena of antioxidants is new and there is nothing definitive to warrant the current cost or tumult, at least not for skin care and definitely not for any one specific ingredient. They won't get rid of wrinkles or replace sunscreen, so calm down!

They can offer increased sun protection, which is important, but that's for UVB protection—not UVA protection—and that's about as much as we know. Of course, that doesn't stop the companies selling products that contain all kinds of ingredients from making claims about reversing aging, building collagen, feeding the skin, and healing sun damage, despite the fact that, as everyone in the industry knows but wants consumers to remain ignorant of, there are no conclusive studies indicating the effectiveness of any antioxidant product or ingredient on wrinkles. I know everyone is looking for the best antiwrinkle product, but other than sunscreen, there isn't one.

## Retinol vs. Retin-A and Renova

Retinol has become a standard buzzword in the world of antiwrinkle ingredients. All the attention revolves around retinol's association with the active ingredient in Retin-A and Renova, which are both prescription medications. Retin-A and Renova both have the same active ingredient: tretinoin. What is the connection between retinol and tretinoin? Retinol is the technical name for (preformed) vitamin A (vitamin A is created in the body from beta-carotene). Tretinoin (or technically all-trans retinoic acid) is the acid form of vitamin A. This seemingly close relationship between retinol and tretinoin has a lot of companies hoping to prove and convince those in search of an antiwrinkle cure that retinol can do the same thing as tretinoin without any of the side effects.

It is interesting to note that retinol was first introduced as a miracle skin-care ingredient in the late 1980s. It faded away by the early 1990s and then was resurrected with a marketing vengeance proclaiming it to be *the* ingredient (along with vitamin C) for fighting wrinkles in the late 1990s. Doesn't this sort of make you wonder what all the renewed clamor is about? If retinol didn't work back in the '80s (because if it had worked, it would have stuck around), why should it work now? Great question.

What is unquestionably clear and well established is the vast amount of research showing tretinoin to be effective in changing abnormal cell production (caused primarily by sun damage) back to some level of normalcy. Tretinoin's effect on cell production is truly astounding and it should be a serious consideration for anyone wanting a functional, valid method of addressing wrinkles and overall improvement in cell production in the layers of skin. Applying tretinoin doesn't produce miraculous results, but the positive outcome in terms of skin health is indisputable. *However*, the potential for irritation from using tretinoin on the skin (from products like Retin-A or Renova) is significant and many people cannot tolerate this side effect. Irritation aside, a lot of people don't want to bother seeing a dermatologist to get a prescription for Retin-A or Renova.

Given the irritating side effects of tretinoin and the bother of making an appointment with a physician to obtain a product that contains it, wouldn't it be nice if some nonprescription form of vitamin A could have the same effect as tretinoin? So while tretinoin and other acid forms of vitamin A exist in the realm of prescription medication, retinol and retinyl palmitate (a distant cousin of vitamin A) exist in the world of cosmetics. Cosmetics companies from Estee Lauder to Neutrogena, Avon, and hundreds of others all have their assortment of products containing retinol or retinyl palmitate, and their claims for these mirror those made for Retin-A. But can cosmetics containing retinol or retinyl palmitate perform like tretinoin? The answer is, we truly don't know, but probably not. In the skin, tretinoin is all-trans retinoic acid. All-trans retinoic acid is the component that can affect actual cell production. Retinol needs to be altered to become all-trans retinoic acid, and that process requires a series of steps. The possibility that the tiny amounts of retinol being used in cosmetics can be converted into all-trans retinoic acid is remote. It is even more improbable for this to happen with the ingredient retinyl palmitate. Retinyl palmitate is an ester of vitamin A. An ester is a compound several generations removed from the original form. This means that while retinol has to go through several steps to become all-trans retinoic acid in the skin, retinyl palmitate has to through even more of a change. If that is even possible, no one knows.

What is especially interesting in the hoopla around retinol is that Johnson & Johnson, the very makers of Retin-A and Renova, also happen to own Neutrogena, who sell a retinol product called Healthy Skin Anti-Wrinkle Cream. The claims on the Neutrogena product sound quite similar to the claims for Retin-A and Renova. Healthy Skin Anti-Wrinkle Cream with retinol claims it "visibly reduces the appearance of fine lines, wrinkles, and age spots . . . works deeper within the skin's surface to visibly reduce past sun damage." Gee, that sure sounds just like what Retin-A and Renova are supposed to do. If retinol and tretinoin can do the same thing, and are being sold by the same parent company with apparently similar claims, why would anyone bother making an appointment with their dermatologist to get a prescription for Retin-A or Renova (or some other prescription tretinoin) when all they'd need to do is buy an over-the-counter retinol product like Neutrogena's? It seemed like a good idea to talk to Johnson & Johnson directly and to ask them about this conflict. So I did.

I was able to arrange an interview with Rachel Grossman, M.D., World Wide Director of Medical Affairs for Johnson & Johnson consumer products, and Stanley Shapiro, Ph.D., World Wide Director of Preclinical Research for Johnson & Johnson Consumer Products. From their viewpoint, no retinol product, not even theirs, is a direct substitute for Renova and Retin-A. Tretinoin is still, by far, the best option for combating sun damage. The studies proving what tretinoin can do for skin are copious, while retinol, by comparison, has been minimally studied. Retinol has been investigated for improvement of the appearance of skin (just like tons of skin-care products), but there have been no studies comparing it to the functionality and activity of tretinoin. According to Shapiro, "Retinol can theoretically become all-trans retinoic acid in the skin" but the process isn't direct. Retinol absorbs into the skin and if conditions are right (meaning the presence of enzymes) it would then take some steps for it to be converted to all-trans retinoic acid. Shapiro said, "Retinol can get into skin, but whether or not it is being converted into all-trans retinoic acid has not been demonstrated." And that's the point.

The studies I've seen, particularly three from the Department of Dermatology at the University of Michigan, Ann Arbor, two of which were published in the *Journal for Investigative Dermatology*, were done on small groups of women; the studies were done by a team who has done work for Johnson & Johnson before, and the results were not compared to other types of moisturizing formulations. In other words, would you have gotten the same results with a moisturizer that contained vitamin E or vitamin C? Good question, but that's not what the studies looked at.

Still, both Shapiro and Grossman felt retinol was an option if someone can't tolerate Retin-A and Renova. Whether or not it's an option that is any better than vitamin C products or other antioxidants is a complete unknown.

For now, all products with retinol, such as Neutrogena's, Estee Lauder's Diminish, or Alpha Hydrox's Retinol Night ResQ Anti-Wrinkle Firming Complex, use anywhere from about 0.1% to 0.33%. That amount doesn't appear to have any potential of being effective in the way tretinoin is (when used in those same amounts in the prescription products of Renova and Retin-A). In other words, if retinol has to go through a process to become all-trans retinoic acid in the skin, it would take a significantly larger amount of retinol to break down and be converted to the active form of the ingredient. All this doesn't make these products bad, but they are not the antiwrinkle cure the ads would lead you to believe.

I would strongly encourage the use of Retin-A or Renova or another prescription topical tretinoin as a first line of offense against wrinkles (after a sunscreen, that is). If you do decide to use a retinol product (and with all the marketing inducement and propaganda, you probably will), please keep in mind that there are many inexpensive options that have the same retinol content as the expensive versions. Moreover, because retinol is incredibly unstable, the kind of packaging it comes in is very significant. Retinol, like all antioxidants, can deteriorate on exposure to air and sunlight. This means the packaging for retinol products must be opaque and airtight. A clear or transparent container (such as Nu Skin's and Estee Lauder's retinol products have) assures that you are not getting an effective retinol product.

# Vitamin K

This might seem to be an intriguing product to consider, especially if you are aware that a study published in the December 1999 issue of *Cosmetic Dermatology* seemed to demonstrate that vitamin K could reduce dark circles under the eye. However, what you may not know is that the study's results are, at best, questionable, having been conducted by the company that manufactures the ingredient, and by the doctor, Melvin Elson, who holds the patent for it. The study merely looked at 28 women who applied this vitamin K cream and then a few weeks later reported on how they liked it. That isn't a scientific study by any standard; it isn't double-blind, nor were the results measured by any known protocols. It's nice when a woman says her skin looks better, but lots of women feel their skin looks better after using new products. As it stands, there is no independent research showing vitamin K to be effective for any aspect of skin care.

Previously, Elson's research (also questionable and not substantiated by any independent source) pointed to vitamin K for improving the appearance of surfaced capillaries. It didn't work for that problem, and other than being a good moisturizer this version won't fare any better at reducing dark circles.

Vitamin K's reputation, when taken orally, relates to its primary function for promoting blood clotting. Like vitamins A, D, and E, vitamin K is fat soluble, meaning that it can be stored in the body and that it's possible to overdose on powerful supplements. In the worst-case scenario, that might mean brain or liver damage, jaundice, or the destruction of red blood cells. But there are problems of a different sort, too. Patients on anticoagulants (a standard medication for those with heart disease) should cut down on foods high in vitamin K and avoid multivitamin pills containing vitamin K, because these cancel out the effects of the medication. Of course none of this is a concern for any of the topically applied vitamins because they don't work like vitamins (meaning nutrients) on the surface or even below the surface of skin.

# Green Tea or Grape Juice?

You may have seen headlines showcasing the antioxidant benefits of grape juice and tea (specifically green and black teas). Forget coffee and soda pop; the drinks to consider for the millennium are green tea and grape juice! With some interesting research and data under their collective belts, researchers claim that these two beverages have healthy benefits. Articles in *Consumer Reports* magazine reported how topically applied green tea reduced cancerous mouth lesions in 39 out of 50 volunteers. Also according to *Consumer Reports*, grape juice ranked highest in antioxidant powers, with green tea just behind it. I've been told that Europeans are so taken with grape juice and wine for skin care that there are spas being created dedicated to treatments focused on grapes, wine, grape extract, grape seed oil, and the like. I hope that's true, not because the research shows this is finally the true skin healer (any more than vitamin C, retinol, or a horde of other ingredients is the answer for skin), but if grape-juice spas abound in Europe, perhaps the spas specializing in sheep placenta will go the way of all useless fads and leave the poor sheep to graze blissfully away from the insatiable needs of those fighting wrinkles. But back to the teas and grape juice.

The article in *Consumer Reports* was primarily concerned with oral consumption of green tea, and its use in animal studies. A cover story in *USA Today* on February 2, 2000, confirmed my caution about getting too excited about any of this, especially from any considerations for its topical use, stating, "It's too early to put so much faith in tea, many scientists say. Most of the studies have been done on animals and in the test tube, and full-scale clinical studies on humans are needed to find out whether tea can deliver on those preliminary promises."

From a health point of view, I think consuming grape juice or green and black teas is an excellent idea (along with blueberries, which were rated just as high as the teas and grape juice—so you can probably expect blueberry extracts showing up in skin-care products too); however, how that translates into skin care is unknown. There is still no proof from any arena of the efficacy of these substances for skin or wrinkles. Animal studies are intriguing, but as many animal-rights activists and medical experts would tell you, animal studies don't always translate to the way a human would react or tell how much is needed to gain benefit. The fractional amounts used in cosmetic products wouldn't be enough to be beneficial for skin, although they do appear to be beneficial for marketing strategies.

Antioxidants are a big issue, and I do feel strongly that the millennium will see incredible strides in this area. Right now, to suggest we know how much (if any) of this is helpful for skin is like talking about the benefits of vitamin C (and keep in mind that vitamin C was last year's big antioxidant miracle!). The answer is that no one knows.

## Coenzyme Q10

What is fascinating about coenzyme Q10 has nothing to do with wrinkles. Rather, it is a well-researched nutrient with many studies demonstrating what it can do to improve health. CoQ10 has received particular attention in the prevention and treatment of various forms of cardiovascular disease, strokes, and hypertension. It has also been shown in a small number of studies to increase the metabolism of fat and to increase brain activity. It turns out that CoQ10 resides primarily in organs, particularly the heart, with its presence peaking around age 20 and declining after that. I've seen articles in *Health News* and *International Health News* suggesting CoQ10 should be taken with vitamin E, with a meal containing some fat, or in combination with soy or vegetable oil, which enhances its absorption quite substantially. "CoQ10 supplements are readily absorbed by the body and no toxic effects have been reported for daily dosages as high as 300 mg," according to Dr. Andrew Weil. Weil, the guru of the dietary supplement world, says that 100 mg is considered plenty—check out his Web site at www.drweil.com. He also notes that because "the safety of CoQ10 has not been established in pregnancy and lactation, . . . caution is advised here until more data becomes available."

What about wrinkles? The only studies I've seen concerning coenzyme Q10 and its effect on skin are from cosmetics companies claiming the following: after ten weeks of use, the appearance of wrinkles around the eyes and face decreased by 34%. But all cosmetics companies have that same study for their products, regardless of the ingredient. Even more frustrating is that a "34% improvement" doesn't tell you what it was improved from. What was the condition of the skin before the product was applied? What were the improvements compared to? These and a plethora of other questions aren't addressed in a statement like "34% improvement." Coenzyme Q10 isn't a bad ingredient but whether it can help skin in any way, shape, or form is simply unknown.

## Copper

Copper (in a form typically called "blue" copper) and other copper derivatives are showing up in skin-care products. Yet there is little to no evidence that they are effective for any form of normal skin care. There are presently four published placebo-controlled studies on the use of blue copper in skin care. These studies have focused on wound healing and allergic reactions, and not wrinkles or skin firmness. One particular study looked at three groups of people: one a control group (meaning nothing was applied to the skin), one getting a placebo (using the base formula without the blue copper stuff), and a third using the same base formula with the blue copper ingredient. While the study seems to be on the up-and-up (meaning double-blind and the use of a placebo vehicle for comparison), the only information you can garner from it is that, as an ingredient, copper seems to help skin heal. However, the study did not compare other ingredients such as vitamin C, vitamin A, superoxide dismutase (copper stimulates the production of superoxide dismutase), a range of other antioxidants, or even a silicone-based product to the copper formula. Do those other ingredients in their base formula do the same thing? That wasn't part of the study, so there is no way to know. All the study showed is that the base formula didn't work as well without the copper. In the long run, damaged skin can use some help healing, and I suspect there are lots of ingredients that can help that process; copper is possibly one such ingredient.

As is typical in the cosmetics industry, the blue copper craze sounds a lot like the one that happened when the concept of using oxygen to promote healing of some ulcerated wounds got picked up and translated into a miracle cure for wrinkles, when it does nothing of the kind.

# *Human Growth Factors (HGF)*

To suggest that the topic of human growth factors (HGF) is complicated is a gross understatement. The complexity of this issue defies anything this book can delve into adequately, though even if I could devote the extensive space needed to shed light on this topic, the physiological intricacy of these substances defies a layperson's comprehension. Nonetheless, because the use of HGF seems to be a direction some skin-care companies are taking (Ré Vive, Jan Marini, Osmotics, and Kinerase are the ones that come to mind for this edition), it deserves comment so you can understand some of the concerns and realities behind the claims being made. For this section, I will explore the claims made by Ré Vive, a line of skin-care products being sold at Neiman Marcus and on the Internet at www.revivecosmetics.com.

There is no doubt that the founder of Ré Vive, Dr. Greg Brown, has some impressive credentials. According to his curriculum vitae, he is a board-certified general and plastic surgeon, who trained at Vanderbilt, Harvard, and Emory Universities, and received his medical degree from the University of Louisville. Given this esteemed medical background and the products he is marketing, he can join the ranks of Dr. Howard Murad (of Murad infomerical fame), Dr. Sheldon Pinnell (of Cellex-C and SkinCeuticals), and Dr. N.V. Perricone (with products bearing his name) as a physician turned skin-care salesperson. Now there is one more doctor telling you his research is the way to go for the fountain of youth, and it will cost you a pretty penny (lots of pretty pennies) if you decide this one's got the answer.

Brown says that the answer to "rejuvenated, young-looking skin is bioengineered products." The Web site for Ré Vive products describes Brown's "experiments using human Epidermal Growing [sic] Factor (EGF) to stimulate wounds to heal faster. 'I saw evidence of absolute [healing] acceleration the first day and I became impassioned.' " Wow, sounds great. These products must be flying out of Neiman Marcus, where they're being sold, but that's only because cosmetics companies don't have to tell you the rest of the story.

According to Dr. Bruce A. Mast, M.D., Division of Plastic and Reconstructive Surgery, Department of Surgery, at the University of Florida, Gainesville, in material for his class on wound healing, "Brown's research, done at the University of Louisville back in 1989 [published in the *New England Journal of Medicine* at that time], did show Epidermal Growth Factor (EGF) to have a positive effect on wound healing, however, a study from from the University of West Virginia by Dr. I. Kellman Cohen; et al., showed no positive effect on wound healing with EGF." Mast went on to say that "as a result of the contradictory information the research on EGF for wound healing has gone by the wayside and the primary research for wound healing is looking at TGF-A, TGF-B, and PDGF."

Note: EGF promotes proliferation of epithelial (skin) cells; TGF-A (Tranforming Growth Factor-Alpha) may be important for normal wound healing; TGF-B (Transforming Growth Factor-Beta) promotes the growth of fibroblasts (collagen); PDGF (Platelet Derived Growth Factor) promotes the growth of blood clotting factor. The more well known HGFs for skin are EGF, TGF-A, and TGF-B (there are at least 100 different family members for TGF-B).

So what is Epidermal Growth Factor (EGF) anyway? It is a cytokine. I know, what's a cytokine? Cytokines are any substances released by a cell or cells that cause an action to take place on another cell or cells. EGF is part of a much larger group of cytokines known as Human Growth Factors (HGFs). HGFs are proteins (proteins are primary components of all living cells and include many substances, such as enzymes, hormones, and antibodies, that are necessary for all life functions). These HGF proteins bind to receptor sites on the cell surface (receptor sites are the way cells communicate with any substance). HGFs need to communicate with cells to instruct them to activate the production of new cells or to tell a cell to create new cells that have different functions. Many HGFs are quite versatile, with the ability to stimulate cellular division in numerous different cell types, while other HGFs are specific to a particular cell type, like blood cells or bone cells.

The main problem with HGFs, when they are taken internally as in certain cancer treatments (Interleukin and Interferon are cytokines), is that they can be highly mitogenic (causing cell division) and at certain concentrations and lengths of application can cause cells to overproliferate, resulting in problems that can include cancer.

But what happens when you put EGFs on skin? According to Dr. Mast, "The biggest reason not to use these [EGFs] is that they could accelerate the growth of skin cancer by stimulating the overproduction of skin cells." Another reason not to use them, Mast says, is because "TGF-B primarily stimulates fibroblasts [collagen] which can encourage scarring. Scars are excessive collagen, [so] if you make too much collagen you get a scar or a knot on the skin."

All of the research on the issue of HGFs for skin has primarily looked at the issue of wound healing for skin. But Ré Vive and other product lines purporting to use these substances aren't just talking about wound healing and short-term use, they're talking about wrinkles. Ré Vive wants you to believe that EGF "stimulates skin cells to revert to their adolescent renewal pattern." Now if that isn't the fountain of youth, I don't know what is. Despite this outlandish statement, there are no studies showing this to be even remotely possible. According to Mast (and many other phsicians I've interviewed), "Wound healing is unrelated to wrinkles."

There is one other body of research concerning the HGFs that are being brandished as answers for wrinkles. Here is what the research shows. Based on established scientific protocol, you can create "living" skin cells in a petri dish. It is known that normal human skin cells divide a predictable number of times and then die. Skin cells grow and divide rapidly early on, then the division rate slows as we age. Finally the cells cease replicating. In vitro, you can re-create the skin cell's life process and accelerate the effect so you can watch the growth process of cells in a short period of time (weeks as opposed to a normal person's life span). If you leave these skin cells alone they go through a normal life span and eventually stop replicating. However, when you add some forms of growth factors (GFs) the skin cells live far longer than they would on their own. While that sounds like your skin would stay young forever, the other part of the picture is that if you add *too* much GF the skin cells die off sooner than they would if you hadn't added any. This part of the information is often left out of the impressive data companies like to use when touting their products.

The research into HGFs and GFs is without question intriguing, but if these products really do work, the risk to skin is just too great. Basically, what I suspect and believe to be true is that these products can't even remotely do what they claim.

## *Battling Hormones: Is Progesterone in Skin-Care Products the Answer?*

Most women in their mid-40s and beyond have become familiar with the terms "peri-menopausal" (the changes in a woman's menstrual cycle that take place before menopause) and "menopausal" (when a woman's menstrual cycle actually stops). Personally, I know these terms better than I ever thought I would! The multifaceted and controversial changes a woman experiences, both physiologically and emotionally, during this fundamental life process are far more complex than this book can hope to cover. However, I would like to provide a bit of insight on the area where menopause and skin care cross paths, and offer some suggestions and resources so you will be better equipped to make informed decisions. One of the primary areas where they cross paths is for progesterone creams, which are not regulated as drugs but rather are nothing more than cosmetics, just like any other moisturizer being sold.

For years, women have relied on Estrogen Replacement Therapy (ERT) as their major remedy to ward off peri-menopausal and menopausal symptoms such as hot flashes, vaginal dryness, osteoporosis, and changes in skin texture. For many women (including my mother and other close friends of mine in their 60s and 70s), ERT was nothing short of a blessing. It eliminated hot flashes, kept osteoporosis at bay, and kept them feeling and looking young. However, recent studies have brought to light the serious risks associated with ERT in regard to an increased risk of breast cancer. According to a study conducted by the Fred Hutchinson Research Center in Seattle, Washington, and a study published in the *Journal of the American Medical*

*Association*, January 26, 2000, there is a correlation between use of ERT and increased risk of heart attack (as opposed to what was once thought to be a decrease in heart-attack risk, as reported in an article published by the American Heart Association, *Estrogen and Cardiovascular Disease in Women*), and an association to endometrial cancer, though this is not conclusive due to conflicting research. The National Cancer Institute Information Resources, November 1999, released the following statement: "Because reports have shown that estrogen increases the risk of developing endometrial cancer … the National Cancer Institute is sponsoring a clinical trial to determine the effects of estrogen in women treated for early stage endometrial cancer."

When you couple these ERT drawbacks with a societal attitude that anything natural must be good for you, you can understand the desire to want a natural alternative that could effectively deal with peri-menopausal and menopausal symptoms was inevitable.

At the forefront of the female hormone battle is a Dr. John Lee, with his books *What Your Doctor May Not Tell You About Menopause: The Breakthrough Book on Natural Progesterone* (Warner Books, 1996) and *What Your Doctor May Not Tell You About Premenopause* [peri-menopause]: *Balance Your Hormones and Your Life from Thirty to Fifty* (Warner Books, 1999). Lee's primary thesis is that ERT was flawed for many reasons. On one level, Lee feels ERT is problematic because it utilizes synthetic estrogen and/or synthetic progesterone. But a matter of more concern to Lee is that ERT (without progesterone, as it was typically prescribed for years) puts the emphasis on the wrong hormone, namely estrogen, instead of progesterone. Lee's research suggests that too much estrogen, or "estrogen dominance" as he calls it, is the problem, and that natural progesterone is the only option to combat a woman's hormonal changes.

So what is the difference between progesterone and estrogen? Progesterone is manufactured in the body from the steroid hormone pregnenolone, and is the source or precursor of other steroid hormones, including cortisol, androstenedione, estrogens, and testosterone. For women, progesterone and estrogen work together in a subtle symphonic harmony. This hormonal balance creates the rhythm of the menstrual cycle and when that harmony gets out of tune, particularly during peri-menopausal and menopausal years, the problems for women are significant. Estrogen levels drop by 40% to 60% at menopause, which is just enough to stop the menstrual cycle. But progesterone levels drop too, and for some women, they may drop to being almost nonexistent. According to Lee, "Because progesterone is the precursor to so many other steroid hormones, its use can greatly enhance overall hormone balance after menopause, even for estrogen …" although estrogen cannot affect progesterone levels.

Menstruation depends on what is taking place in the ovaries and uterus, the hormones generated by the hypothalamus and pituitary gland in the brain, and the corpus luteum in the ovary. During the first half of the menstrual cycle, as an egg follicle grows in the ovary, estrogen is manufactured and released into the blood. As the egg follicle matures in the lining of the ovary, a hormone called luteinizing hormone (LH) causes the egg to be released directly into the ovary. The ovary then starts producing progesterone while estrogen production declines. Progesterone's role is to help the egg to mature even faster, increasing fertility. As you may know, this hormonal fluctuation in the production of estrogen versus progesterone takes place at midcycle, when a woman is the most fertile. Not surprisingly, the increased progesterone levels correspond to a surge in a woman's sexual drive (after all you can't get pregnant if your libido—brain—doesn't want to have sex). If fertilization does not occur, ovarian production of progesterone falls dramatically. It is this sudden decline in progesterone levels that triggers the shedding of the uterine lining that results in a menstrual cycle. In essence, estrogen encourages the growth of endometrial tissue in the uterus, and progesterone causes this lining to be shed.

In a recent interview with Dr. John Lee, he told me that he "wants people to understand that natural progesterone brings everything back into balance. Around the time when progesterone is low in women, approximately age 45, there is an estrogen dominance occurring in the body which causes such things as auto-immune disorders, hair loss because there are more androgens [in the body not counterbalanced with progesterone], risk of breast cancer, and a low libido." Lee went on to explain that "natural" progesterone "is the same identical hormone found in women as opposed to the use of synthetic forms of progesterone (progestins) found in prescription-only drugs that merely mimic the effect progesterone has on the body."

So, if Lee is right, why is the research about natural progesterone so controversial? According to Lee it's because "natural progesterone cannot be patented, it is available to everyone and anyone who wants to put it into any lotion or cream they make. Pharmaceutical companies do not fund research that has no likelihood of netting a profit. Therefore, pharmaceutical companies put a lot of money into researching synthetic hormones that … can be patented and sold exclusively by the patent holder. It follows that there is a lot of research out there to show that synthetic progesterone and synthetic estrogen works and [explains] why there is little research about the use of natural progesterone [there is simply no profit in the latter]. Pharmaceutical companies do not even broach the issue of natural hormonal options versus synthetic ones with physicians because there is no financial motivation to do otherwise."

There is also controversy among physicians as to whether or not progesterone applied topically can provide the body with the same amounts as synthetic forms of progesterone taken orally. Physicians point out that anecdotal information about positive results from natural progesterone is flawed, because in double-blind studies the placebo effect for hot flashes or other physical improvements is about 40% when compared to a test vehicle. Further, when actual blood levels of progesterone are measured, physicians find low levels of natural progesterone, confirming their suspicion that not enough of the natural progesterone is being absorbed through the skin. Lee is frustrated by this finding because the medical profession will not accept that "natural" progesterone levels are best tested in saliva and not in blood serum, the way synthetic progesterone is measured. Lee's saliva tests indicate that the natural progesterone creams do produce normal levels of progesterone that can be accurately read.

Is there any risk to applying natural progesterone topically? Lee said he has not seen adverse effects since he began studying it over 20 years ago. This is one aspect of Lee's work that is wanting. While Lee may not have seen any problems, that doesn't mean they don't exist. After all, Lee would not be the doctor to see; if problems occurred, women would turn to other doctors for uterine or breast difficulties (he was a family physician). What Lee does acknowledge is that there is a risk of hyperplasia (an abnormal increase in the number of cells in an organ or a tissue with resulting swelling) and a feeling of lightheadedness and lethargy. However, Lee also points out that "during pregnancy, the placenta produces 300 to 400 milligrams of natural progesterone daily during the last few months of pregnancy, so we know that such levels are safe for the developing baby. But [synthetic progesterones—progestins] even at fractions of this dose, can cause birth defects."

Clearly, more research is needed to settle the issue, but without question, this is a growing option for treating hormonal changes. Understanding the options and risks, and separating the truth from what is truly intense hype, both by the "believers" in natural progesterone cream and the "believers" in pharmaceutical or synthetic hormonal therapy, is imperative for woman facing this change in their bodies.

And there are lots of formidable believers on both sides of the coin. Typing the term "natural progesterone" into a search engine on the Web brings up over 40,000 hits (and most of those are from companies or doctor's offices selling natural progesterone creams), and searching for "Estrogen Replacement Therapy" brings up just about the same number from medical professionals prescribing ERT. When it comes to natural progesterone products, Lee explained that right now there are about 140 companies marketing natural progesterone creams that come from 20 different labs. And with the baby boomers coming full fledged into their peri-menopausal and menopausal years, there will probably be more and more coming to market. Given that natural progesterone creams are not regulated in any way by the FDA, and that they are, in actuality, merely cosmetics, that means anyone can put them into any product they want to.

According to an associate of Lee's, David Zava, Ph.D., Director of Research for ZRT Laboratory in Portland, Oregon, "nearly all of the [natural] progesterone cream products are formulated to deliver about 15 to 30 milligrams of USP grade progesterone per 1/4 teaspoon of cream." For peri-menopausal women, Lee recommends 15 to 24 milligrams applied daily for 14 days before the menstrual cycle is expected to begin and then stopping the day before the menstrual cycle starts. For menopausal and postmenopausal women, he suggests reducing the application to 15 milligrams per day for 25 days and then not using it for five days. Lee states that 15 to 20 milligrams "… is the same amount the ovaries make naturally."

A study published in the *American Journal of Obstetrics and Gynecology*, June, 1999, volume 180, concurs with Lee's position, stating that "In order to obtain the proper (effective) serum levels with use of a progesterone cream, the cream needs to have an adequate amount of progesterone in it [at least 30 milligrams per gram]. Many over the counter creams have little [example, 5 milligrams per ounce] or none at all. The creams that are made from Mexican yams are not metabolized to progesterone by women. The cream used in the above study (Pro-Gest) contains pure United States Pharmacopeia [USP] progesterone." Ironically, Pro-Gest was the only cream around at the time Lee started his research.

Lee explains that "The USP progesterone used for hormone replacement comes from plant fats and oils, usually a substance called diosgenin, which is extracted from a very specific type of wild yam that grows in Mexico, or from soybeans. In the laboratory, diosgenin is chemically synthesized into real human progesterone. Some companies are trying to sell … 'wild yam extract' [or other plant extracts]… claiming that the body will then convert it into hormones as needed. While we know this can be done in the laboratory, there is no evidence that this conversion takes place in the human body." Lee is quick to explain that he doesn't sell any of these products and receives no profit from their sale either. He also does NOT recommend natural progesterone creams with any other active hormones or herbs.

So what should you use if you want to give natural progesterone creams a try? Lee recommends creams that contain between 400 and 500 milligrams per ounce of cream. That amount would provide about 20 milligrams per day when applying a 1/4-teaspoon amount of the cream. But before you venture out shopping for natural progesterone creams, I would strongly encourage you to check out Lee's books (available on www.amazon.com and most bookstores) and to visit Lee's Web site at www.johnleemd.com. Lee lists companies that sell products that meet his criteria. There is also a listing of products that meet the recommended amount of USP progesterone provided by Aeron LifeCycles Laboratory, San Leandro, California, on their Web site at www.aeron.com.

# Plants: a Growing Problem

Most all of my comments regarding the efficacy of plant extracts used in products throughout this edition were taken from the following resources. *The PDR [Physician's Desk Reference] Family Guide to Natural Medicines & Healing Therapies*, Ballantine, 1999; *Encyclopedia of Common Natural Ingredients Used in Food, Drugs, and Cosmetics*, second edition, Yeung and Foster, Wiley Inter-Science, 1996; *Botanicals: A Phytocosmetic Desk Reference*, D'Amelio, CRC Press, 1999; the quarterly journal *Healthnotes Review of Complementary and Integrative Medicine*, Healthnotes, Portland, Oregon; Winter's *A Consumer's Dictionary of Cosmetic Ingredients,* fifth edition, Three Rivers Press, 1999; *Concise Science Dictionary,* third edition, Oxford University Press, 1996; www.herb.com; www.vitamins.com/encyclopedia/Index; http:// metalab.unc.edu/herbmed/eclectic/kings/main.html; www.healthlink.com.au/ nat_lib/index.htm; http://BoDD.cf.ac.uk/BoDDHomePage.html (Botanical Dermatology Database); and http://onhealth.com/alternative/resource/herbs/.

**Please see the Dictionary Appendix for a listing of the plant extracts used in products reviewed in this book.**

The use of plants and the claims about "all natural" have only gotten worse since the last edition of this book. The cosmetics industry wants women to believe that a plant extract of any kind, short of rubbing broccoli or asparagus on our faces, must be good for skin, and that synthetic ingredients must be bad. It doesn't matter if it's a completely unknown plant; if it grows, there must be an excellent reason to use it. It also doesn't matter that the plant ingredients are less than 0.5% to 3% of the total product and the other unnatural ingredients account for more than 47% (the rest being water) of the contents. Regardless of these facts, the image of plants in cosmetics is an overpowering one for the consumer. Aveda has made a religion out of plants and The Body Shop has turned it into a political issue.

But why use *Prunus persica* (peach extract) over *Hordeum distichon* (barley extract), *Betula alba* (birch extract) rather than *Brassica oleracea capitata* (cabbage extract), or *Cananga odorata* (ylang-ylang oil) instead of *Anthemis nobilis* (chamomile extract) or *Pseudopterogorgia elisabethae* (sea whip extract—actually this one is a marine invertebrate, but you get my drift)? There are literally thousands and thousands of potential extracts that can be used in cosmetics. Do they all perform equally well, or at all? And what about overdoing it? Can you overdose on plant extracts?

The issue of natural versus synthetic is one I've written about extensively over the years. To sum it up succinctly, natural does not mean good and synthetic does not mean bad. Each group has its shortcomings and strengths, but I would no sooner accept any plant as automatically being good for my skin than I would walk naked through a patch of poison ivy assuming that because it's a plant, it must be OK.

"Natural" simply defines the source of the ingredient; it tells you nothing about the ingredient's effectiveness or risks. Menthol and peppermint may have a natural source, but both are serious skin irritants and absolutely terrible for the skin. Ingredients like silicone and stearyl alcohol are synthetic but they are remarkably silky-soft ingredients, vital to a vast array of cosmetic formulations. Licorice extract (in the form of glycyrrhetinic acid) is an excellent anti-irritant but it functions on skin as a corticosteroid; does that mean repeated use of this ingredient on skin can cause thinning and wrinkles, the same effect as any topical steroid? C16-14 olefin sodium sulfate and sodium lauryl sulfate are both detergent cleansing agents derived from coconut, but that doesn't make them good for skin.

"Synthetic" merely tells you that the ingredient was derived in a laboratory, and although that kind of origin may sound unhealthy, it often means that the resulting ingredient is going to be purer than a natural ingredient. Natural ingredients can be made up of hundreds of known and unknown ingredients and not all those components may be good for skin. Plus, the ingredients it took to create the plant extract—the chemical processes used to extract the oil or other natural substance from the plant— are almost always completely synthetic and unnatural.

None of this should be taken to suggest that plants don't have benefit in skin-care products. But the notion that watercress, comfrey, lavender, or green tea, and on and on, have any antiaging properties, can change one wrinkle on your face, or heal acne, especially the way they are used in cosmetics, is completely without substantiation or proof of any kind.

Some plants really do have benefits to offer, and where the research is clear on this, I make clear in my review. But to imply that a pure tincture of a plant can have the same effect when mixed into a cosmetic is, more times than not, a stretch of the imagination.

Having scoured through the research regarding plant extracts, here's what I can say unequivocally:

1. Most plant extracts in products either have minimal or no research establishing their efficacy.

2. When research does exist it is usually for the pure plant extract, not a watered-down version used in fractional amounts, mixed into a cosmetic of some kind.

3. Most research that establishes a plant's efficacy doesn't take into consideration that plant extracts are highly unstable. Think about it: how long does a head of lettuce last in your refrigerator? The notion that a plant extract can last and remain effective in a skin-care product is sheer fantasy.

4. While plants are unquestionably loaded with all kinds of substances that may be great when taken internally, the notion that all (or any) of those internal benefits can be transferred to the skin is unlikely. There is no research establish-

ing that rubbing pure green tea or grape juice (both potent antioxidants) directly over your face is helpful for wrinkles or any other aspect of skin care. When taken orally, there are many reasons to consider some of these plants for regular use, but for skin care, the benefit is all theory, and in a skin-care product, the theory is a lot more diluted.

5. **Almost without exception I rate the extracted active substance of the plant as having more efficacy potential than the plant.** For example, bisabolol is the active anti-inflammatory component in chamomile (specifically *Matricaria recutita*). While chamomile in a pure concentration can have that type of effectiveness, the likelihood is that this is lost in a plant extract used in teeny amounts in skin-care products. However, when bisabolol is listed on the label, it means the product uses the isolated active ingredient in chamomile that has anti-inflammatory benefits, and that the skin has a better shot at gaining benefit.

As seductive as it may be to get trapped by the plant craze in cosmetics, please think again. "Natural" doesn't give you any information about the quality of the formulation.

# Battle Plan for Wrinkles

There are no miracles when it comes to helping skin look smoother and reducing the appearance of lines. The classic treatment for sun damage, one with fairly impressive, well-researched, substantiated results, involves the following products.

1. **Retin-A or Renova,** to change abnormal cell production (caused by repeated sun exposure) back to some level of normalcy.

2. **An effective AHA or BHA product.** For AHA I recommend glycolic or lactic acid with a concentration of 8% to 10%; though higher concentrations exist I do not recommend them, due to the risk of irritation and inflammation. For BHA I recommend salicylic acid, the only effective form of BHA, in a concentration of 0.5% to 2% with 1% being preferred. Both AHA and BHA require a pH of 3 to 4 to be effective to exfoliate the top layer of skin. There are lots of inexpensive ones available. (BHA can exfoliate the surface of skin and inside the pore.) Enzymes are an option for topical exfoliation as well but are not considered as stable or as well researched as AHAs and BHA.

3. **A skin-lightening product** that includes at least 1% to 2% hydroquinone over the counter, and 4% and greater available only from physicians. Hydroquinone improves the appearance of brown discolorations by inhibiting melanin production. AHA or BHA in the formulation is also beneficial to encourage cell turnover, but is not necessary if a separate AHA or BHA product is used. Many plant extracts are now being hyped as being effective in blocking melanin production; however, the research for these extracts is not done on human skin but rather in vitro, and that doesn't translate to effectiveness, much less spending extra money on a product that contains these substances.

**4. A great, reliable sunscreen.** The only way to determine the quality of a sunscreen is to check the SPF number on the label (it must be SPF 15 or greater only), and then check the active ingredient label to be sure it has the UVA-blocking ingredients of either titanium dioxide, zinc oxide, and/or avobenzone (also called Parsol 1789 or butylmethoxydibenzoylmethane), and, outside of the U.S., Mexoryl SX™. This must be used every day, for the rest of your life.

**5. A gentle cleanser** used twice a day won't change wrinkles, but keeping skin irritant-free helps the healing process.

**6. A soothing, lightweight moisturizer** to be used over dry areas. Moisturizers help make skin look smoother, especially if it's dry, but use only the lightest texture that makes the skin feel soft. Overmoisturizing with layers of lotions and serums or using moisturizers that are too emollient and heavy for your skin type can hurt your skin.

All other so-called miracle antiwrinkle products and ingredients are bogus, misleading, and completely without substantiation or proof for their claims. It's not that there aren't great products for skin out there, but they won't change wrinkles. I know you get tempted, but giving up on any of the above recommendations so you can try a new gimmick (which will be replaced by the next skin miracle a few months or weeks later) is a waste of your time and money, and, even worse, possibly damaging to your skin!

## Skin Peels: Renova to Lasers

Most women are looking to achieve smoother skin. To that end, many are aware that exfoliating (removing) layers of unwanted dead skin can produce some pretty impressive results. But where do you go from there? How do you choose which product or service to use to help resurface your face? If you are trying to decide between having an AHA or BHA peel, microdermabrasion, laser resurfacing, or just using an AHA or BHA product, you are not alone. A lot of women wonder the same thing—in fact I would say this is the third most typical question I am asked (the first is about which is the best moisturizer and the second is about battling blemishes).

You may at least be happy to know that I consider all of the above valid options for dealing with wrinkles or some kinds of scarring. You may also be pleased to hear that, in many ways, the decision is less baffling than you may think. That's because it isn't about which method is effective (they are all effective in their way for removing surface layers of skin); rather, it is a question of money, tolerance, how comfortable you are about the risks (if any), and, finally, what results you are hoping to achieve. Once you understand how the answers to those questions affect your choice, you can start shopping for what you want as opposed to being sold a service by a convincing doctor or aesthetician.

For the sake of clarity, I'm going to start with Renova and Retin-A. The reason

I am beginning with these two topical prescription items that contain the same active drug ingredient, tretinoin, is not to consider them as a way to resurface or exfoliate layers of skin (though they are absolutely a consideration for treating sun-damaged skin) but to *eliminate* them as options, because they are not exfoliants! Tretinoin affects actual cell production deep in the dermis, far away from the surface of skin. That can help skin look and feel smoother, but the process is subtle and very different from the concept of removing surface layers of skin to create a smoother texture and appearance. All the other methods listed below affect the surface of the skin (or just below it) by actually ungluing or dissolving layers of dead skin cells. Why all the confusion about the effect these two creams have on the skin? Primarily it's due to the fact that using Renova and Retin-A can cause irritation and inflammation, resulting in the skin becoming flaky and dry. This flaking and dryness is not exfoliation, nor is it a desirable or advantageous result. If either Renova or Retin-A causes your skin to be consistently dry and flaky, it is a problem, and probably they are an option you should avoid for skin care.

**Risk: Minimal to none** except for irritation or allergic reaction, which stops when use is discontinued.

**Cost:** Inexpensive to moderate.

**Results:** A slightly noticeable smoother surface, but wrinkles and scars won't disappear or diminish in any significant way. Has no effect on ice-pick or dented scars from acne or chicken pox. Can have some positive effect in improving stretch marks, though it will not eliminate or change them significantly.

**Duration:** Ongoing while the product is being used.

<u>**AHA or BHA creams, gels, or lotions in concentrations ranging between 1% and 2% of BHA and 5% to 20% of AHA in a pH of 3 to 4.5 (with 3 to 3.5 being preferred).**</u> When it comes to removing surface layers of skin, this is really the place to start. While scrubs are the original topical exfoliants, they can't perform as evenly or smoothly as a well-formulated AHA or BHA topical skin-care product. Some fear that using AHAs and BHA may thin the skin, but that result has never been established. If anything, there is substantial research showing that AHAs or BHA may help produce collagen and improve skin integrity, making skin thicker (which is healthier than the thinning caused by the natural aging process) by removing unhealthy surface layers of skin on an ongoing basis. However, it should be mentioned that this new collagen production and skin thickness is probably caused by the repeated irritation this kind of exfoliation can cause. No one is quite sure why the improvement in skin takes place.

The FDA recently confirmed that there is a risk of UVB sun sensitivity following the use of AHAs and BHA. That makes sense, given that AHAs and BHA work to remove sun-damaged skin, which leaves the skin somewhat more vulnerable. Of course this sensitivity is easily preventable with the diligent use of a sunscreen, but that should be part and parcel of anyone's fight against wrinkles.

AHAs and BHA in skin-care products do have limitations. They don't go very deep (though BHA can be absorbed into a pore, making it preferred over AHA for blemish-prone skin). Their effect is entirely superficial, improving the surface feel of skin and creating minimal to slightly noticeable changes in the appearance of lines and color. Of course once you stop using them, in a short period of time the skin will return to the way it was before. There are negligible negative considerations for this option. These products are safe for most all skin types, skin colors, ages, and skin problems. There is that risk of irritation and sun sensitivity, but it is easily overcome by discontinuing use. Price is also not a problem, because there are great inexpensive options available. (Note that if you are allergic to aspirin, you will probably have difficulty using BHA, because just like aspirin BHA is a salicylate, which could cause a topical allergic reaction.)

**Risk: Minimal to none** except for irritation or allergic reaction, which stop when use of the products is discontinued.

**Cost: Inexpensive to expensive.** Some expensive options are available, but the cost doesn't have any impact on their effectiveness, just on the buyer's ego or belief in exaggerated cosmetic claims.

**Results:** A slightly noticeable smoother surface, but wrinkles and scars won't disappear or diminish in any significant way. Has no effect on ice-pick or dented scars from acne or chicken pox.

**Duration:** Ongoing while the product is being used.

**The next option to consider for skin resurfacing is microdermabrasion.** This relatively new procedure is performed by facialists, dermatologists, and plastic surgeons. It is little more than a deep surface scrub done with a machine that shoots ground mineral crystals onto the skin and then vacuums them back up. There is minimal to moderate risk, but that has little to do with your skin type or color and more to do with your reaction to the procedure and the skill of the technician. For some skin types, the irritation is too much, and some aestheticians get carried away and go over and over an area causing wounds and oozing. In order to obtain any kind of lasting or noticeable results, microdermabrasion needs to be constantly repeated, because once (and even three or four times) is not enough.

The most typical result is a noticeable reduction in the appearance of wrinkles and red skin discolorations (superficial scarring). This takes repeated sessions, and it is felt that the outcome is most likely a reaction to the skin being irritated and not by a change in the surface layers of skin. But that conclusion is open to debate, with most studies substantiating the concern. There is also little downtime associated with microdermabrasion, although some women do get red, dry, and flaky. The price varies widely, but generally the procedure can be pricey—and to get the smooth skin you are looking for, the repeated treatments can go on forever. The results also vary depending on the skill of the technician.

**Risk: Minimal.** Some women can experience redness, flaking, dryness, and irritation, but this usually diminishes within a few days. If you are prone to cold sores *(Herpes simplex)* around your mouth or on your face, this can trigger an outbreak.

**Cost: Expensive.** A series of microdermabrasion treatments can range from $300 to $600 for three treatments. That's pricey, considering the short-term nature of the results, and over a few years the amount can add up.

**Results:** After two to three treatments a noticeably smoother surface, with wrinkles and redness from surface acne scars reduced but not eliminated. Has no effect on ice-pick or dented scars from acne or chicken pox.

**Duration:** Improved appearance can last for one to three months, but treatments must be repeated for improvements to stick around.

**AHA peels ranging between 20% and 40% concentrations in a pH of 2 to 3.** Let me start by stating that there are no effective over-the-counter AHA or BHA peels available to the consumer (though some effective 20% concentration skin-care products are available from M.D. Formulations). There are products making claims that they have a high AHA content, but none of them work to exfoliate the surface of skin. All of those available over the counter have been neutralized and are ineffective for resurfacing the skin. Although cosmetics companies make it sound like you are buying an at-home peel, it is a blessing that these don't work! The risk to your skin of leaving these on too long is frightening to think about.

BHA peels are done strictly by physicians, as are AHA peels using concentrations of over 50%. AHA peels in concentrations of 40% or less are done by both physicians and facialists. There is a vast difference between results and risks at these varying concentrations (see the next section). At lower concentrations, AHA peels are similar in efficacy and results to microdermabrasion, with AHAs having a slight to moderate edge in creating a smoother appearance and less noticeable wrinkles and scars with only one to three applications. However, to obtain more significant, lasting results, it does take subsequent treatments—up to three and six over the period of a year. Both microdermabrasion and low-concentration AHA peels share the need for repeated treatments. While microdermabrasion may not produce the same quality of noticeable results, far fewer risks are associated with it. Even low-concentration AHAs can result in extreme redness, flaking, a burning sensation on the skin, and even some oozing and scabs.

**Risk: Minimal to moderate.** Some women can experience extreme redness, flaking skin that can last for a week, irritation, and dryness, although this usually diminishes in a week or two. If you are prone to cold sores *(Herpes simplex)* around your mouth or on your face, this process can trigger an outbreak.

**Cost: Moderate to expensive.** A series of AHA treatments can range from $300 to $600 for three treatments, and the treatments need to be repeated to maintain the effect.

**Results:** After two to three treatments a noticeably smoother surface, with less noticeable wrinkles and less obvious redness from surface acne scars. Has no effect on ice-pick or dented scars from acne or chicken pox.

**Duration:** Improved appearance can last from two to three months.

<u>**AHA peels ranging between 50% and 70% concentrations in a pH of 2 to 3, or BHA peels at 8% to 13% concentrations in a pH of 3.**</u> These high-concentration peels are performed strictly by physicians—and with good reason: the risk to skin is far higher, with many concerns about hypo- or hyperpigmentation, severe irritation, and risk of infection. As you may suspect, the higher risk goes hand in hand with more impressive, longer-lasting results. These kinds of medical peels can make a significant difference in the appearance of skin. They can fundamentally change the appearance of wrinkles and surface scarring; however, they still won't have an effect on ice-pick or dented scars from acne or chicken pox. Peels like this also have a far longer duration, with the effects lasting between two and three, and up to five, years.

**Risk: Moderate.** Most women will experience severe redness, and flaking, oozing skin, and that can last for one to four weeks. The risk for these effects is reportedly somewhat less with a BHA peel, as BHA's relation to aspirin may provide an analgesic effect along with the peeling action. There is also the possibility of a minimal risk of skin discoloration (either darkened areas of skin or lighter areas of skin—however, when this does occur it often doesn't last and fades with minimal treatment of prescribed skin-lighteners). This risk of discoloration is more significant for those with darker skin tones. If you are prone to cold sores *(Herpes simplex)* around your mouth or on your face, this can trigger an outbreak.

**Cost: Expensive.** A high-concentration AHA or BHA peel can range from $1,000 to $2,500.

**Results:** After healing is completed, the skin will have a markedly smoother appearance, with facial lines and surface scarring being greatly reduced. High-concentration AHA and BHA peels have no effect on ice-pick or dented scars from acne or chicken pox.

**Duration:** Improved appearance can last from two to five years.

<u>**Laser resurfacing.**</u> This is the prince of all peels. Other than a face-lift, this is the last of the effective surface treatments to help reduce the appearance of wrinkles. This procedure is both extremely effective and the most risky. The results can be astounding, but when it's overdone or done with poor pre- and postoperative procedures, it can give the skin a plastic look. When done right, it can smooth out a good deal of wrinkling, uneven skin texture, skin discoloration, and acne scarring. It can't

undo deep folds or heavily sagging skin, but it can retract some sagging. It cannot eliminate dented or ice-pick scars.

Preoperative care, including the use of skin lightener (to reduce the risk of skin discoloration), Renova or Retin-A to improve the skin's healing ability and the general health of the skin, and the use of effective sunscreens, is important, and it can help achieve positive results. It is also essential that the patient stop smoking for as long as possible before treatment (smoking not only causes wrinkles but it can also weaken the skin's immune system enough to put the patient in a higher risk category). Postoperative care varies, but silicone bandages are considered one of the best options, along with antibiotic creams and oral antibiotics. There should be minimal exposure to sun and irritating skin-care products of any kind.

**Risk: Moderate to severe.** Most women will experience severe redness, flaking, and oozing skin, and that can last for two to five weeks. There is also a possible risk of skin discoloration (either darkened areas of skin or lighter areas of skin). This risk of discoloration is more significant for those with darker skin tones. If you are prone to cold sores *(Herpes simplex)* around your mouth or on your face, this can trigger an outbreak.

**Cost: Expensive.** Prices range from $2,500 to $5,000.

**Results:** After healing is completed, the skin will have a markedly smoother appearance, with facial lines and surface scarring greatly reduced and some eliminated altogether. Deep, furrowed lines will not be affected very much. Laser resurfacing can greatly improve and eliminate some acne scarring. It cannot eliminate sagging skin but some retraction will be visible.

**Duration:** Improved appearance can last from three to seven years.

# *SunBelievable*

I have written extensively about issues having to do with sun protection. Those of you who have read my earlier work should all be wearing a sunscreen of SPF 15 or greater every morning regardless of the weather, right? You also keep some in your purse for applying after you wash your hands or after perspiring heavily, right? You apply it 20 minutes before going outside, right? And you've checked the label for those all-important UVA-protecting active ingredients, right?

While the world of skin care is definitely providing better and better sunscreen products, some really bad products are also still out there. This list will also help you handle the myths that are generated as different companies try to defend their products as being the best when they aren't.

1. **There is no such thing as a safe tan,** at least not from the sun or tanning beds. Even if you tan slowly without burning, the damage to the skin is still hazardous to the health of your skin.

2.   UVB radiation describes the sun's burning rays, which have an immediate harmful impact on skin. **Damage from UVB rays takes place the very first minute** (yes, 60 seconds) you walk outside.

3.   **UVA rays are the sun's silent killers;** you don't feel them, but they are the primary cause of skin cancer and wrinkles! (UVA rays also penetrate through clear glass windows.)

4.   Even on a cloudy day, the sun's rays are ever present and ever attacking the skin.

5.   Sitting in the shade or wearing a hat only protects from a small portion of the sun's rays. Plus, other surrounding surfaces such as water, cement, and grass reflect the rays from the ground to your skin, giving you a double whammy of damage.

6.   Altitude is a sun enhancer; for every 1,000-foot increase in altitude, the sun's potency increases by 4%.

7.   According to the FDA, a product's SPF (sunscreen protection factor) number tells you how long you can stay in the sun while wearing it without getting burnt. Here's how it works: if it normally takes you 20 minutes in the sun before you start turning pink, an SPF 15 product will let you stay in the sun for five hours without burning. The formula is 20 (minutes) x 15 (SPF) = 300 (minutes), or five hours. But that five hours applies only if you aren't swimming or perspiring. If you are active or if you get wet, you need to reapply the sunscreen after 60 to 90 minutes.

8.   **SPF is crucial, but it is a measurement that only pertains to sunburn** (UVB rays). There are no numbers to tell you about protection from UVA radiation. For that protection you have to check the active ingredient list to see if either <u>zinc oxide</u>, <u>titanium dioxide</u>, or <u>avobenzone</u> (which may also be listed as Parsol 1789 or butyl methoxydibenzoylmethane) or, outside of the United States, <u>Mexoryl SX</u>™ is one of the active ingredients. If one of those isn't part of the active ingredient listing (it doesn't count if it is just part of the regular ingredients), you will not be getting adequate UVA protection.

9.   Several sunscreen ingredients are approved for use in the United States for sunburn protection, with a wide variety of technical names. While benzophenone and oxybenzone sound like avobenzone, and though they do have some UVA protection to offer, they are not as effective as titanium dioxide, zinc oxide, avobenzone (also called Parsol 1789 or butylmethoxydibenzoylmethane), or Mexoryl SX™. Both oxybenzone and benzophenone protect only up to 350 to 360 nanometers of the UV spectrum, but UVA radiation goes up to 400 nanometers, which means those two ingredients fall short of providing complete protection. Titanium dioxide, zinc oxide, avobenzone (also called Parsol 1789 and butyl methoxydibenzoylmethane), and Mexoryl SX™ all protect up to and over 400 nanometers.

10. For those of you who want more specifics about the issue of UVA versus UVB protection: according to information in the *Skin Therapy Letter* published by

the Division of Dermatology at the University of British Columbia, vol. 2, no. 5, 1997, the "UVA [range is] 315 [through] 400 nanometers" [according to the FDA the UVB range is from 280 to 315]. The range of protection for the following sunscreen ingredients is listed in this article as "Padimate O, 290–315 nanometers; benzophenones, 250–350 nanometers; octyl methoxycinnamate, 290–320 nanometers; avobenzone, 320–400 nanometers; titanium dioxide, 290–700 nanometers; and zinc oxide, 290–700 nanometers."

11. **Waterproof sunscreens are actually not waterproof,** a fact the FDA is trying to impose on sunscreen labeling. However, sunscreens can be *water resistant,* which means they need to be reapplied if you've been swimming or sweating for more than 90 minutes to two hours.

12. An SPF 2 blocks about 50% of the UVB rays, an SPF 10 filters out about 85% of the UVB rays, an SPF 15 stops about 95%, and an SPF 30 through SPF 50 stops about 97%. So even if the SPF number on the label of your sunscreens is an ultra-high SPF 50, it still has limitations, which explains why you still might get some color after prolonged exposure to the sun despite slathering sunscreen on your skin. Another reason you may be getting color despite the use of a good sunscreen is because of the next two pieces of information.

13. **Always apply sunscreen at least 15 to 20 minutes before going outside.** This gives the sunscreen time to be absorbed and to spread over and into the skin.

14. **You must apply sunscreen liberally.** In a study published in the *Archives of Dermatology* "…sunscreen users are only applying 50 percent of the recommended amount, so they are only receiving 50 percent of the SPF protection." What is the right amount? A generous application that spreads a noticeable layer over the entire exposed area of skin, and that is then massaged into the skin until it is absorbed.

15. Because of this issue concerning liberal application, expensive sunscreens can be dangerous to your skin's health. After all, how likely are you to liberally apply a sunscreen from Lancome that costs $32 for 2 ounces or, even more absurdly, a sunscreen from La Prairie that costs $150 for 1 ounce?

16. If you are using AHAs, BHA, Retin-A, Renova, Differin, or any other topical pharmaceutical retinoid, it can make your skin more vulnerable to sun damage due to the surface exfoliation and changes (removing the top layer of sun-damaged skin) caused by using these types of products. This information does not impact those who are already diligent about using sunscreen, but if you are using these products and not being diligent, your skin is even more at risk for sun damage and sunburn with even minimal sun exposure.

17. Getting a sunburn is bad enough, but what you may not know is that **a sunburn continues to develop for 12 to 24 hours after the initial burn takes place!** Treating a sunburn immediately and effectively is the same as treating any other burn. Do not

cover it with thick salves (butter and thick moisturizers are the worst). These will trap the heat and cause more damage. Get the skin in contact with cool water immediately (do not put ice directly on the skin—that's too much cold and can cause a different kind of burn). Keep applying the cool water on and off for several hours.

18. With babies or small children, the issue of sunscreen protection should absolutely be of primary concern. Their delicate skin is even more sensitive to the sun's damaging energy. All sunscreen formulations that have an SPF are regulated closely by the FDA; the formulations don't differ in any way because of the age of the intended user. Of greater concern than the cute packaging kids' products come in is that the formulation you choose must contain one of the UVA-protecting ingredients, either avobenzone (also called Parsol 1789 or butylmethoxydibenzoylmethane), titanium dioxide, or zinc oxide.

19. If you are looking for a less-irritating sunscreen for your kids or yourself, choose one that contains only pure titanium dioxide or zinc oxide as the active ingredient; these will definitely be less irritating than products made with other types of sunscreen agents.

20. If you're determined to tan, the only safe way to do it is with the self-tanning products sold by cosmetics lines of all kinds.

## Applying Sunscreen Is Serious Business

Now that so many products contain sunscreen (foundation, concealers, moisturizers, and even face powders), the question I'm constantly asked is, what about application? That's a great question! Keeping in mind that liberal application is the key element of getting the best protection possible, these other key points give you the rest of the story.

**At what part of a skin-care routine does sunscreen get used?** If you are applying several skin-care products, ranging from toners to acne medications to moisturizers, the rule is that **the last item you apply during the day is your sunscreen.** If you apply sunscreen and then apply, say, your moisturizer or an acne product, you could inadvertently be diluting or breaking down the effectiveness of the sunscreen you've just applied.

**What about applying foundation (one that doesn't contain sunscreen) over the sunscreen you've just applied?** If the foundation is a thin, watery-type foundation or you're using a tinted, lotion-type moisturizer (which doesn't contain sunscreen) you would in all likelihood be reducing the potency of the sunscreen underneath. However, if you are applying a standard liquid foundation, a cream-to-powder foundation, a cream foundation, or a pressed-powder foundation, and as long as you are smoothing that over the skin and not wiping it off or rubbing it too heavily into the skin, there is minimal to no risk that you are affecting the sunscreen underneath.

If you are using more than one product that contains sunscreen, such as an SPF 15 moisturizer and an SPF 8 foundation, it's the one with the higher SPF number that must contain UVA-protecting ingredients. However, two sunscreens with different numbers do not add up to one big SPF number. In other words, an SPF 8 and an SPF 15 do not add up to an SPF 23. Yes, you would be getting an increased SPF value for protection, but there is no way to know what increased protection that would be. If you want to count on getting an SPF 30's worth of protection, that is the SPF number you should look for in one product.

**What if your foundation is the product you've chosen for sun protection?** Then the trick is to be sure you've applied it evenly and liberally. If you apply it too thinly or blend most of it off, you would not be getting the amount of protection listed on the label.

I am concerned about the new pressed powders with SPF ratings. While I don't doubt the validity of the SPF number, I worry that most women don't apply pressed-powder foundations liberally enough to get the amount of protection indicated on the label. **If you lightly dust the powder over the skin, there is no way you will get the SPF protection indicated on the label.** You must be sure you are applying the pressed powder in a manner that completely and evenly covers the face. I feel that pressed powders are an iffy way to get sun protection for the face, but they are a great way to touch up your makeup during the day and reapply sunscreen at the same time! Olay has an excellent SPF 15–rated pressed powder and so does Neutrogena with an SPF 30!

Because it bears repeating, as I mentioned above, **you must apply sunscreen liberally.** In a study published in the *Archives of Dermatology* ". . . sunscreen users are only applying 50 percent of the recommended amount, so they are only receiving 50 percent of the SPF protection." That means a generous amount must be used to get the protection indicated by the SPF number.

## Sunscreens for Oily Skin?

The search for a sunscreen that is appropriate for oily skin can be a frustrating, lifelong pursuit. Even those I've created for my line can have problems for some people. The difficulties are several-fold. The types of ingredients that can be used to suspend sunscreen agents are not exactly the best for oily skin. Regardless of the claim on the label, there is a risk that the base formulation can clog pores or feel slippery or greasy on the skin. There's also the problem that the sunscreen ingredients themselves can cause an irritated breakout reaction from the synthetically derived sunscreen agents. (Regrettably, that is the nature of almost all active ingredients used in cosmetics—"active" meaning they actually do something on the skin. Whether they are AHAs, Renova, benzoyl peroxide, hydroquinone, or sunscreen ingredients, they can be irritating.) In the case of titanium dioxide and zinc oxide, even though they are relatively innocuous and have minimal to no risk of irritation on skin, they can still clog pores, being the thick, creamy ingredients that they are. Finally, given the wide variety in formulations, there is no way to quantify which ingredients are more problematic than others for causing problems.

What to do? The only true answer is to experiment. I wish there was a slam-dunk solution I could offer, but there are no product lines that can legitimately make the claim that their sunscreen won't cause breakouts (but those of you with this problem already know that).

## *Battle Plans for Blemishes*

Regardless of your age, from puberty to menopause and beyond, there are no real mysteries about how a pimple is created. A pimple starts with some amount of oil, usually too much oil, being produced in the pore. That oil is controlled and regulated primarily by your hormones. The oil, for many reasons, cannot get out of the pore in an even flow. This restricted oil flow is more than likely caused by a pore that has a thickened lining that prevents the oil from easily moving out of the pore. The backed-up oil creates a clogged pore. The next element needed to create a pimple is bacteria (typically propiobacterium) sitting in the pore and living on the oil. Together the inflammation and bacteria proliferation result in a pimple.

The steps listed below address each of the factors that cause pimples. These are the best options for absorbing oil production (though you can't affect the hormonal cause of oil production from the outside in), the best options for disinfecting the skin (to reduce or eliminate the presence of the bacteria causing the pimple), and the best options for improving exfoliation within the pore (which can improve the shape of the pore lining, preventing oil production from getting backed up). Finding the combination that works for you is the goal, and that takes experimentation. However, it is essential to address all the issues—just using a disinfectant or an exfoliant or an oil-absorbing mask alone won't cut it. It's the combination of these that produces the desired results.

To find the right combination of products that works for you is to always be certain you are addressing each of the issues that create a pimple and that the products you use tackle each of those blemish triggers. For example, if you choose plan A but find 3% hydrogen peroxide (the disinfectant) is not effective and you want to try something else, switch to another option for disinfecting blemishes, such as a benzoyl peroxide product or a prescription topical antibiotic (disinfectant). If you decide to try plan C but find Retin-A (a retinoid that can improve skin-cell production, thereby making the shape of the pore more normal) too irritating, switch to a different prescription retinoid, such as Differin or a topical exfoliant like Azelex (azelaic acid) that can also improve the shape of the pore.

**Cleaning the face:** Using a water-soluble cleanser that gently cleans your skin without stimulating the oil glands, increasing redness, or creating dryness is fundamental. This step is standard for any skin-care routine because it makes an instant difference in the appearance and feel of the skin, and it is essential for reducing breakouts. Specifically with regard to breakouts, using drying or irritating skin-care products hurts the skin's healing process, making scarring worse and encouraging proliferation of the bacteria that cause pimples. Further, using cleansers with pore-clogging ingredients like soaps or bar cleansers (the ingredients that keep bar cleansers in their bar form can clog pores) can make matters worse.

If you are using an ultra-matte-finish foundation or a cream-to-powder foundation, it may be necessary to use a washcloth with your cleanser to be sure you are getting all your makeup off every night. To prevent bacteria growth, use a clean washcloth every time you wash your face.

**Exfoliating:** Using an 8% alpha hydroxy acid (AHA) product or a 1% to 2% beta hydroxy acid (BHA) product is a crucial over-the-counter starting point for exfoliating the skin to prevent skin-cell buildup and to reshape the pore itself so oil can flow more evenly, preventing clogged pores. I recommend using AHAs or BHA in gel, liquid, or thin lotion form, because they are unlikely to contain thickening agents or emollients that can clog pores. For all forms of breakouts, BHA is preferred over AHA because AHA is not as effective at cutting through the oil inside the pore. Getting into the pore is necessary to exfoliating the pore lining in order to effect a more normal pore shape. However, because some people can't use BHA, AHA is the next option to consider.

If you are seeing a physician, you will probably want to supplement this step with, or exclusively use, a retinoid such as Retin-A, Differin, or perhaps Azelex (contains azelaic acid, which is not a retinoid but more like an AHA with some antimicrobial activity; it is prescription-only). If you choose to use both a retinoid and an AHA or BHA, you can use the AHA or BHA during the day and the Retin-A, Differin, or Azelex at night. Some dermatologists recommend applying an AHA or BHA product first and then applying Retin-A, Differin, or Azelex directly over that. The thought is that the AHA or BHA boosts the effectiveness and penetration of the other products. Again, experiment to see what works best for your skin.

Also, don't forget good old reliable baking soda, used as a mechanical exfoliant over breakouts and blemishes. It's not as gentle or as "smooth" an exfoliant as AHA, BHA, Retin-A, Differin, or Azelex, but many people still find it a handy option for exfoliating dead skin cells and for removing the surface of blemishes without damaging the skin.

**Note:** Benzoyl peroxide and hydrogen peroxide negate the effectiveness of retinoids and therefore cannot be used at the same time. To get both effects, you can use a topical prescription antibiotic or benzoyl peroxide in the morning and the retinoid in the evening.

**Disinfecting:** There aren't many options when it comes to disinfecting the skin. Alcohol (when used in the right concentrations, and very few products ever contain the right amount) and sulfur can be good disinfectants, but they are too drying and irritating, and that ends up generating more breakouts by hurting the skin's healing process, which in turn encourages the production of more bacteria. (Other irritating ingredients that repeatedly show up in products for problem skin, such as lemon, grapefruit, acetone, witch hazel, peppermint, menthol, eucalyptus, and camphor, have no effect at all on bacteria and cause more problems by hurting the skin's healing process.) Currently popular plant-derived disinfectants such as tea tree oil (melaleuca) are not present in high enough concentrations to reliably kill bacteria (further explained below).

For quite some time, I have been recommending 3% hydrogen peroxide as a disinfectant, and it is a great starting point in your battle plan. If 3% hydrogen peroxide doesn't prove effective, the next option is benzoyl peroxide at a 2.5% strength, then 5%, and then 10%. To see what works best, begin with the lowest strength and work up. However, be careful with peroxides, as they can lighten the hair on and surrounding your face (including eyebrows and sideburns). If those products fail to have the effect you want, a topical antibiotic or even an oral antibiotic prescribed by a doctor may be the only options left to kill stubborn blemish-causing bacteria, but an oral antibiotic should be a last resort. Oral antibiotics can indeed kill blemish-causing bacteria, but they also kill good bacteria in the body, cause yeast infections, bring about stomach problems, and yellow the teeth. As bothersome and problematic as all those side effects are, the most serious side effect is that your body will adapt to the antibiotic. That means the antibiotic eventually will no longer be effective for fighting acne bacteria or any other bacterial infection you might get. And that can pose a dangerous threat to your long-term health.

**Absorbing excess oil:** While most people think clay masks are the only way to absorb excess oil on the skin, these are my last choice for that purpose. Using milk of magnesia as a facial mask is by far the best way to absorb oil I have ever found or personally used. Milk of magnesia is nothing more than liquid magnesium hydroxide, which is known to soothe skin and reduce irritation, and it has incredible oil-absorbing properties. Magnesium absorbs more oil than clay, and clay has no disinfecting or soothing properties. How often you use the milk of magnesia depends on how oily your skin is. Some use it every day; others, once a week. Only you and your skin can determine what frequency works best for you.

**When all else fails:** If your breakouts persist after you've tried these over-the-counter and prescription options for gentle cleansing, disinfecting, exfoliating, and absorbing excess oil, it may be necessary to consider more serious drugs that can affect hormonal production, such as hormone blockers or birth-control pills designed to reduce breakouts. Accutane is one of the last options in this lineup only because of its serious side effects if a woman becomes pregnant while using it (I discuss these options at length in my book *The Beauty Bible*). However, **Accutane is the only option that can potentially cure breakouts.** All other methods simply keep the problem reduced or at bay. More than 50% of the people who take Accutane once never break out again, and it eliminates oily skin altogether. Those odds are increased significantly for some people who take it a second time.

The following battle plans are presented in order, starting with the most commonly available products with the least potential for side effects such as irritation, and working up to stronger products, some available only by prescription. The first battle plan may be all that is required to heal your skin. As you see how your skin responds, you can experiment with the various options for each category. **The most important element for all these skin-care battle plans is consistency. It takes a minimum of six weeks to see a consistent improvement in your skin.** Remember, spot treatment doesn't work. You have to maintain consistent gentle cleansing, exfoliation, disinfecting, and oil absorption to change the way your skin behaves.

If irritation or skin sensitivity occurs, you may need to cut back on the exfoliant, disinfectant, and/or facial mask you are using. It doesn't mean the skin-care routine isn't or won't eventually work for you, but perhaps your skin can't handle the frequency of application, at least not in the beginning. In that case you may need to reduce how often you apply the AHA, Retin-A, or Differin from twice a day to once a day or every other day, and the same is true with the disinfectant and facial mask.

**Plan A.** Gentle cleanser; baking-soda scrub over blemishes; 3% hydrogen peroxide used as a disinfectant over blemishes; and milk of magnesia as a facial mask to absorb excess oil.

**Plan B.** Gentle cleanser; 8% AHA gel or liquid; 2.5% or 5% benzoyl peroxide liquid or gel; and milk of magnesia as a facial mask.

**Plan C.** Gentle cleanser; 1% or 2% BHA gel or liquid; 2.5% or 5% benzoyl peroxide liquid or gel; and milk of magnesia as a facial mask.

**Plan D.** Gentle cleanser; 8% AHA gel or liquid in the morning and Retin-A or Differin at night; 2.5% benzoyl peroxide liquid or gel or 3% hydrogen peroxide *(Note: you cannot apply benzoyl peroxide at the same time as Retin-A or Differin; you would apply the Differin or Retin-A in the evening and the benzoyl peroxide in the morning);* and milk of magnesia as a facial mask.

**Plan E.** Gentle cleanser; 1% or 2% BHA gel or liquid in the morning and Retin-A or Differin at night; 2.5% or 5% benzoyl peroxide liquid or gel *(Note: you cannot apply benzoyl peroxide at the same time as Retin-A or Differin; you would apply the*

*Differin or Retin-A in the evening and the benzoyl peroxide in the morning);* and milk of magnesia as a facial mask.

**Plan F.** Gentle cleanser; Retin-A, Differin, or Azelex; a topical prescription antibiotic; and milk of magnesia as a facial mask.

**Plan G.** Gentle cleanser; Retin-A, Differin, or Azelex; a topical prescription antibiotic; an oral antibiotic; and milk of magnesia as a facial mask.

**Plan H.** Gentle cleanser; and hormone blockers or low-dose birth-control pills (discussed in my book *The Beauty Bible)* to control hormone levels that cause breakouts.

**Plan I.** When all else fails, Accutane can be a consideration. It is a serious prescription drug, with potentially unsafe side effects for pregnant women, but it has a good success rate for curing acne and oily skin. Recurrence can happen for a percentage of those who take Accutane but that can take years to happen and a second series can nip that in the bud.

**Order of Application:** The best option for application of skin-care products with active ingredients (both over the counter and prescription) is as follows: After cleansing and toning (the toner part is optional but it can be helpful to remove the last traces of makeup), you would apply an AHA or BHA product. Next you can apply a topical disinfectant such as a 2.5% or 5% benzoyl peroxide product. You can also apply an AHA or BHA product and then apply a topical retinoid such as Retin-A or Differin. The reason for this order is because the exfoliating properties of AHAs and BHA "open up" the skin and the pores, allowing the other active ingredients to penetrate the skin better. The only exception is that you cannot apply peroxides and retinoid at the same time.

## *Tea Tree Oil/Melaleuca*

There are skin-care lines based solely on proclaiming the astonishing benefits of tea tree oil. The most typical claim for tea tree oil (from the plant *Melaleuca alterniflora)* is that it is a good option for treating acne, and better than pharmaceutical versions. After all, it's a plant. But according to the *Healthnotes Review of Complementary and Integrative Medicine* that is not the case. The *Healthnotes Review of Complementary and Integrative Medicine* (for subscription information call 503-234-4092) presents a compilation of published (meaning objective and peer-reviewed) scientific research concerning the effectiveness of herbal preparations. One of the issues addressed in the *Review*'s summer 1998 issue is the use of tea tree oil versus benzoyl peroxide for the treatment of acne. A study of 119 patients using 5% tea tree oil in a gel base versus 5% benzoyl peroxide lotion was discussed. There were 61 in the benzoyl peroxide group and 58 in the tea tree oil group. The conclusion was "both treatments were effective in reducing the number of inflamed lesions throughout the trial, with a significantly better result for benzoyl peroxide when compared to the tea tree oil.

Skin oiliness was lessened significantly in the benzoyl peroxide group versus the tea tree oil group." However, while the reduction of breakouts was greater for the benzoyl peroxide group, side effects of dryness, stinging, and burning were also greater—"79% of the benzoyl peroxide group versus 49% of the tea tree oil group."

It seems clear that a 2.5% strength benzoyl peroxide solution would be better to start with to see if it is effective, rather than jumping to the more potent and more irritating 5% concentration. If you were interested in using a 5% strength tea tree oil solution to see if that would be effective, I know of no products that claim to contain that amount. From what I can tell, most all tea tree oil products being sold contain less than a 1% concentration, not enough to really help breakouts, at least not based on this research.

## Getting Rid of Blackheads

A lot of people are unclear (pun intended) about how to win the fight against blackheads and whiteheads (technically, whiteheads are called *milia*). Why all the confusion? Primarily it's due to the myriad products that claim they can rid the face of these insidious, tiny white and black dots that mar its appearance, yet don't make them go away—and sometimes even make them worse. In essence, the truth about blackheads (usually accompanied by oily skin) and whiteheads (usually accompanied by dry skin) is hard to accept. What is the truth? The truth is they are just hard to get rid of. It is hard to win the battle against clogged pores.

Normally working pores produce a normal amount of sebum (oil) and easily distribute the oil to the surface of skin. The amount of sebum production is regulated almost exclusively by hormones. When a regular amount of oil is produced, it effortlessly moves through the pore and out onto the surface of skin, where it melts into an imperceptible film that forms a protective barrier over the face.

When hormones cause too much oil to be produced, or skin cells block the path of the oil, or when for genetic reasons you happen to have pores that are malformed, the tendency is to get blackheads or whiteheads. Further exacerbating these conditions is the buildup in the pore of skin-care or makeup products along with skin cells that can get trapped in the sticky sebum sitting in the pore. When the sebum and skin cells are sitting in a pore that is not covered over by skin, they are exposed to the air, which causes the sebum and skin cells to oxidize and turn black. When the sebum and skin cells are sitting in a pore that is covered by skin, the sebum and skin cells are not exposed to air and therefore stay clear, but form a slight white bump under the skin.

The never-ending questions are: Why do some people get whiteheads and not blackheads? Why does the problem occur in some areas of the face but not others? What causes some products to make people break out but *not* give them blackheads?

And finally, what makes some products cause blackheads but not acne? Those questions have no specific answers. It seems to be primarily a genetic predisposition accompanied by the right conditions (mentioned above) randomly taking place in any one of the thousands of pores we have on our face. Not to mention an unknown reaction to the over 50,000 cosmetic ingredients we may come in contact with from the products we use.

To clear up (again, pun intended) the confusion, this is as good a time as any to go over the battle plans against blackheads and whiteheads, because with some effort they can be reduced, and, depending on how your skin reacts, may even be eliminated.

Other than avoiding products that are too emollient (meaning thick or greasy creams) and not using moisturizers when you don't need them, there are really only three essentials for dealing with whiteheads and blackheads:

**1. Gentle, water-soluble cleansers** (and avoiding bar soap). The ingredients that keep bar soap in its bar form can clog pores, and irritation can cause skin cells to flake off before they're ready and thus accumulate in the pore.

There are lots of gentle cleansers to consider, ranging from Alpha Hydrox, Basis, Cetaphil, Neutrogena, and Olay to Paula's Choice. It's actually getting more and more difficult to find a cleanser that isn't gentle. The only different approach would be for someone with dry skin to use a slightly more moisturizing cleanser—but be careful: cleansers that are too emollient leave a greasy film on the skin and that can cause further problems.

**2. Gentle exfoliants** that can both remove the excess skin cells on the surface of the face (so they don't build up in the pore) and exfoliate inside the pore (to improve the shape of the pore, allowing a more even flow of oil through it). Keep in mind that the structure of the pore itself is lined with skin cells that can build up, creating a narrowed shape that doesn't allow natural oil flow. But don't get carried away with this step. Removing too many skin cells (overdoing it) can cause problems and hurt skin. Exfoliation is essential for both dry and oily skin to try to eliminate blackheads or whiteheads. The only difference is that someone with dry skin will want an exfoliant that has a more moisturizing base.

The best option for a good exfoliant is a 1% or 2% BHA gel, liquid, or lotion. There are still only limited options for this one, including: Paula's Choice 1% or 2% Beta Hydroxy Acid, Serious Skin Care Clarifying Treatment with 2% Salicylic Acid, Oxy Balance Night Watch Maximum Strength with 2% Salicylic Acid, and Neutrogena Clear Pore Treatment with 2% Salicylic Acid.

*By the way, topical disinfectants such as benzoyl peroxide or topical antibiotics available by prescription are unwarranted in the treatment of blackheads and milia because there is no bacterial involvement related to these conditions.*

**3. Absorbing excess oil.** This step is more for those with oily skin and is really not an option for those with whiteheads and dry skin, because with milia, *excess* oil isn't as much the problem as *trapped* oil. For those with oily skin, you all know I prefer milk of magnesia (a few companies, including mine, have cosmetic versions of this step. Smash Box has Anti Shine, a magnesium-based solution for absorbing oil). Clay masks are an option. Though they're not my favorite, some women do like these, and as long as they don't contain other irritants, they can have a positive effect in absorbing oil. The handful of silicone-based oil-absorbing products meant to be worn under makeup, from companies like Lancome and Clinique, get mixed reviews from women and I find them fairly ineffective for really oily skin. Still, they are always worth a trial run.

**4. Effective but optional considerations** for all skin types are Retin-A, Renova, or Differin. These can be used on their own or with a BHA product. Research has definitely established that Retin-A, Renova, and Differin have positive effects on how pores function, and these products should be a consideration for very stubborn cases or when blackheads are accompanied by breakouts.

For those with oily-skin troubles, hormone blockers or certain low-dose birth-control pills to reduce the hormone levels that create the excess oil that is at the root of the problem may be an option. And, when all else fails, Accutane can be a consideration. Though many doctors are reluctant to prescribe Accutane for "merely" oily skin and blackheads, for those with that kind of persistent skin problem, it does not feel like a "mere" problem in the least and Accutane can be a cure.

For all skin types, AHA peels, microdermabrasion, and laser resurfacing can have some impact on the appearance of blackheads and milia; however, they don't improve pore functioning—rather they temporarily get rid of the surface problem, making things look better.

**Please note:** This isn't a pretty topic, but it is a fact of life and human nature that just leaving a blemish or blackhead alone is almost impossible. Fortunately, gently removing a blackhead or blemish with light-handed squeezing can actually help the skin. Removing the stuff inside a blackhead or especially a pimple relieves the pressure and reduces further damage. Yes, squeezing can be detrimental to the skin, but how you squeeze determines whether you inflict harm. If you oversqueeze, pinch the skin, scrape the skin with your nails, or press too hard, you are absolutely doing more damage than good. Gentle is the key word and, when done right, squeezing with minimal pressure is the best, if not only, way to clean out a blackhead or blemish.

*Although I never recommend steaming the face (heat can overstimulate oil production, cause spider veins to surface, and create irritation), a tepid to slightly warm compress over the face can help soften the blackhead or blemish, making removal easier. First, wash your face with a water-soluble cleanser. Pat the skin dry, then place a slightly warm, wet cloth over your face for approximately 10 to 15 minutes. Once that's done, pat the skin dry again. Using a tissue over each finger to keep you from slipping and tearing the skin, apply even, soft pressure to the sides of the blemish area, gently pressing down and then up around the lesion. Do this once or twice only. If nothing happens, that means the blemish cannot be removed, and continuing will bruise the skin, risk making the infection or lesion worse, and cause scarring. Again, only use gentle pressure, protect your skin by using tissue around your fingers, and do not oversqueeze.*

**One more note:** What about pore strips? What has me most concerned about these so-called pore removing strips is that they are accompanied by a list of strong warnings such as not to use them over any area other than the nose and not to use them over inflamed, swollen, sunburned, or excessively dry skin. It also states that if the strip is too painful to remove, you should wet it and then carefully remove it. What a warning! You may at first be impressed with what comes off your nose. (Well, if you have very black-looking blackheads, there is no question: you will be impressed.) Most people do have some oil sitting at the top of their oil glands (most of the face's oil glands are located on the nose), and whether you use these strips or a piece of tape, black dots and some skin will be removed. Is that helpful? Only momentarily, but if you use these repeatedly, they will not eliminate the problem and the ingredient on the strip can eventually irritate skin and potentially trigger further breakouts.

Also, despite the warning on the package, most women will try these strips wherever they see breakouts. If I didn't know better, I know I would. The way these strips adhere, they can absolutely injure or tear skin and cause spider veins to surface. They are especially unsafe if you've been using Retin-A, Renova, AHAs, or BHA; having facial peels or taking Accutane; or if you have naturally thin skin or any skin disorder such as rosacea, psoriasis, or seborrhea.

## What About Empty, Enlarged Pores?

Once a pore is emptied and the unsightly blackhead is removed, it can take a period of time for the pore to heal and close up. Maintaining the regimen of gentle cleansing, exfoliating, and absorbing oil can go a long way to making this happen. If your skin can tolerate Retin-A, Renova, or Differin, that can also help promote healing by further improving cell production in the pore. However, even after all this, an empty, open, but permanently damaged pore can remain and be an unattractive byproduct of the original problem. If you have patiently adhered to all the right steps, there is very little else that can be done to change the damage. Time will tell if the effect of improving pore function can shrink a pore, but it does take time, and not everyone will have the same results. Microdermabrasion, AHA or BHA peels, and laser resurfacing can improve the appearance of pores, but this is considered a temporary fix and is not noted for actually changing or correcting the problem. Most likely, the improvement is caused from the skin's swelling and making the pores look smaller. Again, it is hard to determine success rates, because very few long-term published results are available.

The struggle to cover large pores is nothing less than maddening. The very nature of a depression in the skin makes it difficult if not impossible to keep the indentation from showing. Especially if your skin is still oily, and even if you use an extremely matte foundation like Revlon's ColorStay Lite or regular ColorStay, Lancome Teint Idole or Eau de Teint, or Estee Lauder's Double Wear or Double Matte, the oil can still make for some shifting, creating a look of pooled foundation in the pore.

I apologize for sounding dismal about this, but there are limitations in the skin *and* in the world of makeup, and searching for better options or alternatives can waste money and only increase your frustration. Here is a game plan to tackle the problem. It isn't foolproof and it won't work for everyone, but these are the best options available:

1. **Avoid moisturizer over the open-pore areas of the face before applying makeup.** Even if you have dry skin. Any extra "slip" on the skin will cause makeup to pool in the pore. If the skin is dry and flaky, be more diligent in the evening about treating dry skin, and in the morning use a toner with water-binding agents that can help soothe skin and reduce any dry feeling but not add anything that can make skin feel slippery. That means it is essential that your foundation contain your sunscreen, because an additional sunscreen under the foundation will almost certainly cause slippage.

2. **Do use a matte or ultra-matte foundation.** Even if you have dry skin, these stay on far better than any other foundations, are somewhat impervious to oil production, and therefore prevent slippage of the foundation into the pore.

3. **Consider wearing a tiny amount of milk of magnesia under your foundation over the open-pore area.** This is a bit like applying spackle that has minimal to no movement. It can absorb oil at the same time, and the foundation glides over it, creating an even surface. This works better under matte foundations as opposed to ultra-matte foundations.

4. **For more stubborn problems, touch up your makeup several times during the day with oil-blotting papers.** Then dust the face with a pressed powder designed to be worn as a foundation. These tend to apply a slightly thicker layer of powder that can better hide the pore. But only do this with a brush; never use a sponge or pad to apply powder because they can place way too much product on the face, making things look cakey and thick.

## "Oil-Free" Is a Bad Joke

But the joke is on us, because "oil-free" is a meaningless claim and may mislead consumers into buying products that can clog pores. There are plenty of ingredients that don't sound like oils but can absolutely aggravate breakouts. **Almost all cosmet-**

ics contain waxlike thickening agents or fluids (slip agents) that are notorious for clogging pores or making skin feel oily. Simple, standard moisturizing ingredients that are great for dry skin can wreak havoc on someone with oily skin or breakouts. Triglycerides, palmitates, stearates, myristates, stearic acid, plant oils, plant waxes, shea butter, vitamin E, acrylates, and many other ingredients can all clog pores. These ingredients are used in moisturizers because they duplicate the natural lipids (sebum/ oil) in our skin, and that's great. But if you happen to be having problems with the sebum being created in your pores, adding more of the same kind of substance will only make things worse. Despite the problems these ingredients can cause, they show up in lots and lots of so-called "oil-free" products. However, reading labels doesn't tell you much about the amount of an ingredient used, which plays a vital role in whether or not any of these ingredients, including oils, will be a problem. But I'll get into that more in the following section.

Above and beyond the claim of being oil-free, label after label promises that the product is "noncomedogenic" or "nonacnegenic." Most of us have bought products with this assurance, only to find that they did cause breakouts. The terms "non-comedogenic" and "nonacnegenic" have slowly but surely begun to replace "hypo-allergenic" on cosmetics labels. Those are all meaningless marketing words, just like "oil-free." The ingredients list is the place to check out whether a product may put your skin at risk.

## Will It Make Me Break Out?

I have received an amazing number of questions lately asking whether or not a specific product will or won't cause breakouts. It seems there is an explosion of curiosity about finding out which comedogenic ingredients (meaning ingredients known to clog pores) to avoid. The confusion warrants a quick review of the issues. Some of the information you may already be aware of, but it bears repeating.

First of all, you can't trust any product that makes the claim that it's *not* comedogenic, because there is no approved or regulated standard for that assertion. Aside from the regulatory aspect of this bogus claim, I'm certain all of us have used products promising not to cause breakouts and yet we still broke out. What many women already know from experience is that trying to guess how their skin will react based on a product's promises, especially when it comes to blemishes, is truly a lost cause—or at the very least, a difficult problem with no easy, slam-dunk answers. Why does it seem to be so impossible to find products that won't cause breakouts? It's because almost any and all the ingredients used in cosmetics (except for water) can cause breakouts, depending on your skin type.

While there is some evidence that some specific ingredients can trigger breakouts, there are no absolutes. I wish there were but there aren't. As I mention in my newsletter, there are some Web sites showcasing lists of comedogenic ingredients, with the major source of information most likely being *Dr. Fulton's Step by Step Guide to Acne,* published in 1983 by Harper & Row. At the time (and 1983 is long time ago), Fulton's research regarding the causes for breakouts was unprecedented. Fulton applied cosmetic ingredients to rabbits' ears and waited to see what happened. As promising as this research was, it has never been repeated, and is rarely cited in later research (except when it suits a company's marketing agenda). There are many reasons why listings of this kind are unreliable.

First, the methodology looked at pure concentrations of the ingredient, not how the ingredient is used in actual cosmetic formulations, which is usually a fractional amount. It also didn't address the issue of usage and application. Ingredients in a cleanser left on the skin for a few seconds versus a lotion or liquid left on the skin for hours have very different exposure risks. The research also didn't look at the host of plant extracts or sunscreens in cosmetics that were introduced later than the early '80s. To call this list out-of-date and inconclusive would be an understatement.

I have to admit that I'm also to blame for some of the confusion. In my books I have included a listing of ingredients that may cause breakouts. I based this on the emollient or waxlike characteristics of the ingredients, and on findings in the occasional more contemporary research when it was available. I warned against products that contain ingredient groups such as triglycerides, myristates, and palmitates, but I'm now wondering if this was a wise listing to include, because in some ways it is also misleading information. For example, isopropyl palmitate is a waxy thickening agent used to bind other ingredients together, has an emollient feel on skin, and is used most frequently in moisturizers for dry skin. On the other hand, ascorbyl palmitate is a stable form of vitamin C and is used in small amounts in skin-care products, and is rarely a problem for skin. So much for following the rule about palmitates! Further, depending on the ingredient, just because it is present in a formulation may mean nothing. If it is toward the end of the ingredient list it probably won't do much, whereas if it's the second, third, or fourth ingredient, it may be problematic. Yet that may not be true if many of these kinds of ingredients are strewn across a label. Also, keep in mind that even the most notorious ingredients (such as isopropyl myristate) won't cause problems for everyone. Just because an ingredient *may* cause breakouts doesn't mean that it *will.*

Another point these kinds of lists can't account for is that there are thousands and thousands of cosmetic ingredients being used in skin-care and makeup products today! A lot of them are emollients, waxy thickening agents, or irritants that can cause skin problems, but whether they do or not is completely dependent on the amount used and the nature of the individual ingredient (some ingredients cause problems in far smaller amounts than other ingredients, while others cause problems in various combinations). A comprehensive listing would not only be impossible, it would be nothing more than guesswork.

I know; there are no easy answers for this one, but you can understand that trying to research, categorize, classify, and make absolute conclusions about 50,000+ ingredients with an infinite number of possible combinations is just not humanly possible. So what's a woman to do when trying to fend off blemishes and still use skin-care and makeup products? While I still think some ingredients are more problematic than others, I think the easiest and most reliable practice for a consumer to consider is consistency. The thicker the product (meaning a high, creamy viscosity), the more likely it is to cause problems. That means you can feel more safe with a gel or serum (meaning these have a low or watery viscosity).

It is also safe to assume that although a product with plant or mineral oils of any kind high up on the ingredient listing might make the skin feel greasy, greasiness doesn't necessarily trigger breakouts. And finally, do watch out for irritating ingredients. It doesn't take much alcohol, menthol, peppermint, balm mint, eucalyptus, camphor, lemon, grapefruit, or lime to cause a negative skin reaction that can hurt the skin's healing process—and that won't help heal blemishes.

## *Getting Worse Before It Gets Better*

The notion that skin has to get worse before it gets better is generally not true. It is also a complete fiction that the skin is breaking out because the new products are somehow purging toxins lurking in the pore or under the skin, making skin worse before it can get better. Women have heard this repeatedly from cosmetics salespeople, and even from some dermatologists who either don't know any better or haven't taken the time to explain what may really be happening to the skin. As a result, this long-standing myth puts women in a position to tolerate bad or ineffective skin-care products longer than they need to. Here's what can happen:

Typically, breakouts occur from a new skin-care routine because it is just bad for the skin and probably contains ingredients that trigger blemishes, or are ineffective or irritating, causing a rashlike breakout. However, the most common cause of breakouts from a new skin-care routine is really one of coincidence that has nothing to do with the new products you are using. If you have a skin type that tends to break out, you could very easily start a new skin-care regimen at a time when you may be going through a normal breakout phase. Remember that effective acne-treatment products can take two to three weeks to show an effect, so there wouldn't be time for them to have an impact on the new cycle of breakouts you just happened to be going through.

On occasion, for some skin types, it is true that an effective skin-care routine can cause breakouts. This is particularly true when you are using disinfectants, exfoliants, and Retin-A; however, that isn't a necessary phase. Rather it may be due to the initial effect of the active ingredients, which can be irritating and cause breakouts, and then the skin may need a while to adapt. If the skin doesn't adapt and the irritation and redness continue, other options need to be considered.

## Is It Good for Sensitive Skin?

Allergic reactions, irritation, and skin sensitivities are not technically the same thing, but they can feel the same on your skin. Regardless of the physiologically precise definition, almost everyone has used some type of cosmetic that caused their skin to burn, tingle, swell, flake, redden, itch, blister, break out, dry up, or just feel bad. How could this happen? Given how many products we use and the diversity of ingredients, I'm shocked it doesn't happen more frequently. Skin-care products are a notorious source of skin sensitivities, allergic reactions, and irritation. Just think about the number of cosmetics most women use daily. The average woman uses at least 12 different skin-care, makeup, and hair-care products a day, with each one, on average, containing about 15 to 20 different ingredients. That means her skin is exposed to anywhere from 100 to 180 different cosmetic ingredients on any given day. The fact that any of us have skin left is a testimony to the skin's resiliency and the talent of cosmetics chemists. Whether we like it or not, most of us have sensitive skin to one degree or another.

Fragrance and preservatives are often thought to be the major culprits when our skin reacts to a cosmetic. Preservatives are almost impossible to avoid: How many of us want to use a moldy, contaminated skin-care or makeup product? This is what would happen to an unpreserved cosmetic. However, you can and should stay away from cosmetics, particularly skin-care products, that contain fragrance.

The cosmetics industry knows that most women emotionally and psychologically prefer cosmetics that smell nice, even if they say they want to avoid fragrance. But if a cosmetics company produces products without fragrance, you will instead get the scent of the ingredients, which simply are not as appealing as an added aromatic fragrance. So despite the fact that fragrance is problematic for skin care, cosmetics companies continue to add fragrance to products.

You could easily avoid products that add the word "fragrance" to the ingredient label but unfortunately there are other sources of fragrance to be concerned about. As lovely as essential oils sound, they are almost all volatile, fragrant oils that can prove quite irritating and sensitizing to skin. So when you don't see the word "fragrance" on the list, you may approvingly think that wintergreen, lemon, cardamom, ylang-ylang, lavender, cinnamon, citrus, lemon, or bergamot may sound pleasant and healthy, and then find your skin responding disapprovingly.

There are many more factors that can trigger allergic, irritating, or sensitizing skin reactions. Plant extracts can cause reactions like this (if you suffer from hay fever, plants are the last thing you want in abundance in skin-care products), and stimulating and drying ingredients like sodium lauryl sulfate, SD alcohol, mints, menthol, camphor, eucalyptus, and citruses can all cause skin irritation. Emollients like lanolin and vitamin E, and fragrant plant oils can cause allergic reactions in some people. And sunscreen agents are among the many more-common irritating (or pore-clogging) ingredients in cosmetics.

Is there one line of cosmetics that's best for sensitive skin? It would be great if there were, but it just doesn't exist. Skin reactions are amazingly random and dissimilar. What you're allergic to has little to do with what someone else reacts to, and then there's the intricacy of ingredients being combined on the face. The culprit may not be the product you think caused the problem. You may think a new moisturizer made your eyes swell, but it could turn out that the nail polish you were wearing in combination with the new moisturizer triggered the problem. What you can do to avoid the risk of irritation is to avoid those irritating ingredients that are unnecessary and useless for skin.

Preventing skin irritation, regardless of skin type, is the course of action I recommend throughout this book in each and every review. Of course, some skin types can and should try to tolerate certain potentially irritating ingredients—such as a topical disinfectant (2.5% benzoyl peroxide or a topical antibiotic, for instance) for someone with acne, a BHA solution (a salicylic acid exfoliant) for someone with blackheads, an AHA (an alpha hydroxy acid product to exfoliate), or Retin-A or Renova (to improve cell formation) for someone with sun-damaged skin. And the use of sunscreen is indispensable for healthy skin. But aside from those limited departures from the gentleness rule, if something is irritating it can be detrimental for all skin types. If it is bad for sensitive skin, it is probably bad for oily skin, acned skin, combination skin, dry skin, or mature skin. As you begin to integrate this gentleness philosophy into your skin-care routine, you will slowly solve many skin problems you may have been experiencing.

## Choosing a Really Great Skin-Care Routine

Most skin-care regimens are at best unrealistic. They are either too complicated (too many steps, such as two or three cleansing steps), too contrived (such as layering products or applying too many moisturizers, which can clog pores and make skin look dull), too irritating (toners that contain alcohol, lotions that contain peppermint or menthol, which can obstruct the skin's healing process), or absurdly and unnecessarily expensive. Choosing a really great skin-care routine isn't about the proverbial notion of getting back to basics, because what is the definition of basic? A lot of women think of soap as basic, but the pH of most soaps increases bacteria in the skin, and the same ingredients that keep the bar in its form can clog pores. Is sun protection part of getting back to basics? And what about exfoliation with an AHA or BHA or the use of a retinoid like Renova or Retin-A to improve cell production for those with sun-damaged skin? Skin care doesn't have to be complicated, but it does have to address what is best for *your* skin, and, depending on your skin type, that can be complicated.

Choosing a really great skin-care routine also doesn't mean looking for plants and natural ingredients. There are lots and lots of natural ingredients that can be damaging to skin, and for the most part adding plants or foods to a cosmetic just increases the need for it to have a stronger preservative base and more fragrance to mask the smell of rancid, molding ingredients. After all, how long do plants of any kind last in your refrigerator?

Choosing a really great skin-care routine means doing what it takes to be good to your skin without wasting money, and buying only products that live up to their claims. The following is a realistic, viable skin-care routine that's free from gimmicks and selling techniques.

## Step 1

Even at night, when you're removing makeup, always wash your face with a gentle, water-soluble cleanser that rinses off completely and doesn't irritate the eyes. Your eye makeup should come off with the same water-soluble cleanser that cleans your face. Do not use an extra product to wipe across the eye, pulling the skin and eyelashes unnecessarily. (Wiping off makeup is never good for the skin; it pulls at the skin, and rubbing with a tissue or washcloth, no matter how gentle you try to be, can irritate skin.)

Use only tepid to slightly warm water. Hot water burns the skin, and cold water shocks it. Repeated use of hot water, saunas, or Jacuzzis can cause broken capillaries to surface on the nose and cheeks and cause unwanted irritation that damages skin and depletes the skin's healing ability.

If you are wearing one of the new ultra-matte foundations, you may need to use a washcloth to help remove makeup. This is an exception to the rule but may be necessary for the new breed of stubborn foundations that are very effective for oily skin types.

## Step 2

Exfoliating the skin helps unclog pores and removes dead skin cells, benefiting both dry and oily skin. There are two ways to exfoliate: with a mechanical exfoliant such as a scrub and with a chemical exfoliant such as AHAs or BHA. For many skin types only one of these two types of exfoliant is necessary. Overdoing the exfoliation bit with scrubs and several AHA or BHA products is at best overkill, and I do mean kill. You only have so much skin, and too much exfoliation can start causing damage and negate any of the positive effects you were hoping for.

*Chemical exfoliants:* There are many reasons why exfoliating the skin is helpful. If you have breakouts, exfoliating the skin and the pore lining can reduce or eliminate clogged pores. If you have sun-damaged skin, the outer layer of skin becomes thickened and exfoliation can reduce that leathery, rough appearance. For this purpose AHAs (preferably in the form of glycolic acid or lactic acid) or BHA (in the form of salicylic acid) are the most researched of all the exfoliants being sold in the world of skin care, so we know the most about their risks and performance requirements. AHAs are most effective in concentrations of 5% or greater in a pH of 3 to 4. BHA is most effective in concentrations of 1% to 2% in a pH of 3 to 4. (AHAs and BHA products with an emollient base can double as moisturizers or can be the only product your skin needs besides a cleanser and sunscreen.) The AHA or BHA product is applied after the face is washed and dried (see Step 4 below).

*Scrubs:* Scrubs are a way to mechanically exfoliate the skin and are still an option for some skin types, particularly those that tend to break out, but must be used sparingly if you are using an effective AHA or BHA. Overexfoliating the skin is not helpful and can cause problems such as irritation or a rashlike breakout. Mechanical exfoliation comes after using your cleanser. One of my favorite scrubs is baking soda with a gentle, water-soluble cleanser. While your face is still wet, pour a scant handful of baking soda into the palm of your hand. Add a small amount of water to create a paste, gently massage your entire face with this paste, then rinse generously with tepid water. (You can also mix 1 or 2 teaspoons of baking soda with 1 or 2 tablespoons of a good, water-soluble cleanser such as Cetaphil Gentle Skin Cleanser. This alternative is good for any skin type.) Be extra careful not to get carried away: overscrubbing can cause more problems than it solves. The important word to remember for all skin care is "gentle."

If you have combination skin, massage only those areas that tend to break out, and avoid the areas that are dry. If you have normal skin, use the baking soda scrub only two to three times a week. If you have dry skin, use the baking soda mixed with Cetaphil Gentle Skin Cleanser only about once or twice a week, and rinse very well. If you have extremely dry skin, follow the advice for dry skin, but use more Cetaphil Gentle Skin Cleanser and just a pinch of baking soda in your mixture, and be very, very gentle when massaging your face.

## Step 3

Once your face is clean, occasionally and gently squeeze any blackheads or blemishes you want to remove. Blackheads usually don't leave on their own. They can be stubborn even if you are using a good AHA or BHA product or Retin-A. For pimples, though they can heal on their own, relieving the pressure and removing the contents can help them heal faster and prevent further swelling, which can cause scarring. If you are shocked by this suggestion, that's OK; you don't have to do this, but it does help. This is what most facialists do best for your skin; however, it's cheaper to do it yourself. Many people worry about making matters worse. The only way to prevent that from happening is to NEVER, absolutely NEVER, oversqueeze. If the blemish or blackhead does not respond easily, stop and leave it alone. Squeezing does not cause problems on the face; in fact, it is one of the best ways to clean out the skin and remove pressure from a swollen lesion. The problems occur when you massacre the skin by squeezing until you create scabs and sores.

## Step 4

Toners are an optional step after the cleanser and scrub. Depending on your skin type and the one you choose, a toner can remove last traces of makeup, help soothe skin, and add some good water-binding agents to the skin. For someone with normal to oily skin, it can be the only moisturizer needed. For someone with normal to dry skin, it can be a good addition to your regular moisturizer. If you have acne or blemish-prone skin, this toner needs to be soothing or to contain an effective disinfectant to kill blemish-causing bacteria.

When your face is completely rinsed and dried, take a cotton ball and apply the appropriate toner for your skin type. Please keep in mind that toners (as well as any skin-care product that comes near your face or body) need to be as irritant-free as possible. There are many irritant-free toners to choose from, but the more-expensive ones are absolutely not worth their exorbitant price tags, especially when you consider that their basic ingredients are almost always the same as those in the less-expensive versions.

## Step 5

If you have extremely oily skin or skin that breaks out frequently, try a facial mask of plain Phillips' Milk of Magnesia (the stuff in the blue bottle that you normally take for indigestion; just ask your pharmacist). Milk of magnesia is a mixture of magnesium hydroxide and water. Magnesium is a good disinfectant, and it can absorb oil. The clay masks for oily skin have no disinfecting properties, and their ingredients cannot absorb oil as well as magnesium can. Your skin type and reaction to the mask will determine how often you can use it. Those with severely oily skin can use it every day; those with slightly oily skin may need to use it only once a week.

## Step 6

After your face is clean (cleanser and scrub) and you've applied the toner, this is the time to apply an AHA or BHA product or Retin-A and Renova. If you have chosen to use both an AHA and Retin-A or Renova, the AHA is applied first and then the Retin-A or Renova. This can be done once or twice a day or every other day, depending on your skin type.

## Step 7

Moisturizing is the step in skin care most women obsess over, and the cosmetics industry is certainly glad they do. Loading up on moisturizers and antiwrinkle potions is big business. Yet, in truth, you only need to wear a moisturizer if you have dry skin. In short, not everyone needs a moisturizer! The biggest myth you've been sold by the cosmetics industry is that there are wrinkle creams and moisturizers out there that will undo or prevent wrinkles. It just isn't true. Every month a host of new antiwrinkle creams are launched with more promises and supposedly newfangled formulations. And every few months our hope is renewed—until the next round of lies and misleading claims are thrown at us. You can choose not to believe me on this one, but unless you have dry skin or want to improve the appearance of your wrinkles (not change them), it is not necessary to wear a moisturizer!

Even more to the point, dry skin and wrinkles are not associated. Yes, moisturizers help to make skin look smoother, but they don't alter wrinkles, their effect is gone the next day, and no moisturizer supplants the need for sunscreen (sunscreens come in moisturizing bases, so you only need one product, not two). During the day, if you have dry skin, wear a moisturizer with a reliable SPF. At night, if you choose to wear a moisturizer, it is only necessary over dry areas. Do not use moisturizer of any kind over areas that tend to break out. Oil-free moisturizers still contain waxy thickening agents that can clog pores. Heavy, rich, creamy moisturizers are best only for extremely dry skin. Try the less-expensive moisturizers before you venture into the higher-priced brands. The price doesn't relate to what ingredients are in a formulation! For more specifics about formulations, see the section "What Makes a Good Moisturizer?"

At night, if you want to use an AHA or BHA product that comes in a moisturizing base, apply it after the toner. If you use a liquid- or gel-type AHA product, apply it after the toner but before the moisturizer.

## Step 8

During the day, it is essential to wear a sunscreen with an SPF of 15 that contains UVA protection. You must be certain that the product you choose contains one of the following in the list of active ingredients: avobenzone (also called Parsol 1789 or butylmethoxydibenzoylmethane), zinc oxide, or titanium dioxide. If you have normal to dry skin, wear a sunscreen that comes in a moisturizing base (actually, most sunscreens come in a moisturizing base). If you have normal to oily skin, you do not need a moisturizer, but you still must wear a sunscreen with an SPF of 15 that includes UVA protection. In this instance you can choose a matte foundation with an effective sunscreen. **Remember: The only way to prevent wrinkles is sun protec-**

tion. It is also essential to remember that your sunscreen is always the last product to apply. If you are applying several skin-care products, in order not to dilute the effectiveness of the sunscreen, it must be the last product you apply to skin.

## Step 9

If you have melasma or chloasma, which are brown or ashen discolorations caused by sun damage or hormonal changes (usually the result of birth-control pills), then you may want to consider adding a skin-lightening product to your routine. These products need to contain at least 1% to 2% hydroquinone, available over the counter, or 4% or greater, available from physicians. This step would come after the toner and AHA or BHA product steps, but before the Retin-A, Renova, or sunscreen. This layering process can be tricky for some skin types, but it can prove to be quite effective in the lightening process. Please keep in mind that no lightening process works if you do not use an effective sunscreen day in and day out.

# *Animal Testing*

The National Anti-Vivisection Society (NAVS) is a not-for-profit educational group that opposes the use of animals in product testing, research, and education for any purpose. While I find some of their policies and agendas to be rather extreme and radical, I still support many of their efforts to stop unnecessary animal testing and prevent animal cruelty in all forms. NAVS and I differ in that I do not oppose the use of animal testing for health-care research of afflictions such as breast cancer, Alzheimer's, and heart disease, and I am not vegan (NAVS and PETA, People for the Ethical Treatment of Animals, are both opposed to the use of animals for any medical or food use). However, I do oppose the inhumane treatment of animals (no animal should suffer in the pursuit of helping humankind), as well as the testing of standard cosmetic formulations and ingredients on animals. In this regard, NAVS and I agree.

The definitive book on the issue that lists which cosmetics companies do and do not test on animals is NAVS's *Personal Care for People Who Care,* now in its tenth edition. This is a must-read source for any consumer interested in purchasing products that have not been tested on animals. You can obtain the book by calling NAVS at (800) 888-NAVS; communicating via e-mail at navs@navs.org; or by writing them at P.O. Box 94020, Palatine, IL 60094-9834. It is a 200-page book listing companies that do and do not test their products on animals, at a cost of $6.95 per book. Visit their Web site at www.navs.org.

**Please note:** When a company's label states that they don't test on animals and they report this information to NAVS for the listing they ultimately use in their book *Personal Care for People Who Care,* there is every reason to believe that information is correct. However, it is naïve to assume that means animal testing information was not an integral part of creating the product. All sunscreen ingredients and most all of the new antioxidant ingredients currently used in cosmetics, including vitamin C, vitamin A, and many plant extracts, have all been tested on animals. In reality, what we know about the efficacy of these ingredients was first obtained from animal testing. I have broached this apparent double standard with NAVS several times but they refuse to acknowledge the challenge to their criteria. So, while the label on a skin-care product may indeed be accurate in regard to the company's policy of animal testing, what it does not represent is the vast group of ingredient manufacturers and university research facilities that use animal testing to determine the basic efficacy of cosmetic ingredients.

The August 1999 issue of *Cosmetics & Toiletries* magazine reported on a new in vitro testing alternative that can further reduce the need for animal testing. It was approved by the Inter-Agency Coordinating Committee for the Validation of Alternative Methods (ICCVAM). The new "Corrositex assay [test] determines skin corrosivity of a chemical by placing it on a layer of collagen, the same material that holds skin together. As the chemical penetrates the collagen barrier, a material underneath changes color. Corrosivity is rated according to the time it takes the chemical to penetrate and by the color change of the material beneath the barrier."

I am proud to say that my skin-care company, Paula's Choice, does not test any aspect of its products on animals, and I donate a portion of my company's earnings to The Humane Society of the United States (HSUS) every year and particularly during the April Prevention of Cruelty to Animals month. Please check out HSUS's Web site at www.hsus.org. Their mailing address is: The Humane Society of the United States, 2100 L Street NW, Washington, DC 20037 (they can use your financial help as well).

HSUS's approach to the issue of animal rights and animal testing is one I agree with most strongly. The spring 1998 issue of *HSUS News* stated, "The HSUS shares with these scientists [the many who are opposed to or are uncomfortable with animal testing] the desire to eliminate the harmful use of animals in laboratories. In the meantime The HSUS is planning a campaign to urge the scientific community to adopt, as a priority goal, the elimination of all animal pain and distress in the laboratory. The HSUS believes that an emphasis on humane issues will lead to good science and will benefit, rather than harm, the advance of human knowledge."

# CHAPTER THREE

# Product-by-Product Reviews

## *The Process*

You may well be wondering how I go about deciding what distinguishes a terrible product from a great one, or a good product from a fantastic product. Above all, you need to know that I do not base any decision on my own personal experience, or let my personal feelings about a particular company blur my judgment. In other words, just because I like the way a cleanser feels on my skin doesn't translate to how thousands of other skin types will feel about it. Rather, I base my decision on the individual product's formulation via published research about the ingredients that are being used and their possible resulting interactions with the skin. From that I can assess the potential for irritation, dryness, breakouts, sensitivities, greasiness, and other issues of texture and performance. If I think a company is absurdly overcharging for its products or is exceedingly dishonest in its claims and literature, no matter how unethical I find it, that won't prevent me from saying its product is good for a particular skin type (though I do often say, "This is a good product but what a shame the price has to be so absurd and the claims so offensive!").

Almost without exception, my evaluation process for this edition was the same as for previous editions of this book. I reviewed each cosmetics line for several different elements. The first consideration was overall presentation and how user-friendly the displays or company literature were. For those lines available at retail locations, I always considered it an asset if their display units were set up with convenient color groupings, such as colors divided into warm (yellow) and cool (blue) tones, or were easily accessible. Skin-care and makeup products that were convenient to sample without the help of a salesperson were also rated high. For drugstore lines, colors had to be easy to see, and samples or tester units were also considered a bonus.

For infomercial and in-home shopping channel companies, my major criterion was the organization of their skin-care routines. Generally, ordering from sources like these means you are buying a set of products, not picking and selecting from what is being offered. If these prefab kits do not include an adequate sunscreen, or the kit for someone with breakouts is only minimally different from the kit for dry skin, then the overall rating went down dramatically (skin-care products with ingredients that are good for someone with dry skin are never suited for someone with oily, acne-prone skin).

I was also leery of any company's claim of being the best or having state-of-the art formulations if they did not have a sunscreen of SPF 15 or greater with UVA-protecting ingredients as part of their daily skin-care regimen. Any company purporting to have worthwhile products or well-researched formulations could not possibly be telling the truth if they were not even aware of the well-known and easily accessible information on sunscreens.

The fundamental determination for each individual product's rating was based on specific criteria I've established for each product category. Every category, from blushes to eyeshadows, concealers, foundations, cleansers, toners, scrubs, moisturizers, facial masks, AHA products, brushes, and wrinkle creams, has its own standards for garnering a happy, unhappy, or neutral (meaning unimpressive but not bad) face.

**Makeup products** were assessed mostly on texture (was it silky-smooth or grainy and hard?), color (was a wide range of colors available, and was there an adequate selection for women of color?), application (could it be applied easily or was it difficult to spread or blend?), ease of use (was the container poorly designed, were colors placed too close together in an eyeshadow set, was foundation put in a pump container that squirted too much product or didn't reach to the bottom of the jar?), and, finally, price.

**Skin-care products** were evaluated almost exclusively on the basis of content versus claim. If a product said it was good for sensitive skin, it couldn't contain irritants, skin sensitizers, or drying ingredients.

I also asked the following questions to see if a product could hold up to its claims, based on established research: (1) Given the ingredient list, could the product do what it promised? (2) How did the product differ from other products? (3) If a special ingredient or ingredients were showcased, how much of them were actually in the product, and was there independent research verifying the claim? (4) Did the product contain problematic preservatives, fragrances, coloring agents, plants, or other questionable ingredients? (5) How far-fetched were the product's claims? (6) Did I feel this product was safe? Were there risks such as allergic reactions or increased sun sensitivity?

**I wish I had the space to challenge and explain every single exaggerated claim and lofty explanation that accompanied the products listed in this chapter, but there was just not enough room (or time) to tackle that prodigious task.** I tried to cover many of the distortions and some of the hyperbole about products in my book *The Beauty Bible*, but even that book can't keep up with the hundreds and hundreds of skin-care ingredients with miraculous-claims, much less the vast number of available products claiming miraculous-results. For this book, I chose to include all the information I could to overcome the sales and advertising pitches so you can focus on a product's quality, realistic performance, and feel.

## Can You Judge a Product by Its Label?

Many people wonder whether I can judge a skin care product by its label. You may be thinking, "Wouldn't that be like judging a food just by the ingredients in it? What about taste?" As it turns out, I absolutely judge food by its ingredient list. It is no longer wise for any of us to consume any food without a clear understanding of how much fat, sodium, preservatives, coloring agents, or calories it contains, along with many other details pertinent to our health. Without that information, regardless of taste (and everyone has their own bias), you would never know what you were putting in your body. You could be causing yourself harm by eating more fat, calories, or salt than you should, leading to weight gain, cancer, high blood pressure, and so on. If you don't eat enough fiber, you could end up with gastrointestinal distress or other serious problems. If you aren't getting appropriate nourishment you could get very sick. And what about food allergies or sensitivities? How would you ever know what you were doing to yourself? The food label is every consumer's best friend, whether you're shopping at a discount grocery store or the fanciest gourmet shop.

Food labels are incredibly important, as are skin-care labels. If a skin-care product says it is good for sensitive skin or won't cause breakouts but contains ingredients known to cause irritation or breakouts, that is essential information. If a skin-care product sells for $100 but contains the same ingredients as a product that costs $10, that is, to say the least, very important information. Perhaps even more significant, if a $100 product contains fewer or less effective ingredients than a $10 version, I think that is crucial consumer information.

The ingredient list helps you sort through the jungle of choices. Besides, it is a far better starting point than basing decisions strictly on advertising mumbo jumbo or promises that are never delivered.

## Evaluation of Makeup Products

**FOUNDATION:** My fundamental expectation for any foundation, regardless of type (liquid, pressed powder, loose powder, stick, or cream-to-powder), was that it not be any shade or tone of orange, peach, pink, rose, green, or ash—because there are no people with that color of skin. Consistency, coverage, and feel were also important. All foundations, regardless of texture, needed to go on smoothly and evenly, not separate or turn color, and be easy to blend. Foundations that claim to be matte or ultra-matte must be truly matte, meaning no shine or glossy finish, and they have to have the potential to last most of the day. Foundations that claim to moisturize have to contain ingredients that could do that. Many foundations that claim to be oil-free contain silicone, which is an ingredient that has a definitely slippery, somewhat oily feel. It is most unlikely that silicone will cause breakouts, but in some formulations it can leave a slippery or slightly greasy feel on the skin.

There is a new generation of shiny, iridescent foundations on the market today from many cosmetics lines. They come either in a sheer, moisturizing-type formula or with a slight amount of tint. What they provide is some amount of iridescence or sparkle on the face. While I generally do not care for sparkly makeup, especially for daytime, these products were rated on ease of use, how well they lasted, how much they flaked (controlling where the shine is placed is important—you don't want sparkles falling on your clothes), and how sheer and easy they were to blend.

Foundations that contain sunscreens were held to the same standards as any other sunscreen, which means they had to have at least an SPF 15 and had to include a UVA-protecting ingredient listed as one of the active ingredients on the label. The only acceptable UVA-protecting ingredients are titanium dioxide, zinc oxide, or avobenzone (also called Parsol 1789 or butyl methoxydibenzoylmethane). In the reviews, you will notice that foundations with poor or inadequate sunscreens were criticized severely but may still have received a happy face. In these situations, the performance of the foundations was considered excellent but the foundation could not be relied on for sun protection.

**Beauty Note:** Color suggestions for all makeup products were often based on tester units available at the cosmetics counter, or samples (including gifts with a purchase or discounted promotions), but mainly from products that were purchased. The color, shade, or tone of a particular product can fluctuate for a number of reasons. If I referred to a particular foundation as being "too peach" and you find that it's just right, it may be that we simply disagree, or it may be that the product I tested or bought was different from the one you ended up buying.

<u>CONCEALER:</u> Concealers should never be any shade of orange, peach, pink, rose, green, or ash, and they should not slip into the lines around the eye. I looked for creamy, smooth textures that went on easily without pulling the skin, didn't look dry and pasty, and, perhaps most important, did not crease into lines. I generally do not recommend using concealers over blemishes, but there is rarely a problem with using most concealers on other parts of the face if they match the skin.

I don't recommend medicated concealers because they are rarely, if ever, "medicated" with ingredients or formulations that can affect breakouts. In order for medicated concealers to work, they would need to contain an effective exfoliant or an effective disinfectant, and I have yet to test one that met those criteria and had a color that anyone would dare put on her face.

Despite claims a product may make that recommend it for oily skin versus dry skin, please keep in mind that companies can make these claims regardless of ingredient content. In general, the thicker and greasier the product, the more likely it is to be problematic for oily, acne-prone skin. However, anything you apply over skin can cause problems. Just because a product does or doesn't contain oil is no guarantee one way or the other that it won't cause problems for the skin. There are lots of ingredients that don't sound like oil that can cause problems for skin. Generally, a matte-finish product is best for oily skin, but that still won't assure a lack of breakouts.

**COLOR CORRECTOR:** I am not a fan of color correctors in any form. Color correctors are usually a group of concealers you apply before you apply your foundation color. They generally come in shades of yellow, mauve, pink, or green. Color correctors are marketed as a way to change skin color, so that if your skin has pink undertones, a yellow color corrector is supposed to even that out. All these products do is give the skin a strange hue. Does anyone think the colored layer isn't noticeable? That yellow or mauve layer then mixes with your foundation, giving it a strange color. Another problem with this kind of product is that it adds another layer on the skin, and the buildup of cosmetic ingredients on the face can be pore-clogging. A well-chosen foundation color and blush can easily provide the color balance you are looking for without adding another layer of strange makeup colors on the skin.

**POWDER:** Finishing or setting powders come in two basic forms: pressed and loose. I evaluated them on the basis of whether they went on sheer, chalky, or heavy and whether they were too pink, peach, ash, or rose. I consistently gave higher marks to powders that went on sheer and had a silky-soft texture with a natural beige, tan, or rich brown finish. Talc is the most frequently used ingredient in powders in all price ranges, and it is probably one of the best for absorbing oil and giving a smooth finish to the face. Some companies make claims about their grade of talc being better than another's. The issue of a grade difference cannot be proven and is irrelevant unless the product's feel and performance are affected.

Other minerals are used for the same purpose, and though they may sound more exotic, they are not any better for the skin. Cornstarch or rice starch in powders do help create a beautiful texture and these are interesting substitutes for talc, but they can also be a skin concern, as there is some evidence that they can clog pores and cause breakouts. I tried to screen for these as much as possible.

**Note:** Talc often gets showcased as being an awful cosmetic ingredient that should be avoided, and I do not agree in the least with that assessment for makeup products. The concern about talc is not about how it is used in makeup, but, rather, when it is used in pure, large concentrations in the form of talcum powder. A 1992 Harvard study cited a modest association between talc and ovarian cancer and a 1996 *American Journal of Epidemiology* study found a 50% increased risk of ovarian cancer from vaginal application of talcum powder. The application of talc vaginally is unrelated to how women use face and eye makeup. There is no indication that there is any risk for the face in the amounts used in makeup. That doesn't mean you should not use eyeshadow or face powder with talc, but it absolutely means to consider never using it on your children, or on yourself vaginally.

When it comes to bronzing powders, I generally suggest using them as a contour color and not an all-over face color. Darkening the face almost always looks over-done. After all, if a foundation is supposed to match the skin, how can the use of a powder that darkens the skin be rationalized? The face will be a color decidedly different from the neck, and there will be a line of demarcation where the color starts and stops. Also, most bronzing powders are iridescent. Dusting a color over the face that is darker than your skin tone is bad enough, but why make it more obvious with particles of shine all over, particularly in daylight?

A preponderance of shiny powders are being sold today. These products were rated on ease of use, how well they lasted, how much they flaked, and how sheer and easy they were to blend. Shiny powder as an oil-absorbent was never judged as a good idea. If the idea is to powder down shine, applying more shine doesn't make sense.

Powders are often designated by the cosmetics companies as being for dry or oily skin. Those designations are often bogus; I rated a product as being good for oily skin if it contains minimal waxy or oily ingredients. Cornstarch or rice starch in powders was considered problematic for causing breakouts, despite the dry feel on the skin. I indicated which powders contained these ingredients, as they could be a potential problem for acne-prone skin.

**BLUSH:** I considered it essential for blushes to have a smooth texture and to blend on easily, and the silkier the feel, the better the rating. I don't recommend shiny blushes. Although they don't make cheeks look as crepey or wrinkly as shiny eyeshadows do the eyes, sparkling cheeks look out of place during the day. Blushes that went on with a sheen or shine but did not sparkle were described with a warning and were not rated as highly as matte blushes. This is more a matter of personal preference than a problem; you simply should know exactly what you are buying and what you can and cannot expect.

Cream blushes and cream-to-powder blushes were rated on their blendability, whether they streaked, how greasy they felt, and how well they lasted. I also described which cream blushes tended to work better over foundation and which ones worked better directly on the skin.

**EYESHADOW:** It won't surprise most of you who have read any of my previous books or newsletters to find out that I don't recommend eyeshadows of any shade of blue, violet, green, or red, whether they shine or not. Intense hues may be a personal preference, but I don't encourage anyone to use them. Makeup that speaks louder than you do may be kicky and fun, but it doesn't help empower a woman or help her to be taken seriously. If that's not your goal in life, ignore my color or shine recommendations. Regardless of color or shine, all eyeshadows were evaluated on texture, and ease of application. I pointed out which colors had heavy, grainy textures, because they can be hard to blend and can easily crease. Eyeshadows that were too sheer or powdery were also a problem because the color tended to fade as the day wore on, and they can also be difficult to apply, flaking all over the place. I was also leery of eyeshadow sets that include difficult-to-use color combinations. Many lines have duo, trio, and quad sets of eyeshadows, with the most bizarre color combinations imaginable. Sets of colors must be usable as a set, coordinated in complementary colors; they should never paint a rainbow or kaleidoscope of color across the eye. However, if you are looking for a kaleidoscope, I've pointed them out; they just have an unhappy face next to them. Generally, it is best to buy eyeshadow colors singly, not in sets. That way you can be assured of liking all the colors you buy, not just two out of three or four.

Specialty eyeshadow products such as liquids, creams, powdery or creamy pencils, and loose-powder eyeshadows were evaluated on ease of use, blendability, staying power, and how well they worked over and with other products. My reviews indicate a clear bias toward matte eyeshadow powders as opposed to any other type of eyeshadow. I find liquids and creams hard to control and even more difficult to blend with other colors. However, some women are quite adept at using this kind of product and should balance my preference against theirs.

EYE AND BROW SHAPERS: Basically, all pencils, regardless of brand, have more similarities than differences. Most eye pencils, lip pencils, and eyebrow pencils are manufactured by the same company (meaning the same manufacturing plant) and are then sold to hundreds of different cosmetics lines. Whether they cost $30 from Chanel or $4 from Almay, they are likely to be exactly the same product. Some pencils are greasier or drier than others, but for the most part there are few marked differences among them. Eye pencils that smudged and smeared and eyebrow pencils that went on like a crayon—meaning thick and greasy—were always rated as ineffective, because they can get very messy as the day goes by. (Keep in mind that whether an eye pencil smears along the lower eyelashes depends to a large extent on the number of lines around your eye, how much moisturizer you use around the eye area, the type of under-eye concealer you use, and how greasy the pencil is. The greasier the moisturizer or the under-eye concealer, the more likely any pencil will smear, and you can't blame that on the pencil.)

As a general rule, I do not recommend pencils for filling in the brow. Eyebrow pencil almost always looks matte and artificial next to an eyebrow. I use only powder, and I encourage you to do the same. Any eyeshadow color that matches your eyebrow color as closely as possible can do the trick, applied with a tiny eyeliner or angle brush. The goal is to create a brow that is as natural looking as possible. Brow gel and eyeshadow or brow shadow work superbly together to fill in the brow. A handful of companies make a clear brow gel meant to keep eyebrows in place without adding color or thickness. This works well, but no better than hairspray on a toothbrush brushed through the brow.

**LIPSTICK AND LIP PENCIL:** Every woman has her own needs and preferences when it comes to lipstick. Some women like sheer applications; others prefer glossy or matte finishes. Colors are also difficult to recommend because of the wide variation in taste. Given those limitations, I primarily reviewed the range of colors and textures available, commenting on texture rather than critiquing it, because personal preference is vital to a final decision. The general groupings are glossy or sheer, creamy, creamy with shine or iridescence, matte, and ultra-matte. As a matter of preference, because of staying power and coverage, I gave highest marks to creamy or semi-matte lipsticks that go on evenly and aren't glossy, sticky, thick, or drying. The ultra-matte lipsticks (introduced first by Ultima II with its LipSexxxy and then made overwhelmingly popular by Revlon's ColorStay, which is virtually identical to the former) were unique because of their dry, flat finish, and because they didn't easily come off on coffee cups or teeth. I evaluated them for how dry their finish was, how much they chipped and peeled, and how well they lasted during the day. Please note that ultra-matte lipsticks can dry out the lips and peel off during the day. I usually don't recommend lip glosses, because they don't stay on longer than an hour or two, while most women want long-lasting lip makeup. I evaluated lip pencils according to whether they go on smoothly without being greasy or dry.

**MASCARA:** Mascaras should go on easily and quickly while building length and thickness. Brush shape has improved phenomenally over the years. A brush can be awkward to use if it is too big or too small. Mascara should never smear or flake, regardless of its price. A $4 mascara is no bargain if it doesn't go on well. However, no mascara can hold up to a heavy layer of moisturizer around the eyes. If you pile on any kind of moisturizer, whether it be oil-free, a gel, or a product designed especially for the eyes, your mascara will be affected.

Except for swimming and special occasions that may produce tears, I don't recommend waterproof mascaras. All that pulling and wiping to get waterproof mascara off isn't good for the skin and tends to pull lashes out. There are dozens of waterproof mascaras out there, but only a handful are truly reliable. Plus, waterproof mascaras do not stay on any better than water-soluble ones, given that both break down in contact with emollients from moisturizers, sunscreens, under-eye creams, foundations, creamy under-eye concealers, and other specialty products applied around the eye.

**Beauty Note:** I should mention that I have a personal preference for mascaras that produce long, thick lashes. I admit that my own preference in this regard can get in the way of my evaluations, so understand that I got particularly excited about a mascara such as L'Oreal Le Grand Curl that built thick, long lashes fast and easy without smearing, clumping, or flaking.

**BRUSHES:** Brushes are essential to applying makeup correctly and beautifully. Blush and eyeshadow brushes are offered by some of the major cosmetics lines, and most department stores sell brush sets of some kind. Brushes were rated on overall shape and function as well as on the softness and density of the bristles. An eyeshadow or blush brush with scratchy, stiff, or loose bristles was not recommended. Also, let me warn you against buying brush sets. They almost always include brushes you don't need or can't use. It is best to buy brushes individually so you can select the best ones for your needs and for the shape of your face and eyes.

## Evaluation of Skin-Care Products

The following were the criteria I used to evaluate the quality of varying groups of skin-care products. For those of you who are familiar with my reviews, you may notice that I am now much more cautious about products that contain any amount of irritating ingredients, particularly those containing lemon, grapefruit, mint, peppermint, menthol, camphor, eucalyptus, ivy, fragrant oils, and overly drying detergent cleansing agents. My more exacting criteria on this subject relate to the growing research indicating that irritation damages skin and hurts the skin's healing process. In the midst of our daily battle against sun damage, wrinkles, and the causes of breakouts, there is never a reason to unnecessarily irritate the skin with ingredients that provide no benefit whatsoever for the face or body.

My reviews of skin-care products in each line are, with a few exceptions, organized in the following categories: cleanser, eye-makeup remover, exfoliant (scrubs or AHA products), facial mask, toner, moisturizer (all kinds regardless of the claim), eye cream, specialty products (serums), sunscreen, and acne products.

**CLEANSER:** In reviewing facial cleansers, I was primarily interested in how genuinely water-soluble they are. Facial cleansers should have rinsed off easily, without the aid of a washcloth, and been able to remove all traces of makeup, including eye makeup. Once a water-soluble cleanser was rinsed off, it should not have left skin feeling dry, greasy, or filmy. And it should never have burned the eyes, irritated the skin, or tasted bad. Removing makeup with a greasy cleanser is an option for some women with extremely dry skin; however, it is not a preferred method of makeup removal. Wiping at the skin pulls at it and causes the skin to sag. Plus, wiping at the skin with a washcloth or tissue can be irritating. Wiping off makeup with cotton balls is less irritating but the pulling is still problematic.

I do not recommend cleansers that contain effective concentrations of AHAs or BHA or the topical disinfectant benzoyl peroxide. While these ingredients can be quite helpful in other skin-care products, in a cleanser these are rinsed down the drain before they have a chance to have a real effect on skin. It is also a concern that these ingredients can inadvertently get into the eye when rinsing the cleanser off the face. (I should mention that I never found a cleanser that includes an AHA or BHA that contains both an effective concentration and an appropriate pH.)

**EYE-MAKEUP REMOVER:** Using a separate eye-makeup remover more often than not is completely unnecessary. An effective but gentle water-soluble cleanser should take off all your makeup, including eye makeup, without irritating the eyes. The problem with wiping off makeup is simply that you have to wipe and pull at your skin to get the stuff off. That pulling and wiping causes the skin to sag faster than it would otherwise. Another problem is the tendency for makeup to get wiped into the eye itself as opposed to splashed away, and that can cause irritation. Unless you are wearing waterproof mascara or can't get the knack of removing your eye makeup with a water-soluble cleanser, there are many reasons to avoid this step.

Some women who find using a water-soluble cleanser ineffective for removing eye makeup can saturate a large cotton pad with eye-makeup remover, close their eyes, and very gently place it against the eyebrows and eyelids, holding it there for a few seconds. This way, they aren't tugging or pulling but instead loosening and dissolving the eye makeup. Then they follow with a water-soluble cleanser and more easily remove the makeup. Most every eye-makeup remover I've seen was either water with a lightweight surfactant (detergent cleansing agent) or some form of oil. More so than with any other skin-care category, there is no reason to waste money on this group of products. My tendency was to rate these products with a "neutral" face regardless of the product's effectiveness. Almost all of these products were formulated similarly, with no surprises or real cautions needed other than telling you that they are not the best way to remove makeup on a daily basis, although they can be effective and necessary for those with a particular preference for this type of product.

**EXFOLIANT/SCRUB:** With the advent of alpha hydroxy acids (AHAs) and the increased use of beta hydroxy acid (BHA; technical name, salicylic acid), there is little reason to use a mechanical exfoliant on the skin. Mechanical exfoliants are scrubs that remove skin cells as you rub particles over the skin. Even when the scrub particles are small and uniform in size, this can still abrade the skin and be harsher than necessary, causing damage and hurting the skin's healing process. That means the major consideration for any topical scrub was that it was gentle on the skin and not rough or overly abrasive. Some women prefer the feeling of a scrub on the skin, but I've yet to see one that can supersede using plain baking soda mixed with Cetaphil Gentle Skin Cleanser. My strong suggestion, if you do want to try a scrub, is to start with Cetaphil and baking soda mixed together before shopping a cosmetics line for a scrub.

**ALPHA/BETA HYDROXY ACID PRODUCTS:** I expected products containing AHAs or BHA to be exfoliants. Though AHAs and BHA can be effective moisturizing ingredients, no one is expecting that function and, above all, AHAs and BHA excel in exfoliation.

There were very specific criteria for determining whether or not an AHA or BHA product would be an effective exfoliant. I wish you could tell whether an AHA or BHA product would be effective by its label, but that just isn't possible. All the claims and promises on the sticker, and even the ingredient label, won't tell you whether you are purchasing an effective AHA or BHA product. Unfortunately, effectiveness was based not only on ingredient content (which I explain in the next section, "Ingredients in Skin Care), but also on the percentage of the active ingredients (how much of the AHA or BHA was in the product) and the pH level (how acid or alkaline it was). I had two major considerations when reviewing products that contain alpha hydroxy acids (AHAs) and beta hydroxy acid (BHA). First, I assessed the percentage of AHAs or BHA used in the product, with 5% to 10% being preferred for AHAs—more in this regard did not mean better because of the resulting irritation that can cause, but there are effective products that go up to 20% AHAs—and 1% to 2% being preferred for BHA. Then I measured the pH of the product. The pH is significant, because these ingredients can work only when they are in an acid base. If the base is too neutral or too alkaline (a pH over 4), the base becomes more alkaline and ineffective for exfoliating the skin. AHAs and BHA both work best in a pH of 3 to 4. By the way, an AHA or BHA product with a high pH is not a harmful product, just one that's ineffective for exfoliation.

As a general rule I do not recommend products that use AHAs and BHA together. Each has its preferred action and that does not translate to all skin types. AHAs work on the surface of the skin and are best for sun-damaged skin that has developed a thickened outer layer, or for someone with dry skin who has a buildup of layers of skin that make skin look dull and impede cell turnover.

BHA can exfoliate on the surface of skin much like AHAs can, but BHA can also cut through the lipid layer of skin and therefore work better in the pore, helping skin to shed cells and loosen any plugs in there, improving the size and function of the pore. If you don't have breakouts, you don't need that kind of penetration; if you have breakouts, AHAs may help to some extent, but the penetration from the BHA can be more effective.

One word of caution: Anytime you use a well-formulated AHA product that contains more than 5% AHAs, some stinging can occur, though this can diminish as the skin gets used to it. You should not let AHAs or BHA products come in contact with the eyes or any mucous membranes. You may have an irritation or sensitivity to AHAs. Slight stinging is expected, but continued stinging is not. Discontinue use if this should happen.

**FACIAL MASK:** Most facial masks contain claylike ingredients that absorb oil and, to some degree, exfoliate the skin. The problem with many masks is that they contain additional ingredients that are irritating or that can clog pores. Although your face may feel smooth when the mask is first rinsed off, after a short period of time problems may be created by the mask's drying effect. As a rule, I am not fond of recommending many facial masks. The few clay masks that contain emollients and moisturizing ingredients can still be too drying for dry skin and can cause oily skin to break out. There are also a range of masks that contain plasticizing (hairspray-like) ingredients that peel off the face like a layer of plastic. These take a layer of skin off when removed, and that can make skin feel temporarily smoother, but no long-term benefit is gained from this. Another type of facial mask that shows up is the kind with strictly moisturizing ingredients. These don't differ from other moisturizers being sold, but to call the product a mask seems to make women feel like they are doing something special for their skin when they aren't. Despite all these shortcomings, which I pointed out in the individual reviews, there are masks in this book that did get happy faces.

**TONER:** Toners, astringents, fresheners, tonics, and other liquids meant to refresh the skin or remove the last traces of makeup after a cleanser is rinsed off should not contain any irritants whatsoever. I evaluated these products primarily on that basis. Claims that toners can close pores or refine the skin are unachievable, so I ignored such language and looked primarily for toners that left the face feeling smooth and soft, were able to remove any last traces of makeup, and did not irritate the skin. Some toners may also contain water-binding and anti-irritant ingredients, and these were listed as being preferred for normal to dry skin. Toners with lightweight detergent cleansing agents, lightweight water-binding agents, and anti-irritants were rated high for normal to oily skin. However, toners are always considered an optional step for most skin types. For someone with normal to oily skin, they can be the only moisturizer the skin needs; for someone with dry skin, they can be a great lightweight start to add extra water-binding agents to the skin.

**MOISTURIZER:** In spite of all the fuss surrounding wrinkle creams and moisturizers as a way to make skin look and stay young, this category was actually quite easy to review. Wrinkle creams and moisturizers all do the same thing—they keep the skin from looking and feeling dry—so I expected the same thing from all of them: they had to contain ingredients that could smooth and soothe dry skin and keep water in the skin cell. Most other claims were exaggerated and misleading. Remember that dry skin and wrinkles are not associated, so you can't stop or get rid of wrinkles by applying a moisturizer, despite the claims.

Lots of moisturizers boasted that they can penetrate layers of skin cells better than others do, which was a meaningless claim. Skin cells are quite permeable, so claims of penetrating layers of skin would be true for most products if they contained even one drop of water. Nonetheless, it is essential that some moisturizing ingredients be left on the surface of the skin to prevent the air from drinking up the water in your skin cells. My reviews showed a preference for formulas that utilized unique or interesting water-binding agents and antioxidants.

I also listed the ingredients I thought are more hype than help, such as brewer's yeast; bee pollen; gold; animal extracts from thymus, spleen, placenta, and fish collagen; and many plant extracts ranging from algae to flowers, and countless weeds. Additionally, I was interested in what order the "good" or "hyped" ingredients were listed on the container. Often the percentage of the most interesting or the most extolled ingredients was so negligible that those ingredients were practically nonexistent. Just because an ingredient was in there doesn't mean there's enough to make a difference.

There were moisturizers that claimed they were great for combination skin because they were able to release moisturizing ingredients over dry areas and oil-absorbing ingredients over oily areas. This is categorically impossible. A product cannot hold certain ingredients back from the skin—where would they go? Imagine a lotion touching your skin and the ingredients for the oily parts get up and run over here and the ones for the dry area get up and head over there. It just isn't feasible in any way, shape, or form.

Please read over my comments in the section on "What Makes a Good Moisturizer?" where you'll find specifics regarding the use of water-binding agents, anti-irritants and soothing ingredients, emollients, and nonfragrant plant oils; that will give you the background for how I went about determining what made one moisturizer preferred over another.

<u>**MOISTURIZER FOR OILY SKIN:**</u> The only time to use a moisturizer is when you have dry skin; if you don't have dry skin, you don't need to use a moisturizer. When a product, particularly a moisturizer, claims to be "oil-free," more often than not it misleads consumers into thinking they are buying a product that won't clog pores. There are plenty of ingredients that don't sound like oils but can absolutely aggravate breakouts. Almost all cosmetics contain waxlike thickening agents that are notorious for clogging pores. Simple, standard moisturizing ingredients that are great for dry skin can wreak havoc on someone with oily skin or breakouts. Triglycerides, palmitates, stearates, myristates, stearic acid, plant oils, plant waxes, shea butter, vitamin E, acrylates (film-forming agents), and many other ingredients can all clog pores. These ingredients are used in moisturizers because they duplicate the natural lipids (sebum or oil) in our skin, or prevent dehydration, and that's great. But if you have problems with the oil already being created in your pores, adding more of the same kind of substance will only make things worse. Despite the problems these ingredi-

ents can cause, they show up in lots and lots of so-called "oil-free" products. To that end, I've judged all moisturizers on their effectiveness for some level of dry skin. Never use a moisturizer over areas of the face that are oily, that break out, or that have blackheads—it will only make matters worse. Moisturizers are only needed where you have dry skin.

**DAY CREAM VERSUS NIGHT CREAM:** The only difference that should exist between a daytime moisturizer and a nighttime moisturizer is that the daytime one should have an effective SPF (sunscreen) with UVA-protecting ingredients. Other than that, there are no formulation variances that make one preferable over the other. There are many moisturizing formulations that have great sun protection, and that is the only way you should differentiate a daytime product from a nighttime version. All other claims on the label are rhetoric you should ignore.

**EYE, THROAT, CHEST, NECK, AND OTHER SPECIALTY CREAM AND SERUM:** Buying a product for a special area of the face or body, whether it is in the form of a cream, gel, lotion, or serum, is altogether unnecessary. Almost without exception, the ingredient lists and formulations for these products are identical to other creams, gels, serums, and lotions for the face. That doesn't mean there aren't some great products out there for different skin types in the form of some specialty products, especially eye products, but why buy a second moisturizer for the eye area when the one you are already using on the rest of your face is virtually identical? Even more bothersome is the fact that most cosmetics companies give you a tiny amount of the so-called specialty product but charge you much more for it than for an equal amount of nonspecialty face creams, despite the similarities.

What do sometimes show up in eye-care products are irritating ingredients such as witch hazel. These types of ingredients temporarily swell the skin around the eye, creating an appearance of diminished wrinkles. Swollen skin can temporarily look smooth, but the resulting irritation is, in the long run, harmful, not helpful, for the skin.

**SUNSCREEN:** Please refer to Chapter Two, *Face Facts*, for more information about sun care. To sum up, my main criterion for evaluating sun-care products was the SPF rating, with SPF 15 being the standard to meet. Because of the difference between UVA damage and UVB damage, to be assured you are getting adequate UVA protection, your sunscreen must contain one of three UVA-protecting ingredients listed as an **active ingredient** on the label. Those **active ingredients must include avobenzone (also called Parsol 1789 or butyl methoxydibenzoylmethane), titanium dioxide, zinc oxide, or Mexoryl SX™**. No sunscreens received a happy face unless one of those is listed on the active-ingredient part of the ingredient listing, along with an SPF of 15 or greater.

Sunscreen ingredients can be irritating no matter what a product's label says, because the way these ingredients work can cause a reaction on the skin. You just have to experiment to find the one that works best for you. Although sunscreens that use only titanium dioxide or only zinc oxide as the active ingredient are considered almost completely nonirritating, they can still pose problems for someone with oily or acne-prone skin because their occlusive composition can clog pores and aggravate breakouts.

**Although I've said this before, it still bears repeating:** Many products make claims about UVA protection that are truly misleading. While titanium dioxide, zinc oxide, or avobenzone (also called Parsol 1789 or butylmethoxydibenzoylmethane) protect from about 80% to 90% of UVA radiation, other formulations that don't contain these ingredients only protect from about 20% of UVA radiation.

<u>SELF TANNER:</u> For the most part I did not review self-tanning products individually. All of these products, whether you choose one made by Revlon, Clarins, Decleor Paris, or Estee Lauder, are created equal. The active ingredient in every one of these products is dihydroxyacetone. That's what turns the surface layer of skin brown. The ingredient acts on the skin cells and their amino acid content, and that chemical reaction is what turns the skin a darker color. Self tanners do not add a tint of color on top of the skin, though those products that contain tints can help you see where you've applied the product, which can help you make a smoother application.

Your personal preference as to how self tanners make your skin appear actually has less to do with the product itself than with the nature of your own skin cells. The interaction between the active ingredient and your skin is controlled more by your body's chemistry than anything else.

You may not like the smell of one product versus another, but that is merely a function of the fragrance added to the product to mask the smell of the dihydroxyacetone. A masking fragrance might be pleasant, but it doesn't change how the product functions, and the natural odor of the product is transient. Where self tanners do differ is in the amount of dihydroxyactone used. There is no way to judge that from the ingredient list. However, you can assume that those self tanners rated as light, medium, and dark have the correct corresponding amount of dihydroxyacetone. You can also assume that self tanners without any stated level have a light to medium concentration of dihydroxyacetone.

For more specific critiques of self-tanning products, I find the Web site www.sunless.com to be incredibly helpful and I strongly recommend a visit.

<u>ACNE PRODUCTS:</u> From all the research I've seen, particularly in dermatological journals and literature from the American Academy of Dermatology, acne products need to deliver four categories of performance to deal with breakouts: gentle cleansing, effective exfoliation, disinfecting, and absorbing excess oil. I delve into this subject at length in my book *The Beauty Bible*. I based my reviews here on how well over-the-counter products (as opposed to those available by prescription only) responded to those skin-care needs.

**Cleansing:** Using a gentle, water-soluble cleanser is standard for any skin-care routine, but even more so for oily skin because it reduces irritation and redness. After all, what color is acne? Red. So why use any product that makes skin redder? I also never recommend bar soap for acne or breakouts. Bar soaps of any kind are kept in their bar form by ingredients that can absolutely clog pores. Research also shows that high-pH cleansers (soaps are usually over a pH of 8) can increase the presence of bacteria in the skin. To that end, gentle cleansers were rated high if they do not contain irritating or excessively drying ingredients.

**Exfoliating:** For exfoliating the skin with an over-the-counter treatment, it is best to start with either a 5% to 8% alpha hydroxy acid (AHA) product or a 1% to 2% beta hydroxy acid (BHA) product, and these must have a pH of 3 to 4 (pH refers to how alkaline or acid a formulation is). BHA and AHA are effective as exfoliants in a more acidic base, but at much over a pH 4 these types of products lose their acid base and become ineffective for exfoliation. For blemishes or oily skin, these products were rated especially good if they are available in gel or very lightweight lotion form.

When it comes to cosmetic scrubs, I almost never preferred them for exfoliating the skin, because they were almost all formulated with waxy thickening agents that can clog pores and cause breakouts. That's not to say they can't be effective for exfoliation, because they can, but I found most of these formulations troublesome or flawed for blemish- or blackhead-prone skin. For all skin types, if you are looking for a mechanical scrub, I still have yet to find a product that can beat mixing baking soda with Cetaphil Gentle Skin Cleanser.

**Disinfecting:** In order to kill the bacteria in the skin that cause blemishes, you need a reliable disinfectant. There aren't many options when it comes to disinfecting the skin. Alcohol, when used in very high concentrations (more than 60%—thankfully, never found in skin-care products) and sulfur can be good disinfectants, but they are way too drying and irritating for most skin types, and can just make matters worse, because irritation can cause rashlike breakouts and hurt the skin's healing process, making the potential for scarring worse. Other ingredients that repeatedly show up in products for problem skin, such as lemon, grapefruit, acetone, witch hazel, peppermint, menthol, eucalyptus, and camphor, have no effect at all on bacteria and cause unnecessary irritation. The currently popular plant-derived dis- infectants such as tea tree oil (from *Melaleuca alterniflora*) were not present in high enough concentrations to reliably kill bacteria. The best over-the-counter disinfectants are 3% hydrogen peroxide, and 2.5%, 5%, and 10% benzoyl peroxide (but only when no irritating ingredients are added). Only the types of products that contained these ingredients, with no irritating or moisturizing ingredients added, were given high ratings.

**Absorbing excess oil:** There are many types of skin-care and makeup products designed for creating a matte finish or oil-absorbing layer of ingredients on the skin.

These typically use absorbent materials such as talc, silicates (magnesium aluminum silicate is one of the more popular ones), clays, dry-finish silicones (usually cyclomethicone or phenyl trimethicone), and film-forming agents (hairspray-like ingredients). These can all work well to absorb oil. However, none of them can control oil production. Oil production is primarily a result of your hormones, and that can not be affected from the outside in with cosmetics. I often point out my concern that ingredients like rice starch, cornstarch, and other food products are typically considered problematic for breakouts. Food substances can get into pores and encourage bacteria production, which is not the best when your goal is fighting off bacteria.

Clay masks are also a popular option for absorbing excess oil on the skin, and while these can help, they often contain other ingredients that are skin irritants or can clog pores. I typically recommend as a starting point that you try milk of magnesia (yes, like the Phillips' Milk of Magnesia that you take for indigestion) as a facial mask. It is by far one of the best ways to absorb oil. Milk of magnesia is nothing more than liquid magnesium hydroxide, which is known to soothe skin and reduce irritation, and it has incredible oil-absorbing properties. Magnesium absorbs more oil than clay, and clay has no disinfecting or soothing properties. How often you use the milk of magnesia has to do with how oily your skin is. Some use it every day; others, once a week. Only you and your skin can determine what frequency works best for you.

SKIN-LIGHTENING PRODUCTS: The surge in skin-care products making claims about lightening skin and depigmenting skin discolorations caused by sun exposure is nothing less than astounding. Until a few years ago, these products were almost exclusively bought by Asian women who culturally are concerned about having whiter skin, or by darker-skin-tone women concerned about facial discolorations or uneven, ashy skin tones. Now that baby boomers are aging and brown patches (caused primarily from sun damage—they are not liver spots or age related at all) are beginning to turn up on hands and faces, skin-lightening products are basic to any antiaging skincare routine. To convince consumers that these products are different and natural, lots of plant extracts are thrown into the mix, ranging from mulberry extract to kojic acid (extracted from a fungus grown on rice or soybeans). While those ingredients have some research showing them to be effective, mulberry extract has minimal effectiveness and then only in pure concentrations (not mixed into a moisturizer), and kojic aicd can be a skin irritant and is an unstable ingredient. It also turns out that those plant extracts are highly unstable and have little to no efficacy when mixed into skin-care products.

**Hydroquinone has by far the most extensive research in regard to its ability to inhibit hyper-melanin production. Hydroquinone products containing 1% to 2% concentrations, available over the counter, and products with a concentration of 4% or greater, available from physicians, were the only ones I rated highly.**

I am aware that there is some concern about hydroquinone being potentially carcinogenic. Back in 1995, Mark Green, New York City's consumer affairs commissioner, was trying to ban 11 leading skin-bleaching creams (containing hydroquinone) that were being marketed primarily to African Americans (*Drug and Cosmetic Industry* magazine, April 1996). However, nothing ever came of that attempt, because what was true back then is still true now: the single in vitro (test-tube) study showing a cellular problem was never duplicated and never shown to be true in vivo. According to Howard I. Maibach, M.D., Professor of Dermatology at the University of California School of Medicine, San Francisco, "Overall, adverse events reported with the use of hydroquinone .... have been relatively few and minor in nature. ... To date there is no evidence of adverse systemic reactions following the use of hydroquinone" and it has been around for over 30 years in skin-care products. Maibach has also stated that "hydroquinone is undoubtedly the most active and safest skin-depigmenting substance." Research supporting Maibach's contentions was published in the *Journal of Toxicology and Environmental Health,* 1998, pages 301–17.

## The Ingredients for Skin Care

While I wanted to emphasize the extent of the misleading portrayals of skin-care products made by the cosmetics industry, I also wanted to underscore that great products *do* exist for all skin types. However, it was difficult for me to describe my elation or enthusiasm about any product without always being careful to let you know what can really be expected and how out-of-line the price often was for what you are getting. Just because I thought a formula can be amazing for dry skin, that doesn't mean I concurred with its claims about firming, lifting, undoing or preventing wrinkling, reducing lines, fighting stress, erasing cellulite, building collagen, and on and on and on. . . .

Every skin-care product was evaluated on the basis of what it contained. The ingredients are the basis for whether a claim can be verified. Unlike earlier editions of *Don't Go to the Cosmetics Counter Without Me,* **I did not summarize the ingredient listing for every skin-care product** in this edition. I wanted to include as many new lines as possible, and the repetitive "this product contains" listing—which was not everyone's cup of tea—took up an astounding amount of room. Unless I felt this kind of information was needed to help understand a product's performance, I provided just a general summary of the product's contents and then described what it could and couldn't do. When I did describe a product's ingredients, it was always **in the order they appeared on the ingredient list.** I also let you know how it compared to similar products that cost much less. Of course, you will have to test for yourself how any specific product feels on your skin and how you react to its fragrance or lack thereof.

When I did describe a product's contents in the product reviews, I frequently used the phrase "contains mostly," often followed by one or all of the following terms: **thickener** or **thickening agent, slip agent, water-binding agent, film former, scrub agent, absorbent, detergent cleansing agent** or **standard detergent cleanser, preservative, fragrance, plant extract** or **plant oil, vitamin, antioxidant,** and **anti-irritant.** It was easiest to summarize groups of ingredients by using these general terms, but they need more explanation before you read the reviews.

**Beauty Note:** When reading ingredient lists, remember that the closer a specific ingredient is to a preservative (such as methylparaben, propylparaben, ethylparaben, imidazolidinyl urea, or quaternium-15) or a fragrance (listed as fragrance or often as an individual essential oil like lavender or bergamot oil), or the closer it is to the end of the ingredient list, the less likely it is that any significant amount is present in the product.

When I used the term "**thickeners**" to describe an ingredient, the term refers to those components that add texture, thickness, viscosity, spreadability, and stability to a product. Thickeners are also vital for helping to keep other ingredients mixed together. **Thickening agents** often have a waxlike texture or a creamy, emollient feel, and can be great lubricants. There are literally thousands of ingredients in this category, and they are the staples of every skin-care product out there, regardless of the product's price or claims about "natural" ingredients.

**Slip agents** help other ingredients spread over or penetrate the skin and they also have humectant properties. Slip agents include propylene glycol, butylene glycol, hexylene glycol, methyl gluceth-10, polysorbates, and glycerin, to name only a few. They are as basic to the world of skin care as water.

**Water-binding agents** are known for their ability to help the skin retain water. These ingredients range from the mundane glycerin to the more exotic hyaluronic acid, sodium hyaluronate, mucopolysaccharides, sodium PCA, glycerin, collagen, elastin, proteins, amino acids (of which there are dozens), cholesterol, glucose, sucrose, fructose, glycogen, antioxidants, phospholipids, glycosphingolipids, and on and on. For the most part, they all work equally well. Looking for a specific one is a waste of your time and energy. They are what they are: good water-binding ingredients.

**Scrub** or **abrasive** ingredients are found in cleansing products meant to remove dead skin cells, as an extra cleaning step. The most typical scrub particles used are almond meal, cornmeal, ground apricot or almond pits, and polyethylene. Polyethylene is the most common form of plastic used in the world and the most popular scrub agent. It is flexible and has a smooth, waxy feel. When ground up, the small particles are used in scrubs as a fairly gentle abrasive. Seashells (listed as diatomaceous earth on the ingredient label) are also used as abrasive substances in scrubs, but they can be extremely rough on skin.

**Absorbents** are ingredients used in skin-care and makeup products designed for creating a matte finish or oil-absorbing film layer on the skin. These absorbent materials are typically talc, silicates (such as magnesium aluminum silicate), clays, dry-finish silicones (usually cyclomethicone or phenyl trimethicone), nylon-12, and film-forming agents (hairspray-like ingredients). They can all work well to absorb oil. Some have drier finishes than others, but that is very dependent on the specific formulation and amount of the ingredient used. I often point out my concern that ingredients like rice starch, cornstarch, and other food products are typically considered problematic for breakouts. Food substances can get into pores and encourage bacteria production, which is not the best when fighting off bacteria is the goal.

**Film formers** are ingredients such as polyvinyl pyrrolidone, methylacrylate, and the polyglycerylacrylates presently being used in a vast number of moisturizers, wrinkle creams, and eye gels to help the skin look smoother. Film formers are usually found in hairsprays and hairstyling products like gels and mousses because they place a thin, transparent, plastic-like layer over the hair (and skin). In the past, the kinds of film formers used were problematic for some skin types; today, with the advent of new polymers, these film-forming ingredients do a good job of keeping moisture in the skin and are generally used in such tiny amounts that they are unlikely to be a problem for most skin types. They can also work to absorb oil in some formulations. When these film-forming ingredients are found higher up on a product's ingredient list, they can leave a slightly tacky feeling on the skin.

For products such as skin cleansers, in which an ingredient is included primarily for its sudsing or degreasing ability, I used the phrase "**detergent cleansing agent**" or "**standard detergent cleanser.**" Ingredients in this category include sodium lauryl sulfate, sodium laureth sulfate, TEA-lauryl sulfate, cocamide DEA, ammonium laureth sulfate, and ammonium lauryl sulfate, to name a few (though these tend to be the most typical). Because sodium lauryl sulfate, TEA-lauryl sulfate, and sodium C14-16 olefin sulfate are very strong detergent cleansing agents and are known for their irritation potential, I warned against using a product that contained these ingredients when they appeared in the first part of its ingredient list.

There are **preservatives** that some people feel are more problematic than others. I have not included specific warnings for preservatives such as quaternium-15, 2-bromo-2-nitropane-1,3-diol, phenoxyethylanol, or dmdm hydantoin. There is research indicating that these ingredients pose a higher potential for irritation than other preservatives. Recent data, however, strongly dispute that conclusion. After discussing this matter with several cosmetics chemists, I have concluded that all preservatives can be a problem for many different types of skin, so it would be unfair and misleading to pinpoint one or two specific preservatives as problems. If you are concerned, you can easily avoid any of these ingredients; however, as several cosmetics chemists warned me, a reliable preservative system is better for the skin because microbial contamination of a product can cause more problems for the eyes, lips, and skin than the risk of a reaction to a preservative.

On a related matter, some of you may be familiar with research that warns against using cosmetics that contain DEA, triethanolamine, or TEA-lauryl sulfate mixed in the same product along with formaldehyde-releasing preservatives such as imidazolidinyl urea, quaternium-15, 2-bromo-2-nitropane-1,3-diol, or dmdm hydantoin. There is evidence that suggests these combinations can form nitrosamines in a cosmetic, creating a potential carcinogen (nitrosamines, as you may recall, are carcinogenic substances). There is substantial disagreement among the cosmetics chemists I spoke to as to how significant a problem this is for the skin (or whether it even is a problem). They suggested that going out of the house without a sunscreen or sitting in a bar exposed to secondhand cigarette smoke poses more risk to the skin than any combination of skin-care ingredients ever could. However, you should be aware that there are those who consider this nonchalant attitude to be mere apologetics for and sidestepping around a very serious question. As someone who has looked at this issue for some time, I actually understand both viewpoints and have no definitive position to share. To that end, I leave the final decision up to you. All you need to do is check the ingredient list of any product you are considering to determine whether it excludes amines as well as the questionable preservatives mentioned above.

When **fragrances** were listed in the ingredients, I indicated this simply by stating it as such. Fragrance is used in cosmetics either to mask the smell of a product's ingredients or to add a specific fragrance. My strong recommendation is that skin-care products not contain fragrance. Fragrances of all kinds, including essential oils, are irritants and serve no function for skin. Because of that I would prefer that all skin-care products be fragrance-free. Nevertheless, women like their products to smell nice. It is up to every woman to make her own decision on that matter. Even if I thought fragrance was OK in a skin-care product, fragrance is still a very tricky thing to comment on because smell is such a personal experience. Avoiding fragrance is easy to do by checking the ingredient label (you can't trust the term "unscented," because the product may still contain a masking fragrance). If fragrance (listed as "fragrance" on the ingredient label) or individual fragrant essential oils like lavender, cardamom, lemon, ylang-ylang, bergamot, and cinnamon, among others, are listed on an ingredient label, you know it has fragrance and you can choose what to do: either make your nose happy or make your skin happy; unfortunately, you can't do both.

It is impossible to list all the individual **plant extracts** used in cosmetics. As far as the world of cosmetics is concerned, if it grows, it can change skin. Yet there is no consensus on which plant is the most amazing. According to the various cosmetics companies, the plants they use have the most astonishing merits. When plants were an issue in a skin-care product, I pointed out those plants' known benefits; otherwise, I mentioned all plants only under the generic category of plant extracts.

**Plant oils** (other than those called essential oils) are almost always beneficial as emollients and lubricants. The debate whether or not emu, mink, sunflower, canola, or a myriad of other oils or blends of oils are superior is a marketing game to showcase a product; it has nothing to do with the structure of skin or reliable skin care.

Some plant oils, often referred to as essential oils, are highly fragrant, volatile oils and are almost always irritants or photosensitizers, and I indicated when this was the case. However, I attributed no superiority to one over another, because there is none. **Essential oils** are nothing more than a way to get fragrance into a skin-care product. The cosmetics industry knows that many women are aware that fragrance can be a strong source of skin irritation and sensitivities, so they use the term "essential oils" as a way to put fragrance in a product without saying "fragrance." Women may know that fragrance ingredients are bad, but they still want their products to smell nice. Caught between a rock and a hard place, the cosmetics industry came up with essential oils as the way around the dilemma. But the notion that plants can save the skin from wrinkles, stress, sun damage, scars, and a host of other skin ills is sheer fantasy and has no legitimate substantiation. That doesn't mean that natural ingredients can't be helpful, but they can't perform the miracles attributed to them by sales pitches, and fragrant oils such as clove, peppermint, citrus, ylang-ylang, cinnamon, coriander, and lavender, among many others, can cause irritation.

I often listed the exact name of any **vitamin** included in a product. Regardless of the individual vitamin—whether it is vitamin A, C, or E—vitamins in skin-care products can't feed the skin. However, they can work as antioxidants when the product contained enough of them, and theoretically that can benefit the skin.

When specific antioxidant ingredients such as superoxide dismutase, selenium, glutathione, vitamin E, vitamin A, and vitamin C were included, I sometimes referred to these specifically as **antioxidants**. While research indicates that antioxidants may have much benefit for the skin, a vast amount is still not known. For example, even if antioxidants do have definitive benefits, there are no amounts established for effectiveness. Is 0.25% enough or 3% too much? Is there such a thing as too much? Should we be putting vitamins only on the skin? What about oral supplements? For many of the more popular antioxidants, like vitamin A or vitamin C, and other plant extracts that can work as antioxidants, stability is a problem. Vitamin C deteriorates in the presence of air or sunlight and doesn't mix well with other ingredients. Ascorbic acid is considered a poor antioxidant because of its irritating effect on the skin. Until there is more information, we can only assume that antioxidants are good guys because they keep the drying effect of the air off the skin and help protect skin cells. Other than that, it is all guessing and hoping.

If you are still sold on the hype around antioxidants, don't worry; most cosmetics in all price ranges contain them. These aren't secret ingredients to which only some cosmetics companies have access. Everyone knows about them and they are widely used in the industry.

**Anti-irritants** are **soothing ingredients** known for their ability to reduce inflammation on the skin. A small group of ingredients can perform this function and they do so quite nicely. When these types of ingredients—such as bisabolol, allantoin, burdock root, aloe, licorice root, or green tea—are present in a product, I refer to them by the term "anti-irritant(s)."

Many products use an assortment of exclusive-sounding adjectives—**deionized, purified, triple-purified, demineralized, fossilized**—to describe what is nothing more than just plain **water.** These terms indicate that the water has gone through some kind of purification process or been taken from a specific water source, which is standard for cosmetics. You will also find phrases such as "infusions of" or "aqueous extracts of," followed by the name of one or more plants. That means you're getting plant tea, or plant juice and water. Though descriptions like this indicate that you are getting mostly water and a hint of plant, they sound so pure and natural that they create the impression that they must be better for the skin. Well, water is water. The kind of water used does not affect the skin or the final product. After the water is combined with other ingredients, its original status is unimportant.

**Silicone** is a skin-friendly ingredient that shows up repeatedly in skin-care, makeup, and hair-care products. I would venture a guess that the ubiquitous silicone appears in about 80% of all cosmetic products being sold. In the past, I have referred to silicone as silicone oil, which I have recently learned is incorrect terminology. While silicone may look, act, and feel like oil, and though every cosmetics chemist I've spoken to refers to it as silicone oil, this ingredient is still not an oil. Technically speaking, silicone as a chemical compound is related to fluid technology. Either way, regardless of the precise name, silicone is an elegant skin-care ingredient that has an exquisite, silky, somewhat slippery feel. Its popularity in formulations reflects its versatility and the finish it gives products. It is also a cheap ingredient, and standard to all kinds of cosmetics in all kinds of price ranges. **For someone with oily or acne-prone skin, silicone is not necessarily a problem, at least when it comes to breakouts, though it can leave a residue behind on the skin that someone with oily skin might not like.**

**Antibacterial ingredients:** While cleanliness has merit, there are limitations to how clean a person can be. In the battle against germs and other loathsome microorganisms floating about our environment, the desire to wash with zest is valid (do not take that as a plug for Zest bar soap; I just couldn't resist the pun). We are also greatly influenced by news programs that ballyhoo the horror of bacteria being spread through less-than-scrupulous ablutions. It isn't surprising, then, to hear that antibacterial soaps have recently had an upsurge in sales. Unfortunately, this attention to antiseptic skin care is misplaced. It's not that I'm against cleanliness—far from it—and it goes without saying that disinfecting the skin is absolutely necessary in the battle against acne. The problem is that antibacterial cleansers of any kind, even the kind used in a doctor's office, and regardless of the active ingredient, can't really kill germs and bacteria. At least, not any better than regular soaps and cleansers.

Here's the issue. In order for any disinfectant to work, it must be in contact with the skin for at least several minutes, and ten minutes or more is best. How many of us scrub our hands and face for that long with an antibacterial cleanser? Hopefully, none of us, because that much contact with such potent disinfecting cleansers would destroy the skin in short order. But that's what it takes for antibacterial cleansers to do their job. When physicians scrub up for a surgical procedure, they wash their hands vigorously for several minutes, depending on the type of wash they use. They know that contact and scrubbing are the key to effectively disinfecting the skin. They also know that it makes their skin raw and dry, but there is no way around this one. Washing your hands and face with an antibacterial cleanser for a few seconds is fine, but don't expect your skin to be totally disinfected.

I'm not encouraging everyone to start scrubbing, because it is certainly detrimental to anyone's skin in the long haul, and for many skin types in the short haul. It hurts the intercellular layer of skin (the mortar that holds skin together), and that, ironically, is what keeps bacteria and germs out. Generally speaking, I do not encourage the use of antibacterial products for the face if you don't have a problem with breakouts. If you do have a problem with breakouts, I still think bar cleansers are a poor option because, though you may be getting some minimal benefit from the disinfecting ingredient, you're stuck with the ingredients that keep the bar soap in its bar form, which can clog pores. Liquid or lotion water-soluble antibacterial cleansers are an option, but again, the contact with the antibacterial agent is so brief that I find it a poor option, given the other types of topical disinfectants available.

Further, it is interesting to note that in the April 19, 1999, issue of the *Journal of Biological Chemistry*, researchers at St. Jude Children's Research concluded that the ability of *E. coli* "to acquire genetic resistance to **triclosan** [the antibacterial agent found in many antibacterial hand creams and toothpastes] ... suggests that the widespread use of this drug will lead to the appearance of resistant organisms that will compromise the usefulness of triclosan."

**Alpha hydroxy acids** and **beta hydroxy acid:** I absolutely do not recommend products that claim an association with AHAs or BHA but contain ingredients such as fruit extracts or sugarcane extracts, which sound like they can work like AHAs or BHA, but cannot. There are a host of legitimate AHA ingredients, the two most popular and most well researched being glycolic acid and lactic acid. While glycolic acid is indeed derived from sugarcane, assuming that sugarcane will net you the same result as glycolic acid would be like assuming you could write on a tree the way you can on paper. Paper is derived from wood but that doesn't mean you can write on the original wood. The same analogy holds true for lactic acid, which is derived from milk. If milk were as acid as lactic acid, you would not be able to drink it without serious complications. There is a vast difference between the isolated ingredient and the original form.

The only acceptable BHA ingredient is salicylic acid. Salicylic acid is derived from willow bark; many products use willow bark and claim they contain an effective form of BHA. Willow bark extract contains salicin, a substance that when taken orally is converted by the digestive process to salicylic acid. The process of converting willow bark to salicylic acid requires the presence of enzymes to take the salicin and turn it into salicylic acid. And the digestive conversion process that turns salicin into saligenin, and then into salicylic acid, is complicated. Further, salicin, much like salicylic acid, is stable only under acidic conditions. The likelihood that willow bark in the tiny amount used in these products can mimic the effectiveness of salicylic acid is at best problematic, and in all likelihood probably impossible. However, willow bark may indeed have some anti-inflammatory benefits for skin because in this form it appears to retain more of its aspirin-like composition. That is nice for skin but it's definitely not better than other anti-inflammatories used in cosmetics, and it doesn't deliver the same exfoliating benefit as BHA.

Aside from glycolic acid and lactic acid, the following are considered acceptable forms of AHA on an ingredient label: malic acid, ammonium glycolate, alphahydroxyethanoic acid, ammonium alphahydroxyethanoate, alphahydroxyoctanoic acid, alphahydroxycaprylic acid, 2-hydroxydodecanoic acid, and hydroxycaprylic acid.

**Just a reminder:** Anytime you use a well-formulated AHA product that contains more than 5% AHAs, some stinging can occur; also, you should not let the product come in contact with the eyes or any mucous membranes. You may have an irritation or sensitivity to AHAs. Slight stinging is expected, but continued stinging is not. Discontinue use if this should happen.

## Before You Read the Reviews: The Ratings

The following are the rating symbols for the products reviewed in this book. These simple but succinct (and cute) symbols depict my approval or disapproval of a specific product.

For those who are more familiar with my reviews and ratings from past editions of my books and newsletters, this edition has incorporated a major shift in what constitutes an expensive and reasonably priced product and what constitutes a product that is well-formulated and state of the art.

☺ This smiling face indicates a great product that I recommend highly and that is also low in price. This smiling face means the product is definitely worth checking into and potentially worth buying.

☻ This neutral face indicates an OK but unimpressive product, or an OK product that can cause problems for certain skin types. I often use this face to portray a dated or old-fashioned product formulation. That doesn't mean it's a bad or poorly formulated product, but one that just isn't very interesting or is lacking some of the newer water-binding ingredients, antioxidants, anti-irritants, emollients, or nonirritating ingredients for dry skin. I also use the neutral face to reflect a makeup product that isn't really bad, but that is completely unnecessary, or unnecessarily overpriced for such an ordinary product that could easily be replaced with a far less-expensive version from the drugstore. Depending on your personal preferences, products rated with this face may be worth checking out but they're nothing to get excited about.

☹ For many reasons, this frowning face reflects a product that is truly bad for skin or appearance from almost every standpoint, including price, performance, application, texture, potential for irritation, skin reactions, and breakouts.

☺ $$$ This symbol designates a great product that I would recommend without a doubt were it not so absurdly overpriced, either in comparison to similar products or in relation to what you are getting for the money.

☻ $$$ This symbol indicates an ordinary, boring product whose excessive price makes it ludicrous to consider. For skin care it usually lacks interesting or a significant amount of water-binding agents, anti-irritants, emollients, antioxidants, effective exfoliants, or gentle cleansing agents. For makeup it reflects a performance that pales in comparison to other far better formulations but still can look OK when applied.

**Prices:** Because the cost of drugstore cosmetics often fluctuates from store to store, and because cosmetics companies often change prices every six months, the prices listed in this book may not be up-to-date or match what you find when you are shopping. Use the prices as a basis for comparison, but realize that they may not precisely reflect what you will find when you go shopping.

**Up-to-date information:** My staff and I struggle to make sure all the information we have is accurate and current. **However, cosmetics companies frequently and without notice change or reformulate their products, sometimes in a minor way and sometimes extensively.** To keep abreast of these changes that cannot be kept current in a book, I report all revisions and new product launches that occurred after this book went to press in my newsletter, *Cosmetics Counter Update*.

**Foreign names:** For the most part, I give only the English names of foreign-produced products. The French and Italian names are pretty, but they don't tell you anything about the product if you don't speak the language.

**No endorsements:** Neither the information nor the evaluations included in any of my work are to be misconstrued as endorsements, nor do they represent a particular company's sponsorship. None of the cosmetics companies paid me for my remarks or critiques. This includes the listing of my own products. While I clearly like my products, they are only options—just like any of the other products I've reviewed for this book—and I do not recommend them above any others. All "Best Choices" are just that, choices, with the final decision up to you.

**Order of presentation:** The cosmetics are listed alphabetically by brand names, so the order in which they appear does not represent my preference. There is no implied winner among any of the cosmetics companies included, and no one line has all the answers or the majority of great products. Almost every line has its strong and weak points.

**Don't go shopping without me:** I encourage you to take this book with you on shopping trips to the cosmetics counters or the drugstore. Then you will have all the information you'll need readily at hand. There is no way you can remember the details of each product, color, and brand. Do try to be discreet at the department-store cosmetics counters—and don't be surprised if you find that using the book in clear view of the salespeople makes them defensive or irritated. There are always risks when a consumer comes prepared with information that disagrees with the salesperson. I urge you to persevere. Nothing will change at the cosmetics counters if you don't change first.

# *The Reviews A–Z*

I decided early on in organizing this book that the best way to arrange the list of companies was alphabetically (except for baby and men's products, which are included in a separate chapter). There were many reasons for this, but primarily it was because women instinctively turn first to the products they are using to see if I agree with their impressions, and following the alphabet is the easiest way to make your way through a list. The second major reason is that an alphabetical sequence implies no hierarchy of preference, which is how I truly feel.

Please be aware that you may not and need not agree with all my reviews to obtain benefit from this book. As you read my comments, you may very well find yourself disagreeing with me. That is perfectly understandable and as it should be, because the criteria you use to evaluate cosmetics may differ from mine. Or, for any one of a dozen reasons (personal preference, different expectations, actual usage—once a week versus twice a day), a product I dislike may work well for you, or just the opposite can be true: you may hate a product I rate highly. What I cannot account for is how millions of women will feel about a particular product.

You may also notice that in this edition the reviews of products have changed from previous editions. There are several reasons why this happens: I have acquired new research that supports a different evaluation; the company changed the product since I last tested it; I've changed my criteria, based on new information or research, to include a perspective different from what I did when I last updated this book—this is particularly true for moisturizers and the use of plant extracts; or I was wrong the first time I checked out the product and have corrected that error. The other typical reason for differences in reviews is the actual age of the product. Because cosmetics don't have to be stamped with the date of manufacture, there is no way to know how long they have been sitting on a shelf. I may have previously tested an older or newer product (or one different from the one a consumer buys), and that can greatly affect the performance. This is particularly true for mascaras and foundations. When mascara sits on a shelf for a long period of time, it can dry up and perform poorly, and an old foundation that has been on the shelf way past its manufacture date can have a color change.

One of the dilemmas of doing a consumer product guide about the cosmetics industry (aside from the sheer plethora of products) is that products and product lines change. Every month new items are added to and deleted from almost every line out there. That means if I finished researching a line in, say, January, by August, when I finish this manuscript, newly launched products or product changes occurring after those dates won't be in this edition. That is why I do my newsletter—the cosmetics industry is ever changing, and for those of you who want to keep abreast of all those changes, my newsletter, *Cosmetics Counter Update*, is an option you may want to consider. To view a copy please visit my Web site at www.cosmeticscop.com or call (800) 831-4088.

What I present in the following pages are merely guidelines, based on my extensive research and experience about what works and what doesn't. If you decide to follow any of my suggestions, be aware that my recommendations are not a guarantee, but a suggestion as to how to narrow down the endless options the cosmetics industry sells. It is my earnest desire to help you chose from this very crowded field so you can make the best choices possible. The final choice is up to you.

# 5S

5S is Shiseido's trademark and this line is their stab at joining the niche arena of the boutique cosmetics shop. Along the lines of Aveda or The Body Shop, 5S is a stand-alone store with a bevy of products. 5S stands for the five senses of well-being: energizing, purifying, calming, adoring, and nurturing. Somehow the products have an effect on each of these. We are talking makeup and skin care, right?

When it comes to skin care, this is some of the most innovative marketing smoke and mirrors I've ever seen. For example the cleanser formulations (and there are ten of them) are virtually identical, with the only differences between them being fragrance or the addition of peppermint or menthol! The categories of energizing and purifying sound alluring and different, but here too the products end up being almost mirror images of each other, with only changes of fragrance or different color additives—and descriptions that sound like poetry—yet the products end up being anything but poetry. Overall, the skin-care line is strikingly disappointing, with not one, and I mean not *one* redeeming factor (and that comment even ignores the fact that this line doesn't include a sunscreen of any kind).

The real twist for 5S is that almost all of the makeup products are multipurpose and can be used anywhere. So if you think the red liner would look great on your eyes, the concept is that the formulation is as safe for that area as it is for the mouth. If you want to use the powder colors on your lips or all over your face, go for it. For some color choices that is a clever alternative, but for the most part pencils don't work on eyes or cheeks.

The line also has its quota of herbal extracts that are played up and celebrated as a motivation for the consumer, but the minimal amounts of plants in here are hardly worth mentioning. These otherwise very basic formulas have textures that are both exemplary (the powder colors) and uninspired (the stick and the blush shades). The large array of makeup colors is organized into, you guessed it, five groups, from the 100s, which are the light pastel tones, to the 200s, which are called subtle; the 300s, which are neutral (this group has the fewest options); the 400s, which are deep shades; and the 500s, which are the more bold, vivid shades.

The tester unit at the counter is well structured and the salespeople encourage you to play to your heart's content. There's even a row of chairs and mirrors set up at their "mingle table," which is very inviting. For now, there is not a lot to recommend unless you prefer shiny eyeshadows, blushes, and do-nothing mascaras for brow or hair only. Perhaps with time the color selection will branch out to provide some suitable matte shades and less greasy textures. Until then, it may be best to admire 5S from afar and hope that other lines adopt their open-play policy. For more information about 5S, call (800)-PHONE5S or visit their Web site at www.five-s.com.

# 5S Skin Care

☹ **Adoring: Charm Foam Cleanser** *($11 for 3.3 ounces)* is a standard, detergent-based water-soluble cleanser that can be drying for most skin types. This would only be appropriate for someone with oily skin.

☹ **Adoring: Mattifying Foam Cleanser with Cleansing and Scrubbing Granules** *($11 for 3.3 ounces)* is almost identical to the one above, only this one includes synthetic scrub particles of polyethylene. It also contains menthol, which can be too irritating for most skin types.

☹ **Calming: Cool Foam Cleanser** *($11 for 3.3 ounces)* is virtually identical to the Adoring Charm Foam Cleanser only this version contains menthol and that makes it a problem for most skin types. This product also contains *Scutellaria baicalensis* extract, from a plant used in China to treat burns. While this may be helpful in its pure form, in the teeny amount used in this cleanser it is just useless.

☹ **Calming: Quiet Foam Cleanser** *($11 for 3.3 ounces)* is virtually identical to the Adoring Charm Foam Cleanser and the same comments apply.

☹ **Energizing: Empowering Foam Cleanser** *($11 for 3.3 ounces)* is virtually identical to the Calming Cool Foam Cleanser above only this one adds peppermint to the mix, which only makes matters worse.

☹ **Energizing: Toning Foam Cleanser** *($11 for 3.3 ounces)* is virtually identical to the Calming Cool Foam Cleanser above and the same comments apply.

☹ **Nurturing: Rebirth Foam Cleanser** *($11 for 3.3 ounces)* is virtually identical to the Adoring Charm Foam Cleanser and the same comments apply.

☹ **Nurturing: Rehydrate Foam Cleanser** *($11 for 3.3 ounces)* uses sodium lauryl sulfate as the second ingredient and that is an irritation waiting to happen.

☹ **Purifying: Equalizing Foam Cleanser** *($11 for 3.3 ounces)* is virtually identical to the Rehydrate version above and the same comments apply.

☹ **Purifying: Refreshing Foam Cleanser** *($11 for 3.3 ounces)* is virtually identical to the Adoring Charm Foam Cleanser only this version contains menthol, and that makes it even more of a problem for most skin types.

☺ **Makeup Eraser** *($9 for 2 ounces)* is great for removing makeup but it can feel slippery and slightly greasy on the skin.

☹ **Adoring: Charm Basic Solution** *($17 for 6 ounces)* has alcohol as the second ingredient, and is not recommended for any skin type.

☹ **Adoring: Mattifying Basic Solution** *($17 for 6 ounces)* is virtually identical to the Charm Basic version above and the same comments apply.

☹ **Calming: Cool Basic Solution** *($17 for 6 ounces)* is virtually identical to the Charm Basic version above only this one adds camphor and menthol, which make this anything but calming.

☹ **Calming: Quiet Basic Solution** *($17 for 6 ounces)* uses alcohol as the third ingredient, which is still too drying and irritating for most all skin types.

☹ **Energizing: Empowering Basic Solution** *($17 for 6 ounces)* contains alcohol as the second ingredient, and further down the list are camphor, eucalyptus, peppermint, and menthol—Ouch!

☹ **Energizing: Toning Basic Solution** *($17 for 6 ounces)* contains alcohol as the second ingredient with menthol further down the list. That isn't energizing, it's irritating.

☺ **Nurturing: Rebirth Basic Solution** *($17 for 6 ounces)*. Finally, a 5S toner-like product that isn't irritating, though for the money it's a real burn. There are far more interesting toners to consider than this one.

☺ **Nurturing: Rehydrate Basic Solution** *($17 for 6 ounces)* is similar to the one above and the same comments apply.

☺ **Purifying: Equalizing Basic Solution** *($17 for 6 ounces)* is similar to the one above and the same comments apply.

☹ **Purifying: Refreshing Basic Solution** *($17 for 6 ounces)* has alcohol as the second ingredient and that is too drying and irritating for all skin types.

☺ **$$$ Wrinkle Cream** *($25 for 1 ounce)* pretty much misses the boat in the world of wrinkle creams. There aren't even any trendy ingredients in this one to help it attempt to be something it's not. This product does contain a minuscule amount of *Rubus suavissimus* (Chinese blackberry), which has no research establishing it for any use. But just so you know, in Chinese herbal lore this blackberry is believed to be "yin" and associated with female functions.

☹ **Eye Gel** *($15 for 0.5 ounce)*. If you're looking for irritation and dry skin, this is an option.

☹ **Aloe Hydrating Essence** *($25 for 0.8 ounce)* has alcohol as the third ingredient, and the amount of aloe present is less than 0.1%. This is a shockingly bad product with a completely misleading name.

☺ **$$$ Blemish Treatment** *($13 for 0.5 ounce)* is a clay-based, masklike product that uses sulfur as the active ingredient. While sulfur is a good disinfectant it is also extremely irritating and drying and not the best option for daily use. This product does contain *Phellodendron amurense* (corktree) extract, used in China as a disinfectant and for wound healing. Even if that research was valid, the amount used in this product is negligible.

☹ **Lightening Essence** *($25 for 0.8 ounce)* has alcohol as the second ingredient, which can be drying and irritating for all skin types. There is some vitamin C but there is scant evidence that this can lighten skin. Even if it could, there are far less-expensive vitamin C products out there to consider. The quantity of geranium extract in here is so minute that even if it could affect the color of skin (it can't) there's not enough to change one skin cell.

☹ **Oil Controller** *($13 for 1 ounce)* lists alcohol as the second ingredient. That can be drying and irritating for all skin types and it won't control oil in the least. This product also contains cornstarch, which can potentially clog pores.

☹ **Pore Peel** *($13 for 1.7 ounces)* is a polyvinyl mask that goes on in a sticky mess. When it dries, it's supposed to be rubbed off, and comes off in rolled-up balls. That can take off a layer of skin, but there are better and more gentle ways to do that than by peeling a layer of vinyl off the face. The third ingredient is alcohol, and that's harsh for the face.

☺ **$$$ Skin Smoother** *($13 for 1.7 ounces)* does feel soft on the skin but it is so boring and basic it is truly shocking.

☹ **Spray Refresher** *($10 for 3.8 ounces)*. There is nothing in here refreshing other than the water. This do-nothing product is just shocking.

# 5S Makeup

☺ <u>FOUNDATION:</u> **Base Color SPF 12** *($15)* is a very sheer, gel-like foundation with titanium dioxide as the active sunscreen agent, and a somewhat disappointing SPF. This is meant to be used as a foundation, concealer, or highlighter, but works best as a lightweight foundation. There are some color-correcting shades to avoid (#171, #172, and #376), but most of the remaining 11 shades are neutral and have a soft matte finish. The shades numbered 373, 374, 377, and 380 are too peach for most skin tones. Also, #571 is iridescent and best avoided unless a shiny face is what you're after.

☺ <u>POWDER:</u> **Powder Color** *($11)* comes in 36 different colors and is meant for use on eyes, cheeks, or all over the face. There are almost no colors appropriate for powder, since all of these have a slight to high shine (some have more of a sheen, which is subtler, but can still look obvious in daylight and negates the purpose of using powder to remove shine). The texture is velvety-smooth and the colors go on sheer, making it almost a travesty to not include any true matte options. For nighttime, these are options for eyeshadow but make sure you try them on first to see how the shine agrees with you.

<u>BLUSH:</u> ☹ **Tube Color** *($12)* is creamy, slick, and very shiny. It can be used everywhere, including the lips, but I wouldn't recommend using these 14 colors anywhere, unless messy, short-lived makeup is your goal.

☺ **Stick Color** *($12)* is packaged in a thin lipstick tube and comes in a rainbow of 45 different colors. Within these colors, there are four finishes to choose from: **Creamy** (these are more greasy than creamy), **Pearl** (greasy with iridescence), **Sheer** (less pigment, still greasy), and **Matte** (more creamy than matte, but with by far the longest lasting, most attractive texture and finish). There are some concealer colors in the line's 300 range, but they are too greasy and the colors are poor. If you decide to try these, for the best results stick with those that are designated as mattes.

☺ <u>EYE, BROW, AND LIP SHAPER:</u> **Pencil Color** *($10)* are standard pencils that require sharpening. There are 30 colors available, and most of them are the wide (or chubby-style) pencils. The rest are regular narrow pencils, and neither type will last, as the company claims, "as long as you do," unless you typically fade away early in the day. Numbers 257, 253, 456, 458, 554, and 557 are designated for eyes and cheeks only, and have a drier, powdery texture. The rest are much creamier and glide well but are hardly a first choice when it comes to all-in-one makeup if longevity is important to you.

☹ <u>MASCARA:</u> **Brush Color** *($10)* is 5S's all-purpose mascara, but it doesn't end up working out that way. First it fails as mascara, building no length or thickness. Then, as a brow tint, it goes on too thick and heavy, and the same is true for your hair, making a thick, sticky mess. The ten shades are an interesting selection but the performance is abysmal. Number 493 is billed as being waterproof, and it is, but it still has the same problems with length and thickness.

☹ <u>BRUSHES:</u> The **Brushes** *($3 to $15)* at 5S are synthetic, which is great for animals but not that great for you when it comes to reliability for applying your makeup. The collection is a poor assortment of travel-sized brushes that are modestly priced, but not worth any attention when compared to the fine brush collections of many other department-store lines. For really great synthetic brushes consider Origins, Paula Dorf (some synthetic brushes), or Shu Uemura.

# Acne-Statin (Skin Care Only)

This line has been around for years and is still being sold. Does that indicate a modicum of success? Yes, at least financially for the company, but does that mean it's good for you? I doubt it. How does Acne-Statin claim to deal with acne? Well, not very directly, that's for sure, because Acne-Statin doesn't list ingredients on its label. Thanks to a grandfather clause in the FDA's mandatory rules for listing ingredients, Acne-Statin doesn't have to list any of its nonactive ingredients. Nevertheless, it does have to list the active ingredients. The other 99.5% is composed of standard cosmetic ingredients that hold no hope for acne sufferers, and the thick consistency makes me suspect it contains ingredients that are probably not the best for someone with breakouts or oily skin.

It turns out the Federal Trade Commission (FTC) seems to agree with my conclusions. According to a press release from the FTC on July 31, 1998, "Acne-Statin ... has agreed to pay a $200,000 civil penalty to settle Federal Trade Commission charges that ads touting the product as an effective treatment for severe or cystic acne were deceptive. The claims also violate a 1979 order prohibiting Dr. Atida H. Karr from making unsubstantiated claims about the effectiveness or superiority of any acne preparation she markets, the agency alleges. Karr and her Beverly Hills, California, based companies sold Acne-Statin and currently sell the Acne-Statin Kit.

"The 1979 order prohibits Karr and her firms from advertising the effectiveness or superiority of any acne preparation unless the claims are supported by competent and reliable scientific or medical evidence. Karr paid $175,000 into a consumer refund account as part of the 1979 settlement of the initial case."

Acne-Statin's claims sound sweeping and impressive. But as consumers, we are given only advertising and hype to help us make a decision. The ingredient list, the only verifiable truth on any cosmetics label, is kept a secret. If the Acne-Statin products could cure acne, as the ads and infomercial claim, who would have acne? Bottom line: The active ingredients listed can't do what the product claims they can do, and moreover, despite the age of these formulations (they've been around for more than a decade), they haven't been updated either.

☹ **Skin Cleanser and Moisturizer** *($39.95 for 4 ounces)* contains 0.5% triclosan, a standard disinfectant found in many antibacterial products.

☹ **Cream** *($39.95 for 4 ounces)* contains 0.5% salicylic acid (which is almost useless an amount for exfoliation) but otherwise is the same as the Skin Cleanser and Moisturizer, and the same comments apply.

# Adrien Arpel/Signature Club A (Skin Care Only)

Not much has changed for Arpel since I last reviewed this line. It is still true that Adrien Arpel sold both her department-store line and the right to use her name in any publicity or marketing ventures. So, when Arpel started selling a new line of cosmetics on the Home Shopping Network, she legally could not use her own name for endorsement purposes, hence her infomercial line is called "Signature Club A." It is interesting to note that whenever Arpel is on HSN, she is never introduced as "Adrien Arpel." She is always introduced as just "Adrien." Due to this legal technicality "Adrien Arpel" has nothing to do with the line bearing her name. These days, the original Arpel line is sold primarily via mail order. Arpel's Signature Club A is available via mail order through the Home Shopping Network (HSN).

Like most infomercial lines, Arpel promises her Signature Club A products will cure your skin-care woes, especially by erasing wrinkles. Arpel sells her products as miracles that deliver newly smooth, flawless skin with instant success. But there are no miracles to be found in this line, and I have yet to hear Arpel discuss sunscreens. To find so many instant-lift products with no sunscreens is about as funny as finding cars without brakes. Maybe even funnier is the vacuum machine with a rotation device and pumice head for massage, and a suction device for who knows what. Either way, the trauma this machine delivers to the skin is problematic. Over-manipulating and scrubbing the face isn't anything I would ever recommend, and that's what this vacuum machine does. The pumice stone might as well be sandpaper; the skin just doesn't need that kind of abrasion. The risk of surfaced capillaries not to mention irritation is unwarranted.

Arpel also promotes the effectiveness of her Big "7" Wondercover Compact as being the only skin perfecting makeup you need. This group of seven concealers in colors that range from blue to mauve, peach, shiny, beige, medium beige, and dark tan is a greasy mess that may be OK for very dry skin, but that will easily crease if you place it around the eyes or other lined areas of the face. Mauve, peach, and blue only give the skin a strange cast; to cover face problems, all it takes is one concealer and one good foundation that doesn't crease.

For more information about Signature Club A call (800) 247-2868 or visit HSN's Web site at www.hsn.com.

For more information about Adrien Arpel's original line, now owned by Color Me Beautiful, call (800) 627-9126 or visit the Web site at www.adrienarpel.com.

## *Signature Club A by Adrien Arpel*

☺ $$$ **French Vanilla Meltdown, Cleansing Creme for Face & Eyes** *($18 for 4 ounces)* is just a wipe-off, cold cream–type cleanser with a tiny amount of vitamin A thrown in for effect. Even if the vitamin could help, you would be wiping it away before it had a chance to work. This can be an option for someone with dry skin, but it is easily replaced with far less expensive options. It does contain fragrance.

☺ **AHA Daily Face Wash** *($15.50 for 6 ounces)* is a standard, detergent-based water-soluble cleanser that can be somewhat drying depending on your skin type. It has an assortment of AHAs and some vitamins thrown in, but the pH is wrong for it to be an effective AHA, and even if any of the ingredients were effective they would be rinsed off before they had a chance to have any effect. It does contain fragrance.

☹ **AHA Toner** *($15.50 for 6 ounces)*. Between the salt and the mints that this product contains, the irritation for the face would be significant. Salt should never be left on the skin.

☹ **Soft Resurfacing Peel** *($14.50 for 2 ounces)* contains mostly very thick, heavy waxes. Rubbing wax over the skin can take off skin cells, but it can also clog pores and cause breakouts. There are much better ways to exfoliate the skin than with this product.

☺ **Alpha Hydroxy and Retinol Soft Scrub with Vanilla Bean** *($14.50 for 2 ounces)*. Not another AHA product? But don't worry, the pH isn't right for the AHAs to be effective. This is a standard, water-soluble cleanser, and the scrub particles in it come from ground-up vanilla beans. This is an option for a topical scrub for someone with normal to dry skin. It does contain fragrance.

☹ **Instant Lift & Hold for Face and Neck** *($21.95 for eight vials)* contains plenty of alcohol, so the resulting slight swelling (due to irritation) should make your skin look smoother. Other than that, this is just plant extracts and water-binding agents; it won't lift or hold any part of your skin anywhere.

☹ **Instant Lift & Hold for Eyes** *($24.95 for eight 0.8-ounce vials and a compact with a concealer)* comes with two shades of concealer in the compact, both very un-skin-like shades of peach and orange, not to mention that the consistency is exceptionally greasy and will crease easily into lines. The vials of liquid contain mostly alcohol, which can't hold anything, though it can be drying and irritating. They also contain some fairly irritating plant extracts, including balm mint and mistletoe.

☺ **Peaches & Cream Facial Cleanser** *($32.50 in a set that includes 8-ounce cleanser, 8-ounce toner, and 9-ounce body cream )* is a standard, detergent-based water-soluble cleanser that also contains some emollients. That makes it a good option for someone with normal to dry skin. It does contain fragrance and coloring agents.

☺ **Peaches & Cream Toner** *($32.50 in a set that includes 8-ounce cleanser, 8-ounce toner, and 9-ounce body cream).* The minuscule amount of vitamins in here don't have much of an impact on skin, and the vitamin K can't live up to the claims about affecting surfaced capillaries. It is a good, fairly nonirritating toner that would work well for most skin types, if the fragrance doesn't knock you over first.

☹ **Peaches & Cream Body Cream** *($32.50 in a set that includes 8-ounce cleanser, 8-ounce toner, and 9-ounce body cream)* has a fragrance that will knock you over, and while it is best not to put fragrance on any part of the skin, it is definitely only an option for the neck down.

☹ **The 5 Essentials Creme** *($24.95 for 4.5 ounces)* is a two-part container, with one on top of the other. There is nothing essential about any of this. Without sunscreen, it leaves much to be desired for daytime. The Face Cream is just a good moisturizer for dry skin; it falls down on many aspects of the claims made about it. It's supposed to be an AHA product but both the amount of AHA and the pH make it ineffective for exfoliation. It contains a small amount of retinol, but the packaging guarantees it will decompose, as it is not airtight and retinol is highly unstable. The vitamin C in here is ascorbic acid, also considered to be unstable and a skin irritant. It does have some good water-binding agents and emollients, but that's about it. The Eye Cream is almost identical, only for some impractical reason it contains several irritating plant extracts, including lemon, sage, lavender, and orange.

☹ **$$$ CR2 Wrinkle Softening Stick with Vitamin C and Retinol** *($18 for 0.24 ounce).* This lipstick-like moisturizer is greasy stuff and somewhat sticky, but it would work for dry skin. The pH and amount of AHA aren't right for it to be effective as an exfoliant, the vitamin C is ascorbic acid, which is unstable and potentially irritating, and the packaging makes the retinol decompose because it isn't airtight.

☹ **C3 High Potency Moisturizing Triple-Cream Mask with Vitamin C Plus Ginkgo & Ginseng** *($22.50 for 4.5 ounces).* The amount of laughter this product caused in my office is almost a first. The mask is this plastic contraption filled with water and orange glitter (the glitter got all over the face despite the apparent seal). You're supposed to place this in the microwave, which definitely makes it warm, and then place it on your face over the accompanying moisturizer. And women are buying this stuff?!!! A warm mask doesn't help skin, though if you have surfaced capillaries it can make them look worse. Other than that, this is just an exceptionally standard moisturizer with some water-binding agents—a negligible amount, as they come well after the preservatives. This product is a joke, but the joke is on the consumer who buys this.

☹ **Glow from Within Moisturizer SPF 15** *($22.50 for 2 ounces)* doesn't contain the UVA-protecting ingredients of titanium dioxide, zinc oxide, or avobenzone, and is not recommended.

☹ **High Potent-C Anti-Wrinkle Age Defying Capsules** *($26.50 for 0.5 ounce)* does contain vitamin C but it uses ascorbic acid, which is not the most effective form it is considered to be irritating. (The preferred form is magnesium ascorbyl palmitate.) It also contains some irritating ingredients that don't belong in a moisturizing-type product, including aluminum starch (octenylsuccinate) and ginseng extract.

☺ **$$$ Morning Eye Gel & Night Eye Creme** *($24 for 0.75 ounce of Eye Gel and 0.75 ounce of Eye Creme).* The eye gel is a good lightweight moisturizer, but there is nothing in here that will live up to the anti-sagging claims. Without sunscreen, this product is a serious problem for daytime. The Night Eye Creme is a good emollient moisturizer for dry skin but that's about it. Both products contain minuscule amounts of caviar, and while some fish eggs may be great to eat, none have any benefit on skin.

☺ **Morning Pearl Creme with Caviar Extract & Microsphere Night Creme with Caviar Extract, Anti-Sag Extra Firming Cremes** *($28.50 for 4 total ounces)* contain nothing that can affect any aspect of the skin's sagging. These are just moisturizers and there isn't even one fish egg's worth of caviar in here; even if there were more, caviar has no effect on skin. The Morning Pearl Creme is a problem to rely on for daytime since there are no sunscreen agents in here. The Microsphere Night Creme is similar to the Morning version, and the same comments apply, though the night version contains teeny amounts of antioxidants.

☺ **Vitamin C Complex, Illumination Source** *($24.50 for 6 ounces)* is OK, but don't expect much from the vitamins in this one. The vitamin C used here is ascorbic acid, which is not one of the forms recommended in the research I've seen. Other than that, it shouldn't be a problem, but it also won't be of much use.

**Flower Acid Wrinkle Remedy Help Line** *($49.95 for five-piece kit)* includes the following:

☺ **Flower Acid Wrinkle Remedy Day Eye Creme** *(1 ounce)* is a good moisturizer for dry skin but there is no "flower acid" of any kind in here.

☺ **Flower Acid Wrinkle Remedy Day Face Creme with Sunscreen SPF 20** *(2 ounces)* is a good in-part avobenzone-based sunscreen in a very standard moisturizing base.

☺ **Flower Acid Wrinkle Remedy Neck, Throat, and Breast Creme** *(2 ounces)* has sodium polystyrene sulfate as the third ingredient, a film former that is not the best for skin. Other than that, this is similar to the moisturizing base in the sunscreen above, OK but very basic.

☺ **Flower Acid Wrinkle Remedy Night Eye Ointment** *(1 ounce)*. The name is far more exotic than this very standard moisturizer for very dry skin could ever live up to.

☺ **Flower Acid Wrinkle Remedy Night Face Creme** *(2 ounces)* is similar to the Flower Acid Day Eye Cream above and the same basic comments apply.

☹ **The Big "7" Wondercover Wheel** *($20)* is a group of seven concealers in colors that range from blue to mauve, peach, shiny, beige, medium beige, and dark tan. This is a greasy mess that may be OK for very dry skin. Even so, if you place it around the eyes or other lined areas of the face it will easily crease and it tends to feel opaque and slippery on the skin. Mauve, peach, and blue only give the skin a strange cast; to cover face problems, all it takes is one concealer and one good foundation that doesn't crease.

☹ **Hide-A-Line Putty** *($19.50)* won't hide anything because no one's skin color looks like this shade of peach, and the greasy consistency will make it crease into lines and make them look more noticeable.

# Adrien Arpel

☺ **$$$ Oily Skin Sea Foam Gel Cleanser** *($19 for 4 ounces)* is a standard, detergent-based water-soluble cleanser that would work well for someone with normal to oily skin. It does contain fragrance and coloring agents.

☺ **$$$ Aromafleur Petal Daily Cleanser** *($22.50 for 4.5 ounces)* is a detergent-based water-soluble cleanser that would work well for someone with normal to oily skin. It has its share of plant extracts, which are at the end of the ingredient list, but even if they could benefit the skin (they can't) it wouldn't matter, since they all get washed down the drain. It does contain fragrance and coloring agents.

☹ **Foam Cleanser** *($20 for 8 ounces)* is a plant oil–based cleanser that doesn't quite take off all the makeup and can leave a greasy film on the face. It has its share of interesting plant extracts and water-binding agents, but any benefit from these is washed away. It also contains peppermint, which can cause significant skin irritation.

☹ **Freeze-Dried Collagen Protein Cleanser, Super Dry Skin Formula** *($20 for 4 ounces)* has changed its name; it was "Embryonic Collagen," though the ingredient listing has remained identical. I imagine the notion of associating an embryo with younger skin is no longer something a consumer can swallow. Regardless, this is merely a detergent-based water-soluble cleanser that uses sodium lauryl sulfate, known for causing irritation. There are also several thickening agents that are difficult to rinse off without a washcloth. The showcase ingredient is calfskin, and although it may be a good water-binding agent, any benefit is washed down the drain.

☺ **$$$ Sea Kelp Cleanser** *($20 for 4 ounces)* is a fairly greasy scrub that uses a rather formidable abrasive. Despite the name, there's only a small amount of sea kelp, and the mineral oil and petrolatum can leave a greasy residue on the skin. It does contain fragrance and coloring agents.

☺ $$$ **Coconut Cleanser** *($20 for 4 ounces)* is a cold cream that contains mostly water, plant oils, and some lanolin. This is a wipe-off cleanser that can leave a greasy film on the skin, but for very dry skin it can be an option. It does contain fragrance.

☹ **Honey and Almond Scrub** *($32 for 5 ounces)* has ground almonds that will help slough skin; however, any gentle cleanser mixed with baking soda and a little water will do the same thing for a lot less. The lemon in this product can be a significant skin irritant. For this amount of money you could just buy several pounds of crushed almonds and use that without the other irritating extras.

☹ **Lemon & Lime Freshener** *($18.50 for 8 ounces)* is a freshener that is alcohol-free and instead delivers several other potential skin irritants, including balm mint, lemon peel, and lime extract. Ouch!

☹ **Flower Extract Freshener** *($18.50 for 8 ounces)* is nothing more than witch hazel and plant extracts, several of which, such as lemon flower, lemongrass, and geranium flower, can be skin irritants.

☺ $$$ **Bio-Cellular Night Cream with AHA** *($35 for 1.25 ounces)* contains about 2% AHAs and an entire arsenal of water-binding agents. It is a far better moisturizer for dry skin than it is an AHA exfoliant. The scientific name won't impress your skin cells and the price is unwarranted for what you get.

☺ $$$ **Bio-Cellular Anti-Aging Serum with Alpha Hydroxy Complex** *($52.50 for ten 0.23-ounce vials)* is essentially some thickener agents, AHAs, and water-binding agents. Much like the Night Cream above, this serum doesn't have the right pH to make it an effective exfoliant, though it can be a good lightweight moisturizer for someone with dry skin.

☺ $$$ **Bio-Cellular Night Eye Gelee with AHA Complex** *($26 for 0.4 ounce)* makes me ask, How many AHA products does one face need? Thankfully, none of these are effective exfoliants, so don't worry. Basically this product is the "greasy kid stuff." If you have extremely dry skin, this product would be just fine.

☹ **Eyelastic Lift** *($40 for 30 capsules and 0.5 ounce of the creme)* is a two-part product: you're supposed to mix the **Extra Strength Puff Deflator Capsules** with the **Eyelastic Lift and Firm Creme**. It won't lift the eye anywhere. The Puff Deflator (do you believe that name?) contains mostly silicone, water-binding agents, placental extract (doesn't say whose, but whatever kind of placenta it is, give me a break), and preservatives. The rather common ingredients make for a good moisturizer, but that's about it. Placenta extract can't make your skin one hour younger, no matter where it comes from. The Lift and Firm Creme contains mostly water, water-binding agent, silicone, mineral oil, oat flour, plant extract, and more thickeners. It works as a paste and contains some moisturizing ingredients. All this is a complete waste of time and money.

☺ $$$ **Skinlastic Lift Daily Transparent Tightening & Firming Lift** *($40 for 1.7 ounces in 18 individual vials)* is a good lightweight moisturizer for normal to slightly dry skin, but that's about it. Most of the plant extracts in here can function as anti-irritants but it also contains arnica, which can be a skin irritant.

☺ **Skin Correction Complex Four Cremes in One with Alpha Hydroxy Complex** *($34.50 for 2 ounces)* calls itself "the only creme you will ever need." It isn't. What about a sunscreen? It also contains *minimal* AHAs. This is an overpriced but good moisturizer for someone with dry skin.

☺ $$$ **Clear & Even Skintone Complex** *($45.95 for 1.7 ounces)* is an exceptionally overpriced moisturizer with AHAs. Though it contains about 6% AHAs, the pH of 5 makes this only minimally effective as an exfoliant, and there are no other skin-lightening (meaning melanin-inhibiting) ingredients in this product to make it effective for that purpose. It's a very good moisturizer for dry skin but that's about it.

☹ $$$ **Swiss Formula Day Cream #12 with Collagen** *($50 for 1 ounce)* is a very ordinary but good emollient, rich moisturizer for someone with very dry skin. It claims to be nongreasy, but that doesn't jibe with the inclusion of mineral oil, lanolin, and a form of tallow, all fairly greasy ingredients. It also contains teeny amounts of brewer's yeast and placenta, but that has no effect on wrinkles.

☹ $$$ **Swiss Formula #12 Day Eye Creme, with Vitamin A Palmitate and Collagen** *($27.50 for 0.5 ounce)* is similar to the cream above, only with a tiny amount of vitamin A added, and the same review applies. Vitamin A is many generations removed from retinol, which is a few generations away from Renova, and it does not have the same effect on skin.

☹ **Adult Oily Skin Detoxifying Spray** *($18.50 for 8 ounces)* is a toner that won't detox anything, but it is OK for normal to dry skin and slightly oily skin.

☺ $$$ **Aromafleur Flower Petal and Botanical Extract Masque** *($24 for 4 ounces)* does contain plenty of plant extracts, so if you have allergies this mask could be a problem, though they may also have some anti-irritant benefits. Other than that, it is an OK lightweight mask.

☹ **Aromafleur Flower Petal Mini-Facial in a Jar** *($29.50 for 4.5 ounces)* is just a good moisturizer with several plant extracts that can be more of a problem than a help for skin; some can cause irritation, though a few can be helpful as anti-irritants.

☺ $$$ **Bio-Cellular Lip Line Cream with Alpha Hydroxy Complex** *($22.50 for 0.5 ounce)*. No one needs a specialty AHA product just for around the lips, but then this one doesn't contain enough AHAs or have the right pH to qualify, so it doesn't matter anyway. This is just a very emollient moisturizer for any part of the face.

☹ $$$ **Clear & Even Skintone Complex** *($45.95 for 1.7 ounces)* is a decent 7%

AHA product using lactic acid in a good emollient base for someone with dry skin. However, AHA is not the best option for reducing the appearance of brown spots on the skin. This product does contain magnesium ascorbyl phosphate, which has been shown in 10% concentration to inhibit melanin production, but the amount in here is less than 1% so it has no real effect on skin.

☺ $$$ **Freeze-Dried Protein Lip Peel and Salve** *($39.50 for 1 ounce of peel and 0.25 ounce of salve)* is a two-part system quite similar to BeautiControl's Lip Apeel that I have recommended quite often (and which is also half the price of this one), and my line has a similar one for slightly less. All of these work the same; the peel is a wax you rub over the lip and the salve is just a good lip gloss. It's great for preventing dry lips but none of these will do anything for wrinkles.

☹ **Sea Mud Mask** *($24.50 for 4 ounces)* is just clay, alcohol, and film former. To sum it up, this is a lot of money for potentially irritating results.

☹ **Vegetable Peel Off** *($20 for 2 ounces)* does peel off, but that serves no function, and it contains peppermint, which is a potent skin irritant.

## *Ahava (Skin Care Only)*

Ahava is the Hebrew word for love and also the name for this group of skin-care products imported from Israel. Other than the endearing title, the gimmick here is that Ahava products contain salts and minerals from the Dead Sea in Israel. So is your skin going to love these products containing Dead Sea water? Supposedly Cleopatra did, and of course she must have been a skin-care enthusiast or Mark Anthony wouldn't have risked everything for her. Isn't that a good enough reason to consider these for your skin-care routine? I hope not. Aside from the folklore, there is little truth behind the hype.

The Dead Sea is one of the most saline bodies of water in the world. Its composition includes magnesium, sodium, potassium, calcium, bromine, sulfur, and potash. But it is predominantly the sulfur you notice when you're standing close by. And you don't have to get all that close to the Dead Sea to appreciate the intense wafting smell of rotten eggs emanating from it. What does seem to be authentic about Dead Sea water is that it can bring about temporary relief from psoriasis and other severe skin rashes. Studies done by the Department of Medicine and Department of Epidemiology and Dermatology at the Soroka Medical Center of Kupat-Holim in Israel and Ben-Gurion University of the Negev found that "improvement [in skin] was found when patients soaked in two pounds (one kilo) for three baths per week, for a period of six weeks." That's a lot of Dead Sea water and that improvement is only for serious skin rashes. If you are looking for Dead Sea water to heal wrinkles, which are completely unrelated to skin rashes, you're better off saving your money. Even if Dead Sea salts could benefit normal skin in some way, the amounts found in the Ahava products are infinitesimally small in comparison with what the published studies cite.

Is there anything else in these products worth considering? Ahava products are about as standard and boring as they come. For more information about Ahava call (800) 252-4282 or visit the Web site at www.ahava.com.

☺ **$$$ Advanced Deep Cleanser for All Skin Types** (*$20 for 2.5 ounces*) is a standard, detergent-based water-soluble cleanser that would work well for most skin types. The plant oil in here can be a problem for someone with oily skin. For this kind of standard cleanser formulation, the price is completely unwarranted.

☺ **$$$ Advanced Facial Cleansing Milk for Normal to Dry Skin** (*$20 for 2.5 ounces*) is more of a cold cream than anything else. It would need to be wiped off, and can leave a greasy film on the skin.

☺ **Advanced Facial Cleansing Milk for Oily Skin** (*$24 for 8.5 ounces*) contains several ingredients that are problematic for oily skin, including octyl palmitate and myristyl myristate. While those are good for dry skin, these standard thickening agents can leave a greasy feel on the skin.

☹ **Dead Sea Mineral Glycerin Soap for Dry and Sensitive Skin** (*$6 for 100 grams*) is soap, and that can be drying and irritating for most skin types.

☹ **Dead Sea Mineral Mud Soap for Oily and Problematic Skin** (*$6 for 100 grams*) is soap, and that can be drying and irritating for most skin types.

☹ **Dead Sea Mineral Salt Soap for All Skin Types** (*$6 for 100 grams*) is soap, and that can be drying and irritating for most skin types.

☺ **$$$ Advanced Gentle Mud Exfoliator for All Skin Types** (*$24 for 3.4 ounces*) is a standard, detergent-based water-soluble cleanser that uses Dead Sea mud (salts) as the scrub agent. It is a decent exfoliator for someone with normal to dry skin. The emollients in here make it problematic for someone with normal to oily skin.

☺ **$$$ Eye Makeup Remover** (*$18 for 4 ounces*) is a standard, detergent-based eye-makeup remover that works well enough to remove makeup. It does contain fragrance and coloring agents.

☺ **Advanced Facial Toner for Normal to Dry Skin** (*$21 for 8 ounces*) isn't advanced in the least. It is minimally beneficial for skin but basically it offers no real benefit for dry skin except to help remove leftover makeup.

☹ **Advanced Facial Toner for Oily Skin** (*$21 for 8 ounces*) lists alcohol as the second ingredient, which makes it too irritating and drying for all skin types.

☺ **$$$ Advanced Eye & Neck Cream for All Skin Types** (*$40 for 1 ounce*) is an incredibly overpriced moisturizer that would be very good for dry skin.

☺ **Advanced Moisturizer for Normal to Dry Skin** (*$26 for 2.5 ounces*) is a standard moisturizer that would be good for dry skin, but mostly it's boring and not worth the money.

☺ **$$$ Advanced Nourishing Cream for Normal to Dry Skin** *($40 for 1.7 ounces)* is even more boring than the one above, but it would be good for someone with normal to dry skin.

☺ **Advanced Moisturizer for Very Dry Skin** *($26 for 2.5 ounces)* is a good, but standard, moisturizer for normal to dry skin.

☺ **Advanced Moisturizer for Oily Skin** *($26 for 2.5 ounces)* is a good light-weight moisturizer for normal to slightly dry skin. It should not be worn over oily or blemish-prone areas unless those areas are dry. This does contain a tiny bit of balm mint that may be slightly irritating.

☺ **$$$ Advanced Mineral Beauty Serum for Very Dry Skin** *($60 for 1 ounce)* would be a good lightweight moisturizer for normal to slightly dry skin. Several of the plant extracts in here, including orange and lemon, are potential skin irritants. But the price? They've got to be kidding!

☺ **$$$ Advanced Mineral Beauty Masque for Very Dry Skin** *($28 for 4.2 ounces)*. Most of the ingredients are actually quite good for dry skin, but why anyone with dry skin would want to put mud on their skin to absorb the very moisturizing ingredients dry skin needs is beyond me.

☺ **$$$ Advanced Mud Masque for Oily Skin** *($28 for 4.2 ounces)* is a standard clay mask that would work well for normal to oily skin, although it can't surpass the price and oil-absorbing properties of plain milk of magnesia.

☺ **$$$ Advanced Mud Masque for Normal to Dry Skin** *($28 for 4.2 ounces)* is almost identical to the oily version above and the same comments apply.

# *Alexandra de Markoff*

Alexandra de Markoff has had ownership problems during the past several years. It was owned by Revlon, who then sold it to a small company called Parlex, was again sold to Cosmetic Essence in 1998, and is now owned by a company called Irving Rice. All of this leapfrogging and different ownership has caused a lack of direction that has hurt the line, and the number of stores carrying it has declined. Despite this line's apparent stagnation, for some women Alexandra de Markoff has retained its image as a prestige line of cosmetics offering the same illusion of affluence as do Chanel and Christian Dior. However, as was true in the last edition of this book, there isn't much that's new here. There are no AHAs or BHA, and none of the sunscreens offer reliable UVA protection. The makeup has basically stayed the same, with its one strong point being some excellent foundation choices for those with very dry skin and the weak points being some pretty awful colors and finishes that are way too shiny.

For some unknown reason Markoff has retained a longtime older clientele who must like the elegant mental picture this line still exudes for them. Many of the salescounter personnel confirm that these clients are steadfastly devoted to the line, even though there are clearly many products out there that are more modern and effective. In general, this line has limited appeal and, for the money, is relatively unimpressive. For more information about Alexandra de Markoff, call (800) 366-7470 or visit them on the Web at www.eve.com.

## *Alexandra de Markoff Skin Care*

☺ $$$ **Balancing Cleanser** *($28.50 for 6 ounces)* is a mineral oil–based cleanser that also contains a detergent cleansing agent, thickeners, and a group of fragrant oils. This can be a good cleanser for someone with very dry skin, but it may leave skin feeling greasy. The fragrant oils can be a problem for sensitive skin.

☺ $$$ **Comfort Cleanser** *($40 for 4 ounces)* is a standard, mineral oil–based wipe-off cleanser. This is a lot of money for oil and standard waxy thickeners. The cleanser also contains protein and elastin, which are good water-binding agents but won't affect the collagen and elastin in your skin. There are also antioxidants but they have no real impact on skin.

☺ $$$ **Complete Foaming Cleanser with Ivy and Birch** *($28.50 for 6 ounces)* is a standard, detergent-based wash-off cleanser. Several of the cleansing agents are fairly drying and irritating, which makes this cleanser more of a problem than most. There are a host of fragrant oils in here, including clove oil and galbanum, which can be skin sensitizers.

☹ **Luxury Cream Cleanser, with Aloe and Rosewater** *($40 for 6 ounces)* is a cold cream–type cleanser with a host of thickening agents, plant extracts, and vitamins. Even if the plant extracts could have an effect they would be wiped away, but these plants are mostly fragrant and potential skin irritants.

☹ **Luxury Facial Cleansing Bar** *($20 for 4 ounces)* is a very overpriced, standard bar cleanser. The ingredients that keep bar cleansers in their form can clog pores and the cleansing agents can be drying for most skin types.

☺ $$$ **Eye Makeup Remover Pads** *($18 for 60 pads)* is a standard, detergent-based eye-makeup remover with plant extracts. Several of the plant extracts can be anti-irritants, but this also contains witch hazel, which can be a skin irritant.

☹ **Fresh Solution with Sage and Witch Hazel** *($26 for 7.5 ounces)* contains mostly water, water-binding agent, calamine, clay, witch hazel, plant extracts, more water-binding agents, vitamin B, mineral salts, thickeners, plant oils, and preservatives. This is a lot of money for what is essentially calamine lotion. Calamine is zinc, while calamine lotion is zinc mixed with an amount of phenol, which is extremely toxic. While zinc by itself is not a problem, and this version probably does not use calamine lotion, several ingredients in here—clove oil, witch hazel, galbanum, rose oil, and sandalwood oil—are serious potential irritants. The minerals in here can be skin irritants.

☺ **$$$ Luxury Skin Toner, with Aloe Vera and Comfrey** *($28.50 for 6 ounces)* is a very good irritant-free toner with a handful of plant extracts that can be anti-irritants and water-binding agents. It also contains fragrance and coloring agents.

☺ **$$$ Soothing Lotion, Alcohol Free, for Dry or Sensitive Skins** *($48 for 4 ounces)* is a very good, irritant-free toner, with a handful of plant extracts that can be anti-irritants and water-binding agents. It does contain coloring agents and preservatives.

☺ **$$$ Compensation Skin Serum** *($65 for 2 ounces)* is a very good emollient for someone with very dry skin. It does contain antioxidants and some good water-binding agents, but the $65 price tag just doesn't make sense for what you get.

☹ **Countess Isserlyn Moisture 364 +, with SPF 15** *($45 for 1.8 ounces)* doesn't contain titanium dioxide, zinc oxide, or avobenzone, and is not recommended.

☺ **$$$ Daytime Moisturizer** *($32 for 2 ounces)* has isopropyl myristate as the first ingredient, which can cause breakouts or clogged pores in this amount. Otherwise, this just a standard ordinary moisturizer for dry skin. Lubriderm and L'Oreal have far better formulations than this. Because this product does not contain sunscreen it is best to wear it only at night.

☺ **$$$ Fresh Moisture Lotion** *($45 for 4 ounces)* is an OK lightweight moisturizer for someone with normal to slightly dry skin, and it contains a small quantity of antioxidants, but there are several fragrant oils in this product that can be problem for sensitive skin types.

☹ **Moisture Reserve Cream SPF 8** *($55 for 2.25 ounces)* does not contain titanium dioxide, zinc oxide, or avobenzone for UVA damage prevention, and the SPF 8 is an unreliable number for sun-damage protection. This product is not recommended.

☹ **Oil-Free Matte Moisture** *($38 for 4 ounces)* is a confused product. The talc in here can absorb oil, but that's what pressed powder is for. All this product does is lay down some waxy ingredients that aren't needed for oily skin, while the talc probably just ends up absorbing the emollients in the product.

☺ **$$$ Skin Renewal Therapy Restorative Eye Cream** *($42 for 0.5 ounce)* won't renew anything, but it can be a good, though absurdly expensive, moisturizer.

☺ **$$$ Skin Tight Firming Eye Cream** *($50 for 0.4 ounce)* won't firm skin, but it is very emollient—good for someone with dry skin.

☺ **$$$ Sleep Tight Firming Night Cream with Comfrey** *($60 for 1.7 ounces)* doesn't contain enough comfrey to warrant a mention. It is a standard moisturizer. It also has a long list of fragrant oils, of which several are strong potential skin sensitizers.

☹ **Vital 10 New Age Skin Complex with Marigold, SPF 6** *($65 for 2 ounces)* isn't vital, it's pointless. SPF 6 isn't adequate to protect the skin from sun, and it doesn't contain titanium dioxide, zinc oxide, or avobenzone for UVA protection.

☹ **Weekly Revitalizing Clay Mask, with Green Tea and Sage** *($30 for 2 ounces)* is a fairly standard clay mask that contains peppermint, which can be a skin irritant.

☺ **$$$ Weekly Revitalizing Exfoliating Mask, with Pineapple and Papaya** *($30 for 2 ounces).* The plant extracts here are supposed to sound like they are related to AHAs and enzymes. They aren't, although they can be skin irritants. This is just a mask with little benefit.

☹ **Weekly Revitalizing Moisture Mask, with Jasmine and Avocado** *($30 for 2 ounces)* is a moisturizer with some talc and some very irritating plant oils, including menthol, clove, and rose oil. This mask is not recommended.

☹ **Extra Help Gel for Lips** *($20 for 1 ounce)* offers minimal help for dry lips. It has almost no emollients or skin-softening ingredients. It can put a film over the lips to make them look smooth temporarily but it won't feel very good, particularly in the winter.

# Alexandra de Markoff Makeup

**FOUNDATION:** There are a lot of poor shades to wade through here, with nothing suitable for darker skin tones. Thankfully, they are nicely organized on a revolving tester unit and numbered according to the shade's undertone. The #70s are mostly pink, the #80s are supposedly neutral but there are still colors to watch out for, and the #90s have a golden undertone, with the exception of numbers 94 to 97, all of which are extremely rose and do not resemble real skin in the least.

☹ **Countess Isserlyn Liquid Makeup** *($47.50)* comes in 20 shades and is oil-based. The formula is dual-phase, meaning the oil and pigments are separate and this needs to be shaken vigorously to blend the two parts. Expect this separation to translate onto the skin and cause streaking. Even though this can blend on smoothly and provides light to medium coverage, it leaves a slick, moist finish appropriate only for very dry skin. These shades are undeniably too peach or rose for all skin tones: $72^1/_2$, $76^1/_2$, $86^1/_2$, $89^1/_2$, 94, 95, 96, $96^1/_2$, 97, and $97^1/_2$.

☺ **$$$ Countess Isserlyn Matte Makeup** *($47.50)* is hardly passable as matte; it has only a slightly lighter texture than the one above due to the silicone instead of mineral oil in the base. The silicone adds a lighter feel, but this foundation is meant for oily skin, and most would assuredly reject this as being too greasy and slick. Normal to dry skin would fare better, and this offers light to medium coverage. This is also a dual-phase formula and the same separation issue applies here as well. You'll find some neutral colors within the 12 shades, but consider avoiding $71^1/_2$, $72^1/_2$, $76^1/_2$, $86^1/_2$, and $96^1/_2$.

☺ **$$$ Countess Isserlyn Creme Makeup** *($47.50)* is an exceptionally thick, emollient foundation that is suitable only for very dry skin and those who prefer medium to full coverage and a moist, satin finish. It blends on better than you might expect, but is very moist and slightly greasy. Of the 11 shades, over half, including

71½, 72½, 76½, 86½, 92½, and 96½ are too glaringly peach, pink, or rose for most skin tones. Colors to consider are 81½, 88½, and 91½.

☺ $$$ **Countess Isserlyn Powder Finish Creme Makeup** *($35)* is a cream-to-powder makeup that has a definite creamy texture that tends to stay that way on the skin. This could still be an option for normal to dry skin that prefers medium to full coverage and a minimal powdered finish. There are ten shades, and again, half are nowhere near flesh-toned colors. Avoid these shades: 71½, 72½, 92½, 96½, and 98½.

☹ <u>CONCEALER:</u> **Disguise for Eyes** *($22)* comes in a tube with a wand applicator and has a rather greasy but opaque texture that will surely crease. Of the three shades, only Neutral is a noteworthy option. **Countess Isserlyn Concealer** *($19.50)* has a very smooth cream texture and a greasy finish that gravitates into any lines around the eye. The colors are inadequate, and make this a problem for most skin tones.

☺ $$$ <u>POWDER:</u> **Countess Isserlyn Loose Powdermist** *($40)* has the same pleasingly soft, dry texture found in numerous other talc-based powders in all price ranges. If opulent packaging appeals to you, be aware that it's what you're paying for with this one. **Countess Isserlyn Pressed Powdermist** *($35)* is identical to the Loose Powdermist except this one has a bit more coverage (as most pressed powders do) and a slightly better finish. The colors for both are acceptable.

<u>BLUSH:</u> ☹ **Outlasting Moisturizing Powder Blush** *($31.50)* has a great, smooth texture but all of the colors take shine to new heights and are not recommended unless making your cheeks as shiny as possible is your goal.

☺ $$$ **Outlasting Cream Blush** *($31.50)* is a traditional cream blush, meaning it is indeed creamy with a dewy, moist, and sheer finish. The four shades are fine; it's the price tag that's hard to applaud.

☹ <u>EYESHADOW:</u> **Disguise for Eyes Eyelid Foundation** *($27)* is nothing more than a semi-opaque, pale-pink liquid that claims to solve every eyeshadow pitfall. It just puts another layer on the eyelid that isn't necessary. The pitfall these eyeshadows try to make up for is de Markoff's greasy foundations, but that is better solved with a dusting of powder and not a concealer. If concealing was the objective, then a good concealer, which this line doesn't have, would be better. **Eye Defining Shadow** *($20)* is sold as single eyeshadows and almost every one of them is ultra-shiny, in colors that are makeup mistakes waiting to happen. For an older clientele, these products are inappropriate.

☺ $$$ <u>EYE AND BROW SHAPER:</u> **Eye Defining Pencil** *($18.50)* is a standard pencil with a princess-pleasing price. **Brow Defining Pencil** *($18.50)* is also standard and overpriced but does have a very nice, soft texture that applies easily and should stay put. There is a brow brush on the end to soften the line. **Professional Secrets Liquid Eyeliner** *($19)* has a good firm brush that is capable of drawing a thin line. The formula dries quickly and is quite tenacious. Caution: Heathered Taupe dries to an iridescent finish.

**LIPSTICK AND LIP PENCIL:** ☺ **$$$ Lasting Luxury Lipstick** *($18.50)* makes the claim of having "unique liposomes that constantly release pigment and moisturizers." That's hard enough to swallow, but considering this lipstick's greasy texture, it's unlikely to stay on long enough for the liposomes to do much of anything anyway. ☺ **$$$ Lip Defining Pencil** *($18.50)* is a standard pencil with a creamy application and soft powder finish. Nothing exceptional, and not worth the imperious price tag.

☹ **Undercolor for Lips** *($26.50)* has a jaw-dropping price for what amounts to a sheer peach, silicone-based tint that smoothes over the lips. This one claims to prevent lipstick from feathering and, unbelievably, that it will make any lipstick transfer-resistant—both of which it absolutely cannot do.

**MASCARA:** ☺ **$$$ Professional Secrets Mascara** *($20)* builds decent length with a good amount of thickness and no clumping or smearing, but for the money I wouldn't run out and make this my choice. There are far more impressive mascaras around to consider.

☹ **Lash Amplifier** *($18.50)* is a clear mascara that is supposed to enhance the lashes, but it's no better than an extra coat of mascara. Besides, if the regular mascara is any good, why would it need an amplifier in the first place?

# *Almay*

Almay has a long-standing reputation for being one of the few lines that is 100% hypoallergenic. Given that the FDA has never issued specific guidelines about which ingredients are likely to cause allergic reactions, this is an admirable marketing feat. However, what's true is that Almay's attempts to eliminate certain irritants and allergens has become a mixed bag. On the one hand, it does a good job of screening out well-known irritants and allergens, such as fragrances, lauryl sulfate, formaldehyde compounds, and lanolin. Yet more than a few products contain universal irritants such as menthol and alcohol. To add to that contradiction, it can also be asserted that certain allergens Almay leaves out may not be the ingredients likely to cause your particular skin problem.

Almay does excel in several areas. Within its makeup you'll find some good mascaras, great blushes and lipsticks, two excellent concealers, and some reliable foundations. Many of the older foundations with poor colors are gone, although Almay would do well to introduce testers or sample packets of its existing foundations so its customers can avoid mistakes (and so it can better compete with Olay, which has one of the best makeup tester displays at the drugstore). The Amazing Lasting products are truly ultra-matte and some of the best around—not surprising, considering Almay is owned by Revlon, which originated the ultra-matte technology. Again, many of the unfavorable Amazing Lasting products have been done away with, no doubt because they were simply too difficult to use and dried up quickly.

This line has some excellent skin-care products and one of the largest selection of them in the business. Unfortunately, many of the products listed are not reliably found at every drugstore, which can make finding the items you're interested in a 50/50 proposition. For more information about Almay, call (800) 473-8566 or visit its section on www.drugstore.com. As this book went to press, Almay's own Web site, www.almay.com, was under construction.

# Almay Skin Care

☺ **Moisture Balance Cleansing Lotion for Normal/Combination Skin** (*$7.69 for 7.25 ounces*) is a mineral oil–based cleanser that does not rinse off well without the aid of a washcloth, and it leaves some makeup behind. If you have normal or combination skin you will find this cleanser somewhat greasy. If you have extremely dry skin and use a washcloth, it is an option.

☺ **Moisture Renew Cleansing Cream for Dry Skin** (*$6.29 for 3.75 ounces*) is similar to the Moisture Balance Cleansing Lotion above, and the same review applies.

☺ **Time-Off Age Smoothing Cleansing Lotion** (*$7.99 for 7.25 ounces*) is similar to the Moisture Balance Cleansing Lotion above, and the same review applies.

☺ **Moisturizing Eye Makeup Remover Lotion** (*$4.39 for 2 ounces*) and **Moisturizing Eye Makeup Remover Pads** (*$3.29 for 35 pads*) are just mineral oil and some slip agents. They will wipe off eye makeup, but they also make a greasy mess and are no different from just using plain mineral oil.

☺ **Moisturizing Gentle Gel Eye Makeup Remover** (*$4.49 for 1.5 ounces*) is similar to the Moisturizing Eye Makeup Remover Lotion above, only in gel form. It's still mineral oil, and it's still fairly greasy. It does contain vitamins that are antioxidants but that isn't helpful in a wipe-off product.

☺ **Non-Oily Eye Makeup Remover Lotion** (*$4.49 for 2 ounces*) is indeed non-oily; it is just a lightweight detergent cleansing agent that can cut through makeup. This is good and would work well if you are looking for a wipe-off, nongreasy makeup remover.

☺ **Non-Oily Eye Makeup Remover Gel** (*$4.03 for 1.5 ounces*) is similar to the lotion above only in gel form, and the same review applies.

☺ **Non-Oily Eye Makeup Remover Pads** (*$2.80 for 35 pads*) is similar to the lotion above only in a pad, and the same review applies.

☹ **Moisture Renew Balance Toner for Dry Skin** (*$7.69 for 7.25 ounces*) contains mostly water and alcohol, and the only thing it can do for the skin is cause irritation.

☹ **Moisture Balance Toner for Normal Skin** (*$7.69 for 7.25 ounces*) contains ingredients almost identical to those in the Renew toner above, and it too can irritate the skin. It's a completely useless product.

☺ **Time-Off Age Smoothing Toner** *($8.39 for 7.25 ounces)* would be a rather soothing toner with its methoxypropylgluconamide (among several other good, water-binding agents), but the second ingredient is witch hazel, and that may be a skin irritant.

☺ **Moisture Balance Eye Cream for Normal Skin** *($6.79 for 0.5 ounce)* is a very good petrolatum-based moisturizer with antioxidants that would be good for someone with very dry skin.

☺ **Moisture Balance Moisture Lotion for Normal/Combination Skin** *($9.99 for 4 ounces)* lists mineral oil as the second ingredient, and also contains several thickeners, film former, plant oil, vitamins, and even a small amount of petrolatum. Now, who in the world with combination skin would be happy with this formula? It could be good, though very standard, for someone with dry skin, though.

☺ **Moisture Balance Night Cream for Normal/Combination Skin** *($10.39 for 2 ounces)* is similar to the Moisture Lotion above and the same review applies.

☹ **Moisture Balance Moisture Lotion SPF 15 for Normal/Combination Skin** *($7.39 for 4 ounces)* doesn't contain zinc oxide, titanium dioxide, or avobenzone, and is not recommended.

☺ **Moisture Renew Cream for Dry Skin** *($7.99 for 2 ounces)* is a standard, very ordinary mineral oil–based moisturizer with small amounts of vitamin A and water-binding agents. This would be a good moisturizer for someone with dry skin. The label suggests that it is greaseless, but calling mineral oil greaseless is just not accurate.

☺ **Moisture Renew Moisture Lotion for Dry Skin** *($9.99 for 4 ounces)* is almost identical to the Renew cream above, and the same comments apply.

☺ **Moisture Renew Eye Cream for Dry Skin** *($6.79 for 0.5 ounce)* is a very good moisturizer for dry skin.

☹ **Moisture Renew Moisture Lotion for Dry Skin SPF 15** *($10.59 for 4 ounces)* doesn't contain zinc oxide, titanium dioxide, or avobenzone, and is not recommended.

☺ **Moisture Renew Night Cream for Dry Skin** *($7 for 2 ounces)* is almost identical to the Renew creams above, and the same comments apply.

☺ **Time-Off Age Smoothing Moisture Lotion** *($10.59 for 2 ounces)* is a rather good, lightweight moisturizer for someone with normal to dry skin.

☺ **Time-Off Age Smoothing Eye Cream** *($8.49 for 0.5 ounce)* is similar to the Moisture Lotion above only in cream form.

☺ **Time-Off Age Smoothing Night Cream** *($9.69 for 2 ounces)* is similar to the Moisture Lotion above and the same basic comments apply.

☺ **$$$ Time Off Revitalizer Daily Solution** *($18 for 0.72 ounce)* contains a good concentration (about 1%) of salicylic acid (BHA), at the correct pH, to make it a good, reliable exfoliant. However, it comes in a mineral-oil base, which isn't great for someone with oily or combination skin. This would be an option for someone with normal to dry skin who tends to break out. It also works on the surface of skin as an exfoliant.

☺ $$$ **Time Off Daily Solution Pads** *($18 for 112 pads)* is similar to the Revitalizer Daily Solution above, only this one doesn't contain mineral oil and is far better for someone with normal to oily skin.

☹ **Time-Off Wrinkle Defense Cream SPF 15** *($12.49 for 2 ounces).* The sunscreen ingredients in this one do not include UVA-protecting ingredients of titanium dioxide, zinc oxide, or avobenzone and is not recommended.

☺ **Time-Off Lasting Moisture SPF 25** *($14.99 for 3.8 ounces)* is a good sunscreen that uses part titanium dioxide for UVA protection, for someone with dry skin. It has a similar base as the Time Off Age Smoothing Moisture Lotion above. It contains salicylic acid, but the pH isn't low enough for it to be effective as an exfoliant.

☺ **Stay Clean Medicated Pore Strips** *($5.94 for five strips),* like all pore strips, is basically gauze and a form of hairspray (film former). Almay's contains a bit of silicone, probably to help with sticking, as well as salicylic acid (BHA). These can make a difference if you have noticeable black dots on your face, but they do not eliminate the problem. Please be aware that all pore strips have five to six user warnings that include the possibility of skin tearing, as well as directions not to use them over blemishes or if you are on certain acne medications. Ironically, one of the medications that can be a problem with pore strips is BHA. BHA exfoliates skin and makes it more susceptible to "tearing." But that's not really a problem as these strips aren't left on long enough to let the BHA do that. Still, it is confusing for the consumer. If you are curious about pore strips, stick with the originator, Biore. All these other Johnny-come-latelys are trying to get your attention but are not making their products any better.

## Almay Makeup

<u>FOUNDATION:</u> ☺ **Clear Complexion Light and Perfect Compact Makeup SPF 8** *($8.37)* has a too-low titanium dioxide–based SPF, but is a good cream-to-powder makeup that comes in eight colors. With no testers around, and even with neutral shades, if you get the color wrong, it just looks bad. If Almay would invest in some testers, this one would be wholeheartedly recommended as an option for normal to slightly dry skin as long as you wear an appropriate sunscreen underneath.

☺ **Amazing Lasting Makeup SPF 6** *($10.49)* comes awfully close to being amazing, at least in terms of staying power and color selection, but the titanium dioxide–based SPF 6 is a very unamazing number. Other than that, the ten colors, though limited to light and medium skin tones, are (except for Warm) wonderfully neutral.

This provides a dry, unmovable, ultra-matte finish. If the SPF was bumped up to 10 or 12 (15 would be superb), I would give this one a much better rating, but as is, for someone with oily skin (who this makeup is really the best for) it would require an additional sunscreen underneath, thus negating the ultra-matte finish.

☺ **Amazing Lasting Sheer Makeup SPF 12** *($10.49)* is definitely sheer—actually it's beyond sheer to almost nonexistent. The titanium dioxide–based sunscreen is fine and the application smooth and even. The appearance is so sheer it would be hard to make a mistake with this stuff, but the tradeoff is you don't get any meaningful coverage. If you want transparent coverage with a slightly sticky texture (similar to Revlon's ColorStay foundations), with a decent SPF (though SPF 15 would be the best) and no moisturizing feel whatsoever, this one is a great option, but that is definitely a narrow range of requirements. Most of the ten colors are superior, just watch out for Pale, Naked, and Warm.

☺ **Time Off Age-Smoothing Makeup SPF 12** *($9.39)* has a great light texture and a smooth, seamless finish that provides medium coverage. The SPF is pure titanium dioxide, which is excellent, though an SPF 15 would have been even better. There are eight shades, but many of them are too pink or peach for most skin tones, and they tend to go on darker than you would expect. Without testers, that makes this one pretty risky. These shades are best avoided: Honey Beige, Soft Beige, Almond Beige, and Ivory Beige.

☺ **One Coat Light and Easy Makeup** *($12.49)* is a great option for foundation in the now popular stick form. It has a smooth, creamy application and a sheer, light powder finish. There are ten decent shades to select from, and though all have a slight peach hue, they are still worth considering for some skin tones. The one real drawback is that you can't see the colors. The swatch on the package is no help at all—it's an amazingly poor representation at best—so again, choosing is all guesswork. This also has a sponge tip for blending. It's a clever idea but it's actually more of a contrivance, as it is too tiny to really be effective for a smooth, even application. As is true for most all stick foundations, this one is best for normal to slightly dry or slightly oily skin.

☹ **Skin Stays Clean Oil Free Foundation** *($10.89)* contains menthol, and you will notice the burning sensation when you apply it anywhere near the eyes. There is no reason to put menthol into a skin-care product—it provides no benefit whatsoever—and that's why this foundation is not recommended.

☺ **Skin Stays Clean Foundation** *($12.89)* has almost the same name as the one above, but this is a cream-to-powder version that claims somewhat indirectly that it can prevent breakouts (the label doesn't state that clearly but it is indeed implied and most consumers will read it that way). First, wearing foundation isn't all that clean in and of itself, plus the thickening agents in here can potentially clog pores, which can cause breakouts. Although this contains salicylic acid, the pH is too high for it to be effective. Having said all that, this does have a great, smooth application that dries to a soft matte finish. It is an option for normal to partly dry or partly oily skins, and the ten colors are quite nice, except that you cannot see them without breaking open the box, so you're left in the aisle alone to guess your shade. One caution: this one also contains menthol, but I suspect the amount is so small it shouldn't be a problem for the skin.

☹ **Moisture Tint Sports Formula SPF 6** *($7.19)* has an extremely low SPF with no UVA protection. It might have passed muster as a standard tinted moisturizer if the two available colors weren't so peachy-pink.

☺ <u>CONCEALER:</u> **Cover-Up Stick** *($5.79)* is a good concealer that comes in three workable shades: Light, Medium, and Dark. The lipstick-like applicator helps it go on creamy, but not greasy, and it tends not to crease in the lines around the eyes. This one is definitely worth looking into, although the consistency may be too moist for someone with oily skin. **Extra Moisturizing Undereye Cover Cream** *($5.73)* comes in three excellent shades: Light, Medium, and Dark. It goes on somewhat greasy, though it is anything but extra-moisturizing. It dries to a matte, almost powdery finish. It isn't best if you have lines around the eyes or dry skin (it can look too dry and make wrinkles more obvious), but it doesn't crease in the lines and that's great. **Time-Off Age Smoothing Concealer** *($6.69)* doesn't erase wrinkles, but it goes on smoothly and doesn't crease. The color selection, though small, is terrific. **Amazing Lasting Concealer** *($6.69)* is amazing. It doesn't crease and it goes on smoothly and evenly! **Sensitive Care Concealer** *($6.69)* is actually a decent concealer with good color choices, but nothing about it makes it any better for sensitive eyes than any other concealer.

<u>POWDER:</u> ☺ **Moisture Balance Pressed Powder for Normal to Combination Skin** *($6.06)*, **Moisture Balance Oil Control Oil Blotting Powder for Oily Skin** *($7.19)*, **Time Off Age Smoothing Pressed Powder** *($9.19)*, and **Clear Complexion Light and Perfect Pressed Powder** *($8.59)* are all good, talc-based powders, with similar smooth finishes and decent color choices. The problem is that each is packaged in a box that prevents you from getting a peek at the real color. Without at least seeing the real color, you can absolutely end up with the wrong one and that is not attractive or a money-saver.

☺ **Skin Stays Clean Powder** *($10.98)* is a talc-based powder with an exceptionally silky, somewhat thick feel. That can work as well as any powder for coverage, but the claims for this one are the same as for the Skin Stays Clean Foundation above and most of the same comments apply.

☺ **Amazing Lasting Powder SPF 4** *($8.37)* has an extremely poor SPF number; it is titanium dioxide–based, but relying on any powder to provide significant sun protection is a bad idea. This does have staying power, at least more so than your average powder, but the cream-to-powder application does not work well over dry skin because any flakes will look exaggerated, and it's also tricky to blend on evenly. It has a lot of slip initially, leaving some areas streaked if you're not careful, but once this stuff dries into place it doesn't move and can make skin very tight. This can be both good and bad. If you have normal to oily skin and want a real matte finish from a powder, the three shades are a definite option, but one to check very carefully in the daylight before you decide to wear it in public. Keep in mind that it does not work well over foundation.

☺ **Luxury Finish Loose Powder** *($9.19)* has a very satiny, shiny finish. If you're using loose powder to reduce shine, this would not be the way to go about it. However, if a shiny powder is what you're looking for, this will work nicely.

☺ **BLUSH: Cheek Color** *($5.73)* is a small group of standard powder blushes, all with a perfectly matte, soft texture. **Beyond Powder Blush** *($8.49)* has an extraordinarily silky feel, and applies beautifully. However, all of the colors go on extremely sheer and half of them have a sparkle that is quite evident in daylight. Still, this is an option for very pale to light skin tones.

**EYESHADOW:** ☹ **Amazing Lasting Eye Color** *($5.47)* does have amazing staying power, at least more so than your average powder shadows—these actually stick to the skin. The application is another story. The eyeshadows have a cream-to-powder finish with a strong stain and tend to streak when applied. Unless you love frustration, these are not recommended.

☺ **Beyond Powder Eyeshadow** *($3.59 singles; $5.99 quads)* has a silky, ultra-soft texture that is almost identical to the Beyond Powder Blush reviewed above. They apply and blend well, but almost all of the colors are shiny and offer a sheer finish that takes some effort to build any intensity. The quads offer some suitable color combinations, but at least one shade in each is very shiny. If shine doesn't bother you, they are an affordable option.

☺ **EYE AND BROW SHAPER: I-Liner** *($6.69)* is a good liquid liner that goes on smoothly and easily, creating a thick, dramatic line without flaking or looking crinkled, and I think you will find it identical in performance to many department-store liquid liners. **Amazing Lasting Eye Pencil** *($6.69)* is a standard pencil formula with a twist-up, no-sharpen pen applicator. It's nice but hardly amazing. **One Coat Gel Eye Pencil** *($5.69)* is similar to Almay's discontinued Gel Eye Colors. This pencil goes on slightly less smoothly, but still somewhat wet, then dries to a matte, powdery finish that doesn't smear. In fact, don't ask me how they do it, but these last all day without smearing! The colors are OK, and there is no way to see the real color without buying the product, which is a shortcoming. Hint: you have to clean off the tip from the powder it picks up while applying to retain a smooth application.

**LIPSTICK AND LIP PENCIL:** ☺ **One Coat Lip Color** *($8.49)* is just a very greasy lipstick. It works well enough but doesn't go on any more reliably in one application than any other lipstick with the same glossy finish. **One Coat Lip Shine** *($6.99)* is a standard but very emollient and shiny lip gloss with a misleading name. If one-coat coverage is what you like, you can put on one coat of most any lip product. If you like more, then you have to apply more. Simple, right? **Amazing Lasting Lip Color** *($8.49)* is Almay's rendition of an ultra-matte-finish lipstick, and this is one of the better ones to consider. **Amazing Lasting Lip Liner** *($7.19)* is just a good, standard, automatic pencil–style lip liner. It doesn't last longer than any other lip liner.

☺ **One Coat Lip Cream SPF 15** *($8.69)* doesn't have adequate UVA-protecting ingredients and is otherwise just a fairly glossy, standard lipstick with a large range of colors to choose from. The finish is rather sheer, especially if you stick with just "one coat." **One Coat 3-in-1 Color Stick** *($8.69)* is an oversize, fat crayon–type pencil that can be used over the eyes and cheeks, but that's essentially just for the lips. If you thought Chanel's Triple Colour Crayon ($30) was a cool idea, this one is another, virtually identical option to consider. These can be tricky to apply to the cheeks, and Almay's selection of shades does make for an interesting eyeshadow look, but the slightly greasy, sheer application can smear over the eye and just looks greasy on the cheeks. These can be hard to sharpen and are not too practical, but for a monochromatic, kicky look, they can be considered convenient.

☹ **Stay Smooth Lip Color SPF 25** *($9.19)* doesn't contain UVA protection and is not recommended for sun protection, but it does contain menthol, which can cause irritation and chapped lips, and is not what I would call a smooth move. **Stay Smooth Medicated Lip Color SPF 25** *($8.49)* also does not have any reliable UVA protectants and is a split product, with one half being a lip balm and the other half a lightweight lip color that merits the same warnings as the one above. **Stay Smooth Anti-Chap Lip Liner** *($7.29)* has a name that cannot live up to its irritating performance. Although this is indeed a smooth, automatic pencil, it burns and tingles on the lips for some time after it has been applied. There is no ingredient list on the product, but I suspect the tingling is more menthol coming back to wreak havoc and *encourage* chapping.

**MASCARA:** ☺ **Stay Smooth Mascara** *($7.49)* is really a packaging gimmick rather than a new mascara formulation. This one does stay on well during the day and applies easily, building decent length, but it also tends to clump. To help smooth out those clumps there is a built-in lash comb. It's cute and can be of help, but mascara that didn't clump would be more helpful. **One Coat Color and Curl Mascara** *($6.69)* is just OK. You'll notice little to nothing in terms of curl, and minimal thickness. With some effort, you'll get long lashes with a soft, natural appearance that doesn't flake or clump. But the curved brush is not all that easy to use. **Super**

Rich Mascara *($6.49)* is just average—but why bother with middle-of-the-road when there are so many great mascaras out there? **Perfect Definition Mascara** *($6.23)* is slow going. It takes forever to get even a little thickness, but if length and thickness aren't your goal, this can be a good mascara. **Stay Smooth Waterproof Mascara** *($7.49)* builds some length and definition but makes the lashes stick together and look almost brittle. It is waterproof, but there are other choices that are far more flattering.

☺ **One Coat Mascara Lengthening** *($6.69)* is a superior mascara that applies beautifully and builds lashes that get decidedly thicker as opposed to longer. You will definitely get some length, but don't be fooled by the name—it makes lashes thick too. **One Coat Mascara Thickening** *($6.69)* builds much greater length and thickness, and applies a bit unevenly with minor clumps, even after wiping down the wand. By the way, for both of these mascaras, the "one coat" term is meaningless. You will find it necessary to apply a few coats to get a truly defined, separated look, as is true for all mascara, no matter the price or quality. **Longest Lashes Mascara** *($6.23)* is a good mascara, but not as good as the Thickening and Lengthening versions. **The Insider** *($6.85)* is supposed to nourish lashes and make them stronger. It can't do that any more than hair care products can do that for your tresses. This is just mascara and an OK one at that. It does build decent, though not exciting length but no thickness. For a softer mascara look it works fine and it doesn't smear or clump.

☹ **Amazing Lash** *($6.69)* is, at best, unreliable. Purchasing several different tubes from various stores proved that each one performed differently. They all built some amount of length, but with this much inconsistency, I don't quite know what to say except that it's best to not take the risk with so many other more reliable Almay options. **One Coat Waterproof Mascara** *($6.69)* is not a one-coat mascara in the least. It can take many coats and then you still won't look like you have any lashes. Plus, the lashes tend to clump together when wet—not the best look from waterproof mascara. **Amazing Lash Waterproof Mascara** *($6.69)* isn't amazing, unless you're amazed by a mascara that claims it's waterproof but only builds little length and then comes off with mere drops of water.

# Aloette (Skin Care Only)

Clearly aloe is at the heart of these formulas. As a cosmetic ingredient, it may have some benefit for the skin as an anti-irritant, but not a great deal more. In the summer of 2000, Aloette revamped its product line and for some products those changes have been for the better. What is interesting to me about the changes is that I received a great number of complaints from Aloette salespeople and executives regarding my comments on their original product line. They insisted I was wrong and that these products were the best ever. If they were the best ever, then why reformulate? It seems somewhere along the line management got the idea that the Aloette formulations were exceptionally dated and that aloe alone wasn't enough for skin care. Several of the new formulations include good water-binding agents, plant oils, and anti-irritants (and not just aloe), but some of the products still include alcohol and irritating plant extracts. There are definitely some inexpensive options to consider in this line, as well as ones to stay away from.

For more information call (905) 336-6590 or (800) 256-3883 or visit the Web site at www.aloettecosmetics.com.

☺ $$$ **Aloepure Essential Cleansing Oil** *($15.50 for 2 ounces)* contains, as the name implies, some plant oils, but thankfully none of them are volatile oils—just safflower, sesame, peanut, sunflower, olive, avocado, and mineral oils. This can leave a greasy film on the face, though it can be an option for very dry skin. While the mix of oils seems interesting, you could get the same effect with a single oil from your kitchen cabinet for far less money.

☺ **Aloepure Foaming Citrus Cleanser** *($13 for 6 ounces)* is a standard, detergent-based water-soluble cleanser that would be an option for someone with normal to oily skin. The cleansing agents in here are more drying than most. It does contain fragrance and coloring agents.

☺ **Aloepure Gentle Citrus Scrub** *($13.50 for 4 ounces)* can work as a scrub but the clay makes it hard to rinse off, and in the long run plain almond meal would do the same thing minus the preservatives and fragrance found here.

☺ **Aloepure Alcohol-Free Toner** *($13.50 for 8 ounces)* is definitely a good, irritant-free toner that would work well for most skin types. What a shame the other toners in the line didn't go the same route.

☹ **Aloepure Skin Refining Toner** *($13.50 for 8 ounces)* lists alcohol as the second ingredient and that makes this too drying and irritating for all skin types.

☹ **Aloepure Oil Control Toner** *($13.50 for 8 ounces)* is similar to the one above only with more irritating ingredients that include camphor and lime peel.

☺ **Aloepure Line Control Eye Gel** *($12 for 0.5 ounce)* includes nothing that will change one wrinkle on your face, but it is a good, lightweight moisturizer for slightly dry skin. It does contain yeast, which can be a good antioxidant but also a skin irritant, however, the amount in here is so tiny as to almost be not worth mentioning.

☺ **Aloepure Nutri-C Moisture Cream** *($15 for 3 ounces)* is a good but rather standard moisturizer for normal to dry skin.

☺ **Aloepure Nutri-Moisture Lotion** *($15 for 3 ounces)* is similar to the cream above, only this one contains ginseng, which can be a skin irritant, and a far more boring ingredient listing.

☹ **Aloepure Nutrition Vitamin Complex** *($16.50 for 8 ounces)* has alcohol as the third ingredient, which makes this potentially drying and irritating for all skin types.

☹ **Aloepure Time Repair Anti-Wrinkle Serum** (*$40 for 1 ounce*) contains lime extract high up on the ingredient list, which is a skin irritant and a potentially problematic thickening agent as well. It also contains willow bark, something that is distantly related to BHA, but too distant to have exfoliating properties. This is a rather ordinary moisturizer with more problems than positives.

## Alpha Hydrox (Skin Care Only)

Alpha Hydrox Lotion and Alpha Hydrox Face Creme were two of the more effective and reasonably priced alpha hydroxy acid products that first appeared on the market when the AHA craze was launched back in 1992. While other companies often hedge when telling you how much AHA their products contain, Alpha Hydrox is one of the few companies that is more than forthcoming about their contents. The AHA in its products is glycolic acid, which is considered one of the best, and the pH of the products is a level that makes AHAs effective. If you are interested in trying an AHA in a moisturizing or gel base, this is a great place to start. The prices and the product quality are excellent. One word of caution: To capitalize on the success of its two showcase products, Alpha Hydrox has introduced an additional 15-plus products to its line, including several that have no AHA content, though it does now have a good retinol and an OK BHA product. So while the non-AHA products are nowhere near as impressive, there are some interesting and reasonably priced products to check out. For more information about Alpha Hydrox, call (800) 447-1919 or visit the Web site at www.alphahydrox.com.

☺ **Foaming Face Wash, for All Skin types** (*$5.57 for 6 ounces*) is a standard, detergent-based water-soluble cleanser that does not contain AHAs. It can be good for someone with normal to oily skin, but may be too drying for other skin types.

☹ **Toner-Astringent for Normal to Oily Skin** (*$5.50 for 8 ounces*) contains alcohol and menthol, and that makes it too irritating and drying for all skin types.

☺ **AHA Creme, 8% AHA Facial Treatment for Normal Skin** (*$7.64 for 2 ounces*) is a very good and effective AHA exfoliant, in a standard moisturizing base for normal to dry skin types.

☺ **AHA Enhanced Creme, 10% AHA Facial Treatment, for Dry to Normal Skin** (*$8.41 for 2 ounces*) is similar to the 8% AHA Facial Treatment above only this one contains more AHA; the same basic comments apply.

☺ **AHA Lotion, 8% AHA Facial Treatment, for Dry Skin** (*$8.64 for 6 ounces*) is a very good 8% AHA exfoliant in a very standard, ordinary moisturizing base, best for someone with normal to dry skin.

☺ **AHA Sensitive Skin Creme, 5% AHA Facial Treatment** (*$7.64 for 2 ounces*) is similar to the Enhanced Creme, 10% above, only this one has half the amount of AHA, which does make it better for sensitive skin.

☺ **Extra Strength AHA Oil-Free Formula, 10% AHA Facial Treatment** *($8.53 for 1.7 ounces)* is virtually free of any ingredients that could clog pores and is a very good option for an AHA exfoliant for someone with normal to oily skin.

☹ **SPF 15 Moisturizing Daily Lotion** *($7.58 for 4 ounces)* does not contain avobenzone, titanium dioxide, or zinc oxide, and is not recommended.

☺ **Night Replenishing Creme for Normal to Dry Skin** *($7.95 for 2 ounces)* would be a good, though standard, moisturizer for someone with normal to dry skin.

☺ **Oxygenated Moisturizer** *($12.29 for 2 ounces)* contains oxidized corn oil, but the notion that this can release oxygen to the skin in any way is a stretch of the imagination. Even if it were possible it doesn't answer the question about oxygen causing free-radical damage. This is a good standard moisturizer for dry skin, and the claims about oxygen being beneficial for skin care are not valid.

☺ **Multi-Performance Eye Therapy Creme** *($8.99 for 0.5 ounce)* is a good moisturizer for normal to dry skin.

☺ **Fade Cream** *($8.99 for 3.5 ounces)* is a very good 2% hydroquinone-based skin lightener in a fairly standard moisturizer base for normal to dry skin. Hydroquinone is considered by all standards to be the most effective ingredient for reducing hypermelanin production. However, without the diligent use of a sunscreen, all skin-lightening products are useless.

☺ **Purifying Clay Masque 4% AHA Facial Masque, for Normal to Oily Skin** *($8.35 for 4 ounces)* is a standard clay mask with a small amount of AHA but the pH is too high for it to be effective as an exfoliant. Regardless, keep in mind that you don't need more than one effective AHA product. Using several is just overkill—after all, you only have so much skin that needs to be exfoliated. And it's best to use only one effective AHA product on a regular basis, rather than in a face mask you use once or twice a week. This is a good clay mask for normal to oily skin.

☹ **Lasting Lip Treatment, SPF 8 Sunscreen, All-in-One Care** *($3.85 for 0.35 ounce)* doesn't contain avobenzone, titanium dioxide, or zinc oxide, and the SPF 8 is not reliable protection, so this product is not recommended.

☹ **Vanishing Blemish Solution** *($7.99 for 0.5 ounce)* would be an excellent 2% salicylic acid (BHA) product if the second ingredient weren't alcohol (ethanol to be exact). I have much respect for Alpha Hydrox and its AHA formulations, but the alcohol in here is just not necessary for skin.

☺ **Retinol Night ResQ Anti-Wrinkle Firming Complex** *($11.99 for 1.05 ounces)*. If you are interested in finding out if all the talk about retinol is true (I'm referring to the notion that vitamin A can work just as well as the active ingredient in Retin-A or Renova), for content and price this is one of the better options you will find!

# AlphaMax (Skin Care Only)

This is a line of products that touts the AHA they contain, and is AHA overkill at best. At least three of the five products contain the correct pH and a decent amount of glycolic and lactic acid, but the face needs only one competent AHA product. There are a lot of excellent AHA products available from many venues for less than this. To add insult to injury, the AlphaMax brochure presents consumer questions about its products that are answered by two dermatologists who endorse the line. Here is an example. "**Q.** Can AlphaMax be used with Retin-A? **A.** Personally, we think AlphaMax is comparable to Retin-A and Renova in effectiveness." Retin-A and Renova are prescription items that can alter cellular growth, have detailed safety studies, and can increase collagen (to what extent is still under dispute) after two years of use. AHAs have no such supportive studies or effectiveness. Moreover, the doctors literally don't answer the question asked: "Can this product be used WITH Retin-A . . ."

Here is another gem. "**Q.** Will the use of AlphaMax result in increased sun sensitivity of my skin? **A.** There is no ingredient in the AlphaMax program that would make your skin sensitive to the sun." That statement is incredibly misleading. Yes, there are no ingredients that would create a phototoxic reaction, but continued use of effective AHAs absolutely makes the skin more susceptible to sun damage because it removes older skin that can be a protective layer. This issue is a serious concern of the FDA. AlphaMax's doctors' suggestions to the contrary are unconscionable. You can order by calling (800) 810-6299 or visit the Web site at www.thane.com.

☹ **$$$ Collagen and Elastin Facial Cleanser** *(2 ounces as part of the $139.97 kit)* is a standard, detergent-based water-soluble cleanser that can feel drying to some skin types. It contains a tiny amount of collagen and elastin, but even if there were more, these two ingredients can't change a wrinkle on anyone's face. You are supposed to use this cleanser with a sponge like Buf-Puf. Clearly, this company thinks skin can handle a large amount of abuse. It can't. Between this cleanser and the sponge, watch out for some serious dryness and irritation.

☹ **$$$ Intensive Exfoliator Pads** *($49.97 for six pads when sold separately from the kit)* is a series of six pads, each one soaked with a different concentration of AHAs, although the company is not forthcoming about what those concentrations are. I was not able to test the pH because the liquid took the color off my pH paper! I assume it is a decent enough pH to make the pads effective, but since I don't know the concentrations, I worry that this product may deliver more irritation than a face needs. If it is a high concentration, as they suggest—high enough to eliminate the need for a peel—you should not be using these pads at home. Of course, I doubt that this company would take the risk of selling a product with that high a concentration, but who knows? They've said many things that have led me to believe they are not interested in truthful information.

☺ $$$ **Weekly Intensive Exfoliator** *(60 pads as part of the $139.97 kit)* is similar to the above product and the same review applies.

☺ **Daily Renewal Lotion with AHA and SPF 15** *($29.97 for 2 ounces)* is a decent mix of AHAs and sunscreen. It even has a pH low enough to make the AHAs effective. For someone with normal to dry skin, this is one of the first products I've seen that contains a good UVA-protecting sunscreen formula (titanium dioxide is one of the active ingredients) and glycolic acid with a pH of 3 to 4. This lotion is worth considering if you want to try to kill two birds with one stone. Keep in mind, though, that when you can't separate your AHA product from your sunscreen, night-time use becomes an issue, and you may not want to use AHAs twice a day. I should mention that this cream has a noticeable medicinal smell that lingers for some time.

☺ **Moisturizing Cream** *($19.97 for 1.7 ounces)* contains mostly water, glycerin, several thickeners, aloe, silicone, anti-irritant, more thickener, plant oil, still more thickeners, vitamins, plant extracts, and preservatives. This is an OK but rather ordinary moisturizer for someone with normal to slightly dry skin. The amount of vitamins and plants in it is too minuscule to have any real effect on the skin.

☺ $$$ **Renewal Eye Cream with AHA** *($19.97 for 0.5 ounce)* doesn't have a low enough pH to make it effective. That's a relief, especially when it comes to causing irritation to the eye area.

☺ **Intensive Hand and Body Lotion with AHA and SPF 15** *($14.97 for 6 ounces)* is a good sunscreen with titanium dioxide for someone with normal to dry skin. It does contain a tiny amount of glycolic acid and a handful of plant extracts, and the label makes them sound like AHAs when they aren't. Glycolic acid is the only one that counts, but in this tiny amount it won't help exfoliate the skin.

☺ $$$ **Fade Out with Kojic Acid** *($22.97 for 1 ounce)* is an interesting product. Research has found that kojic acid can help lighten skin by inhibiting melanin production; but hydroquinone, which is not included in this product, is still considered the best ingredient for performing this function, especially when combined with kojic acid.

# *Amway*

There are a lot of people selling Amway products throughout the world, and unless you have been living in a shell or on a mountaintop, someone by now has likely approached you with the opportunity to either share in the theoretical wealth or at least become a customer. Talk about company loyalty! As one Amway sales representative said to me, "Why would the company make anything that wasn't wonderful?" Obviously, no cosmetics line is perfect, or they wouldn't discontinue "old" products and introduce "new" ones as this line has done, particularly for makeup. If you want to shop in the privacy of your own home and enjoy being able to test the products, there are things I encourage you to consider taking a look at in Amway's skin-care and makeup lines. I hope this doesn't mean I've unleashed a monster on any of you who have an Amway representative in your area because you will be recruited to become an Amway salesperson with declarations of making lots of money even while you sleep. Make it clear from the beginning that you are interested only in buying products and not in becoming an Amway representative.

As was true last time I reviewed this line, the price increase for these products is startling. This line is not a bargain in the least—it is up there in price with the high-end department stores. It is worth noting that there have been some improvements in the Amway line, particularly in foundations and moisturizers. There are some good products here, but watch out for the shiny eyeshadows and blushes, overpriced moisturizers, and the concealers. For more information about Amway call (616) 787-6000 or (800) 992-6929 or visit the Web sites at www.amway-usa.com or www.quixtar.com.

# Artistry by Amway Skin Care

☺ **Moisture Rich Cleansing Creme for Normal to Dry Skin** *($15.60 for 4.2 ounces)* is a standard, mineral oil–based cleanser that needs to be wiped off, and that can leave a greasy residue on the skin. It also contains coloring agents and fragrance.

☺ **Moisture Rich Toner for Normal to Dry Skin** *($16.60 for 8.1 ounces)* is a very good, irritant-free toner. Ignore the avocado and rose extracts—they are window dressing, have little impact on skin, and may actually be sensitizing. The same is true of the essential oils at the end of the ingredient list, which add fragrance to this product and a risk of irritation for sensitive skin types. It also contains coloring agents.

☹ **Moisture Rich Moisturizer for Normal to Dry Skin SPF 15** *($21.15 for 2.5 ounces)* does not include UVA-protecting ingredients of avobenzone, zinc oxide, or titanium dioxide, and is not recommended.

☺ **Clarifying Cleansing Gel for Normal to Oily Skin** *($15.60 for 4.2 ounces)* is a very good, detergent-based facial cleanser for most skin types (except very dry skin) that cleans well without drying out the skin or irritating the eyes, and can remove all of your makeup. It does contain fragrance and coloring agents.

☹ **Clarifying Astringent Toner for Normal to Oily Skin** *($16.60 for 8.1 ounces)* is a standard, alcohol-based toner and that is too irritating and drying for all skin types.

☹ **Clarifying Moisturizer for Normal to Oily Skin SPF 15** *($21.15 for 2.5 ounces)* does not include UVA-protecting ingredients of avobenzone, zinc oxide, or titanium dioxide, and is not recommended.

☺ **Delicate Care Cleanser for Sensitive Skin Types** *($15.60 for 4.2 ounces)* is a good cleanser for sensitive skin though it does take a washcloth to help get makeup off. It doesn't contain fragrance, coloring agents, or irritating plant extracts. For the money it is actually almost identical to Neutrogena's Extra Gentle Cleanser ($7.29 for 6.7 ounces).

☹ **Delicate Care Toner for Sensitive Skin Types** *($16.60 for 8.1 ounces)* lists the third ingredient as benzyl alcohol, which is a skin irritant and not something I would recommend for any skin type, much less someone with sensitive skin.

☺ **Delicate Care Hydrating Fluid for Sensitive Skin Types** *($21.15 for 2.3 ounces)* is a very good moisturizer for dry skin. It does not contain coloring agents or fragrance.

☺ **Eye & Lip Makeup Remover** *($12.50 for 4 ounces)* is a standard silicone-based makeup remover that also contains plant extracts and detergent-cleansing agents. It will work as well as any.

☺ **$$$ Exfoliating Scrub** *($21.05 for 3.4 ounces)* is a mineral oil– and petrolatum-based cleanser that contains some synthetic scrub particles. It will exfoliate the skin gently, but it can leave a greasy film on the skin.

☺ **$$$ Alpha Hydroxy Serum Plus** *($40.20 for 1 ounce)* is an AHA lotion at about a 6% concentration with a pH of 4 in a gel-like lotion with good water-binding agents and no coloring agents or fragrance. That makes it a good AHA solution—but the price is nonsense; there are formulations equally as good, if not better, available for far less.

☺ **$$$ Time Defiance Nighttime Renewal Creme** *($59.95 for 1 ounce)* is supposed to be "the first and only antioxidant complex designed to delay signs of aging caused by free radicals …" Not only is there no research demonstrating that antioxidants can do this, but there isn't one ingredient in this product unique to Amway's Artistry line; these show up in lots of skin care products. However, there are good antioxidants in here but they won't change skin. This moisturizer is a good option for normal to dry skin, but all the other claims are bogus.

☺ **$$$ Time Defiance Nighttime Renewal Lotion** *($59.95 for 1 ounce)* is similar to the Creme version above and the same comments apply, though this one is better for normal to slightly dry skin.

☺ **$$$ Bright Idea Illuminating Essence** *($49.21 for 1 ounce)* is supposed to be a skin lightener for sun-damaged discolorations, but it is unlikely to do that. This product contains bearberry extract, which primarily has antibacterial properties for skin. However, bearberry also contains arbutin, which has been shown to inhibit melanin but only in vitro (meaning not on human skin). The amount of bearberry extract used in here is too tiny to affect melanin in skin or in a petri dish.

☺ **$$$ Advanced Daily Eye Creme** *($20.30 for 0.5 ounce)* is a very good moisturizer for dry skin. There is nothing about this product unique for the eye area.

☹ **$$$ Hydrating Masque** *($17.10 for 2.6 ounces)* is an emollient, though standard face mask for someone with dry skin; it's more a moisturizer than a traditional mask.

☺ **$$$ Deep Cleansing Masque** *($16.15 for 3.3 ounces)* is a standard clay mask that also contains a small amount of alcohol, but probably not enough to be a problem for the skin. It does contain fragrance.

☻ **Vitamin C + Wild Yam Treatment** *($36.30 for 0.68 ounce)* may contain wild yam, but wild yam does not contain progesterone nor anything else that would act like progesterone. According to *The PDR Family Guide to Natural Medicines & Healing Therapies,* wild yam "is used in the production of artificial [synthetic] progesterone but it will not yield the hormone in the absence of a chemical conversion process that the body can't supply." It has no effect on skin, plus this product does not contain vitamin C.

# Artistry by Amway Makeup

**FOUNDATION:** ☺ **Absolute Oil Control Foundation SPF 15** *($24.25)* is a good liquid foundation with a fairly matte finish that has light to medium coverage. It can be an option for someone with normal to oily skin. It does contain zinc oxide as one of the sunscreen agents, which is great, but don't count on this product to control seriously oily skin in the least. Avoid these colors because they are too peach, pink, or rose: Honey Beige, Shell Bisque, Warm Amber, and Cappuccino.

☺ **Versatile Matte Pressed Powder Foundation** *($18.20)* is really a standard, talc-based pressed powder that has a silky-smooth feel, though it can appear a bit too powdery if you have dry skin. Using it wet is an option but it can look streaky and uneven so be careful. All but one of the shades are excellent; only Shell Bisque may be too peach. For Amway, these are both pressed powder as well as an option for foundation, but they are best as pressed powders.

☺ **Self-Defining Sheer Foundation SPF 15** *($22.45)* doesn't contain UVA-protecting ingredients of titanium dioxide, zinc oxide, or avobenzone so you can't rely on the SPF for complete sun protection. It is a liquid foundation with a soft matte finish and light coverage. Many of the colors do look like real skin so this is an option for normal to slightly dry or slightly oily skin, but only if you wear a good sunscreen underneath.

☺ **Featherlight Maximum Coverage** *($23.25)* may be good for someone with dry skin, but it tends to be greasy and very thick; there is nothing featherlight about this product. Most of the colors have a slight peach tone, but only slightly, so they may be an option for some skin tones.

<u>CONCEALER:</u> ☺ **Enhancing Concealer** *($14.55)* is a stick concealer with four decent shades, though it does tend to crease into lines around the eyes. **$$$ Ultimate Coverage Concealer** *($16.85)* comes in a squeeze tube and has three shades.

☺ **$$$ <u>POWDER:</u>** The **Loose Powder** *($17.50)* is a standard, talc-based powder with three good color choices, though three is definitely a limited selection. It has a dry, smooth finish.

☺ <u>EYESHADOW AND BLUSH:</u> Amway's eyeshadows and blushes come in individual tins that are placed into a compact you purchase separately, either a **Two Pan Compact** *($11.25)* or a **Four Pan Compact** *($12.85)*. That means you can create your own makeup-collection compact that includes blushes and eyeshadows. It's a nice idea. The prices given below for the Powder Blush and Eye Colour are for the tins only, without a compact. Unfortunately, the blush and eye colors all have some amount of shine. The handful of **Powder Blush** *($11 refills)* colors have a silky texture that goes on soft and even, but all the colors have some amount of shine, as do the **Eye Colour** *($7.30 refills)* eyeshadows, which have a lovely soft texture and go on smoothly and evenly; here even the so-called matte ones have shine.

☺ <u>EYE AND BROW SHAPER:</u> **Softstick for Eyes** *($12.40)* are standard pencils in seven good shades, though these aren't all that soft. One end of the stick has a sponge applicator to soften hard lines. A brow pencil called **Softstick for Brows** *($9.35)* is available in five colors identical to the pencils for eyes. **Fine Liner** *($13.45)* is just a standard tube liquid liner that goes on smooth and doesn't chip or flake; it comes in only two shades.

☺ <u>LIPSTICK AND LIP PENCIL:</u> **Perfect Moisture Lip Colour** *($12.90)* are standard creamy lipsticks with a slight glossy finish. The color selection is decent. **Lip Sheer Colour SPF 15** *($12.90)* are standard glossy finish lipsticks but the SPF 15 doesn't include UVA-protecting ingredients. **SoftStick for Lips** *($11.10)* are just standard lip pencils with a creamy application and a good color selection, but these do require sharpening.

☺ **Jumbo Lip Pencil** *($12.50)* is a very soft lipstick in pencil form. This one may be too soft, can smush down to nothing fairly fast, and isn't the most reliable option for applying lipstick or lip liner.

☺ <u>MASCARA:</u> **Smudgeproof Mascara 200** *($14.50)* builds decent length and thickness quite quickly and doesn't smudge or smear.

☹ **Waterproof Mascara 200** *($14.50)* builds great length and some amount of thickness but it isn't all that waterproof. It can start coming off after a few splashes with water, and it easily smears even when you aren't wet.

☹ <u>BRUSHES:</u> The **Cosmetic Brush Set** *($32.95)* is disappointing and shockingly overpriced for what you get. It comes with six brushes, of which three are OK; the other three are not worth the money. The powder brush is fine, but the bristles are a little too loose, so the powder can be hard to control on the face. The eyeshadow and angle brushes are also OK and usable. The eyebrow/eyelash comb is like those found everywhere; an old toothbrush would work equally well. The lipstick brush is a good 6 inches long and wouldn't fit easily in most makeup bags; the smaller, retractable lipstick brushes are much better. The blush brush is too small to be suited to anyone's cheeks.

## Anna Sui Makeup

Joining the ranks of fashion designers who have cosmetics lines bearing their name is Anna Sui. Much as Tommy Hilfiger, Calvin Klein, and, from way back, Christian Dior have found, a designer logo can sell just about anything—so why not makeup? If you aren't familiar with Anna Sui, it may be because her more unconventional designs are not exactly what you would call mainstream. What then do Anna Sui's eccentricities bring to her makeup line? Basically what you'll find is a lot of style with very little substance. Sui's makeup line can only be described as gothic. Her all black, scallop-shelled containers and black tester units look like they would be right at home on the vanity of Morticia Addams (this is not the "Chanel" black-lacquer look). I'm not quite sure who this line is supposed to appeal to—even teenagers and 20-somethings who are known to be attracted to glitter and vivid colors would soon realize that all the shine in the world won't make up for poorly formulated, hard-to-apply products.

Many of the products are confusing to the consumer, such as the Face Powder, which includes both skin-tone shades and blush colors, and there's an Eye Gloss, which is little more than Vaseline with color.

Far be it from me to dispel anyone's right to artistic expression, but when all is said and done, as far as makeup is concerned, Anna Sui should stay with her day job. Anna Sui makeup is available at Sephora, some Nordstrom stores, or on the Web at www.eve.com.

**FOUNDATION:** ☹ **Liquid Foundation** *($35)* is a sheer-coverage, light matte foundation that would be OK for normal to oily skin. It blends out smoothly but there are only four shades, and from that token assortment the only neutral color to even consider is #700. The other three shades are either too pink or iridescent.

☺ **Compact Powdery Foundation** *($25 for powder; $8.50 for compact)* is a standard pressed powder with slightly more coverage, so it can be used as a foundation. It offers a far better color selection than the Liquid Foundation, with six shades to choose from, and all are neutral with some great options for very light skin tones. Pressed-powder foundations are best for normal to slightly dry skin (they can be too drying for dry skin) and for normal to slightly oily skin (because they can become thick and caked over truly oily skin).

POWDER: ☺ $$$ Face Powder *($33)* has only four colors, and all of them are shiny. This is definitely overpriced for what amounts to nothing more than a standard talc-based loose powder. The shine negates the intended effect of powdering, which is to take down shine and set makeup.

☹ Pressed Face Powder *($23.50)* is a very chalky, grainy powder texture that features an odd assortment of colors. The shades are divided into accent, nuance, or base colors, but that only slightly helps determine how you use them. The only colors to consider for powdering the face are #701, 702, 703, and 704, although these all have a slight shine. All of the others are either too yellow, peach, pink, white, lavender, or green (these are supposed to be for nuance or accent but they don't add anything but a strange color to the skin). The puff that comes with this powder is ridiculously small for practical use.

☺ $$$ BLUSH: Face Colors *($22)* are the blush colors in this line and they are pretty disappointing. Of the seven shades, only #400 would work for a soft daytime look. All of the others are quite vivid and almost borderline greasy. This is a shame because the texture and blendability are nice.

☺ $$$ EYESHADOW: The Eye Color *($17)* has a grainy, powdery texture that would ensure flaking onto the skin while you're applying it. The colors are quite sheer, but they tend to deposit color unevenly. Looking at the available colors, I'm not sure any other criterion was followed except for making sure every shade had lots of shine and glitter. Eye Gloss *($17)* is a greasy, sparkly (of course) product that is supposed to add a "wet look" to the eye. If you really want to try this, Vaseline would produce the same smeary, messy effect used over any iridescent eyeshadow you already own.

☹ EYE AND BROW SHAPERS: Eyeliner *($16)* is a chubby pencil with a creamy, smear-prone formula. This borders on greasy and is not recommended. The Eyebrow Pencil *($16)* offers a dry, hard texture that would pull the skin and create a harsh line. There are countless other options to look toward before even considering this overpriced selection.

LIPSTICK AND LIP PENCIL: ☺ $$$ The Lipsticks *($19)* have a greasy feel and high-shine, opaque finish. So as not to break the pattern, many of the lipsticks have glitter galore, although there are some good red and red-brown shades to consider. ☺ Lip Gel *($13)* is a fairly standard gloss with a light feel and some opaque color choices accented with lots of glitter. Enough with the glitter already!

☺ $$$ MASCARA: Anna Sui does have a decent Mascara *($19)*, which lengthens and defines lashes nicely, but there are dozens of other superlative mascaras available that outperform this one for far less.

☺ BRUSHES: There is a small and strange collection of Brushes *($8 to $16)* that have very little to offer. The **Finishing Brush** *($8)* is, quite literally, a tufted cotton ball on a stick. This is as useless a blending tool as you'll find and is easily replaced by a far less expensive, disposable powder puff you buy at the drugstore. The **Eye Color Applicator** *($8)* is a sponge tip on a stick for applying shadow, which is identical to the free sponge applicators many eyeshadows come packaged with. There is a synthetic **Eyeshadow Brush** *($16)*, which is stiff and not as reliable as natural hair, and a **Lip Brush** *($14)*, which is oversize and fluffy—definitely not suitable for applying anything creamy, and that includes lipstick!

☺ **SPECIALTY PRODUCTS:** Perhaps the biggest attention-getter here is the huge assortment of **Nail Colors** *($13)*. These tend to be the focus of the line's visual presentation. There are over 40 colors with most having the same glitter content as Revlon's Street Wear, which costs far less.

# Aqua Glycolic (Skin Care Only)

Herald Pharmacal has a small line of drugstore AHA products called Aqua Glycolic. Aqua Glycolic products are, for the most part, a disappointment. The only option is the Advanced Smoothing Cream for someone with normal to dry skin. Of the other two products, one has skin-irritating ingredients and the other is a risk for the eyes. For information, call Aqua Glycolic at (800) 253-9499 or visit www. drugstore.com or www.plantrx.com.

☹ **Facial Cleanser Advanced Cleansing Care 12% Glycolic Compound** *($9.99 for 8 ounces)* resembles Cetaphil Gentle Skin Cleanser, but with a strong concentration of AHAs. I do not recommend washing the face with an AHA product because of the risk it poses for the eyes. Additionally, if you do want the exfoliation effect from an AHA, in a cleanser most of the potential is simply washed away before it has a chance to have an effect.

☹ **Astringent Advanced Oily Skin Therapy 11% Glycolic Compound** *($7.09 for 8 ounces)* is an alcohol-based AHA product; the alcohol compounds the irritation of the glycolic acid. It also contains eucalyptus oil, another seriously irritating skin-care ingredient.

☺ **Face Cream Advanced Smoothing Therapy 10% Glycolic Compound** *($11.29 for 2 ounces)* is a good basic AHA in a lightweight moisturizing base. It would be suitable for someone with normal to somewhat dry skin.

# Aquanil

☺ **Aquanil Lotion** *($6.99 for 8 ounces)* is a very good cleanser for normal to dry, sensitive skin.

# Aquaphor

☺ **Aquaphor Healing Ointment** *($5.69 for 1.75 ounces)* is one of the more cost-effective options for very dry skin. It isn't fancy and it can feel heavy but it works.

# Arbonne

This is one exceedingly expensive line, ranking up there with those found at many department stores, yet the offerings are not all that impressive and are definitely not worth the cost. Like many in-home sales lines from Nu Skin USA to Shaklee, Arbonne boasts more about what its products do not contain than about what they do. That isn't necessarily good or bad, but I happen to like some of the ingredients Arbonne warns against. Much of its literature states that things such as mineral oil, lanolin, collagen, artificial fragrances, and artificial colors are *not* used in any Arbonne products. I disagree strongly with Arbonne's argument that mineral oil, petrolatum, and collagen are inherently bad for the skin because (it claims) their molecular structure is too large to be absorbed into the skin, and therefore they can clog pores, cause blemishes, and interfere with skin respiration. The molecular structure of many other cosmetic ingredients, including elastin, mucopolysaccharides, waxes, and other thickeners, is also too large to permit absorption into the skin. Yet one of the best ways to prevent dehydration is to keep air off the face, and one of the best ways to do that is with a cosmetic ingredient that works as a barrier between your skin and the air. If everything were absorbed into the skin, what would be left on top to keep air off the face? Mineral oil, petrolatum, and collagen are not so totally occlusive that the skin suffocates, they simply protect it from the air. Besides, just because a cosmetic ingredient is absorbed into the skin doesn't mean it won't clog pores. Quite the contrary: once inside the pore, the ingredient is trapped and can't easily be washed or wiped away.

Arbonne also doesn't like beeswax. The company's theory is that because beeswax is sticky, bacteria and dirt will stick to the skin. However, like many waxes in cosmetics, beeswax is just another thickener, and there is rarely very much of it in a product. Moreover, beeswax isn't all that different from the synthetic waxes used in cosmetics to keep the product blended. Arbonne's products contain ingredients such as myristyl myristate and cetyl alcohol, which are quite similar to beeswax.

I do agree with Arbonne's recommendation against alcohol because of its drying and irritating effect on the skin. If only the company excluded all other irritants, such as witch hazel and certain plant extracts, the line would be even better.

I could go on, but to sum up, none of my reservations mean I don't like some of these products, and I am glad that Arbonne does not use animal products or perform animal testing. But the rather misleading marketing language is not convincing. All of the natural-sounding ingredients in the world can't keep you from reacting to an irritating preservative or fragrance or from breaking out due to cosmetic waxes such as stearic acid or myristyl myristate. For more information about Arbonne International, call (800) ARBONNE or visit the Web site at www.arbonne.com.

## *Arbonne Skin Care*

☺ $$$ **Bio-Matte Oil-Free Cleanser** *($16 for 2 ounces)* is a good detergent-based water-soluble cleanser that would work well for most skin types. The plant extracts in here are a strange mix of irritants and anti-irritants, which doesn't help skin in the least. It does contain fragrance.

☹ $$$ **Cleansing Lotion** *($14.50 for 3.25 ounces)* is supposed to be a water-soluble cleanser, but it can leave a film on the skin and doesn't take makeup off very well without the help of a washcloth. It can still be an option for someone with normal to dry skin. The plant extracts in here are a strange mix of irritants and anti-irritants, which doesn't help skin in the least.

☹ $$$ **Cleansing Cream** *($15.50 for 2 ounces)* is a fairly greasy cleanser that leave a film on the skin and doesn't take off all makeup without the aid of a washcloth, but it can still be an option for someone with dry skin. The plant extracts in here are a strange mix of irritants and anti-irritants, which doesn't help skin in the least.

☹ $$$ **Bio-Hydria Gentle Exfoliant** *($23 for 2 ounces)*. The plant extracts in here are a strange mix of irritants (clover and ginseng) and anti-irritants (comfrey and watercress), which doesn't help skin in the least. The scrub particles are fairly gentle on skin but there are better options for exfoliating skin than this.

☹ **Facial Scrub** *($17 for 2 ounces)*. The plants and vitamin E come well after the preservatives and are barely present. This is an OK scrub, but ground nuts are not the best way to exfoliate because they can scratch the skin and the peppermint in here can add to the irritation.

☹ **Bio-Matte Oil Free Toner** *($15 for 4 ounces)* contains witch hazel, balm mint, and ivy, which makes it too potentially irritating for all skin types.

☹ **Freshener** *($18.50 for 8 ounces)*. The witch hazel in here is an irritant and several of the plant extracts in here can be as well—and that's a problem for all skin types.

☹ **Toner** *($18.50 for 8 ounces)*. Witch hazel, peppermint, and lemon are very irritating and drying, and they won't change the amount of oil your skin produces.

☹ **Bio-Matte Oil Free Moisture for Day, SPF 8** *($20 for 2 ounces)* has a dismal SPF, doesn't contain UVA-protecting ingredients of avobenzone, zinc oxide, or titanium dioxide, and is not recommended.

☹ **Bio-Matte Oil Free Moisture for Night** *($20 for 2 ounces)* contains several ingredients that are problematic for someone with oily skin and several of the plant extracts can be irritants. This is a mediocre moisturizer for someone with dry skin. It has more problems than benefits.

☹ **Bio Hydra Alpha Complex SPF 8** *($34.50 for 2 ounces)* has a dismal SPF, doesn't contain UVA-protecting ingredients of avobenzone, zinc oxide, or titanium dioxide, and is not recommended.

☺ **$$$ Bio Hydria Night Energizing Cream** *($58 for 2 ounces)* is a good emollient moisturizer for someone with dry skin, but it won't energize the skin or "retard the formation of wrinkles," as the label claims. And the price tag is completely ludicrous for what you get. Plus, several of the plant extracts in here can be irritants, which negates the effectiveness of the anti-irritant ingredients this product contains.

☺ **$$$ Bio Hydria Eye Cream** *($24.50 for 0.75 ounce)* is very similar to the cream above, and the same review applies.

☺ **Moisture Cream Normal to Dry Skin** *($18.50 for 2 ounces)* is a very good moisturizer for dry skin. The plant extracts in here are good anti-irritants.

☹ **Moisture Cream Normal to Oily Skin** *($18.50 for 2 ounces)* is similar to the Normal to Dry version above only this one also has peppermint oil, a completely unnecessary skin irritant, adding up to a formula that is completely inappropriate for any skin type but especially not oily skin.

☺ **Night Cream for Normal to Dry Skin** *($20.50 for 2 ounces)* is similar to the Moisture Cream Normal to Dry Skin above and the same comments apply.

☹ **Night Cream for Normal to Oily Skin** *($20.50 for 2 ounces)* is almost identical to the Moisture Cream for Normal to Oily Skin, and the same comments apply.

☺ **Rejuvenating Cream for All Skin Types** *($30 for 2 ounces)* is almost identical to the Moisture Cream Normal to Dry Skin above and the same comments apply.

☺ **Skin Conditioning Oil** *($16 for 1 ounce)* is a blend of several plant oils as well as aloe vera, vitamin E, and some plant extracts. For someone with very dry skin, this would be a nice extra for problem areas, but any plant oil from your kitchen cabinet would work as well for far less money.

☺ **$$$ NutriMin C Night Cream with Bio-Hydria** *($58 for 2 ounces)*. This moisturizer is mostly water, wax, and fragrance; the good ingredients are so far down the list it makes this one a waste of time. Plus the plant extracts in here are a mix of irritants (ginseng, watercress, and clover) and anti-irritants (comfrey), which is a problem for skin.

☺ **$$$ NutriMin C Night Serum with Bio-Hydria** *($38 for 1 ounce)* is supposed to contain AHAs, but the lactic acid in here is only about 2%, which is too small a concentration to be effective as an exfoliant. Sugarcane extract is not AHA. The salicylic acid in here (about 0.5%) could potentially exfoliate but the amount and pH of this product makes that unlikely. There are several plant extracts in here that can be irritants, including lemon, orange, ginseng, clover, and watercress.

☺ $$$ **Bio-Hydria Alpha-Complex Hydrating Masque** *($29.50 for 2 ounces)* contains a mix of plant extracts with some being anti-irritants (comfrey) and others irritants (watercress, clover, and ginseng). It also contains a film former that places a layer of plastic over the skin. Peeling that off can make skin feel temporarily smoother but that's about it. The sugarcane and citrus extracts in here are not related to AHAs, despite the claims made about them.

☹ **Bio-Hydria Naturesomes** *($38 for 0.95 ounce)* contains a mix of plant extracts with some being fairly potent irritants, including arnica, watercress, clover, and ginseng.

☹ **Lip Protector SPF 15** *($5 for 0.12 ounce)* doesn't contain UVA-protecting ingredients of avobenzone, zinc oxide, or titanium dioxide, and is not recommended.

☹ **Take Cover Face SPF 15** *($15 for 2 ounces)* doesn't contain UVA-protecting ingredients of avobenzone, zinc oxide, or titanium dioxide, and is not recommended.

☺ **Mild Masque** *($17 for 5 ounces)*. For a clay mask, this is indeed fairly mild, but it is still just a clay mask. It can leave the skin feeling soft, but it could also make extremely dry skin feel even drier. The plant extracts in here are a strange mix of irritants and anti-irritants, which makes them a complete waste.

☺ **Extra Strength Masque** *($17 for 5 ounces)* is a fairly standard clay mask. Someone with oily skin won't be pleased with the oil in this product, and the grains can be rough on the skin. The ginseng can be a skin irritant, which negates the anti-irritant comfrey. This can be an option but be careful.

# *Arbonne Makeup*

**FOUNDATION:** ☹ **Match Perfect Oil-Free Foundation SPF 8** *($20)* is a cream-to-powder foundation with a more creamy than powdery finish. It is a titanium dioxide–based sunscreen, which is great, but the SPF number is too low for it to be taken seriously for sun protection. The compact for this foundation comes packaged with two colors that are supposed to be blended together to create your perfect skin color. That's a tricky thing to have to do every morning, and for most of the duo sets one of the shades is either too peach or too ash.

☺ **True Colour Soft Finish Makeup SPF 8** *($17)* is a liquid foundation with a titanium dioxide–based SPF 8. While the titanium dioxide is great, the SPF number is too low to be considered reliable sun protection. Of the 12 shades available, most have a peach tone. The best colors are Beige, Taupe, Toasty, and Mahogany.

☹ **CONCEALER:** **Cream Concealer** *($11.50)* comes in only one shade and it is exceedingly pink.

POWDER: ☺ $$$ **Translucent Pressed Powder** *($16)* has a soft, smooth, slightly powdery finish; the choices for color (two) are limited, though they are good.

☹ **Translucent Finishing Powder** *($18.50)* comes in two shades; both are fairly peach. **Bio Matte Oil-Free Powder Personalizer** *($21)* is a strange shade of green that contains mostly clay, oat flour, and wheat starch. While it does have a dry finish, the green builds a strange color on the skin, and the oat flour and wheat starch are not the best idea for preventing breakouts—it's sort of like feeding the bacteria that cause the problem.

☺ **BLUSH: Global Color Blushes** *($12.50)* have an impressive array of blush colors that go on smoothly though slightly powdery.

☺ **EYESHADOW: Global Color Eyeshadows** *($12.50)* come in an impressive range of matte shades in very workable, soft, more natural-toned colors. Be careful, some of the shiny shades are hard to detect. These colors are excellent (but don't ask me to explain the bizarre names): Techno Tokyo, China Silk, California Raisin, Thunder Down Under, London Fog, Valencia Grape, German Chocolate, Seville Suede, Klondike, Havana Road, and Irish Cream.

☺ $$$ **EYE SHAPER: Global Color Eye Pencils** *($8.50)* are standard pencils with a somewhat dry texture that will need sharpening.

**LIPSTICK AND LIP LINER:** ☺ **Global Color Lipsticks** *($12)* have a great creamy texture, with only a slightly glossy finish. The colors have a slight stain that helps keep the shades around somewhat longer than normal. ☹ **Sheer Shine** *($12)* is just a very standard, overpriced lip gloss. ☺ **Global Color Lip Pencils** *($8.50)* have a great range of colors and an application that is soft and easy.

☺ **MASCARA: Lash Colour Mascara** *($11.50)* is an excellent mascara that creates long lashes and some amount of thickness without clumping or smearing.

# Ashley Skin Care

Depending on where you live, you may have seen a full-page ad in your local newspaper for a group of skin-care products called Ashley of Beverly Hills/Ashley Skin Care. Interestingly, the woman pictured in the ads is Veronica Barton, who claims that these products are the best in the world. And she does indeed look all of 20 years old although the ad trumpets her age to be 50. To say that this is powerful advertising is an understatement. Clearly there are lots of women who believe that this woman must look the way she does in the picture and that what gives her that youthful visage are these products. But it turns out that Veronica Barton has a salon called The Veronica Skin & Body Center in Malibu, California (also at www.veronicaskincare.com, (310) 456-8883), where she not only sells her own product line, called Veronica, but also products from Guinot, Decleor Paris, and Murad, to name a few. So which group of products gets the credit for her apparently phenom-enal skin-care success? According to Fox TV news reporter Deborah Sherman, it's none of the above. Sherman spoke to Barton, who admitted that a very digitally enhanced picture was used. What a shock!

This line has several other misleading aspects. While Ashley may be from Beverly Hills (she's the daughter of one of the owners, according to the salesperson I talked to), the company is based in Austin, Texas (500 N Loop 360, Bldg. 6, Austin, TX 78746-3302, (512) 327-7130). Evidently Austin isn't as sexy or elite sounding as Beverly Hills. Further, the salesperson on the phone said the products themselves are from neither Austin nor Beverly Hills, but from Switzerland. Of course, where a product happens to come from is irrelevant to its efficacy or formulation. Moreover, the Better Business Bureau in Austin, Texas, has had a lot of complaints against Ashley Skin Care, and supposedly the company has apologized for misleading con-sumers and will be pulling their ads.

An interesting ingredient listed in these products is something called tissue res-piratory factor. It is touted by many cosmetics companies as having a "therapeutic effect by bringing oxygen to connective tissue." Though there is research establishing that some dietary supplements can perform this function, in skin-care products tis-sue respiratory factor is merely a protein offering some water-binding benefits; there is no evidence it has any other function on skin, and it absolutely cannot help skin breathe when applied topically. Aside from the fact that getting oxygen delivered into skin tissue is not possible topically, if it were, then you'd risk free-radical damage from the extra oxygen, and that problem isn't addressed. Further, what can have an effect on the inside of the body rarely translates to the surface of the skin. But what good is any of this without a good sunscreen? The prices listed below are for the individual products, but you can buy the products in kits that are shipped to you every two months for a reduced price. For more information about Ashley Skin Care call (800) 964-0670.

☺ $$$ **pH Balancing Cleanser** *($26 for 6 ounces)* is a standard, detergent-based water-soluble cleanser that would work well for most skin types. It contains mostly water, detergent cleansing agents, thickeners, fragrant oil, and preservatives.

☺ $$$ **Gentle Exfoliating Polish** *($32 for 6 ounces)* is a good standard scrub that would work better for someone with normal to dry skin. The oil and thickeners make it a problem for normal to oily skin.

☹ **Nutraceutical Toner** *($46 for 6 ounces)* contains alcohol as the second ingre-dient, which is too irritating and drying for all skin types.

☺ $$$ **Hyaluronic Serum** *($48 for 1.01 ounces)* is a good lightweight moistur-izer for normal to slightly dry skin. While sodium hyaluronate is the second ingredient, it is simply a good water-binding agent and that's about it; it's not any better than lots of other good water-binding agents. This product also contains something called tissue respiratory factor but, as I explained above, there is no evidence that this helps topically on skin.

☺ $$$ **Vitamin Complex** *($56 for 1.01 ounces)*. The pH of this product is too high for the BHA to be effective as an exfoliant, but if you are looking for a vitamin C product, this one is an option.

☺ $$$ **Dermaceutical Eye Lift** *($40 for 1.01 ounces)* is a good moisturizer for normal to slightly dry skin, and the film former can make skin appear temporarily lifted.

## Aubrey Organics (Skin Care Only)

If you haven't heard of Gale Hayman, Zia Natural Skin Care, Rachel Perry, or Aubrey Organics, you haven't been paying attention to the world of natural cosmetics, which of course is fine by me. The products manufactured under the names of this group of "natural" notability contain enough plants and herbs to make me wonder how anything can still be growing on this Earth. These gurus of the "natural" skin-care and makeup craze sell a plethora of foliage-based concoctions that are supposed to deliver every woman's deepest desire for her face—namely, flawless skin. Of course, none of their formulas are the same. Each company has its own "natural" recipes that guarantee wrinkle-free, acne-free, smooth, even-toned, glowing skin.

If there is any such thing as a "natural" true believer, Aubrey Hampton is indeed one. His books *Natural Organic Hair and Skin Care* (Organica Press) and *What's in Your Cosmetics* (Odonian Press) articulately express his convictions. Foremost is his philosophic position regarding his products: "For almost 30 years I have collected herbs from around the world and combined them in 100% natural hair- and skin-care products. I make my natural shampoos, conditioners, soaps, lotions, masks, and so forth the way my mother taught me almost 50 years ago—without chemicals, using herbs known to be beneficial to the hair and skin." And yes, every plant is a miracle and every synthetic ingredient that he doesn't use is bad.

If Hampton is relying on information that is over 50 years old, people using his products are in a lot of trouble. What we know about sun protection we've only learned about over the past few years, and cell turnover, the life-and-death process of every skin cell, is a recent discovery. The whole complex physiology of skin (the formation of the intercellular layer and its functions), along with the nature of skin disease, are still being investigated, but very current data can, and does, fill volumes, and these volumes are being rewritten almost monthly as new research reveals astonishing information that has altered everything we once thought to be true about the skin. It's nice to think Mom knew it all, but I wouldn't make a skin-care decision based on such obsolete and fanciful thinking.

Hampton also lauds his position on animal testing: "I don't believe in animal testing and never use it. None of my products are formulated with data obtained from animal testing, and yet I know they're safe to use because they contain ingredients that have been used for hundreds, sometimes thousands, of years by people all over the world. That's the best track record, don't you think?"

Well, I don't think so in the least. As nice as all that sounds, in some ways it's actually dangerous. By his own admission, Hampton has only anecdotal past history to go by, and that is just too risky for my taste. "Natural" powders laced with "natural" lead were used by fashionably correct women centuries ago, causing necrotic skin and sometimes death. And what about sun exposure, which causes skin cancer and pervasive wrinkling? No one knew about that until very recently. So much for history being an arbiter of good health. Furthermore, while I abhor animal testing, scientists over the past 20 years have ascertained the benefits of most new skin-care ingredients, from water-binding agents and the new anti-irritants to AHAs, BHA, Retin-A, and sunscreens that provide UVA protection, mostly based on animal research. If Hampton is truly telling us that he ignores all that information, his products would be risky to use and some of the most dated in the industry.

Another Hampton phobia, shared by many other "natural" eccentrics in the world, has to do with petrochemicals. (I assume Hampton doesn't drive a car, take a taxi, or fly anywhere.) He states, "Petrochemicals, [which] are infinitely cheaper and much more convenient for mass manufacturers to use . . . [make] our hair and skin suffer as a result. What's worse, the long-term effects of these harsh chemicals on both the body and the environment are still unknown . . . "

Suggesting that all petrochemicals are harsh and all plants are good is as uninformed as thinking that eating any plant you encounter in the wild won't kill you because it is natural. Besides, petrochemicals have a decidedly natural source: they come from decomposed plant and animal life! But I've belabored these subjects before. More to the point is Aubrey Organics' arsenal of skin-care recommendations.

One of the steps in Hampton's skin-care routine is steaming the face. "Applying steam is an excellent way to detoxify and deep-cleanse your skin. Pour boiling water into a heat-proof glass bowl and add 4 tablespoons of Face Flowers [an Aubrey Organics product]." Nowhere does Hampton mention what kind of toxins are sweated out of the skin, nor does he discuss the potential for damage from overheating the face, such as causing surfaced capillaries to occur or look worse.

I am also very skeptical of the way Hampton handles his skin-care ingredient lists. They make no mention of standard cosmetic preservatives, and the ones that are listed—vitamins C, A, and E—have their own stability problems, with vitamin C being the most unreliable. Cosmetics chemists I have interviewed, including some who formulate "natural" skin-care products, suggest Hampton isn't revealing everything. If he is, product stability is a serious concern and the type of base he is using is questionable. But that's not surprising given this item in *The Rose Sheet* for March 15, 1999, stating that Aubrey Organics was "in violation of catalog mislabeling and Good Manufacturing Practices. ... [The] FDA investigators also determined several Aubrey products ... bear labeling that is not in compliance."

Setting aside my continuing concern about the far-fetched hype and unsubstantiated claims surrounding natural products (though Hampton is one of the few who seems to glory in the lack of real evidence), I must point out that Aubrey Organics is one of the most reasonably priced "natural" skin-care lines around, almost to the point of being cheap! If you are one of the myriad "natural" skin-care seekers out there, this line won't hurt your pocketbook. Of course, I question what it can really do for skin, but that's what my reviews will reveal. For more information, call (813) 877-4186 or (800) 237-4270, or visit the Web site at www.aubrey-organics.com.

☺ **Blue Green Algae Herbal Antioxidant Cleansing Cream** *($7.50 for 4 ounces)* contains detergent cleansing agents that can be fairly drying for most skin types. The shea butter and evening primrose oil are nice emollients but they won't undo the dryness from the soap. It does contain fragrance.

☺ **Evening Primrose & Lavender Skin Care Bar** *($5.50 for a 3.6-ounce bar)* contains detergent cleansing agents that can be fairly drying for most skin types. The shea butter and peanut oil are nice emollients but they won't undo the dryness from the cleansing agents. It does contain fragrance.

☺ **Honeysuckle & Rose Vegetal Soap** *($5.50 for a 3.6-ounce bar)* is similar to the Evening Primrose version above and the same comments apply. It does contain fragrance.

☺ **Green Tea Facial Cleansing Lotion** *($7.25 for 4 ounces)* is a standard, detergent-based water-soluble cleanser that can be drying for the skin. Green tea is a good anti-irritant, but then why would anyone add irritating ingredients like lemon peel that could irritate the eyes? It does contain fragrance.

☺ **Mandarin Magic Mandarin & Cucumber Facial Cleanser** *($11.40 for 8 ounces)* is a standard, detergent-based water-soluble cleanser that can be drying for the skin. The plant extracts in here are mostly fragrant and can be skin irritants. It does contain fragrance.

☺ **Rosa Mosqueta Moisturizing Cleansing Bar Normal to Dry Skin** *($5.35 for a 3.6-ounce bar)* is a standard soap with coconut fatty acids (standard detergent cleansing agents) like those found in most bar cleansers. It also contains some good plant oils but that won't undo the drying effect of the cleansing agent. It does contain fragrance.

☺ **Rosa Mosqueta Moisturizing Cleansing Bar** *($5.29 for a 3.6-ounce bar)* contains detergent cleansing agents that can be fairly drying for most skin types. The emollient peanut oil in here is nice but it won't undo the dryness from the soap. It does contain fragrance.

☹ **Rosa Mosqueta Rose Hip Complexion and Body Soap** *($8.99 for 8 ounces)* contains peppermint oil, which is an irritant for all skin types. It does contain fragrance.

☺ **Sea Buckthorn Facial Cleansing Cream with Ester-C** *($8.25 for 4 ounces)* contains detergent cleansing agents that can be fairly drying for most skin types. The emollients in here are nice but they won't undo the dryness from the cleansing agents. It does contain fragrance.

☺ **Sea Buckthorn Skin Care Bar with Sandalwood** *($5.75 for 3.6 ounces)* is similar to the Sea Buckthorn Facial Cleansing cream above and the same comments apply.

☹ **Sea Wonders Seasoap Face & Body Cleansing Cream** *($6.99 for 8 ounces)* contains peppermint oil, which is an irritant for all skin types. It does contain fragrance.

☺ **White Camellia & Jasmine Emollient Soap** *($5.50 for a 3.6-ounce bar)* is similar to the Sea Buckthorn Facial Cleansing Cream above and the same comments apply.

☹ **White Camellia & Jasmine Mint Facial Cleanser** *($6.95 for 4 ounces)* contains eucalyptus, menthol, and lemongrass, all of which are potential skin irritants.

☹ **Meals & Herbs Exfoliation Skin Care Bar Normal to Dry Skin** *($4.55 for 3.6 ounces)* is similar to the bar soap above, but with almond and walnut meal. While exfoliating the skin with crushed nuts is an option, it can cause problems. Nuts can scratch the skin, and a mechanical scrub affects only the very surface of the skin. While AHAs can produce a somewhat deeper, more even exfoliation and BHA can affect exfoliation in the pore, nuts can do neither.

☹ **Jojoba Meal and Oatmeal Facial Scrub and Mask** *($7.69 for 4 ounces)* contains eucalyptus, menthol, and lemon oil, which makes it too irritating and drying for all skin types.

☹ **Green Tea & Ginkgo Facial Toner** *($7.29 for 4 ounces)* contains witch hazel, lemon peel, and balm mint, which are irritants for all skin types.

☹ **Herbal Facial Astringent Normal to Oily Skin** *($8.29 for 8 ounces)* is mostly witch hazel with some plant extracts. The nettle, rosemary, and balm-mint extracts, like the witch hazel (which is part alcohol), can be irritating or sensitizing for many skin types.

☹ **Rosa Mosqueta & English Lavender Toner Normal to Dry Skin** *($8.75 for 8 ounces)* contains mostly witch hazel, lemon peel, coltsfoot, arnica, and several other plant extracts that are potentially irritating and damaging to skin.

☹ **Apricot & Amidroxy Toning Moisturizer** *($19.95 for 4 ounces)* contains several potentially problematic plant extracts, including witch hazel, coltsfoot, and grapefruit.

☺ **Celltherapy Cellular Night Repair Cream** *($20.85 for 1 ounce)*. The lack of preservatives (at least there are none listed on the label) and the animal source indicated make this product problematic in terms of contamination. Aside from that, there is no evidence that tissue extracts have any effect on human skin whatsoever. It still may be a good moisturizer for dry skin, but the ingredient label leaves much to be desired.

☺ **Collagen Therapeutic Cream Moisturizer** *($12.89 for 2 ounces)* is similar to the Celltherapy above and the same comments apply.

☺ **Elastin Natural Moisturizing Factor** *($12.89 for 2 ounces)* is similar to the Celltherapy above and the same comments apply.

☺ **Honeysuckle Rose Complexion & Body Moisturizer** *($15.35 for 4 ounces)* can be a good moisturizer for normal to dry skin, but the coltsfoot extract in here is problematic as a skin irritant and sensitizer.

☹ **Maintenance for Young Skin Moisturizer** *($11.75 for 2 ounces)* contains balsam, coltsfoot, and balm mint, which are all potential skin irritants.

☹ **Mandarin Magic Moisturizer** *($14.35 for 1 ounce)* includes several extracts that can be skin irritants and sensitizers, including ginseng, lavender, and angelica.

☺ **Rejeunesse Moisturizing Cream** *($19.35 for 1 ounce)* contains mostly thickeners, aloe, plant oil, emollient, water-binding agents, fruit acids, fragrant plant extracts, and vitamins.

☺ **Rosa Mosqueta Rose Hip Moisturizing Cream Normal to Dry Skin** *($14.35 for 4 ounces)* is indeed an emollient moisturizer for someone with dry skin, but it also contains coltsfoot, which can be a skin irritant and sensitizer.

☺ **Sea Buckthorn Ester-C Silky Smooth Moisturizer** *($15.99 for 4 ounces)* is an OK but standard moisturizer.

☹ **Vegacell Herbal Cellular Complex** *($15.60 for 1 ounce)* contains several plant extracts that are problematic for skin, including lime tree, pine tree, lemon, and arnica.

☹ **Vegecol TMC (Therapeutic Moisturizing Cream)** *($12.89 for 2 ounces)* contains coltsfoot extract, which can be a skin irritant and sensitizer.

☹ **Green Tea & Ginkgo Daily Moisturizer SPF 15** *($14.90 for 4 ounces)* does not contain avobenzone, zinc oxide, or titanium dioxide, and is not recommended. It also contains irritating and sensitizing plants.

☹ **Green Tea Sunblock for Children SPF 25** *($7.99 for 4 ounces)* does not contain avobenzone, zinc oxide, or titanium dioxide, and is not recommended. It also contains irritating and sensitizing plants.

☹ **Nature Tan SPF 4, Easy Tan Formula** *($6.95 for 4 ounces)*. A skin-care company selling tanning products is like an oncologist giving you cigarettes. How pathetic!

☹ **Rosa Mosqueta Sun Protection Herbal Butter SPF 15** *($6.95 for 4 ounces)* does not contain avobenzone, zinc oxide, or titanium dioxide, and is not recommended.

☹ **Saving Face SPF 15 Sunblock Spray** *($6.95 for 4 ounces)* does not contain avobenzone, zinc oxide, or titanium dioxide, and is not recommended.

⊗ **Sun Shade 15** *($6.95 for 4 ounces)* does not contain avobenzone, zinc oxide, or titanium dioxide, and is not recommended.

⊗ **Swimmers Moisturizer SPF 15** *($8.75 for 4 ounces)* does not contain avobenzone, zinc oxide, or titanium dioxide, and is not recommended.

⊗ **Titania Full Spectrum Natural Herbal Sunblock SPF 25** *($7.69 for 4 ounces)* does not contain avobenzone, zinc oxide, or titanium dioxide, according to the active ingredient list, and this product is not recommended. It says it contains titanium dioxide, but if that is not on the active list there is no way to know if the amount needed for sun protection is in here.

⊗ **Ultra 15 Natural Herbal Sunblock SPF 15** *($7.45 for 4 ounces)* contains in-part titanium dioxide, but it also uses PABA, although Aubrey lists this as a plant extract. How did this one get by the FDA? No plant form of PABA is on the list of FDA-approved sunscreen ingredients. Separate from the labeling, PABA (para-aminobenzoic acid) is considered one of the more sensitizing sunscreen agents and is rarely used by anyone in the industry.

⊗ **Winterizer WPF 15 Skin Protection** *($9.25 for 4 ounces)* does not contain avobenzone, zinc oxide, or titanium dioxide, and is not recommended. It also contains several irritating plant extracts that add insult to the injury caused by this product.

⊗ **Sunshade 15 Sunblock SPF 15** *($6.75 for 4 ounces)* does not contain avobenzone, zinc oxide, or titanium dioxide, and is not recommended.

⊗ **Amino Derm Gel Oily and Problem Skin Treatment** *($7.69 for 2 ounces)* contains witch hazel, lemon, ivy, and zinc, which are all potential skin irritants.

⊗ **Blue Green Algae Herbal Antioxidant Clay Mask with Grape Seed Extract** *($8.75 for 43 ounces)* contains arnica, lemon, ivy, lime tree, and zinc, which are all potential skin irritants.

⊗ **Rosa Mosqueta Herbal Mask** *($8.15 for 4 ounces)* contains coltsfoot, peppermint, and eucalyptus, which are all potent skin irritants.

⊗ **Sea Wonders SeaClay Mask** *($7.99 for 4 ounces)* contains peppermint, a potential skin irritant.

⊗ **Herbessence Complexion Oil with Rosa Mosqueta, Borage Oil, and Alfalfa** *($6.69 for 2 ounces)* contains arnica, which is a serious potential skin irritant.

☺ **Green Tea & Green Clay Rejuvenating Facial Mask** *($8.50 for 4 ounces)* is a standard clay mask and because of the oils it can be OK for someone with normal to dry skin. It does contain lemon oil, which can be a skin irritant or sensitizer.

# *Aveda*

Aveda's brochure poses the question, "Would you moisturize with petroleum? Enjoy the sweet smell of methyl-octine-carbonate? [Or] accentuate your eyes with a coat of tar? That's just what you do with many mainstream health and beauty products. Aveda's products are grown from a simple premise: what you put on your body should be as healthy and natural as what you'd put into it." I imagine Aveda never took a look at its own ingredient listings. Who would want to eat isostearyl benzoate, polyglyceryl-6 deoleate, diazolidinyl urea (a formaldehyde-releasing preservative), or octyl methoxycinnamate (a synthetic sunscreen ingredient)? I could go on, but you get my drift. Petroleum starts to sound pretty good in comparison to this lineup, and ends up being far better for the skin than many of the irritating and skin sensitizing-plants in Aveda's products.

What is even more mind-boggling to comprehend is that Aveda was purchased by Estee Lauder in 1997. Given the kind of ingredients that Lauder uses, I imagine that Aveda's brochures will either be toned down over the next couple of years, or there will be a lot of questions about hypocrisy to answer.

Beyond the claims made about these products, a consistent draw for many consumers is the fragrance of Aveda's products. As a bystander in an Aveda store, it is interesting to note how many customers are lured in by the smell alone, and often make a purchasing decision based on that single criterion. As nice as that sounds, in the end it only shortchanges the consumer. Regardless of whether or not a product's fragrance is natural or synthetic, the potential for irritation and a host of other problems is still there. In fact, many of the "essential" oils used in Aveda products have a known history of unpleasant side effects, including allergies and dermatitis. Aveda would truly like you to believe that it is in fact the flower and plant essences in its products that are doing the "work." Alas, one only has to look at the ingredients to realize that Aveda utilizes many of the same industry-standard ingredients as everyone else. Many of the "special" ingredients merely contribute to the fragrance of the products, which is an obvious draw, but not enough to ensure a great (or even good) product. It has also been well established that once many of these "organically derived" plants and oils are purified and processed for use in cosmetics, they retain very little of their original benefit.

Aveda has created a line of skin-care and hair-care products called All Sensitive. Whenever I see products described as being good for sensitive skin, I am curious about how that was determined, given that there are no established guidelines for this. Some think that no fragrance, milder preservatives, and fewer ingredients (no more than eight to ten) are a basic standard for products aimed at those with sensitive skin. When I started researching Aveda's All Sensitive products, I was struck by four things: the ingredient lists are huge, they contain several potentially irritating ingredients, they use a mixture of plant extracts (which increases the amount of preservative needed and risks irritation for anyone with plant allergies), and they contain fragrance (ingredients like geranium oil and sandalwood are highly fragrant and have a high potential for causing skin reactions). If you are still in the process of experimenting, this line is not one I would encourage you to check out.

Having said all of that, I do think that Aveda has some good products to consider. I also want to applaud Aveda for demonstrating such concern for the environment and animals. In many ways, it has been an industry leader in the effort to streamline packaging and utilize recycled materials. Now if it would only turn down the "natural" rhetoric and work to eliminate some of the hyperbole surrounding its "wild kingdom" of ingredients, we would all be able to see the forest for the trees! For more information about Aveda, call (800) 328-0849 or visit www.aveda.com.

# Aveda Skin Care

☺ **$$$ All Sensitive Cleanser** (*$19 for 5.5 ounces*) is a standard, detergent-based water-soluble cleanser. It can be drying for some skin types and the plant extracts are hardly good for sensitive skin.

☺ **Purifying Cream Cleanser** (*$18 for 5.5 ounces*) is a lightweight, detergent-based cleanser that is supposed to be water soluble but can definitely leave a film on the face. It may be OK for someone with normal to dry skin who prefers a creamy feel and is not sensitive to plant extracts.

☺ **Purifying Gel Cleanser** (*$18 for 5.5 ounces*) is a good, detergent-based water-soluble cleanser that is best for someone with normal to oily skin.

☺ **$$$ Pure Gel Eye Makeup Remover** (*$15 for 3.7 ounces*) is a standard gel-based makeup remover that contains detergent cleansing agents. The plants in here are problematic for the eye area.

☹ **Exfoliant** (*$16 for 5.5 ounces*) could have been a good BHA exfoliant except it contains alcohol and other plant extracts that can be skin irritants.

☺ **All Sensitive Toner** (*$18 for 5.5 ounces*) is definitely not appropriate for sensitive skin due to the long list of plant extracts, of which several can be skin irritants—including sandalwood, spikenard, cardamom, and vetiver. Mainly, this is a good basic toner that contains tea water, glycerin, water-binding agents, anti-irritant, slip agents, detergent cleansing agents, and preservatives.

☺ **Skin Firming/Toning Agent** (*$18 for 5.5 ounces*) is a simple rosewater toner. This would be an option for someone with normal to dry skin.

☹ **Toning Mist** (*$16 for 5.5 ounces*) contains a host of irritating ingredients, including alcohol and peppermint. Aveda recommends this for oilier skins, but this is best avoided by any skin type, unless irritation is the goal!

☺ **All Sensitive Moisturizer** (*$30 for 5.5 ounces*). Several of the plant extracts in here can be a problem for sensitive skin, including vetiver, cardamom, and sandalwood. Other than that, this just a very basic, ordinary moisturizer for normal to dry skin.

☺ **$$$ Firming Fluid** (*$32 for 1 ounce*) does contain vitamin C, but that won't firm skin, nor will the other vitamins or the algae extracts in here. This is a good moisturizer for normal to dry skin, but that's it.

☺ **Hydrating Lotion** *($28 for 5.5 ounces)* is a good, rather ordinary moisturizer for normal to dry skin.

☺ $$$ **Night Nutrients** *($38 for 1 ounce)* is a silky, silicone-based moisturizer that also contains several emollient plant oils and some vitamins. This would be a good moisturizer for dry to very dry skin. Although it will not rejuvenate the skin from daily damage and it can't feed skin as the label claims, it is one of the few Aveda products that are aroma- and fragrance-free!

☺ **Oil-Free Hydraderm** *($26 for 5 ounces)* is a gel-based moisturizer. It is a good, lightweight moisturizer for someone with normal to slightly oily skin, though the plant water does contain some potential skin irritants.

☺ $$$ **Pure Vital Moisture Eye Creme** *($25 for 0.5 ounce)* is a good moisturizer for someone with normal to dry skin, but most of the really interesting ingredients are at the end of the ingredient list and don't add up to much.

☺ **Daily Light Guard SPF 15** *($16.50 for 5 ounces)* is a titanium dioxide–based sunscreen that would be very good for someone with dry skin.

☺ **Sun Source** *($16.58 for 5 ounces),* like all self-tanning products, uses dihydroxyacetone to turn skin a shade of brown, but this doesn't work any better than far less expensive versions.

☺ **Tourmaline Charged Hydrating Creme** *($30 for 1.7 ounces).* This relatively standard moisturizer has its share of plant extracts, but thankfully ones like huang qi, a vasodilator that can cause surface capillaries, are in such minute amounts they aren't much of an issue. Aveda's claim for this product is that the tourmaline crystals in here (and there's less than 0.1% of them) "galvanize marine and plant ingredients to highest efficacy." There is no known efficacy on skin for minuscule amounts of plankton and algae. By the way, the process of galvanizing has to do with coating iron or steel with a layer of zinc to prevent it from rusting. There is no way to coat plants with tourmaline, nor is there any reason to do so.

☺ $$$ **Balancing Infusion for Dry Skin** *($18 for 0.33 ounce)* is a blend of several plant oils that would benefit dry skin nicely, but given that these are just plant oils, you'd be better off using almond oil or canola oil from your kitchen cabinet; you'd get the same results.

☹ **Balancing Infusion for Oily Skin** *($18 for 0.33 ounce)* contains 0.5% salicylic acid as well as jojoba oil, plant oil, and silicone (which has a slippery texture). Even if this form of BHA had the right pH to work as an exfoliant (it doesn't), the other ingredients can feel greasy and that is absolutely not the best on oily skin!

☺ $$$ **Balancing Infusion for Sensitive Skin** *($18 for 0.33 ounce).* What would have been preferred is for Aveda to leave out all the other irritating plant extracts in its other products.

☹ **Bio-Molecular Perfecting Fluid** *($28 for 1 ounce)* is about a 5% AHA and

BHA product combined; however, the pH of the product isn't low enough for it to be an effective exfoliant. The presence of alcohol, lemon, and ylang-ylang make this potentially irritating for most all skin types.

☺ $$$ **Deep Cleansing Herbal Clay Masque** *($19 for 4.5 ounces)* is a standard clay masque that is also recommended as a cleanser. Clay is too drying and is ineffective in a facial cleanser that needs to be rinsed off. Although this masque has enough glycerin and emollients to make it more "comfortable" than many other clay masks, these emollients sort of negate the oil-absorbing effect of the clay, which is what clay does best for skin. For normal to dry skin this would be an option.

☺ $$$ **Intensive Hydrating Masque** *($19 for 5.5 ounces)* can be a very soothing mask or moisturizer for normal to dry skin. It contains a "tissue respiratory factor," described on the label as biofermentation of corn. Fermentation in this instance means the action of bacteria on corn. The bacteria breaks down the corn, resulting in the release of gases such as hydrogen sulfide and carbon dioxide. It sounds better when you don't know what it really is, doesn't it? And none of this helps skin breathe.

☹ **Active Composition** *($19 for 2 ounces)* contains menthol, camphor oil, peppermint oil, and eucalyptus oil, which makes this actively irritating and drying for skin.

☹ **Lip Saver SPF 15** *($7.50 for 0.15 ounce)* doesn't contain avobenzone, titanium dioxide, or zinc oxide, and is not recommended.

## Aveda Makeup

**FOUNDATION:** ☺ **Cooling Calming Cover Sheer Face Tint** *($18)* is Aveda's version of a stick foundation, only with a stay-put finish. The application is similar to both Dior's Teint Glace *($35)* and Olay's All Day Moisture Stick Foundation *($13.59)*. The texture of these makes them suitable for normal to oily skin, as they go on rather wet and quickly dry to a light matte finish with light to medium coverage, depending on your blending. Aveda's is a bit trickier than Dior's and Olay's because once it dries, it has no slip. That means any streaks or uneven blending stay that way all day (so if you get it right, that can be great for someone with oily skin). But keep in mind that any attempts at evening out mistakes will only make matters worse. If you get this blended on well, it provides sheer to light coverage in six very good colors. Regrettably, there is nothing for very light or very dark skin tones.

☺ **Base Plus Balance** *($20.50)* is a very good foundation for normal to slightly dry or slightly oily skin. The colors are, for the most part, neutral and the application is smooth. Thanks to the talc it contains, this foundation leaves a semi-matte finish. However, oilier skin types will find this formula rather heavy and any breakthrough shine will be noticeable shortly after application. The only colors to watch out for are Wheat and Amber, which can turn slightly orange.

☺ **Dual Base Minus Oil** *($19.50 without compact, $30 with)* is an excellent pressed-powder foundation that goes on lighter than most. It is supposedly good for both wet and dry use, but to avoid streakiness use it dry and blend it well. The colors are all quite workable and soft; only Teak can be too orange on the skin. This base can be layered for an ultra-matte, full-coverage look. It's not the most natural, but for some skin types this may be an option. Keep in mind that pressed-powder foundations work best for normal to slightly dry or slightly oily skin.

☺ **Moisture Plus Tint SPF 15** *($25)* is an ultra-sheer foundation that offers an excellent titanium dioxide–based sunscreen! Although the color selection is limited to three shades, I am told this will change soon. There are currently no color options for very fair skin. The formula is best for normal to dry skin, as it contains several emollients that would not please oily skin types. The coverage is truly sheer, with excellent blendability.

<u>CONCEALER:</u> ☺ **Conceal Plus Protect** *($13.50)* goes on and on about the vitamins it contains, as do most of the Aveda makeup products. Too bad there aren't enough of them in any of the formulations to really make much, if any, difference for your skin. This concealer does go on smoothly and covers well, with minimal to no chance of creasing, but may need to be layered for very dark circles or redness. The application is more cream-to-powder than cream, so any drier areas will look cakey or flaky unless moisturized first. The color selection is workable, and Aveda has wisely added two new shades (a light and dark tone) to satisfy a wider range of skin tones.

☺ $$$ <u>POWDER:</u> **Pressed Powder Plus Antioxidants** *($17.50 without compact, $29 with)* and **Pure Finish Loose Powder Plus Antioxidants** *($18 in tub with puff)* are standard, talc-based powders with a silky, dry, translucent finish. The color selection is beautiful and the application sheer and soft.

<u>BLUSH:</u> ☺ **Blush Minus Mineral Oil** *($11)* comes in an attractive selection of seven very good, subtle shades. The application is soft and quite blendable, although darker skin tones may have to layer quite a bit to get the extra intensity needed to complement them. Of the seven colors, all except Vapor are matte, and Nutmeg is excellent as a bronzer or contour color.

☺ $$$ **Cooling Calming Color** *($18)* is identical to the Cooling Calming Cover Sheer Tint foundation reviewed above, only these colors are attractive blush shades. The same problems for blending and streaking exist for this version as well. You can use this one on the cheeks or eyes. Of the four colors available, two are soft and matte and two are softly shiny. This formula is best for normal to oily skin types.

☹ **Bronzer Minus Sun** *($11)* offers two shades of cream-to-powder colors, one warm (and very orange) and the other cool (an acceptable mauve/brown). What a shame both shades are quite shiny, and best for more of a fun look, if at all.

**EYESHADOW:** ☺ **Shadow Plus Vitamins** *($11)* has a decent selection of both matte and shimmer shades. The matte shades are wonderfully neutral and soft, with more of a translucent coverage and minimal to moderate intensity. The shimmer shades are easily identified and ignored or fawned over, depending on your tastes. There are a handful of matte shades that make excellent eye lining or brow-filling shadows as well.

☺ **Onecolor Plus Two** *($14.50)* is an assortment of the chubby pencils made popular by Aveda's sister companies, Origins and Clinique. These feature two colors on each end, and are certainly clever. If looks alone counted, they would be fine, but performance is the issue here, and these can drag and pull. Aveda says they are for eyes, lips, and cheeks, and that can be an option, but the texture is too dry for lips and too creamy to function for long as an eye color. Add all of this to the fact that these need regular sharpening and you are looking at a clever inconvenience. Of all the pencils, each has at least one shiny color, and that's just too many strikes on my score pad.

☺ **EYE & BROW SHAPER:** **Eye Liner Minus Petro Waxes** *($11)* are nothing special, just a nice selection of standard pencils. For the pencil devotee, these should please. By the way, most all pencils being sold in the United States don't contain "petro" waxes, meaning petroleum-derived. However, there is nothing bad about petroleum-derived ingredients; after all, their origin—oil from the ground—is about as natural a source as it gets.

**LIPSTICK AND LIP PENCIL:** ☺ **Lip Satin Plus Fresh Essence** *($14.50)* is a beautiful collection of creamy lipsticks that do offer more staying power than many others in this class. Some shades are quite iridescent, but the reds and neutrals have excellent color and coverage. There are some sheer colors as well. If you are at all sensitive to peppermint, cinnamon, or anise (they can be sensitizing on skin), beware: these lipsticks are flavored with all three.

☺ **Lip Satin Plus Uruku** *($14.50)* is Aveda's attempt at an "all natural" lipstick. While uruku is indeed a plant pigment used to make annatto and other colors, one only has to read the ingredient list to see that these stack up the same as any other pigmented lip product—meaning that the same standard, unnatural-sounding pigments are right there with the uruku, offering their color support. **Lip Gloss Minus Lanolin** *($11.50)* is typical lip gloss in a pot—nothing remarkable—and comes in a very limited color selection seemingly aimed at a younger crowd. Unless you are sensitive to lanolin, avoiding it as an ingredient in lip products does not make much sense because it is excellent for dry skin.

☹ **MASCARA:** **Mascara Plus Rose** *($11)* can be a clumpy, smeary mess. This is a very creamy mascara that, with effort, will build OK length and some thickness—but the side effects of the formula are most unattractive, and for the most part it is a poor performer.

☺ **BRUSHES:** Aveda has updated its brush collection from good to superb. The hair being used has switched from ox/goat (which can feel too scratchy) to the much softer pony/sable hair. Brush thickness and shape have improved as well, which is excellent. Of particular note are the **Powder Brush** *($27.50)*, which is more stable and streamlined for better control, the **Blush Brush** *($25)*, which is much denser and cut to fit the contours of the face, and the **Eyeshadow Brushes** *($15, $11, and $9, depending on size)*, which are more rounded as opposed to tapered and offer greater ease in deft blending of shadows. The **Lip Brush** *($19)* still has a handle most would find inconvenient, although it may be an option for concealer application. Aveda has, inexplicably, discontinued its much better **Retractable Lip Brush** *($9.95)*. Overall though, the improvements make these a definite option for a reliable, professional collection of essential makeup tools.

## Aveeno (Skin Care Only)

Aveeno uses colloidal oatmeal (colloidal refers to the oatmeal being ground up and suspended in a base) in its products. Oatmeal is known for being an anti-irritant and soothing agent. While that may be true, many of the other ingredients in the products are irritants and potentially problematic for skin, undoing any benefit the oatmeal may provide. For more information about Aveeno products, call (877) 298-2525 or visit the Web site at www.drugstore.com.

☹ **Gentle Skin Cleanser** *($5.99 for 6 ounces)* is a standard, detergent-based water-soluble cleanser that contains oat flour, but it also contains hydrogenated tallow glyceride, which may be irritating and can clog pores.

☹ **Natural Colloidal Oatmeal Cleansing Bar for Combination Skin** *($2.99 for 3 ounces)* is a standard, detergent-based bar cleanser that contains about 38% oatmeal, and that can be soothing. Though this is a fairly gentle bar cleanser, it is still more drying for the face than a gentle, water-soluble cleanser would be.

☹ **Natural Colloidal Oatmeal Cleansing Bar Moisturizing for Dry Skin** *($2.39 for 3 ounces)* is similar to the Combination Skin version above only with the inclusion of plant oil. That can be better for dry skin, but less-drying cleansing ingredients would be better yet.

☹ **Natural Colloidal Oatmeal Cleansing Bar, Oil Control Formula for Acne Prone Skin** *($2.99 for 3 ounces)* is similar to the Combination Skin version above only with the inclusion of BHA; in a cleanser, that would just be rinsed off the face, plus the pH for this product is too high for it to be effective as an exfoliant.

☻ **Medicated Acne Cleanser** *($5.60 for 6 ounces)* contains about 2% BHA. In a cleanser, however, it would just be rinsed off the face, plus the pH is too high for it to be effective as an exfoliant, and the tallow in here can clog pores. This just doesn't make sense for skin.

# Avon

Avon has gone to great lengths over the past few years to modernize its products and image from the 1970s ad campaign of "Avon calling" to its current direction of "Let's Talk Avon." The ads embody Avon's attempt to appeal to savvy, beauty-conscious women who prefer the attraction and status of "department store quality" makeup. For the most part, Avon is succeeding, as it continues to be one of the top-volume cosmetics companies in the world.

The most telling transformation is Avon's Web site, www.avon.com. It is state of the art for on-line cosmetics shopping, including accurate ingredient listings and easy navigation (though its search engine is one of the worst, with no ability to find what you type in even when the product exists). Avon has also opened kiosk-style stores at several malls across the country. Add to this the improvement in the quality of its skin-care products and Avon is a player to contend with in the world of cosmetics. The complaint that still lingers for Avon is its sales force. Though they try hard, most of them are little more than order-takers. In fact, most of the representatives I talked to were quite honest about how much they didn't know about makeup or skin care, or specifics about the products they were selling. None of the Avon women I spoke to even had samples or testers. And there is often a great deal of confusion about what products are available during a given "campaign." If you have the wrong book or the products aren't up on the Web site, you're out of luck. That's not just confusing, it's frustrating.

Adding to the confusion is the astonishing number of Avon products. I doubt that any salesperson could keep track of them all anyway, or afford to. In addition, most of the women who work for Avon do it part-time, to earn extra money, not as a major source of income. (The average sales representative earns about $5,000 a year, top sellers earn about $10,000, and only the rare exceptions earn more than $20,000 a year.) That constitutes a sales force whose main interest is not necessarily Avon. (Avon does guarantee 100% satisfaction, and it is true to that policy.)

However, if you know what you want, there are some incredible bargains, particularly within the selections of lip and eye pencils, mascaras, lipsticks, and some very good skin-care products, particularly the water-soluble cleansers and moisturizers for dry skin. Do keep in mind that there are also plenty of poorly formulated and lackluster products that aren't a bargain at any price.

By the way, Avon's line of AHA products, called Anew, went through quite an overhaul that has eliminated the reliability of these products. While it now offers more products than ever before, for the most part the AHA content is missing, and some of the sunscreen additions contain no UVA protection. That isn't an improvement in the least.

I must praise Avon's commitment to consumer information. The operators at its ordering number—(800) 233-2866—and its consumer information center number—(800) 445-2866—were quite helpful. No matter how many products I requested ingredient lists for, they provided them without hesitation or question. Thank you, Avon, for great customer service. Avon's Web site is www.avon.com.

## Avon Skin Care

☺ **Anew Ultra Force Hydrating Cleanser** *($14 for 4 ounces)* is more of a wipe-off cleanser than anything else. It would be OK for someone with normal to dry, sensitive skin, but it won't take off makeup very well and you'll need a washcloth to really clean the face. For the money, Neutrogena's Extra Gentle Cleanser ($7.29 for 6.7 ounces).

☺ **Anew Perfect Cleanser** *($14 for 5.1 ounces)* isn't perfect, it is merely a standard, detergent-based water-soluble cleanser that can be good for most skin types. It does contains a small amount of fragrant oils, which can be skin irritants, but that is true for all fragrance additives.

☺ **Anew O2 Energizer Clarifying Essence** *($14.50 for 4.2 ounces)* has no extra oxygen, unless you count the minuscule amount of yeast in this product that in fermentation lets off air (but not in a cosmetic). Even if it did and could defy physiology and get in the skin, the amount is so minute as to be absurd. This is just an exceptionally ordinary toner of water and glycerin, very basic and very overpriced.

☺ **$$$ Anew Day Force Vertical Lifting Force SPF 15** *($20 for 1 ounce)* won't do anything to get rid of wrinkles, but it is a very good, though very overpriced, moisturizing sunscreen with avobenzone. Both Ombrelle and Lancome (as well as my line) have avobenzone-based sunscreens for far less money.

☹ **Anew Advanced All-in-One Self-Adjusting Perfecting Lotion SPF 15** *($17 for 1.7 ounces)* and ☹ **Anew Advanced All-in-One Self-Adjusting Perfecting Cream SPF 15** *($17 for 1 ounce)* are Avon's attempt to do more revamping of its Anew (AHA) line of products. Why couldn't they just leave well enough alone? These two overly blue-colored moisturizers pale in comparison with other current additions to the line. "Pale" is actually an understatement: these are just very poorly formulated moisturizers from every perspective. Neither of these has UVA protection, and the AHA content is in a pH of about 4.5 to 5, which isn't low enough to make them effective as exfoliators. They don't even come close to the effectiveness of Avon's own Luminosity Skin Brightener SPF 15, Avon Age Block SPF 15, or Anew Day Force Vertical Lifting Force SPF 15.

☹ **Anew Clearly C 10% Vitamin C Serum** *($20 for 1 ounce)* contains mostly alcohol, which is clearly drying and a skin irritant. It does contain ascorbic acid, a form of vitamin C, but that is considered one of the more irritating and least stable forms of this vitamin when it comes to antioxidant properties.

☹ **Anew Direct C Vitamin C Facial Patches** *($15 for 16 patches)* is similar to the Vitamin C Serum above, although this version does leave out the alcohol.

☺ **Anew Formula C Treatment Capsules** *($19 for 30 0.41-ounce capsules)* is a pricey way to get ascorbic acid to the skin. The encapsulation does make it more stable, but it is still irritating and there are other forms of vitamin C that are considered better for skin. If you need vitamin C, though, there is no reason to consider this ingredient the answer for skin—there are less expensive and better ways to do it.

☺ **$$$ Anew Eye Force Vertical Lifting Complex** *($18 for 0.5 ounce)* is a good lightweight moisturizer. From my point of view, this formula is very close to Clinique's Stop Signs, even the inclusion of caffeine. In some ways, this product has better moisturizing ingredients (meaning ingredients that mimic the skin's own structure) than Clinique's does. However, in terms of price, they end up being about the same. In fact, ounce for ounce, Avon's is about $4 more expensive than Clinique's.

☺ **$$$ Anew Instant Eye Smoother** *($16 for 0.5 ounce)* is a good, silicone-based moisturizer for normal to dry skin and would work well to smooth and soothe. It is in many ways quite similar to Clinique's All About Eyes.

☹ **$$$ Intensive Line Minimizer** *($12.50 for 0.13 ounce)* comes with a wand applicator, the most inefficient, overpriced way to use an AHA product. While it does have a good concentration of AHA (glycolic acid) and a low pH, the price is bizarre: it ends up being almost $100 for an ounce of this stuff. That makes this one of the most expensive AHA products on the market and absolutely not worth it.

☺ **Luminosity Skin Brightener SPF 15** *($20 for 1.7 ounces)* is a good, avobenzone-based sunscreen for normal to slightly dry skin. That makes it a mediocre moisturizer for normal to dry skin (assuming the amount of alcohol is so minor it would not be irritating for skin). It also contains a form of AHA but only about 2%, which isn't enough for it to work as an exfoliant (though it acts as a good water-binding agent). The plant extracts of bilberry, licorice, and mulberry are supposed to reduce brown patches, but the research is minimal for these, and especially not in a cosmetic (as opposed to their pure form). What this product does contain is a good group of antioxidants with very technical long names extracted from curcumin.

☺ **Anew Moisture Supply Day Cream** *($16 for 1.7 ounces)* is a very good moisturizer for dry skin, but for daytime you would need to add a sunscreen.

☺ **Anew Moisture Supply Night Cream** *($16 for 1.7 ounces)* is just a simple moisturizer. It would be good for someone with dry skin, but the Supply Day Cream version above is a more state-of-the-art formulation.

☺ **Anew Night Force Vertical Lifting Complex** *($20 for 1.7 ounces)*. From my point of view, this formula is very close to Clinique's Stop Signs, even the inclusion of caffeine. In some ways, this product has better moisturizing ingredients (meaning ingredients that mimic the skin's own structure) than Clinique's does. However, in terms of price, they end up being about the same. In fact, ounce for ounce, Avon's is about $4 more expensive than Clinique's.

☺ Anew Night Force Vertical Lifting Complex *($20 for 1.7 ounces)* does have two new ingredients that I haven't seen anywhere else that show up in several Avon products: ammonium trioxaundecanedioate and trioxaundecanedioic acid. At this writing, I can't find independently confirmed information about what they do, but I suspect they are some kind of thickening agent and possibly a peeling agent; right now, no research or sources describing what these do is anywhere to be found.

☺ Anew Perfect Eye Care Cream SPF 15 *($13.50 for 0.53 ounce)* is a product containing about 2% AHAs with a pH of 6, which makes it a poor exfoliant. Though the AHA part is misleading, part of the SPF 15 is titanium dioxide, and that's good. This is a good moisturizer.

☺ $$$ Anew Perfecting Lotion for Problem Skin *($16 for 1.7 ounces)* is a standard lotion-based product that also contains about 0.5% BHA and about 2% AHA. There isn't enough AHA in here for that to be effective, and the BHA amount is small but can be of help for exfoliation. This is minimally an option for exfoliating within the pore for most skin types to reduce clogged pores.

☺ Anew Retinol Recovery Complex P.M. Treatment *($17.50 for 1 ounce)* is just a good standard moisturizer for someone with normal to dry skin, and that's it. Research does show that retinol, a vitamin A derivative, can benefit the skin; however, it takes a lot more retinol than this product contains. Still, if you're looking for a retinol product, this one is as good as any being sold and the packaging is appropriate to keep the retinol stable.

☺ Anew Skintrition Multi-Vitamin Skin Primer *($20 for 1.7 ounces)*. If you were looking for every vitamin and mineral under the sun, this product contains them (well, almost). The amounts are negligible but no one has any information about how much the skin needs of any of this stuff anyway, so it doesn't really matter. This lightweight, silicone-based moisturizer would be good for normal to slightly dry skin and it competes nicely with Estee Lauder's Nutritious Bio Protein *($45 for 1.7 ounces)* and Origins Night-A-Mins *($27.50 for 1.7 ounces)*. Avon's version contains mostly water, silicones, slip agents, salt, thickener, lots of vitamins and minerals, plant oil, preservatives, and fragrance.

☹ Anew Alpha Peel Off Facial Mask *($13 for 2.5 ounces)* contains a film former in an alcohol base that hardens and then is peeled off. It also contains about 4% AHA, but in a pH of 5, which is too high for the AHA to work as an exfoliant. This is a mask that can cause irritation and dryness, and though the peeling effect may produce a temporary smooth feel, the risks outweigh that brief positive.

☹ **Clearskin Cleansing Pads for Sensitive Skin** *($3.99 for 42 pads)* contains alcohol and menthol, which makes the product too irritating and drying for all skin types, especially for sensitive skin.

☹ **Clearskin Maximum Strength Cleansing Pads** *($3.49 for 42 pads)* is even more irritating than the Cleansing Pads above.

☹ **Clearskin Antibacterial Cleansing Scrub** *($3.49 for 2.5 ounces).* As a scrub this is OK, but the oils are not great for anyone with oily skin, and the menthol and alcohol are irritating for any skin type.

☺ **Clearskin 10% Benzoyl Peroxide Vanishing Cream** *($3.99 for 0.75 ounce)* is a good topical disinfectant for blemishes and would work well for most skin types.

☹ **Clearskin Overnight Acne Treatment** *($3.49 for 2 ounces)* contains alcohol as the second ingredient, which makes it too irritating and drying for all skin types.

☹ **Clearskin Clay Mask** *($3.99 for 3 ounces)* is a standard clay mask with alcohol and cornstarch, two very problematic ingredients for acne-prone skin.

☹ **Clearskin Clearbreeze Astringent** *($3.49 for 8 ounces).* The number of irritating ingredients in this product is astounding and none of them are beneficial for the skin.

☹ **Clearskin Astringent Cleansing Extra-Strength Cleansing Lotion** *($3.99 for 8 ounces)* contains more alcohol than anyone should even consider allowing near their face.

☺ **$$$ Purifying Pore Patch Deep Cleansing Face Strips** *($6),* like all pore strips, is basically gauze and a form of hairspray (film former). Avon's contains a bit of silicone, probably to help with sticking, as well as salicylic acid (BHA). These can make a difference if you have noticeable black dots on your face, but they do not eliminate the problem. Please be aware that all pore strips have five to six user warnings that include the possibility of skin tearing, as well as directions not to use them over blemishes or if you are taking certain acne medications.

☹ **Pore Reducer Beauty Treatment Mask** *($8.50 for 3.4 ounces)* contains alcohol as the second ingredient as well as balm mint, and that makes it too irritating and drying for all skin types.

☺ **$$$ Naturally Almond Cleansing Milk** *($20 for 5 ounces)* is a very standard cold cream–like lotion that can leave a greasy film on the skin. It would be OK for someone with dry skin but it takes a washcloth to get this stuff off and this is pricey for what you get.

☺ **$$$ Ultra-Cleansing Deep Pore Cleanser** *($17 for 3.4 ounces)* uses sodium lauryl sulfate as the main cleansing agent, which can be too irritating and sensitizing for all skin types.

☺ **Daily Balance Everyday Toner** *($17 for 8.4 ounces)* is a good, but very basic toner for normal to dry skin.

☹ **Positive Improvement Toning Serum** *($20 for 1.7 ounces)* lists the second ingredient as alcohol and it also contains ivy and lemon, which makes this one positively irritating.

☺ **Positivity Recharging P.M. Replenisher** *($25 for 1 ounce)* has over 57 ingredients, and so you might hope something in here could live up to the promise of reducing hot flashes for those having warm moments in their middle years. This 2% AHA product won't do it. The plant extracts are nice but have no effect on the hormonal rush or change in skin texture that a lack of estrogen can cause. One of the plant extracts is soy, which can contain phytoestrogen (meaning a plant source of estrogen). However, the minuscule amount of soy in here does not have any potential of having estrogenic effects on the skin. Positivity also contains saw palmetto. Saw palmetto's primary reputation is for reducing the presence of dihydrotestosterone, the male hormone responsible for hair loss, though this has not been proven, and is strictly theory. There is some anecdotal information that saw palmetto can have an estrogenic effect, but that is unlikely, and is highly improbable when applied topically. This is a good basic moisturizer. It's OK, but not worth the money or effort.

☺ **Positivity Empowering A.M. Fortifier SPF 15** *($25 for 1 ounce)* definitely has avobenzone, but the third ingredient is alcohol, which makes this potentially drying and irritating for most skin types. With all the good avobenzone-based sunscreens available now, it is possible to be more critical of less-satisfactory formulations. The claims about it improving menopause are the same as for the P.M. version above.

☹ **Positivity Empowering Spritz** *($15 for 1 ounce)*. With alcohol, menthol, and ginseng being the first ingredients, you will get a cooling sensation but you will also get dryness and irritation too.

☹ **7 Day Wonder Intensive Skin Moisture Ampoules** *($35 for seven 0.08-ounce capsules)* list the second ingredient as alcohol, which makes this one wonderfully irritating.

☺ **Age Block Daytime Defense Cream SPF 15 UVA/UVB Protection** *($12.50 for 1.7 ounces)* definitely has avobenzone for UVA protection, but the third and fifth ingredients are forms of alcohol, which makes this potentially drying and irritating for most skin types. With all the good avobenzone-based sunscreens available now, it is possible to be more critical of general formulations like this. Age Block is a disappointment, because the other ingredients in the listing are actually quite good. But the entire contents should be good for skin, not just some of them.

☺ **Eye Block Environmental Protection Cream** *($12.50 for 0.5 ounce)* is almost identical to the Age Block above only this version has slightly less alcohol; that is still too much for the skin, however, especially the area around the eye.

☹ **Eye Perfector Soothing Eye Gel with Liposomes** *($9 for 0.5 ounce)* lists witch hazel as the second ingredient; it also contain ginseng, which can be drying and irritating for the skin. It does contain several anti-irritants, but why add any irritating ingredients to the eye area at all?

☺ **Hydrofirming Cream Night Treatment** *($11 for 1.7 ounces)* is a good emollient moisturizer with antioxidants and good water-binding agents for someone with dry skin. The cream won't firm anything, but it is an excellent emollient moisturizer for someone with dry skin.

☺ **Hydrofirming Eye Treatment** *($9.50 for 0.5 ounce)* is a good emollient moisturizer with antioxidants and good water-binding agents for someone with dry skin. The cream won't firm anything, but it is an excellent emollient moisturizer for someone with dry skin.

☹ **Hydrofirming Day Cream SPF 15** *($11.50 for 1.7 ounces)* doesn't contain titanium dioxide, zinc oxide, or avobenzone, and is not recommended.

☹ **Hydrofirming Day Lotion SPF 15** *($11.50 for 1.7 ounces)* doesn't contain titanium dioxide, zinc oxide, or avobenzone, and is not recommended.

☺ **$$$ Refraiche Me Cleansing Foam** *($20 for 5 ounces)* is an exceptionally standard, detergent-based water-soluble cleanser that would work well for someone with normal to oily skin, though it is probably too drying for those with normal to dry skin. It does contain fragrance.

☺ **$$$ Refraiche Me Re-Texturizing Moisture Treatment** *($20 for 1.7 ounces)*. Some of the plant extracts can be good anti-irritants, while others can be irritants. Other than that, this is a good basic moisturizer for normal to dry skin.

☺ **$$$ Refraiche Me Re-Texturizing Moisture Lotion** *($20 for 1.7 ounces)*. The Treatment version above is far more interesting than this one, though it is still a good moisturizer for someone with normal to dry skin.

☹ **$$$ Facial Renewal Gel Mask** *($17 for 2.5 ounces)* is little more than a gel moisturizer. This do-nothing mask contains several plant extracts that can be skin irritants.

☺ **Lighten Up Undereye Treatment** *($14.50 for 0.5 ounce)* is supposed to reduce dark circles and diminish lines, just what most women want from an eye product. It is a very good emollient moisturizer for any area of the face, but it contains nothing that makes it better for the eye area and nothing that will lighten the eye area anymore than hundreds of other moisturizers. This one does contain magnesium ascorbyl phosphate, a form of vitamin C, but there is no evidence this can lighten any area of skin.

☺ **Banishing Cream Skin Lightening Treatment** *($8.50 for 2.5 ounces)* can have an effect on darkened patches of skin. It uses 2% hydroquinone in a fairly standard moisturizing base of water, thickeners, petrolatum, and preservatives. Like all hydroquinone-based skin-lightening products, it can improve pigment problems if you are using a reliable sunscreen every day; just don't expect the dark areas to go away completely.

☺ $$$ On Everyone's Lips Daily Lip Refiner *($8.50 for 0.5 ounce)* won't refine anything, but it is a good "lip filler." To help hold lipstick in place, it is minimally effective. The AHAs in here are not in the right pH or amount to be effective as exfoliants.

☺ Skin–So–Soft Kids Sunblock SPF 40 *($9 for 4.2 ounces)* is a good, part-avobenzone-based sunscreen. It would work well for someone with normal to slightly dry or slightly oily skin.

☺ Stress Shield Serum *($12.50 for 1 ounce)* is a good 5% AHA product, but that has nothing to do with fighting or preventing stress.

☹ Skin–So–Soft Bug Guard Mosquito Repellent SPF 15 Moisturizing Sunblock Spray *($9.95 for 4 ounces)* doesn't contain avobenzone, zinc oxide, or titanium dioxide, and is not recommended. What about repelling bugs? It does contain the biochemical pesticides butylacetylaminopropionate and butylacetylaminopropionic. While these will keep bugs away, they are also potent chemicals and can be problematic for skin and mucous membranes.

☺ Sun–So–Soft Kids Sunblock SPF 40 *($9 for 4.2 ounces)* does contain in part avobenzone, and that makes it a great sunscreen for UVA and UVB protection, and not just for kids. However, if the issue is one of skin sensitivity, then the synthetic sunscreen agents, though effective, are not the most gentle for skin. For that you would need a sunscreen that used only titanium dioxide or/and zinc oxide as the active agent and that didn't include fragrance. This would be good for normal to slightly dry or oily skin.

☺ Sun–So–Soft Moisturizing Suncare Plus SPF 15 *($9 for 4.2 ounces)* is similar to the SPF 40 above and the same comments apply.

☺ Sun–So–Soft Moisturizing Suncare Plus SPF 30 *($9 for 4.2 ounces)* is similar to the SPF 40 above and the same comments apply.

☺ Sun–So–Soft SPF 25 Sunscreen Stick *($7.50 for 0.42 ounce)* is a very good in-part avobenzone-based sunscreen in stick form. This is definitely an emollient sunscreen that contains mostly plant oil (mostly castor oil, which can feel sticky), thickeners, plant oils, aloe, vitamins, antioxidant, plant extracts, and fragrance.

☹ Sun–So–Soft SPF 8 Sunscreen Spray Lotion *($7.50 for 4.2 ounces)*, with its pitiful SPF 8 and no UVA-protecting ingredients, is not recommended.

☹ Sun–So–Soft SPF 15 Lip Balm *($1.50 for 0.15 ounce)* doesn't contain UVA-protecting ingredients and is not recommend.

☺ New Figure Cellulite Body Cream *($10 for 2 ounces)* is supposed to "improve the appearance of skin in cellulite-prone areas and smooth skin in areas subject to stretch marks. And it's been clinically proven to show results in as few as four weeks." All that for $10. My, oh, my! Of course, the copy doesn't say it will get rid of cellulite or stretch marks, just improve their appearance, which any moisturizer could. Salicylic acid can help exfoliate skin, but won't change a bump on your body.

# Avon Makeup

**FOUNDATION:** ☹ **Perfect Wear Foundation SPF 6** *($10)* does have a titanium dioxide–based sunscreen, but the dismal SPF 6 makes it pretty useless. This is Avon's version of a stay-put foundation, and it does work OK although the texture leaves much to be desired, having a dry feel and an almost sticky finish. Also, all of these colors have some amount of sparkle. What is shine doing in a product meant to have a matte, transfer-resistant finish? Of the 16 shades, these colors are too peach, pink, or rose for most skin tones: Honey Beige, Soft Bisque, Ivory Beige, Cocoa, Warm Bronze, Almond Beige, Rose Beige, Blush Tint, and Toasted Brown.

☺ **Hydra Finish Stick Foundation SPF 8** *($9)* is a water-to-powder stick foundation (much like Olay's All Day Moisture Stick) that has a cool, wet application and quickly dries to a reasonably solid powder finish. The texture is light, though blending takes some practice for even application and to prevent streaks, but it can be an option for normal to slightly oily skins that wish to use a stick foundation and want a sheer finish. There are 16 shades with options for very light but not very dark skin tones, and the SPF, though too low for reliable, all-day protection, does contain titanium dioxide. These colors are too peach, pink, or rose for most skin tones: Honey Beige, Rich Copper, Warmest Beige, Rich Honey, Cappuccino, Blush Beige, and Natural Cream.

☹ **Beyond Color Vertical Lift Foundation SPF 8** *($12)* has a reliable titanium-dioxide sunscreen but an unimpressive SPF, so it should not be relied on for daily protection. It comes with statistics and percentages showing how improved your skin will look after using it. Yet after using this product with such a paltry SPF, there is no way that you are going to have improved skin. Basically, this is just a very lightweight, sheer, silicone-based foundation with a matte, almost staining finish, which would be fine except the colors are some of the worst I've seen in a long time. For the most part, all of the 16 shades are too peach or pink to consider, and I mean *really* peach or pink. The only ones worth considering are Natural Cream, Classic Ivory, Honey Beige, Toast, Rich Honey, and Cappuccino (good for dark skins). One more warning: the fragrance of this is so sickly sweet I almost couldn't finish this review.

☺ **Face Lift Moisture Firm Foundation** *($9)* is a light, creamy foundation that would work well for someone with dry skin. It doesn't lift skin anywhere, but does blend smoothly and provides light-to-medium coverage. There are 18 shades, and some of them are decent options, but consider avoiding these shades: Natural Fawn, Bisque, Ivory Beige, Rich Honey, Honey Beige, Almond Beige, Rose Tint Beige, Copper, Toast, Cocoa, and Cool Copper.

☺ **Clear Finish Oil Free Foundation Anti Acne Treatment** *($5.25)* gets its anti-acne effects with salicylic acid (BHA). BHA isn't a treatment, it's an exfoliant, and it works better in skin-care products in which the pH is around 3 and you have better control over where and how often your skin needs it. This foundation has a pH of 5, which means the BHA won't even exfoliate well. Still, this does have a lightweight texture and leaves a soft matte finish. There are 19 shades to choose from, and these are the ones to steer clear of due to overtones of peach, rose, or pink: Creamy Beige, Ivory Beige, True Beige, Soft Bisque, Blush Beige, Rose Tint Beige, Honey Beige, Warmest Beige, Cool Copper, Toasted Tan, Rich Copper, and Cocoa.

☹ **Triple Finish Cream to Powder Foundation** *($8)* is a terrible option for cream-to-powder makeup. Not only does this have a dry, almost rough powdery finish, it applies unevenly, and virtually all of the 16 colors are glaringly peach, pink, or rose. The few possible colors are hurt by this makeup's unpleasant texture.

☹ **Sunny Outlook Liquid Face Bronzer** *($7)* is as far removed from bronzer as broccoli is from chocolate cake. It is a sheer liquid whose color is an unsuitable orangy-pink!

<u>CONCEALER:</u> ☹ **Perfect Wear Concealer** *($6.50)* comes in a tube with a wand applicator and has an awful, runny texture and colors that significantly darken once they dry into place—just the opposite of what a concealer is supposed to do.

☺ **Concealing Stick** *($4.25)* has a far superior texture and finish than the one above, but it is still lacking in shade selection. Only Light Clair is worth considering, and then only if you have light skin.

☺ **Big Cover Up Concealer Pen** *($4.75)* is actually a decent concealer that goes on somewhat thick but blends out smooth and even with minimal to no creasing. Unfortunately, this thick pencil-style of application is made more difficult because sharpening is so time-consuming and messy.

<u>POWDER:</u> ☺ **Translucent Loose Powder** *($8)* has a very agreeable soft, silky texture and a nice (improved) matte finish. The container features a unique way to minimize loose powder's messy tendencies, as once you take the top off you twist the container and a small amount of powder is pushed up from below. Very clever and helpful, but it would be even better if this came in more than two colors! **Translucent Pressed Powder** *($8)* also has a pleasant texture and dry finish. It comes in six colors, and the only one to avoid is Deep 2, which is too orange and doesn't look anything like skin.

☹ **Bronzing Powder** *($6.75)* comes in three shades, and all of them are slightly too intensely shiny. Also, the powdery texture can be messy while applying this one.

<u>BLUSH:</u> ☺ **True Color Powder Blush** *($8)* has a sheer, powdery texture and some amount of shine. These could work for an evening look, but iridescent cheeks look out of place in daylight or at the office. **Natural Radiance Blush Stick** *($5)* is a cream blush in a twist-up stick. You can swipe this fairly greasy, somewhat iridescent blush over the cheeks and blend it out fairly sheer.

☹ **Perfect Wear Blush** *($9.50)* is only perfect if left alone. This has a do-nothing, dry texture that takes a lot of effort and patience to apply, and the aftermath is less than stellar. **Hydra Finish Cheek Color** *($9.50)* is a two-part product—at least Avon was kind enough to separate the one with shine. In addition to the shiny cream highlighter side (which is the same color for every blush shade), there is a cream-to-powder blush part that blends on very sheer but can still look spotted and uneven, which is not a good look for anyone. **Bronzing Stick** *($7.50)* comes in two shades, with more shine than any face should be asked to handle and a greasy texture to boot.

☹ <u>EYESHADOW</u>: **True Color Powder Eyeshadow Quad** *($5.50)* is conveniently separated out into cool and warm tones, and there are some attractive, soft neutral shades. These are further labeled as matte or shiny, but most of the colors labeled as matte are indeed shiny, which is very disappointing for those who don't wish to make their eyelids look wrinkly. **Perfect Wear Eye Color** *($6.50)* are wind-up cream eyeshadow sticks with a creamy/waxy texture and an unpleasant finish. The fact that most of these are shiny adds nothing to their limited appeal. **Beyond Color Triple Benefit Eyeshadow** *($6.50)* doesn't have one benefit. It has a creamy, almost greasy texture with way too much slip for even, controlled blending and colors that are high-wattage shine that will put the spotlight on any and all wrinkles. **Hydra Finish Eye Color** *($6.50)* is another poor option for shadow. These water-based (and very shiny) colors come in a pot and tend to dry out quickly, which makes them very difficult to use, ensuring a choppy application.

<u>EYE AND BROW SHAPER:</u> ☺ **Perfect Wear Eye Liner** *($6.50)* is an automatic pencil that has a creamy, slightly sticky texture. There are much better options available in this price range at the drugstore that aren't this greasy. **Brow Shaper** *($6)* is tinted brow gel with an OK brush and two decent colors, with nothing for lighter brows. It has a non-sticky texture. **Brow Powder** *($6)* is matte powder for the brows, and works as well as any, although these do go on very sheer, so be prepared to experiment until you achieve the intensity you prefer.

☹ **Duplicity Wet/Dry Eyeliner** *($4)* are standard pencils that can be used wet or dry. The texture is greasy when applied without water, and runny and streaky when used with water. What a shame, because it's an intriguing concept and the price is right! **Hydra Finish Gel Eye Pencil** *($6.50)* has a very slick, smooth application that is supposed to be a cross between pencil and liquid liner. It ends up being too creamy to stay put, and the point is too soft and wide for a thin line. By the way, this is a reformulated version of Avon's overhyped Hydro Liner Liquid Eye Gel Pencil. **Perfect Wear Liquid Eyeliner Pen** *($6.29)* has a stiff brush that isn't the best if you want to create a controlled, even line. It goes on fairly wet, dries to a matte finish, and doesn't chip—yet the color can look uneven and streaky when it has dried.

☺ **Glimmerstick Eye Liner** *($5.50)* and **Glimmerstick Brow Definer** *($5.50)* are both automatic pencils with standard textures that are indistinguishable from each other and work as well as any pencil you will find but do beware of the blue, green, and shiny colors.

LIPSTICK AND LIP PENCIL: ☺ **Beyond Color Triple Benefit Lipstick SPF 12** *($7.50)* and **Color Rich Renewable Lipstick** *($7.50)* are virtually identical. They are both very emollient, mostly glossy lipsticks that come in an extensive range of colors. They do have enough stain to keep the color around longer than some. The Beyond Color's SPF is without good UVA protection. **Satin Moisture 15 Lipstick SPF 15** *($5.50)* is more of a sheer gloss than a lipstick, and does not have adequate UVA protection. **Marbelized Lip Color** *($6)* is a split-side lipstick, with half being creamy and semi-opaque and half being sheer and frosted. It's eye-catching but still just a glossy lipstick. **Glazewear Liquid Lip Color** *($7)* is similar to Revlon's ColorStay Liquid Lip, in that both are basically heavily pigmented glosses that go on slick and stay wet-looking without the usual fleeting quality seen in traditional gloss. **Beyond Bronze Split Lipstick SPF 15** *($6)* is identical to the Marbelized Lip Color, only this one has added a UVA-deficient sunscreen and the colors are bronze tones. **Perfect Wear Lip Liner** *($6)* is an automatic pencil that goes on thick and creamy and is nearly identical to the **Glimmerstick Lip Liner** *($5.50)*, which has a slightly softer texture.

☹ **Perfect Wear Double Performance Lipstick** *($7.50)* is Avon's ultra-matte lipstick, but it is not all that matte. Rather, it has a very slick texture and a slightly creamy finish. These do have a lot of stain, which makes for longer wear, but be careful: most of the colors are frosted. **Hydra Finish Lip Color** *($8)* is just a moist, greasy lipstick that feels slippery and would not be a good choice if you have any lines around your mouth or need your lipstick to last.

MASCARA: ☹ **Hydra Finish Soft 'N Natural Mascara** *($5.50)* is a watery mascara that takes forever to build the least amount of length and no thickness. **One Great Mascara** *($6.50)* isn't all that great. It does start out with great promise of building long lashes, but it tends to clump and look sparse, creating little thickness or lash definition. However, for minimal length it is an option as it doesn't smear or flake. **Voluptuous Full-Figured Mascara** *($5.50)* is a decent mascara that claims it "dramatically increases the dimensions of lashes" but doesn't come close, and can also go on spiky. **Incredible Lengths Long and Strong Mascara** *($5.50)* is a thick, clumpy, do-nothing mascara, and **Beyond Color Triple Benefit Lash Conditioner** *($5.50)* is a standard lash primer that adds unnecessary weight to fragile lashes and is not required if you are using any of the superior mascaras (not Avon's) available.

# *Awake*

The makeup collection from this relatively new cosmetic line from Japan called Awake is worth getting up for. All of the requisite products are here, from foundations to mascara, and many of them have enviable textures that apply evenly. The same philosophies extolled in its skin-care products are here as well, which are little more than marketing hype and not what is giving you the product's end result. One point of interest is Awake's assertion that it uses specially treated pigments in its makeup to "reduce irritation." Treated pigments are pretty much the standard throughout the cosmetics industry, and are chiefly used to make colors more stable, thus enhancing their longevity. Awake uses this claim with the angle that its cosmetics are more suited to sensitive skin, but there is no proof for this assertion. Regardless of claims, you will find some excellent options within Awake's range of foundations, as well as excellent mascaras. The tester unit is user-friendly, but the colors would benefit from a better organizational scheme.

When it comes to skin care, Awake should wake up to some basic information about irritation and skin sensitivity. The cleansers are fairly strong, lots of the products contain potentially irritating or sensitizing plant extracts, and there are no real options for very dry skin or for those with blemish-prone skin. Some of the comments made about the products defy logic: "skin rejuvenates by retaining oxygen and protecting cells from free radicals." But since oxygen causes free-radical damage, how does it help to have the skin retain the very thing that is causing the problem? Awake's brochure explains that "glycine is an amino acid that makes up 33% of collagen" and implies that therefore glycine can somehow affect the production of collagen in skin. It can't. Protein is a complex structure made up of an intricate network of amino acids, and triggering just one won't get the collagen to change. The technology for these products is not advanced in the least and actually leaves much to be desired.

For more information about Awake, call (212) 598-4400 or visit the Web site at www.awakecosmetics.com.

# Awake Skin Care

☹ **$$$ Clear Cream Wash for Dry Skin** *($25 for 4.2 ounces)* is a standard, detergent-based water-soluble cleanser that could work well for normal to dry skin but the cleaning agents and several plant extracts can be irritating and sensitizing for the skin.

☹ **$$$ Clear Cream Wash for Oily Skin** *($25 for 4.2 ounces)* is similar to the Dry Skin version above and the same concerns apply.

☹ **$$$ Clear Gel Wash for Combination Skin** *($25 for 4.2 ounces)* is similar to the Dry Skin version above and the same concerns apply.

☹ **$$$ Point Makeup Remover (Eye and Lip)** *($25 for 2.1 ounces)* is basically mineral oil with some film former, slip agent, and preservatives. If you want this kind of product, your skin and pocketbook would be far happier with just plain mineral oil!

☹ **Lotion Refresher** *($25 for 6.3 ounces)*. Several of the plant extracts in here can be irritating or sensitizing for skin, including ivy, lemon, pine cone, and sage.

☹ **Lotion Exfolizer** *($30 for 3.3 ounces)* lists its second ingredient as alcohol, which makes it a problem for all skin types.

☺ $$$ **Direct Nutrition** *($65 for 1 ounce)* is just a good, basic moisturizer for normal to dry skin that would work well but is absurdly overpriced for what you get. Avon has moisturizers with more interesting formulations than this one.

☺ $$$ **Hydro Plus** *($40 for 1.4 ounces)*. The amount of plant extracts in here is not even worth mentioning. Some of the plant extracts can be anti-irritants while others are skin sensitizers—what a waste. Other than that, it is just a good, light-weight moisturizer for normal to slightly dry skin. It would work well, but Avon has moisturizers with more interesting formulations than this one.

☹ **Hydro-Plus Eyes** *($40 for 0.7 ounce)* contains far too many irritating ingredients to make this a benefit for skin, including alcohol, lemon, ginseng, pine cone, and sage.

☹ **Nano Essence** *($60 for 0.8 ounce)* is similar to the Hydro Plus above and the same basic comments apply.

☺ $$$ **Nano Essence AX Dry Skin** *($60 for 0.8 ounce)* is a good, lightweight moisturizer for normal to slightly dry skin, with good antioxidants, but there is no reason it would change anything and the price is the only thing really significant about this product. The yeast in here won't provide oxygen to the skin as claimed, and the serine, an amino acid, won't affect collagen in skin.

☹ **Nano Lotion White** *($40 for 2.1 ounces)* lists its second ingredient as alcohol, which is a problem for all skin types and doesn't help to lighten skin.

☹ **Lotion Whitener** *($40 for 6 ounces)* has alcohol as the second ingredient, and that will only serve to irritate the skin. There are several plant extracts in here but none that will reduce melanin production. Actually the plant extracts are the same as in all of the Awake products, and they can mostly be skin irritants.

☺ $$$ **Skin Renovation** *($95 for 1 ounce)* is a very good, lightweight moisturizer for normal to slightly dry skin, but it won't renovate anything and the price is the only thing really significant about this product. The yeast in here won't provide oxygen to the skin as claimed, and the serine, an amino acid, won't affect collagen in skin.

☹ $$$ **Skin Renovation Eye** *($90 for 0.7 ounce)* is about as basic a moisturizer as you can find, and for those who can read ingredient listings it would only make your eyes hurt to realize what your money is buying. Alcohol is rather high up on the ingredient listing and is probably here as the preservative, which means the interesting ingredients are in short supply. This is more of a toner serum than anything else and won't renovate anything.

☹ **True-Matte Fresh** *($40 for 2.1 ounces)* lists its second ingredient as alcohol, and it also contains lemon, menthol, ivy, sage, and pine cone, making it a very expensive way to irritate the skin.

☹ **Cream Exfolizer** *($35 for 1 ounce)*. There is nothing in this product that can exfoliate skin, but there are several plant extracts that can be irritating, including ivy, lemon, pine cone, sage, and soapwort.

☺ **$$$ Eye Concentrate Mask** *($50 for 0.7 ounce and 20 sheets)*. What makes this product unique is that you get a really small vial of a lotion and 20 sheets of a material that you soak with the lotion. You then place them on the face and the sheets become clear. You are supposed to believe that the sheets are like skin and that they help heal and cure whatever is taking place in your skin. What a concept! But the sheets aren't like skin in the least and the ingredients don't add up to much. It does contain soybean extract, which can be an antioxidant and possibly soothing for skin, but the estrogenic effects it can have when taken orally cannot be absorbed through skin.

☺ **Gentle Day Protection SPF 16 Sunscreen** *($30 for 1 ounce)* is a very good, pure titanium dioxide–based sunscreen in a very basic moisturizing base. Several of the plant extracts in here are potential skin irritants. There is nothing this product offers that Neutrogena's Sensitive Skin UVA/UVB Block SPF 17 *($8.99 for 4 ounces)* and Sensitive Skin UVA/UVB Block SPF 30 *($8.99 for 4 ounces)*, both pure titanium-dioxide sunblocks, don't do far better without the irritating ingredients and for far less money.

☹ **Pop-Out Mask** *($15 for 24 pieces)* is an expanding sponge material that becomes a full sheet when soaked with Awake's Lotion Refresher or Lotion Whitener. This just absorbs and wastes a lot more product than your skin needs.

☹ **Sebum Clear Mask** *($40 for 2.1 ounces)* has a hairspray ingredient (film former) first on its ingredient list, the third is alcohol, and the plant extracts in here can be skin irritants, so in general this product is more of a problem than it could ever be a help.

☹ **Smooth Clear Mask** *($40 for 2.8 ounces)* is almost identical to the Sebum Clear Mask above and the same comments apply.

☺ **$$$ Vital Express** *($60 for four 0.14-ounce capsules)* does contain vitamin C (magnesium ascorbyl palmitate) with some slip agents, but that's about it. If you want vitamin C, this is an option, but this won't help skin, and the dent in your pocketbook for what you get is painful.

## Awake Makeup

**FOUNDATION:** Although I like Awake's foundation textures very much, many of the colors have a slight peach tone to them and there are no suitable colors for very dark skin tones.

☺ $$$ **Hydro-Touch Foundation SPF 18** *($40 with compact; $30 for refills)* is very similar to Vincent Longo's Water Canvas Foundation, probably because they are made by the same manufacturer. Awake's version (which it claims is superior to the ones in other lines) has a reliable in-part titanium dioxide–based sunscreen and maintains a slightly less wet feel than Longo's. But both have a wet, cool application and then dry to a matte finish that provides sheer to light coverage. This one requires deft, quick blending, as the formula tends to dry quickly into place and is then not easy to move. This new breed of water-to-powder foundation (as opposed to cream-to-powder) works best on normal to oily skin (the cream versions contain ingredients that are problematic for oily or blemish-prone skin). This foundation has nine mostly neutral shades to choose from, with options for very light skin tones. Peach and Ecru can be too peach for most skin tones.

☺ $$$ **Oil Free Foundation** *($32)* is a very sheer, liquidy foundation that has a smooth texture and a soft, natural finish. For those who prefer slight coverage and have normal to slightly oily skin, this is an option and blends out effortlessly. Of the ten shades, five are too orange or peach to recommend: Buff, Peach, Sand, Beige, and Dark Tan. There are some very light shades to consider, but nothing suitable for darker skin.

☺ $$$ **Fine Finish Foundation** *($38 with compact; $28 refill; $4 for sponge)* is Awake's rendition of a wet/dry powder foundation, which is nothing more than a talc-based pressed powder. It does have an incredibly smooth, silky texture. This would be best for normal to slightly dry skin or slightly oily skin, but the emollient feel this imparts would not be great over oily skin and the powder part can be drying for dry skin types. As usual, wet application of this type of foundation can produce streaks and an uneven finish, but used dry it is beautiful. Of the ten shades, these three are too peach for most skin tones: Sand, Beige, and Dark Tan.

☺ $$$ <u>CONCEALER:</u> **Concealer** *($18)* comes in a compact; it has a rather tacky feel and a slightly greasy application, but it does dry to a natural matte finish with minimal risk of creasing. The one drawback is that this only provides moderate coverage, and if you layer more on to get the results you may need, it can end up looking heavy or dry. The six shades are quite workable, with the exception of Ecru and Bronze, which are too peach for most skin tones.

<u>POWDER:</u> ☺ $$$ **Loose Powder** *($28)* is a standard, talc-based powder that has a very silky texture and a sheer finish. The container it comes in can make applying this even messier than it usually is for loose powder. The five shades are mostly neutral; Ivory and Nude are extremely light and great for pale skin tones.

☺ $$$ **Nuance Veil** *($35)* is a compact-type pressed powder with four colors swirled together in either a pale flesh tone or a bronzer. Both products come off as one color on the skin and have a noticeable shiny finish.

☺ **$$$ BLUSH:** The powder **Blush** *($18)* comes in ten predominantly warm-toned shades and has a lovely, soft texture. There are some shiny shades here, but nothing too intense.

☹ **$$$ EYESHADOW: Multidimension Eye** *($36)* is a set of three shadows, all sheer and very shimmery. Their texture is gorgeous, but the color combinations are hardly amenable to an understated look. **Eye Shadow** *($16)* has a large collection of single, somewhat powdery shadows, all with a smooth texture. About half of the shades are shiny, and there are a number of blues and greens to ignore, but the matte shades are worth a try.

☹ **EYE AND BROW SHAPER:** Both the **Eye Pencil** *($15)* and the **Brow Pencil** *($15)* are standard fare, with a dry texture and a soft powder finish. The Brow Pencil is very easy to apply, and is worth considering if you prefer pencil to powder.

☺ **LIPSTICK AND LIP PENCIL: $$$** The standard **Lipstick** *($17.50)* is very creamy and smooth, with medium to sheer coverage and a slightly glossy finish. The color selection is quite nice but overall there is nothing about these that makes them preferable to any other (far less expensive) lipsticks. **Lip Color Palette** *($12)* is a mini-compact with six lip colors that are fairly creamy and have a slightly glossy finish. If you don't mind having to apply your lip color with a brush all the time, this is an option, but you only get a tiny amount of each color. **$$$ Lip Gloss** *($16)* is basic gloss with a wand applicator and a pleasant, non-sticky texture, but it's nothing to consider over anything you may find at the drugstore for a quarter of the price. **Lip Pencil** *($15)* is as standard as they come and it needs to be sharpened, but for this price it should be self-sharpening. It does have a creamy texture that is almost too soft for a controlled, fine line. ☹ **$$$ Lipscape** *($16)* is a small group of silky, powdery colors that can be used on lips, cheeks, or eyes. These are mostly shiny and yet claim to leave a matte texture. Who do they think they're fooling?

**MASCARA:** ☺ **Volumizing Mascara** *($15)* is an excellent mascara that builds incredible length and thickness without clumping or smearing. Lancome look out—this is one that can give the best of your mascaras a run for the money.

☹ **Lengthening Mascara** *($15)* has small fibers in the formula that are supposed to help with lengthening, but they don't help much in that regard. If you get the wand too close to the eye, the small fibers easily fall off and can get into the eye, causing irritation. I thought they did away with fiber mascaras years ago for this very reason.

**BRUSHES:** The ☹ **$$$ Brushes** *($11 to $80)* at Awake need to work out a few kinks. Obviously well intentioned, most of them are either absurdly small or too big to work with on a variety of face shapes and features. If price is not a concern, these are the best ones to consider: ☺ **Retractable Lip Brush** *($15)* has an excellent full but tapered cut; the ☺ **Eyebrow Brush** *($20)* is firm without being scratchy; the **Eye**

Shadow #3 brush *($18)* is adequately sized for detailed work, and the ☺ **Eye Shadow #4** *($20)* brush is full and soft, with a squared-off tip for stronger contouring.

# Bain de Soleil (Sun Care Only)

For more information on Bain de Soleil, call (800) 543-1745 or visit the Web site at www.pfizer.com.

☺ **UV Sense SPF 50** *($9.89 for 3.12 ounces)* and **Bebe Block SPF 50** *($9.89 for 3.12 ounces)* are identical despite the different names. Bebe Block is aimed at kids, but there is nothing particularly kid-oriented in the formulation. What counts for both adults and kids is the protection, and it is significant, if not a bit excessive—after all, there is only so much sunshine on any given day. Both contain titanium dioxide in a waterproof formula claiming eight hours of protection, a good option for long days out in the sun. One word of warning: several ingredients in these products could be problematic for sensitive skin.

☺ **All Day Extended Protection Sunscreen SPF 30** *($9.19 for 4 ounces)* is a very good titanium dioxide–based sunscreen for normal to slightly dry skin.

☺ **All Day Extended Protection Sunblock SPF 15** *($6.99 for 4 ounces)* is similar to the sunscreen above only with an SPF 15, and the same review applies.

☺ **All Day Waterproof Sunblock SPF 15** *($9.19 for 4 ounces)* is a very good titanium dioxide–based sunscreen for normal to slightly dry skin.

☺ **Gentle Block Sunblock SPF 30** *($8.99 for 4 ounces)* is similar to those above, which makes it a good sunscreen, although there is nothing gentle about it.

☺ **Mademoiselle Sunblock SPF 15** *($6.99 for 4 ounces)* is similar to those above and the same basic comments apply.

☹ **All Day Extended Protection Sunscreen SPF 8** *($6.99 for 4 ounces)* is a serious disappointment. An SPF 8 is not extended protection by anyone's definition and is a dangerous risk for skin, leaving it vulnerable to all the negative effects of sun damage. It also does not contain titanium dioxide, zinc oxide, or avobenzone to protect adequately from UVA damage.

☹ **Sand Resistant Oil Sunfilter SPF 2** *($5.09 for 4 ounces)* ) is similar to the SPF 8 version above and the same comments apply.

☹ **Apres Soleil After Sun Moisture Replenishing Lotion** *($6.99 for 8 ounces)* is a good, though standard, moisturizer for dry skin, but that's about it. It contains mostly water, mineral oil, slip agent, thickeners, soothing agent, plant oil, water-binding agents, and preservatives.

☹ **Apres Soleil After Sun Revitalizing Aloe Mist** *($6.99 for 8 ounces)* lists the third ingredient as alcohol, which is drying and irritating and doesn't revitalize anything.

☹ **Orange Gelee SPF 28** *($7.99 for 3.9 ounces)* does not contain avobenzone, zinc oxide, or titanium dioxide, and is not recommended.

☹ **Orange Gelee Sunscreen SPF 15** *($8.65 for 3.12 ounces)* does not contain avobenzone, zinc oxide, or titanium dioxide, and is not recommended.

☹ **Orange Gelee Sunscreen SPF 8** *($8.65 for 3.12 ounces)* does not contain avobenzone, zinc oxide, or titanium dioxide, and is not recommended; the SPF 8 makes this a serious problem for skin.

☹ **Orange Gelee Sunscreen SPF 4** *($8.65 for 3.12 ounces)* does not contain avobenzone, zinc oxide, or titanium dioxide, and is not recommended; the SPF 4 makes this a serious problem for skin.

☺ **Kids Sunblock SPF 30** *($8.99 for 4 ounces)* in part is titanium dioxide and works well to prevent sun damage. It has a fairly light, fairly nongreasy feel.

☺ **Sunless Tanning Spray** *($7.99 for 3.5 ounces)* comes in Dark and Very Dark, and both are worth checking out for a tan with all of the color and none of the damage.

☺ **Sunless Tanning Creme Light** *($7.99 for 3.5 ounces)*, like all self tanners, contains dihydroxyacetone, which can affect skin color. However this version also includes eucalyptus, an unnecessary skin irritant that just isn't worth the risk given how many good self tanners there are without irritating ingredients.

☺ **Sunless Tanning Creme Dark** *($7.99 for 3.5 ounces)* is similar to the Creme Light version above and the same comments apply.

☺ **Sunless Tanning Creme Deep Dark** *($7.99 for 3.5 ounces)* is similar to the Creme Light version above and the same comments apply.

☺ **Sunless Tanning Spray Dark** *($7.99 for 3.5 ounces)* is similar to the Creme Light version above and the same comments apply.

☺ **Sunless Tanning Spray Deep Dark** *($7.99 for 3.5 ounces)* is similar to the Creme Light version above and the same comments apply.

☺ **Streak Guard Dark** *($7.99 for 3.5 ounces)* is similar to the Creme Light version above and the same comments apply.

☺ **Streak Guard Deep Dark** *($7.99 for 3.5 ounces)* is similar to the Creme Light version above and the same comments apply.

## *bare escentuals*

In terms of cosmetics boutique appeal, bare escentuals is a store concept quite similar in style to Aveda, The Body Shop, and Garden Botanika. While lots of women may never have heard of bare escentuals, many women have heard of its bareMinerals loose powder eyeshadows, blushes, and face powders. That popularity is due to QVC, where bare escentuals' bareMinerals products are sold. QVC reaches lots of women with its rapturous praise for everything it sells. As a result, thousands of women want to know if bareMinerals work as amazingly and purely as the spokesperson asserts.

Of course, nothing ever works as well as they say in ads, though these powders are unique in their coverage, application, and simple formulation, and, depending on your point of view, they are an interesting way to apply face and eye makeup. See the reviews below for details.

QVC also sells a skin-care line from bare escentuals called Cush. There is nothing cushy about peppermint oil in every skin-care product you put on your face, because that's just an irritation waiting to happen. Cush is a line you can easily avoid.

If you are shopping at the bare escentuals store, you'll find a huge range of products, including the bareMinerals products and a skin-care line called Habit, as well as a wide range of other fragrant bath, body, and aromatherapy products. None of this is very exciting; it's just an Aveda or Garden Botanika wannabe with one hook— loose powder makeup. For more information about bare escentuals, call (800) 227-3990 or visit the Web sites at www.bareescentuals.com or www.bareescentuals. qvc.com.

## bare escentuals Cush Skin Care

☹ **Deep Sea Foaming Seaweed Cleanser** *($20 for 6.5 ounces)* contains sage oil, lavender oil, and peppermint oil, and while these all may smell nice they are extremely irritating and sensitizing for skin.

☹ **Equilibrium Sea Facial Tonic** *($20 for 6.5 ounces)* contains sandalwood oil, lavender oil, and peppermint oil, and while these all may smell nice they are extremely irritating and sensitizing for skin.

☹ **Turning Tide Fresh Face Exfoliator** *($36 for 2.3 ounces)* contains sandalwood oil, spearmint oil, and peppermint oil, all of which are potential skin irritants.

☹ **Life Source Time Peeling Serum** *($36 for 1 ounce)* contains witch hazel and peppermint oil, which are potential skin irritants.

☹ **Sea Life Nutritious Marine Moisturizer** *($32 for 2.1 ounces)* is finally one Cush product without peppermint! But the number of fragrant plant oils high up on the ingredient list is a problem for skin.

## bare escentuals Habit Skin Care

☺ **Rose Geranium Cleansing Lotion Normal to Dry Skin** *($18 for 5 ounces)* is mostly plant oil, thickeners, and preservatives. This is a standard, wipe-off cleanser that can leave a greasy film behind on the skin.

☹ **Lavender & Wild Thyme Cleanser Normal to Oily Skin** *($18 for 5 ounces).* The plant oil and thickeners in here can clog pores and be a problem for oily skin. The amount of tea tree oil is so small it probably wouldn't be a problem for the eyes.

☺ **$$$ Tea Tree Foaming Cleanser Normal to Oily Skin** *($18 for 5 ounces)* is a standard, detergent-based water-soluble cleanser that can be drying for some skin types. The tea tree oil can be a problem for the eye area.

☺ **Rosewater & Lactic Acid Time Balm Normal to Dry Skin** *($29 for 2 ounces)* is a good emollient moisturizer for dry skin; while it does contain lactic acid, the pH is too high for it to be an effective exfoliant.

☹ **Rose & Neroli Freshener Normal to Dry Skin** *($18 for 5 ounces)* is mostly water, witch hazel, glycerin, and fragrance. Witch hazel is an unnecessary skin irritant that can be a problem for most skin types.

☹ **Cypress & Rosemary Toner Normal to Oily Skin** *($18 for 5 ounces)* is similar to the one above and the same review applies.

☺ **Rose & Royal Jelly Anti-Oxidant Moisturizer Normal to Dry Skin** *($32 for 2 ounces)* isn't much of an antioxidant—there is only a tiny amount of vitamin E in here. This is a fairly standard but good moisturizer for dry skin.

☹ **Tea Tree & Lavender Oil Control Moisturizer Normal to Oily Skin** *($24 for 2 ounces)* includes several plant oils that would be a problem for someone with oily skin.

☹ **Tea Tree Spot Treatment Normal to Oily Skin** *($12 for 1 ounce)* contains a teeny amount of tea tree oil and a lot of plant oils, including lemon oil. Plant oils aren't best for oily skin and lemon oil is a skin irritant.

☺ **$$$ Eye Makeup Remover** *($12 for 3 ounces)* is a standard, detergent-based eye-makeup remover. Wiping off makeup is a problem for skin.

☺ **Bare Aloe Vera** *($8 for 2 ounces)*. For this kind of product you would be better off going to the health food store and purchasing a huge bottle of pure aloe vera gel for half the price.

☺ **$$$ Papaya Enzyme Peel Mask** *($16 for 2 ounces)* is a standard clay mask. Papain has some exfoliating properties but is considered unstable and becomes ineffective after a short period of time.

☹ **Seaweed Clay Mask** *($16 for 2 ounces)* contains menthol, which is a skin irritant and a problem for all skin types.

☺ **Firming Eye Gel** *($14 for 1 ounce)* isn't all that firming or moisturizing, it is just a lightweight gel. It would only be OK if you weren't worried about dry skin.

☹ **Chamomile & Mallow Exfoliator** *($16 for 2 ounces)* is a fairly scratchy scrub that uses ground-up shells. This can be hard on skin.

☹ **Wisdom Glycolic Acid Multi-Vitamin SPF 15** *($20 for 2.3 ounces)* doesn't contain avobenzone, zinc oxide, or titanium dioxide, and is not recommended. Moreover the pH is too high for the glycolic acid in here to work as an exfoliant.

# *bare escentuals Makeup*

All of the **bareMinerals** powders, whether for foundation, eyeshadow, or blush, are loose powders that are applied with a brush. The products boast that they don't contain fragrance, oil, binders, surfactants, emulsifiers, or any other problematic ingredients. While that is the case according to their ingredient list (though I strongly doubt it, given the number of shades from blue to red displayed in the stores, because there just aren't natural dyes available that can create this range of colors), that doesn't make these products problem-free. Bismuth oxychloride is a major ingredient in all the powder formulations and it can cause skin irritation, while the other minerals can be drying. Aside from the bogus claim about natural being good, loose powders are as messy as it gets in terms of your vanity (counter top not ego) and your makeup bag. The powder just gets all over the place! Additionally, while there are nicely neutral soft shades, and some fairly exotic shades as well, all are extremely shiny and make any amount of crepey skin look more so. The face powder does provide some amount of opaque coverage, but the shine and the thickness can be a bit much. The eyeshadows and blush apply in a somewhat lighter way, though they still give good coverage. If you find the loose powder concept and the shine intriguing, these are an option, but I feel fairly safe in suggesting they will end up as one of those cosmetics whims that you never use more than a few times.

☺ $$$ <u>FOUNDATION:</u> **bareMinerals Foundation** *($24).* For a review, see my comments above. **liquid insurance** *($16)* is a fairly thick foundation that grabs the skin better than most, but all of the shades are shiny, and several of the eight shades are too peach or pink for most skin tones; stay away from 2, 3, 6, and 7. A word of warning: the salespeople I spoke to all claimed these foundations had a high SPF even though no SPF number is attributed to them. Not only is this information illegal, it is unethical: you cannot rely on any of these foundations—or any product for that matter—for sunscreen protection without an SPF rating and UVA-protecting ingredients in the active list.

☹ <u>CONCEALER:</u> **Concealer** *($12)* comes in a tube, and all of the colors are extremely peach or pink and not recommended for any skin tone.

☺ $$$ <u>POWDER:</u> **bareMinerals mineral veil** *($18)* is a loose powder with a softer and lighter consistency than the bareMinerals Foundation and doesn't have shine! It has a sheer but dry powder finish, and is best for someone with normal to oily skin. **pressed mineral veil** *($18)* is a standard pressed powder with a soft, sheer finish that is extremely translucent and quite nice.

☺ $$$ <u>BLUSH:</u> **bareMinerals blush** *($16)* has the same basic texture as the foundation, and the comments about its being messy and hard to control are the same. There are some matte shades for this product, and the application is soft and beautiful. It's hard for me to encourage this option but I'm sure some women will love it. I would try it before buying.

☺ **pressed minerals blush** *($11)* has a limited color selection, and they are all mostly in the rose and pink color family. They do have a soft, even finish.

☺ **EYESHADOW AND EYE PENCIL:** bareMinerals eyeshadow *($11)* is similar to the blush and foundation reviewed above. All of these colors are slightly shiny, though there are some great neutral shades. I still don't get the advantage of opting for this kind of messy, flaky application, but for some women it is an option. **bareMinerals Glimmer** *($12)* is the same as the mineral foundation and blush except that these are ultra-shiny. This is about personal preference and style, though I don't recommend this look except for evening wear. **pressed minerals eyeshadow** *($12)* is just eyeshadow with some amount of shine and a nice color selection. **Eye Pencil** *($10)* is a standard, twist-up eye pencil that comes in a limited number of shades.

☺ **LIPSTICK AND LIP PENCIL:** Lipstick *($14)* has a creamy, opaque, slightly glossy finish. **Lip Gloss** *($12)* is a standard tube lip gloss, nice but ordinary. **Lip Liner** *($10)* is a standard, twist-up eye pencil that comes in a limited number of shades.

☹ **MASCARA:** Mascara *($13)* is a terrible mascara that builds almost no length or definition. It's a definite waste of money.

☺ **BRUSHES:** The **Brushes** *(from $12 to $24)* for the most part are soft and easy to use. The sizes offered definitely depend on your preference for application. For example there are two eyeshadow brushes, one that is rather oversize and the other that is almost too small. I would prefer two brushes in sizes right between these. The **Powder Brush** is a great size but the **Blush Brush** is probably too large for most cheeks.

## Basis (Skin Care Only)

If you are looking for some good, inexpensive sunscreens, this is the line to consider. Other than that, there isn't much in this skin-care line, at least not when it comes to gentle skin care. It is available in most drugstores across the country. For more information on Basis products call (800) 227-4703 or visit its section on the Web at www.planetrx.com.

☹ **All Clear Bar** *($2.69 for 4 ounces)* contains a tiny amount of triclosan, an OK disinfectant, but its effectiveness is washed down the drain before it can affect the skin. It contains several ingredients that could be drying and irritating, including sodium xylenesulfonate, lemon, sage, lime, and sodium lauryl sulfate.

☹ **Cleaner Clean Face Wash** *($4.99 for 6 ounces)* is a standard, water-soluble cleanser that also contains lemon and spearmint. These can irritate and burn the eye area, and this cleanser is absolutely not recommended for anyone's face.

☺ **Comfortably Clean Face Wash** *($4.09 for 6 ounces)* is a standard, water-soluble cleanser that can be quite good for someone with normal to oily skin. It has a terrible taste and can be drying for some skin types. It does contain fragrance.

☹ **Sensitive Skin Bar** *($2.69 for 4 ounces)* is a fairly standard bar cleanser that contains tallowate and detergent cleansing agents. Tallowate can be a skin irritant and could cause breakouts and dermatitis.

☹ **Vitamin Bar** *($1.99 for 4 ounces)* makes no sense. Even if vitamins could affect the skin, this way they are washed away before they have a chance. This is nothing more than a standard bar cleanser with ingredients that can dry the skin and potentially clog pores.

☺ **So Refreshing Cleansing Towelettes** *($4.99 for 30 cloths)* is just a standard detergent-based makeup remover presoaked on towelettes. It works, though fragrance-free baby wipes do the same thing, and without the fragrance.

☺ **Face the Day Lotion SPF 15** *($6.55 for 4 ounces)* is a very good in-part zinc oxide–based sunscreen for someone with normal to dry skin, and it includes antioxidants and anti-irritants.

☺ **One Step Face Cream SPF 15** *($6.55 for 1.5 ounces)* is a good moisturizing sunscreen (with part zinc oxide), but it is a poor AHA product.

☺ **$$$ All Night Face Cream** *($6.55 for 2 ounces)* is a good moisturizer for someone with normal to dry skin, but a poor AHA product.

## *Bath & Body Works*

The general appearance of the Bath & Body Works stores is similar to their neighboring mall competitors—The Body Shop, H₂O Plus, and Garden Botanika. In addition to the wafting fragrance and herbal-natural influence they share, all of these stores have open display units and encourage makeup testing. Bath & Body Works takes this a step further with a notably friendly environment and a take-your-time demeanor. Where Bath & Body Works has a slight edge over the others is in the makeup area, where it has a wide range of color options, many with attractive textures. There are more than enough beautiful, inexpensive options to consider. For skin care, as this book goes to print in August 2000, Bath & Body Works was once again reformulating its product line so it is not reviewed here. It will be interesting to see if this ends up being an improvement or not (its last change over two years ago was a mixed bag of good and bad products). I will report on the changes as soon as they take place in an issue of my newsletter, *Cosmetics Counter Update*.

For more information about Bath & Body Works, call its customer service number at (800) 395-1001 or visit the Web site at www.intimatebrands.com.

## *Bath & Body Works Makeup*

**FOUNDATION:** ☺ **Fresh Face Liquid Makeup SPF 15** *($10)* would be a steal if it only provided reliable UVA protection. Alas, it does not, but it is a very smooth-textured foundation with a sheer, natural finish that would be suitable for normal to dry skin. There are 15 shades, with impressive colors for both light and dark skin tones (but nothing for very light or very dark tones). These are the only ones to avoid: True Bronze (too rosy) and Ginger (ash).

☺ **Complexion Perfection Creme to Powder Makeup SPF 10** *($13)* does not contain effective UVA-blocking ingredients and the SPF is below what is needed for a full day of protection, but this is still a decent cream-to-powder makeup with a smooth texture that dries quickly to a powdery finish. The creamy ingredients can be too greasy for oily skin and the powder finish too drying for dry skin, so that makes it best for normal to slightly dry or slightly oily skin. The eight shades are a mixed bag, with Natural Beige, Fresh Beige, and Almond all being too peach for most skin tones. There are no colors for very light or very dark skin.

☺ **Fast Fix Makeup SPF 10** *($12)* is a stick foundation that would work best for normal to slightly dry skin. It has a texture and finish almost identical to the Creme to Powder version above (and is best for the skin types above). This one does have an in-part zinc oxide–based sunscreen, but what a shame the SPF isn't 15; this way you can't rely on it for all-day sun protection. It features eight fairly good shades but be cautious of Golden Honey and Toffee—both can be too peach for most skin tones.

☺ **CONCEALER: Imperfection Correction Creme** *($7)* is a great, lightweight concealer with a smooth finish and minimal chance of creasing into lines. There are three beautifully neutral flesh-toned colors and two color correctors in yellow and green, but you can just ignore those.

**POWDER:** ☺ **Once Over Pressed Powder** *($11.50)* has a silky, dry texture and softly sheer finish. It is talc-based and comes in seven praiseworthy colors.

☹ **Sunny Side Up Bronzing Powder** *($13)* is an OK bronzing powder with three shades, two of which are shiny and look artificial. The one to consider (for fair skins only) is Morning Glow. Note: this is a seasonal item, and tends to come into the stores and then out accordingly.

**BLUSH:** ☺ **First Blush Cheek Color** *($8)* comes in an impressive range of colors and has a velvety-smooth texture that applies evenly without streaking or grabbing. Some of the colors have a slight amount of shine, but it's almost too negligible to even mention.

☹ **You're Blushing Creme Color** *($11)* is a twist-up stick blush that has a typical cream-blush texture and six very shiny colors. If the shine was gone or muted, these would be great for normal to dry skin and those who prefer this kind of creamy blush application.

☹ **EYESHADOW: Catch My Eyeshadow** *($6.50)* is a large range of eyeshadow colors that have too many problems to make them a consideration; all of the colors are shiny, the texture is powdery, and the application flaky and uneven.

**EYE AND BROW SHAPER:** ☹ **Defining Moment Eyeliner** *($7)* has a very sticky, almost greasy application and is not recommended. ☹ **Shape-Up Brow Pencil** *($7)* comes in only two shades, and has a dry, almost stiff application. ☹ **Fixed**

Image Waterproof Eye Pencil *($7)* is a standard pencil that comes in two colors and is reasonably waterproof as far as pencils go, but I wouldn't swim with it on! **Eye Drama Liquid Liner** *($7)* has a suitably firm brush but only draws a wide line. Most of the colors are shiny and take far too long to dry. **Tint and Tame Brow Color** *($7)* is a group of tinted brow products whose colors perplex me; who has metallic copper, silver, lilac, or charcoal brows? That's what you'll end up with if you attempt to use these. The brush is great, but who thought up those colors?

☺ <u>LIPSTICK AND LIP PENCIL:</u> **Feel Good Lip Color** *($8)* is just to the greasy side of creamy; that feels good, but don't count on much longevity. **See-Thru Lip Color SPF 15** *($8)* is very greasy and offers no UVA protection. **Draw-On Lip Crayon** *($6.50)* is a standard chubby pencil that need sharpening. This is far from a practical or helpful way to apply lip color because sharpening is tricky and then you get a point that easily smushes and is unreliable for shaping the mouth. **Here to Stay Lip Color** *($10.50)* is not an improvement over Revlon's ColorStay lipsticks. This one has an OK color selection and a slick, opaque application.

☺ **Jewel Finish Lip Polish** *($8)* is simply a sheer liquid lip color in a tube with a wand applicator that has a very emollient and glossy finish. **Color Kissed Lip Gloss** *($5.50)* is just routine gloss with a handful of good colors, though most are iridescent. **To the Point Lip Pencil** *($6.50)* is an affordable, standard pencil that has a smooth application and a soft, dry finish.

☹ **Smooth Talkin' Lip Buffer** *($5.50)* is a greasy, twist-up lip exfoliator that uses walnut-shell particles as the abrasive agent. It won't do much for lips other than feel sticky and mildly gritty.

☹ <u>MASCARA:</u> **All Out Volumizing Mascara** *($7)* and **All Out Lengthening Mascara** *($7)* are two of the worst mascaras I've tested in a long time. They didn't build any length or volume; in fact, I swear they made my lashes look shorter and sparser, leaving me all-out disappointed.

☺ <u>BRUSHES:</u> Bath & Body Works has a nice array of brushes to choose from, with great prices too. They aren't the softest brushes you'll find, but they are very good and very workable, earning smiles overall. **Powder Brush** *($9.50)*, **Blush Brush** *($8)*, and **Large Eyeshadow Brush** *($6.50)* may be too large for some faces; the **Small Eyeshadow Brush** *($5.50)* is a good option for the crease area. The **Brow Brush** *($5)* is just a toothbrush and not worth the expense, and the **Retractable Lip Brush** *($7)* is as basic as they come.

# *BeautiControl*

BeautiControl, now owned by Tupperware, tries very hard to be all things to all women. The company not only gives you information about skin care and makeup application when you book a free consultation with one of its sales representatives, but they also analyze your wardrobe and tell you which colors look best on you and which clothing styles complement your body shape. Unfortunately, as always, you must depend on the expertise of the salesperson, but several of the sales representatives I met seemed to be in dire need of wardrobe counseling themselves and had little to no technical information about skin care and makeup. The color information is helpful, but it takes skill and training to translate it into a total look.

For the makeup, there are strong and weak points. For example, while there are three types of foundation, none is appropriate for someone with dry skin; one is oil-free, the second is a very thick cream-to-powder, and the third is a powder meant to be used as a foundation. That isn't a bad selection, but it's limited.

All of the colors are divided into warm and cool groups, which is helpful, but there are almost twice as many cool colors as warm. If I were an Autumn or Spring, that would be a serious shortcoming. On the other hand, a Winter or Summer might be quite pleased.

Several of the skin-care products are rather impressive, and the average price for many of these products is under $12. As you would expect, the wrinkle products are all absurdly expensive (and unnecessary), but if you stay away from them you won't get soaked. One word of caution: the company claims that your skin type and product needs are determined by a "precise, scientific … dermatologist-tested, proven Skin Condition Analysis." There is nothing precise or necessarily scientific about it. Little pieces of sticky paper the company calls "sensors" are stuck on different cleansed areas of your face. What comes off on these strips determines the products you are to use. Depending on the time of day I had the test done, I received different evaluations, which makes sense: my skin isn't the same in the morning as it is at the end of the day. Also, the sensors ripped off skin and left irritation and rough spots. The results aren't surprising and are often wrong. Skin isn't static: it changes with the seasons, your menstrual cycle, stress, and your environment. The idea is cute, but I wouldn't choose skin-care products based on this analysis alone.

BeautiControl's All Clear Skin is a group of four products with one purpose in mind: combating acne. Does this line of defense work? I wish I could say yes, but BeautiControl's battle plan falls short for several reasons: there is no product to absorb excess oil, some of the products are potentially irritating, and there is no disinfectant to kill the bacteria that cause breakouts. That won't help reduce breakouts.

For more information about BeautiControl call (800) BEAUTI-1 or (800) 872-0601 or visit the Web site at www.beauti.com (though you can't gain access to most of the Web site without getting a password from a BeautiControl representative first).

# *BeautiControl Skin Care*

## *System C for Combination Skin*

☺ **Chamomile Balancing Cleansing Lotion for Combination Skin** *($13.50 for 8 ounces)* is a mineral oil–based cleanser that also contains some detergent cleansing agents. It can leave a greasy film but could be good for someone with dry skin. It also has orange, mandarin, and lemon, which are irritating ingredients included for fragrance.

☺ **Balancing Scrub for Combination Skin** *($14 for 3 ounces)* is a standard, detergent-based scrub that uses synthetic particles (ground-up plastic) as the abrasive. This works as well as any scrub for most skin types except dry skin. It does contain fragrance.

☹ **Balancing Tonic for Combination Skin** *($14 for 8 ounces)* is an alcohol-based toner that can be irritating and drying for most skin types.

☺ **Balancing Moisturizer** *($15.50 for 4.5 ounces)* is a good emollient moisturizer for normal to dry skin. This is recommended for someone with combination skin, but the oils in it aren't good for that skin type.

## *System D for Dry Skin*

☺ **Mild Rosemary Cleansing Fluide for Dry Skin** *($13.50 for 8 ounces)* is a mineral oil– and lanolin oil–based cleanser that must be wiped off. This is fairly greasy stuff and absolutely requires a washcloth to get it off. However, for ultra-dry skin it may be an option. It does contain fragrant citrus extracts.

☺ **Renewing Scrub/Masque** *($14 for 3 ounces)* is a detergent-based water-soluble cleanser that contains synthetic scrub particles (ground-up plastic). This would work well for most skin types but not for someone with dry skin. It does contains coloring agents and fragrance.

☹ **Soothing Chamomile Tonic** *($14 for 8 ounces)* contains witch hazel, which can be drying and a skin irritant. It also contains fragrance and a form of menthol, and none of that is soothing.

☺ **Essential Moisture Lotion** *($15.50 for 4.5 ounces)* is a very good emollient moisturizer for normal to dry skin.

## *System O for Oily Skin*

☺ **Purifying Cleansing Gel** *($12 for 8 ounces)* is a standard detergent cleanser that can be good for normal to oily skin. It does contain fragrant citrus extracts.

☺ **Almond Clarifying Scrub/Masque** *($14 for 3 ounces)* is a standard clay mask that also contains apricot seeds and almond meal along with thickening agents, preservatives, fragrance, and coloring agents. It is a fairly scratchy scrub and the thickening agents aren't the best for blemish-prone skin.

☹ **Clarifying Mallow Tonic** *($14 for 8 ounces)* is an alcohol-based toner that can be quite irritating and drying for most skin types.

☺ **Oil-Free Moisture Supplement** *($14 for 4.5 ounces)* is supposed to be oil-absorbing, but it won't absorb oil very well. This is a good moisturizer for someone with normal to dry skin, but it is way too emollient for someone with oily skin. It does contain a few plant extracts that are potential irritants but the amounts are so minuscule they probably have no impact whatsoever on the skin.

## All Clear Skin Products

☺ **All Clear Skin Wash** *($12 for 6 ounces)* is a standard, detergent-based water-soluble cleanser that would be great for normal to oily skin. It does contain a tiny amount of salicylic acid (BHA) but the pH of this cleanser is too high for it to be effective as an exfoliant. It does contain fragrance.

☹ **All Clear Skin Scrub** *($13 for 4 ounces)* contains synthetic scrub particles suspended in alcohol, slip agents, thickeners, and fragrance. Alcohol as the second ingredient makes this potentially irritating and drying for all skin types.

☹ **All Clear Skin Solution** *($15.50 for 6 ounces)* is the most interesting of these products. It is merely 2% salicylic acid suspended in alcohol and witch hazel. It could be an option for a good exfoliating BHA product (it has a pH of 3) if the alcohol weren't in here. The exfoliation from the salicylic acid can be irritating enough for the skin without the presence of the alcohol.

☹ **All Clear Skin Moisture** *($14 for 4 ounces)*. Someone with acne will want to consider avoiding the emollients in this product, but it is a good BHA exfoliant for someone with normal to slightly dry or slightly oily skin.

## Regeneration Products

☺ **Regeneration for Oily Skin** *($31 for 2 ounces)* contains about 4% to 5% AHAs in an effective pH and can be an option for someone with normal to dry or slightly oily skin; however, the amount of AHA and the somewhat emollient base aren't the best for oily skin. The goal is to move from this version to Regeneration 2 for Oily Skin. That may be helpful, but generally BHA is considered better for oily skin due to its ability to penetrate through oil.

☺ **Regeneration 2 for Oily Skin** *($31 for 2 ounces)* is similar to the Oily Skin version above only this one contains about 6% to 7% AHAs; the same basic comments still apply.

☺ **Regeneration Face and Neck Creme** *($31 for 2 ounces)* is about a 5% AHA product using lactic acid. It is an option for exfoliation but it doesn't regenerate anything.

☺ **Regeneration 2 Face and Neck Crème** *($31 for 2 ounces)* is almost identical to the Face and Neck Creme above and the same comments apply.

☺ **Regeneration Extreme Repair for Dry and Damaged Skin** *($30 for 4 ounces)*. It isn't very typical for skin-care products to utilize urea as a main ingredient. Urea is derived from urine, although only synthetic forms are used in cosmetics. As unpleasant as this ingredient might sound, it is actually a very good humectant (along the lines of propylene glycol and glycerin), and it also has keratolytic action (loosens skin and helps with exfoliation) much like an AHA. Generally, urea is used for parts of the body other than the face, but there is no reason not to consider it as an alternative to AHA.

☹ **Regeneration Blemish Duo** *($14.50 for 0.11 ounce of Blemish Gel and 0.12 ounce of Blemish Cover-Up)* is a tube with **Oil-Free Blemish Cover-Up**, which is nothing more than foundation (it comes in two colors, neither of which matches most skin tones) at one end, and **Blemish Gel**, which is mostly alcohol, and that's irritating and not helpful for any skin type. It does contain salicylic acid (BHA), but that is for exfoliating and it takes exfoliating *and* disinfecting (topical antibiotic or benzoyl peroxide) to deal with blemishes.

☺ **$$$ Regeneration Gold** *($55 for 1.8 ounces)* is another AHA moisturizer, this time with 7% lactic acid. This one is similar to the ones above and other than costing more money it adds no other benefit. It does contain a minuscule amount of coral extract that has no known benefit for skin.

☺ **$$$ Regeneration Gold Eye Repair** *($25 for 0.5 ounce)* is a good moisturizer for normal to slightly dry skin (though the amount of film formers in here can be problematic for sensitive skin types). This does contain soy flour but it has no estrogenic effects when applied topically. There is also only about 1% AHA and a truly insignificant amount of BHA, but even if there were more, the pH is too high for it be effective as an exfoliant.

☺ **$$$ Regeneration Gold Lip Therapy** *($20 for 0.12 ounce)* is just an emollient lipstick. The pH of this product is too high for the AHA or BHA to be effective as exfoliants.

☺ **$$$ Regeneration Retinol PM** *($35 for 1 ounce)*. This addition to the Regeneration line is surprising. Given how miraculous all the other Regeneration products were supposed to be, why would you need this? The BeautiControl brochure states: "Enjoy all the benefit of leading retinol products without a prescription." The notion that retinol can work like the active ingredient in Renova or Retin-A is absolutely not proven and is a stretch of the imagination. This version does contain retinol in a good moisturizing base but if you're looking for retinol in a product, L'Oreal's Line Eraser Pure Retinol Concentrate *($12.49 for 1 ounce)* and Alpha Hydrox Retinol Night ResQ Anti-Wrinkle Firming Complex *($11.99 for 1.05 ounces)* contain it too, and for far less.

☹ **Cell Block-C SPF 20** *($25 for 1 ounce)* doesn't contain the UVA-protecting ingredients titanium dioxide, zinc oxide, or avobenzone, and is not recommended.

☹ **Cell Block-C P.M. Cell Protection** *($30 for 0.95 ounce)*. While this product does contain a form of vitamin C, the amount is so teeny as to be almost not present. It also contains boric acid, which is not recommended for use on skin by the American Medical Association. While vitamin C is hardly the answer to wrinkles (though it is the latest fad), if you must have it there are other versions to consider for less money that are far better formulated than this one.

☺ **Microderm Oxygenating Firming Gel** *($29.50 for 2 ounces)* is a good, lightweight moisturizer for normal to slightly dry or slightly oily skin. It does contain superoxide dismutase, an ingredient that doesn't give oxygen (no product can do that anyway) but is considered a very good antioxidant. Did anyone at BeautiControl read the ingredient listing? If they had, they would have seen that the components make this a good anti-oxygenating product, not an oxygenating one.

☺ **Microderm Eye-X-Cel Daily Therapy Creme** *($19 for 0.75 ounce)* is a extremely standard moisturizer for normal to dry skin with nothing special for the eye area or skin in general. Several of the plant extracts can be potential skin irritants.

☺ **Lash & Lid Bath** *($9 for 4 ounces)* is a standard, water-soluble, wipe-off eye-makeup remover and it is a definite option for those wanting to wipe off eye makeup. It does not contain fragrance and that's a plus.

☹ **Herbal Hydrating Mist** *($8 for 8 ounces)* contains arnica, a potent skin irritant, and is not recommended. What a shame, because otherwise this would be a good toner for most skin types.

☺ **Oil Controller Oil Absorbing Formula** *($15.50 for 4.5 ounces)*. There is very little in this product that can control oil, and the thickening agents can clog pores.

☺ **$$$ Lip Apeel** *($16 for 1.25 ounces)* is a two-part product (peel and balm) that helps peel dry skin off the lips and then places a thick gloss on them afterward. The peel is a bit of wax, clay, and silicate that can indeed rub off dead skin. The balm is simply a very emollient, thick lip gloss of castor oil, petrolatum, and lanolin. It does the trick and is one of my favorite winter products for lips.

☺ **Corticulture Comfort Lotion** *($25 for 4 ounces)* is a good cortisone cream. Cortisone is fine for small irritations if you use it only occasionally; repeated use of cortisone can break down the skin's support structure. You can get the same effect from Lanacort and Cortaid at the drugstore.

☺ **Tone Corrector, Skin Tone Normalizer** *($20 for 6 ounces)*. The pH of this product is too high for the AHA to be effective as an exfoliant. It does contain a tiny amount of bearberry extract (this contains arbutin, related to hydroquinone), which can inhibit melanin production. However, in the amount used here (and allowing for the distant relationship between bearberry and arbutin) it's unlikely to have any effect on skin color.

☺ **Skin Hydrator Anti-Ash Creme** *($12 for 4.5 ounces)* is a very good moisturizer for very dry skin, but it is also very ordinary and standard.

☹ **Sunlogics Sun Shield Lotion SPF 15** *($13 for 4.5 ounces)* doesn't contain avobenzone, zinc oxide, or titanium dioxide, and is not recommended.

☹ **Sunlogics Tanning Mist SPF 8** *($14 for 8 ounces)* doesn't contain avobenzone, zinc oxide, or titanium dioxide, and is not recommended. The name of this product is accurate, it *is* a tanning product, because SPF 8 is not enough sun-damage protection.

☹ **Sunlogics UV Lip+Eye Stick SPF 15** *($9.50 for .06 ounce)* doesn't contain avobenzone, zinc oxide, or titanium dioxide, and is not recommended.

☹ **Sunlogics Water-Resistant Sunblock SPF 30** *($15 for 4.5 ounces)* doesn't contain avobenzone, zinc oxide, or titanium dioxide, and is not recommended.

## *BeautiControl Makeup*

FOUNDATION: ☺ **Sheer Protection Oil-Free Liquid Foundation** *($10.50)* is a lightweight foundation that provides light to medium coverage and has a soft matte finish. All of the shades are divided into cool and warm tones, but most are too pink or peach. Someone with warm skin tones should not wear a vivid peach foundation, nor should someone with cool skin tones wear a vivid pink foundation. Another caution: there are definitely ingredients in this product that could trigger breakouts and that you might want to avoid. These are the only colors to consider: Nude, Natural, Alabaster, Buff, Porcelain Beige, Tawny, and Mahogany. These colors are too pink or peach: Ivory, Bisque, Beige, Golden Honey, Peaches & Cream, Sunglow, Bronze, Desert Tan, Caramel, Nutmeg, Toffee, and Mocha.

☹ **Perfecting Creme to Powder Finish Foundation** *($12.50)* is a very thick, greasy foundation that does have a powder finish but never loses its greasy feel. Its claim to be waterproof is pretty accurate, but it is almost cleanser-proof too. It can easily clog pores if you're not careful.

☺ **Perfecting Wet/Dry Finish Foundation** *($20.50)* is a standard, talc-based pressed powder that has a decent color selection and covers softly and smoothly. The texture and finish are great. It's supposed to be able to diffuse light in order to minimize lines, but it can't do that. Most of the colors in the large selection are reliable and neutral. The only colors to avoid are: Peaches & Cream, Bisque, Golden Honey, Sunglow, Dark, and Bronze.

☹ **Creme Sheer Protection** *($12)* is more like a creamy pancake makeup and is very greasy, containing mineral oil, heavy wax, and lanolin, which is a lot for the skin to handle. It is recommended for dry skin but it is really heavy for that skin type. The colors tend to be on the peach side.

☺ **Color Freeze Liquid Makeup SPF 12** *($19.50)* is an excellent matte-finish foundation that is great for oily skin types. The SPF 12 is decent and it does contain titanium dioxide. This is definitely an option and one of the better foundations of this type. The only colors to avoid are: Peaches & Cream, Bisque, Golden Honey, Sunglow, Dark, and Bronze.

☹ <u>CONCEALER:</u> **Extra-Help Concealer** *($5.50)* blends on easily and provides good medium coverage, but it is fairly greasy and can crease into lines around the eyes moments after being applied and continue to do so the rest of the day; the Light and Medium shades can be too peach for most skin tones.

☹ **Color Perfectors** *($10)* are standard skin-color correctors that come in three shades: Mint, Mauve, and Lilac. They can't change skin tone convincingly, can wreak havoc when you choose a foundation, and layer on more makeup than any woman needs.

<u>POWDER:</u> ☺ **Loose Perfecting Powder** *($10.50)* is a standard, talc-based powder that has a soft, dry texture and comes in three colors. Medium can be too peach for some skin tones. **Oil-Free Translucent Pressed Powder** *($11.50)* has a soft, somewhat dry texture. The colors are very neutral and would work well for someone with normal to oily/combination skin.

☺ <u>BLUSH:</u> The **Unbelievable Blush** *($13.50)* shades all have some amount of shine, but not enough to be a problem for most skin types. (Someone with oily skin may not be happy.) The colors are beautiful and the texture is soft and smooth. But be careful: the colors are fairly vivid and pastel, and there aren't many neutral shades.

<u>EYESHADOW:</u> ☹ **Sensuous Shadows** *($13.50)* come in compacts of three shades, but some of the combinations are poor, and the colors range from somewhat shiny to very shiny; if you have any lines on your eyelids, shine will make them look worse. **Tinted Shadow Control Creme** *($7)* does help to keep your eyeshadow on, without creasing, for the entire day. There are six colors, but, like the eyeshadows, they are all shiny.

☺ **Color Freeze Eyeshadow Pencils** *($12)*. Although the color does "freeze" into place, sharpening the pencils isn't fun. Also, most of the colors in this group are shiny, which may be fun, but it makes wrinkles more evident.

<u>EYE AND BROW SHAPER:</u> ☺ **Eye Defining Pencils** and **Eye Brow Pencils** *($7.50)* are standard pencils that come in a nice range of colors. They tend to be on the dry side, which makes them a little harder to apply, but they also tend to last longer. **Color Freeze Eye Liner** *($9.50)* comes in a twist-up container and does have better staying power than the Eye Defining Pencils.

☹ **Brow Control Creme** *($7.50)* comes in a squeeze tube that you apply to a mascara-like wand and then roll through the brow. I like making brows look fuller, but this is a messy option. Similar products come with the brush inside, so the color is evenly distributed.

<u>LIPSTICK AND LIP PENCIL:</u> ☺ **Lasting Lip Color** *($9)* is a very creamy, slightly greasy lipstick that doesn't last all that long, but the color selection is attrac-

tive. The colors are divided into cremes and frosts, which helps prevent the acciden-
tal purchase of an iridescent lip color if that's not what you're looking for. **Lip Control
Creme** *($7)* is excellent. It prevents even greasy lipstick from feathering into the lines
around the mouth; however, it would be better if it came in an easier-to-use applicator rather than having to spread it with your finger or a lipstick brush. **Lip Shaping
Pencils** *($7.50)* are just standard pencils in a nice array of colors that need to be
sharpened. **Color Freeze Lip Liner** *($9.50)* is a twist-up container that does have
better staying power than the Lip Shaping Pencils.

☺ **Color Freeze LipColor** *($9)* performs just like all the other ultra-matte lip-
sticks, only this one is so soft in the tube it smushes and deteriorates with the least
amount of pressure. It isn't a bad product, just not an improvement in price or performance over Revlon ColorStay Lipstick or Maybelline Budgeproof Lip Color.

**MASCARA:** ☺ **Spectaculash Waterproof Mascara** *($7)* comes off easily with
water and cleanser, and it doesn't smear after a long day. It would be a great mascara
if it could build long, thick lashes, but it can't. It's just OK.

☹ **Spectaculash Thickening** *($8.50)* is not what I would call spectacular in the
least. It doesn't make lashes thick and creates minimal length.

# Beauty for All Seasons/Norma Virgin Makeup

The confusing header for this in-home-sales cosmetics line is due to a name
change the company is going through. The makeup end of the business, for some
very confusing reason, is being altered from Beauty for All Seasons to Norma Virgin,
who is Chairman of the Board for Beauty for All Seasons. It seems an unwise business decision, but there it is. What seems even more unwise is why anyone would
want to put their name on makeup that is overwhelmingly outdated and pales to
most any of the color selections at the drugstore or any department store.

Much like Color Me Beautiful, Beauty for All Seasons prides itself on helping
women to choose their best makeup shades by analyzing their skin tone, hair color
and eye color and choosing the best hues that complement their features. Although
this concept, known here as Color Alliance, has some merit, a lot of its success is
dependent on the "expertise" of the salesperson and whether or not you want to be
pigeonholed into wearing specific colors. The truth is that women can wear an array
of colors, especially if their makeup is balanced accordingly. What happens here is
that you can get narrowed down to a slew of pastel blues, greens and/or purples,
which may be OK for clothing but for blush, eyeshadow, and lipstick is just about as
'70s as you can get. A far more versatile approach to building a makeup collection
would be to start with soft, neutral colors and build from there, ignoring the loud,
vivid hues in favor of a classic, proportionate, and understated look that works to

your advantage rather than against it. Any fashion magazine or celebrity sports this very concept.

Regardless of theory, the actual products fall short on many counts. The foundations have mostly terrible un-skin-like colors, the blushes and eyeshadows are almost all shiny with the majority of them being exceptionally vivid and contrasting colors, the pencils are slick and greasy, and the mascara is at best described as an underachiever. The lipsticks are nice, though a tad too greasy and the loose powder is silky, but then again, it's hard to make a bad loose powder.

The skin-care products are slightly more interesting than the makeup, but only slightly. There are OK AHA products and the line does have a sunscreen with UVA protection (though there is only one). The disappointment comes from overly fragranced products, a range of irritating plant extracts that are a problem for all skin types, and toners that contain alcohol.

Overall, this is a line to be wary of and one to approach cautiously. For more information on Beauty for All Seasons/Norma Virgin makeup, call (800) 942-4336 or visit the Web site at www.bfas.com.

## Beauty for All Seasons Skin Care

☺ **AlphaCeuticals Wash** *($11.50 for 4 ounces)* is a standard detergent-based water-soluble cleanser that would work well for most skin types. There are some problematic plant extracts so irritation is a risk. This does contain fragrance.

☹ **Gentle Azulene Cleanse** *($14.50 for 6 ounces)* contains a host of skin-irritating ingredients including spruce needle, lime, peppermint, and mandarin. Calling this gentle is a joke.

☹ **Orange Blossom Foaming Cleanse** *($14.50 for 6 ounces)* contains a host of skin-irritating ingredients including orange peel, sage, lemon, balm mint, coltsfoot, citrus, and juniper.

☹ **Cucumber Eye Makeup Remover Gel** *($13.50 for 4 ounces)* is a very standard detergent-based makeup remover. Unfortunately, one of the cleansing agents is sodium lauryl sulfate and using this in an eye makeup–removing product is just unbelievable, given its high potential for irritation and a sensitizing skin reaction.

☹ **AlphaCeuticals Toner** *($10.50 for 4 ounces)* contains mostly alcohol along with other problematic plant extracts, including lemon and lime.

☹ **Bergamot Active Astringent** *($13 for 4 ounces)* contains several problematic ingredients that are irritating and drying for skin including bergamot, peppermint, eucalyptus, camphor, and lemon. Ouch!

☹ **Gentle Neroli Freshener** *($13 for 4 ounces)* contains way too much fragrance to be called gentle. Actually this is more like putting fragrance on your skin than any beneficial skin-care ingredients. It contains mostly geranium oil, orange oil, and cardamom oil, which are all potential skin sensitizers.

☺ **AlphaCeuticals Serum 5** *($33 for 2 ounces)* is a decent lightweight glycolic acid–based gel-like lotion with a 5% concentration of AHA. The pH is just borderline, meaning it is not really a low enough pH to be effective as an exfoliant. For the stronger strength AHA Serums below, that's good news because AHA concentration of 15% and 20% can be overkill for many skin types.

☺ **AlphaCeuticals Serum 10** *($33 for 2 ounces)* is similar to the Serum 5 and the same basic comments apply.

☺ **AlphaCeuticals Serum 15** *($33 for 2 ounces)* is similar to the Serum 5 and the same basic comments apply.

☺ **AlphaCeuticals Serum 20** *($33 for 2 ounces)* is similar to the Serum 5 and the same basic comments apply.

☺ **Skin Clarifier with Glycolic Acid** *($38.50 for 2 ounces)* is a moisturizer with about 5% AHA (glycolic acid); though the pH is too high for it to be effective as an exfoliant, it is a good moisturizer for normal to dry skin but that's about it.

☺ **AlphaCeuticals Hydro-Gel with Antioxidants** *($12.50 for 1.3 ounces)* is a good, though rather standard lightweight moisturizer for someone with normal to slightly dry skin. The vitamins in here are antioxidants but the amount is so minor as to be hardly worth mentioning.

☺ **AlphaCeuticals Moisture Creme with Antioxidants** *($12.50 for 1.3 ounces)* is a standard moisturizer for normal to dry skin. The vitamins in here are antioxidants but the amount is so minor as to be hardly worth mentioning.

☺ **AlphaCeuticals Eye Gel** *($10 for 0.5 ounce)* is an OK gel for slightly dry skin but the formula is incredibly boring, with all of the interesting ingredients coming well after the preservative. The pH of this product is not low enough to be an effective exfoliant.

☺ **AlphaCeuticals Eye Creme** *($10 for 0.5 ounce)*. The amount of glycolic acid in here is less than 2% and it isn't effective as an exfoliant in that amount. Other than that, this is just a very standard moisturizer. The vitamins and water-binding agent are barely present and can't have much impact on the skin, though the form of vitamin C in here is magnesium ascorbyl phosphate, and that's considered one of the better ones for antioxidant properties.

☹ **French Botanical Creme with Liposomes** *($16 for 2 ounces)* contains way too much fragrance as well as arnica and ivy, which makes it a problem for many skin types.

☹ **Ginseng Moisture Boost with Vitamin A** *($17.50 for 1 ounce)*. The plant extracts in here of mandarin orange, mandarin orange oil, and ginseng are irritating and not helpful for skin.

☺ **Golden Ginseng Oil with Vitamin A** *($20 for 1 ounce)*. The tiny amount of ginger in this product probably won't be a problem for most skin types. Other than that, this is mostly silicone and plant oils. Given that it is mostly just safflower oil, you can just use that from your kitchen for far less money.

☺ **Moisturessence SPF 18** *($20 for 4 ounces)* is a very good, in-part avobenzone-based sunscreen in a rather standard moisturizing base that would be good for someone with normal to dry skin.

☹ **Original Moisturessence** *($16 for 4 ounces)* is a very boring lotion. It would work for someone with normal to slightly dry skin but this is rather unexciting.

☺ **ReVive Extra-Dry Skin Treatment** *($16 for 2 ounces)* is a good, though boring emollient moisturizer for normal to dry skin. It contains mostly water, thickeners, Vaseline, glycerin, plant oils, and preservatives.

☺ **Chamomile Calming Eye Gel** *($10.50 for 0.5 ounce)* would be an option for someone with normal to slightly dry skin.

☹ **Vitamin E Stick SPF 12** *($9 for 0.12 ounce)* doesn't contain UVA-protecting ingredients of titanium dioxide, zinc oxide, or avobenzone and is not recommended.

☹ **ElastiShield** *($16.50 for 1 ounce)* contains several seriously irritating plant extracts including lemon peel, eucalyptus oil, geranium oil, and orange oil and is not recommended.

☹ **Mir'Cle Vitamin C Treatment** *($33 for set that includes 1-ounce solution and 0.4-ounce powder)*. The form of vitamin C in this product is ascorbic acid, which is considered to be the least stable and the most irritating to use. If you are looking for vitamin C, this is not the product to consider.

☹ **$$$ Mud Treatment from the Sea** *($23 for 2.5 ounces)* is a standard clay mask that is overly fragranced. Still, for a basic clay mask it's an option for oily skin. There is nothing about sea clay that is better for skin.

☹ **Papaya Peel with Glycolic Acid** *($23.50 for 2.5 ounces)* does contain papain, which is an enzyme that can exfoliate skin, although it is considered to be a fairly unstable skin-care ingredient so the effectiveness of this product in that regard is questionable. However, the real exfoliation comes from the walnut shell powder, which definitely scrubs skin. The amount of glycolic acid in here is less than 2%, so it isn't effective in that aspect either.

☹ **VitaBeauty Firm 'n' Tone** *($19 for 4 ounces)* does contain aminophylline, which was the ingredient used when the cellulite cream craze hit about ten years ago. There was, and still is, no proof that it has any effect on skin. The caffeine in this product can constrict skin, which temporarily may make skin look smoother, but it can cause irritation. Keep in mind that when consumed in coffee, caffeine can be a strong diuretic, but there is no evidence that effect can take place when caffeine is applied to skin. Given how much coffee many of us drink, it clearly hasn't changed cellulite one iota. This product also contains *Ephedra sinica* extract, the Chinese herb

Ma Huang. While there is evidence that orally it may be of help for weight loss, there is no known benefit for skin.

☹ **VitaBeauty Wild Yam Creme** *($13.50 for 2 ounces)*. Wild yam extract does not contain progesterone or anything else that would act like progesterone. According to *The PDR Family Guide to Natural Medicines & Healing Therapies* and the *American Journal of Obstetrics and Gynecology*, volume 18, 1999, wild yam is used in the production of artificial [synthetic] progesterone but it will not yield the hormone in the absence of a chemical conversion process that the body can't supply, though it can be created in a laboratory.

## Norma Virgin Makeup

☹ FOUNDATION: **Powder Crème Foundation** *($13; $5.50 for compact)* has a standard cream-to-powder texture and an even application but the three shades are just too pink, peach, or ash to recommend. **Makeup Base Regular** *($12.50)* is a dewy-finish liquid foundation whose ten colors leave much to be desired (with the exception of Beige Ivory) and there is really no reason to try this or the **Makeup Base Oil-Free** *($12.50)*, which is lighter in texture and has fewer shades, but what're available are not realistic skin shades in the least. **Flawless Finish** *($12.50)* is a foundation intended for women of color, but the six shades all have overtones of peach, copper or red that may work for a small percentage of those with darker skin tones, but I wouldn't consider these over the foundations from Black Opal or Iman. **Perfect Finish Foundation SPF 15** *($12)* does not contain reliable UVA protection and an otherwise nice texture and finish are forfeited to four rosy-ash shades.

☹ CONCEALER: **Color Perfection Crème** *($9.50)* are small compacts of greasy, sheer color correctors that add a strange cast and crease-prone finish to the skin. **Shadow Concealer** *($9.50)* is virtually identical to the one above, only the color is closer to real skin tone. The same texture and creasing problems are found here as well as in the **Concealer Stick** *($9.50)*, a standard, heavy-textured lipstick-style concealer that comes in one shade. How much more limiting can you get?

POWDER: ☺ $$$ **Line-Diffusing MicroPowder** *($17.50)* is a standard talc-based loose powder that has a silky feel and soft matte finish. The three colors are very nice although Dark may be too peach for some skin tones.

☹ $$$ **Vivid Translucent Powder** *($17.50)* is identical in formulation to the Line-Diffusing version above; this one is intended for darker skin tones, though it's a bit too coppery-red to look like a real skin color.

☹ **Pressed Powder** *($12)* is talc-based and features three colors that may work for some skin tones; I just can't think of whose because they are so overly peach and rose.

☹ BLUSH: **Smooth Velvety Dry Blush** *($9.75)* is accurately named. The large assortment of colors is divided into Spring/Summer (warm) and Autumn/Winter (cool) tones, and that's helpful but doesn't explain the preponderance of shiny, ultra-vivid colors. If it weren't for the shine, the deeper shades would be a viable option for darker skin tones.

☹ EYESHADOW: **Long Lasting Eyeshadows** *($6.75)* are sold as singles and there aren't many lines left that are displaying so many green, blue, purple, orange, pink, and violet shadows. These colors may somehow complement your eye color, but wearing them on the eyelid or underbrow area does little to reflect the purpose of eyeshadow, which is to shape and define the eye. Not to mention that blending such vivid hues is extremely tricky and mostly not worth the effort. There are some matte, neutral colors to consider, but nothing that can't be found several times over elsewhere and without having to wade through the otherwise dated color selection.

EYE AND BROW SHAPER: ☹ **Refillable Ultra-Soft Eye Liner** *($11; $7.50 refills)* are standard twist-up retractable pencils that have a slick, greasy texture that just invites smudging.

☺ **Cake Eyeliner** *($9.50)* is standard cake liner that is best used wet; dry application tends to not go on as smoothly. This one goes on sheerer than most.

☺ **Artistic Eyes** *($12)* is your everyday liquid eyeliner, with a soft but firm brush that applies color swiftly and evenly. **Natural Brow** *($10.50)* is a fairly dry-texture matte-finish pressed powder for brows. There are three duos, each with a realistic light and dark tone. For those inclined to mix colors, these will provide that option, but I have a feeling most women will settle with one of the two shades and ignore the other one, which is not smooth enough to double as eyeshadow, but may work for liner. **Controla Brow** *($10.50)* is a good, basic clear brow gel that applies cleanly and has a non-sticky finish to help keep brows in place.

☺ LIPSTICK AND LIP PENCIL: **Super Creamy Lipstick** *($10)* goes past creamy all the way to greasy. The colors are bold and opaque, and many have a fair amount of iridescence, but this is not the one to consider if you're at all prone to lipstick feathering or bleeding. **LipSheers SPF 15** *($10)* are creamy, sheer lip colors with a glossy finish and no adequate UVA-protecting ingredients. **Refillable Ultra-Soft Lip Liner** *($10)* are automatic, twist-up pencils that have a very soft, almost too creamy texture. Don't count on these to help in the fight against lip colors feathering.

☹ **Color Seal for Lips** *($6)* is a hairspray-type sealant for the lips that never really sets and remains sticky to the touch. The consultant I spoke with felt the same way and told me she doesn't even order it anymore. Ditto for the **Color Bind for Lips** *($11.50),* a lip primer gel that is supposed to help prevent feathering but just stays gummy and tacky on the lips, which makes applying a lipstick over this (as the instructions say to do) a messy endeavor.

MASCARA: ☺ **Marvelous Mascara** *($10.50)* is hardly marvelous. It's mundane mascara that, if you're willing to wield the wand repeatedly, will manage to build some length but no significant thickness. If you decide to try this, avoid the Teal and Eggplant shades.

☹ **Fat Lash Mascara** *($15.50)* is basically just another lash primer that tends to go on clumpy and makes a mess that is truly avoidable with a superior mascara.

# Beauty Without Cruelty (Skin Care Only)

Many companies proudly boast that they do not test their products on animals. However, it isn't always clear whether the products contain animal-derived ingredients or whether individual ingredients were ever tested on animals. Some companies, including The Body Shop, have a self-imposed five-year "grandfather clause," which means they use ingredients previously tested on animals as long as the testing took place five years prior to the date the raw ingredient was purchased. Beauty Without Cruelty is one of the few companies with a strict, rigorously defined position concerning animal testing. Its products are not tested on animals, none of its products contain animal by-products, and not one of the ingredients it uses has been tested on animals since 1965. The ethics of this company in this regard are admirable.

Of course, the company makes elaborate claims about the benefits of its plant extracts, but if you ignore that and look for the ingredients that really make a difference, you can find some very good products. They are typically distributed in health food stores and in drugstores such as RiteAid and Long's. You can also order direct by calling (707) 769-5120 or (800) 227-5120 or on-line at www.vitamins.com.

☺ **Extra Gentle Facial Cleansing Milk Dry/Mature Skin Types** *($7.49 for 8.5 ounces)* is a fairly standard wipe-off cleanser that can leave a greasy film on the skin, though it may be an option for those with very dry skin. The vitamins are just wiped away and the amount is so insignificant it doesn't matter anyway.

☺ **Herbal Cream Facial Cleanser Normal/Dry Skin** *($7.49 for 8.5 ounces)* is a detergent-based water-soluble cleanser that also contains some plant oils. This can be a very good cleanser for someone with normal to dry skin. It does contain fragrance.

☺ **3% Alpha Hydroxy Facial Cleanser Normal/Oily Skin Types** *($7.49 for 8.5 ounces)* is a standard, detergent-based water-soluble cleanser that can be very good for someone with normal to oily skin. There isn't much AHA in here and the type isn't even delineated, so it isn't significant one way or the other. This does contain fragrance, and several of the plant extracts can be skin irritants.

☺ **Extra Gentle Eye Makeup Remover** *($5.89 for 4 ounces)* is a fairly standard eye-makeup remover, though the tea water contains some witch hazel, which may be a problem for the eye area.

☺ **Extra Gentle Facial Smoother** *($7.49 for 4 ounces)* can be an OK facial scrub for someone with normal to dry skin. Several of the plant extracts can be skin irritants.

☺ **Balancing Facial Toner for All Skin Types** *($7.49 for 8.5 ounces)* is a good, almost irritant-free toner. Some of the plant extracts in here can be a problem for sensitive skin types.

☺ **Renewal Moisture Cream 3% Alpha Hydroxy Complex for All Skin Types** *($13.49 for 4 ounces)* doesn't contain enough AHA in a low enough pH to make it a good AHA product for exfoliation, but other than that it is a good moisturizer for normal to dry skin. The amount of vitamins is insignificant.

☺ **All Day Moisturizer Normal/Dry Skin** *($12.49 for 2 ounces)* doesn't contain a sunscreen, which makes it a poor choice for all day, but it can be a very good, emollient nighttime moisturizer for someone with dry skin.

☺ **Green Tea Nourishing Eye Gel** *($14.49 for 1 ounce)* is a very good light-weight moisturizer that can be used on the entire face. This does not contain fragrance.

☺ **Maximum Moisture Cream Benefits Dry/Mature Skin** *($14.49 for 2 ounces)* is a very good moisturizer for someone with very dry skin.

☹ **Oil-Free Facial Moisturizer** *($12.49 for 2 ounces)* contains several plant extracts that can be skin irritants. However, it could be a good lightweight moisturizer for someone with normal to slightly dry skin.

☺ **Vitamin C Renewal Cream** *($18.95 for 2 ounces)* is a good emollient moisturizer for normal to dry skin. It does contain a good form of vitamin C (magnesium ascorbyl palmitate) but that is nothing more than an antioxidant; that's helpful, but it won't get rid of one wrinkle on your face.

☺ **Vitamin C Vitality Serum** *($24.95 for 1 ounce)* is similar to the Renewal Cream above only in a light lotion form, which makes it better for someone with normal to slightly dry skin.

☹ **Vitamin C SPF 15 Moisture Plus** *($14.95 for 4 ounces)* doesn't contain the UVA-protecting ingredients titanium dioxide, zinc oxide, or avobenzone, and is not recommended.

☺ **SPF 15 Daily Facial Lotion, Benefits All Skin Types** *($9.49 for 4 ounces)* is a very good, titanium dioxide–based sunscreen for someone with normal to dry skin.

☺ **Purifying Facial Mask** *($8.49 for 4 ounces)* is a standard clay mask. This is as good an irritant-free clay mask as any you will find.

# *BeneFit*

BeneFit was developed by twins Jean Danielson and Jane Blackford, whose brief claim to fame was a stint as the Calgon twins back in the 1960s. They opened their first cosmetics store in San Francisco around 1976. When BeneFit was purchased by the LVMH group, the parent company of the Sephora chain of stores, BeneFit traded a bit of its independence, but vowed to stay true to the zany irreverence that put it on the map. Fortunately the change hasn't eroded Benefit's makeup philosophy, which is outrageously fun, or its product arsenal centered around impossibly cute names and a lexicon aimed at teenagers. "Zaparella, feared foe of the Evil Blemish, sweeps night skies" and "Do the bags under your eyes look like carry-ons? Unload those bags …" are hardly your typical scientific, elegance-laden skin-care selling points. You'll find the standard promises of curing wrinkles and blemishes are here but with a large dose of misleading and erroneous information. The cuteness aside, most of these products simply can't do what they say. The blemish products contain irritating ingredients that can make breakouts worse; products claiming not to contain fragrance blatantly contain extremely fragrant plant oils and plant extracts that are all potential skin irritants; and the label describes several decidedly unnatural ingredients as being natural. Here is one of the more maddening examples: "…moisturize or you'll break out more!" Sorry, moisturizers cannot prevent breakouts in any way, shape, or form.

The strong points here lie in the excellent, reasonably priced brushes and a vast collection of lipsticks with a color range that would satisfy everyone from a debutante to a malcontent. The rest of the line tries its best to entice you, and I must admit the products are almost irresistible, but does anyone really need seven products to take care of the lips? However, there is nothing here that is worthy of too much attention or that can't be found in many other lines that offer the shine and glitz of BeneFit along with a healthy dose of real-world shades and exemplary textures.

For more information about BeneFit, call (800) 781-2336 or visit the Web site at www.benefitcosmetics.com.

## BeneFit Skin Care

☺ **All Types Skin Wash** *($14 for 4 ounces)* is about as close a knockoff of Cetaphil Gentle Skin Cleanser as I've seen. At least they're on the right track for a sensitive-skin cleanser, but they're charging twice as much as Cetaphil.

☹ **Fantasy Mint Wash, for Combo/Oily Skin** *($24 for 4 ounces)* contains mint, which can be a skin irritant, especially for the eyes, for all skin types. This product also contains emollients that would be problematic for combination and oily skin.

☺ **Clean Sweep** *($14 for 4 ounces)* is a very standard, detergent-based eye-makeup remover. It will indeed wipe off your eye makeup.

☹ **Alpha Clean 5% AHA** *($18 for 5.56 ounces)* doesn't list the form of AHA used, which doesn't meet FDA requirements for ingredient listings. Plus the scrub particles in here are scratchy and potentially irritating. Even if the AHA in here was effective, it would just be washed down the drain in this strangely formulated cleanser.

☺ **Honey … Snap Out of It! Scrub, for All Skin Types** *($17 for 5 ounces)* is an almond meal–based scrub with a great enticing name and an overwrought price tag.

You would be better off with Cetaphil Gentle Skin Cleanser and baking soda or just plain almond meal (the scrub source for this product). The clay and rye flour in this product can be hard to rinse off.

☹ **Azulene Tonic** *($14 for 4 ounces)*. Several of the plant extracts in this product can be skin irritants including witch hazel, arnica, ivy, pellitory, and rose oil. Azulene is a chamomile extract but it is used primarily as a coloring agent in cosmetics and has few of chamomile's anti-irritant properties.

☹ **Rosewater Tonic** *($14 for 4 ounces)*. The witch hazel in here can be a skin irritant. The urea in here can work like an AHA as an exfoliant and a humectant.

☹ **Alpha Smooth 5% AHA Toner** *($18 for 5.56 ounces)* doesn't have a low enough pH to be an effective exfoliant, plus the source of the AHA is not listed so not only does the ingredient label not meet FDA standards, but also you can't rely on it for information about what you're putting on your skin.

☺ **$$$ Seven % Fine Wrinkle Line Remover** *($36 for 1 ounce)* doesn't contain a low enough pH to be an effective exfoliant, plus the label doesn't indicate what kind of AHA is used, so this is definitely not in compliance with FDA regulations. Other than that this is a good moisturizer for normal to dry skin.

☺ **$$$ Dr. Feel Good** *($24)* is supposed to be worn either alone or over makeup to "smooth pores and fine lines leaving skin silky, flawless and matte to the touch." And because it contains vitamins A, C, and E, "it repairs skin without a prescription." Wow! Who wouldn't want this product? It turns out that Dr. Feel Good is an extremely thick pot of wax resembling a thick lip balm or clear shoe polish more than anything else. I guess you could also call this product spackle, because that is exactly how it works. The wax melts over the skin and then fills in the flaws (at least somewhat). I didn't notice a difference in my wrinkles, but over the long haul I would be very concerned about clogged pores because this is really thick, heavy stuff.

☺ **Eye Lift** *($25 for 1 ounce)* is a rather standard moisturizer for normal to dry skin, and nothing about it will lift the eye.

☹ **In the Shade, SPF 15** *($24 for 2.5 ounces)* doesn't contain avobenzone, titanium dioxide, or zinc oxide, and is not recommended.

☺ **Daily Hyaluronic Creme** *($22 for 2 ounces)*. The amount of vitamin E and pollen extract in this product is at best a dusting; however, it is still a good emollient cream for someone with dry skin. Hyaluronic acid is a good water-binding agent, but no better than dozens of other such ingredients.

☺ **Daily Vitamin Creme** *($25 for 2 ounces)* doesn't contain enough vitamins to be a daily dose of anything. This is a just a good lightweight moisturizer for someone with slightly dry skin.

☺ **Daily Vitamin Creme for Sensitive/Dry Skin** *($22 for 2 ounces)* is a good moisturizer for someone with dry skin, and if you want antioxidants, they're in here.

☹ **ReEyedrate Aromatherapy, for Eyes** *($30 for 1 ounce)* includes rose and citrus, which can irritate the eye area. The chamomile can be a good anti-irritant but these other two ingredients get in the way of that.

☹ **RePair Aromatherapy, for Sun Damage** *($30 for 1 ounce)* contains no ingredients that can repair sun-damaged skin. This is a very misleading product that insinuates that you can get sun damage and then reverse it, when you can't. The plant extracts in here, including lavender, artemesia, and other fragrance additives, can be skin irritants.

☹ **ReBalance Aromatherapy, for Combo Skin** *($30 for 1 ounce)* contains a bunch of plants that have no effect whatsoever on breakouts or skin tone.

☹ **ReVitalize Aromatherapy, for Combo Skin** *($30 for 1 ounce)* may smell nice, but there are no ingredients in it that can stimulate cell generation.

☺ $$$ **"Aruba in a Tuba" Ultra Sunless Tan** *($22 for 5 ounces)* is a sunless tanner that uses the exact same active ingredient to turn the skin brown that all other sunless tanners use: dihydroxyacetone.

☹ **Boo-Boo Zap** *($16 for 0.25 ounce)* contains mostly water, two types of alcohol, witch hazel, and styrene. This doesn't help blemishes in the least, in fact it can cause more irritation and redness and make skin dry and inflamed.

☹ **Buh-Bye! Nighttime Blemish Blaster** *($21 for 0.25 ounce)* is a blemish product that contains Vaseline as the third ingredient. Unbelievable! But it's just one of the many problems for this product. It also contains pineapple juice and eucalyptus oil, which can be irritating and won't help blemishes, plus sanguinaria (bloodroot) extract; that has some antimicrobial properties, but whether or not it has any impact on blemishes or is effective in the teeny amount used in this product is unlikely.

☺ $$$ **Shrink Wrap Mask, for Combo/Oily Skin** *($26 for 2 ounces)* is a good mask for most all skin types.

☺ $$$ **Smoooch** *($15 for 0.25 ounce)* is just a very good, though standard, clear lip gloss in a tube applicator. It would work as well as any.

☹ **Thigh Hopes** *($23 for 8 ounces)* lists the second ingredient as sodium lauryl sulfate, which can be a skin irritant. It does contain aminophylline, the substance originally hyped as being able to get rid of cellulite, but a later exposé proved the research to be faulty and biased (the researchers owned the very product being tested).

## BeneFit Makeup

<u>FOUNDATION:</u> ☺ $$$ **PlaySticks** *($30)* is a strictly cream-to-powder foundation in stick form that must be blended quickly as it dries to a powder finish almost immediately, and it does have a soft matte finish in the long run. Coverage can go from light to medium and the drier finish makes this suitable for normal to

slightly oily skins only, but it won't hold up as the day goes by for those with very oily skin. All of the colors are soft and neutral.

☺ $$$ **Sheer Genius** *($26)* is a standard, pressed-powder foundation with a limited number of shades. This does provide smooth, sheer coverage and has a slightly dry finish. The available shades are all fine.

☹ **Out and About Tinted Moisturizer** *($18 for 2.5 ounces)* has a tint that is too peach for most skin tones.

☺ $$$ <u>CONCEALER:</u> **Boi-ing** *($16)* is for those "yucky dark circles" and it does provide fairly opaque coverage. However, the cream-to-powder texture may not last through the day without fading or creasing, and the two colors available are slightly pink or peach. Still, this may work for some skin tones. **Ooo La Lift** *($18)* is an "instant eye lift that firms and tightens!" or so BeneFit would like you to believe. This is just a pale-pink liquid highlighter with a smooth texture and a slight shine. There is absolutely nothing in here to support the "lift, firm, and tighten" claims.

☹ **It-Stick** *($16)* is a thick pencil concealer intended to "pop out" expression lines. There is only one color, a pale peach, which won't work on most skin tones, and the creamy texture dries to an unflattering chalky finish. ☹ **Eye Bright** *($16)* is a pale-pink, slightly greasy pencil meant to be used on the dark inner corners of the eyes. It is completely unnecessary (any neutral-shade concealer can do the same without the somewhat odd pink tint).

<u>POWDER:</u> ☺ $$$ **Powder Tint** *($22)* is a very drying, almost chalk-like face powder that comes in seven colors. There are a few shades to steer clear of: Coast is a ghost-like white, Chamois is too yellow (it is meant to even out redness, but it just looks slightly jaundiced on the skin), and White Lavender (a pale purple) serves no known purpose for skin. The other four are excellent neutral shades and very good for someone with exceptionally oily skin.

☹ **Get Even** *($24)* is a standard pressed powder with two shades of yellow. This is supposed to invisibly get rid of shine and discoloration. Yellow powder on the face is hardly invisible; all it does is alter the color of your foundation to a strange, unattractive hue.

☺ $$$ <u>BLUSH:</u> **Color Wash** *($24)* is a loose powders in blushlike colors that are an exceedingly messy and inconvenient way to use blush. With so many excellent blush options at other counters, this is a total waste of time and money. ☺ **BeneTint** *($26)* gets an absurd amount of press in the fashion magazines when it is nothing more than a rose-tinted, watery cheek color that, while sheer, is only best on flawless, smooth skin. ☺ **Glamazon** *($26)* is virtually identical to the BeneTint, only this is a sheer (though liquidy) believable bronze tint. If your skin is perfectly smooth and even, it will work well. **Nine One One** *($18)* is a soft, brownish-pink tint in a tube applicator meant to be used for the eyes, lips, and cheeks. It has a slightly sticky texture and a creamy finish that works best on the lips. If you're prone to breakouts, the greasy feel isn't best for the cheeks and if you have any problem with eyeshadows creasing, this will make matters worse.

☺ <u>EYESHADOW</u>: **$$$ Creaseless Crème Eyeshadow** *($14)* has a creamy, slick feel with a soft powder finish. These actually do a great job of not creasing, but the colors, though sheer and relatively easy to apply, are almost all shiny. I would suggest that it is easier to start off with a powder in the first place, but if you are interested in cream eyeshadows this is a definite option. **$$$ Lemon Aid** *($16)* is an unnecessary pale-yellow eyeshadow base that has a thick texture; it does not work as well as a neutral foundation for minimizing discoloration. **$$$ FY ... eye** *($20)* is an over-priced, peach-toned eyeshadow base that adds a subtle, strange tone to the eye area. Again, your foundation will do fine instead. **Powder Eyeshadow** *($10)* is unimpressive with mostly shiny colors that can't hold a candle to the generous offerings from M.A.C. or countless other lines. **Show-offs** *($14)* are small vials of iridescent loose powder that are pretty to look at but messy to apply. For intense shine and sloppy application, these are hard to beat. **Swingin' Sweetie Eye Sparkle** *($14)* are small pots of very shiny, loose-powder eyeshadow. Both the color and shine are potent enough, but why put up with such a messy product when countless pressed (shiny) eyeshadows exist?

☹ <u>EYE AND BROW SHAPER</u>: **Babe Cakes** *($15)* are standard cake eyeliners that go on wet and then dry to a dramatic, shiny finish. **Bad Gal, Gilded,** and **Mr. Frosty** *($15)* are standard chunky pencils that are all shiny and creamy enough to consistently smear. **Flash** *($11)* is a shiny beige pencil that you are supposed to place on the rim of your lower lid. Please do not place anything that near to your eye. It is not only irritating, it is unhealthy and potentially damaging to the eye.

☺ **Eye Pencils** *($12)* go on well, with a slightly dry texture. They're standard but nice, and there's a nice assortment of soft colors. ☺ **$$$ Brow Zings** *($20)* are brow colors that are a cross between a waxy pencil and a powder applied with a stiff brush. They are meant to tame brows, but they can make the brow look matted. For longevity and ease of use, these are not preferred over a good matte powder.

☹ **$$$ She-Laq** *($16)* is a thick liquid with hairspray ingredients that is meant as a sealant for lipstick, eyeliner, or brow color. This should not go anywhere near the eye, as the irritation potential is just too high, and is otherwise just an expensive variation on brow gel.

☺ <u>LIPSTICK AND LIP PENCIL</u>: BeneFit's **Lipstick** *($14)* has some great colors to choose from. Although they are unspecified (which is confusing), there are **creams** that are indeed creamy with a glossy finish, and **mattes** that are almost matte, but do have a slight creamy finish. **Lip Gloss** *($13)* has a slippery, non-sticky texture and most of the colors are opaque. Nice, but overpriced. **Lip Pencil** *($12)* has a rich, creamy texture but is otherwise standard and ho-hum. **Smoooch** *($15)* is simply lip balm in a tube. It's emollient and feels nice, but why spend this much for something so boring and basic when many other lines have identical versions for far less?

☹ **Protectints SPF 15** *($14)* are sheer, greasy lipsticks with no active sunscreen agent listed, and are not recommended.

☺ **It's a Girl/It's a Boy** *($14)* are, for some reason, set apart from the regular lipsticks—but aside from extra iridescence these are identical to the Protectints listed above. ☺ **depth change** *($14)* and **light switch** *($14)* are lipsticks you apply over other lipsticks you want to make lighter or darker. Basically, they are light and dark lipsticks just to the greasy side of creamy, and as any light or dark lipstick shade can, it will change the color of a lipstick you want to alter. ☺ $$$ **Dancing Darlings Lip Sparkle** *($16)* are just standard lip glosses in pots with a handful of colors infused with sparkles. For glittery lips at a premium price, these will do. ☺ $$$ **De-groovie** *($21)* is supposed to prevent lipstick from feathering. It does do an OK job, but just OK.

☹ **Lip Plump** *($16)* is a lightweight concealer for the lips that gets almost as much beauty press as the BeneTint. It slightly, and I mean *slightly*, fills in the lines on your lips, but breaks down almost immediately after you apply your lipstick, meaning the difference is barely discernible.

☺ **MASCARA:** BeneFit's **Mascara** *($13)* is an OK mascara that can work for lengthening, but don't expect much thickness. It applies nicely and tends to not smear, which is always a plus. There is also clear mascara that could work as a brow gel.

☺ **BRUSHES:** There is much to like about BeneFit's **Brushes** *($11 to $27)*, including the down-to-earth prices. You will find that most of these are beautifully shaped and appropriate for a variety of looks. Check these out if you happen upon them! There are really only two to avoid: **Get Bent Eyeliner** *($13)* has a fun name and it is bent, but the brush itself is long and splays too easily to get a controlled line. **Sheer Powdering** *($16)* is a sparse, fan-shaped brush whose purpose has never been adequately explained to me, and whatever the intended effect is, it can surely be created with a more traditional brush.

☺ $$$ **SPECIALTY PRODUCTS:** Because BeneFit's image emphasizes fun and frivolity, you'll find some additional products that can be a brief departure from the norm for special occasions. **Lightning** *($20)* is an intense, golden shimmer body lotion. **Flamingo Fancy** *($20)* is almost identical to Lightning, only it has a coral-bronze shimmer color. **Kitten** *($24)* is nothing more than adorably packaged, shiny, talc-based loose powder for the body, incredibly overpriced but decidedly sexy. And **High Beam** *($18)* comes in a nail-polish bottle and is applied to the face in a similar manner. It is just a shiny moisturizer that dries to a matte finish, leaving the shine behind. Cute, definitely cute!

# Bioelements (Skin Care Only)

You may have seen this line of skin-care products being sold at the salon where you get your hair cut or nails done. It is very attractive and uses all the current buzzwords that the cosmetics industry loves to bandy about. The brochure states, "Your skin is a mirror that reflects your inner well-being. Visible surface problems like premature wrinkles, dryness, excess oil, irritation, and blemishes are often visual reflections of deeper, below-the-surface imbalances. These imbalances occur when your body is thrown out of sync by the normal everyday challenges of air pollution, chemicals, the sun, poor nutrition, or emotional upsets. ... [This] stress[es] your system's inner balance."

That sounds great, but none of it is true. The aging process is much more complicated than this diatribe on inner peace and health lets on. The one thing it is right about is that the effects of the sun are potent, and for that it does have a good SPF 15 sunscreen. The rest of the products are on the hokey side, as are the claims that you can give extra oxygen to the skin to slow down visible signs of aging, or detoxify the skin with antioxidants. For more information on this line, call (800) 433-6550 or visit the Web site at www.bioelements.com.

☺ **Decongestant Cleanser** *($18.50 for 6 ounces)* is a standard, detergent-based water-soluble cleanser. It would be good for someone with oily to combination skin. It does contain fragrance.

☺ **Moisture Positive Cleanser** *($18.50 for 6 ounces)* can be a good cleanser for someone with dry skin, though it doesn't remove makeup well without the help of a washcloth. It does contain fragrance. However, to save money and forgo the fragrance, Neutrogena's Extra Gentle Cleanser ($6.06 for 6.7 ounces) is almost identical for almost a third the price.

☹ **Twice Daily Bar Gentle Non-Soap Cleanser** *($16.50 for 5 ounces)* is one expensive bar of soap. It is indeed far more gentle than regular soap, but the detergent cleansing agents can still be drying and the ingredients that keep it in a bar form can potentially clog pores. It does contain fragrance.

☹ **Makeup Dissolver, Oil-Free Formula for Your Eyes** *($15.50 for 6 ounces and a sponge)* has witch hazel as the first ingredient, and that can be a skin irritant, especially around the eye area.

☺ **$$$ Measured Micrograins** *($21.50 for 2.5 ounces)* is a standard scrub that uses little pieces of polyethylene (plastic) for the scrub particles. It does contain fragrance. It would work well enough as a scrub for normal to dry skin, it's just overly expensive for what you get.

☺ **Equalizer** *($17.50 for 6 ounces)* is an OK (but very ordinary) toner for most skin types. Some of the plant extracts in here can be skin irritants, including ginseng and sumac.

☹ **Quick Refiner with AlphaBlend** *($40 for 3 ounces)* is an alcohol-based AHA toner. AHAs can be irritating enough without adding further irritation from the alcohol. Not only are there cheaper AHA products available, but there are much less irritating ones.

☹ **Everyday Protector SPF 8** *($29.50 for 6 ounces)* is not recommended due to the low SPF. With the amount of sun damage possible on a daily basis, and all the wonderful SPF 15s available, there is no reason to use anything less. What a shame, because this one has both titanium dioxide and zinc oxide, both of which offer great UVA protection when there's enough of them.

☺ **$$$ Sun Diffusing Protector SPF 15** *($29.50 for 6 ounces)* is a zinc oxide– and titanium dioxide–based sunscreen in a rather ordinary but OK base of thickeners, with minute amounts of plant extracts.

☺ **Absolute Moisture** *($29.50 for 2.5 ounces)* is a good moisturizer, but only for someone with normal to dry skin.

☹ **Beyond Hydration Moisturizer** *($29.50 for 2.5 ounces)* contains several problematic plant extracts, including peppermint, sage, sumac, and ginseng. There is never a reason to put any irritating ingredients on the skin, and especially not when the goal is moisturizing.

☹ **Crucial Moisture** *($29.50 for 2.5 ounces)*. There is nothing crucial or even very interesting about this product. It would be a good, though ordinary, moisturizer for someone with normal to slightly dry skin.

☹ **$$$ Eye Area with AlphaBlend** *($31.50 for 1 ounce)*. The pH of this product makes it a poor exfoliant, but it is also an exceedingly boring moisturizer as well.

☹ **$$$ Instant Emollient** *($8.50 for 0.14 ounce)* is more of a clear lipstick than anything else. It's emollient, but also greasy and heavy.

☹ **$$$ Cremetherapy Very Emollient Mask** *($23 for 2.5 ounces)*. Because there are so many emollients in this product and so little clay, it could be a fine mask for someone with dry skin. What a shame that it also contains several irritating plant extracts, including peppermint, sage, ginseng, and sumac.

☺ **$$$ Immediate Comfort 1% Hydrocortisone Lotion** *($22 for 1 ounce)* is a version of other over-the-counter cortisone creams such as Lanacort and Cortaid. Given the similarity, it's up to you to choose whether you want to spend $3 for 1 ounce or $22 for 1 ounce for almost identical products.

☺ **$$$ Jet Travel** *($31.50 for 1 ounce)* is a good, toner-like product that would work well for someone with normal to slightly dry skin.

☺ **$$$ Stress Solution** *($31.50 for 1 ounce)* is similar to the Jet Travel above and the same comments apply.

☺ **$$$ Urban Detox** *($31.50 for 1 ounce)* is similar to the Jet Travel above only this version contains a good antioxidant.

☺ **$$$ Oxygen Cocktail Natural Defense Against Visible Skin Aging** *($31.50 for 1 ounce)* contains something called tissue respiratory factors. That may be a water-binding agent for this product, but it can't provide oxygen for skin. Even if it could provide oxygen, doesn't that negate the idea of using antioxidants, which several of the BioElements products contain? Regardless, this is similar to Jet Travel above and the same comments apply.

☺ **$$$ Pigment Discourager** *($18.50 for 0.5 ounce)* is a standard 1% hydroquinone skin-lightening product. Hydroquinone can improve skin discolorations but not without the help of a sunscreen or a skin exfoliant, plus there are far less expensive products like this available.

☹ **$$$ Breakout Control** *($31.50 for 1 ounce)*. Benzoyl peroxide is a good disinfectant and can help reduce breakouts, though the standard waxy cosmetic thickeners used in this product could clog pores and are not the best when you're fighting breakouts.

☹ **T-Zone Monitor** *($31.50 for 1 ounce)* contains lemon, sage, and eucalyptus, which are all skin irritants that will only hurt skin, not help it.

☺ **$$$ Restorative Clay Active Treatment Mask** *($21.50 for 2.5 ounces)*. If you have dry skin and want to try a clay mask, the oils in here can help soften the drying effects of the clay.

☹ **Yang Aromatherapy Oil** *($19.50 for 2 ounces)* contains a number of potentially irritating plant oils. If you like the way this smells, that's great; just don't put it on your face.

☹ **Yin Aromatherapy Oil** *($19.50 for 2 ounces)* contains a number of potentially irritating plant oils. If you like the way this smells, that's great; just don't put it on your face.

## Biogime (Skin Care Only)

Just the name alone conveys a message of plants, science, and cleanliness. But though the name has great appeal, the information regarding these products is a mixed bag. On one hand the brochure states concisely that "there are no miracles" but then the rest of the facts about skin care are just sheer fantasy. For example, the information about oily skin goes like this: "How do people with oily skin normally combat this excess oil? They use alcohol or alcohol-based products. …the message sent to the oil gland is, I'm dry up here on the surface, send more oil." That isn't true in the least. If all it took was having dry skin to create oil production, then those with naturally dry skin would have richly flowing oil glands, and they don't. Oil is almost 95% generated by hormonal activity, and that can't be affected from the outside in.

Here's another Biogime gem, for sensitive skin: "Finding a maintenance program is difficult since staying away from perfumes or fragrances, collagen, elastin,

SD alcohol, and other known irritants is critical to proper care of your skin type." Yet several of Biogime's products contain fragrance (lemon and bergamot oils are fragrances), witch hazel (which contains alcohol), and extremely irritating and sensitizing cleansing ingredients such as sodium C14-16 olefin sulfate and sodium lauryl sulfate. Didn't Biogime read its own ingredient labels? Further, Biogime states that its "Skin Care System is perfect for all skin types because it allows you the flexibility to customize the system for your particular concerns." Yet this line contains no topical disinfectants for breakouts and only one effective sunscreen—and that certainly won't work for all skin types.

Its claim regarding the pure and natural content of the products is also bogus. All the products contain their share of very unnatural preservatives, chemical emulsifiers, and synthetically derived detergent cleansing agents. That doesn't make these products bad, but it's one more example of the kind of ersatz claim cosmetics companies love to perpetrate so the consumer can never know for certain what she is really buying. For more information call (800) 952-6226 or visit the Web site at www. biogime.com.

☺ **Colloidal Cleanser** (*$15.95 for 6 ounces*) is a mostly standard wipe-off cleanser that contains sunflower oil instead of mineral oil. It can still leave a greasy film on the skin. Biogime's suggestion is to use this cleanser to wipe off the makeup, and then follow up with the Lathering Cleanser. A two-step makeup-removing process should not be necessary. There are plenty of gentle, water-soluble cleansers that can take off everything, so a wipe-off makeup remover is rarely necessary.

☹ **Lathering Cleanser** (*$17.95 for 6 ounces*) contains sodium lauryl sulfate as the first ingredient, which, in this amount, can be seriously irritating for most skin types.

☹ **Oil Absorbing Cleanser** (*$18.95 for 6 ounces*) is a standard, detergent-based water-soluble cleanser with several irritating ingredients, including lemon oil, mandarin oil, lime oil, orange oil, and grapefruit extract, that make it a problem for all skin types.

☹ **Gentle Facial Buff** (*$17.95 for 4 ounces*) is extremely scratchy and potentially irritating to all skin types. The diatomaceous earth (seashells) in the scrub may sound natural, but it is incredibly rough on the skin. This product also contains spearmint oil, which adds more irritation.

☹ **Oil Absorbing Citrus Scrub** (*$19.95 for 4 ounces*) is even more of a problem than the one above. This one also contains diatomaceous earth, plus it uses sodium C14-16 olefin sulfate as the cleansing agent, and that is extremely drying and irritating for all skin types. The lemon oil, mandarin oil, lime oil, and orange oil just add fuel to the fire.

☺ **Essential Toner** (*$22.50 for 8 ounces*) is an OK, relatively irritant-free toner that could work for most skin types. It is mostly just water, slip agents, and detergent cleansing agent. It does contain some arnica and witch hazel; they are far enough down in the ingredient listing so they probably won't be sensitizing, but be careful.

☹ **Oil Controlling Toner** *($19.95 for 6 ounces)* contains mostly witch hazel, and that can be irritating for most all skin types.

☺ **Protective Toner** *($19.95 for 6 ounces)* is an extremely ordinary toner. This would be a good, though standard, irritant-free toner for most skin types.

☺ **Natural Conditioner** *($22.45 for 6 ounces)* contains mostly sunflower oil, thickeners, preservatives, and vitamins. This is almost identical to the Colloidal Cleanser, so the extra cost is only a marketing gimmick. It is a good, though exceptionally ordinary moisturizer for someone with normal to dry skin. The amount of vitamins is almost negligible.

☹ **Oil-Free Gel Conditioner** *($22.95 for 4 ounces)* is indeed oil-free but the second ingredient is witch hazel, which means it isn't irritant-free.

☺ **Skin Perfection with Retinol Palmitate and Lipsosomes** *($34.95 for 4 ounces)* is almost identical to the Natural Conditioner above and Ultimate Conditioner below, only in cream form, and the same reviews apply. There is vitamin A in here, which is OK as an antioxidant, but the amount is so negligible as to be barely present.

☺ **Ultimate Conditioner** *($23.45 for 6 ounces)* is almost identical to the Natural Conditioner and the same review applies.

☺ **$$$ Youthful Eye Gel** *($39.95 for 0.5 ounce)* is mostly film former (hairspray) with a small amount of glycerin. It would deliver minimal moisturizing benefit for the skin, but the film former can make things look temporarily smoother. The plants are listed after the preservative, making their quantity completely insignificant.

☺ **Sun Protector SPF 15** *($17.95 for 4 ounces)* is a good, in-part titanium dioxide–based sunscreen. This one would be good for someone with normal to dry skin.

☹ **Aerobic Fitness Facial Kit** *($34.95 for 2 ounces with a small glass bowl and brush)* is supposed to rebuild tissue while tightening your 55 facial muscles. Nothing in here can rebuild tissue or tone facial muscles, although several ingredients could irritate the skin. It contains mostly egg white and cornstarch. The minuscule amount of RNA in here has minimal effect only as a water-binding agent.

☺ **$$$ Refining Sea Mud** *($36.95 for 5.5 ounces)* is decent clay mask for normal to slightly dry skin. The oils in here are problematic for someone with oily skin.

# *BioMedic*

Dermatologists are selling skin-care products these days, lots of them. Not surprisingly, the number of lines marketed to dermatologists has increased more than 100% over the past ten years. But there is nothing medical about these (or any) products being sold at a doctor's office. Every skin-care and makeup line being sold at doctors' offices comes under the FDA's guidelines regulating cosmetics, and that means they legally don't have to provide accurate or viable claim substantiation. Just like the rest of the industry, the ingredients these products contain can only be those approved for cosmetic or over-the-counter use.

The benefit touted by physicians in defense of their selling skin-care products is, who else is better able to prescribe products for someone's skin? I find that a plausible argument, except when I see the price tags and the types of products these doctors are selling. When a physician sells expensive sunscreens (such as the ones from the BioMedic line) that have formulas and efficacy similar to drugstore brands, knowing that this might mean improper application will be used, I simply don't buy the premise of "better recommendations." (As I've stated in my newsletter, most people aren't willing to liberally apply a 2-ounce sunscreen that costs $30 the way they do a 6- or 8-ounce sunscreen costing $10.) And when doctors recommend their product lines by filling out a prescription, when similar or identical products are available from other lines for far less, that's a problem.

There is also a problem when some of the information being merchandized to the physician and then sold to the consumer is distorted information. It's one thing when that kind of misleading marketing is from a regular cosmetics line, but when you're buying products from a dermatologist or plastic surgeon, different ethics come into play. I find it extremely questionable and unethical when doctors make the same foolish claims as the rest of the cosmetics world.

For example, here is information from the BioMedic brochure. "Acne is basically good skin that is out of balance ... The sebaceous oil glands become overactive from internal factors such as the hormonal surge or external factors like pollution and sun exposure." The first part is true, the second part is bogus. There is no evidence that pollution or sun damage have any influence on oil production.

Another excerpt from the BioMedic information packet made this presentation to doctors: "the cleanser and conditioner will last two to three months. The gels, creams, and sunblocks will last four to six months." The cleansers come in 6-ounce containers; the sunscreens in 2-ounce containers, and the self tanner in a 4-ounce container. If that much self tanner and cleanser last more than a month you would be doling them out in minute amounts, and if you used the sunscreen for more than a month you'd be seriously hurting your skin by not using the product liberally enough, which is required for adequate protection. Doctors who sell expensive sunscreens are setting their patients up for problems.

One other issue is that the BioMedic line sells three types of retinol creams with supposedly different strengths of retinol. The real question is, why sell a retinol product at all when the medical literature barely suggests it is useful for skin? It's not that retinol isn't a good skin-care ingredient—but to sell it as a special wrinkle cream that can take the place of Retin-A, the way the BioMedic brochure sells it, is misleading. BioMedic even goes so far as to suggest that retinyl palmitate can work like Retin-A. Retinyl palmitate is so far removed even from retinol (much less Retin-A or Renova) that claiming any potential relation for it is just that much more unlikely.

Despite some really poor misinformation, the BioMedic line, while expensive, does provide reliable information regarding hyperpigmentation problems (though the product designed for this purpose is not recommended), and there are some well-formulated products too. It is also refreshing to see that most of the products are fragrance-free (except for one or two products where they snuck lavender oil or fragrant plant extracts in) and that coloring agents have been omitted. For these, the only thing that is really disconcerting is the price. A typical skin-care routine from BioMedic costs $150 to $200. There is nothing in this line worth that expenditure, or that you can't get elsewhere for far less.

BioMedic's true claim to fame is its MicroPeel, which carries a bit more panache and allure. The MicroPeel is a light, acid-type peel with concentrations ranging between 15% and 30% (as opposed to deeper peels with concentrations of 50% to 70%). The light acid peels can be performed by an aesthetician, and like all AHA peels there can be immediate benefits; however these light peels are not long-lasting. Even the BioMedic brochure states that "only the advanced chemical peels [TCA or phenol] effectively treat wrinkles. In no way do we feel the results of the BioMedic MicroPeel Procedures are equivalent to that of an advanced [deep] peel." That is true and completely honest. Because the results are fleeting, many aestheticians or doctors perform these peels in sets of four and six. I am concerned about the repetitive deep irritation and the limited duration of the benefits. I often wonder why women would get light-AHA peels (15% to 30%) instead of the higher-concentration versions or other peels, or even laser resurfacing, which is longer-lasting and only needs to be done once every several years.

For more information about BioMedic, call (800) 736-5155 or visit the Web site at www.biomedic.com.

☺ $$$ **Purifying Cleanser** *($25 for 6 ounces)* is a standard, detergent-based water-soluble cleanser that can be good for normal to oily skin. It contains a tiny amount of AHA (less than 1%), which is not enough for it to be effective as an exfoliant even though the BioMedic information claims otherwise.

☹ **Gentle Cleansing Gelee** *($25 for 6 ounces)* uses TEA-lauryl sulfate as the main detergent cleansing agent, which is a strong possible skin irritant for all skin types.

☹ **Micro Massage Exfoliating Wash** *($20 for 6 ounces)* is a fairly abrasive scrub that uses ground-up shells. It also contains grapefruit, orange, and lemon, which are about the most inane ingredients I've ever seen in a scrub.

☺ **Gentle Soothing Toner** (*$20 for 6 ounces*) is as standard a toner as you will find. This is not worth the money, though it would be fine for someone with normal to dry skin.

☺ **Conditioning Gel** (*$25 for 2 ounces*) and **Conditioning Gel Plus** (*$30 for 2 ounces*) are two skin-lightening products with various concentrations of hydroquinone, AHA, BHA, and kojic acid (Gel Plus has 2% hydroquinone and the Gel has 1%). These are both valid options for skin lightening, being good state-of-the-art formulations. However, the second ingredient is alcohol and that can be drying and irritating; given the other potent active ingredients, it can make using these products extremely difficult on the skin.

☹ **Conditioning Solution** (*$20 for 6 ounces*) is a toner form of AHA with 5% glycolic acid and 0.5% BHA, only this one contains a lot of alcohol and eucalyptus. This product is an irritation waiting to happen.

☺ **Conditioning Cream** (*$27 for 2 ounces*) is a very standard, 8% glycolic acid moisturizer. The pH is great and makes it very effective for exfoliation, but the other ingredients are no different from what you would find at the drugstore in Alpha Hydrox's AHA products.

☺ **Phospholipid Lotion** (*$30 for 2 ounces*) is an 8% to 10% AHA lotion in a very simple moisturizing base. Lipids are fats, and "phosphate" is a way of making them more lightweight, which makes them good, standard moisturizing ingredients. This is a good option for normal to dry skin.

☺ **Phospholipid Gel** (*$30 for 2 ounces*) has the same AHA content as the one above only in gel form. It contains minimal emollients and would be an option for someone with normal to oily skin.

☺ $$$ **Microencapsulated Retinol Cream 15, 30, or 60** (*15: $30 for 1.05 ounces; 30: $32 for 1.05 ounces; 60: $35 for 1.05 ounces*). These are good moisturizers, although there's no reason to spend money on products boasting about their retinol content. If you want retinol, you would be just as well off using Neutrogena's version.

☺ $$$ **Maximum C** (*$20 for 0.25 ounce*) contains magnesium ascorbyl palmitate, which is the form of vitamin C of interest to those who want to be on the vitamin C bandwagon. It can have some benefit for inhibiting melanin production, but probably not at the minimal amount this product contains.

☺ $$$ **Ultra C Protection** (*$45 for 1 ounce*) is similar to the one above and the same comments apply.

☹ **Damage C Control** (*$32 for 0.5 ounce*) does contain vitamin C, only this one uses ascorbic acid, which is considered to be an irritating and unstable ingredient. This version does contain sulfur, which can be a skin irritant. Overall this isn't the vitamin C product to consider.

☺ **Pure Enzyme** (*$30 for 1 ounce*). Enzymes can provide some exfoliation, but they are not as stable or as reliable as AHAs or BHA. This is an option if you are interested in trying an enzyme-type product, but why bother?

☹ **Acne Control** *($20 for 0.5 ounce)* contains mostly alcohol along with grapefruit and sage oil, which makes this extremely irritating for all skin types.

☹ **Antibac Protection** *($30 for 1 ounce)* has no antibacterial agent. It is simply an ordinary, otherwise boring moisturizer. What a misnamed product.

☺ **Extra Mild Protection** *($27 for 2 ounces)* is an extremely standard moisturizer. It would be fine for normal to dry skin.

☺ **Facial Shield SPF 20** *($30 for 2 ounces)* does contain an in-part titanium dioxide–based sunscreen and is an option for sun protection, but the expense is unwarranted. There are many similar and far less expensive versions, and with them you are more apt to use the right amount so you get complete sun protection.

☺ **Pigment Shield SPF 18** *($30 for 2 ounces)* does contain in-part zinc oxide and is an option for sun protection, but the expense is unwarranted and there are far less expensive options with zinc oxide at the drugstore.

☹ **Gentle Day Block SPF 30** *($18 for 2 ounces)* doesn't contain UVA-protecting ingredients, and is not recommended.

☺ **Hydro Active Emulsion** *($27 for 2 ounces)* is a good, extremely standard moisturizer for dry skin. The tiny amount of vitamins in here is window dressing.

☻ **Hydrating Fluid** *($32 for 2 ounces)*. Even if there were a benefit from beta-carotene for the skin, this lightweight moisturizer contains eucalyptus, an unnecessary skin irritant.

☺ **$$$ Conditioning Eye Cream** *($25 for 0.5 ounce)* is by far the most elegantly formulated of any of the moisturizers in the BioMedic line, and is filled with state-of-the-art water-binding agents.

☺ **Extra Rich Moisturizer** *($30 for 1 ounce)* is similar to the one above, and the same comments apply.

☺ **High Density Gel** *($26 for 2 ounces)* is a very good, extremely lightweight moisturizer for normal to oily skin.

☹ **Pigment Control** *($20 for 0.5 ounce)* lists alcohol as the second ingredient, which makes it too drying and irritating for all skin types. It does contain kojic acid, which can have some impact on melanin production, but this has only been demonstrated in vitro and not on skin.

# *Biore (Skin Care Only)*

Many skin-care lines are launched with a specific gimmick to grab the consumer's attention, and Biore is in this category. The gimmick is Biore's **Pore Perfect Deep Cleansing Strips** *($5.99 for six nose strips)*. This product is supposed to instantly clean pores. All you do is place a piece of cloth with an incredibly sticky substance on it over your nose, as you might do with a Band-Aid, wait 15 minutes for it to dry, and then rip it off. Along with some amount of skin, blackheads are supposed to stick to it and come right out of the skin on your nose. What does this miracle product contain? The main ingredient on the strip is polyquaternium-37, a film-forming hairspray ingredient—so it's basically a piece of gauze with a form of hairspray on it.

What has me most concerned about these so-called Cleansing Strips is that they are accompanied by a strong warning not to use them over any area other than the nose and not to use them over inflamed, swollen, sunburned, or excessively dry skin. It also states that if the strip is too painful to remove, you should wet it and then carefully remove it. What a warning!

You may at first be impressed with what comes off your nose. (Well, there is no question: you will be impressed.) Most people do have some oil sitting at the top of their oil glands (most of the face's oil glands are located on the nose), and whether you use these strips or a piece of tape, black dots and some skin will be removed. Is that helpful? Only momentarily, but if you use the Biore product, the plastic-forming agent can get into the pores and possibly cause breakouts and irritation.

Also, despite the warning on the package, most women will try these strips wherever they see breakouts. If I didn't know better, I know I would. The way these strips adhere, they can absolutely injure or tear skin and cause spider veins to surface. They are especially unsafe if you've been using Retin-A, Renova, AHAs, or BHA; having facial peels; or taking Accutane; or if you have naturally thin skin or any skin disorder such as rosacea, psoriasis, or seborrhea.

Biore's brochure claims this product can pull an entire blackhead plug out of the skin. It can't. If you could grab a blackhead out of the skin, your skin would be left with an empty hole (and there is nothing in this product that will close it up), but that's not what happens. Instead, just the top layer of the blackhead is removed, and then the blackhead returns because the source of the problem was never corrected. Nothing was done to reduce irritation, exfoliate skin cells, help keep oil flow normal, or close the pore. What about the rest of Biore's products? Here's my review, but clearly this line is based on these strips and little else. Biore is being sold in drugstores across the country. For more information call (888) BIORE-11 or visit the Web site at www.biore.com.

☹ **Blemish Fighting Cleanser** *($6.99 for 5 ounces)* is a standard, detergent-based water-soluble cleanser that would be an option except that the fourth ingredient is alcohol, and that can be drying and irritating for skin. This also contains a minimal amount of BHA (0.5%), which would be a problem in a cleanser for the eyes, but the pH of this cleanser makes it ineffective as an exfoliant.

☹ **Warming Deep Pore Cleanser** *($6.99 for 5 ounces)* does feel warm, but heat on the skin has no benefit for breakouts. If anything, the heat can make already red-looking blemishes even redder.

☹ **Facial Cleansing Cloths** *($7.19 for 34 cloths)* contain mostly alcohol, and that's too drying and irritating for all skin types.

☺ **Cleansing Gel, Non-Foaming** *($5.99 for 5 ounces)* is a very good, water-soluble cleanser for someone with normal to dry skin, but it may not remove makeup very well. The brochure states that this cleanser and the one below use sorbitol, a natural plant extract, to dissolve dirt and remove pollutants. Didn't anyone at Biore read the ingredient lists for these products? They contain standard detergent cleansing agents, just like thousands of other water-soluble cleansers. Besides, sorbitol isn't a cleansing agent; it is a good but ordinary cosmetic thickening agent.

☺ **Foaming Cleanser** *($5.99 for 5 ounces)* is almost identical to the cleanser above, but with stronger cleansing agents and foaming agents. It can be a very good, water-soluble cleanser for someone with normal to oily skin.

☹ **Facial Cleansing Cloths** *($5.97 for 34 cloths)*. Why does this contain alcohol? Someone please tell me what the purpose of the alcohol is! Why can't the cosmetics industry just stop this one? It's not like it's a big secret to anyone that alcohol is irritating and drying, and burns on raw skin. Whoops, I started ranting didn't I? Sorry. This product is not recommended.

☺ **Mild Daily Cleansing Scrub** *($4.94 for 5 ounces)* is a standard, detergent-based water-soluble cleanser that uses synthetic scrub particles (polyethylene, a form of plastic) for the abrasive. This would work as well as any for most skin types. It does contain fragrance.

☹ **Self-Heating Mask** *($5.12 for six packets)* is a standard clay mask that does get warm when applied to the skin, but the heating effect doesn't help skin—if anything heat can make inflamed skin look more red and irritated.

☹ **Self-Heating Moisture Mask** *($5.99 for six packets)* is similar to the one above only without the clay. This is fairly emollient for dry skin, but the heating effect can be problematic for skin.

☹ **Pore Perfect Toner** *($4.94 for 5.5 ounces)* has three different types of alcohol in it, including the alcohol in witch hazel. What in the world were they thinking?

☹ **Blemish Bomb** *($6.99 for ten packets)* contains way too much alcohol to make it anything other than a real bomb for the face.

☹ **Balancing Moisturizer, Oil Free** *($8.99 for 3.5 ounces)* won't balance anything, and actually feels rather sticky and tacky when applied. The foam dispenser is cool, which is the only thing of interest.

☹ **Hydrating Moisturizer** *($8.99 for 4 ounces)* is a fairly sticky, useless moisturizer for any skin type.

☹ **Hydrating Moisturizer SPF 6** *($8.99 for 4 ounces)* is not recommended. The SPF 6 is dismal, and it doesn't contain titanium dioxide, zinc oxide, or avobenzone, which are necessary for adequate UVA protection.

⊗ **Fine Line Gel Patches** (*$12.49 for six pairs of patches*) won't change a wrinkle and the film former can be irritating for some skin types.

⊗ **Pore Perfect Ultra Strip** (*$6.99 for six strips*). Aside from my feeling that any pore strips can be problematic for skin, this version contains menthol, adding (ouch!) *more* irritation to the risk of using these.

## BioTherm

BioTherm is one of the many companies owned by L'Oreal USA that has a vast array of products. In many ways this line isn't as elegant or interesting as L'Oreal or Lancome (also owned by L'Oreal). Though BioTherm's claims are wrapped around the exotic spa concept, the products are far from unique or specially formulated. One ingredient BioTherm utilizes to gain your attention is something they call "biotechnological thermal plankton." For your information, plankton are microscopic plants and animals that are adrift in fresh and salt water. They come in many forms, including one-celled amoebas, tiny jellyfish, fish larvae, and some forms of algae. I imagine the thermal reference is that they were somehow heated before being stuck in some of these products. What can plankton do for your skin? That's anyone's guess. I have yet to see any research suggesting that this is the cosmetic ingredient you've been waiting for. However, if thermal plankton is supposed to be so remarkable, why don't the other L'Oreal product lines use it?

"Naturally purifying extracts" is another phrase BioTherm likes to use. While these products do indeed contain a handful of plant extracts, they are neither purifying nor essential. Actually, a strong point for BioTherm is that it uses minimal amounts of plant extracts, which reduces the risk of allergens and irritation. Several of the products do contain decent antioxidants, including vitamin E and superoxide dismutase, and, outside of the United States, it has excellent suncare products. The strengths of this line are some very good cleansers and well-formulated moisturizers. BioTherm also has a spa gimmick—its added a group of mineral salts, including magnesium, zinc, copper, manganese, potassium chloride, and regular table salt, to its products. However, minerals can't be absorbed by the skin, and they may cause irritation when left on the skin instead of being rinsed off.

BioTherm's makeup still consists only of foundations, and to some extent, these have improved. Some new light shades have been added and these are right on target with neutral colors, but there are no colors for very light or darker skin tones. What's objectionable is the very strong fragrance wafting from all of the makeup—there is no skin-care benefit from overly perfumed products, regardless of the source of the fragrance components, and the chance of irritation and allergic reactions is magnified. For more information on BioTherm, call (212) 818-1500, or visit the Web site at www.biotherm.com.

☺ **$$$ Biosensitive High Tolerance Fluid Cleansing Milk** *($20 for 5 ounces)* is mostly glycerin and thickening agents. That makes it an exceptionally ordinary cleanser that requires a washcloth to help get makeup off.

☺ **$$$ Biosensitive Self-Foaming Gentle Cleanser** *($19 for 5 ounces)* is a standard, very ordinary, detergent-based cleanser that would work well for most skin types. It does contain fragrance. It also contains something called vitreoscilla ferment, a bacteria culture, but there is no research indicating this to be of any help for skin.

☹ **Biosource Express Cleansing Fluid** *($20 for 8.5 ounces)* is a lightweight, water-soluble cleanser that doesn't remove makeup very well, although it may be OK for someone with dry, sensitive skin. The minerals may have antibacterial benefit but they can also be skin irritants.

☺ **Biosource Foaming Gel Cleanser** *($15 for 5 ounces)* is a detergent-based water-soluble cleanser that would work well for most skin types.

☹ **Biosource Instant Cleansing Foam** *($15.50 for 5 ounces)* uses fairly drying and irritating cleansing agents and is not recommended.

☹ **Biosource Invigorating Cleansing Milk** *($19 for 8.5 ounces)* is a mineral oil–based cleanser that also contains a small amount of detergent cleansing agents. This would be an option for someone with normal to dry skin, though it can leave a greasy feel on the skin. It does contain fragrance.

☹ **Biosource Softening Cleansing Milk** *($19 for 8.5 ounces)* is almost identical to the Invigorating version above and the same comments apply.

☹ **Biosource Softening Cleansing Mousse** *($15.50 for 5 ounces)* uses fairly drying and irritating cleansing agents and is not recommended.

☹ **$$$ Biocils Soothing Eye Make-up Remover** *($17 for 4.2 ounces)* is a standard eye-makeup remover with slip agents and detergent cleansing agents. The amount of detergent cleansing agents in this one can be problematic for the eye area.

☺ **$$$ Biocils Waterproof Eye Make-up Remover** *($18 for 4.2 ounces)* is a silicone-based eye-makeup remover and it works well to remove waterproof makeup.

☹ **$$$ Biosource Softening Exfoliating Cream** *($18 for 2.5 ounces)* is a mineral oil–based cleanser that also contains several other emollients and crushed seashells. It works as a scrub but can feel somewhat scratchy and irritating.

☹ **$$$ Biosource Clarifying Exfoliating Gel** *($18 for 2.5 ounces)* is similar to the Cream version above only with detergent cleansing agents. The same basic comments apply.

☹ **$$$ Biosensitive Calming Thermal Spring Spray** *($20 for 5 ounces)*. The microscopic amount of plankton in here is barely worth mentioning. It does contain fragrance.

☹ **$$$ Biosource Invigorating Toner** *($19 for 8.5 ounces)*. The mixture of good ingredients and potentially irritating ingredients makes this a confused product for the skin.

☺ **Biosource Softening Toner** *($19 for 8.5 ounces)* is almost identical to the Invigorating version above, only minus the witch hazel. That makes it a decent option for a toner, though the minerals can be potentially irritating for skin. It does contain fragrance.

☹ **Biosource Clean Skin Peel-Off Mask** *($23 for 2.5 ounces)* is basically alcohol and film former. It will peel off and make the skin feel temporarily smooth, but the risk of irritation is a problem.

☺ **Aquasource Oligo-Thermal Moisturizing Gel for Dry Skin** *($29 for 1.7 ounces)* is a good moisturizer for normal to dry skin. The alcohol in here is an insignificant amount (along with the remaining interesting ingredients) so it isn't a problem for skin.

☺ **Aquasource Oligo-Thermal Moisturizing Gel for Normal Skin** *($29 for 1.7 ounces)* is almost identical to the Dry Skin version above and the same comments apply.

☺ **Biojeunesse Skin Refining Day Cream** *($35 for 1.7 ounces)* is a good, though standard moisturizer for nighttime (no sunscreen means it is dangerous to use during the day). It does contain a teeny amount of salicylic acid, but the pH is too high for the BHA to have any exfoliating effect on the skin.

☺ **Bionuit Overnight Visibly Effective Skin Treatment** *($35 for 1.7 ounces)* is a very good moisturizer for normal to dry skin.

☺ **Biosensitive Calming Regulating Daily Cream** *($27 for 1.7 ounces)*. This standard moisturizer would be good for someone with normal to dry skin but the interesting ingredients come well after the preservative.

☹ **Biosensitive Calming Regulating Oil-Free Lotion SPF 12** *($30 for 1.7 ounces)* doesn't contain any of the UVA-protecting ingredients—titanium dioxide, zinc oxide, or avobenzone—and is not recommended.

☺ **$$$ Biosensitive Yeux Calming Eye Cream** *($35 for 0.5 ounce)* would be a good moisturizer for normal to dry skin but it contains a plant extract from *Terminalia sericea,* which can be a skin irritant or cause contact dermatitis.

☹ **D-Stress Fortifying Anti-Fatigue Radiance Essence** *($40 for 1 ounce)* lists alcohol as the second ingredient, which makes this potentially drying and irritating for all skin types.

☹ **D-Stress Fortifying Anti-Fatigue Radiance Gel for Normal/Combination Skin** *($37.50 for 1.7 ounces)* is similar to the version above and the same comments apply.

☺ **$$$ D-Stress Fortifying Anti-Fatigue Radiance Gel/Cream for Dry Skin** *($37.50 for 1.7 ounces)* is a good moisturizer for someone with normal to dry skin.

☺ **$$$ Hydra-Detox Yeux Moisturizing Eye Gel** *($25 for 0.5 ounce)* would be a good moisturizer for normal to dry skin but it contains a plant extract from *Terminalia sericea* and caffeine, which can be skin irritants or cause contact dermatitis.

☺ **Hydra-Detox Daily Moisturizing Cream** *($35 for 1.7 ounces)* can't "detox" the skin, though it is a good moisturizer for someone with dry skin. It has one of the longest ingredient lists in the line, but it adds up to a good, silicone-based moisturizer. Without sunscreen, it is not appropriate for "daily" use.

☺ **Hydro-Detox Daily Moisturizing Lotion** *($35 for 1.7 ounces)* is similar to the product above, only in lotion form.

☹ **Hydra Detox Moisturizing Detoxifying Mask** *($20 for 2.53 ounces)* contains alcohol, menthol, and a plant extract from *Terminalia sericea*, which can all be problems for most skin types.

☺ **Reducteur Rides Anti-Wrinkle and Firming Cream, for Dry Skin** *($37 for 1.7 ounces)* is a standard mineral oil– and Vaseline–based moisturizer that also contains thickeners, fragrance, and preservatives. This is an extremely ordinary moisturizer that won't get rid of one wrinkle and has nothing of interest that Lubriderm or Cetaphil moisturizers can't replace for far less.

☺ **$$$ Reducteur Rides Anti-Wrinkle and Firming Eye Creme** *($30 for 0.5 ounce)* is similar to the product above, and the same review applies.

☹ **Reducteur Rides Tensing Wrinkle and Firming Essence** *($52 for 1 ounce)* has alcohol as its second ingredient, which makes it potentially irritating and drying for the skin.

☺ **$$$ Retinol Re-Pulp Smoothing Anti-Wrinkle Care** *($45 for 1 ounce)* does contain retinol, but is virtually identical to L'Oreal's Line Eraser Pure Retinol Concentrate ($12.49 for 1 ounce). If you're looking for retinol, there is no reason to spend this kind of money.

☺ **$$$ Symbiose Daily Aging Treatment Liposome Gel** *($45 for 1.7 ounces)* would be a good lightweight moisturizer for someone with normal to slightly dry skin.

☺ **BioPur Pure Cleansing Gel** *($15 for 5 ounces)* is a decent (though truly standard) detergent-based water-soluble cleanser that would work well for most skin types. It has a small amount of copper and zinc gluconate. Zinc gluconate can have antibacterial or antiviral benefit, while copper has no known benefit; however, copper negates the effectiveness of zinc, at least internally. Even if these did have some benefit topically, in a cleanser they would just be rinsed away. It does contain fragrance.

☺ **$$$ BioPur Double Purifying Exfoliator** *($15.5 for 2.53 ounces)* is a standard, detergent-based water-soluble cleanser that uses synthetic scrub particles (polyethylene—ground-up plastic) as well as seashells as the abrasive. This can be a fairly irritating way to scrub the skin. Baking soda with a gentle cleanser would do the same thing for far less. This does contain fragrance and coloring agents.

☹ **BioPur Mattifying Astringent Lotion** *($20 for 8.5 ounces)* lists the second ingredient as alcohol and that is too irritating and drying for all skin types.

☹ **BioPur Clarifying Balancing Night Gel** *($30 for 1.7 ounces)* won't balance anyone's skin. It contains a group of standard thickening agents (several that could cause breakouts) and some clay. It also contains a small amount of salicylic acid, but the pH is too high to make this an effective exfoliant. This product is a waste of time and money.

☹ **BioPur Matte Hydrating Fluid** *($24 for 1.7 ounces)* definitely has a matte finish because the fourth and fifth ingredients are aluminum starch (octenylsuccinate) and clay. With the oil-absorbing ingredients here negated by the silicone and thickening agents it contains, this is a confused product. There is a small amount of BHA in here but the pH is too high for it to work as an exfoliant.

☺ **$$$ BioPur Balancing Purifying Mask** *($20 for 2.5 ounces)* contains wheat starch, which can be problematic for people prone to breakouts. Other than that, it is a basic clay mask that can't balance or purify.

☹ **BioPur Emergency Anti-Imperfection with AHA** *($18 for 0.5 ounce)* contains too little AHA and BHA and doesn't have the right pH to be an effective exfoliant. It does contain several thickening agents that can cause breakouts. The second ingredient in this cream is zinc oxide and the third is clay. That makes it more like spackle than anything else.

☹ **BioPur Ultra-Matte T-Zone Essence** *($24 for 1.7 ounces)* lists alcohol as the second ingredient, which makes this too irritating and drying for most skin types.

☺ **Sunscreen Lotion SPF 30** *($15 for 5 ounces)* is a good, in-part titanium dioxide–based sunscreen. It contains aluminum starch (octenylsuccinate) as the fourth ingredient, which would give it a fairly matte finish but also a small risk of causing irritation. It does contain fragrance.

☺ **Ecran Total Sunblock for Face SPF 30** *($15 for 1.7 ounces)* is almost identical to the Lotion SPF 30 above and the same comments apply.

☺ **Hydrating Sunscreen Gel SPF 15** *($15 for 5 ounces)* is a good, in-part avobenzone-based sunscreen. The second ingredient is alcohol, which makes it better for the neck down and not for the face.

☹ **Soothing After Sun Gel for Face and Body** *($17 for 2.6 ounces)* lists the second ingredient as alcohol, which doesn't make this soothing, though it can be drying and irritating for most skin types.

## *BioTherm Makeup*

**FOUNDATION:** ☺ **Base Magic Makeup Beautifier** *($15.50)* is a standard silicone-based gel that makes the skin feel incredibly silky and supposedly acts as a primer to your foundation. That may work for some drier skin types who don't want a heavy feel, but this one's orange tint and strong orange scent are big turn-offs in my book.

☺ **Aqua Teint Fixe Non-Transfer Fluid Makeup** *($20)* has a very slick, smooth texture that dries to a satiny finish. This is an ultra-matte foundation in the sense that it almost stains the skin, but the formula never quite dries to a true matte finish.

The nine colors are a mixed bag; the lighter shades are fine, but these medium to dark colors should be avoided by most skin tones: 05, 07, 20, 55, and 85.

☺ **Naturel Perfection Foundation with Fruit Extracts** *($19)* has four new lighter shades that are very good, though the remaining four shades are too peach or rose for most skin tones. The application is sheer and appropriate for normal to dry skin. The fruit acids are not the right kind to exfoliate the skin, and even if they were, the pH of this product is too high for exfoliation to occur, so this one loses on both counts.

☺ **BioPerfection Liposome Treatment Makeup** *($20)* starts off moist and dries to a natural matte finish with light to medium coverage that would be an option for normal to dry skin. However, of the six shades, only the lighter ones (01 and 02) look like real skin color. Most skin tones would do well to avoid 03, 04, 05, and 06.

☺ **Aqua Teint Mat Fluid Makeup** *($19)* has a silky, silicone-based texture that must be blended quickly to ensure an even application. It has a good matte finish without feeling heavy or thick, yet there is enough slip in the formulation to allow shine to break through quickly on someone who is very oily. The seven shades are surprisingly good; the only ones to watch out for are 40, 55, and 85.

☹ **Dual Perfection Foundation** *($22.50)* is a standard, talc-based powder foundation with a smooth texture that is still rather awkward to blend. It's very sheer and the powder doesn't pick up and hold the product the way most every other powder foundation does, so applying it is time consuming and, in light of the countless other options, futile.

☺ **Ecran Naturel Eye Block Concealer SPF 15** *($12)* lists titanium dioxide as the active sunscreen, which is great—but there is nothing about this formula that makes it better suited to the eye area; the consistency and coverage is more akin to foundation than concealer, and it stays creamy on the skin. Of the two shades, Pale is acceptable while Nude is too peach.

# *Black Opal*

Black Opal is a cosmetics line aimed at African American women. The skin-care products, although reasonably priced, have some problems. They were supposedly designed by a dermatologist, but either the dermatologist didn't do all the chemistry homework necessary to design a skin-care line or there were terrible oversights. When a skin-care line boasts about its plant extracts, I wonder exactly what a dermatologist could be thinking, given the potential for allergic reaction and the lack of evidence that these types of ingredients provide a benefit for the skin. Lastly, the designer of the skin-care line seems to think that women of color have only oily or combination skin and that darker skin tones can tolerate irritating ingredients. They can't. If anything, drying, irritating products can increase skin discolorations by causing more dead skin cells to accumulate on the surface of the skin.

Black Opal's makeup offers women of color the richly pigmented products they need to perform beautifully on deep skin tones. You'll find a pleasing (but dwindling) array of velvety-textured eyeshadows, although many have taken on a shiny edge that is not as attractive on any skin tone as matte shades can be. Where Black Opal excels is its foundations. The textures and finishes may not be universally appealing but the shades are in line with true skin tones, with very few to avoid. The selection isn't as big as Prescriptives, but for the money this is a color line that women with medium to very dark skin tones on a budget would be mistaken to overlook. For more information about Black Opal, call (800) 554-8012 or visit the Web site www.planetrx.com.

# Black Opal Skin Care

☹ **Blemish Control Complexion Bar** *($3.50 for 3.5 ounces)* contains the same ingredients that keep all bar cleansers in their bar form and that can exacerbate breakouts, while the cleansing agents can be drying for skin. This product is not recommended.

☹ **Blemish Control Wash** *($5.95 for 6 ounces)* has sodium lauryl sulfate, a strong skin irritant, as the main detergent cleansing agent. This cleanser also contains several other serious skin irritants, including camphor, menthol, eucalyptus oil, and peppermint oil. This product is absolutely not recommended.

☺ **Oil Free Cleansing Gel** *($4.51 for 6 ounces)* is a standard, detergent-based water-soluble cleanser that can be good for someone with oily skin. It can be drying for some skin types.

☹ **Pre-Fade Complexion Bar** *($3.50 for 3.5 ounces)* contains ingredients that keep bar cleansers in their bar form (in this case, tallow), and that can exacerbate breakouts. There is nothing in this product that will help fade skin discolorations; if anything, the drying effect of the cleansing agents can make skin look more ashen. This product is not recommended.

☹ **Blemish Control Astringent** *($4.79 for 6 ounces)* contains mostly alcohol but it also has arnica, menthol, eucalyptus, peppermint, and camphor, which makes this an irritation waiting to happen.

☺ **Purifying Astringent** *($3.99 for 6 ounces)* won't purify anything, but it is a good irritant-free toner that contains mostly water, glycerin, slip agent, anti-irritants, more plant extracts, aloe, and preservatives.

☺ **Oil Free Moisturizing Lotion** *($3.99 for 1.75 ounces)* is a good, though ordinary moisturizer for someone with normal to slightly dry skin.

☹ **Revitalizing Eye Gel with Undereye Lighteners** *($8.95 for 0.6 ounce)* contains several ingredients including lemon, grapefruit, and witch hazel, that can be skin irritants, and that will only make puffiness worse.

☺ **Skin Retexturizing Complex with Alpha-Hydroxy Acids** *($9.95 for 1 ounce)* would be a very good 7% AHA product for most skin types.

☹ **Maximum Moisture Night to Day Face Creme** *($6.95 for 6 ounces)*. Several of the plant extracts in this product, such as arnica extract, ginseng, pine extract, and lemongrass oil, can cause skin irritation.

☹ **SPF 15 Daily Protection for Photosensitive Skin** *($3.99 for 2.25 ounces)* doesn't contain the UVA-protecting ingredients of titanium dioxide, zinc oxide, or avobenzone, and is not recommended.

☺ **Advanced Dual Phase Fade Creme with Sunscreen** *($11.95 for 1.75 ounces)* doesn't contain avobenzone, zinc oxide, or titanium dioxide, and can't be recommended for a sunscreen, especially in conjunction with a fade cream, in which sun protection is so crucial for the skin-lightening ingredients to have an effect. However, it does contain 2% hydroquinone, which makes it an effective skin lightener in a very good moisturizing base.

☺ **Advanced Dual Complex Fade Gel** *($11.95 for 0.75 ounce)* is a standard 2% hydroquinone gel that would work well for someone with normal to oily skin.

☹ **Blemish Control Gel** *($5.95 for 0.35 ounce)* contains resorcinol, a disinfectant. Though it is considered fairly irritating, it would be worth a try—only this gel also contains camphor, menthol, eucalyptus oil, and peppermint oil, which serve no purpose for skin except to create irritation and dryness.

☺ **Skin Refining Peel** *($3.99 for 1.75 ounces)* is a standard clay mask with some wax, thickeners, glycerin, silicone, and preservatives. It would be a good clay mask for someone who likes this skin-care step.

# *Black Opal Makeup*

**FOUNDATION:** ☹ **Cream Stick Foundation SPF 8** *($6.99)* comes in a stick form and looks like it would go on quite greasy but in fact just the opposite is true. It goes on smooth and then dries to a soft, matte finish. It does tend to stay in place once it's on, so blending can be tricky. There are only a handful of colors that are quite good for the most part, but some are too orange. Without testers, it is hard to recommend the Black Opal foundations, though if you find this line at Sears, testers are usually on hand. The SPF is not only too low, but has no UVA protection.

☹ **Cream to Powder Foundation SPF 8** *($6.99)* not only doesn't have any UVA protection, but the nine colors are either too red or peach for most skin tones, and the consistency of this will cause the colors to turn on oilier skins.

☺ **True Color Maximum Coverage Foundation** *($8.39)* is a thick, stay-put foundation that offers truly opaque coverage and a soft matte finish yet doesn't leave a heavy after-feel. The six shades are mostly excellent, but watch out for Heavenly

Honey, which is too peach for most skin tones. **True Color Liquid Foundation Oil Free** *($6.99)* goes on quite smooth and sheer, drying to a matte finish. It can feel very dry on the skin and is best for oily skins. The nine shades are mostly good options, but avoid Cinnamon Toast and Sandalwood, which are too rosy-red for most skin tones.

☺ **CONCEALER: Flawless Concealer** *($3.89)* is a lipstick-style concealer that comes in four workable shades. It has a thick, creamy texture that covers well and leaves a minimal powder finish. The four shades are slightly orange but may work for some skin tones, and creasing shouldn't be a major problem.

**POWDER:** ☺ **Oil Absorbing Pressed Powder** *($6.99)* is a standard, talc-based powder that comes in a small assortment of colors; it has a silky texture that blends on easily. Cafe Au Lait and Cappuccino can both be too peach for most skin tones, but Mocha is a great option. **Color Fusion Pressed Powder** *($9.89)* comes in one "shade," which is actually several colors swirled together that come off as one sheer brown color on the skin. It's talc-based and may work for some skin tones, but test it first. **Color Fusion Bronzer** *($9.49)* is similar in appearance to the Color Fusion Powder above but this comes in matte and shimmer options, with the matte strongly preferred even though it is not deep enough for truly dark skin tones.

☹ **Deluxe Finishing Loose Powder** *($6.99)* has an unfriendly assortment of peach and rosy-red shades that are best avoided.

**BLUSH:** ☹ **Color Fusion Blush** *($9.89)* tries to please all skin tones by combining fragments of peach, rose, red, pink, purple, and plum tones in one compact. It's more of a contrivance, and the color you get is no substitute for Black Opal's single-color blush options. ☺ **Natural Color Blush** *($2.85)* comes in eight beautiful matte shades that go on silky and impart rich, lasting color. These are a real find for darker skin tones—if you can find them. While these are hard to come by at the drugstore, you may have luck finding them at Sears.

**EYESHADOW:** ☺ **Color Rich Eyeshadows** *($4.89)* have an exceptional matte finish and are richly pigmented, but are hard to find in most stores. What is widely available are several eyeshadow duos, called ☹ **Double Takes Eyeshadows** *($6.49)*, that are very shiny or are infused with brightly colored shiny particles that tend to flake off on the skin. These require precise blending, as they tend to grab on the skin and are hard to move.

☺ **EYE AND BROW SHAPER: Dual Ended Eye Pencil** *($4.99)* is a standard pencil with one end having a matte finish and the other end being outrageously shiny. **Precision Eye Definers** *($4.89)* are standard pencils with a more traditional selection of non-shiny colors.

☺ **LIPSTICK AND LIP PENCIL: Matte Plus Moisture Lipstick** *($4.99)* isn't all that matte and is actually rather creamy with an almost glossy finish. The color selection is small but wonderful for darker skin tones. **True Tone Vitamin Rich Lipstick** *($4.99)* is more emollient than matte, but not in the least bit greasy. Again, the shade selection is on par with the needs of deeper skin tones. **Simply Sheer Lipstick SPF 15** *($4.99)* is, as the name implies, a sheer, more glossy lipstick with no UVA protection, which is a shame as this used to have an in-part titanium dioxide base. **Double Features Lip Gloss** *($6.49)* is a two-sided lip gloss that has a very slick texture, with one end being standard wet gloss and the other end being glittery gloss. **Lip Gloss** *($3.49)* is a very greasy gloss that comes in a pot and features some excellent deep colors, but they are mostly iridescent. **Precision Lip Definer Pencil** *($3.99)* is a standard lip pencil with some great colors to complement dark lipsticks. At this price, if you love pencils, buy them all!

☺ <u>MASCARA:</u> **Lash Defining Mascara** *($3.99)* still has one of the strangest brush shapes I've ever seen for mascara. It definitely doesn't aid in making lashes longer, and takes a while to build much length or thickness. It doesn't clump or smear, but that brush is not deserving of a happy face.

## Blistex (Lip Care Only)

How this small line of lip products has achieved the status of being the solution for cold sores or chapped lips eludes me. These lip products contain enough irritating ingredients to chap anyone's lips. Lots of lip products claim to be medicated, but "medicated" is a dubious term at best, with no regulated meaning. As Blistex does, these types of products often contain camphor, peppermint oil, eucalyptus, or menthol, but these are not medicines for dry lips; they make dry skin worse. Products like Blistex can include 0.5% phenol, a potent disinfectant, but phenol is strong stuff and can actually trigger some serious problems, the least of which are dryness and irritation. It is not something I would recommend for anything but extremely limited use. You may have heard a rumor that lips can adapt to or get used to lip balm. It isn't possible. So if the lip balm you are using contains irritating ingredients, your lips will stay dried up. For more information about Blistex call (630) 571-2870.

☹ **Medicated Lip Ointment** *($1.50 for 0.21 ounce)* contains menthol, camphor, and phenol in a base of Vaseline and alcohol. Everything but the petrolatum is too irritating for the lips—or any part of the body, for that matter.

☹ **Lip Medex** *($0.86 for 0.25 ounce)* is similar to the one above, only with large quantities of the irritating ingredients.

☹ **Lip Balm SPF 10** *($0.99 for 0.15 ounce)* doesn't contain avobenzone, zinc oxide, or titanium dioxide, and is not recommended.

☹ **Daily Conditioning Treatment SPF 20** *($1.50 for 0.25 ounce)* doesn't contain avobenzone, zinc oxide, or titanium dioxide, and is not recommended.

☺ **Lip Revitalizer** *($1.59 for 0.25 ounce)*. At least this version doesn't contain irritants, which makes it a good emollient balm for lips.

☹ **Lip Tone SPF 15** *($1.59 for 0.15 ounce)* doesn't contain avobenzone, zinc oxide, or titanium dioxide, and is not recommended.

☺ **Medicated Lip Balm Berry, SPF 10** *($1.49 for 0.21 ounce)*, although it doesn't contain UVA-protecting ingredients, is still a good emollient lip balm for dry lips that contains mostly thickeners, emollient, lanolin, mineral oil, and Vaseline.

# *Bobbi Brown*

Bobbi Brown has been one of the most quoted and referred-to makeup artists in fashion magazines for several years now, and her handiwork has graced the faces of countless models and celebrities. Brown's product line established her reputation as the source of the natural neutral palette. As women lined up to see what her line had to offer, no one seemed to notice the striking similarities to M.A.C., at least as far as the blush and eyeshadows were concerned, and that many of her foundation colors were strongly yellow.

Although classic, neutral colors were once Brown's only mantra, her line has grown by leaps and bounds under the watchful eye of parent company and owner Estee Lauder. On the plus side, the foundation colors have been toned down to true neutrals and the product options are impressive, with great eyeshadows, cream-to-powder blushes, a tinted moisturizers with SPF, a workable brow gel, and attractive lipstick choices. On the other hand, Brown's color palette has also grown to embrace all the trendy makeup gimmicks Brown previously eschewed. Her line now includes everything from shiny eyeshadows to glitter-infused lipsticks. This is a curious development from a woman whose company once proclaimed, "Bobbi Brown shuns the trendy and unwearable for a muted spectrum of sophisticated shades. ..." That sounded great but no doubt left Brown's line in the dust when it came to all the latest bells and whistles other lines offered. To compensate, Brown launched ColorOptions, an ancillary collection of bold, bright, and shiny colors. Jumping on bandwagons, even when it doesn't agree with your philosophy about beauty, appears to be a good business maneuver.

In the beginning Brown's line sported only makeup products, but her skin-care product line has expanded too. Although many of the products are absurdly overpriced, there are some good options, but these are more of an afterthought than anything of consequence for taking care of the skin.

Where this line excels is in its original offerings of superior foundations, true matte blushes and eyeshadows, and all of the other basics that really *are* essential to a woman's classic makeup wardrobe. All of these are certainly worth checking out and win this line high marks. For more information on Bobbi Brown and ColorOptions, call (212)-572-4200 or visit the Web site at www.bobbibrowncosmetics.com.

# Bobbi Brown Skin Care

☹ **Face Cleanser** *($27 for 6 ounces)*. There are some fairly irritating plant extracts in this product, including arnica, pine, kiwi, and lemon, which can all be too irritating for the eyes and for most skin types.

☹ **Gel Cleanser** *($27 for 6 ounces)* is a standard, detergent-based water-soluble cleanser that would work well for someone with normal to oily skin. It includes a tiny quantity of plant extracts that are potentially irritating but the amount isn't enough to be a problem. It does contain coloring agents.

☺ **$$$ Gentle Foaming Cleanser** *($27 for 5 ounces)* is a standard, detergent-based water-soluble cleanser that would work well for most skin types, and without fragrance and coloring agents it is more gentle than the one above. It does contain a teeny amount of witch hazel, though not enough to be a problem for skin.

☺ **$$$ Eye Makeup Remover** *($16.50 for 4 ounces)* is a fairly standard, detergent-based eye-makeup remover, like hundreds of others. It works as well as any.

☺ **$$$ Waterproof Eye Makeup Remover** *($16.50 for 3.4 ounces)* is a version that uses silicone instead of mineral oil; it works well and has a great slippery finish that quickly dissipates.

☹ **Exfoliating Face Wash** *($18.50 for 3.5 ounces)* contains menthol, camphor, eucalyptus oil, peppermint oil, and grapefruit oil, all of which are extremely irritating and pose problems of dryness and inflammation for the skin.

☺ **Face Lotion** *($38 for 2 ounces)* is about a 6% AHA product with a good pH, which would be fine for someone with normal to dry skin. However, for the money, it can't hold a candle to Pond's or Alpha Hydrox's versions at the drugstore.

☺ **$$$ Hydrating Face Cream** *($38 for 1.7 ounces)* contains mostly water, silicone, slip agents, thickeners, water-binding agents, vitamins, fragrance, film former, and preservatives. This is a good but extremely ordinary moisturizer for dry skin.

☺ **$$$ Eye Cream** *($32.50 for 0.65 ounce)* would be a good, though very standard moisturizer for normal to dry skin. The amount of vitamins and water-binding agents in here barely amount to anything.

☺ **$$$ Revitalizing Eye Gel** *($32.50 for 0.5 ounce)* is a good, lightweight moisturizer for normal to slightly dry skin. The caffeine and cucumber in here will not revitalize the eyes.

☺ **$$$ Shine Control Hydrating Face Gel** *($38 for 1.7 ounces)* is a good, matte-finish moisturizer for normal to slightly oily skin, though it won't hold up for oily skin types. It does contain BHA (salicylic acid) but the pH isn't low enough for it to be effective as an exfoliant.

☺ **$$$ SPF 15 Face Lotion** *($38 for 1.7 ounces)* is a good titanium dioxide–based sunscreen for normal to dry skin. It does contain anti-irritants and vitamins, which is nice but not special.

☺ **$$$ Intensified Moisture Cream** *($42.50 for 1.7 ounces)* is indeed an emollient moisturizer. This would work great for someone with normal to dry skin.

☹ **$$$ Intensified Moisture Mask** *($25 for 2.5 ounces)* is an extremely standard moisturizer. This would work for dry skin but it is extremely ordinary and not as helpful as many better formulated moisturizers.

☹ **Purifying Clay Mask** *($25 for 2.5 ounces)* contains several irritating ingredients, including peppermint and menthol, and while those won't purify skin in the least, they can cause irritation and inflammation. Ironically, this product does contain other ingredients that work as anti-irritants, so why negate the effectiveness of those by adding problems to the mix?

# Bobbi Brown Makeup

☺ **$$$ <u>FOUNDATION</u>:** Bobbi Brown offers four different foundations, and all of them have strong points and a good selection of colors. **Moisturizing Foundation** *($35)* is a wonderful foundation for someone with for normal to dry skin seeking light to medium coverage. This blends on beautifully and leaves a natural finish. The only colors to avoid are Honey (slightly orange) and Almond (too pink). There are some excellent options here for darker skin tones. **Oil-Free Foundation** *($35)* is a great choice for normal to oily skins in need of a true matte finish. The coverage is on the medium to full side, but this has enough slip to blend out well. Avoid Honey (slightly orange) and Walnut (too red). Again, there are some good options for darker skin tones, particularly Chestnut and Espresso. **Fresh Glow Cream Foundation** *($35)* is best for normal to slightly dry or slightly oily skins. This has a whipped texture and a thicker consistency but blends on better that you might expect. The coverage is medium to full, with a semi-matte finish, meaning those with very dry skin expecting a rich foundation will not be happy with this one. Avoid these colors: Chestnut (too red), Almond (too pink), and Golden (too orange).

☺ **$$$ Foundation Stick** *($35)* bills itself as "foundation and concealer in one." It falls short on both counts, especially in comparison with Brown's other foundations. This is fairly greasy and could easily crease into lines around the eyes or mouth. The coverage is light to medium with a creamy finish, making this best for normal to dry skin. Most of the colors are quite neutral and not nearly as yellow as they originally were. Avoid Walnut (too red) and Honey (too orange).

☺ **$$$ SPF 15 Tinted Moisturizer** *($35)* is just that: a lightweight, sheer-coverage moisturizer with a good, part titanium dioxide–based sunscreen. All three shades are excellent.

☹ **$$$ CONCEALER:** The **Professional Concealer** *($22.50)* is a thick, opaque concealer in a compact. The colors are all fine but the texture of this will eventually crease into any lines around the eyes. Bobbi Brown recommends setting this with lots of powder; that will help prevent creasing, but it will also make the eye area look dry, and any wrinkles will seem more prominent. This is way too thick to use over any blemishes, but would work well to cover other discolorations beyond the eye area.

☹ **$$$ POWDER:** Bobbi Brown's loose **Face Powder** *($29)* is a standard, talc-based powder that has a light, silky texture and a dry finish. The colors are a mixed bag: half are just too orange or yellow (sallow) to recommend. If you're considering trying one of these, proceed with caution and double check the color in natural light. **Pressed Powder** *($26)* is virtually identical to the loose powder, with the same colors and same warnings. For both powders, avoid Sunny Beige, Golden Orange, and Pale. **Sparkledust** *($20)* is a very shiny, overpriced loose powder meant to be used anywhere on the face. The colors are decidedly not neutral: green, lavender, blue, and pure white with glitter are best used for a fun nighttime look, if at all, and are easily replaced with far less expensive versions from Maybelline, L'Oreal, or Revlon StreetWear.

☺ **$$$ BLUSH:** The powder **Blush** *($19)* features gorgeous colors that apply and blend evenly with a smooth matte finish. The only color to think twice about is Soft Pink, which is shiny. **Cream Blush Stick** *($25)* is a sheer, slightly greasy cream blush that remains creamy on the skin. Blending takes some time, and this is really best for flawless normal to dry skin, as it is too greasy for oily skin types. The only color to be careful with is Warm Peach, which can be too orange for most skin tones. **Bronzing Stick** *($28)* is the same texture as the Cream Blush Stick, only these are great bronze tones that are an option for creating a sun-kissed look. All three shades are quite sheer, with no shine to be found! **Bronzing Powder** *($26)* would be a better choice for most skin types than the Bronzing Stick. This one is richer in pigment but easier to apply and to control the intensity since you would use this with a brush. All three shades are beautiful and matte.

☺ **$$$ EYESHADOW:** Bobbi Brown's **Eyeshadows** *($17)* have a silky-smooth blending texture and all of the colors are beautifully matte. There are some great choices here for darker skin tones, and many of these shades would work well for lining the eyes. **Shimmer Eyeshadow** *($18)* are at least named accurately, because these are three very shiny cream-to-powder eye colors that you may want to sidestep. Conversely, the shine is soft, making these wearable for a special evening look.

☹ **$$$ Shimmer Wash Eyeshadow** *($17)* is a collection of sheer, iridescent colors that are set apart from the matte colors on the tester unit, making them easy to avoid. The shiny particles in here tend to flake on the skin—not the desired effect but a reality nonetheless.

☹ **Cream Shadow Stick** *($20)* is a creamy eyeshadow in a roll-up stick form. These may be an option for some, but they do tend to go on choppy and are difficult to blend out evenly. Plus, the texture of this starts smooth but once it has set, it remains sticky!

☺ $$$ <u>EYE & BROW SHAPER:</u> **Eye Pencil** *($15.50)* is a standard pencil with good colors that is slightly creamy but can drag over the skin. Check out Brown's excellent matte eyeshadows for lining instead or opt for the exact same or better pencil from L'Oreal or Neutrogena for one-third the price. **Natural Brow Shaper & Hair Touch-Up Mascara** *($16.50)* is a great way to groom and shade your eyebrows with natural-looking color. This is truly best for the brows only; it applies well and dries quickly, yet the bristles on the brush aren't long enough to reach down to the roots of any gray hair you may wish to conceal. The colors aren't the best for very dark brown or black hair but there is a nice range for lighter hair shades.

☺ $$$ <u>LIPSTICK AND LIP PENCIL</u> Most makeup-artists' cosmetics lines have a plethora of lip options, and Bobbi Brown's is no exception. The **Lipstick** *($16)* is another so-called "creamy matte formula." This is strictly a cream lipstick with a nice opaque coverage and great colors, most of which are brown-based. **Lip Shimmer** *($17.50)* is basically the same as the regular lipsticks, only with iridescence. Why these are $1.50 more is a mystery. **Lip Stain** *($16)* is more of a gloss in lipstick form than anything else, and these are too sheer to leave any trace of a stain. **SPF 15 Lip Shine** *($17.50)* is a creamy, shiny lipstick that is overpriced for what you get and the sunscreen has no UVA protectants.

☺ The **Lip Gloss** and **Shimmer Lip Gloss** *(both $18)* are extremely overpriced, standard, stick glosses with a poor brush that tends to splay after a few uses; the Shimmer version just adds sparkle. **Lip Lacquer** *($18)* is part of Brown's ColorOptions line, and it is slightly less sticky and more pigmented than the other glosses. As far as innovation goes, this is nothing to jump up and down about. **Lip Pencil** *($15.50)* has a slightly dry texture but otherwise is indistinguishable from anyone else's pencils—many of them are far less expensive.

☺ $$$ <u>Artstick</u> *($25)* is a copycat version of everyone else's jumbo pencils for lips and cheeks. This is too greasy to work well as cheek color because application can be streaky and blending tricky. As a lipstick, it may be OK, but at this price a regular lipstick is far easier and doesn't need to be sharpened. **Lip Glimmer** *($17.50)* is Brown's attempt to compete with Urban Decay or Hard Candy—these are brightly colored lipsticks speckled with chunks of glitter.

☺ $$$ <u>MASCARA:</u> The **Defining Mascara** *($16)* is Bobbi Brown's original mascara that does a decent job with lengthening and tends to not clump or smear. **Thickening Mascara** *($16)* is not thickening in the least but could work for a natural, defined lash look. Avoid Plum, which is obviously purple. Neither of these are worth the price tag. **Lash Lustre Waterproof Mascara** *($16)* is a very good mascara that builds some length but very little thickness. It is indeed waterproof, but the brush tends to stick the lashes together while you're applying it, so be careful.

☺ $$$ <u>**BRUSHES:**</u> Brown's **Brushes** *($18.50 to $62.50)* are quite nice, with well-tapered edges and dense bristles. As an added bonus, all of the brushes are available in either a travel (4-inch) or professional (6-inch) length. There are some to carefully consider, and some to ignore altogether, and these are the **Loose Powder Brush** *($62.50)*, which for this amount of money should be perfect but is too floppy and soft to apply powder well. The same holds true for the **Blush Brush** *($42.50)*, also too floppy and soft for controlled application. The **Brow Brush** *($18.50)* is very stiff and scratchy, and the **Contour Brush** *($29)* and **Eye Shader Brush** *($26)* are both too big for most women's eye area, again making control and placement of color an issue. The rest of the collection is worth a look for some nice additions or extras for your makeup tool kit.

# The Body Shop

The Body Shop's makeup line is known as Colourings, and over the years it has gone through several transformations. At one point it was an attractive range of soft, neutral colors and clever, fun products aimed at young women with an eco-consciousness. Its recent incarnation as a slew of shiny, trendy products that are clearly being marketed toward adolescents is disappointing. This latest attempt by The Body Shop at revamping its makeup collection was apparently done to ensure that this target demographic has access to what everyone else is pushing, which is shine, shine, and more shine. What's frustrating is that it is getting harder to find the reliable, basic products that used to be the backbone of Colourings. True, there are still agreeable foundations, concealers, and pressed powders, but from the eyeshadows to the brushes there are many items to avoid. You will find a paltry selection of matte eyeshadows and the brushes are scratchy and stiff, and are now hardly worth mentioning. Several salespeople told me that the inclusion of shine and shimmer is going to continue, while many of the classic colors were on the way out. In fact, in the next year or so Colourings is getting another overhaul, and although I am keeping my fingers crossed that there will be some sort of return to more useable day-to-day colors and textures, that doesn't seem to be the trend right now.

A few of The Body Shop's original strong points remain. The Body Shop wants you to know that they are not only about beauty but about saving our environment and ending cruelty to animals. Brochures describing the horrors of animal testing, the efforts of Amnesty International, the educational impact of The Body Shop in Harlem, and the beauty philosophy of the Woodabe tribe of Africa are prominent. Plus, its prices are still very reasonable and the tester units are open for experimenting. There isn't much room to spread out and the mirrors are awkward, but the sales pressure is low-key. For the most part, you should find the staff quite knowledgeable on the products.

You already know that almost all of the natural ingredients being touted as The Body Shop's point of difference really make no difference at all (except to add potential irritation and fragrance), right? But to check out each plant included in these products is a task worse than making your way through the rain forest. Plus, for all the natural boasting, these products contain lots of unnatural ingredients, and many of the sunscreens lack UVA-protecting ingredients.

For more information about The Body Shop and Colourings, call (800) 541-2535 or visit the Web site at www.usa.the-body-shop.com.

## *The Body Shop Skin Care*

☹ **Aloe Vera Face Soap** *($3.70 for 3.5 ounces)* is a standard soap that also contains aloe, but aloe can't undo the drying effect of the soap. It does contain fragrance and coloring agents.

☺ **Balancing Cleansing Gel for Normal to Oily Skin** *($9 for 6.76 ounces)* is a standard, detergent-based water-soluble cleanser that could be good for someone with normal to oily skin. It does contain a small amount of witch hazel, which may be a slight problem for some sensitive skin types.

☺ **Cucumber Cleansing Milk for Normal to Dry Skin** *($8.15 for 8.4 ounces)* is little more than just using plain mineral oil, which would be better because that would leave out the coloring agents and preservatives. Lanolin can be an allergen for some skin types. This must be wiped off with either a washcloth or a tissue, and it definitely leaves a greasy residue on the skin.

☺ **Foaming Cleansing Cream for Normal to Dry Skin** *($9 for 6.7 ounces)* is a standard, detergent-based water-soluble cleanser that contains some emollients that make it better for someone with normal to slightly dry skin. It contains preservatives but no fragrance.

☹ **Glycerin & Oatmeal Facial Lather for Normal to Dry Skin** *($9.70 for 1.7 ounces)* is a potassium hydroxide–based cleanser that can be fairly drying for most skin types.

☺ **Honey Cream Cleanser for Dry Skin** *($9.70 for 3.5 ounces)* is a fairly emollient, wipe-off cleanser. It can leave a greasy film on the skin but can be an option for someone with very dry skin.

☺ **Orchid Cleansing Milk for Normal to Dry Skin** *($8.15 for 8.4 ounces)*. Skip the fragrance and preservatives and just use plain almond oil; it would work the same and you'd omit the irritation potential from these other additives. Regardless, this cleanser must be wiped off with a washcloth or tissue, and it can leave a greasy residue on the skin, though that may be an option for someone with very dry skin.

☹ **Pineapple Facial Wash for Normal to Oily Skin** *($9.70 for 3.5 ounces)* is an OK, detergent-based water-soluble cleanser that can take off all the makeup, but because it contains some plant oils and problematic thickening agents that can clog pores, it is not recommended for oily skin as its name implies. Plus the pineapple juice can be a skin irritant.

☺ **Passion Fruit Cleansing Gel for Normal to Oily Skin** *($8.15 for 8.4 ounces)* is a good, water-soluble cleanser that can be slightly drying to sensitive or dry skin types.

☹ **Oil-Free Cleansing Wash for Oily Skin** *($9 for 6.76 ounces)* contains mint, which can be a skin irritant, causing problems for all skin types.

☹ **Rich Cleansing Cream for Dry Skin** *($9 for 6.7 ounces)* is basically a cold cream–type wipe-off cleanser that can leave a greasy film on the skin, though it can be an option for someone with very dry skin.

☺ **Japanese Washing Grains for All Skin Types** *($4.75 for 1.7 ounces)* contains ground azuki beans; if that sounds like a good scrub, then these will work, but so will baking soda or almond meal for far less.

☹ **Peachy Clean Exfoliating Wash** *($10 for 3.4 ounces)* is a standard, detergent-based water-soluble cleanser that used peach-pit granules as the scrub. It would work as an exfoliant, though it can be harsh for sensitive or dry skin types. It does contain fragrance, preservatives, and coloring agents.

☹ **Conditioning Cream Scrub for Normal to Dry & Dry Skin** *($12 for 3.7 ounces)*. It's not much of a conditioner; it can leave a greasy residue on the skin, and the cornstarch, orange oil, and orange fruit can be skin irritants.

☹ **Foaming Gel Scrub for Normal to Oily & Oily Skin** *($12 for 3.7 ounces)* is basically a detergent-based water-soluble cleanser that contains walnut shells and olive pits as the scrub agent. It can be fairly abrasive, though it is an option for normal to slightly dry or slightly oily skin types. It does contain fragrance.

☺ **Chamomile Eye Makeup Remover** *($10.95 for 8.4 ounces)* is about as standard a detergent-based makeup remover as you'll find. It does work well, though wiping off makeup is not the best option for skin. It does not contain fragrance.

☺ **Soothing Eye Makeup Remover Gel** *($9 for 3.38 ounces)* would work well to remove makeup though it can leave a slightly slick feel on the skin.

☹ **Cucumber Freshener for Normal to Oily Skin** *($8.55 for 8.4 ounces)* contains alcohol, which is an irritant and drying agent for all skin types.

☹ **Equalizing Freshener for Normal to Oily & Oily Skin** *($8 for 6.76 ounces)* contains witch hazel, peppermint, and mint extracts, adding up to irritation and inflammation for all skin types.

☹ **Grapefruit Freshener Toner** *($9 for 8.4 ounces)* contains alcohol and menthol, which can cause dryness and irritation.

☺ **Hydrating Freshener for Normal to Dry & Dry Skin** *($8 for 6.76 ounces)* is a very good, irritant-free toner for most skin types.

☺ **Orchid and Calendula Freshener for Normal to Dry Skin** *($8.55 for 8.4 ounces)* is a very ordinary but OK, irritant-free toner.

☺ **Honey Water** *($5 for 4.2 ounces)* is an irritant-free toner. It is pretty standard, and fine for most skin types.

☺ **Aloe Vera Moisture Cream** *($9.50 for 1.8 ounces)* is an emollient moisturizer for dry skin. It's fairly standard, though effective.

☺ **Carrot Moisture Cream** *($9.50 for 1.8 ounces)* is similar to the Aloe Vera version above and the same basic comments apply.

☺ **Hydrating Moisture Lotion for Normal to Dry Skin** *($16 for 3.38 ounces)* would be a very good moisturizer for someone with dry skin. There are tiny, insignificant amounts of vitamins at the end of the ingredient list.

☺ **Light Moisture Lotion for Normal to Oily Skin** *($16 for 3.38 ounces)* is indeed light, but that doesn't mean oily skin needs moisturizers. This is only appropriate for dry areas.

☹ **Oil-Free Moisture Gel for Oily Skin** *($16 for 3.38 ounces)* contains peppermint, mint, and witch hazel, which are too irritating for all skin types.

☺ **Night Supplement for All Skin Types** *($14 for 1 ounce)* contains a small amount of AHA that isn't enough to make it much of an exfoliant. Otherwise it is just an average moisturizer for normal to dry skin. There are a handful of interesting ingredients, but they come far after the preservatives and that means they are barely present.

☺ **Rich Night Cream with Vitamin E** *($9.50 for 1.4 ounces).* The amount of vitamin E in the cream is hardly worth mentioning. This is a very emollient (though ordinary) moisturizer for someone with very dry skin who doesn't have a problem with breakouts.

☺ **Rich Moisture Cream for Dry Skin** *($16 for 3.52 ounces)* is similar to the Night Cream version above and the same comments apply.

☹ **Elderflower Eye Gel** *($5.95 for 0.4 ounce).* Witch hazel is a skin irritant, and so is the alcohol this product contains. This is one of the last products I would consider putting around the eye area.

☺ **Eye Supplement for All Skin Types** *($12 for 0.5 ounce)* is a good lightweight moisturizer, but it is very standard and doesn't add much of anything to the skin.

☺ **Undereye Cream** *($6.05 for 0.5 ounce)* is a very standard, very heavy moisturizer for dry skin.

☹ **Exfoliating Lotion for All Skin Types** *($9 for 6.76 ounces)* contains alcohol as the second ingredient, and it also has mint, both of which are drying and irritating for skin. It does contain willow bark, which is distantly related to BHA (salicylic acid), but this has minimal to no effect on the skin as an exfoliant.

☺ **Vitamin C Hydrating Cleanser** *($12 for 8 ounces)* contains a teeny amount of vitamin C in a cold cream–type cleanser that needs to be wiped off. It is an option for normal to dry skin, but if you're looking to get vitamin C on your skin, this trace amount isn't the way to do it. It does contain fragrance.

☺ **Vitamin C Energizing Face Spritz** *($8 for 4 ounces)* is a toner that does contain a small amount of ascorbic acid (a form of vitamin C) in a base of rose water (glycerin and fragrance). Ascorbic acid is considered to be one of the least stable and more irritating forms of vitamin C to use. If you want to consider a vitamin C product, this is not the one.

☺ **Vitamin C Intensive Night Repair** *($18 for 1.25 ounces)* is ascorbic acid in a silicone base. The same basic comments for the Face Spritz above apply for this one.

☺ **Vitamin C Protective Daywear Moisturizer with SPF 15** *($12 for 2.5 ounces)* is a good in-part titanium dioxide–based sunscreen that would work well for someone with normal to dry skin. The teeny amount of vitamin C in here is hardly worth mentioning, but the other emollients and water-binding agents are great.

☺ **Vitamin C Super Charged Serum** *($18 for 1 ounce)* is a good emollient moisturizer for someone with normal to dry skin, but the amount of vitamin C in here is barely worth mentioning.

☺ **$$$ Vitamin C Stimulating Mask** *($15 for 2.5 ounces)* could have been a good emollient facial mask for dry skin, but the inclusion of menthol, though only a tiny amount, can add unnecessary irritation (not stimulation) for the skin.

☹ **Vitamin E Cleansing Bar** *($3.50 for 3.5 ounces)* is made with the same ingredients that keep all bar cleansers in their bar form, which can clog pores, and the detergent cleansing agents are drying. The amount of vitamin E in here is insignificant.

☺ **Vitamin E Moisture Cream** *($9.50 for 1.8 ounces)*. The amount of vitamin E in this cream is hardly worth mentioning, but it is a very emollient moisturizer for someone with very dry skin who doesn't have a problem with breakouts.

☺ **Vitamin E Face Mist** *($10 for 3.2 ounces)* is a very standard, ordinary toner that would work well for most skin types.

☺ **Vitamin E Under Eye Cream** *($10 for 0.5 ounce)* is a good though fairly standard moisturizer for normal to dry skin.

☹ **Vitamin E Lip Care SPF 15** *($2.50 for 0.15 ounce)* does not contain avobenzone, zinc oxide, or titanium dioxide, and is not recommended.

☺ **Facial Sun Stick SPF 30** *($6.50 for 0.6 ounce)* is a fairly expensive way to apply sunscreen, but this is a good in-part zinc oxide–based sunscreen. It does contain some thick, waxy ingredients that are notorious for clogging pores.

☹ **Sun Lotion, Very High Protection SPF 15** *($8.50 for 5.2 ounces)* does not contain avobenzone, zinc oxide, or titanium dioxide, and is not recommended.

☹ **Sun Block, Ultra Protection SPF 25** *($9.50 for 5.2 ounces)* does not contain avobenzone, zinc oxide, or titanium dioxide, and is not recommended.

☹ **Sun Lotion SPF 8** *($8.50 for 5.2 ounces)* does contain zinc oxide for UVA protection, but its SPF 8 is not adequate.

☹ **Sun Spray SPF 6** *($8.50 for 6 ounces)* is sun damage waiting to happen and is not recommended. SPF 15 is considered the standard to meet for daily protection, plus this one doesn't contain UVA-protecting ingredients, which makes it a significant problem for skin every which way you look at.

☹ **Watermelon Spray SPF 6** *($8.50 for 6 ounces)* is similar to the one above and the same comments apply.

☺ **Blue Corn Scrub Mask** *($9.95 for 4.3 ounces)* is a fairly standard clay mask that uses blue corn powder as the scrub. This can be fairly abrasive but it does work as an exfoliant for someone with oily skin. It also contains fragrance.

☺ **$$$ Honey & Oatmeal Scrub Mask for Dry Skin** *($11.25 for 2.4 ounces)* is a standard clay mask that uses oatmeal as a scrub agent. Clay is very dehydrating for dry skin and there are no other emollients in here to offset that effect. This would work for someone with oily skin.

☺ **Passion Flower Massage Mask** *($11 for 3.5 ounces)* is more of a good moisturizer than anything else and would work well for dry skin.

☹ **Warming Mineral Mask, for All Skin Types** *($12 for 5.1 ounces)* really seems warm on the skin because of the cinnamon and ginger oil, sort of like the way Red Hot candies heat up your mouth. However, these can be skin irritants, and they don't do much for the skin. This is just a standard clay mask with a gimmick that can hurt your skin.

☺ **Intense Moisture Mask for All Skin Types** *($12 for 3.38 ounces)*. I wouldn't call this intense moisture in the least, but it is an OK mask for someone with normal to slightly dry skin.

☹ **Tea Tree Oil Soap** *($3.70 for 3.5 ounces)* is a standard bar soap with a tiny amount of tea tree oil. Soap is drying and the ingredients that keep soap in its bar form can clog pores. Tea tree oil in concentrations of 5% can be a good topical disinfectant, but the amount in here is far below that.

☺ **Tea Tree Oil Facial Wash** *($3 for 2 ounces)* is a standard, detergent-based water-soluble cleanser with a small amount of tea tree oil. Tea tree oil in concentrations of 5% can be a good topical disinfectant, but the amount in here is far below that.

☹ **Tea Tree Oil Freshener, for Oily or Blemished Skin** *($8 for 8.4 ounces)* includes tea tree oil, and while there is one study showing that can have some benefit similar to benzoyl peroxide, there isn't enough tea tree oil in here to come close to the 5% level needed. Besides, this version contains witch hazel and alcohol, which can cause unnecessary irritation, and that won't help breakouts in the least.

☹ **Tea Tree Oil** *($3.95 for 0.34 ounce)* The Body Shop claims this is a 15% concentration of tea tree oil, which would make it more effective for disinfecting blemishes, but the alcohol concentration in here and the strength of the tea tree oil make it fairly irritating and drying for all skin types and is not recommended.

☺ **Tea Tree Oil Facial Moisture Concentrate for Oily or Blemished Skin** *($6.50 for 1.7 ounces)* does contain tea tree oil but the amount's too small for it to work as a disinfectant for breakouts. The moisturizer base can be a problem for someone with breakouts or oily skin.

☺ **Tea Tree Oil Moisturizing Gel, for Oily or Blemished Skin** *($13.50 for 8.4 ounces)* has too small an amount of tea tree oil for it to work as a disinfectant for breakouts, but the gel base in this one makes it a far better option for normal to oily blemish-prone skin.

☹ **Tea Tree Oil Blemish Stick** *($4.50)* won't help anything. Even if the tea tree oil could help breakouts, the alcohol in this product would just cause irritation and dryness.

☺ **Tea Tree Oil Facial Mask** *($8 for 4.8 ounces)* is a standard clay mask that contains several emollients that would be a problem for someone with blemishes, though it could be an option for someone with dry skin. It does contain a teeny amount of tea tree oil but not enough to work as a disinfectant for blemishes.

☹ **Sage & Comfrey Blemish Gel** *($6 for 1.5 ounces)* contains mostly alcohol, witch hazel, plant extracts, thickeners, and preservatives (need I say more?)

## *The Body Shop Makeup*

☺ **FOUNDATION:** The Body Shop's foundations have been whittled down from six formulas to four, which is certainly limiting, but not terrible. Most of these have a soft finish and texture; however, the shades in each group mostly cater to fair and medium skin tones only. In fact, most of the darkest shades aren't going to be around much longer. What's here is still worth a look, and the prices should please you. **All-in-One Face Base** *($15; refills $11)* offers six very good shades of traditional wet/dry powder foundation. The texture is very smooth and blends flawlessly to a matte finish with light to moderate coverage. You will get better results from using this type of product dry. When wet, the color tends to streak. The only color to be cautious with here is Tan, which is slightly orange. **Everyday Foundation** *($10)* is a good creamy foundation in a tube that works best on normal to dry skin. This provides a smooth, even finish and medium coverage, although the colors have gotten worse, with only 01 and 02 being neutral. 001 may work for some skin tones, but it is slightly peach, while 03, 04, and 05 are all too peach or orange to recommend. The previous Oil Control Foundation has been reformulated and is now known as **Oil-Free Liquid Foundation SPF 8** *($12.50)*. This is an improvement over the old version and offers a matte finish with light to medium coverage. The sunscreen is titanium dioxide–based, but SPF 8 is exceedingly disappointing. SPF 15 is the standard, so this one leaves the skin still in need of protection. If you have fair coloring and oily skin that isn't prone to breakouts, give this one a try. Of the ten available shades, half are too pink, orange, or red to recommend. Avoid 02, 06, 07, 08, and 09. **Skin Treat Foundation SPF 8** *($15)* comes in a bottle with a pump applicator, which does take some getting used to. This is a great choice for normal to dry skin, as it is creamy and dries to a lovely satin-matte finish with light to medium coverage. All six shades are excellent, but even if it is titanium dioxide–based, this SPF is too low to consider for complete protection.

<u>CONCEALER:</u> ☺ **Liquid Concealer** *($8.50)* has a wand applicator and gives great opaque coverage and a soft matte finish; the colors are mostly neutral (watch out for Honey and Almond—both can be too orange for most skin tones). The texture of this one makes it a poor choice if you have many wrinkles, as this type of finish will only accentuate them, but otherwise it holds up well and doesn't crease.

☺ **Everyday Concealer** *($7.50)* is a creamy, medium-coverage, lipstick-type concealer with OK colors. This goes on creamy and stays that way, so creasing will be a problem.

☹ **Lightening Touch** *($10)* supposedly "brings radiance" to the skin. It looks like shine to me, and the two colors are disappointingly pink and peach. These have a light finish, but the shine is uncalled for. **Tea Tree Oil Cover Stick** *($6)* is meant as a blemish cover-up, but the color is too golden to look anything but obvious. Besides, this is too waxy to put on a blemish, and the amount of tea tree oil isn't enough to work as a disinfectant.

<u>POWDER:</u> ☺ **Translucent Loose Powder** *($10)* is available in two workable shades, but having only two shades is almost laughable. It has a soft, dry finish and comes in a saltshaker container, which looks cute but tends to create a mess when you're trying to get it on your brush. **Pressed Face Powder** *($10)* is almost identical to the one above in terms of feel and texture, only in compact form. This one has only three shades and none are for medium to dark skin tones. **Tinted Bronzing Powder** *($11)* is a slight improvement over the one above, as this is a pressed bronzing powder that goes on sheer and matte, but it's still a little too dry for most skin types. $$$ **Multi-Swirl Bronzer** *($16.50)* is several different bronze tones pressed in a compact. The end result is a sheer, tan finish with slight shine.

☺ **Brush-On Bronze** *($13.50)* consists of three different shades of powder beads that you swirl a brush over and dust on. This is a clever concept but the end result is a shiny powder with a chalky, dry finish.

☺ <u>BLUSH:</u> **Powder Blusher** *($8)* features a beautiful assortment of soft colors that apply evenly and have a slight, barely perceptible shine. **Complete Colour Bronze** *($10)* is what's left of the Complete Colour range. It's a wind-up stick that can be used as blush, eye, and lip color, but it tends to blend on choppy and is not worth the effort. **Twist & Blush** *($10)* and **Twist & Bronze** *($13.50)* both have a brush that twists up into a layer of pressed color that you then apply to the face. It goes on rather soft and slightly shiny. Yes, it is gimmicky but sometimes you just have to concede to that.

☹ **Translucent Bronzer SPF 4** *($7.50)* has a pitiful SPF with no UVA protection, but can work as a sheer bronze gel with a slight orange tone. This works best on normal, flawless skin and the formula is relatively easy to blend, but it has more shortcomings than positives, which makes it a waste of money.

☹ <u>EYESHADOW</u>: If you just can't get enough of shine and shimmer, here is a treasure trove of sparkle for you. **Special Edition Eye Shadow** *($8)* is a small group of pale pastel, shiny eyeshadows that all tend to have a gray cast and lose their pastel appearance on the skin. **Shadow Lustre Crayon** *($7.50)* is a collection of chubby, standard pencils that have a waxy feel and a creamy finish. All of them are very shiny, and the tip wears down in no time. These look more convenient to use than they end up being. **Eye Shine** *($7.50)* is self-explanatory. This is a shiny liquid eyeshadow that dries to an opaque powder finish. **Highlighter Sticks** *($10)* are cream-to-powder eyeshadow in stick form, and yes, they're shiny too. **Spartacles Eye Colours** *($8)* are tiny pots of very small colored-powder beads that, of course, are all shiny. In addition, these come with a small sponge that adds to the mess this product makes. **Glitter Bug** *($10)* is shiny loose powder with flecks of glitter; if that's not glitter enough for you, there's **Silver Shimmer Gel Enhancer** *($10)* and **Enhancer** *($12.50)*. Both are ultra-shiny; one is a gel and the other is a cream-to-powder formula in a compact. **Quickshadows** *($9)* are cream-to-powder eye colors that apply well; they're all sheer and have a slight to obvious shine.

☺ The regular **Eyeshadows** *($7)* offer a decent choice of very soft, sheer colors that blend well. Unfortunately, there are only a handful of true matte shades and the shine is very apparent and not smooth or soft. **Continual Eye Colour** *($10)* is another cream-to-powder formula, but this one has a wand applicator and just two matte shades to choose from! Although this type of product can be hard to blend with other colors, by itself it works fine and holds up well with no fading or creasing.

☺ <u>EYE AND BROW SHAPER:</u> **Eye Definer** *($7)* is a standard pencil with a slightly dry application and a creamy finish. Of course, there are shiny shades but there are some mattes to consider. **Eyebrow Powder Pencil** *($7)* does indeed have a powdery feel and three good, soft colors. If you prefer a pencil to powder, give this one a whirl. **Eyebrow Powder Makeup** *($8)* also offers three soft, matte shades but the texture is very dry, which makes a smooth, even application difficult to achieve.

☺ **Eye Liner Pen** *($10)* is a liquid liner that would be great if the brush weren't so stiff. That can make application uneven, and liquid liner is hard enough to apply even with a superior brush! It comes in three shades and dries smooth. Still, if you're a pro at it and love the look, this one is worth a try. **Brow and Lash Gel** *($8)* is a standard, clear, hairspray-like formula that should work fine for taming the brows and lightly grooming the lashes. The texture is smooth and it dries slowly, but it's not sticky.

☺ **LIPSTICK AND LIP PENCIL:** Colourings used to have a beautiful range of creamy lipsticks, many of which had enough stain to somewhat live up to their "long-lasting" claim. Now, many of these classic, creamy lipsticks have been replaced by greasy, iridescent colors! There are still some winners here, and shine on the lips is a much better alternative than shine elsewhere. **Hi-Shine Lipstick** *($8)* is a sheer, slightly greasy lipstick with a small group of iridescent colors. **Colourings Lipstick** *($8)* is creamy with a glossy finish and semi-opaque coverage. This one has the best color options. **Lip Treat SPF 20** *($9.50)* is a greasy, sheer lip color with no UVA protection and I would only recommend it for use as a gloss. **Lipstick SPF 20** *($9.50)* provides very good UVA protection with a zinc oxide base and has a creamy texture and slightly greasy finish. There are only a handful of colors and they won't last too long, but for sun protection they win high marks. **Colour-Proof Lipstick** *($10)* has an opaque, matte finish that should hold up well but may feel dry on the lips. There are only four colors to choose from, but they're all contenders. **Fragrance Colour Sticks** *($7.50)* are The Body Shop's version of the chubby lip pencils. These have a waxy, sticky texture and smell like various foods—cute but not for everyone. **Lip Tints** *($8)* are standard, non-sticky gloss with sheer colors. **Lip Balm** *($4.35)* is a selection of very slick, sheer, fruit-scented balms that will take you back to early adolescence. **Lip Definer** *($7)* is a standard pencil with an adequate creamy feel and decent colors.

☺ **MASCARA: Lash Build Mascara** *($8.50)* is just an OK mascara that takes some effort to build much length or thickness, but it does stay on well with minimal smearing. **Definitive Mascara** *($8.50)* is at best described as mediocre. It takes forever to build any noticeable length and thickness and is not worth the effort. **Conditioning Mascara** *($8.50)* is a good mascara that does an OK job of lengthening without clumping, but it adds minimal thickness. **Waterproof Mascara** *($8.50)* goes on well and adds some length but not much thickness. What's great is that it really is waterproof and does not chip off!

☹ **BRUSHES:** The Body Shop's brushes have slowly gone from wonderful to woeful, and that's a shame. The prices were (and still are) great, but it's no bargain if the quality is poor. The existing **Brushes** *($4.50 to $12)* are insufficient for most makeup application needs. The face and blush brushes are too loose and the hair too long to get a controlled application, and all of the eye-makeup brushes are either too stiff, too big, or just unnecessary. There are much better options out there that cost a little more, yet in the long run are more than worth the extra expense. Perhaps The Body Shop will rethink these brushes when Colourings gets its impending face-lift.

## Bonne Bell (Makeup Only)

Bonne Bell was one of the first drugstore lines with products aimed specifically at the teen market. The skin care, though minimal, was tightly linked to "will it ruin my date?" acne anxiety, while the makeup sported a decidedly youthful look, from flavored lip glosses to shine-stopping powders. The line has been revamped more than once, and its latest incarnation is somewhat of a return to its roots, with many of the makeup items that had a more "vanilla wrapper" look replaced by a group of products with a more upbeat, kid-oriented look called Gear Bonne Bell.

It is apparent that Bonne Bell is simply trying to keep up with other teen lines such as Revlon StreetWear and Jane, as there are more glittery, ultra-shiny products here than ever before. For anyone not satisfied with just a few lip balms, Bonne Bell's options will seem like a pot of gold at the end of a candy-scented rainbow.

For more information about Bonne Bell products, call (216) 221-0800 or visit the Web. site at www.bonnebell.com.

☺ **Gel Bronze Face and Body Bronzer** *($3.49)* is a unique way to go about changing the color of skin. I generally never recommend any kind of makeup cover that alters (as opposed to matches) skin color, but this is a lightweight gel formulation that spreads beautifully over the skin and gives it a rather natural-looking, extremely sheer tan appearance. It has no after-feel, so it works great for someone with normal to oily skin who doesn't want a feeling of makeup on the skin. One major drawback of this product is that it tints the skin, which means once in place it doesn't come off until it sloughs off along with your skin cells, and that can look choppy and uneven.

<u>FOUNDATION:</u> ☺ **Cream Bronze Face Bronze** *($3.49)* is one of the most convincing matte-finish bronzing products I've reviewed. This lotion-like formula has a believable-looking tan color that blends easily into the skin, leaving a slightly moist finish appropriate for normal to dry skin. **Powder Bronze** *($3.49)* isn't as nice as others in this price range (including Wet 'n' Wild's bronzing powders), but is nevertheless a consideration. There are two shades, both with a matte finish and a dry texture that goes on with more color than you may think, so be careful.

<u>POWDER:</u> ☹ **Cosmic Cheeks Glitter Gel** *($2.89)* is simply flecks of glitter suspended in a gel base. Because of the application, it doesn't work well over other makeup colors (the gel would smear or rub off the other products), and if you want

to apply other products over it, the glitter can chip off. If you want glitter on the face, there are better ways to do that than with this one. **Iridescent Highlights** *($3.49)* is exactly named. These are ultra-shiny, gel highlighters that, for shine, will get you all you want, though the same application warning exists for this one as the Cosmic Cheek version above. **Glimmer Dust Loose Shimmer** *($3.49)* is an assortment of very shiny loose powder. If shine really speaks to you, this is the better way to control application, but brushing on shiny loose powder can still be a messy undertaking.

EYESHADOW: ☺ **Eye Shades** *($3.49)* are sheer cream-to-powder eye shadows that produce a moderate amount of shimmer. These have a bit of a slick finish, which can make them crease easily, but if shine is the goal and duration isn't, then these would work.

☺ **Powder Pak** *($1.99 for two shadows; $1.09 for compact)* are powdery eyeshadows in a small selection of colors that are sold in sets of two. They are extremely sheer but have a soft, blendable texture.

EYE AND BROW SHAPER: ☺ **Eye Definer** and **Lip Definer** *($2.29 each)* are standard pencils with a selection of 12 shades each. Being standard is not equivalent to being bad—quite the contrary; these are an excellent option for lining, especially for lips, with a diverse color range that is undeniably worthwhile.

LIPSTICK AND LIP PENCIL: ☺ All manner of lip balms and glosses set Bonne Bell apart from the "adult" side of the cosmetics world. Almost every lip product here has some kind of sweet candy- or berry-flavored taste. **Lip Lix** *($2.19)* are very emollient, greasy lipstick/glosses that are good for dry lips. **Lip Lites** *($3.49)* are greasy glosses in a tube with flavors ranging from raspberry to chocolaty mud pie. **Lip Burst** *($3.49)* is a very sheer, tinted, oily gloss available in various food flavors. **Flip Gloss** *($3.49)* is a non-sticky sheer gloss in a unique package that opens the cap and draws up the lip color with one stroke. Very clever but still just gloss! **FlipSticks SPF 15** *($3.49)* do not indicate any sun-protecting ingredients so I can't comment on the SPF and you shouldn't rely on it either, but otherwise they are standard, sheer lipstick with the same flip-up packaging as the one above. **Lip Sheers** *($3.39)* are basic, greasy, glossy lip colors. **Lip Shake** *($3.49)* is swirled, iridescent lip gloss that has a slick and greasy texture and the flavors that are a staple at Bonne Bell. **Shimmer** *($3.49)* comes in a Chap-Stick–style applicator and is just shiny, waxy color for lips or wherever you please. **Lip Smackers** *($1.49 to $2.89)* are standard lip balms that will nicely moisturize dry lips while adding flavor and shine. Included in this mix are **Jewel Lips, Cosmic Lips, Original Flavored,** and **Roll-On Shiner.** All in all, the choices are vast and this is clearly a cornerstone of the Bonne Bell line. **Sun Smackers SPF 24** *($1.99 each; $4.19 for three)* are the basic Lip Smacker formula with no UVA-protecting ingredients, making them a poor choice for sunscreen.

☹ **Smackers Sponge-On Sparkler** *($2.89)* is a very glossy, utterly shiny, and sticky lip gloss. Any of the regular Lip Smackers have a texture preferable to this one.

# Borghese

Borghese has been bought and sold more times than I can keep track of. Given the tumultuous history I wasn't surprised when I called the company soon after beginning research for this edition and was told that Borghese has been pulled from most department stores where it was being sold. Over the past several weeks as this book is getting ready to go to press, I noticed that Borghese's products were being discounted at several department stores by more than 60% (something you almost never see for high-end cosmetic lines). Since most women won't be able to find Borghese products that are still available (or on the Internet) I decided not to include a review in this edition. If distribution for Borghese changes, I will review those additions in my newsletter, *Cosmetics Counter Update*.

# Burt's Bees (Skin Care Only)

Almost all the skin-care lines in the world prefer to identify themselves as companies established to create elegant, scientific formulations conceived with an in-depth understanding of the skin's functions and needs. I say almost, because Burt's Bees makes no such admission. Quite the contrary; this line is about as unglamorous and as unscientific as it gets (the picture of Burt on the label made me think I was buying fishing gear). Talk about being an iconoclast!

This is how the company gives its history on its Web site, "I guess you could say it all started because there weren't many jobs up there north of Bangor. Though we found, grew, or traded for most of what we needed, I figure a person's got to have at least 3,000 dollars a year in actual greenbacks to survive in this old world, especially if you've got kids. I'd been let go from my last three part-time waitressing jobs at Dottie's ... Burt was enjoying similar commercial success selling quarts of honey off the tailgate of his Datsun pick-up ... By the end of summer we got around to the heart of the matter, which was the beeswax. Well, how we got started making lip balm ... is another story. ..." This is a skin-care line?

Aside from its humble, amorphous beginning, Burt's Bees is about natural, earth-friendly skin-care products, as well as overly fragranced, products. Its philosophy in this respect is fetching and sincere: "We believe that Mother Nature has the answers and She teaches by example...[I know they don't mean tornados or earthquakes, right?]. Our ingredients are the best that Mother Nature has to offer."

For those seeking a line of skin-care products with truly natural ingredients, this line is one of the few that steadfastly adheres to its commitment; there is no hypocrisy here. If the ingredient lists are accurate, and there is no reason to assume otherwise, then you will not find preservatives or synthetically derived ingredients of any kind. Just from the all-natural point of view, there will definitely be people who will be excited about these products, but I'm not one of them. Many of the plant extracts and oils used in these products including orange oil, cinnamon oil, clove oil, lemon oil, orange peel, eucalyptus oil, pine tar, alcohol, lime oil, and balsam peru, are problematic for skin and present a significant risk of irritation or a sensitizing reaction. Ouch! Plus you can't rely on the entire line as there are no sunscreens of any kind, no products for oily skin, and definitely none for blemish-prone skin. An intriguing philosophy and inexpensive products are both attractive but it takes more than that to establish reliable products that are good for skin.

I know that most people are attracted by fragrance and in this regard these products excel. They are also notable for the lack of preservatives (that may be an issue for product stability—but I did not have these products tested for contamination), which can be beneficial for those who can't tolerate preservatives. But for any other skin-care need, I suggest you use your wisdom and recognize that while Mother Nature is assuredly wise about the Earth, *She* does not have everything the skin needs. In fact, Mother Nature offers up many problematic things for skin including the sun and poison ivy.

For more information call (800) 849-7112 or visit the Web site at www.burts bees.com.

☹ **Baby Bee Buttermilk Soap** *($5 for a 3.5-ounce bar)* is indeed soap, which gives it an incredibly high pH of over 10. That extreme alkaline base is very drying and irritating for all skin types.

☹ **Bay Rum Exfoliating Soap** *($5 for a 3.25-ounce bar)* is much like all the soaps in this line; its alkaline base with a pH of over 10 makes this very drying and irritating. To make matters worse, this product contains orange, cinnamon, clove, and lemon oils. It smells nice, but for skin it is problematic.

☹ **Burt's Beeswax and Honey Face Soap** *($5 for a 1.9-ounce bar)* doesn't contain the irritating extracts of the Bay Rum soap, but there is still an unspecified wafting fragrance and the pH is still over 10, which makes it very drying and irritating for skin.

☹ **Farmer's Friend Gardener's Soap** *($5 for a 5.25-ounce bar)* has an alkaline base with a pH of over 10 and it contains eucalyptus oil, and that makes it drying and potentially irritating for skin.

☺ **Farmer's Market Orange Essence Cleansing Creme** *($9 for 4 ounces)* is a fairly standard cold cream, with plant oils, lanolin, and plant extracts. It is still highly fragrant, but for a cold cream it is just fine. It can leave a greasy film behind on the skin.

☹ **Ocean Potion Detox Soap** *($5 for a 3.5-ounce bar)* is just soap with a pH over 10, which makes it drying and irritating for all skin types. The spruce oil and fir needle oil don't "detox" anything; they do make it smell nice but can also cause skin sensitivity.

☺ **Farmer's Market Citrus Facial Scrub** *($7 for 2 ounces)*. You would be far better off just buying some ground-up almonds and using that rather than risking the irritation from the orange peel, orange oil, and clove powder this product contains.

☹ **Burt's Complexion Mist, Chamomile** *($6 for 4 ounces)* is just water and fragrant plant oils. You might as well put perfume on your face.

☹ **Burt's Complexion Mist, Grapefruit** *($6 for 4 ounces)* is similar to the Chamomile version above only this one uses lime, lemon, and grapefruit oil, which are all potential skin irritants.

☹ **Burt's Complexion Mist, Lavender** *($6 for 4 ounces)* is just water and fragrant plant oils, and the lavender oil in here is a photosensitizer.

☹ **Farmer's Market Complexion Mist with Carrot Seed Oil** *($7 for 4 ounces)* is similar to the Chamomile version above and the same comments apply.

☹ **Garden Tomato Toner** *($9 for 8 ounces)* has alcohol as the second ingredient, which makes it too irritating for all skin types.

☺ **Baby Bees Skin Creme** *($11 for 2 ounces)*. The clay in here can be drying and sort of negates the emollients. This is a bit of a confused product and may be problematic for dry skin, and completely inappropriate for combination or oily skin.

☺ **Burt's Beeswax Moisturizing Creme** *($12 for 2 ounces)* is similar to the Skin Creme above and the same comments apply.

☺ **Burt's Jasmine Decollete Creme** *($18 for 3.5 ounces)* contains nothing special for the neck area, as Burt must certainly know. This is similar to the Skin Creme above, and the same comments apply. This one does contain a teeny amount of royal jelly, but I have yet to see research of any kind indicating that it is somehow a preferred skin-care ingredient. It is a good water-binding agent but that's about it.

☺ **Farmer's Market Carrot Nutritive Creme** *($10 for 1 ounce)* is a very good, basic moisturizer for dry skin.

☺ **Burt's Beeswax & Bee Pollen Night Creme** *($8.50 for 0.5 ounce)* is a very good, basic moisturizer for dry skin. There is no research to show that bee pollen, especially in meager amounts, has any benefit for skin.

☺ **$$$ Burt's Beeswax & Royal Jelly Eye Creme** *($11 for 0.25 ounce)*. The clay in here is such a tiny amount it won't have much if any an effect on skin, but it seems strange to put such a drying ingredient in a moisturizer. Aside from that, this is fairly emollient and would be good for normal to dry skin.

☺ **Wise Woman Comfrey Comfort Salve** *($4 for 0.6 ounce)* is a very emollient moisturizer that would be good for very dry skin. What would really be wise is if one of Burt's products contained a sunscreen with UVA-protecting ingredients.

☹ **Green Goddess Clay Mask** *($7 for 1.4 ounces)* contains peppermint as the second ingredient and that serves no purpose but to irritate the skin; it also contains eucalyptus, which just adds to the problem.

☹ **Burt's Beeswax Lip Balm, Lifeguard's Choice** *($2.50 for 0.15 ounce)* has no sunscreen, and without that there is nothing about this appropriate for daytime, much less for use at the beach! It also contains peppermint oil, which can be irritating and drying for the lips in the long run.

☹ **Burt's Beeswax Lip Balm** (*$2.50 for a tin or tube*) is almost identical to the version above and the same comments apply.

☺ **Wings of Love All-Natural Lipstick** (*$9.50*) is, as the name implies, all natural, and for a lipstick with a creamy, somewhat glossy finish it is actually quite nice. Unfortunately, it contains peppermint, which can irritate the skin; if your lips are at all chapped or dry, watch out—this can sting. By the way, a decided departure for Burt's Bees are the pictures of the women on the packages for the lipsticks. The model-like visages were either a compromise, or Burt determined that his face might not sell a lot of lipsticks.

☺ **Wings of Love Powdered Facial Tissue** (*$3 for 65 sheets*) are small pieces of rice paper dusted with cornstarch. This is an option for absorbing oil during the day, but depending on how oily your skin is, these can set down uneven splotches of powder on the face. And though cornstarch is very absorbent and drying, it can also be problematic for breakouts. But for those who prefer this way of taking care of shine during the day, these are an option, and far cheaper than those sold by Shiseido at three times the price.

# Calvin Klein

I just had to run to the store and check out Calvin Klein's reintroduction into the world of makeup. I am perhaps one of the few makeup artists around who remembers when Klein launched an unsuccessful makeup line back in the late '70s. For me, it was the first line of makeup I ever sold at a department store! And what a distinguished line it was back then, not to mention way ahead of its time, which probably explains its demise. Klein had no skin care in those days, and only matte eyeshadows and blushes, all in neutral shades, with nary a blue, green, or pink to be found (such colors were unheard of back then). Now this clothing and marketing genius is returning to the cosmetics fray to join the company of all the other designers out there clamoring for your cosmetics dollars.

If you happen to be around a Saks Fifth Avenue or Nordstrom, the new CK manifestation may be worth a visit—it was for me, at least for a strong whiff of nostalgia—but what about the line's makeup and skin-care quality? The skin care has some interesting gimmicks and good sunscreens, but that's about it. The strong points of the line are without question the concealers, foundation, powders, lip colors, and blush! Klein's line is the first that I've seen to formulate a foundation with avobenzone, and the SPF 20 is great. What you can ignore are some of the trendy products, shiny eyeshadows, and the very standard lip and eye pencils and lip glosses. Calvin Klein is owned by Unilever. For more information call (800) 715-4023 or (212) 759-8888.

# Calvin Klein Skin Care

☹ **Toning Gel Cleanser** *($20 for 6 ounces)* is a standard, detergent-based water-soluble cleanser that contains both arnica and eucalyptus, and is not recommended.

☺ **Balancing Milk Cleanser** *($20 for 6 ounces)* is just a standard creamy cleanser that can leave a slightly emollient feel on skin, which can work well for someone with normal to dry skin. You would need a washcloth to remove makeup effectively.

☺ **$$$ Micro-Exfoliator** *($22 for 4 ounces)*. The buzz on this product is that it contains the same gritty substance used in microdermabrasion machines. Well, yes and no. Microdermabrasion utilizes a pure form of alumina called corundum. In either form alumina is abrasive, and this can be hard for some skin types; it's especially not a good idea for someone with normal to dry or sensitive skin. It could also be a problem if used on a regular basis, but it does work as a scrub, and it is in a lightweight base that isn't waxy or thick, so it would be an option for someone with oily, durable skin.

☺ **$$$ Makeup Remover** *($16 for 4 ounces)* is a standard, detergent-based makeup remover that will allow you to wipe off makeup, but this step wouldn't be necessary if the other two cleansers were any good.

☺ **$$$ Protective Moisture Cream SPF 15** *($30 for 1.7 ounces)* is an overpriced but good avobenzone-based moisturizer. It would work well for dry skin, but there is no reason to consider this formulation over other far less expensive avobenzone-based sunscreens.

☺ **$$$ Protective Moisture Lotion SPF 15** *($30 for 1.7 ounces)* is a good in-part avobenzone-based sunscreen. The price is absurd for what you get, but this silicone-based sunscreen would be an option for most skin types although not for someone with dry skin.

☺ **$$$ Oil Control Hydrator** *($30 for 1.7 ounces)* is a standard, silicone-based gel that has a light matte feel, though it won't control oily skin. It is more just a good lightweight moisturizer for normal to slightly oily skin, leaving it feeling soft and smooth.

# Calvin Klein Makeup

**FOUNDATION:** ☺ **$$$ Sheer Foundation with SPF 20** *($29)* has an excellent SPF 20 with avobenzone as part of its active sunscreen ingredients, which means it has UVA protection! That can be good news for someone with oily skin, though the formulation isn't all that matte. The name is actually quite accurate; this is a very sheer foundation that would be excellent as a moisturizing, sheer tint with sunscreen for someone with normal to dry skin. If you have problems with titanium dioxide as a sunscreen ingredient and want to get sunscreen in your foundation, this is one to try. The eight shades are beautifully neutral.

☺ **$$$ Light Coverage Foundation with SPF 8** *($29)* comes in 15 shades with a disappointing SPF 8. It does have titanium dioxide as part of the SPF, but the low SPF number just doesn't swing. The coverage is almost as sheer as the Sheer Coverage version above, and the colors are almost all wonderfully neutral except for Toffee and Cinnamon, which may be too peach for most skin tones.

☹ $$$ **Medium Coverage Foundation with SPF 8** *($38)* is a cream-to-powder foundation that is more creamy than powdery. The 12 shades are mostly neutral and would work great for normal skin to slightly dry skin types, with the only shades to avoid being Ivory, Linen, Toffee, and Cinnamon. The SPF 8 is in part titanium dioxide, but the low SPF number is just a waste and an absurd oversight for a new line with supposedly the latest information about sun protection. Actually, the need for an SPF 15 is old skin-care news.

☺ $$$ **Pressed Powder** *($27)* and **Loose Powder** *($32)* are standard, talc-based powders with a lovely neutral selection of six shades each. The texture is silky-smooth with a sheer application.

**CONCEALER:** ☺ $$$ **Concealer** *($18)* is a tube concealer that comes in four very skin-friendly shades. It has a terrific soft matte finish with minimal risk of creasing.

☹ **Eye Color Wash** *($14)* is a great name for just a very ordinary cream eyeshadow with shine that comes in a squeeze tube. This is a messy way to apply eyeshadow, because it's very hard to control color placement, plus it creases easily and needs to be set with powder to get it to stay. But why bother with the powder over these when a powder eyeshadow would have been all you needed in the first place?

**BLUSH:** ☺ $$$ **Blush** *($24)* comes in a beautiful array of colors that have a soft, silky finish, although the price is absurd for what you get. It's easily replaced by far less expensive options at the drugstore.

☹ $$$ **Cheek Color Wash** *($23)* is a fairly standard cream blush with a sheer finish that leaves a good deal of shine on the cheek.

**EYESHADOW:** ☹ **Eye Shadow** *($15)* shares one of the true shortcomings of this line, because these are predominantly shiny with only a handful of matte options. The shine is somewhat sparkly, but the application does go on rather smooth and the color options are attractive.

**EYE SHAPER:** ☺ **Eye Definer** *($14)* is a standard pencil with a sponge tip at one end. It does have a good smooth application in comparison to many that tend to be more greasy and thick than smooth.

☹ **Eye Gloss** *($14)* is, just as the name implies, a lip gloss for the eyes. This greasy mess is supposed to look good, but I don't get this trend. It makes everything you've just applied slide around and crease almost immediately. I'm sure there's a reason for this look, but I have no idea what it is.

**LIPSTICK:** ☺ $$$ **Lip Color** *($16)* is a very good, though standard, cream lipstick with a smooth, relatively nongreasy finish and opaque coverage. The huge range of 40 colors is exquisite. **Lip Gloss** *($17)* is a very standard lip gloss with a good amount of iridescence and comes in six shades.

☺ **Lip Color Wash** *($15)* is a great name for a standard glossy-finish lipstick. **Lip Definer** *($14)* is a standard lip pencil with a lip brush on one end. It does have a good creamy finish.

**MASCARA:** ☹ $$$ **Mascara** *($16)* comes in four shades and is just OK. This builds minimal length and no real thickness, though it doesn't clump or smear. It's just lackluster all the way around.

**BRUSHES:** ☺ $$$ **Brushes** *($16 to $38)*. With all the superior brushes available from neighboring lines at the department stores, ranging from M.A.C. to McEvoy, and Bobbi Brown to Stila, there is no reason to consider these. The bristles are soft but not as soft and densely packed as most, plus the shapes for the large eye shadow, powder, and blush brush are clumsy and not the best for most face shapes. The only brushes to consider are the **Eyeliner** and **Small Eye Shadow Brush**.

# CamoCare (Skin Care Only)

If you are looking for chamomile, then this line is the one to consider because it is the showcase ingredient—ergo the name CamoCare. But should you be looking for chamomile in your products? Is this the be-all and end-all for good skin care? Hardly. Chamomile is a good anti-irritant and soothing agent, but it is scarcely the only one—in fact there are dozens and dozens of other effective ingredients used in cosmetics for the purpose of reducing irritation and inflammation. Showcasing one ingredient is always a problem for a skin-care line because when newer research comes along establishing that other options exist, using them sort of takes the wind out of the original marketing premise.

It is interesting to note that while chamomile is a good anti-irritant, CamoCare products include several plant extracts that are known for causing irritation, including lemon, peppermint, orange extract, lavender, and tangerine. That mixture negates the purpose of concentrating on the chamomile in the first place, which is to counteract the irritation caused by environmental factors (primarily sun damage) and not the irritation from the product itself.

And here's another point to keep in mind. The CamoCare Web site cites three studies from the University of Bonn, Germany, proving that the CamoCare products are superior to two other options. Though these three studies are not published or even dated, if you assume that the results are accurate (though they're clearly not unbiased), it is nice to know that these products are soothing when compared to some other cream. However, what the study didn't look at were other creams that contained equally good or better topical anti-irritants. Not to mention that the studies only looked at a small group of women and only for the issue of irritation. There are a lot of skin-care issues besides irritation.

Aside from chamomile, CamoCare has jumped on other bandwagons (I guess chamomile isn't enough). The first one is AHA and BHA, though its products only contain plant extracts and not the actual source, which means these are not really effective for exfoliation (which is what AHAs and BHAs are for). Several of the products contain alpha lipoic acid, the showcase ingredient (along with vitamin C) in Dr. N.V. Perricone's products (reviewed in this edition). Alpha lipoic acid is a good antioxidant, but again, the same issue applies for it as for chamomile—there are lots of good antioxidants, and alpha lipoic acid is not the best or the only one. However, for the money, if you were looking for a topical alpha lipoic acid product, this is by far a cheaper way to get it.

The last bandwagon is the addition of vitamin C products. CamoCare's ingredient of choice is calcium ascorbate. It is indeed a source of vitamin C and according to CamoCare it is the best one. Everyone seems to have the best one, but whether or not you want to believe this company or someone else is up to you. The entire vitamin C craze will be a thing of the past in short order anyway.

The only bandwagon CamoCare has completely overlooked are sunscreens. Now that would be a bandwagon worthy of its attention!

For more information call (800) 226-6227 or visit the Web site at www.camo care.com.

☺ **Camomile Light Foaming Cleanser** *($9.95 for 4 ounces)* is a standard, detergent-based water-soluble cleanser that includes some plant extracts that can be anti-irritants, though their effect would just be rinsed down the drain in a cleanser. This would work well for most skin types, except for very dry skin. It does contain fragrance and preservatives.

☺ **Camomile Moisturizing Cleanser** *($9.95 for 4 ounces)* is a standard, cold cream–type cleanser that needs to be wiped off and can leave a greasy feel on the skin. It can work for very dry skin. It contains the antioxidant alpha lipoic acid, which is nice, but it won't change a wrinkle or the nature of skin.

☺ **Camomile Oil Free Toner** *($8.95 for 4 ounces)*. The fragrant plant extracts in here negate the effectiveness of the plant extracts that can be anti-irritants. Willow bark is a distant relative of BHA, but has no exfoliating effect in this form. This product is a mixed bag with very few strong points, but it isn't a bad product.

☺ **Camomile Stimulating Toner** *($8.95 for 4 ounces)*. The fragrant plant extracts in here negate the effectiveness of the plant extracts that can be anti-irritants. Still, this is a good toner for most all skin types.

☺ **8% Alpha + Beta Hydroxy Face Lift Refining Cream for Normal to Dry Skin** *($20.95 for 1 ounce)* contains some plant extracts that are distantly related to AHA and BHA; however, even if they worked, the pH is too high for this to be effective as an exfoliant. It also contains several plant extracts that can be skin

The Reviews C

irritants. Otherwise, this is a good, though ordinary moisturizer for normal to dry skin.

☺ **8% Alpha + Beta Hydroxy Daily Treatment Pads** *($18.95 for 2 ounces)* is similar to the 8% version above and the same comments apply.

☺ **12% Alpha + Beta Hydroxy Face Lift Refining Cream for Normal to Dry Skin** *($21.95 for 1 ounce)* is similar to the 8% version above and the same comments apply.

☹ **12% Alpha +Beta Hydroxy Intense Treatment** *($19.95 for 2 ounces)* is similar to the 8% version above and the same comments apply. This one also contains additional peppermint, which makes it even more problematic for skin.

☺ **$$$ Eye Lifting Moisture Cream** *($17.59 for 0.5 ounce).* The minuscule amount of interesting ingredients in this product makes it little more than a standard moisturizer for dry skin.

☺ **Facial Therapy** *($20 for 2.4 ounces)* is a very good emollient moisturizer for very dry skin.

☺ **Intense Facial Therapy** *($20.69 for 1 ounce)* is similar to the Facial Therapy above only without the lanolin oil, which makes this better for normal to dry skin.

☺ **Light Facial Therapy** *($13.39 for 1 ounce)* is almost identical to the Facial Therapy above and the same basic comments apply.

☹ **Under Eye Therapy** *($14.49 for 0.25 ounce)* contains lemon and witch hazel, which can cause irritation—and that won't reduce puffiness.

☹ **Clear Solution** *($11 for 0.5 ounce)* is supposed to clear up blemishes, but all it contains is chamomile extract and alpha lipoic acid—at least, that's what's on the label, which I suspect is absolutely not complete. Regardless of what I believe CamoCare isn't disclosing, neither of those two ingredients has any impact on the causes of blemishes.

☺ **$$$ Day Skin Firmer (with Ester-C Topical)** *($38.79 for 1 ounce)* contains several irritating plant extracts, including lemon and orange extract. It does contain vitamin C, but that doesn't make it a miracle for skin any more than the other products in this line. This is a fairly standard, ordinary moisturizer for normal to slightly dry skin.

☺ **$$$ Night Skin Firmer (with Ester-C Topical)** *($41.39 for 1 ounce)* is similar to the Day Skin Firmer above, only this one contains more plant oil, which makes it somewhat better for normal to dry skin.

☺ **$$$ Revitalizing Mask** *($13.39 for 2 ounces)* is a standard clay mask with glycerin and a teeny amount of alpha lipoic acid. It would work well for someone with normal to oily skin.

☺ **Soothing Cream** *($6.19 for 0.71 ounce)* is a very ordinary emollient moisturizer.

# Cargo

Eyeing the success of the M.A.C. line, several Canadian companies have tried to emulate the makeup-artist perspective with makeup lines that have that professional allure. Cargo is just such a Canadian launch. With the impressive colors and textures for most of its products—there's a large range of colors and smooth, silky textures—Cargo is a line of makeup worth checking out. While the products are standouts, the packaging is also eye-catching, with attractive metal tins and metal-looking compacts. The prices aren't outrageous, and some of the products come in ample amounts, but this isn't exactly a bargain either. Cargo is available on www.sephora.com or www.eve.com, and it is also available at Sephora stores, some Macy's stores, and some Barney's and Nordstrom stores. The Web address is www.cargocosmetics.com.

**FOUNDATION:** ☺ **Liquid Foundation** *($22)* comes in ten exceptionally neutral shades (though there are none for very light skin tones), all named after planets and one constellation—clever, but not helpful for identifying shades! It has a silicone and talc–based, soft matte finish that has sheer to light coverage. Don't expect this one to work well for oily skin, though; the amount of silicone in here can feel too oily or slippery, despite the fact it is not technically an oil. The talc adds to the matte finish but it isn't enough to hold back the slip feel. This works best for someone with normal to dry skin.

☺ **Wet/Dry Powder Foundation** *($22)* is a standard, talc-based powder with shine, and that makes it problematic for reducing shine. Plus, the formulation is fairly emollient, which explains the slightly heavy, emollient-feeling coverage, at least in comparison to other pressed powders. It would work well for normal to dry skin but should be avoided by anyone prone to blemishes or oily skin. The same color names apply to these as for the Liquid Foundation, and the colors are all equally excellent. The feel is silky soft, and the application gives sheer to light coverage.

☺ $$$ **CONCEALER:** **Concealer** *($16)* comes in three great neutral shades. The formulation goes on rather greasy and creases easily.

☺ $$$ **POWDER:** **Loose Powder** *($22)* is a standard, talc-based powder that does contain plant oil and mineral oil, so while it does have a silky-smooth feel it is also best for normal to dry skin and not oily skin. The five shades are good, though Powder #2 is definitely on the yellow side, which can add a strange cast to the skin. **Pressed Powder** *($22)* is a standard, talc-based powder that has a drier, sheerer finish than the Wet/Dry version above. There are five good neutral shades. **Glitter** *($19)* is aptly described by its name. This is iridescent loose powder that comes in small vials and are messy to use, as it tends to get all over the place and is almost impossible to apply with any accuracy.

☺ $$$ **BLUSH:** **Blush** *($19)* is packaged in a large tin and the shades are attractive; most of them with a good matte finish. The pigment color is dense, similar to

M.A.C., so you need a deft hand to apply it evenly. **ColorTube** *($24)* is a version of the three-in-one type color sticks from companies such as Chanel and Almay that are meant to be used for the eyes, cheeks, and lips. ColorTube's difference is that it is a thick, pasty cream that comes in a tube, and with five shades. For those who like creamy blushes and greasy eyeshadows that match their lipstick color, this is a product worth playing with, and since it needs no sharpening it has advantages over the pencil versions of these products.

☺ <u>EYESHADOW:</u> **Eyeshadow** *($14)* is a large range of eyeshadows that have a great, smooth application. There are shiny shades to wade through as well as several blue tones, but the neutral shades, though slightly iridescent, go on easy and have great color density. The matte shades are great.

☺ <u>EYE AND BROW SHAPER:</u> **Eye/Brow Pencil** *($13)* is available in only three shades. This pencil goes on creamier than most, which means it can tend to smear, but it can also be easier to line over eyeshadows. It does require sharpening.

☺ <u>LIPSTICK AND LIP PENCIL:</u> **Lipstick** *($15)* is a standard group of lipsticks with a selection of **Sheers** that are fairly greasy, **Creams** that are more glossy than creamy, **Frosts** that are iridescent, and **Mattes** that are more creamy than matte. The color selection is small in each category, but the overall color selection is impressive. **Lip Liner Pencil** *($13)* are standard lip pencils that require sharpening. These are creamier than most, and so are not as helpful in preventing lipstick from feathering. There is a nice range of eight shades to choose from. **Lip Gloss** *($15)* is a group of fairly standard glosses that come two shades to a container, and the container holds a rather generous amount as far as glosses go. **Lip Gloss/Conditioner** *($15)* is simply half gloss and half lip balm, and for lovers of both, it is convenient.

☹ <u>MASCARA:</u> **Mascara** *($15)* takes forever to build any length, and then there is little difference to be seen—and it tends to clump. There are definitely better mascaras available.

☺ $$$ <u>BRUSHES:</u> The **Brushes** in this line are somewhat overpriced (especially the Super Powder Brush) but for the most part have a soft, smooth feel with good density and thickness and come in very workable sizes. The following are all worth feeling and checking out to see if the size and form are what meets your face or eye shape. The **Brow Angle Brush** *($12)*, **Dome Brush** *($68)*, **Eye Liner Brush** *($12)*, **Flat Lip Brush** *($15)*, **Fluff Brush Large** *($34)*, **Fluff Brush Jumbo** *($28)*, **Crease Brush** *($28)*, **Super Powder Brush** *($60)*, and **Medium Fluff Blush** *($28)* are all great! The **Angle Liner Brush** *($18)* and **Concealer Brush** *($22)* are synthetic bristles that can feel stiff and scratchy on the face but for some makeup applications are an option. The **Small Fluff Blush** *($22)* is OK for soft detail work but is almost too small to be considered practical. There are also a few **Brush Kits** *($75–$99)* that feature a grouping of brushes for face, eyes, or basic starter sets.

# Cellex-C (Skin Care Only)

Cellex-C is more of a political yarn than a good skin-care story. I'm not sure where to start with this combative vitamin C saga. You wouldn't think that one nebulous little ingredient would cause so much commotion, but then we're talking about the cosmetics industry, where it only takes one ingredient to start a furor. And especially one ingredient that promises instant youth. Vitamin C is such an ingredient. The drama started with Dr. Sheldon Pinnell from Duke University, who looked at the effect of sun exposure in relation to applying L-ascorbic acid (a specific form of vitamin C) on hairless pigs. It seems the pigs with L-ascorbic acid applied did not get sunburnt. From this study it was assumed that L-ascorbic acid was an exceptional antioxidant. It was also known at the time that L-ascorbic acid was an exceptionally unstable ingredient. Following the study, in an alliance with Cellex-C, Pinnell started representing a skin-care line. But Pinnell knew his L-ascorbic acid was unstable. That's why Cellex-C, the little $70-an-ounce container of L-ascorbic acid, comes in a brown bottle. Even so, when exposed to air, sun, or heat, it decomposes. In essence, Cellex-C loses its vitamin C content after just a couple of weeks.

An interesting side note is that women were experiencing smoother skin from using Cellex-C. In light of the fact that a woman would probably never notice the effect of reduced sun damage on her skin (after all, that's all we know about the effects of L-ascorbic acid; there is no clinical research about how it affects wrinkles or aging on people), how could this be? As it turns out, Cellex-C is formulated with a pH of 2.5. That gives it a highly acidic base that may be stimulating some of the positive effects. Some dermatologists conjecture that a pH of 2.5 may swell the skin slightly, making it look smoother, and increase cell turnover (something like AHAs do). Of course, there are no studies checking this probability out, but then Cellex-C is classified as a cosmetic, and as long as women are buying it, who cares if it really works?

The story became more complicated when Pinnell disassociated himself from Cellex-C in 1997 and started another skin-care company called SkinCeuticals. The angle for SkinCeuticals is that it uses a stable form of L-ascorbic acid, leaving Cellex-C with the original unstable version. (Why we should believe Pinnell now when he let us buy an unstable version previously is a question I can't answer.)

In the meantime, without getting into the convoluted politics between Pinnell and Cellex-C (who were in the midst of a lawsuit suing each other as this book went to press), the bottom line for this company is that the L-ascorbic acid it uses is less desirable, because you can't get the ingredient to last. Further, regardless of what is true for any single ingredient, skin aging is more complicated than just the loss of vitamin C or any other vitamin, enzyme, protein, or fatty acid in the skin. It is the whole picture we should be concerned about, not just one small aspect. Besides, there are many other antioxidants that are as good as or even more impressive than vitamin C, including beta glucan, vitamin E, and superoxide dismutase, to name a few.

The original question I posed some time ago is this: Why, if the little bottle of Cellex-C is supposed to be so amazing—with mesmerizing before-and-after pictures—do there have to be all these other products making more miraculous claims? Why would you need AHAs, toners, and other wrinkle creams if one product was doing all the work? And the before-and-after pictures that Cellex-C has been using date back to when this line was first launched almost ten years ago, making you wonder if those are the only success stories.

It now seems that vitamin C, AHAs, and all the other earlier Cellex-C bells and whistles are not enough because Cellex-C has now introduced Betaplex, to include BHA as a necessary skin-care ingredient. But what Betaplex uses for its source of BHA is willow bark. Willow bark contains salicin, a substance that when taken orally is converted by the enzymes present in the digestion process to salicylic acid. And the digestive conversion process that turns salicin into saligenin, and then into salicylic acid, is complicated. Further, salicin, much like salicylic acid, is stable only under acidic conditions. The likelihood that willow bark in the tiny amount used in these products can mimic the effectiveness of salicylic acid is at best problematic, and in all likelihood impossible. However, willow bark may indeed have some anti-inflammatory benefits for skin because in this form it appears to retain more of its aspirin-like composition. That is nice for skin, but definitely not better than other anti-inflammatories used in cosmetics and not at all the same as the exfoliating benefit of BHA. In the long run, for AHAs this line is a consideration, but even so it goes without saying that there are far less expensive versions of AHAs available.

For more information about Cellex-C, call (800) CELLEX-C or visit the Web site at www.cellex-c.com.

☺ $$$ **Fruitaplex Purifying Clay Mask for All Skin Types** (*$33 for 2 ounces*) is just an OK clay mask; it won't purify anything. It contains mostly water, thickeners, clay, mixed fruit extracts (which is meaningless for identifying AHA), silicone, and preservatives. This contains several ingredients that would be problematic for someone with oily skin, including zinc oxide, titanium dioxide, and triglycerides.

☺ $$$ **G.L.A. Dry Skin Cream for Dry Skin** (*$48 for 2 ounces*) adds another miracle ingredient to the Cellex-C stable. Now the big cure for wrinkles is gamma linolenic acid (GLA). While linolenic acid is a good fatty acid, it isn't going to cure wrinkles anymore than L-ascorbic acid can. Again, it seems bizarre to find that if L-ascorbic acid is supposed to be such a miracle ingredient, the skin needs still more miracles to get results. This ends up being a very good emollient moisturizer for dry skin. It does contain a tiny amount of lemon oil as fragrance.

☺ $$$ **G.L.A. Extra Moist Cream for Excessively Dry Skin** (*$55 for 2 ounces*).

The same comments about GLA described above apply here. This is a good moisturizer for normal to dry skin.

☺ $$$ **G.L.A. Eye Balm for Dry Skin** *($44 for 1 ounce)* is a very good moisturizer for dry skin. The same comments about GLA described above apply here. This product contains a small amount of lemon oil as fragrance.

☹ $$$ **Cellex-C Serum** *($75 for 1 ounce)* is a combination of vitamin C (L-ascorbic acid), water-binding agent, zinc, and tyrosine, an amino acid and a water-binding agent. If you do decide to give it a try, just keep in mind that once you open it, it stops being effective after two weeks, or possibly even sooner, depending on where you store it. Plus, if you feel these are the ingredients for skin, you shouldn't need any of these other products.

☹ $$$ **Cellex-C Eye Contour Gel for Normal to Oily Skin** *($42 for 0.5 ounce)* is virtually identical to the serum above, and the same review applies.

☹ $$$ **Cellex-C Skin Firming Cream Plus** *($95 for 2 ounces)* has the same showcased ingredients as the Serum only in a basic moisturizing base. The same basic comments for the Serum apply for this version.

☹ $$$ **Cellex-C Eye Contour Cream Plus for Sensitive, Dry Mature Skin** *($58 for 1 ounce)* is almost identical to the Skin Firming Cream, and the same review applies.

☺ $$$ **Seline-E Cream, for Normal Skin** *($48 for 2 ounces)*. Selenium is a good antioxidant, but the amount in here is barely noticeable. This is a good, though very standard moisturizer for dry skin but that's about it.

☹ $$$ **AlphaShade SPF 8 for All Skin Types** *($53 for 2 ounces)* includes both titanium dioxide and zinc oxide as the active sunscreen ingredients, but the low SPF number is absurd from a line claiming to know so much about skin care. How come it doesn't know the American Academy of Dermatology and the Skin Care Institute both recommend at least an SPF 15?

☺ $$$ **Bio-Botanical Cream for Normal to Oily Skin** *($45 for 2 ounces)*. There are several ingredients in here that would *not* be great for someone with oily skin, but this can be an overpriced option for someone with dry skin. Given that this doesn't contain any of the heralded ingredients Cellex-C brags about as miracles for skin, why would you spend the money for this one?

☺ $$$ **Hydra 5 B-Complex Moisture Enhancing Gel for All Skin Types** *($55 for 1 ounce)* contains a tiny amount of vitamin B, and that's a good antioxidant, but it's not anything essential for skin care much less at this kind of price. The water-binding agent is hyaluronic acid, and while it is very good for skin there are lots of other excellent water-binding agents used in this line and many other lines as well. This is a good lightweight moisturizer, but the price could cause your skin to crawl.

☺ $$$ **Salicea Gel for All Skin Types** *($45 for 1 ounce)* is a lightweight gel. It is almost identical to the Hydra 5 above and the same basic comments apply.

☺ **$$$ Betaplex Gentle Cleansing Milk** (*$23.20 for 3 ounces*). While AHA and willow bark may be helpful for skin, in a cleanser they would just be rinsed down the drain before they could have an effect. This is more of a cold cream with a minimal detergent cleansing agent, which could make it better for someone with normal to dry skin.

☺ **$$$ Betaplex Gentle Foaming Cleanser** (*$23.20 for 3 ounces*) is a standard, detergent-based water-soluble cleanser that also contains AHA and willow bark extract, plus coloring agents. While AHA and willow bark may be helpful for skin, in a cleanser they would just be rinsed down the drain before they could have an effect. It would be an option for someone with normal to dry skin, but the price is absurd for what you get.

☹ **Betaplex Facial Firming Water** (*$23.20 for 3 ounces*) has alcohol as the fourth ingredient and it also contains peppermint oil, which makes it too irritating and drying for all skin types.

☹ **Betaplex Fresh Complex Mist** (*$23.20 for 3 ounces*) is almost identical to the Firming Water above and the same comments apply.

☺ **$$$ Betaplex Line Smoother** (*$47.20 for 0.5 ounce*) contains about 8% AHA and little else, with a pH of 4.5. It would be a good, toner-style AHA product for use by itself or under a moisturizer for exfoliating the skin.

☺ **$$$ Betaplex Smooth Skin Complex** (*$47.20 for 1 ounce*) would be a good moisturizer with AHA for someone with normal to dry skin. There is little reason to consider this one over versions from Pond's to Alpha Hydrox.

☺ **$$$ Betaplex Complexion Cream** (*$47.20 for 1 ounce*) contains about 8% AHA. It is similar to the Skin Complex above and the same comments apply.

## Cetaphil (Skin Care Only)

Galderma is the company that manufactures Cetaphil Gentle Skin Cleanser. Those of you who have been familiar with my work from the beginning know that Cetaphil Gentle Skin Cleanser is a facial cleanser I have been impressed with for quite some time. In 1983, when I first discovered this obscure little cleanser, I was almost alone in recommending it, because no one else knew about it. Back then there were very few good products available for women to clean their faces with. Until recently, the only options were cold cream or cold cream–like products, which had to be wiped off and left the face greasy, and bar cleansers or soaps, which left the face dried out and irritated. Cetaphil Gentle Skin Cleanser was one of the only water-soluble cleansers available that cleaned the face without drying it out or leaving it feeling greasy. Times have changed, of course, and there are now many more alternatives for cleaning the face, but Cetaphil Gentle Skin Cleanser remains a primary option for women with dry, sensitive skin who don't wear much makeup. Unfortunately, Cetaphil Gentle Skin Cleanser is not very good for removing makeup, but it is dynamite in the morning or if you wear minimal makeup, and now they have Cetaphil Oily Skin Cleanser that can be used to remove makeup no matter what your skin type may be. For more information about Cetaphil products, call (800) 582-8225 or visit the Web site at www.cetaphil.com.

☺ **Cetaphil Gentle Skin Cleanser** *($8.31 for 16 ounces)* is a very good cleanser for someone with dry, sensitive skin. It is a simple formulation containing thickeners and a detergent cleansing agent. One word of warning: it doesn't remove makeup very well, so it is best for daytime or at night if you use minimal to no foundation. This does contain sodium lauryl sulfate, but it is less than 1% concentration and therefore has minimal to no risk of irritation.

☺ **Cetaphil Oily Skin Cleanser** *($5.50 for 2 ounces)*. Finally Cetaphil has an oily skin version, although it is really an all-skin cleanser. It removes makeup nicely, far better than the original Cetaphil Gentle Skin Cleanser, and doesn't irritate the eyes or dry out the skin. The price and amount are hard to understand, but you don't need very much when you use it and I've been told the pricing will change for the better.

☹ **Cetaphil Gentle Cleansing Bar for Dry, Sensitive Skin** *($3.29 for 4.5 ounces)* is a standard bar cleanser that uses a detergent cleansing agent. It does contain tallow, which can cause breakouts. It is best used from the neck down.

☺ **Cetaphil Moisturizing Lotion** *($7.49 for 16 ounces)* contains mostly water, glycerin, thickeners, plant oil, silicone, more thickeners, and preservatives. This is a good moisturizer for someone with sensitive, normal to dry skin.

☺ **Cetaphil Daily Facial Moisturizer SPF 15** *($7.99 for 4 ounces)* is a great addition to the Cetaphil line of products. This part avobenzone-based sunscreen comes in a rather standard but moisturizing base that is good for someone with normal to slightly dry skin. It contains mostly water, thickeners, silicone, slip agents, glycerin, preservatives, and vitamin E. This isn't a very elegant formula, but for sun protection it is one to consider, and it doesn't have to be used just on the face!

# *Chanel*

As far as Chanel's makeup products are concerned, not much has changed since the last edition of this book. The elegant, black-lacquered, urbane image is still intact but its shiny eyeshadows, poor concealer, and overpriced blushes are there too, offering little to extol. While Chanel does have some great foundation textures and decent colors, its SPFs are disappointing. Its lipsticks are wonderful, but lots of lines have wonderful lipsticks for far less. Its powders have an excellent texture, yet some of the colors are strange and the loose powders in both matte and dry-skin formulas are iridescent, while the pencils are very standard and commonplace. In general, there is little about this makeup line that warrants the price tag. All of the products have far less expensive counterparts that easily outperform Chanel's. One thing that has changed for the better is that at many Chanel counters, particularly those featuring "open sell" units, most everything is accessible, and that's a vast improvement over the previous hands-off, towering black display unit.

A major change for Chanel came in mid-1999, when the company launched a completely reformulated line of skin-care products. I found that an intriguing situation. After all, when you sell some of the more expensive skin-care products around, and make great claims about being the best, it takes a lot to say, "No, those really weren't the best, *now* we're selling you the best." I imagine a lot of Chanel women are going to be wondering what to do. I assure you that there is nothing precise or spectacular about this repackaging and remarketing venture. Chanel does seem to have used the "kitchen sink" approach to skin care, throwing in every ingredient under the sun so it can make a ton of claims and promises. Some of these products contain more than 75 different ingredients. Is that better for skin? That depends on your point of view. The notion that several types of antioxidant are better than just one or two effective ones is not established in the least. Plus, the longer the ingredient list, the higher your chance of irritation or allergic reaction. However, on the positive side, having a large group of ingredients does cover a lot of bases, especially for those looking for a little bit of everything (with the emphasis on *a little bit*, because many of the interesting ingredients are present in negligible amounts). From my perspective, if Chanel was going to go to all the trouble of creating a new line, it could have really set a new standard for excellence and let go of the coloring agents and fragrance. Now that would have been really impressive.

Nevertheless, what is definitely impressive is the inclusion of an SPF 15 sunscreen with UVA protection. Finally! It's ironic to consider that just a few years ago Chanel was sending me letters taking me to task for criticizing its SPF 8 products without UVA protection. How sad it took Chanel so long, and that in the meantime so many women wasted so much money and put their skin at risk. It's great that Chanel has come around at last.

For more information about Chanel, call (212) 688-5055 or visit the Web site at www.chanel.com.

## Chanel Skin Care

☺ $$$ **Aquamousse Foaming Cream Face Wash** *($28.50 for 5 ounces)* is a rather strong, detergent-based water-soluble cleanser that uses myristic acid, sodium methyl cocoyl laurate, and potassium hydroxide as the main cleansing agents. That can be drying and irritating for the skin. This standard formulation is wildly overpriced.

☺ $$$ **Gel Purete Foaming Gel Face Wash** *($30 for 5 ounces)* is an exceptionally standard but good detergent-based water-soluble cleanser that would work well for normal to oily skin.

☺ $$$ **Gel Tendre Non-Foaming Makeup Remover Face and Eyes** *($30 for 5 ounces)* is almost identical to the Gel Face Wash above only minus the foaming ingredients; other than that the same comments apply.

☹ $$$ **Lait Tendre Gentle Makeup Remover Face and Eyes** *($28.50 for 6.8 ounces)*. What a price tag for mineral oil! It works, and it would be gentle, but it would be more gentle without the fragrance and preservatives, much as using plain mineral oil would be.

☹ $$$ **Demaquillant Yeux Intense Gentle Biphase Eye Makeup Remover** *($22.50 for 3.4 ounces)* is less greasy than the one above, and silicone does feel nice on skin, but the price for this formulation is nonsense.

☻ **Lotion Purete Purifying Toner** *($28.50 for 6.8 ounces)*, with witch hazel, lemon, and grapefruit high up on the ingredient list, is a problem waiting to happen. They won't purify anything, but these ingredients can cause irritation, dryness, and redness.

☺ $$$ **Lotion Tendre Soothing Toner** *($28.50 for 6.8 ounces)* is a good non-irritating toner that's far better for all skin types than the one above. The price tag is bizarre and the formulation rather standard, but if price is no object and you like the new containers, why not?

☺ $$$ **Hydra Max Balanced Hydrating Cream** *($40 for 1.7 ounces)* is a very good moisturizer for dry skin, but that's about it.

☺ $$$ **HydraMax Balanced Hydrating Gel** *($40 for 1.7 ounces)* is a silicone-based gel moisturizer that would work well for normal to dry skin.

☹ $$$ **HydraMax Oil-Free Hydrating Gel** *($40 for 1.7 ounces)* is basically identical to the Balanced version above, only this one includes clay and aluminum starch (octenylsuccinate). That can definitely leave a matte finish on the skin but the aluminum starch can be irritating for some skin types. You have to ask yourself, why bother applying a moisturizer with ingredients that absorb moisture?

☺ $$$ **Rectiface Day Lift Refining Cream SPF 15** *($60 for 1.7 ounces)* is a very good sunscreen with avobenzone for UVA protection. Of course it was Chanel that sent me letters several years back when I complained about its products with SPF 8. I guess they've finally seen the light. This formulation would work well for normal to dry skin. The pH of this product is too high for the AHA or BHA to be effective as exfoliants.

☺ $$$ **Rectiface Day Lift Refining Lotion SPF 15** *($50 for 1.7 ounces)* is similar to the one above, only in lotion form. The same basic comments apply.

☺ $$$ **Rectiface Day Lift Refining Oil-Free Lotion SPF 15** *($50 for 1.7

*ounces)* is similar to the lotion form above, only in a far more matte finish. It does contain witch hazel, and that can be drying; it also uses aluminum starch (octenylsuccinate) to help create the matte finish, which is helpful, but it can also be slightly irritating.

☺ **$$$ Rectifiance Nuit Night Lift Restoring Cream** *($50 for 1.7 ounces)* is another lifting product—what a shock. This won't lift your face any better than Chanel's version before the line renovation, called **Complexe Intensif Night Lift Cream** *($31 for 1 ounce),* but at least the pricing isn't worse. This product does have one of the longest ingredient listings I've ever seen. The need for all this rests with you, but aside from the incredible redundancy, this turns out to be a good moisturizer for dry skin. The pH of the cream isn't low enough for the AHA or BHA to work as an exfoliant (it has a pH of 5).

☹ **$$$ Rectifiance Nuit Night Lift Restoring Lotion** *($60 for 1.7 ounces)* is similar to the cream above only in lotion form, plus it contains aluminum starch (octenylsuccinate). That can definitely leave a matte finish on the skin, but the aluminum starch can be irritating for some skin types. Plus, as I mentioned above, you have to ask yourself, why apply a moisturizer with ingredients that absorb moisture?

☺ **$$$ Source Extreme Dual Benefit Complex** *($65 for 1.7 ounces).* There is nothing extreme about this moisturizer; it would work well for normal to dry skin.

☺ **$$$ Eye Correction Anti-Wrinkle Firming Eye Cream** *($50 for 0.5 ounce)* is a good moisturizer for dry skin but there is nothing about this product that makes it preferable for the eyes. If anything, the other moisturizers in this line have better antioxidant concentrations and far more interesting water-binding agents.

☹ **Eye Lift Anti-Puffiness/Dark Circle Eye Lotion** *($48 for 0.5 ounce)* contains nothing that can change dark circles or puffiness, but the third ingredient, witch hazel, can be drying and irritating to the eye area.

☹ **$$$ Controle Imperfections Blemish Control** *($25 for 0.5 ounce)* is the tiniest quantity and the most expensive BHA product I've seen, plus the concentration of BHA is only 0.5%. The somewhat emollient gel base is fine for normal to dry skin, but the pH isn't low enough for it to be effective as an exfoliant (it has a pH of 5), so why bother?

☹ **T-Mat Shine Control** *($25 for 1 ounce)* contains alcohol and witch hazel as the second and third ingredients. This is too drying and potentially irritating for all skin types.

☺ **Fluide Multi-Protection Daily Protection Lotion SPF 25** *($25 for 1 ounce)* is a good in-part titanium dioxide–based sunscreen. It has a matte finish due to the inclusion of ammonium starch (octenylsuccinate) high up on the ingredient listing. It would work well for someone with normal to slightly oily skin, but the price is a problem if it keeps you from applying it generously.

☹ $$$ **Lip Correction Lip Cure** *($27.50 for 0.5 ounce)* includes a group of ingredients that can't cure anything. This is basically just emollients with talc. It goes on greasy and then dries to a matte finish. That's nice, but it doesn't do much for lips and only minimally helps prevent lipstick from feathering.

☹ $$$ **Estompe Taches Anti-Dark Spot Serum** *($50 for 1 ounce)* has no ingredients that will change a single melanin discoloration. All of the ingredients are moisturizing, which is good, but the claim is bogus. It does contain a form of vitamin C that is helpful as an antioxidant, but that doesn't affect melanin production. There is some research showing that mulberry extract (another ingredient in here) can be helpful, but that research has only been in a petri dish and never on real people. One concern is that this product contains mint extract, which can be a skin irritant, but I suspect it also makes the user feel like something is working.

☹ $$$ **Hydra Serum Vitamin Moisture Boost** *($50 for 1 ounce)* has alcohol as its third ingredient. That's confusing for a product claiming to be a moisturizer boost.

☺ $$$ **Lift Serum Extreme Anti-Wrinkle Firming Complex** *($70 for 1 ounce).* If the collagen and elastin in this product were so great for preventing wrinkles, why aren't they in any of the other products? After all, collagen and elastin are just water-binding agents; they can't affect the collagen or elastin in your skin.

☺ **Solution Destressante Calming Emulsion** *($30 for 3.4 ounces)* is similar to many of the moisturizers in the new Chanel lineup, only with different claims.

☺ $$$ **Masque Lift Express** *($32.50 for 2.6 ounces)* won't lift the skin anywhere, but it is a good moisturizer for normal to dry skin.

☺ $$$ **Masque Force Hydratante** *($28.50 for 2.6 ounces).* While this is a very good moisturizer for normal to dry skin, the mask part isn't adding any benefit.

☹ $$$ **Masque Purete** *($28.50 for 2.6 ounces)* is a standard clay mask. The pH of this mask is too high for the BHA to have any exfoliating properties.

## Chanel Makeup

**FOUNDATION:** ☹ $$$ **Teint Pur Matte SPF 8** *($47.50)* does not offer any UVA protection and even if it did, the SPF rating is below the standards set by the American Academy of Dermatology. Despite the disappointing SPF, it does provide a smooth, even matte finish and light to medium coverage suitable for normal to oily skins. Of the nine shades, four are too peach, pink, or rose for most skin tones, including Warm Beige, Natural Beige, Golden Beige, and Ivory.

☹ $$$ **Teint Naturel SPF 8** *($50)* has a gorgeous, lightly creamy texture and an impeccable, natural finish that provides light to medium coverage. If this had an SPF 15 with appropriate UVA-protecting ingredients (it fails on both counts), it would be a great option despite the unwarranted price tag. The nine shades are mostly fine, except Warm Beige, Golden Beige and Tawny Beige.

☺ $$$ **Teint Lift Eclat SPF 8** *($50)* is a resounding disappointment if you are hoping to hide a few wrinkles behind your foundation. It doesn't diminish wrinkles in the least, and the SPF 8 is not the best (though it is titanium dioxide–based); an SPF 15 would be far better. If wrinkles aren't your problem, this is a silky-soft, matte, slightly powdery finish foundation with good light-to-medium coverage; it's good for someone with oily to combination skin, but a problem for someone with dry or sun-damaged skin. There are 11 shades available, with options for very light but not very dark skin tones. These shades are too peach or rose for most skin tones: Warm Bisque, Clear Beige, Golden Honey, and Warm Honey.

☺ $$$ **Teint Extreme Lumiere with Non-Chemical SPF 8** *($50)* is a rather standard emollient foundation that provides medium to full coverage, a creamy finish, and has nothing luminescent or extreme about it. For dry skin it's an option, but the SPF number is too low to rely on for all-day protection. Of the six colors, three are suspect as too peach or rose: Opal, Buff, and Soft Beige.

☺ $$$ **Double Perfection Makeup SPF 8** *($42)* has reliable UVA protection but it's doubtful you'll work up to the SPF 8 (which is not adequate for all-day protection) with a powder foundation, given that it requires complete coverage to get the amount of protection promised. But this is still a great pressed powder, with a silky-smooth, seamless finish and 12 excellent, fairly neutral shades. This type of foundation is often recommended to be used with a wet application, but that tends to make it look streaked and choppy.

☹ $$$ **Sheer Brilliance** *($35)* is a generous (for Chanel) sized bottle of liquid golden shimmer that can be used anywhere but is recommended for the face, with or without foundation. It has a definite shine that I'll leave up to your taste.

<u>CONCEALER:</u> ☹ **Correction Perfection** *($55)* is a compact with a concealer, a yellow color corrector, a shiny bronze "luminizer," a creamy, very shiny highlighter, an itty-bitty wrinkle-fill-in pencil called **Line Perfector,** and an equally small nylon brush. It is ridiculously overpriced and all the worse for the creamy, thick texture of the concealer and corrector (both will crease) and the notion that a peach-toned pencil will somehow fill in facial lines. There is only one set of colors and they are suited to fair/light skin tones, in spite of Chanel's "one size fits all" decree. **Corrective Concealer** *($28.50)* is a greasy, lipstick-style concealer with poor colors that can easily crease into lines around the eye. **Estompe Extreme Cover Up** *($31)* comes in a tube and has a smooth, creamy texture, but the two shades are noticeably peach and pink, and they tend to easily crease into the lines around the eyes.

☺ $$$ **Quick Cover** *($32.50)* has a silky, light texture and offers even, opaque coverage. This one could easily take the place of Chanel's other concealers. It is available in three shades that hold up well and are relatively waterproof.

☹ $$$ **Eyeshadow Base** *($25)* is a standard matte-finish base tinted a pale pink that does help eyeshadow stay on better, although a matte-finish foundation would work just as well and eliminate the need for this single-purpose product.

POWDER: ☺ $$$ **Perfecting Pressed Powder** *($38.50)* tends to go on dry in spite of its silky texture. It is a very basic, talc-based powder with good colors and a price that is unwarranted for what you get. **Luxury Compact** *($100)* is a stunning gold compact that would be worth this much money if it were a necklace, but it's not. It is refillable with the small assortment of Chanel's pressed powder.

☹ $$$ **Perfecting Loose Powder** *($42)* comes in three shades that are supposed to have "light-reflecting properties," but they are just shiny powders; the shine sort of negates the purpose of using a finishing powder, doesn't it? For an evening look it can be fine but the sparkles on your face in daylight just look too noticeable.

☹ **Powderlights** *($45)* is all about packaging. It comes in an awkward container with a powder brush attached to the base of the container as part of the cap. You have to remove the cap and then get the powder onto the brush, either by shaking the powder onto the brush, which is messy, or shaking some of the powder onto a tissue and then using the brush to pick up some of the powder. Why anyone would want to bother with this contrivance, the five shiny colors, and the cost is beyond me.

☺ $$$ **Perfecting Bronzing Powder SPF 8** *($38.50)* is available in one shade, a tannish-red that is not flattering to many skin tones, particularly light skins. It is matte and blends nicely but don't count on it for sun protection with its measly SPF 8 and no UVA-protecting ingredients.

☺ $$$ BLUSH: **Powder Blush** *($36)* goes on very smoothly and features 13 rich shades. Some of these are obviously shiny, but there are enough matte shades here to merit a look. Price-wise, I would encourage anyone to check out Maybelline's Pure Blush *($6.29)*, whose sublime texture and soft application are identical if not superior to Chanel's. **Face Brights** *($35)* is worth checking out. This twist-up stick blush, eyeshadow, and lipstick in one has an interesting cream-to-powder finish that dries to an almost tintlike, sheer finish with a slight amount of shine. The lipstick application requires a brush, but for an all-in-one look I think you might want to give it a test drive.

☺ $$$ EYESHADOW: Chanel still has a thing for shiny eyeshadows. Haven't they noticed how well other lines are doing with matte shadows? What is the fascination with having the eyes glitter? And what a shame, too, because the textures are quite lovely and smooth. **Quadra Eyeshadow** *($50)* has some options where you will find that three out of four shades are matte, such as **Dunes** and **Variations**. Otherwise, shine is the theme, and many of the Quadra sets have sharply contrasting color combinations that won't make artful blending any easier. **Shadow Light Double Effect Eye Color** *($25 each)* are single eyeshadow colors, weighing in heavily on the shiny side, so any and all wrinkles will look more prominent. They do go on wet or dry, but the shine tends to flake! **Satin Eye Color** *($30)* is more shine for eyes, this time taking the form of a cream to (shiny) powder eye color applied with a wand. The number of shades has been greatly reduced, so don't be surprised if they're all gone for good quite soon. **Basic Eye Color** *($42)* is a compact of eyeshadows with three similarly toned shades in varying depths of color. One shade in each is shiny. The color combinations have improved since the last edition of this book, but there are far better ways to put together a collection of color for your eyes.

☺ $$$ <u>EYE AND BROW SHAPER:</u> **Precision Eye Definer** *($28)* is a very expensive, utterly standard pencil that has a slightly dry finish and an angled sponge tip for blending—they can't be serious about the price? **Eyelines** *($45)* is a compact with four cake-eyeliner tablets and a brush. If cake eyeliner appeals to you, there are much less exorbitant ways to use it, the least of which would be as a deeply pigmented matte eyeshadow applied with a damp brush. **Double Effect Eye Pencil** *($23.50)* can be an interesting way to do a dramatic line—the double effect refers to the fact that these pencils can be used wet or dry. When wet, the result is similar in intensity to liquid liner, while the dry application is reminiscent of every other standard pencil around. There are more shades to choose from than before, but why spend this much for something so ordinary? **Eye Liner Duo** *($27.50)* is a double-ended, automatic, twist-up pencil that can also be retracted. One end is a matte shade and the other is shiny. Both ends have a creamy texture and slight powder finish that can easily smudge and smear unless you're very careful. **Precision Brow Definer** *($28)* has a price that demands some pretty fancy window-dressing for such a boringly standard brow pencil. The brush at the end is a nice touch, but not nearly enough to make this worthwhile.

☺ $$$ **Sculpting Brow Pencil** *($25.50)* is a very good option for brow pencil, with a smooth powder texture that allows for a soft, natural look. What a shame the price will assuredly raise some brows! **Brow Shaper** *($28.50)* is a brow gel with a small color selection: Soft Brown, Taupe, Black, and Clear. There are no shades for brunettes, blondes, or redheads, but brows definitely stay in place and the gel goes on easily, without smearing, which is very important for this type of product.

☹ **Liquid Eyelines** *($27.50)* has a flimsy brush and most of the colors are shiny, plus this stays wet for far too long. **Perfect Brows** *($60)* is a set of three powdered brow colors: a taupe, a medium brown, and a brownish-black, plus Smurf-sized tweezers and a grooming brush. The intent is for women to mix and match between the three shades to achieve their "Perfect Brow," but this ends up being useless for anyone with light hair (all blondes), who could only use the lightest color, and what are brunettes supposed to do with two dark colors, one of which will undoubtedly make the brows look severe? I could go on, but you get the idea. I admit, the concept has merit; no one's brows are all one color. But there are dozens upon dozens of suitable brow powders and eyeshadows that perform beautifully and aren't so insultingly expensive.

☺ $$$ <u>LIPSTICK AND LIP PENCIL:</u> **Metallic Creme Lipstick** *($21)* is a creamy lipstick with a slightly greasy finish. Each color is sheathed in a layer of metallic glitter that mixes with the base color and creates a soft glittery look that's not quite as gaudy as it sounds. **Hydrabase Creme Lipstick** *($21)* has an excellent creamy, opaque texture and a nice variety of colors. It's not worth this amount of money, but do women buy Chanel for performance or the image? **Hydracaresse HydraTreatment Lipstick SPF 15** *($22.50)* does not offer any UVA-protecting ingredients but it is a very emollient, greasy lipstick with rich, opaque colors that leave a slight stain. The print ads make this appear to have a natural matte finish, but in reality this appears quite different. **Triple Colour Crayon** *($30)* is an extra-thick jumbo pencil that actually works quite well as a fairly sheer color for lips, cheeks, and eyes. The colors all have slight to moderate shine, but they do blend on well. If the price doesn't sit well with you, try Jane's One-for-Alls *($2.99)*, available at most drugstores and remarkably similar to Chanel's version. **Lip Intensities** *($47.50)* is a compact of lip color divided into four sections. The four quadrants all have the same shade, but with different textures. One-quarter of the compact has a creamy consistency; the others are matte, glossy, and sheer. It's hardly convenient. It is far easier to use a lipstick tube and quickly sweep color across the lips instead of having to use a brush. Although it sounds nice to have the texture of your choice, most women prefer one over the others. If you like variations on a theme, this is one of the more interesting ways to get it. **Precision Lip Definer** *($25.50)* is shockingly similar to dozens of other lip pencils and absolutely not worth the fee, when everyone from Max Factor to Revlon has their version (with a brush) for so much less. **Lip Liner Duo** *($27.50)* is identical in concept and packaging to the Eye Liner Duo above. There is a matte and a shiny side, and other than the cleverness, they are pretty standard.

☹ **Protective Lip Color** *($26.50)* looks like a lipstick but is sold as a clear base to use prior to applying lipstick. It supposedly allows the lip color to stay true by preventing the acidic nature of skin (which lips don't have because they don't have oil glands) from changing the lipstick's color. There is nothing in here that can do that, and no one at the Chanel counters could explain what allowed it to allegedly work as stated.

☺ $$$ **Crystal Lip Gloss** *($28.50)* is a set of two shiny, slippery glosses in one compact. You won't be able to tell the difference between these and the glosses from Bonne Bell or Jane at the drugstore. **Glossimer** *($22.50)* has a sumptuous name but that does little to make this very standard, sticky gloss deserve such a jaw-dropping price. **HydraSoleil Lipstick SPF 6** *($20)* is a small group of sheer, greasy lipsticks with no UVA-protecting ingredients and an abysmal SPF 6.

☺ $$$ <u>MASCARA:</u> **Instant Lash Mascara** *($20)* builds long, thick lashes fairly fast, so the name is apropos, and you'll be able to achieve this with no smudging or smearing. **Sculpting Mascara Extreme Length** *($20)* and **Extreme Length Fine Lashes** *($20)* consist of a single mascara formula that comes packaged with two different brush options. The Extreme Length Fine Lashes contains a very small, tiny-thin brush that built exceptionally long lashes with no clumping. The Extreme Length mascara has a full round brush that was far less impressive at building long lashes but still delivered a decent mascara. **Extreme Wear Waterproof Mascara** *($20)* lengthens well and thickens minimally. It goes on smoothly with no clumps or flakes and is nicely waterproof but removes easily with the appropriate waterproof makeup remover (which is usually just mineral oil).

☺ $$$ **Extreme Cils Drama Lash Mascara** *($20).* The only thing dramatic about this mascara is how wet and clumpy it goes on. However, it does build very impressive length. **Maximum Lash Base** *($20)* is a standard, creamy-white lash primer that claims to thicken and create the look of false lashes when used with a mascara. Almost without exception, products like this are unnecessary if you have a good mascara. Of course, if you're intrigued, there are less expensive options to be found.

☺ $$$ <u>BRUSHES:</u> Chanel does present an attractive, satiny, and reasonably priced collection of **brushes** *($22 to $38).* Many of them are very useful, with excellent shapes and sizes. For your consideration, take a look at the **#2 Eyeshadow** *($22)*, **#1 Eyeshadow** *($22)*, and **#11 Eyeshadow** *($25)*, as well as the **Blush** *($38)* and **Powder** *($42)* brushes if you're feeling particularly spendy.

☺ $$$ Avoid the **#4 Shadow/Line Brush** *($22)*, which is scratchy, and the **#15 Lip Brush** *($22)*, which is unrealistically tiny.

# *Chantecaille*

The spin on this line of makeup products being sold at Neiman Marcus and some salons and spas is that it was created by Sylvie Chantecaille, a 20-year employee of the Estee Lauder corporation. The fact that she worked for Lauder is impressive—experience alone means a lot in the crowded, complicated cosmetics industry. So it isn't startling that this veteran cosmetics-marketing executive would claim that her products are "based on the purest most natural ingredients possible" (though I found that isn't vaguely true with just a cursory look at the ingredient listings). But given the way the claim is stated, Chantecaille isn't exactly untruthful either. Ironically, the claim also makes sense, because when it comes to formulating makeup products there just aren't many "possible" natural ingredients to choose from. With that limited number of natural ingredients, I guess they chose the ones they could.

The textures are what is most notable about this makeup collection; they are all impressive, with silky smoothness and even application. The shortcoming is the shine. Almost everything shines, and although that can have a nice effect for evening or special occasions, for daywear it's sort of like wearing a sequined outfit to the office. Chantecaille products are available exclusively at Neiman Marcus and Bergdorf Goodman and some salons around the country. For more information visit Neiman Marcus's Web site at www.neimanmarcus.com.

**FOUNDATION:** ☺ **$$$ Real Skin Foundation** *($47)* is almost identical to Vincent Longo's Water Canvas ($40) foundation (at Sephora's), which is almost identical to Borghese's Molto Bella Liquid Powder Makeup ($35). As I mention in my review of Longo's Water Canvas, all these compact foundations are liquidy powders with a gel-like wet feel that dry to a satiny-smooth, sheer, slightly matte finish. Chantecaille's works well for most skin types and has the sheerest finish of the group, but it also has the fewest color choices, with only four shades that resemble skin, though they do so nicely. The other two are shiny, in either white or pink, and while that can have a nice effect for evening, there are less expensive ways to create a shiny look.

☹ **$$$ Future Skin Foundation** *($55)* has a creamy texture that blends out quite sheer and light. The light-reflecting claim comes from the shiny finish, which is indeed noticeable. The seven shades look at first to be too pink or peach but blend on surprisingly neutral. The only one to consider avoiding (if you can put up with the aforementioned shiny finish) is Sand. By the way, although not labeled on the box or the ingredient list, the jar this comes in claims to have an SPF 10. When I inquired as to why there was no SPF listed as an active ingredient, the company claimed the sun protection came from the seaweed this contains. Anyone who believes that seaweed offers any significant sun protection probably also thinks the Earth is flat.

☺ **$$$ New Stick SPF 8** *($38)* is similar to many of the stick foundations now out on the market, from Lauder's Minute Makeup SPF 15 ($27.50) to Clinique's CityStick SPF 15 ($20), Maybelline's Express 3 in 1 SPF 10 ($6.77), and Prescriptives Matchstick Foundation SPF 15 ($35)—and these are all titanium dioxide–based, too. Chante-caille's colors are great and the application is smooth and even for good medium coverage that would work well for normal to dry skin. But for the money and the sunscreen factor, the Lauder, Clinique, and Prescriptives versions are definitely preferred (interesting that these are all from Chantecaille's alma mater).

☺ **$$$ Compact Makeup** *($45)* is a standard, talc-based pressed powder with a wonderful silky-soft texture and an absurd price. The six shades are nice and they can be used wet (like most pressed powders can be). The claim is that this product is supposed to be hydrating, but it isn't—no powder can be. By its very nature it absorbs oil and water and that's not hydrating in the least.

**POWDER:** ☹ **$$$ Talc-Free Loose Powder** *($45).* Showcasing the fact that this powder is talc-free seems strange given that the Compact Makeup above contains talc. If there is something wrong with talc, why put it in any of these products?

Talc is just fine in makeup; has as silky and smooth a texture as any other face mineral; and, as I've commented in my newsletters, there is no health risk associated with the use of talc in face makeup. The shortcoming here is that all these powders are shiny, which negates using this product to reduce shine on the face. For a shiny dusting it's fine, but for setting makeup or reducing the shine from oil on the face, it's useless.

☺ $$$ <u>BLUSH:</u> **Cheek Shade** *($20)*. With just six shades there isn't much selection, but these do have great, soft, matte, silky textures, and the colors are all quite wearable. But speaking of money, check out the new blush textures from L'Oreal Feel Naturale or Maybelline's Pure Blush for far less expensive yet equivalent performances.

☹ $$$ <u>EYESHADOW:</u> **Lasting Eye Shade** *($20)* and **Shine Eye Shade** *($20)*. The salesperson was trying to help me find the matte shades in this large group of 48 colors. Only eight are supposed to have shine, but it turns out most all of these are shiny. Of the 40 supposed mattes, the shine isn't glaring, but if you were hoping for more matte selections this isn't the line to frequent. Aside from that, the textures are luscious and the most impressive part of the line. These can be used wet or dry.

☺ $$$ <u>LIPSTICK AND LIP PENCIL:</u> **Lip Matte**, **Lip Sheer**, and **Lipstick** *($20)*. The Matte is more like opaque creamy lipstick, the Sheer more like gloss, and the Lipstick just a very standard, nice lipstick. The color range is impressive but there is nothing new here to be excited about. **Lip Definer** *($18)* is awfully expensive for what amounts to the same standard pencil with a creamy application that almost every other line has. **Lip Gloss SPF 15** *($20)* does not contain UVA protection and is just a very standard gloss. It's nice but not worth $20.

☺ $$$ <u>BRUSHES:</u> The **brushes** *($22–$70)* from Chantecaille feature exquisite textures and mostly practical shapes and cuts. The various **Eye Shadow Brushes** *($24–$30)* are pricey but worth a look, while the **Face Brush** *($70)* and **Cheek Brush** *($55)*, though nicely shaped, are too soft and fluffy for much control or ability to hold powders evenly. The **Lip Brush** *($28)* should, at this price, come with a cap or be retractable but does not have either feature.

# *Christian Dior*

What was true about Dior in the last edition of this book is still true today. Dior is a great name when it comes to haute couture, yet as often happens when a fashion house trademark expands to makeup and skin care, something inevitably gets lost in the translation. There is not too much here that is new, and the existing products still fall short in some key areas. For example, many of Dior's foundation colors have limited color choices, offering very little for lighter and darker skin tones; the eyeshadows are almost all shiny, the pencils are overpriced while being below the standard, and the tester unit, though somewhat improved, still leaves the majority of products unorganized and inaccessible. That is a few too many shortcomings in my book. But if price isn't an issue, you will find some of Dior's products, particularly its mascaras (for lashes and hair), lipsticks and blushes, and its new foundation Teint Glace to be very good options.

As is typical of high-end designer lines, the packaging is really the star attraction here. In this realm you will not be disappointed; many Dior products are so bejeweled and ornamental that you may want to wear the packaging and forget what's inside! If this type of showmanship appeals to you, that is what you end up paying for.

Dior has reformulated its skin-care products—well, at least on the surface. Its cleansers and toners sport different names but the formulas are shockingly similar to what was already there. Dior has attempted to stay abreast of the latest gimmicks including vitamin C and vitamin A products but completely missed the influence of AHAs, BHA, and the need for well-formulated sunscreens (SPF 15 with UVA-protecting ingredients is now standard) as part of any reliable or effective skin-care routine. If you have oily skin you will only find irritating products with no ability to disinfect or exfoliate. One last concern: as is true for most all European lines, the fragrance wafting from these products is invasive. If you wouldn't put perfume on your face, think twice about applying it in the form of an expensive skin-care product.

For more information on Christian Dior, call (212) 931-2200 or visit the Web site at www.dior.com.

# *Christian Dior Skin Care*

☺ **$$$ Purifying Wash-Off Cleansing Foam** *($22.50 for 6.8 ounces)* is a standard detergent cleanser that is potentially too drying and irritating for most skin types, though it could be an option for someone with very oily skin. It does contain fragrance.

☺ **$$$ Purifying Cleansing Gelee for Face and Eyes** *($22.50 for 6.8 ounces)* is a makeup remover. This is a very standard, overpriced application of silicone that would work fine for normal to dry skin. As a makeup remover this does little more than wiping mineral oil over the skin would; and mineral oil would be far less expensive!

☹ **Purifying Lotion** *($20 for 6.8 ounces)* lists alcohol as the second ingredient, and it also contains menthol. Neither of those things purify anything but they can be irritating and drying for all skin types.

☹ **Refreshing Wash-Off Cleansing Gel** *($22.50 for 6.8 ounces)*. The second ingredient is sodium C14-16 olefin sulfate, which is too drying and potentially irritating for all skin types.

☺ **$$$ Refreshing Cleansing Water for Face and Eyes** *($22.50 for 6.8 ounces)* is a very standard, boring toner.

☹ **Refreshing Lotion** *($20 for 6.8 ounces)* lists alcohol as the second ingredient, and that isn't refreshing but it is irritating and drying for all skin types.

☺ $$$ **Softening Cleansing Milk for Face and Eyes** *($22.50 for 6.8 ounces)* is a good cold cream–style cleanser that is no different from using Neutrogena's Extra Gentle Cleanser, except Neutrogena's is half the price.

☺ $$$ **Softening Wash-Off Cleansing Creme** *($22.50 for 6.8 ounces)* is virtually identical to the Cleansing Milk above and the same comments apply.

☺ **Softening Lotion—Alcohol Free** *($20 for 6.8 ounces)* is alcohol-free, and I'm glad it is, but all the toners in this line should be. It would be an OK (but boring) option for normal to dry skin.

☺ $$$ **Instant Eye Makeup Remover** *($18.50 for 3.4 ounces)* is a good makeup remover, but there are lots of good makeup removers for far less.

☺ $$$ **Deep Radiance Exfoliating Creme** *($25 for 2.4 ounces)* will work as a scrub but only for someone with normal to dry skin, and be careful: this can be abrasive.

☹ **Clarifying Cleansing Mask** *($25 for 1.9 ounces)* is an exceptionally standard clay mask that would be an option for normal to oily skin except this one contains menthol and camphor, which makes it too irritating for all skin types.

☺ $$$ **Capture Essential Time-Fighting Serum with Pure Micro-Proteins** *($70 for 1.7 ounces)* is a lot of money for what amounts to a good, lightweight moisturizer for normal to slightly dry skin.

☺ $$$ **Capture Eyes Contour Gel** *($45 for 0.5 ounce).* The interesting ingredients are at the end of the ingredient listing, making their presence mere dustings; however it also contains an extract from the plant *Terminalia sericea,* considered to be fairly irritating and sensitizing for the skin.

☹ **Capture Rides Fluide Multi-Action Wrinkle Lotion SPF 8 with Cyclic AHA** *($45 for 1 ounce)* has an SPF 8, but that number is pathetic for good skin care, and this product doesn't contain avobenzone, zinc oxide, or titanium dioxide, and is not recommended.

☹ **Capture Rides Multi-Action Wrinkle Creme SPF 8** *($45 for 1 ounce)* is similar to the one above and the same review applies.

☺ $$$ **Capture Rides Wrinkle Creme for Eyes** *($45 for 0.5 ounce)* is a good, though ordinary, moisturizer for normal to dry skin.

☺ $$$ **Capture Lift Complexe Liposomes** *($62 for 1 ounce)* is a good but rather ordinary moisturizer for normal to dry skin. The "good" ingredients come well after the fragrance and preservatives, and that means they are barely present.

☺ $$$ **Hydra-Star Moisture Creme for Dry Skin** *($46 for 1.7 ounces)* would be a very good moisturizer for someone with dry skin.

☺ $$$ **Hydra-Star Moisture Creme, for Normal and Combination Skin** *($46 for 1.7 ounces)* is almost identical to the Hydra-Star Moisture Creme for Dry Skin above. That makes it unacceptable for someone with combination skin but it is an option for someone with normal to dry skin.

☺ $$$ **Hydra-Star Moisture Lotion for Normal to Combination Skin** *($46 for 1.7 ounces)* is a very lightweight moisturizer. It would be good with antioxidants for normal to slightly dry or combination skin, but is not in the least appropriate for someone with combination skin.

☹ $$$ **Hydra-Star Moisture Lotion for Dry Skin** *($46 for 1.7 ounces)* is identical to the Hydra-Star Moisture Lotion for Normal to Combination Skin above, and except for a slight texture difference, the same basic review applies.

☺ $$$ **Hydra-Star Night Treatment Creme for Dry Skin** *($56 for 1.7 ounces)* is similar to Hydra-Star Moisture Lotion above, only more emollient, and would be a good moisturizer for normal to dry skin.

☺ $$$ **Icone Hypersensitive Skin Emulsion for the Face** *($58 for 1 ounce)* would be a good moisturizer for someone with normal to dry skin, but nothing about it makes it more suitable for sensitive skin.

☺ $$$ **Icone Regulating Crème Dehydrated Skin** *($70 for 1.7 ounce)* is a good though exceptionally overpriced moisturizer for someone with dry skin, and it won't regulate your skin in any way, shape, or form.

☺ $$$ **Icone for Hyper-Sensitive Skin** *($44 for 1 ounce)* is almost identical to the Icone Dehydrated version above and the same comments apply.

☹ $$$ **Icone for Oily Skin** *($44 for 1 ounce)* would be a good lightweight moisturizer for normal to slightly dry skin, but I wouldn't recommend using it to control oil because the product is not all that absorbent.

☺ $$$ **Vitalmine** *($45 for 1.1 ounces)* is one more vitamin C product for you to swallow (well, not literally). This one does contain magnesium ascorbyl palmitate, considered to be one of the more stable forms vitamin C in terms of reliable antioxidants, but the notion that this is the best antioxidant or that it can stop or improve wrinkling is just nonsense. This is a good moisturizer for dry skin.

☹ $$$ **Phenomen-A Double Retinol Wrinkle Treatment** *($50 for 1 ounce)* does have retinol, but other than for the Dior label there is no reason to choose this retinol version over Neutrogena's, RoC's, or Alpha Hydrox's at the drugstore for far less. The amount of retinol here is the same as most.

☺ $$$ **Model Lift** *($45 for 1 ounce)* is a good, silky moisturizer for normal to dry skin, but it is more reminiscent of Avon's Luminosity, which costs half the price; Avon's formula is actually a bit more elegant with more state-of-the-art water-binding agents.

☺ $$$ **UV 30 Ultra UV Face Coat** *($31 for 1 ounce)* is a good in-part titanium dioxide–based sunscreen. This is shockingly overpriced for what amounts to a boring, basic sunscreen that is easily replaced with dozens of others for far less.

☹ **Ultra-Mat Perfect Matte-Finish** *($32 for 0.5 ounce)* is basically an expensive version of the milk of magnesia I recommend as a facial mask. It works to help keep oil in check but, because of the alcohol, the irritation it can cause makes it impossible to recommend.

☹ **Mati-Star Oil-Free Mattifying Moisturizer** *($38.50 for 1.7 ounces)* contains mostly alcohol along with other irritating ingredients, menthol, and camphor. This is an irritation waiting to happen. It does contain a tiny amount of niacinamide (less than 1%). Niacinamide is vitamin B3 and the 1% concentration makes it ineffective for treating breakouts. There are a handful of studies demonstrating that a 4% concentration of niacinamide applied topically in gel form can have similar effects to the topical prescription drug clindomycin. (Clindomycin is a topical antibiotic that kills the bacteria known to cause pimples.) However, this research is primarily from the company that makes this product (Papulex) and it can still cause dryness and inflammation.

# Christian Dior Makeup

**FOUNDATION:** Dior has added some new foundations that have reliable UVA protection. Now if they could just tone down some of their overly peach and rose shades and add larger range of colors, these would be wholeheartedly recommended.

☺ **$$$ Teint Glace** *($35)* has a wonderful, slightly cool, wet application, with a sheer, smooth, soft matte finish. What a shame Teint Glace has only a few shades available (none for darker skin tones), because this is one of the more interesting stick foundations for a sheer, matte finish without the heavy emollients that often get deposited from other types of stick foundations. (By the way, Olay's All Day Moisture Stick Foundation, reviewed in this edition, is virtually identical to this one, and with better color options). Of the five shades available, most are slightly peach to orange, but if you have light skin and want to give this one a test-drive, consider #200 or #202.

☺ **$$$ Teint Dior Compact Lisse SPF 15** *($38.50)* has a soft and powdery finish, with no moist or greasy after-feel. While it claims to be oil-free, it does have waxy thickening agents that can be a problem for blemish-prone or oily skin. Still, the finish is still relatively matte and has good staying power throughout the day. It has an excellent SPF with the active ingredient being titanium dioxide. This would work well for someone with normal to oily skin. Why the low rating then? Dior Teint Compact Lisse comes in nine colors, of which most are fairly peach or pink, and there are definitely no darker shades to choose from. The limited color selection makes it hard to be too excited about this one. This could be an option for normal to slightly oily skins, but three of the six shades are too peach or rose to recommend. Avoid Medium Beige, Medium Golden, and Soft Rose.

☺ **$$$ Teint Diorlight SPF 10** *($38.50)* is an extremely sheer, beautifully smooth foundation with a light-textured, natural finish and a part titanium dioxide sunscreen (though SPF 15 is the number to be looking for). This blends on easily and would be fine for almost all skin types (except very oily) preferring bare minimum coverage. How sad that after all these good points, the colors are almost all too peach for most skin tones. These are the only neutral colors to consider: Ivory, Light Beige, and Linen.

☺ $$$ **Diorlift SPF 10** *($38.50)* is a replacement for Dior's former Tient Actuel foundation. The SPF in here is unreliable for UVA protection, so if you're willing to wear something underneath, this could work. The texture is smooth with a lot of slip, so blending takes a while but leaves a natural finish with light to medium coverage. This would be an option for normal to very dry skin; however, there are no colors for very light or very dark skin tones. By the way, this won't lift your skin anywhere or adequately conceal wrinkles—it's simply a good foundation.

☹ **Teint Dior Eclat Satin** *($42.50)* has a smooth, even texture that blends well, leaving a slightly dewy, emollient finish. Unfortunately, with the exception of Soft Beige, all of the colors are just too peach, pink, rose, or orange to recommend.

☺ $$$ **Teint Dior Eclat Mat** *($42.50)* has a light, semi-creamy texture and dries down to a slightly matte finish. This would be appropriate for normal to slightly dry or oily skin needing medium coverage. One caution: this formula is highly fragranced. Of the eight available shades, five are too peach, pink, or rose to recommend. Consider avoiding Light Rose, Golden, Medium Beige, Beige, and Medium Golden.

☺ $$$ **Teint Dior Poudre Foundation** *($42.50; $29.50 refills)* is a standard, wet/dry, talc-based powder foundation with a soft, very smooth texture that is best used dry for light coverage. This has to be one of the most expensive pressed powders around, yet there's little reason to consider the price tag given that everyone from Clinique to Olay has excellent options. Of Dior's four shades available, all have a very slight peach hue but this shouldn't be a problem since the application is so sheer.

☹ **CONCEALER: Hydrating Concealer** *($19.50)*. Of the shades available, only Light Beige looks like skin color. **Concealer** *($18)* is a creamy, lipstick-style concealer with only two shades, and neither is recommended.

☺ $$$ **POWDER: Poudre Diorlight Loose Powder** *($42.50)* is a standard, talc-based powder with a silky texture and dry finish. This is recommended for oily skins, but the sheen these three colors leave behind will not be of any help toward taking down excess shine. **Diorlight Pressed Powder** *($35)* is a talc-free powder with a drier texture than the loose powder, though the aluminum starch in here may prove to be irritating for some skin types. **Poudre Plus Fine Loose Powder** *($42.50)* has a wonderfully soft, sheer texture and is talc-based, with a soft matte finish. The three colors available are all reliable skin tones. **Poudre Plus Fine Pressed Powder** *($35)* is a talc-free powder that has a more slippery or emollient feel, which could be an option for drier skin types. All of the available colors are fine.

☹ **Terra Bella Sun Powder** *($31)* has a dry, grainy texture and three overly orange, shiny colors.

☺ $$$ <u>BLUSH:</u> You will not be disappointed with the texture and application of Dior's **Blush Final** *($32)*. In a word, it is superlative, and the available colors are mostly excellent though there are some shiny shades to watch out for. Although the **Effets Blush** *($35)* is an interesting option for blush, it is not one to get too excited about. Of the three colors in each set, one is shiny (for highlighting), one is a brown tone (for contouring), and one is a typical shade of blush. They still have a great texture, and the options for defining are interesting, but this isn't something you would want to bother with every day.

<u>EYESHADOW:</u> ☹ $$$ **5-Color Eyeshadow Compact** *($49.50)* comes with five colors in one elegant compact, and as generous as that appears, it is not only unnecessary, but also the particular combinations Dior has opted for are either difficult to use together, too shiny, or too close a match to merit an additional color. The texture of these is like powdered sugar, and while they do blend on smoothly there isn't much reason for the expense. **Single Eyeshadow** *($20)* is a much more current way to choose eyeshadow colors, and the texture of these is identical to the 5-Color compact above. However, the shine is even more apparent on almost all the colors, making them hard to recommend for a daily makeup application.

☹ **Creme Eyeshadow** *($20)* comes in a tube with a wand applicator and all of the colors are iridescent to the extreme. I am starting to wonder if the word "matte" is just not in Dior's vocabulary for eyeshadow!

<u>EYE AND BROW PRODUCTS:</u> ☹ $$$ **Khol Pencil** *($19.50)* is just a standard pencil that is longer than most and has a slight cream-to-powder texture. Don't count on this for long wear—it can smear with minimal effort. **Crayon Eyeliner** *($19.50)* is also a standard pencil, but this version is quite creamy, making smearing almost a certainty.

☺ $$$ **Diorliner** *($30)* is a liquid liner that has a decent brush that makes an even application easy. The bottom of the pen houses the liquid and you have to click the base to feed the brush. If Dior sold refills, this would be an option; since they don't this is absurdly overpriced for what you get. **Brow Gel** *($16)* is standard, hairspray-like brow fixative. The brush is excellent, with both long and very short bristles, so every hair will be tamed.

☹ **Eyebrow Pencil** *($19.50)* has such a dry, hard texture it actually hurts to apply it. **AquaDior Crayon Eyeliner Waterproof** *($19.50)* is a standard pencil that has a heavy, waxy texture that never sets, so it stays sticky and what's worse, it literally dissolves (right before your eyes) with water! This is a mess and is not recommended.

☺ $$$ <u>LIPSTICK AND LIP PENCIL:</u> There are enough colors here to keep a lipstick enthusiast busy for hours, starting with **Diorific** *($22),* which has a creamy, opaque texture and slightly greasy finish. For this amount of money, these should have enough stain to last through a morning coffee break, but I doubt they'd make it past the morning commute. **Rouge Diorever** *($21)* is supposed to have a "velvety, matte finish" and nothing could be further from the truth. In spite of the matte lips of the model on this unit's display, this is actually quite creamy and slick, with a glossy finish. One plus is the lasting stain these have, similar to Dior's **Hydrating Satin Lipstick** *($19.50)*, a very creamy, rich lipstick with full coverage and a glossy finish. **Rouge Transparent** *($19.50)* is a sheer, extra-glossy lipstick, while **Rouge Brilliant** *($19.50)* is about as standard a tube lip gloss as it gets. **Plastic Shine** *($19.50)* features an opaque, deeply pigmented gloss in a supremely luxurious package. The texture is slightly sticky and most of the colors are iridescent, but for intensity and evening glam, this is an option. The **Lip Liner Pencil** *($19.50)* is a fairly standard, creamy-finish lip liner that comes in a nice array of colors and has a lipstick brush at one end. It's exceptionally overpriced for what you get.

☺ $$$ <u>MASCARA</u>: Here is where Dior excels; its reputation for producing superior mascaras is well deserved, and many of them have great options for brunettes (who may not prefer black mascara) and redheads. **Diorcil** *($19)* makes much ado about the cashmere it contains, but there is no cashmere in here that has an effect on your lashes. What this does is lengthen and thicken the lashes without clumping, and it stays that way all day! **Fascination** *($19)* is also excellent. It builds thick, long lashes with minimal effort and holds up well throughout the day. I suppose that's where the "fascination" part comes into play! **Diorific** *($22)* can't hold a Dior-scented candle to the other mascaras, but nevertheless is a good mascara that doesn't clump or smear and the packaging on this is nothing short of pure indulgence.

☹ **Parfait** *($18)* is very creamy and can build full, thick lashes, but tends to smear by the end of the day. **AquaDior Waterproof Mascara** *($19)* is a less-than-stellar addition to Dior's usually top-notch mascaras. This one is indeed waterproof but takes some effort to get any length and tends to stick the lashes together in the process. It almost goes without saying that there are much better waterproof mascaras than this one.

☺ $$$ **Highlights for Hair** *($19.50)* is Dior's major claim to fame in the cosmetics industry and although the clamor for this type of product has subsided, these are still available from the line that started the craze for hair mascara. This is for your hair (it is not safe for use on the eyes, but for hair only), and allows you to paint in highlights, lowlights, or vivid streaks that apply (and wash out) easily. I rarely recommend splurging on cosmetic nonessentials, but if you're in the mood these are just too much fun to pass up.

☺ $$$ <u>BRUSHES</u>: There are indeed brushes here, but they pale in comparison to the excellent options at most every other counter from Lancome to Elizabeth Arden to Lauder.

# Circle of Beauty

Probably the first thing you think of when you hear the name Sears is washing machines, power tools, lawnmowers, or even vacuum cleaners. Call me a snob, but I wouldn't exactly encourage anyone to go there for haute couture cosmetics inspiration. Sears' own line of skin care and makeup, Circle of Beauty (as well as T.I.M.E. and Studio Makeup reviewed elsewhere in this edition) doesn't change that notion. Circle of Beauty is a huge line, with more than 600 items, retailed in a very inviting, very user-friendly display. Appropriately, the counters form a complete circle with the products on the outside. You can play to your heart's content, with easy access to every single product, but you'll never get to all of them.

By far, this line's strong point is that there are several types of foundations that each have a sizable group of shades appropriate for both light and dark skin tones. The rest of the line is composed of all the other requisite cosmetic products; some are exceptional (the lipsticks) while others are merely OK (the blush colors are fine, but not intense enough for anyone beyond a medium skin tone). The mascaras and brushes barely make it across the finish line, and even at Sears' lower price point, these are no substitute for dozens of other far superior options.

The real disappointment is that the line falls abysmally on its face with Skinplicity, Circle of Beauty's skin-care line. There are five "circles" of products for five different skin types: oily, combination/oily, combination/dry, dry, and dehydrated. Yet there isn't much difference between related products in the different groupings. Actually, the number of products for this line is astounding and one of the more crowded in the industry.

One particularly striking aspect of the skin-care line is that almost every product contains three anti-irritants known for their skin-soothing properties: bisabolol, kola nut extract, and green tea extract. Circle of Beauty refers to this as its exclusive "Trisoothal Irritation Shield." These anti-irritants are often rather high on the ingredient list. Unfortunately, many of the products also contain a batch of so-called essential oils that can be skin irritants. Ylang-ylang oil, lemon oil, lavender oil, geranium oil, and bergamot oil are all well-known skin sensitizers. These ingredients are really more of a nuisance than a help, although the consumer usually thinks that the naturalness of these oils means they are good for the skin.

Depending on what you are looking for, there are definite finds at Sears' Circle of Beauty. For more information about Circle of Beauty, call your local Sears store; Sears' Web site does not feature information on Circle of Beauty products.

# Circle of Beauty Skin Care

⊗ **Come Clean Cleanser Oily Type 1** *($8.50 for 6 ounces)* is a standard, detergent-based water-soluble cleanser that uses TEA-lauryl sulfate, which is fairly drying and can be too irritating for most skin types, as the cleansing agent. Several anti-irritants in the product will help the irritation, but not the dryness. This contains several fragrant plant oils that can be irritants.

☹ **Come Clean Cleanser Combination Oily Type 2** *($8.50 for 6 ounces)* is almost identical to the Type 1 cleanser, and the same review applies. However, this one contains sodium hydroxide, which can be more drying and irritating for the skin, and it's high on the ingredient list.

☹ **Come Clean Cleanser Combination Dry Type 3** *($8.50 for 6 ounces)* is almost identical to the Type 1 cleanser, and the same review applies.

☺ **Come Clean Cleanser Dry Type 4** *($8.50 for 6 ounces)* is more a wipe-off cleanser than a water-soluble one. It could be good for someone with dry skin, despite the presence of anti-irritants. It contains several fragrant plant oils that can be irritants.

☺ **Come Clean Cleanser Dehydrated Type 5** *($8.50 for 6 ounces)* is similar to the Type 4 cleanser above only this one includes mineral oil, and the same review applies. Despite the presence of anti-irritants, this also contains several fragrant plant oils that can be irritants.

☺ **Day Life Gentle Action Cleanse + Tone Foam, Combination Oily** *($9.50 for 7 ounces)* is a standard, detergent-based water-soluble cleanser that would work well for normal to oily skin. It does contain a tiny amount of BHA, but the pH of this product isn't low enough to make it effective for exfoliation and the active ingredient would be washed away before it would have an effect even if this was well-formulated. Despite the presence of anti-irritants, this contains several fragrant plant oils that can be irritants.

☺ **Day Life Gentle Action Cleanse + Tone Foam, Oily** *($9.50 for 7 ounces)* is almost identical to the Combination Oily version above and the same comments apply.

☺ **Day Life Gentle Action Cleanse + Tone Foam, Dry** *($9.50 for 7 ounces)* is similar to the Combination Oily version above only this one includes plant oil, which does make it slightly better for dry skin.

☺ **Day Life Gentle Action Cleanse + Tone Foam, Combination Dry** *($9.50 for 7 ounces)* is almost identical to the Dry version above and the same comments apply.

☺ **Day Life Gentle Action Cleanse + Tone Foam, Dehydrated** *($9.50 for 7 ounces)* is almost identical to the Dry version above and the same comments apply.

☺ **Easy Go Eye Make-up Remover** *($8.50 for 6 ounces)* is a standard, detergent-based makeup remover that would work as well as any, and at least this version doesn't contain the irritating fragrance the other products use.

☹ **Be Smooth Face and Body Exfoliator** *($10 for 4 ounces)* is a standard, detergent-based water-soluble cleanser that uses polyethylene (ground-up plastic) as the abrasive agent. It also uses TEA-lauryl sulfate, which is fairly drying and can be too irritating for most skin types, as the cleansing agent.

☹ **Skin Refiner Oily Type 1** *($8.50 for 8 ounces)* is an alcohol-based toner that is too irritating and drying for all skin types.

☹ **Skin Refiner Combination Oily Type 2** *($8.50 for 8 ounces)* is almost identical to the Type 1 refiner, and the same review applies.

☹ **Skin Refiner Combination Dry Type 3** *($8.50 for 8 ounces)* is very similar to the Type 1 refiner, and the same review applies.

☺ **Skin Refiner Dry Type 4** *($8.50 for 8 ounces)*. Some of the plant oils can be skin sensitizers and irritating for the skin, but this can still be a good toner for someone with normal to dry skin.

☺ **Skin Refiner Dehydrated Type 5** *($8.50 for 8 ounces)* is similar to the Type 4 refiner, and the same review applies.

☹ **All Even AHA Skin Serum Type 1, 2, 3, 4, 5** *($15 for 1 ounce)* are serums that do contain lactic acid, but the pH here isn't low enough to permit any of them to work as an exfoliant.

☹ **Action + Moisture Cream Oily Type 1, 2, 3, 4, 5, SPF 8** *($16 for 4 ounces);* and **Action + Moisture Lotion Oily Type 1, 2, 3, 4, 5, SPF 8** *($16 for 4 ounces)*. All of these are a disappointment with a low SPF 8 (SPF 15 is the standard) and none of them contain UVA-protecting ingredients of avobenzone, zinc oxide, or titanium dioxide, and are not recommended.

☺ **Be Firm Face Serum** *($16.50 for 1 ounce)* is a good lightweight moisturizer for someone with normal to slightly dry skin, although it won't firm anything on your face.

☺ $$$ **Be Firm Eye Serum** *($16.50 for 0.5 ounce)*. At least this one leaves out the fragrant oils so rampant in all the Circle of Beauty products, an omission the rest of the line should copy. This is a good emollient moisturizer for someone with normal to dry skin. The film former can make skin look temporarily smoother, but temporary is the operative word here.

☹ **Lighten It Eye Cream** *($8.50 for 0.6 ounce)* is just a mineral oil–based moisturizer with titanium dioxide that leaves a slight white layer behind on the skin. It does contain a tiny amount of vitamin C but that won't lighten skin. It also contains clay, which can be drying and is not best for the eye area.

☹ $$$ **Circles Off Dark Circle Treatment** *($16.50 for 0.5 ounce)* is similar to the Lighten It Eye Cream above, only with some plant extracts that have minimal to no effect on inhibiting melanin production, plus the *Terminalia sericea* in here can be a skin irritant. This product contains mica, which gives this white-looking cream shine, but that doesn't change dark circles.

☺ **Night Life Oxygen-Retinol Repair Cream, Oily** *($15 for 2 ounces)* definitely contains retinol, and the magnesium aluminum silicate is an absorbent that will leave a matte feel on the skin. The other ingredients add up to a good moisturizer with water-binding agents and vitamins. The fragrant oils are a problem but overall for a retinol product it's as good as any, as none of them will repair skin.

☺ **Night Life Oxygen-Retinol Repair Cream, Dry** *($15 for 2 ounces)* is similar to the Oily skin version above in terms of retinol, and the same comments apply. This one is more emollient, with mineral oil and thickening agents, which is better for dry skin. There are fragrant oils in here and it would be a far better product without them.

☺ **Night Life Oxygen-Retinol Repair Cream, Combination Dry** *($15 for 2 ounces)* is similar to the Oily skin version above in terms of retinol, and the same comments apply. Several thickening agents in this version make it a problem for combination skin but it would be an option for dry skin. There are also some fragrant oils and this would be a far better product without them.

☺ **Night Life Oxygen-Retinol Repair Cream, Dehydrated** *($15 for 2 ounces)* is similar to the Oily skin version above in terms of retinol, and the same comments apply. Otherwise, this one is almost identical to the Dry skin version above and the same comments apply.

☺ **Night Life Oxygen-Retinol Repair Cream, Combination Oily** *($15 for 2 ounces)* is similar to the Oily skin version above, and the same comments apply.

☺ **$$$ Overnight Eye Treatment** *($15 for 0.6 ounce)* contains mostly water, thickener, mineral oil, more thickeners, anti-irritants, more thickeners, and preservatives. This isn't much of a treatment, but it is emollient, and the anti-irritants could be good for the eye area.

☹ **Day Life SPF 15 Sunscreen, Oily** *($15 for 2 ounces)* doesn't contain the UVA-protecting ingredients of titanium dioxide, zinc oxide, or avobenzone, and is not recommended.

☹ **Day Life SPF 15 Sunscreen, Dry** *($15 for 2 ounces)* doesn't contain the UVA-protecting ingredients of titanium dioxide, zinc oxide, or avobenzone, and is not recommended.

☹ **Day Life SPF 15 Sunscreen, Oily, Combination Dry** *($15 for 2 ounces)* doesn't contain the UVA-protecting ingredients of titanium dioxide, zinc oxide, or avobenzone, and is not recommended.

☹ **Day Life SPF 15 Sunscreen, Dehydrated** *($15 for 2 ounces)* doesn't contain the UVA-protecting ingredients of titanium dioxide, zinc oxide, or avobenzone, and is not recommended.

☹ **Day Life SPF 15 Sunscreen, Combination Oily** *($15 for 2 ounces)* doesn't contain the UVA-protecting ingredients of titanium dioxide, zinc oxide, or avobenzone, and is not recommended.

☺ **Self Tanner Body Moisturizer** *($12.50 for 4 ounces)* is a standard, dihydroxy-acetone-based self tanner, and it would work as well as any. The fragrant oils in here can be a problem for sensitive skin.

☹ **Moisture Wrap Peel Off Mask** *($8.50 for 5.5 ounces)*. Alcohol and plastic won't moisturize anyone's skin, and the anti-irritants can't stop the irritation caused by the alcohol.

☹ **Over and Out Blemish Cream** *($8.50 for 0.5 ounce)* contains zinc oxide and cornstarch high up on the ingredient list and both of those can clog pores, so this is not great for a blemish product.

☺ **Pore Purge Clay Mask** *($10.50 for 8 ounces)* is a standard clay mask with the same anti-irritants and fragrant plant oils as the rest of the Circle of Beauty Skinplicity products. It would be good for someone with normal to oily skin, but it can't empty pores any better than any other clay mask, which is to say it won't do much.

☹ **Smooth Off Lip Buffer** *($8.50 for 0.12 ounce)* is too abrasive (with its ground walnut shells) for the lips, and the peppermint extract will cause irritation and dryness.

## *Circle of Beauty Makeup*

FOUNDATION: ☺ **Skin Image Soft Matte Makeup SPF 8** *($11.50)*. The SPF is too low (SPF 15 is the standard for true sun protection) and it doesn't offer any UVA protection, so don't count on it for your sunscreen in any way, shape, or form. What it does offer is a fairly thick texture that blends on more easily than expected and dries to a soft, matte, powdery finish. This is a very good option for normal to slightly oily skins opting for medium coverage. The color range is extensive, with some definite choices for all skin tones. The colors to avoid are: Porcelain (can turn pink), Deep Rosewood (too rose), Rich Walnut and Deep Amber (both too peach), and Rich Mahogany (too copper).

☺ **Skin Image Dewy Moist Makeup SPF 8** *($11.50)* also does not offer any UVA protection but is a good, creamy-smooth foundation with medium coverage and a soft, slightly powdery finish. This would be suitable for normal to dry skin, and there are some really nice options for both light and dark skin tones. These colors are best left alone: Deep Amber and Rich Sandalwood (both too peach), Fair Ivory (slight pink), Rich Bronze and Rich Mahogany (too orange).

☹ **Skin Image Wet or Dry Makeup** *($12.50)* is a standard pressed powder foundation that has a smooth, somewhat silky feel, but it is also rather powdery and can easily cake on skin and, for the most part, the colors are too peach for most skin tones. The only two shades to consider are Deep Tan or Deep Fig.

☺ **Skin Image Cream to Powder Makeup** *($12.50)* comes in eight shades aimed at darker skin tones. It has a creamy, thick application though the finish is a slightly sticky matte. Only three of the shades look like real skin color: Rich Toast, Rich Sable, and Rich Nougat.

☺ **On and On Flawless Cover Makeup** *($11.50)* is Sears' contribution to the ultra-matte foundation category. It proves to be a fairly reliable foundation in terms of long wear, but the texture is quite slippery, and although the finish is softly matte there is just too much silicone in here, which means minimal shine control. This is worth a look if you have normal to slightly oily skin and prefer medium coverage, and the color range is on par with the other foundations. These shades are too pink, peach or orange to recommend: Fair Dawn, Rich Cedar, and Deep Olive.

☺ **Advanced Formula Anti-Aging Makeup SPF 15** *($13.50)* is another disappointing option for sun protection, as this also offers no UVA-blocking ingredients. What this does make a big deal about is the vitamin C in here supposedly being able to "lift and restore firmness to skin" and "diminish lines and wrinkles." There is no substantial research to support any of those claims, so you can safely ignore them and focus on the fact that this is a creamy, slick foundation that would be appropriate for dry to very dry skin seeking medium to full coverage. The finish is a bit slippery, so use even more caution when blending this out. Many of the colors are worth considering; the only ones to avoid are Caramel, Pecan, Honey, and Beige.

☹ **HydroVitamin Minimum Makeup SPF 15** *($13.50)* hardly has even a dusting of vitamins, lacks any UVA-protecting ingredients, and comes in six shades that, in spite of their sheerness, have a peachy to yellow cast that just won't work for most skin tones. Sheer Ivory is a possibility, but with no significant UVA protection, why bother?

☹ **Skin Image Primer** *($10)*. Mint green is the only shade available. It is meant to correct a ruddy complexion but all it does is leave a strange green cast on the skin.

☹ **Skin Image Highlighter** *($10)* is a creamy, sparkly, pink-frosty spread of sheer color. It does highlight, but over makeup it can smear the foundation or powder and under makeup it is too sheer to have an effect.

CONCEALER: ☹ **Out of Sight Sponge-On Concealer** *($7)* has a creamy texture and a greasy finish that can crease into lines. The two shades for darker skin tones, Rich Coffee and Rich Mahogany, are too copper or rose to recommend.

☺ **No Flaw Concealer** *($7)* is superior to the one above in terms of texture and finish and the colors are quite good. Of the seven shades available only Sun Tan and Medium Honey are too peach for most skin tones.

☹ POWDER: Both the **Natural Finish Loose Powder** *($12)* and **Natural Finish Pressed Powder** *($9)* have a somewhat dry texture and finish, which would make them an option for oilier skin types, but the colors all have a slight shine and that negates the effectiveness of reducing shine on the face. Most of the colors here are too peach or pink to recommend.

BLUSH: ☺ **Blush Lightly** *($10)* has a smooth, slightly dry texture and finish. The colors are beautiful—many are excellent sheer, matte options. However, the sheerness makes them a problem for darker skin tones; these just aren't pigmented enough to really show on dark skin. These shades are unacceptably shiny: Lightly Peony, Copper, and Nude.

☺ **Sun Pretender Powder** *($10)* is a small group of shiny bronzing powders that will also work as blush or contour, if you can tolerate the shine. I was told these would be discontinued soon, and I think that's a wise decision.

☺ **EYESHADOW**: **Soft Sweep Eyeshadow Duos** *($10.50)* mostly have a soft, silky texture but they end up looking rather chalky on the skin. All of the duos have at least one shiny shade. **Soft Sweep Eyeshadow Quads** *($15)* have the same texture and finish as the Duos, only here you get some truly strange color combinations that are best avoided. There are a couple of neutral options, but consider these only if you will use all of the colors.

☹ **EYE AND BROW SHAPER**: **Eye Defining Pencil** *($7)* is an automatic pencil (that's good) that glides on but smudges easily (that's bad). **Stroke Up Brow Pencil** *($7)* is a twist-up pencil that has a slightly dry finish and waxy texture that makes for a choppy application. **Color Up Brow Cake** *($8)* is a dry, grainy brow powder with some sheer colors that all have a slight shine—not a great option for creating a natural-looking eyebrow.

LIPSTICK AND LIP PENCIL:  Circle of Beauty's lipstick lineup is most impressive. Here you'll find a rainbow of colors and textures that will appeal to a wide range of preferences and tastes. ☺ **Hydro-Vitamin Lipstick** *($8.50)* sounds like a nutritional oasis for your skin but in reality it is just a standard creamy lipstick with a greasy finish. **Rich Lasting Cream Lipstick** *($8.50)* is a very creamy, full-coverage lipstick with a glossy finish. This does have a nice stain for slightly longer wear, and the color range is impressive. Speaking of impressive, **Satin Matte Lipstick** *($8.50)* is quite a find! This one has a smooth, creamy texture, is opaque, and offers a lovely satin finish. The available colors are remarkable, with options for all skin tones. **Lip Defining Pencil** *($8)* is an automatic pencil with a creamy texture and enough stain to hold up well on the lips.

☺ **On and On Lasting Comfort Lipstick** *($8.50)* is Sears' ultra-matte lipstick. It applies slick and slightly greasy but dries to a powdery matte finish. **Sheer Treat Lipstick SPF 15** *($8.50)* offers no UVA protection and is just a very greasy lipstick with barely-there color. **Crystal Cream** *($6)* has a thick, sticky feel and a strong, unpleasant waxy odor.

MASCARA: ☹ **Long and Silky Mascara** *($8)* is inferior to many other mascaras in this price range. Expect to brush this through over and over again, which is the only way that you may begin to see some length. **Velvety Lashes Mascara** *($8)* isn't much better than the one above, and the thickening claim doesn't translate to your lashes. **Curl and Shine Mascara** *($8.50)* has an incredibly thick brush whose bristles are so bushy they tend to grab and stick lashes together, if you can get to your lashes at all, plus it builds no length and flakes. What a mess.

☺ **Waterplay Lashes** *($8)* does stay on underwater and lengthens well but beware of the potential for this to clump.

☺ BRUSHES: If you're on a budget, you may want to consider a few of these brushes *($6.50–$13.50)*. These will do nicely and are inexpensive: **Face Brush** *($13.50)* and the **Shadow Brush** *($6.50)*. The **Blush Brush** *($9.50)* is small and flimsy and the **Retractable Lip Brush** *($12.50)* will work well for those who like taking half an hour to cover their lips with color.

## Clairol Herbal Essences (Skin Care Only)

Clairol is in the skin-care game with the launch of its skin-care line called Herbal Essences Skin Care. I guess its hair-care line of the same name must be doing well, so why not try to garner the same attention with skin care? From what I can tell, this isn't much of an addition; clearly Clairol does hair far better than it does skin care. For more information on Herbal Essences products, call (800) 223-5800 or visit the Web site: www.clairol.com.

☺ **Foaming Face Wash Clarifying for Combination/Oily Skin** *($4.99 for 6.8 ounces)* is a standard, detergent-based water-soluble cleanser that could be quite drying for most skin types, including oily skin (oily skin doesn't need to be dried, it needs to have oil removed without drying out the skin). My one other concern is an ingredient called *Mentha aquatica* extract, which is a form of mint and can be a skin irritant.

☺ **Foaming Face Wash Moisture-Balancing for Normal/Dry Skin** *($4.99 for 6.8 ounces)* is similar to the one above, minus the mint, only this one includes tea tree oil, which isn't appropriate for dry skin. Though that can have some disinfecting properties, it is rather useless in a rinse-off product. There is nothing moisture-balancing about this cleanser; if anything, it could be quite drying.

☹ **Alcohol-Free Toner Moisture-Balancing for Normal/Dry Skin** *($4.99 for 8.5 ounces)* would be a good, though standard, toner for most skin types if it wasn't for the lemon extract in here. The lemon is just unnecessary, not to mention a serious skin irritant.

☹ **Oil-Controlling Astringent Clarifying for Combination/Oily Skin** *($4.99 for 8.5 ounces)* contains mostly alcohol and is absolutely not recommended.

☺ **Moisture Renewal Lotion Moisture-Balancing for Normal/Dry Skin** *($6.99 for 4.23 ounces)* is a rather good moisturizer for dry skin if you can get past the intense fragrance.

☹ **Oil-Free Moisturizer Clarifying for Combination/Oily Skin** *($6.99 for 4.23 ounces)* isn't bad, just not the best. The amount of wax in here can be problematic if used over oily areas of skin.

# *Clarins*

Clarins is a distinctively French line whose beginnings go back to the early 1950s. It was then that Clarins' founder, Jacques Courtin-Clarins, began formulating plant-based treatments for his clients. He parlayed this into a Beauty Institute, and from there, with an all-natural mantra that was slightly ahead of its time, the business grew. Fast-forward to today and you will notice upon visiting the Clarins counter that the plant-based, natural-extract rhetoric is still intact and so thick you may want to bring along a machete to cut through it. Never wavering from its original marketing angle, Clarins has steadfastly held on to the belief that whatever grows from the ground and smells nice must be the cure for every skin ailment from breakouts to the dreaded "sponginess" of cellulite.

Clarins has something for every concern imaginable—from keeping pollution off the face (not possible) to lifting a sagging jawline (not possible without surgery), it would seem there is nothing these supposedly miraculous products can't do. And you'll find a horde of plants here with the promise that this can all come true. However, once you're armed with even a modicum of ingredient knowledge and a fair helping of myth-busting, you'll realize how ridiculously out of whack all of this hype is. That's not to imply that some of these products are bad—there are good ones— and that some of the plant extracts aren't good—because many are very good anti-irritants, emollients, or antibacterials. But there are also many that are potential allergens or skin irritants. Clarins also has its fair share of ordinary, standard, and completely unnecessary products whose claims are at best misleading and at worst downright false, and the products are incredibly overpriced for what you get. What is most startling is the redundancy of these products. There are few differences between the moisturizers and the mask cleansers, and the oil-control products are more re-runs than new alternatives for skin care.

Clarins makeup has not changed much since the last edition of this book. Its counters are still well organized and the classic white with red trim packaging is still attractive. There have been some new color launches, chronicled in my newsletter, but otherwise familiarity reigns. This has its pros and cons. On the pro side, Clarins continues to offer a beautiful selection of lipsticks and blush colors, all nicely grouped by undertone on the tester unit, as well as very good mascara. As for the cons, its foundation shades have stayed the same—mostly a selection of peaches and pinks that must be selling to someone (or why keep them around?), and many of the eyeshadows and other complexion products have jumped headfirst onto the shine bandwagon, with no brakes in sight. You will find some good choices here, but as Clarins continues to tout the wonders of plants and the latest trends, you must be cautious; otherwise you could get so entranced that your pocketbook goes on safari and returns empty!

For more information on Clarins, call (212) 980-1800 or visit the Web site at www.clarins-paris.com.

## Clarins Skin Care

☹ **Cleansing Milk with Alpine Herbs Dry or Normal Skin** (*$25 for 8.6 ounces*) contains mint, arnica, and pine, which can cause skin irritation, and that make this a poor product for any skin type.

☹ **Cleansing Milk with Gentian Oily/Combination Skin** (*$25 for 8.6 ounces*) contains several ingredients that are extremely emollient and problematic for oily skin. What were they thinking when they formulated this one?

☺ **$$$ Extra-Comfort Cleansing Cream with Bio-Ecolia Very Dry or Sensitized Skin** (*$30 for 7 ounces*). This rather ordinary cleanser needs to be wiped off and can leave a greasy film on the skin. The fragrance in here negates this as being an option for someone with sensitive skin.

☹ **Gentle Foaming Cleanser** (*$19 for 4.4 ounces*) is a very drying, water-soluble cleanser for any skin type. It contains strong detergent cleansing agents and potassium hydroxide rather high up on the ingredient list.

☺ **$$$ Gentle Foaming Cleanser for Dry/Sensitive Skin** (*$20 for 4.4 ounces*) is a standard, detergent-based water-soluble cleanser that can be drying for some skin types. It does contain some emollients that counteract the drying effect of the cleansing agents, but it also contains sodium lauryl sulfate, which can be a skin irritant.

☺ **$$$ Oil-Control Cleansing Gel Oily Skin with Breakout Tendencies** (*$18 for 4.4 ounces*) is a standard, detergent-based water-soluble cleanser that can be drying for some skin types. It won't control oil, but it will clean the skin. It contains fragrance.

☺ **$$$ Purifying Cleansing Lotion** (*$18.50 for 4.4 ounces*) is a standard, detergent-based water-soluble cleanser that contains a few problematic ingredients including witch hazel, zinc sulfate, and wintergreen. I suspect the amount of these is so small that it won't have much if any impact on skin. This won't purify anything but it is a good cleanser for normal to oily skin.

☺ $$$ **Purifying Cleansing Gel** *($18.50 for 4.4 ounces)* is a very standard, detergent-based water-soluble cleanser. The second ingredient is witch hazel, which can be a skin irritant. It also contains salicylic acid, but the pH is too high for it to work as an effective exfoliant.

☹ **Purifying Toning Lotion** *($16.50 for 6.8 ounces)* has witch hazel as the second ingredient, and that can be a skin irritant. It also contains BHA, but with a pH that is too high for it to be an effective exfoliant, and orris root, wintergreen, and zinc sulfate, which can all be skin irritants.

☺ $$$ **Purifying Plant Facial Mask** *($23.50 for 1.7 ounces)* won't purify anything, plus the grapefruit and rice starch in here can be skin irritants.

☺ $$$ **Gentle Eye Make-Up Remover Lotion** *($16.50 for 3.4 ounces)* is gentle enough, but pretty ordinary, and not the most effective for removing makeup.

☺ $$$ **Instant Eye Makeup Remover** *($19 for 4.2 ounces)* is more effective than the Gentle version above. This one contains a more effective cleansing agent. It does contain fragrance.

☺ $$$ **Gentle Exfoliating Refiner for Face** *($21 for 1.7 ounces)*. The abrasive particles in here are fairly gritty, but they dissipate quickly and end up being fairly tame. This would work well for someone with normal to dry skin.

☺ $$$ **Gentle Facial Peeling** *($25 for 1.4 ounces)* will exfoliate the skin, something that happens anytime you rub wax or clay over the skin. That isn't bad, but rubbing can be hard on the skin. There are easier ways to exfoliate.

☺ **Extra-Comfort Toning Lotion Very Dry or Sensitized Skin** *($25 for 8.8 ounces)*. Plenty of ingredients in this product can be problematic for sensitive skin including fragrance, linden extract, and coloring agent.

☺ **Alcohol-Free Toning Lotion for Dry to Normal Skin** *($21 for 8.4 ounces)* is a fairly good, irritant-free toner.

☺ **Alcohol-Free Toning Lotion for Oily/Combination Skin** *($21 for 8.4 ounces)* is indeed an alcohol-free toner. However, several of the plant extracts (orris root and guava) as well as the witch hazel are possible irritants and provide no benefit for oily skin.

☹ **Contouring Facial Lift** *($47 for 1.7 ounces)* lists alcohol as its second ingredient, which is a problem for irritation and dryness.

☺ $$$ **Energizing Morning Cream** *($48.50 for 1.7 ounces)* has one of the longest ingredient listings in the industry. Long ingredient listings are a problem because they substantially raise the likelihood that there is something in here you are going to be allergic to. The other issue is, who needs all this stuff? Much of it is either redundant, potentially irritating plant extracts or the emulsifiers needed to keep these kinds of ingredients combined. The minuscule dusting of vitamins and minerals is hardly worth mentioning. The plant extracts such as orange, kiwi, ginseng, and pineapple are potentially irritating. It also contains sodium lauryl sulfate as an emulsifier, though it can still be a skin irritant. This is about as standard a moisturizer as it gets, with a few more problems than benefits.

☺ $$$ **Extra-Firming Day Cream All Skin Types** *($50 for 1.7 ounces)* lacks a sunscreen, and without that it isn't appropriate for daytime, though it is a good emollient moisturizer for someone with dry skin. There is nothing in here that will firm skin. The emollients and thickeners in here are not appropriate for all skin types. Some of the plant extracts in here are potential irritants while others can be anti-irritants; I guess they sort of cancel each other out, but what a waste.

☺ $$$ **Extra-Firming Day Cream for Dry Skin** *($50 for 1.7 ounces)* is, like the one above, not great for daytime because it lacks sunscreen, but it is a good emollient moisturizer for very dry skin, almost identical to the one above.

☺ $$$ **Extra-Firming Day Lotion SPF 15** *($57.50 for 1.7 ounces)* is a good in-part titanium dioxide–based sunscreen, but the very standard moisturizing base makes the price absurd enough to burn your pocketbook.

☹ $$$ **Extra-Firming Eye Contour Cream** *($43.50 for 0.7 ounce)* is similar to the Day Lotion above only minus the sunscreen. It's a good moisturizer but extremely ordinary and not worth the money for what you get.

☹ $$$ **Extra-Firming Eye Contour Serum** *($43.50 for 0.7 ounce)* is similar to the cream version above and the same basic comments apply.

☺ $$$ **Extra-Firming Night Cream All Skin Types** *($60 for 1.7 ounces)* is a good moisturizer for someone with normal to dry skin, but the claims about being extra-firming stretch what these standard cosmetic ingredients can really do.

☺ $$$ **Extra Firming Concentrate** *($52.50 for 1 ounce)* is a liquidy lotion (serum). Amid this rather nice but lightweight moisturizing lotion for normal to slightly dry or combination skin are extracts of mushroom, *Krameria triandra*, *Kigelia africana*, ginseng, *Sequoia giganteum* (has no known benefit for skin), and yeast. This is supposed to be skin firming? Unbelievable. Krameria (a root) and kigelia (sausage tree) are known for their astringent properties, and while that may be irritating, that isn't the same thing as firming. Yeast and retinyl palmitate are a couple of the other interesting-sounding ingredients. But retinyl palmitate is many generations removed from retinol, and retinol is many generations removed from Retin-A, leaving retinyl palmitate out in the cold for any of the retinol hype. The claims surrounding yeast sound miraculous but the amount in here wouldn't affect skin—or a crumb of bread, for that matter.

☹ $$$ **Firming Neck Cream** *($50 for 1.7 ounces)* is said to be for the neck and not the face, but there is nothing in here that makes this different from the others in the Extra-Firming group, nor is there anything in here that will lift the neck. It is a good moisturizer for slightly dry skin.

☺ $$$ **Face Treatment Plant Cream "Blue Orchid" for Dehydrated Skin** *($29 *for 1.7 ounces)* is a good, standard, mineral oil–based moisturizer for dry skin. The blue orchid fragrance may smell nice but the basic formulation is as ordinary as it comes.

☹ **Face Treatment Plant Cream "Lotus" for Combination Skin Prone to Oiliness** *($29 for 1.7 ounces)* is virtually identical to the cream above (but minus the lanolin) and so is still completely inappropriate for someone with combination or oily skin. Plus, several of the ingredients in here, including lemon and grapefruit, can be irritants.

☺ **$$$ Face Treatment Cream for Dry or Reddened Skin** *($29 for 1.7 ounces)* is a good, emollient moisturizer. Nothing about this product makes it special for reddened skin.

☺ **$$$ Face Treatment Plant Cream "Santal" for Dry or Extra Dry Skin** *($29 for 1.7 ounces)* is almost identical to the version above for Reddened Skin, and the same review applies.

☹ **Face Treatment Oil "Blue Orchid" for Dehydrated Skin** *($33 for 1.4 ounces).* The patchouli oil and fragrance can be irritating to the skin, and while the hazelnut oil is emollient and great for dry skin, you would be far better off to use just plain hazelnut oil and forgo the other irritating ingredients.

☹ **Face Treatment Oil "Santal" for Dry or Reddened Skin** *($33 for 1.4 ounces).* Sandalwood, cardamom, parsley, and lavender oils can all cause skin irritation, which isn't great for someone with reddened skin.

☹ **Face Treatment Oil "Lotus" for Combination Skin/Prone to Oiliness** *($33 for 1.4 ounces).* This product is supposed to help "balance" surface oils. What it does is place more oils on the skin, and the chamomile, rosemary, and sage can be irritants. Someone with oily skin could end up with oilier, more irritated skin.

☹ **Face Treatment Oil "Santal" Dry or Extra Dry Skin** *($33 for 1.4 ounces).* The fragrance can be irritating, and you can get hazelnut oil at the grocery store for far less and with no risk of allergic reaction.

☺ **$$$ Gentle Day Cream for Sensitive Skin** *($39 for 1.7 ounces)* is a good but rather ordinary mineral oil–based moisturizer for dry skin. Because it contains no sunscreen, it isn't best for daytime wear, unless your foundation contains one.

☺ **$$$ Gentle Day Lotion** *($44 for 1.7 ounces)* is a good but extremely ordinary moisturizer for normal to dry skin. Without sunscreen it is inappropriate for daytime.

☺ **$$$ Gentle Night Cream for Sensitive Skin** *($49 for 1.7 ounces)* is almost identical to the Day Cream version above, and the same review applies. Vitamins are present in this cream, but only in negligible quantities. Why this product is more expensive than the other is a marketing caprice, nothing more.

☺ **$$$ Hydration-Plus Moisture Lotion SPF 15 for All Skin Types** *($30 for 1.7 ounces)* is an in-part titanium dioxide–based moisturizer for someone with normal to dry skin. Now this is a daytime sunscreen your skin can live with, although the price isn't warranted for what you get, which is a fairly basic moisturizing sunscreen.

☺ $$$ **Multi-Active Day Cream for All Skin Types** *($45 for 1.7 ounces)* is a good though extremely ordinary moisturizer for normal to dry skin.

☺ $$$ **Multi-Active Night Lotion for All Skin Types** *($50 for 1.7 ounces)* is a good moisturizer for someone with dry skin, but other skin types will find the oil and thickening agents too emollient. It does contain a tiny amount of vitamins, but not enough to help your skin in the least.

☹ **Multi-Active Skin Firming Concentrate** *($47.50 for 1 ounce)*. The second ingredient is condurango extract and has no known benefit for skin. It also contains ginseng and pineapple extracts, which can be irritants. This is more of a useless concoction than anything else.

☺ **Oil-Control Night Lotion** *($28.50 for 1.06 ounces)* is an incredibly ordinary, lightweight moisturizer that would be OK for someone with normal to slightly dry skin. It will not control oil in any way, shape, or form. It contains two plant extracts, *Mimosa tenuiflora* (the second ingredient) and *Crataegus monogina,* which can have antibacterial and anti-inflammatory properties. While that may be helpful for skin, it is irrelevant for oil control.

☹ **Oil Control Moisture Lotion** *($25 for 1.06 ounces)* contains little that will control oil, but some ingredients could be problematic for someone with oily skin. It contains orris root, which can be a skin irritant.

☹ **Ultra Matte Concentrate** *($28.50 for 1.06 ounces)* contains several problematic ingredients, including witch hazel (the second ingredient), wintergreen, orris root, and zinc sulfate, all of which can be skin irritants.

☹ **Hydra-Matte Day Lotion** *($32 for 1.7 ounces)* has several of the same problem with plant extracts as the Ultra Matte above and the same basic review applies.

☺ $$$ **Absorbent Mask Oily Skin with Breakout Tendencies** *($19 for 1.7 ounces)* is a very standard clay mask that contains mostly water, clay, thickeners, plant extracts, and preservatives. It will absorb oil, but there are a few irritating additions (orris root and zinc sulfate) that can be problems for skin.

☹ **Blemish Control** *($15 for 0.5 ounce)* contains mostly alcohol, which makes it too irritating for all skin types. It also contains other irritating plant extracts, and that only compounds the problem.

☹ **Minimizing Blemish Cream** *($15 for 0.53 ounce)* is similar to the Blemish Control above, only this one is in cream form.

☺ **Instant Shine Control Gel** *($18.50 for 1.7 ounces)* can help reduce shine, but not for very long, especially if you have very oily skin. This is one to test drive before you buy.

☺ $$$ **Renew-Plus Night Lotion** *($49.50 for 1.7 ounces)*. While this is a good moisturizer for normal to dry skin, it is supposed to contain BHA; however, the form used here is a salt, not an acid, and therefore it's not effective for exfoliation. It also contains papain, an enzyme that can exfoliate skin, but not in the amount used in this product. Finally, it also contains retinyl palmitate, and the same comments about that in the review above for the Extra Firming Concentrate pertain here.

☺ **$$$ Revitalizing Moisture Cream with Plant Marine "Cell Extract"** *($50 for 1.7 ounces)* contains boring ingredients, in contrast to its long, beguiling name. The amount of plant marine extract is so minuscule as to make the company look silly for putting it in the name of the product; the other plant extracts in here can be anti-irritants. This is a good, but exceedingly overpriced, moisturizer for someone with dry skin.

☺ **$$$ Revitalizing Moisture Base with Plant Marine "Cell Extract" for All Skin Types** *($30 for 1.1 ounces)* is similar to the one above, only in a more lotion-like form.

☹ **Beauty Flash Balm** *($30 for 1.7 ounces)* is an extremely average moisturizer. Witch hazel and rice starch can be problematic for most skin types.

☺ **$$$ Double Serum 38 Total Skin Supplement, Plant Based Concentrate Hydro Serum and Lipo Serum** *($70 for two 0.5-ounce bottles)*. One part of this is a mixture of several plant oils ranging from hazelnut to apricot, sesame, walnut, and avocado. A handful of cosmetic thickening agents and some vitamins are also thrown in, but for the most part this is oil straight out of your kitchen cabinet. The other part is mostly rose water (glycerin and fragrance) along with some algae, pollen, and yeast. Pollen can be an allergen for lots of people, and the other ingredients show little to no evidence that they have any effect on skin. The oils can be great for dry skin, but the price is absurd for what you get. You could get the exact same effect by mixing your own plant oils together (nonfragrant types like the ones I've mentioned, to reduce the risk of irritation), or just use pure sesame oil at night over excessively dry areas of your face or body.

☹ **Skin Beauty Repair Concentrate** *($42 for 0.5 ounce)* includes some plant oils, particularly peppermint and lavender oil, that can cause skin irritation, and that doesn't repair anything.

☺ **$$$ Eye Contour Balm** *($30 for 0.7 ounce)* would be an OK but very ordinary moisturizer for dry skin.

☺ **$$$ Eye Contour Gel** *($30 for 0.7 ounce)* is an extremely do-nothing moisturizer for minimally dry skin.

☹ **Normalizing Night Gel** *($28.50 for 1.06 ounces)* contains several problematic ingredients, including witch hazel (the second ingredient), wintergreen, orris root, and zinc sulfate, all of which can be skin irritants.

☺ **$$$ Gentle Soothing Mask** *($30 for 1.7 ounces)* is a good mask for dry skin.

☺ **$$$ Extra Firming Facial Mask** *($40 for 2.7 ounces)* is a good but very standard moisturizing mask for normal to dry skin. Some of the plant extracts in here have astringent properties that are not helpful for dry skin but the amount of these is probably too minuscule to have an effect.

☺ $$$ **Normalizing Facial Mask** *($21 for 1.7 ounces)* is a very standard, but good clay mask for normal to oily skin. It does contain witch hazel and that can be a skin irritant.

☺ $$$ **Revitalizing Moisture Mask with Plant Marine "Cell Extract" for All Skin Types** *($28 for 1.7 ounces)* is a good, though exceptionally ordinary mask with the tiniest amount of algae extract imaginable.

☺ $$$ **Skin-Smoothing Eye Mask with Plant Extracts** *($35 for 1.05 ounces)* is an OK emollient moisturizer for dry skin, nothing less, nothing more. The third ingredient is rice starch, which can be a skin sensitizer for some skin types.

☺ $$$ **Self Tanning Face Cream, SPF 15** *($22 for 2.7 ounces)*, as all self tanners do, uses a form of dihydroxyacetone to turn the skin brown, and this is also a good in-part titanium dioxide–based sunscreen. The emollient base also makes it good a moisturizer for normal to dry skin. However, I do not recommend using self tanners with sunscreen. Instead, it is best to apply self tanner in the evening when you have time to apply it evenly all over and then let it absorb so you don't put clothing over it and risk stains.

☺ $$$ **Self Tanning Gel without Sunscreen** *($21 for 4.4 ounces)*, as all self tanners do, uses a form of dihydroxyacetone to turn the skin brown.

☹ **Sunblock Stick SPF 30** *($18.50 for 0.17 ounce)* doesn't contain the UVA-protecting ingredients of titanium dioxide, zinc oxide, or avobenzone, and is absolutely not recommended.

☹ **Sun Wrinkle Control Cream SPF 15** *($19.50 for 2.7 ounces)* doesn't contain the UVA-protecting ingredients of titanium dioxide, zinc oxide, or avobenzone, and is absolutely not recommended.

☺ **After Sun Gel Ultra Soothing** *($20 for 5.3 ounces)* is a good, ordinary, extremely lightweight gel moisturizer for normal to slightly dry skin. If you're looking for a good after-sun gel, pure aloe from a health food store would be far better than this version.

☺ **After Sun Moisture Supplement** *($23 for 1.4 ounces)* is a good moisturizer. This moisturizer contains talc high up on the ingredient listing, which makes it anything but a moisture supplement. It may be an option for slightly dry skin.

☺ **After Sun Moisturizer** *($20 for 5.3 ounces)* is a good, standard, emollient moisturizer.

☺ **After Sun Moisturizer with Self Tanning Action** *($20 for 5.3 ounces)*, like all self tanners, uses the ingredient dihydroxyacetone to turn the skin brown. This one works as well as any.

☺ $$$ **Lip Beauty Multi-Treatment** *($16.50 for 0.09 ounce)* is a standard emollient lip gloss. It is good for dry lips, but to spend this kind of money on what is basically an ordinary gloss is almost embarrassing.

# Clarins Makeup

**FOUNDATION:** ☹ **Ultra-Satin Finish Foundation** *($31)* comes in a squeeze tube, which is not the best form of packaging for foundation as it is hard to control how much comes out. This is a moisturizing foundation best for someone with normal to dry skin who prefers sheer to light coverage. This blends quite well with a moist finish, but most of the colors are unrelated to skin tones. All of these shades are either too pink or peach to recommend.

☺ $$$ **Matte Finish Foundation** *($31)* has a rather light, creamy consistency that offers light to medium coverage and a soft matte finish. There are some good color choices and this would work well for normal to slightly dry skin. Of the ten shades available, only Beige Sable, Soft Beige, Golden Honey, and Natural Beige are too peach or pink for most skin tones.

☺ $$$ **Smartstick** *($31)* is Clarins's contribution to foundations in stick form. Its version is definitely an option, with a slightly creamy finish that stays somewhat creamy on the skin and ten good colors that blend out nicely for sheer all the way to medium coverage. For a really smart choice, though, take a look at Clinique's CityStick Foundation SPF 15 ($20)—which has a great sunscreen and costs less. With or without sun protection, this type of foundation is recommended for normal to dry skin, as the ingredients that keep the product in stick form can contribute to breakouts and a creamy feel on the face.

☺ $$$ **Oil-Free Ultra Matte Foundation** *($31)* is excellent for normal to oily skin types. It has a light, silky formula that dries down to a true matte finish with medium to full coverage. Sadly, of the eight shades there are only two good ones to consider; those are 02 and 08. The rest of the bunch follows suit with many of the Clarins foundations, being either too peach or pink. If the color problem could be remedied, this would be a very good option for truly oily skins.

☺ $$$ **Ultra Smooth Compact Foundation SPF 15** *($31)* is a powder foundation that goes on quite soft and sheer, with a nice slip and some OK colors. If you prefer this type of foundation, take a look at Petal Beige, Fair Bisque, Silk Beige, Amber Beige, Mahogany, and Chestnut (the last three being good choices for darker skin tones). Don't count on this for adequate sun protection, as this SPF does not offer any UVA-protecting ingredients.

☺ $$$ **Powder Compact Foundation SPF 15** *($30)* is another powder with an SPF rating (see Maybelline True Illusion Pressed Powder SPF 10, reviewed later in this chapter). This one does have a better SPF number but it doesn't have UVA protection, so that makes Maybelline's a far better choice (UVA protection *is* that important over SPF). As a powder, Clarins has a silky-soft texture with a smooth, even application. Of the ten shades available, only Natural Sand and Soft Beige are too peach for most skin tones. However, the color selection doesn't include colors for those with very light skin or darker skin tones.

☺ $$$ **Extra-Firming Foundation** *($34)* claims it offers "surface firming with Ebony extract and Durvillea Antarctica Algae." It would be nice if this was true, but it isn't possible to firm the skin with these or any other plants. Even if the plant does have some tightening effect in its pure form, that is not what you are getting after the final product is mixed, sterilized, and preserved. Claims aside, this is just a rich, fluid foundation for normal to very dry skin. It offers medium coverage and a lot of slip— in fact, it remains slippery on the skin even when blended. If you can tolerate the heavy fragrance, this may be an option, but avoid 06 and 08 (both too pink), and be wary of 14 (may be slightly orange).

☹ **Moisturizing Tint SPF 6** *($28.50)* is a sheer hint of color in a cream base with a poor SPF rating (SPF 6 is about encouraging sun damage, not preventing it). Add this to the fact that three of the four available colors are too orange or red and it's thumbs down for this one.

☹ **Color Veil** *($28.50)* is meant to even out the skin tone with a sheer "kiss of color." The texture is interesting (airy, moist, and powdery) but the colors are hideous. No one's skin tone is that orange or peach! There is also a Shimmer Veil, so you can be orange *and* shiny. Who is buying this?

☹ **CONCEALER: Perfecting Concealer** *($15)* is a tube concealer with a wand applicator, but it has a very creamy consistency that tends to slide around too much— a sure sign of eventual creasing. Plus, the two colors are way too peach to even consider. $$$ **Concealer Plus Corrector** *($17)* seems like quite a deal as it has two shades to work with. Unfortunately, one half of this liquid concealer is mint green, which will only add a strange cast to the skin wherever it is placed, and the other half is a peach tone with a shiny finish. This is a confused product that is a waste on either end.

☺ $$$ **POWDER: Powder Compact Pressed Powder** *($27)* offers only four colors, all on the peach or pink side, but this is so sheer it is not as big an issue as it first appears. The texture of this is very similar to the Ultra-Smooth Compact Foundation above, but this version is slightly more sheer. **Face Powder** *($32)* comes in a huge tub and has a soft, dry texture, but all of the shades are shiny. This may be an option for evening, but otherwise shine defeats the purpose of powdering, so why bother? **Bronzing Duo** *($27)* includes two shades of powder bronzer in a compact. The application is sheer and matte but the colors are too orange for most skin tones.

☺ $$$ **BLUSH: Powder Blush** *($23)* has an incredibly smooth, velvety texture that is just what a good powder blush should feel like. These are definitely worth a look if the price doesn't bother you. All of the colors blend on quite sheer and build nice intensity if need be. There are some shiny shades, but those are easily identified. **Multi-Blush** *($20)* is a cream-to-powder blush that has only a slightly creamy application and then quickly becomes a powder with a soft matte finish on the skin. It has a little bit of shine but the four colors are subtle and beautiful.

EYESHADOW: ☺ $$$ **Duo Eyeshadow Sets** *($23)* are mostly shiny but there are some matte ones to choose from. These all blend on quite soft and sheer for a soft, subtle look (you won't get drama out of these colors). The combinations are actually quite workable; take a closer look at Biscuit/Sable, Toast/Mocha, Nude/Plum, and Wine/Malt.

☺ **Soft Shimmer Eye Colour Singles** *($15)* are a group of very soft, light pastel, and very shiny eyeshadows. I'm sure there is a reason to consider these, I just can't think of one.

☺ $$$ EYE AND BROW SHAPER: The **Eye Liner Pencil** *($13.50)* is a standard pencil that has a soft texture and comes in a nice array of colors. The consistency can be a bit creamy, so watch out for smearing. One end of the pencil has a sponge tip for softening the line. The **Brow Pencil** *($14)* has a firm texture and comes in a small but good group of colors. One end is a brush, which is a nice touch for softening the effect of the pencil.

☺ $$$ LIPSTICK AND LIP PENCIL: Clarins offers four different types of lipsticks whose formulas are designated by their number. The **Sheer Lipstick** *($17.50)* is a standard creamy lipstick with soft colors and a glossy finish. The **Cream Lipstick** *($16.50)* is a nice collection of good, creamy lipsticks with a slightly greasy finish. The **Long Lasting Lipstick** *($17.50)* does last somewhat longer than the others, mostly due to the stain it has. These are not as creamy as the others but definitely more opaque and there are some bold colors (including some great pinks and reds) to choose from. The **Shimmer Lipstick** *($17.50)* is virtually identical to the Sheer Lipstick in coverage and color strength, except these are all very iridescent. **Lip Color Glaze** *($16)* is lip gloss in a bottle with a wand applicator. The colors are fairly vivid and the texture is non-sticky and smooth. ☺ The **Lip Liner Pencil** *($13.50)* is a standard pencil that has a good, easy-to-apply texture and an attractive color selection. One end is a lipstick brush, which is convenient.

MASCARA: ☺ $$$ **Lengthening Mascara** *($17)* is a good option for a light mascara that doesn't do much in the lengthening or thickening departments but does stay on well.

☺ $$$ **Pure Volume Mascara** *($17)* is a great mascara for building dramatic length and reasonable thickness with minimal effort but it can have a tendency to smear, which is disappointing.

☹ **BRUSHES:** Clarins offers a small selection of **brushes** *($14–$25)* that aren't for everyone. In fact, most women will find the **Powder Brush** *($25)* too big, although it is very soft and full; the **Blush Brush** *($22)* is ridiculously undersized for the cheek area; and the **Angle Brush** *($17.50)* is too stiff for doing a soft line on the brow or for shading the eye. The remainder of the brushes are just OK, which means overpriced and not worth considering given the quality and performance.

# Clean & Clear by Johnson & Johnson (Skin Care Only)

When it comes to breakouts, this line has some great options and some real disappointing shockers. For example, it has some wonderfully formulated benzoyl peroxide and salicylic acid (BHA) products that contain no irritants or fragrance. But then it has a cleanser for oily skin that contains Vaseline! Vaseline for blemish-prone skin? What were these people thinking?

For more information about Johnson & Johnson products call (800) 526-3967 or visit the Web site at www.cleanandclear.com.

☹ **Continuous Control Daily Cleanser, 10% Benzoyl Peroxide Acne Medication** *($5.49 for 5 ounces)* only makes me ask, why would anyone put a 10% benzoyl peroxide acne medication in a base that contains primarily petrolatum (Vaseline) and mineral oil as the first two ingredients? This also contains menthol, making it one of the most confused, potentially irritating, and greasy acne products I've ever reviewed. It does contain fragrance.

☹ **Deep Action Cream Cleanser** *($3.49 for 6.5 ounces)*. The menthol in here can be a skin irritant, and salicylic acid in a cleanser is a problem for the eyes. Plus, the pH of this product is too high for the BHA to be an effective exfoliant.

☺ **Sensitive Skin Foaming Facial Cleanser** *($3.79 for 8 ounces)* is good, detergent-based water-soluble cleanser for someone with normal to oily skin. It is definitely more gentle than any of the other cleansers in this line. It does contain fragrance.

☺ **Foaming Facial Cleanser** *($3.49 for 8 ounces)* is a standard, detergent-based water-soluble cleanser. It can be more drying than some, but it would be an option for someone with oily skin. It contains a tiny amount of triclosan, a disinfectant, that could be effective for controlling breakouts, but in a cleanser it would just be washed away. It does contain fragrance.

☺ **Oil Free Daily Pore Cleanser** *($3.49 for 5.5 ounces)* is a standard, detergent-based water-soluble cleanser for someone with normal to oily skin. It does contain fragrance.

☹ **Oil-Fighting Deep Cleaning Astringent** *($2.99 for 8 ounces)* contains alcohol, eucalyptus, camphor, peppermint, and clove, which are all irritants and have no benefit for controlling breakouts; rather, they can create red and inflamed skin, making matters worse.

☹ **Sensitive Skin Astringent** *($8.99 for 5 ounces)* is shockingly similar to the Oil-Fighting version above and the same comments apply.

☹ **Skin-Toning Astringent** *($3.29 for 8 ounces)* is similar to the Oil-Fighting version above and the same comments apply.

☺ **Dual Action Moisturizer** *($3.79 for 4 ounces)* contains 0.5% salicylic acid, which, at this amount, despite the low pH, is minimally effective as an exfoliant. Other than that, it is an exceptionally boring moisturizer of just thickeners, fragrance, and preservatives. I would not recommend this for most skin types.

☺ **Pore Prep Clarifier** *($4.29 for 2 ounces)* contains 2% salicylic acid and is in an impressive nonirritating base; however, the pH of this product is closer to 4.5 than 3. A pH of 3 to 3.5, and possibly 4 is best for optimal exfoliation. However, this is an option, perhaps as a place to start and see how it works for your skin.

☹ **Invisible Blemish Treatment** *($3.49 for 0.75 ounce)* is similar to the Pore Prep above, only this one contains alcohol and is not recommended.

☺ **Persa-Gel 5, Regular Strength** *($3.49 for 1 ounce)* is a very good 5% benzoyl peroxide gel. If you want to try a benzoyl peroxide product, this one would be just fine.

☺ **Persa-Gel 10, Maximum Strength** *($3.49 for 1 ounce)* is a very good 10% benzoyl peroxide liquid. If you want to try a stronger benzoyl peroxide product, this one would be just fine.

☺ **Clear Touch Oil Absorbing Sheets** *($4.95 for 50 sheets)* are an interesting twist on the standard oil-absorbing papers. These are more like soft plastic sheets with a slight rubbery feel (not the rose-petal texture mentioned in the ads). They do work well enough, but it takes several of them to make a difference, just as it does with any of the more standard oil-absorbing papers.

## *Clear LogiX (Skin Care Only)*

This line of acne products is neither logical nor effective, though it can be terribly irritating. How disappointing! For more information about Clear LogiX, call (800) 966-6960 or visit the Web site at www.advreslab.com.

☹ **Deep Cleansing Acne Treatment Pads** *($5.99 for 75 pads)* has the same problems as the other products described below, plus this one also contains ammonium xylenesulfonate, an ingredient used as nail polish solvent!

☺ **Gentle Foaming Acne Cleanser** *($5.99 for 6 ounces)* uses a fairly drying detergent cleansing agent (sodium methyl cocoyl taurate), making this a potential problem for most skin types. The tiny amount of retinol in here is completely ineffective for any purpose, and the glycolic acid would just be washed away.

☹ **Oil Free Medicated Acne Wash** *($5.99 for 8 ounces)* uses sodium C14-16 olefin sulfate as the main detergent cleansing agent; I don't even recommend this ingredient for hair-care products. It also contains AHA and BHA, which are wasted in a cleanser, and eucalyptus, which serves no purpose except to burn the eyes and irritate the skin.

☹ **Deep Cleansing Astringent, Sensitive Skin** *($4.99 for 8 ounces)* lists the second ingredient as alcohol and it also contains menthol, making this an irritating problem for all skin types, but unbelievably inappropriate for someone with sensitive skin.

☹ **Deep Cleansing Astringent, Oily Skin** *($4.99 for 8 ounces)* is almost identical to the Sensitive Skin version above and the same comments apply.

☹ **Acne Night Treatment Serum** *($6.99 for 2 ounces)* does contain salicylic acid, but it also contains lots of alcohol and eucalyptus and is therefore not recommended.

☹ **Acne Spot Treatment** *($5.99 for 0.75 ounce)* has the same problems as the product above, and is not recommended.

☹ **Acne Spot Treatment Tinted Formula** *($5.25 for 0.75 ounce)* has the same ingredients as the product above, but it is tinted a strange shade of peach.

☹ **Oil Absorbent Acne Mask** *($6.14 for 4 ounces)* is a fairly standard clay mask with sulfur and eucalyptus. Sulfur can be an effective disinfectant for breakouts, but when combined with the eucalyptus it is just too irritating to recommend.

# Clearasil (Skin Care Only)

Clearasil has been around as a teenage acne product for decades! Has it cured anyone's acne? Not that I've seen. The products leave much to be desired when it comes to texture, color, and irritation. From what I remember, these products didn't work for anyone when I was a kid and they still don't. For more information about Clearasil call (800) 981-1841 or visit the Web site at www.clearasil.com.

☹ **Antibacterial Soap** *($2.29 for 3.25 ounces)* is a standard, tallow-based soap with a detergent cleansing agent. It contains the disinfectant triclosan, which is minimally effective for breakouts, but its effects are washed away in a soap. The big problem is that this product contains tallow, which can cause breakouts and blackheads.

☺ **Daily Face Wash** *($4.99 for 6.5 ounces)* is a standard, detergent-based water-soluble cleanser that may be OK for someone with oily skin, though the detergent cleansing agents in here can be more drying than most. It contains the disinfectant triclosan, but its effects are washed away in a cleanser.

☹ **Adult Care Acne Medication Cream** *($3.69 for 0.6 ounce)*. Both resorcinol and sulfur are potent disinfectants that can be extremely irritating. Resorcinol is no longer approved by the FDA for disinfecting and preventing acne. Also, one of the thickeners is isopropyl myristate, which can cause breakouts. Aside from being very drying and irritating, this product may also clog pores.

☺ **Tinted Cream Maximum Strength** *($6 for 1 ounce)* is a 10% benzoyl peroxide product with a tint, but few people have skin the color of this tint. You can find similar products without tints that won't look strange on your skin, but the benzoyl peroxide in here is an effective disinfectant.

☺ **Vanishing Cream Maximum Strength** *($6 for 1 ounce)* is unlikely to cause anything to vanish. It is a 10% benzoyl peroxide product that also contains clay and thickeners. One of the thickeners is isopropyl myristate, which can cause breakouts, but the benzoyl peroxide is an effective disinfectant.

☹ **Stay Clear Acne Defense Cleanser** *($4.99 for 6.78 ounces)* is a standard, detergent-based water-soluble cleanser that also contains salicylic acid. It is a problem for salicylic acid to be in a cleanser because it is rinsed down the drain before it has a chance to absorb into skin. Even if that weren't a problem, this one contains menthol and is too irritating for the skin and eyes.

☹ **Stay Clear Deep Clean Astringent** *($3.49 for 8 ounces)* is a 2% salicylic acid toner steeped in alcohol and menthol, and is not recommended for any skin type.

☹ **Stay Clear Deep Clean Pads** *($3.49 for 65 pads)* is similar to the product above minus the menthol, and the same comments apply.

☹ **Stay Clear Zone Control Clearstick** *($4.99 for 1.2 ounces)* is similar to the one above only in stick form and is not recommended.

## *Clinac*

☺ **Clinac Oil Control Gel** *($19.50 for 90 grams)* is a topical gel that uses a film-forming agent that provides a matte feel on the skin and has some absorbent properties. It contains mostly water, slip agent, film formers, thickeners, and preservatives. This product is not unique in the range of matte gel formulations making claims of absorbing oil. However, this one is as good an option as any. The study being touted in ads as demonstrating that this product works was done by the company selling it. If you're interested in learning more, visit www.dermstore.com.

## *Clinique*

Clinique was Estee Lauder's first attempt at expanding its market with a completely separate line and image. Lauder was clearly a mature woman's line and Clinique became known as the indispensable line for the woman under 30 concerned with breakouts and oily skin. Clinique's tremendous success reshaped the way cosmetics lines identified themselves, sending the concept of line loyalty down the drain. Today, cosmetics companies expand their market by either buying already established companies or creating new ones. Of course cosmetics companies keep this multiple-personality identity hidden from the consumer. If the general buying public realized that companies were so intertwined with each other, how could they flaunt their independence and claim that their unparalleled formulations are secret? Unless you think Lauder (or any company) would keep secrets from part of its own ranks.

Clinique's niche launched the notion of cosmetics being "allergy-tested," "hypoallergenic," "100% fragrance-free," and "dermatologist tested." Of those marketing claims the only one that has significance is 100% fragrance free, which, for the most part, Clinique maintains (it does have some fragrant extracts in a few products). But without seeing the testing results, what difference does it make if a product is "allergy-tested"? What if the test showed 20% of the women who used it had a sensitizing reaction, dryness, or irritation? Moreover, "hypoallergenic" is a term not regulated by the FDA, so any product can wear it. "Dermatologist tested" is also bogus, because without published test results, that can easily mean a dermatologist picked up the product and said, "This looks good."

Clinique's products, particularly those for skin care, are aimed at oily or combination skin types, which is probably why Clinique attracts a younger clientele, but many of these products are exceptionally disappointing, such as those that contain a lot of alcohol, which would be drying, or emollient moisturizers that could trigger breakouts. The strong points are the lack of fragrance of any kind in these products, some great moisturizing formulas, and excellent sunscreens.

Overall, Clinique's color line is nothing short of overwhelming. There are more choices than ever (the selection borders on chaos), and some of the product launches have been hit-or-miss in terms of performance and shade selection. Though the blushes and eyeshadows are still lacking in depth for women of color, there are now more foundation choices for darker skin tones than ever before, and many of them are worth a look. Clinique has updated some of its more gimmicky products, such as color rubs and gel rouges, and for the most part it is a nice improvement. I still think many of these products are limited to those with a deft hand at blending (or flawless skin), but for an occasional, frivolous splurge, you could certainly do worse.

One thing you can be sure of at most Clinique counters is service. There always seem to be four to five white-jacketed women dashing around behind those counters. (Those white jackets are supposed to look medical—how contrived can you get!) The color products are arranged into four groupings: Nudes/Naturels (which are not all that nude), Tawnies/Corals, Pinks/Roses, and Violets/Berries. One more plus is that the products are by far more affordable than those of numerous other lines in department stores. For more information about Clinique call (212) 572-3800 or visit the user-friendly Web site at www.clinique.com.

## Clinique Skin Care

☹ **Facial Soap ExtraMild, Mild,** and **Extra Strength** *($8.50 for 6 ounces)* are standard-issue bar soaps, meaning they are mostly lard and lye. This is a lot of money for your average, everyday bar of soap.

☹ **Rinse-Off Foaming Cleanser** *($15.50 for 5 ounces)* is a standard, detergent-based water-soluble cleanser. It uses fairly strong detergent cleansing agents (potassium myristate and potassium palmitate), plus it also contains lemon, pine, and eucalyptus, which makes this too drying and potentially irritating for the skin.

☹ **Wash-Away Gel Cleanser** *($15.50 for 6 ounces)* is similar to the Rinse-Off version above only with milder cleansing agents, though the eucalyptus and lemon in here can still be irritants for skin.

☺ **Water-Dissolve Cream Cleanser** *($15.50 for 5 ounces)* can leave a greasy film on the skin and doesn't take off all makeup without the help of a washcloth but it can still be an option for someone with dry skin.

☺ **$$$ Extremely Gentle Eye Makeup Remover** *($9.50 for 2 ounces)* contains mostly mineral oil, thickeners, slip agent, and preservatives. This is little more than pure mineral oil and it would be gentle, but using plain mineral oil would work the same for far less money.

☺ **Rinse-Off Eye Makeup Solvent** *($12 for 4 ounces)* contains mostly water, detergent cleanser, and slip agents. It is a standard, detergent-based eye-makeup remover.

☺ **Take the Day Off Makeup Remover, for Lids, Lashes and Lips** *($14.50 for 4.2 ounces)* is a silicone- and detergent-based makeup remover. It works, but it needs to be wiped off, and that's not great for any part of the face, especially the eyes.

☺ **$$$ 7 Day Scrub Cream** *($15 for 3.5 ounces)*. This very thick, heavy product can cause the same problems it's trying to eliminate, because the thickening agents can clog pores. The synthetic scrub particles of polyethylene (ground-up plastic) do work as a gentle abrasive.

☺ **$$$ 7 Day Scrub Cream Rinse Off Formula** *($14 for 3.4 ounces)* rinses off far better than the one above, but that's not saying much. It can still leave a film on the skin and contains ingredients that would be a problem for blemish-prone skin.

☺ **Exfoliating Scrub** *($13.50 for 3 ounces)* was probably added to the Clinique line because the other two scrubs make such a creamy mess. This detergent-cleanser scrub definitely rinses better than the two above but it contains menthol, which is an unnecessary irritation for skin.

☺ **Gentle Exfoliator Rinse-Off Formula** *($13.50 for 3 ounces)* cuses the same exfoliant as the ones above and though it is a gentle exfoliant with very little abrasiveness, I wouldn't call it rinseable. The mineral oil leaves a residue on the skin.

☹ **Clarifying Lotions 1, 2, 3, and 4** *($15.50 for 12 ounces)* all contain varying degrees of alcohol, benzalkonium chloride, and menthol, which are all extremely irritating, and none are recommended unless you are looking for red, irritated, dry, and flaky skin. The best thing I can say is that at least Clinique finally took the acetone (nail polish solvent) out of these formulations.

☺ **Mild Clarifying Lotion** *($15.50 for 12 ounces)* contains about a 0.5% concentration of BHA, recommended for dry, sensitive skin. The pH of this toner is about 4, which is good, but BHA is only appropriate for blemish-prone skin because of its ability to penetrate the pore. This can be an option for someone with breakouts, but a pH of 3 to 3.5 would make it more effective.

☺ **$$$ All About Eyes** *($25 for 0.5 ounce)* feels silky when you rub this light lotion into your skin, primarily from the silicone base; silicones are the first two ingredients on the list. That's not bad, but these ingredients aren't about eyes in particular, and so this is just a good lightweight moisturizer that can feel soothing anywhere on the face. The plant extracts can be good anti-irritants and antioxidants. It is a good lightweight moisturizer for dry skin.

☺ **$$$ Daily Eye Benefits** *($25 for 0.5 ounce)*. The plant extracts (such as tannin, which does constrict skin, but when used on a daily basis can be a skin irritant) are supposed to reduce puffiness around the eyes, but it's unlikely your skin would notice. This is a good, standard moisturizer for normal to dry skin.

☹ **$$$ Daily Eye Saver** *($25 for 0.5 ounce)*. The coffee in here can't save eyes and the amount of vitamin C, as an antioxidant, is so minuscule as to be barely present. This is a very standard moisturizer for normal to dry skin.

☺ **Dramatically Different Moisturizing Lotion** *($10.50 for 2 ounces, $19.50 for 4 ounces)* is a basic, boring moisturizer for dry skin that isn't "dramatically different"; rather, it is dramatically out of date and in need of reformulation to get up to speed with the other moisturizers in the Clinique lineup.

☺ **Moisture in Control** *($30 for 1.7 ounces)* won't control anything. There is no way a product can put moisturizing ingredients in a dry area on the face, but keep them off the face in other areas and instead apply ingredients that absorb oil. It would work well for normal to dry skin, but that's about it.

☺ **Moisture On-Call** *($30 for 1.6 ounces)* is supposed to help skin cells "remember" how to produce their own moisture barrier. The company calls this memory-booster effect "mnemonic." In fact, you can achieve the same effect with the daily use of *any* moisturizer, which is the only claim Clinique is really making. It is a very good emollient moisturizer for someone with dry skin, but no more special than hundreds of other moisturizers.

☺ **Moisture on Line** *($30 for 1.7 ounces)* is almost identical to Moisture On-Call, and supposedly can re-educate the skin. There are no moisturizing ingredients anywhere in the world that can change the nature of skin and make skin remember anything. But skin cells can look better if you faithfully reapply the moisturizer every day, which is exactly what the instructions on this moisturizer tell you to do. Separated from the hype, it is a good moisturizer for someone with normal to dry skin. The lactic acid in this product works more as a water-binding agent than as an exfoliant, given that there is only about a 2% to 3% concentration of it.

☺ **Moisture Surge Treatment Formula** *($32.50 for 2 ounces)* is a very good lightweight moisturizer with a nice quantity of water-binding agents and antioxidants. The ginger in here can be a skin irritant.

☺ **Skin Texture Lotion Oil Free Formula** *($19.50 for 1.25 ounces)*. Don't be misled by the term oil-free, there are still thickening agents in here that could cause breakouts and that would be a problem for someone with oily skin. It is a good, though very unimpressive lightweight moisturizer for normal to slightly dry skin.

☹ $$$ **Stop Signs Visible Anti-Aging Serum** *($32.50 for 1 ounce or $50 for 1.7 ounces)*. Caffeine gets a lot of play these days in cosmetics. Caffeine's tannin content is probably why it's used in skin care, as it constricts skin, and that can make it look temporarily smoother, though it can also cause irritation. Stop Signs also makes reference to lightening skin discolorations. It does contain mulberry extract, which has minimally demonstrated some ability to reduce hypermelanin production, but only in vitro and in pure form, not in the teeny amounts found in a moisturizer. Separate from the hype, Stop Signs is for the most part just a good lightweight moisturizer for normal to dry skin. It won't stop a wrinkle and is not a product to consider over Clinique's Weather Everything SPF 15 for daytime, that's for sure.

☺ **Anti-Gravity Firming Lift Cream** *($35 for 1.7 ounces)*. The more than 50 ingredients in this product can't lift one skin cell. This is a good, but relatively unimpressive moisturizer for normal to dry skin. The microscopic amounts of plant extracts, water-binding agents, and vitamins have no real impact on skin (though they may sound impressive when the salesperson carries on about them).

☹ **Turnaround Cream** *($27.50 for 2 ounces)* has a great name; it sounds as if this cream can turn your skin back to a younger time, but it can't (any more than any of the other products in this line or the entire Lauder stable of lines can, for that matter). Salicylic acid (BHA) is an effective exfoliant, but only at a pH of 3 in a concentration of 1% to 2%. There is no information about concentration for any of the Turnaround products, but even if there were, the pH is 5, which makes them ineffective as exfoliants. This is a fairly matte, lightweight moisturizer for normal to slightly dry skin, and that's about it.

☹ **Turnaround Cream for Dry Skin** *($27.50 for 2 ounces)* is much more emollient than the cream above and would definitely be good for someone with dry skin, but the same basic review applies.

☹ **Turnaround Lotion Oil-Free** *($23.50 for 1.7 ounces)*. If you have normal to slightly oily skin, this can be a good lightweight moisturizer, but it is a poor BHA product.

☺ $$$ **Weather Everything SPF 15** *($37.50 for 1.7 ounces)* is an overpriced, titanium dioxide–based sunscreen. It would provide impressive sun protection for someone with dry skin, but I wouldn't recommend it for oily or combination skin. I wish Clinique had brought out a daily sun-care product years ago, but better late than never.

☺ City Block SPF 15 *($13.50 for 1.4 ounces)* is a good, titanium dioxide–based sunscreen for someone with dry skin. There are several ingredients in here, including the titanium dioxide (the sunscreen agent), that can be a problem for someone with oily or blemish-prone skin.

☺ $$$ Super City Block SPF 25 Oil-Free Daily Face Protector *($14.50 for 1.4 ounces)* is a good, titanium dioxide–based sunscreen that would work well for normal to dry skin. Titanium dioxide is not the best for someone with oily skin.

☹ Face Zone Sun Block SPF 30 *($13.50 for 1.7 ounces)* doesn't contain avobenzone, zinc oxide, or titanium dioxide, and is not recommended.

☹ Full-Service Sun Block SPF 15 *($12.50 for 3 ounces)* doesn't contain avobenzone, zinc oxide, or titanium dioxide, and is not recommended.

☹ Full-Service Sun Block SPF 20 *($12.50 for 3 ounces)* doesn't contain avobenzone, zinc oxide, or titanium dioxide, and is not recommended.

☹ Total Cover Sun Block SPF 30 *($12.50 for 3 ounces)* doesn't contain avobenzone, zinc oxide, or titanium dioxide, and is not recommended.

☺ Lip Block SPF 15 *($7.50 for 0.15 ounce)* doesn't contain avobenzone, zinc oxide, or titanium dioxide, and is not recommended.

☹ Oil-Free Sun Block SPF 15 *($12.50 for 4 ounces)* doesn't contain avobenzone, zinc oxide, or titanium dioxide, and is not recommended.

☺ Quick Bronze Tinted Self Tanner *($14.50 for 1.7 ounces)* has a hint of color so you can see where you've applied it and that does help with a more even application. However, the active ingredient is the same that's in all self tanners and performs the same.

☺ $$$ Self-Tanning Face Formula I/II *($14.50 for 1.7 ounces)* is a good, standard, dihydroxyacetone-based self tanner; this one works as well as any of them.

☺ $$$ Self-Tanning Face Formula III/IV *($14.50 for 1.7 ounces)* is the same as the one above and the same comments apply.

☹ Deep Cleansing Emergency Masque *($18.50 for 3.4 ounces)* is a standard clay mask that also contains cornstarch and menthol, which can create emergencies, not help them.

☺ $$$ Exceptionally Soothing Cream for Upset Skin, Anti-Itch Cream *($30 for 1.7 ounces)* and Exceptionally Soothing Lotion for Upset Skin *($30 for 1.7 ounces)* both contain hydrocortisone acetate, which can indeed soothe irritated skin. For years I have been recommending Lanacort and Cortaid (both found at the drugstore for less than $5 an ounce) to deal with minor, transient skin irritations. What Clinique doesn't warn about is that continuous use of hydrocortisone over time can actually cause skin damage by thinning the skin and breaking down the skin's support structure. If you are aware of this very serious shortcoming and plan only occasional use, there are many reasons why you may prefer Clinique's two new products to Lanacort or Cortaid. Even though the active ingredient in these products is the same, the moisturizing base in both Clinique products is a far more elegant one, with soothing agents, silicone, and water-binding agents. However, in the long run, the base shouldn't make that much difference, because you should only be using it for the short run.

☺ $$$ **Skin Calming Moisture Mask** *($18.50 for 3.4 ounces)* is a good moisturizing mask for dry skin but it is not calming in the least.

☹ **Sheer Matteness T-Zone Shine Control** *($12.50 for 0.5 ounce)* is supposed to help skin look less oily. Given its ingredient listing, I suspect it can do that for a brief period of time; after all, the second ingredient is alcohol, which can degrease just about anything. Of course, what you are supposed to do with the resulting dryness and irritation isn't mentioned. This product also contains silicone (I suspect that's to soothe the effect of the alcohol, but it can be a problem for very oily skin types), film former, slip agent, witch hazel, and BHA. There isn't enough BHA here to be effective for exfoliation, but the irritating ingredients make this a problem for any skin type.

☺ **All About Lips** *($20 for 0.5 ounce)* is a good moisturizer (though nothing about it is special for lips), but the pH isn't low enough to make the BHA effective as an exfoliant.

☹ **Acne Solutions Cleansing Foam** *($16.50 for 4.2 ounces)* contains peppermint and is not recommended.

☹ **Acne Solutions Antibacterial Facial Soap** *($8.50 for a 5.2-ounce bar)* is a soap and can be irritating because the cleansing agents are drying. Also, the ingredients that keep soap in its bar form can clog pores. Beyond that, while the antibacterial agent in here can kill the bacteria that can cause breakouts, it would be rinsed away before it had much of a chance to get in the pore and work. There are better ways to disinfect the skin than with soap.

☹ **Acne Solutions Night Treatment Gel** *($15.50 for 1.7 ounces)* has alcohol as the second ingredient, and witch hazel as the fourth, plus it also contains peppermint, and all combined that makes this too irritating to recommend.

☹ **Acne Solutions Spot Healing Gel** *($11 for 0.5 ounce)* has alcohol as the first ingredient, and witch hazel as the second, which combine to make this too potentially irritating to recommend.

## Clinique Makeup

**FOUNDATION:** Clinique's vast stable of foundations run the gamut from barely there to ultra-coverage, and many of them are wonderful and worth considering.

☺ **Almost Makeup SPF 15** *($16.50)* is a very sheer foundation with a good, titanium dioxide–based SPF 15. The colors are limited to four, but what's there is great. This would work well for a normal to dry skin seeking minimal coverage.

☺ **City Stick SPF 15** *($20)* is one of the stick foundations that have changed the face of the cosmetics industry, with most every line having its version. Clinique's is a very good option to consider and the SPF is excellent, with pure titanium dioxide as the only active ingredient. The coverage is sheer to medium with a definite powder finish. As is true for any cream-to-powder type foundation, the powder element can be drying for someone with dry skin, and the cream part can be greasy for someone with combination to oily skin, so that makes it best for someone with normal to slightly dry or slightly oily skin. Of the eight shades, the only one to watch out for is Beige Twist, which can be too peach for most skin tones.

☺ **City Base Compact Foundation SPF 15** *($20)* is similar to the City Stick Foundation only in compact form, but this one leaves a slightly heavier, creamier finish. The finish is still powdery with a slightly silky feel, but not enough to hold back much shine in oilier areas, making this a best bet for normal to slightly dry skin. The ten shades are all excellent and would work for a wide range of skin tones, from light to dark, but not for someone with very light or very dark skin. The SPF 15 is great, containing titanium dioxide as the only active ingredient.

☺ **SuperFit Makeup** *($18.50)* is an excellent option for those with oily skin who have found the ultra-matte formulations from other companies too drying or heavy feeling and way too difficult to remove. This is a great, soft, matte-finish foundation that also has ten excellent, neutral color options (though it lacks a shade for very light skin tones). The only color to avoid is Healthy, which can be too peach. SuperFit blends on easily, has good staying power, and easily washes off, though it isn't as oil-resistant as the ultra-matte-finish products. You will get shine sooner than you would with a product like Almay Amazing Lasting Foundation or Revlon ColorStay Lite SPF 15. If you decide to check out this product, ignore the claims Clinique is making about the SuperFit Makeup containing a multifiber technology that is supposed to wick away moisture and oil—that just doesn't hold up in real life. After all, where are the oil and water going to get "wicked" away to? It isn't going to fall off the face and disappear; it stays on the surface, just as you would expect.

☺ **Superbalanced Makeup** *($16.50)* claims to contain spongelike ingredients that will absorb oil in oily areas but still moisturize dry areas of your face. It ends up doing neither very well. There is no way for any product to differentiate between the oily parts of your face and the dry parts. The so-called sponges in here will absorb any oil they come in contact with (including the moisturizing ingredients in this product or the one you applied to your skin) and the moisturizing ingredients will get deposited over areas you don't want to be moisturized. What that adds up to is a foundation that is best for someone with normal to slightly dry or slightly oily skin. Someone with any amount of oil would not be happy with the finish or with how it wears during the day. Even more disappointing are the colors, which are astonishingly poor, especially for lighter skin tones. Although the darker shades are actually some of the best around, many of the lighter colors are strongly peach to orange! The following colors are best avoided for most all skin tones: Petal, Fair, Ivory, Cream Chamois, Neutral, Linen, Porcelain Beige, Sunny, Warmer, and Honeyed Beige.

☺ **Clarifying Makeup** *($16.50)* finally replaces Clinique's long-standing Pore Minimizer foundation, which was mostly alcohol with talc. The alcohol was irritating and drying and the talc provided streaky, minimal coverage. While Clarifying definitely still contains alcohol as the second ingredient, the foundation application itself is impressive. It has a soft, sheer-to-light coverage and a smooth matte, somewhat transparent finish. The colors are very nice, with most being neutral to yellow-based. Of the nine shades the only ones to avoid are: Perfect Almond, Blushing Buff, Light Beige, and Neutral Spice, all of which can be too peach or pink for most skin tones.

☺ **Balanced Makeup Base** *($14.50)* is one of Clinique's oldest foundations, and is preferred to its SuperBalanced. This is best for a dry to very dry skin, as the consistency is more emollient and creamy, but it blends on well, leaving a natural finish. The coverage is light to medium, and most of the 12 colors are excellent; the only colors to consider avoiding are: Creamy Peach (too peach), Natural Glow (orange), and Honeyed Beige (very pink).

☺ **Continuous Coverage SPF 11** *($14.50)* is a very opaque, full-coverage makeup that will certainly not look natural but will provide good camouflage for irregular pigmentation or birthmarks. The SPF is all titanium dioxide, and this, coupled with the thick, powdery finish, can lend a chalky look to the skin. The five available shades are good, but this is definitely a trade-off of a foundation, and the SPF 11 still leaves your skin needing higher SPF protection.

☺ **Workout Makeup All-Day Wear** *($14.50)* is a creamy foundation that provides medium coverage and a rather heavy application. If you're looking for a foundation that has staying power when you're sweating, this one does have some tenacity, but it doesn't have a lightweight feel and looks like makeup. Of the six shades, three can be a problem for most skin tones: Ivory and Babyskin (too pink), and Beige (orange).

☺ **Stay-True Makeup Oil-Free Formula** *($15.50)* is a very good foundation for fairly opaque, semi-matte coverage. This should work beautifully on very oily or normal to slightly oily skin that is looking for a soft matte (as opposed to an ultramatte) finish. There are some great colors for both light and dark skin tones, but avoid Beige (too pink), True Toffee and True Copper (very orange), and True Bronze (too reddish-pink).

☺ **Soft Finish Makeup** *($18.50)* is quite similar to Clinique's Balanced Makeup Base in terms of consistency and coverage, but this one has greater slip and is slightly more sheer than the Balanced. This also claims to provide a "soft-focus" effect on the skin, but once you see the finish in daylight, you'll know what a false claim that is. This is still a good foundation for normal to very dry skin. Of the nine shades, all are beautifully neutral except Soft Porcelain (too pink).

☺ **Super Powder Double Face Powder Foundation** *($15.50)* is a standard, talc-based pressed powder with a smooth, soft texture. It can be used alone or as a regular finishing powder. The colors are so sheer it's like wearing no makeup at all. There are eight shades, and most of them are excellent. It is often recommended to wear this type of foundation wet. Don't—it only makes it look thick, streaky, and choppy.

☺ **Bronze Gel** *($8 for 1.5 ounces)* is a good, lightweight, very sheer, nonsparkly hint of tan color. It works well to create a veil of color without looking obvious or heavy. However, this works best on flawless skin, as the gel tint can make pores look bigger and darker.

**CONCEALER:** ☹ **Quick Corrector** *($10.50)* comes in a tube with a wand applicator and has a creamy application that smooths on easily and covers well with a soft, minimally shiny finish. The creamy finish can translate into some creasing around the eyes. Avoid Medium (too pink) and Honey (too orange).

☺ **Soft Conceal Corrector** *($11.50)* comes in a squeeze tube and offers smooth, even coverage in a great but small selection of colors. This has a soft powdery finish and only a minimal tendency to crease.

☹ **Advanced Concealer** *($10.50)* comes in a squeeze tube, goes on like a thick cream, but dries to a powder. It comes in two shades, Light and Medium, and both are excellent. But beware: this product works only if the skin under your eyes is smooth; any dry or rough skin will look worse when this type of concealer is placed over it. **City Cover Compact Concealer SPF 15** *($12.50)* is one of the few concealers that has a reliable SPF 15 with UVA protection. The colors here are great and quite workable, but this has a creamy consistency that will crease before you're out the door. If the sun protection appeals to you, make sure you try this at the counter first and see how it wears over a period of time.

☹ **Anti-Acne Control Formula Concealer** *($11.50)* is very thick and heavy. It comes in two shades, Light and Medium, and both are poor color choices. The anti-acne parts of the formula are colloidal sulfur and salicylic acid. BHA is an option for exfoliation but it isn't necessary in makeup, and sulfur is too much of an irritant. There are gentler ways to disinfect without causing irritation. **Concealing Stick** *($12.50)* is a lipstick-style concealer available in only one color, which is too peach for most all skin tones. Even if the color was more neutral, this is a greasy product that easily slips and doesn't have the best coverage.

☺ <u>POWDER:</u> **Blended Face Powder & Brush** *($15.50)* is a very good, talc-based loose powder that comes in an attractive array of colors and has a light, soft finish that clings well without caking. Of the nine shades, avoid Transparency 2 (pink) and Transparency Bronze (nice color, but it is shiny). **Stay Matte Sheer Pressed Powder Oil-Free** *($15.50)* is an excellent powder with a slightly dry finish that is great for oilier skin types. The eight shades are beautiful and there are some good options for light and dark skin tones here. **Soft Finish Pressed Powder** *($15.50)* is intended by Clinique to be used for drier skins, and that makes sense, as this has a creamier, silky feel and smooth, even coverage. The light-diffusing claims are bogus, but there are some great neutral colors to choose from.

☺ <u>BLUSH:</u> All of Clinique's blush colors are on the sheer side, which can be good (light, soft application) or bad (not deep enough to show on darker skin tones), depending on your needs. **Sheer Powder Blusher** *($15.50)* has a great selection of colors but they are so soft and sheer as to be almost nonexistent on the skin when applied. Even after layering some of the "deeper" colors, it was hard to notice any intensity. Some of the colors have a slight amount of shine but is barely noticeable on the skin. This formula contains rice starch as one of the main ingredients, which may exacerbate breakouts, so be cautious. **Soft Pressed Powder Blusher** *($15.50)* does up the ante a bit in terms of depth of color, but these are still quite sheer and darker skin tones will have a hard time getting these to show up. The colors are all fine, with a minimal amount of shine.

☺ $$$ **BlushWear** *($15)* is Clinique's version of a cream-to-powder blush with an unusually dry finish. Even the salesperson warned me that it is helpful if you apply a moisturizer first to help it spread more easily. How to work that out when you're wearing foundation wasn't explained. It is tricky though, and given the mode of application, not that much easier to use than Almay's Amazing Lasting Blush *($7.59)* or Revlon's ColorStay Cheek Color *($7.89)*.

☺ <u>EYESHADOW:</u> **Stay the Day Eyeshadow** *($11)* is supposed to last all day with no fading. You may not notice whether it fades or not because these colors are all quite powdery and go on very sheer. There are some great matte, neutral colors here but the softness of these and their inability to cling well to the skin make them difficult to recommend. **Pair of Shades Eyeshadow Duo** *($14.50)* features 26 differ-ent duos in a formula virtually identical to the Stay the Day shadows. Thus, these tend to have the same problems. Most of the duos have one very shiny shade, and for an everyday look that can be more sparkles than one face needs. **Touch Base for Eyes** *($11)* is one of the better cream-to-powder eyeshadows. This comes in a compact that must be kept closed tightly or the product will dry out and be useless. This may happen even if you follow that guideline, so recommending this is risky. Take a look and try it out first before buying, as there are a couple of matte colors that would work as an eyeshadow base. **Smudgesicles** *($12.50)* gets my vote for one of the cutest makeup names ever, but the enthusiasm stops there. These are cream-to-powder eye colors in stick form that go on relatively smoothly and blend out sheer. They are tricky to use with other colors, and all of these shades are iridescent. For a one-color, quick eye design, these may be an option, but these are more trendy than a real makeup asset.

**EYE AND BROW SHAPERS:** ☺ **Brow Shaper** *($13.50)* is a powder brow color that comes in four excellent shades. The texture is slightly heavy, but these blend onto the brow quite well, even though the brush these come packaged with is too stiff and scratchy. For the money, a matte, brow-toned eyeshadow would work just as well and could also double as an eyeshadow; this version is too heavy for eyeshadow.

☺ **Brow Keeper** *($14.50)* is a brow pencil that comes in three good shades and has a soft, creamy consistency. These tend to stay creamy, and are prone to smudging or fading. Again, powder eyeshadow would do the trick without adding another pencil to sharpen!

☺ **Quickliner for Eyes** *($13.50)* is a standard automatic pencil that got so much press when it first came out you'd think that this was an innovative miracle. It isn't in the least, and is identical to several less-expensive pencils at the drugstore. **Quick Eyes** *($14.50)* is clever: one end is a creamy pencil and the other end houses a powder eyeshadow in the cap that is dispensed onto a smudge tip. While this may seem convenient, the powder shadows are all very shiny and the pencil is too creamy to last the day. **Shadowliner** *($13.50)* is a cream-to-powder, very soft pencil that glides on easily. This may work for a soft, smoky eye but will otherwise go on thick and smudge on its own. **Eye Shading Pencil** *($10)* is a basic pencil with a smooth, creamy feel and some nice colors. Nothing less, nothing more. **Water-Resistant Eyeliner** *($13.50)* is old-fashioned cake liner that you use with a damp brush. These are too softly pigmented to make a dramatic line, but if you prefer this type of product, it's worth a look. Otherwise, a deeply pigmented matte eyeshadow would be brilliant for this.

☹ **Touch Liner** *($12.50)* is a poor liquid liner that has two shiny colors that take forever and a day to dry. The brush tip is also poor, making this a total washout.

**LIPSTICK AND LIP PENCIL:** ☺ Clinique's lipstick collection is stunning, and there are some beautiful textures and shades here, but they do tend to overlap in terms of feel and finish, making me wonder why they don't try to condense these into three or four formulas. **Different Lipstick** *($11.50)* is a standard collection of lipsticks with a semi-sheer, glossy finish. Don't count on this one for long wear or being any different from any other sheer lipstick. **Long Last Soft Shine Lipstick** *($12.50)* has a smooth, even application with a creamy feel and opaque coverage. The color selection is extensive. **Long Last Soft Matte Lipstick** *($12.50)* is my favorite of Clinique's choices. This is a creamy, smooth lipstick with a nice stain and a slightly matte finish that feels great. **Superlast Cream Lipstick** *($13.50)* is Clinique's ultra-matte lipstick and it wins high marks for staying on well without chipping off or balling up on the lips. The texture is smooth and the finish is slightly matte and dry. **Lip Shaping Pencil** *($10)* is a standard pencil with a slightly dry texture. These go on nicely and there's a nice variety of shades to choose from.

☺ **Liquid Lipstick SPF 15** *($12.50)* comes in a tube with a wand applicator and has a glossy, non-sticky finish. These have fairly opaque coverage for a gloss, but the SPF offers no UVA protection, making these hard to recommend. **Almost Lipstick** *($13.50)* is a sheer, glossy lipstick that is similar to the Different Lipstick and nothing special. **Glosswear SPF 8** *($11.50)* has a poor SPF, a sticky texture, and OK colors. This is fine for a standard gloss but not for sun protection. **Quickliner for Lips** *($12.50)* is an automatic pencil that is not preferred over less-expensive options, as this one tends to smudge and is quite creamy. **Chubby Stick** *($12.50)* is a collection of short, fat pencils with a creamy lipstick application, but they are so soft they never stay sharp enough to draw a good line, making this just a gimmicky, rather unreliable lipstick.

MASCARA: ☺ **Naturally Glossy Mascara** *($11)* is a decent mascara that builds some length and minimal thickness. It's fine for a natural, light look. **Full Potential Mascara** *($11)* goes on very well, with no smudging or clumping, and builds nice, thick lashes with minimal effort. **Supermascara** *($11)* is supposedly better for contact lens wearers because it is fiber-free. Well, so are the rest of Clinique's mascaras, so this one just remains a good lengthening mascara that, with some effort, does create super lashes!

☹ **Longstemmed Lashes** *($11.50)* is the latest mascara from Clinique and it pales in comparison with the others. This applies unevenly, flakes off, and tends to clump the lashes together, even if you wipe the wand down before applying.

☺ **Gentle Waterproof Mascara** *($11.50)* is a bit of a misnomer, as waterproof mascara in general is hard on lashes for both wearing and removing. Still, this is a very good mascara that builds nice length and some thickness and is truly waterproof.

# Club Monaco

Most women are intricately aware of the close relationship clothing has to makeup. Somewhere along the path to adulthood, the message was clearly conveyed through many formats (from mothers to media) that it is stylish to coordinate your wardrobe and makeup. A woman who can successfully do this is thought of as beautiful, classic, and always in good taste. Knowing this, it is not surprising that more and more clothing companies and their designers are sporting complete cosmetic lines as an extension of their textiles. Enter Club Monaco cosmetics, another Canadian import (on the heels

The Reviews C

of M.A.C.) now throwing its hat into the makeup ring. Designed with input from noted New York–based fashion makeup artist Denise Markey, Club Monaco has an appealing look and colors that beckon you to put down those Capri pants and try some makeup on instead. According to Markey, the goal of the line was to be "…easy to understand and apply, and to appeal to a broad spectrum of moods and looks." For the most part, Club Monaco meets those criteria. The displays are clearly marked and easy to understand. Colors are categorized according to their texture or finish on the skin, and the testers are out in the open for play, which is always helpful. The colors themselves are, for the most part, soft and sheer. They blend on well and do tend to last, in spite of their softness. In addition, the foundations and concealers feature one of the best truly neutral palettes around, with some excellent choices for darker skin tones. It is not a stretch to say it would be safe to use these colors as a standard against which to measure most other line's foundation shades.

Along with this, there is also more than enough glitter, shine, and grease to illuminate yourself from head to toe. This portion is up to you, but keep in mind that many of these products will, because of their texture, only serve to undo a careful makeup application and will not hold up well throughout the day. Overall, Club Monaco has a nice cache of reasonably priced makeup (at least for a department store line) that features all the components necessary to create a classic (or contrived) makeup look that will correlate with almost any fashion, from office chic to disco queen.

Club Monaco's skin care, on the other hand, appears to be an afterthought, with problematic ingredients, poor separation of skin types, and standard formulations when the products are good. However, if you want to check out its makeup, and if you live in a city where this line is found (Toronto, Seattle, Detroit, Los Angeles, Washington, D.C., San Francisco, New York, or Chicago), it is worth a visit. For more information about Club Monaco, call (800) 281-3395 or visit the Web sites at www.clubmonaco.com or on www.sephora.com and www.eve.com.

## Club Monaco Skin Care

☹ **Face Foaming Wash** *($14 for 6.7 ounces)* is a standard, detergent-based water-soluble cleanser that also contains menthol and peppermint, which are irritating for the skin and the eyes. This cleanser is not recommended.

☺ **Face Lotion Wash** *($14 for 6.7 ounces)* is more of a cold cream than anything else and it would require a washcloth to get all of your makeup off. But at least they left the menthol out of this version.

☹ **Face Soap Wash** *($15 for 5 ounces)* is a standard, detergent-based bar cleanser that also contains sodium xylenesulfonate and sodium lauryl sulfate, and that adds up to irritation.

☺ **Face Soothing Wash** *($17 for 6.7 ounces)* is just a detergent-based water-soluble cleanser that also contains Vaseline. It would work well for dry skin, but the price is high for what you get and it also doesn't replace a lot of other gentle products being sold at the drugstore.

☺ **Eye Color Remover** *($12 for 6.7 ounces)* is a standard eye-makeup remover that contains mostly water, glycerin, slip agent, detergent cleansing agent, more slip agents, thickeners, plant extracts, and preservatives.

☹ **Face Soother** *($15 for 6.7 ounces)* lists its third ingredient as witch hazel, and that is hardly soothing—it is a potential skin irritant.

☹ **Skin Energizing Mist** *($10 for 3.38 ounces)* contains witch hazel as the first ingredient, which can be irritating and drying for most skin types, as well as several irritating plant extracts including peppermint and citrus.

☹ **Face Exfoliant** *($15 for 3.3 ounces)* contains menthol and peppermint, and is not recommended.

☺ **$$$ Face Mild Exfoliant** *($15 for 3.3 ounces)* is definitely milder than the one above. It would work well for normal to dry skin, but for the money and effect, baking soda with Cetaphil works just as well.

☺ **Face Day Protection Fluid SPF 15** *($19 for 1.7 ounces)* is a good, though overpriced, avobenzone-based sunscreen for normal to oily skin types. It definitely contains oil-absorbing ingredients that can be helpful for oily skin, mixed in with thickening agents, silicone, vitamins, preservatives, and plant extracts.

☺ **Face Night Relief Gel Cream** *($26 for 1.7 ounces)* is supposed to be for normal to oily skin but contains too many problematic ingredients for these skin types. It would work well for normal to dry skin as a moisturizer. It also contains minute amounts of vitamins, plant extracts, and some interesting water-binding agents.

☺ **Face Night Relief Cream** *($26 for 1.7 ounces)* is a good emollient moisturizer for dry skin that contains mostly water, silicone, thickeners, emollients, plant oil, vitamins, and preservatives.

☹ **Eye Treatment Gel Cream** *($25 for 0.5 ounce)* has aluminum starch (octenyl succinate) as the second ingredient, which is a substance good for absorbing moisture but not for adding anything to skin. This is a confusing formulation that isn't great to use anywhere near the eye area. It also contains peppermint, a skin irritant. That may swell the skin around the eye but won't help anything.

☹ **Face Blemish Control** *($12 for 0.5 ounce)* contains alcohol as the second ingredient, which makes it too irritating for all skin types.

## Club Monaco Makeup

**FOUNDATION:** Club Monaco discontinued its Liquid Makeup, undoubtedly due to its confusing similarity to its ☺ **Oil-Free Foundation** *($19)*, which remains. Oil-Free Foundation offers an impressive array of shades that are almost all neutral (only Beige 6 is suspect for being slightly orange). It blends on well and the coverage is light to medium, with a natural, soft-matte finish. Sadly, this is not appropriate for oilier skins, as it is too emollient to keep shine at bay. This formula also uses isopropyl myristate as its third ingredient, which is suspect for clogging pores. If you have normal to dry skin, be it light or dark, give this one a test drive.

☺ **Wet/Dry Powder Makeup** *($22)* is a standard powder foundation with a sheer coverage and a soft, dry finish. The colors are slightly peach, but the finish is almost too sheer to notice. You may find this works better for you as a pressed powder, so test it out alone and with foundation if possible.

☺ <u>**CONCEALER:**</u> This **Concealer** *($11)* is a rare find, with a beautiful selection of neutral shades that go on smoothly, cover well, and do not crease! It is a strong option for those who use concealer, but be wary of shade Neutral 4, which can be too ash for most skin tones.

☺ **$$$** <u>**POWDER**</u>: Both the **Loose Powder** *($19)* and **Pressed Powder** *($19)* have a great, seamless finish and a soft, slightly dry texture. Although overpriced, they feature some great colors that serve the purpose of a good powder. Avoid Enhancer 1 (very yellow) and Enhancer 2 (a strong peach). **Bronzers** *($21)* offer three believable tan shades with only a slight shine. They blend on sheer and would work well to mimic "sun-kissed" color on the face or body.

<u>**BLUSH:**</u> If there's one thing "designer" lines seem to have in common, it's good blush. Almost without exception, the textures are smooth and silky and the available shades are quite workable and matte. Club Monaco's ☺ **$$$ Blush** *($16)* follows suit, offering both silky-sheer matte and shiny colors (easily identified). There are some unusual shades here, but they are worth a try.

☹ **Cheek Dew** *($15)* is a cream blush that comes in a pot and is more greasy that creamy. If this look (glossy cheeks) appeals to you, try mixing Vaseline over your regular blush and see how you like it before buying this.

☺ <u>**EYESHADOW:**</u> Club Monaco's **Eyeshadow** *($12)* has a large selection of shades with three distinct finishes. The **Mattes** are almost matte though there is a subtle shine to many of them, but it's hardly noticeable. The **Satins** have more of a sheen than a straight shine and may be an option for evening. The **Frosts** are shiny to the max and are best avoided. These are also less smooth than the Matte or Satin finishes, and may flake off. All three finishes offer a soft, sheer application that blends and builds well to create a subtle eye design.

☹ **Shimmer** *($15)* are small vials of loose, shiny, colored powders. If you want shine, there are plenty of pressed powders around that can provide the same performance without the mess and flaking this product has.

☹ **Eye Grease** *($13)* is, just as the name implies, a very greasy cream eyeshadow. Three of the colors are very dark, in shades of navy, brown, and black. The other three colors are pale shiny colors of gray, white, and gold. I'm sure this creates some kind of current trendy look, but putting on eyeshadows that you know are going to smear and crease on purpose is a look I hope will be a thing of the past in short order.

☺ **EYE AND BROW SHAPER:** **Eye Pencil** *($10)* is a standard, fairly creamy pencil and not worth the money. **Brow Pencil** *($10)* is slightly creamier than the eye pencil but only slightly and also not worth the money.

☺ **LIPSTICK AND LIP PENCIL:** There are four types of lipsticks here, all nicely organized into a dizzying palette of colors. **Cream Lipstick** *($13)* is a standard, good creamy lipstick with a slightly glossy finish. **Sheer Lipsticks** *($13)* are similar to the Cream Lipstick, only more glossy and not as opaque. **Cream Frost** *($13)* is identical to the Creams, but with iridescence. **Matte Lipstick** *($13)* is more creamy than matte, but this is what passes for matte in most makeup collections these days. The Matte Lipsticks offer the richest colors, with full coverage and a creamy finish that has enough stain to allow it to last through your morning coffee break.

☹ **Lip Gloss** *($13)* is about as boringly standard and overpriced as gloss gets. **Lip Pencil** *($10)* has a creamy texture and is not as pigmented as other standard pencils, so don't count on it for longevity.

☺ **MASCARA:** **Mascara** *($12)* provides decent length and thickness but it is not a better option than several less expensive drugstore mascaras, and the brush is almost too small for a quick application.

☺ **$$$ BRUSHES:** Club Monaco's **Brushes** *($12 to $38)* do not disappoint if you are expecting a good selection, and although the bristles are not as soft as some other lines (Stila, Bobbi Brown, and Lancome all have softer ones), the shapes and sizes are well matched to a variety of needs and should work well. The **Fluff Dusting Brush** *($38)*, **Large Angled Contour** *($34)*, **Round Blending Brush** *($22)*, and most of the **Eyeshadow Brushes** *($15 to $30)* are worth a closer look to see if they meet your needs. The rest of the brushes are either too soft, too small, or too floppy to allow for precision application and can be passed up without a worry.

## *Color Me Beautiful*

Carole Jackson hasn't owned this line for some time. The Color Me Beautiful public relations department told me it would probably be best to remove her name from this introduction. Somehow that seems like sacrilege. Carole Jackson introduced the art of wearing the right colors for your skin type to an entire generation of women via her "seasons" theory, which explained what colors work best with a particular skin tone and hair color. Once a woman knew whether she was a Spring (blonde hair and pink skin tones; requires pastel colors with a yellow undertone), Summer (blonde hair and sallow skin tones; requires pastel colors with a blue undertone), Autumn (red hair and pink skin tones; requires yellow-based earth tones), or Winter (brunette or black hair and any skin color; requires vivid blue-toned pastels), she could find colors that enhanced her skin tone instead of draining the color from it. This philosophy has clearly changed the way women shop for clothing and makeup colors.

Ms. Jackson created this makeup line in response to the demand for her color expertise. Sadly, with or without her, the line doesn't deliver the color organization you may be looking for. The color trays are divided into the appropriate seasons, but many of the colors overlap and not all of the appropriate color swatches are represented. Some colors are in both the Winter drawer and the Spring drawer, which doesn't make any sense given Jackson's beliefs about color. Also, some of the eyeshadows and blushes are just too shiny; and some of the foundation colors are overwhelmingly peach and pink, colors that are far from beautiful for any face. The foundation colors are divided into the four seasons groupings, but, because the shades overlap, there are really only two color groupings, not four. Although I agree wholeheartedly with the idea of using color to complement and enhance skin tone, all foundations should be neutral. Dividing these foundations into color groupings doesn't make sense. Just because a woman's skin has pink tones doesn't mean she needs a pink foundation. Her underlying skin color is still neutral. Adding pink to already pink skin only makes the skin look more pink and artificial. And there is never a reason to buy a peach-colored foundation. In fact, when I asked the salespeople if they sold much of the peach-colored foundations, they said no, none at all. What a surprise! For more information about Color Me Beautiful, call (800) 533-5503 or visit the Web site at www.colormebeautiful.com.

## Color Me Beautiful Skin Care

☺ **Creamy Cleanser for Dry Skin** *($15.50 for 6 ounces)* is a very greasy mineral oil– and Vaseline-based wipe-off cleanser. It is more a cold cream than anything, which isn't great for skin, but what is really a problem for skin are the lemon, orange, grapefruit, and lime oils in this product, which are all fairly irritating.

☺ **Foaming Cleanser for Normal/Oily Skin** *($15.50 for 4.5 ounces)* is a standard, detergent-based water-soluble cleanser that would work well for most skin types, though the fragrant oils can be fairly irritating.

☺ **Lathering Cleanser for Normal/Dry Skin** *($15.50 for 4.5 ounces)* is similar to the Foaming version above and the same comments apply.

☹ **Makeup Remover Gel** *($13 for 2 ounces)* contains pine and lemon extracts that can irritate the skin, especially the eye area, though the amount is small enough that they might not be a problem. The other ingredients are minimally passable for working as an effective makeup remover, and all in all, this product just leaves a lot to be desired.

☹ **Balancing Toner for All Skin Types** *($12 for 6 ounces)* contains grapefruit, citronella, and witch hazel, which are too irritating for all skin types.

☹ **Refining Toner for All Skin Types Except Very Oily** *($13 for 6 ounces)* contains a host of irritating plant oils, including lemon, orange, lime, and grapefruit.

☺ $$$ **Visible Results Glycolic Skin Conditioner for All Skin Types** *($18.50 for 1 ounce)* is a very good 8% AHA product for normal to dry skin.

☺ $$$ **Instant Result Mask for All Skin Types** *($16.50 for 4 ounces)*. There isn't enough AHA here for it to work as an exfoliant, but combining scrub particles with a BHA is too irritating for many skin types anyway.

☹ **Multi-Action Booster** *($22.50 for 1 ounce)* is supposed to "fight time with a vitamin-and-mineral-packed anti-wrinkle serum." What it can primarily do for the skin is cause irritation due to the plant extracts and oil of lemon, pine, grapefruit, mandarin, and citronella it contains.

☺ **Thirst Aid Anti-Wrinkle Serum for Dehydrated/Mature Skin** *($24.50 for 1.1 ounces)* contains several potentially irritating plant extracts and oils. Other than that it is a good, though standard moisturizer for someone with normal to slightly dry skin. It does contain emu oil, which is extracted from a large bird native to New Zealand. It is a good emollient and water-binding agent and has anti-inflammatory properties but it is not a miracle for the skin.

☺ **Thirst Aid Intensive Night Treatment for Normal/Dry Skin** *($24.50 for 2 ounces)* is a good emollient moisturizer that thankfully leaves out several of the irritating plant extracts that show up in so many of these products. The pH of this product (and the paltry amount of AHA) makes it ineffective as an exfoliant. For the emu oil here, see the comments above.

☹ **Daily Defense Light SPF 15 for Normal/Combination Skin** *($17.50 for 1.6 ounces)* doesn't contain avobenzone, zinc oxide, or titanium dioxide, and is not recommended.

☹ **Daily Defense Oil-Free SPF 15 for Oily Skin** *($17.50 for 1.6 ounces)* doesn't contain avobenzone, zinc oxide, or titanium dioxide, and is not recommended.

☹ **Daily Defense Rich SPF 15 for Dry Skin** *($17.50 for 1.6 ounces)* doesn't contain avobenzone, zinc oxide, or titanium dioxide, and is not recommended.

☺ $$$ **Triple Action Eye Cream, All Skin Types** *($18.50 for 0.5 ounce)* is a very good moisturizer for dry skin.

☺ $$$ **Eye Lift Firming Gel** *($18.50 for 0.5 ounce)* has the potential of being a good lightweight moisturizer for normal to dry skin. It does contain a teeny amount of arnica, which is a problem when applied over abraded skin. It also contains a teeny amount of vitamin K but that has no effect on dark circles.

☺ $$$ **Retinol PM Capsules, Cellular Recovery Complex** *($22.50 for 30 capsules)* is just silicones, retinol, and fragrance. If you want retinol, this is as good an option as any.

☺ **C-Plex Time Capsules, Facial Age Defying Treatment** *($20 for 30 capsules)* uses ascorbic acid, which is considered to be one of the more irritating forms of vitamin C. If you're looking for vitamin C this isn't the product to consider.

☹ **Fade Away for All Skin Types SPF 15** *($15 for 1.9 ounces)* has an SPF 15 but it doesn't contain UVA-protecting ingredients so it is not recommended for sun protection. However, it does contain 2% hydroquinone, and that can inhibit melanin production. This product also contains sodium lauryl sulfate, which makes it potentially irritating on skin.

## Color Me Beautiful Makeup

**FOUNDATION:** ☺ **Liquid Foundation** *($16)* is quite good with a light, creamy, soft texture, but it is only for someone with normal to dry skin. Some of the 14 colors are quite good, but the ones that are bad are *really* bad. These colors are too intensely peach or pink: Beige Blush, Cool Beige, Peach Blush, Warm Beige, Country Blush, and Mahogany. There are no real options for darker skin tones.

☹ **Soft Focus Skin Perfecting Oil-Free Foundation SPF 8** *($18.50)* has a poor SPF number (SPF 15 is the standard) and it doesn't contain reliable UVA-protecting ingredients. There is nothing else about this formula that warrants the expense. It is not recommended.

☺ **Illusion Age Defying Foundation SPF 15** *($20)* is a very creamy and soft cream-to-powder foundation that has a slippery feel and slightly greasy finish. The SPF is part titanium dioxide, and there is every reason to give this a try if you have normal to slightly dry skin. There are 11 shades, and the ones to avoid for most skin tones include Sand, Cool Beige, Porcelain, Ecru, and Ivory.

☺ **Perfection Microfine Powder Foundation** *($20)* is a pressed powder–type foundation that has a great dry but soft texture and mostly wonderful colors. It's pricey, but worth a look for normal to slightly dry or slightly oily skins. Of the 14 shades, these are too pink for most skin tones: Rosy Glow and Pink Sand.

☹ **Color Adjuster** *($15)* is a light mint green foundation meant to reduce pink skin tones, and is just like any other color corrector in any format: an extra, unnecessary step that can leave a strange hue on the face.

**CONCEALER:** ☺ **Cover Stick** *($9)* is a lipstick style concealer with a greasy texture that blends easily but can also easily slip into lines around the eyes. If you aren't concerned about concealer slipping into lines around the eye then the four shades may be worth a look as they have become more neutral and less pink than when last reviewed.

☹ **Dual Concealer Pencil** *($10)* is a double sided, thick pencil that has a greasy texture and comes in one duo shade set only, and it's noticeably peach. **Eyeshadow Base** *($9.50)* is applied like a concealer over the eye area. It dries to a sticky powder finish, and doesn't hold eyeshadow any better than using nothing at all. The color this comes in won't work for many skin tones and will alter the color of the eyeshadow you apply over it.

POWDER: ☺ **Translucent Loose Powder** *($13.50)* is a standard, talc-based powder that has a smooth, dry finish and a small but good selection of colors.

☹ **$$$ Bronzer Duos** *($16)* are grouped in the tester drawers with the blushes, and in spite of some good color choices, all of them are shiny enough to look obvious in daylight.

☺ BLUSH: **Powder Blush** *($12)* comes in a nice array of colors and has a smooth application. There are some shiny ones to avoid but some decent matte ones to check out. A few of the colors go on strongly and could work for darker skin tones.

☺ EYESHADOW: The **Eyeshadows** *($9)* are sold as singles and have a great silky texture that applies evenly and blends softly. Many of the colors are vivid and/ or shiny, but there are matte shades worth a test drive.

☹ EYE AND BROW SHAPER: **Smudgeliner** *($9.50)* is a standard pencil that has a sponge tip on one end to soften the line, which is a decent option for applying pencil. **Brow Color** *($12)* is a dry eyeshadow for the brows and is a great way to softly define and fill in the brows, although any matte eyeshadow that matches your brow color would work just as well, and this product only has two color choices, which is, to say the least, limiting. **Brow Fixative** *($9.50)* is standard, clear brow gel that can nicely keep brows in place, just like hairspray on a toothbrush can, which costs far less money.

☺ LIPSTICK AND LIP PENCIL: **Cream Lipstick** *($10.50)* comes in a pared- down range of colors, at least since the last time this line was reviewed, and is a good but basic creamy lipstick that has a slightly glossy finish and not much of a stain, so don't expect these to make it past mid morning before needing a touch-up.

☹ **Color Fix Lip Seal** *($10.50)* is an interesting product made up of alcohol and a film former. This places a layer of hairspray over the lips, which can feel strange and irritating—but it does keep lipstick in place longer than if you didn't use it. **Lip Pencil** *($8)* is a ho-hum standard pencil whose colors are merely OK and there aren't many to choose from.

MASCARA: ☺ **Lush Lash** *($9.50)* is an excellent mascara. It goes on easily, doesn't smudge and builds long, relatively thick lashes.

☹ **Sensitive Eyes Mascara** *($9.50)* doesn't go on as well as the Lush Lash and takes a long time to build any length or thickness. It may or may not be better for sensitive eyes— there is little difference between these two mascara's ingredients list— but it isn't better for defining lashes than the Lush Lash above.

## Complex 15 (Skin Care Only)

☺ **Complex 15 Cream** *($5.99 for 2.5 ounces)* and **Complex 15 Lotion** *($5.99 for 8 ounces)* are simple, rather ordinary moisturizers that have been around for a long time. They get recommended by dermatologists a lot, which is the primary reason they stay on the market, but I wonder if any dermatologist has checked out the ingredient labels. They're not bad, just boring. There are far more elegant and interesting formulations out there. Also, without sunscreen, these are only an option for nighttime. For more information about Complex 15, call (800) 842-4090 or visit the Web site at www.drugstore.com.

## Coppertone (Sun Care Only)

Coppertone makes one of the most woefully disappointing groups of sunscreen products around. Except for its **Shade UVA Guard SPF 30** (the first avobenzone-based sunscreen available in the United States that is now under the Coppertone label), all the other sunscreens in its lineup have no real UVA protection—there's no titanium dioxide, zinc oxide, or avobenzone in any of them. Clearly, with the inclusion of products that do contain avobenzone, it's not as if the Coppertone people don't know about the issue. One word of caution: for some reason, Coppertone also has a product called **Shade SPF 45** that does not contain avobenzone or any other UVA-protection ingredients, and that sounds a lot like its **Shade UVA Guard SPF 30**. Coppertone also boasts that its sunscreens for kids are the ones recommended most by pediatricians. If that's true, be sure you find another pediatrician. It would mean your doctor doesn't have the latest information on sun damage from UVA rays, and I would worry about what else he or she wasn't up to date on. For more information on Coppertone, call (908) 604-1640 or (800) 842-4090 or visit the Web site at www.coppertone.com.

☺ **Shade Sunblock Spray Mist SPF 30** *($6.99 for 4 ounces)* is a good in-part avobenzone-based sunscreen. Although you will get UVA protection from this one, it also contains about 80% alcohol, which can be drying and irritating for all skin types.

☺ **Shade UVA Guard Sunblock Lotion with Parsol 1789 SPF 30** *($6.99 for 4 ounces)* is a good, in-part titanium dioxide–based sunscreen for someone with normal to slightly dry skin or slightly oily skin.

☺ **Aloe Aftersun Gel** *($4.49 for 16 ounces)* is mostly aloe, water, slip agent, glycerin, preservatives, and coloring agents. It should feel soothing and minimally moisturizing on skin.

☺ **Cool Beads! Aftersun Aloe Gel, Light, Summertime Fragrance** *( $5.49 for 16 ounces)* is similar to the Aftersun version above and the same comments apply.

☺ **Cool Beads! Aftersun Moisturizer with Vitamins A + E** *($4.99 for 12 ounces)* is similar to the Aftersun version above and the same comments apply.

☺ **Cool Gel Aloe Aftersun** *($5.49 for 16 ounces)* is similar to the Aftersun version above and the same comments apply.

☺ **Gold After Sun Cool Gel, with Vitamin E & Aloe** *($5.29 for 12 ounces)* is similar to the Aftersun version above and the same comments apply.

☹ **After Sun Aloe & Vitamin E Moisturizing Lotion** *($4.79 for 16 ounces)* is a standard mineral oil–based moisturizer that also contains cocoa butter and lanolin. This is very emollient and best for dry skin; do not use this on sunburn, as the occlusive formula could exacerbate the burn effect.

☹ **4 Waterproof UVA/UVB Protection, PABA Free Moisturizing Suntan Lotion** *($4.79 for 4 ounces)*; **8 Waterproof UVA/UVB Protection, Ultra Moisturizing with Aloe & Vitamin E Sunscreen Lotion** *($4.79 for 4 ounces)*; **Bug & Sun Sunscreen with Insect Repellent, Adult Formula, SPF 15** *($6.99 for 4 ounces, $8.59 for 8 ounces)*; **Bug & Sun Sunscreen with Insect Repellent, Kids Formula, SPF 30** *($6.99 for 4 ounces, $8.59 for 8 ounces)*; **Gold Dark Tanning Exotic Oil Spray, with Vitamin E & Aloe** *($5.29 for 8 ounces)*; **Gold SPF 2 Dark Tanning Dry Oil, with Vitamin E & Aloe** *($5.29 for 8 ounces)*; **Gold SPF 4 Dark Tanning Oil, with Vitamin E & Aloe** *($5.29 for 8 ounces)*; **Gold SPF 2 Dark Tanning Exotic Lotion, with Vitamin E & Aloe** *($5.29 for 8 ounces)*; **Gold, Tan Magnifier Intensive Oil Spray** *($5.49 for 8 ounces)*; **Gold Tan Magnifier Intensive Oil, with Vitamin E & Aloe** *($5.29 for 8 ounces)*; **Gold Tan Magnifier Solar Gel, with Vitamin E & Aloe** *($5.29 for 8 ounces)*; **Kids Colorblock Disappearing Purple Sunblock, Waterproof, SPF 40, 6 Hour** *($6.99 for 4 ounces, $8.59 for 8 ounces)*; **Kids Colorblock Disappearing Colored Sunblock Lotion SPF 30** *($7.99 for 8 ounces)*; **Kids Colorblock Disappearing Colored Sunblock Spray SPF 30** *($7.99 for 8 ounces)*; **Kids Colorblock Wacky Foam SPF 40 (4 different scents/colors)**; *($10.99 for 6 ounces)*; **Kids Spray & Splash Sunblock Spray SPF 30** *($7.79 for 8 ounces)*; **Kids Sunblock Lotion SPF 30** *($6.99 for 4 ounces)*; **Kids Sunblock Stick SPF 30** *($3.99 for 0.6 ounce)*; **Kids SPF 40, 6 Hour Waterproof Sunblock Lotion** *($6.99 for 4 ounces, $8.59 for 8 ounces)*; **Little Licks Lip Balm with Sunscreen SPF 30** *($1.99 for 0.15 ounce)*; **Natural Fruit Flavor Lip Balm with Sunscreen SPF 15** *($1.99 for 0.15 ounce)*; **Oil Free Sunblock Lotion SPF 45** *($7.99 for 8 ounces)*; **Oil-Free Waterproof Sunblock, SPF 15** *($6.99 for 4 ounces, $8.59 for 8 ounces)*; **Oil-Free Waterproof Sunblock Lotion, SPF 30** *($6.99 for 4 ounces, $8.59 for 8 ounces)*; **Oil-Free Waterproof Sunscreen Lotion, SPF 8** *($6.99 for 4 ounces)*; **Shade Oil-Free Gel, SPF 30, UVA/UVB Protection** *($6.99 for 4 ounces)*; **Shade Sunblock Stick SPF 30** *($4.69 for 0.6 ounce)*; **Shade Sunblock Lotion, SPF 45, UVA/UVB Protection** *($6.99 for 4 ounces)*; **Sport Stick SPF 30** *($4.99 for 0.6 ounce)*; **Sport Ultra Sweatproof Dry Lotion SPF 15** *($7.99 for 8* *ounces);* **Sport Ultra Sweatproof Dry Lotion SPF 30** *($7.19 for 4 ounces);* **Sport All Day Protection, SPF 48, UVA/UVB Sunblock** *($6.99 for 6 ounces);* **Sport Sunblock Spray SPF 15** *($6.99 for 7 ounces);* **Sport Sunblock Spray SPF 30** *($6.99 for 7 ounces);* **To Go Sunblock Spray SPF 15** *($6.99 for 3.8 ounces);* **To Go Sunblock Spray SPF 30** *($6.99 for 3.8 ounces);* **Water Babies Lotion Spray SPF 30** *($8.99 for 8 ounces);* **Water Babies Lotion Spray SPF 30** *($8.99 for 8 ounces);* **Water Babies UVA/UVB Sunblock Lotion, SPF 30** *($6.99 for 4 ounces, $8.59 for 8 ounces);* **Water Babies UVA/UVB Sunblock Lotion, SPF 45** *($8.59 for 8 ounces);* **Waterproof Ultra-Moisturizing, SPF 15, with Aloe & Vitamin E** *($6.97 for 10.64 ounces);* **Waterproof Ultra-Moisturizing, SPF 30, with Aloe & Vitamin E** *($6.97 for 10.64 ounces);* **Waterproof Ultra-Moisturizing, SPF 45, with Aloe & Vitamin E** *($7.58 for 8 ounces);* and **Aloe & Vitamin Lip Balm with Sunscreen SPF 15** *($1.99 for 0.15 ounce).* All of the preceding products are not recommend either because they do not does not contain the UVA-protecting ingredients of titanium dioxide, zinc oxide, or avobenzone, or because they have SPF numbers under 15, which encourages tanning, causing a serious risk of skin cancer and skin damage.

## Corn Silk (Makeup Only)

How many of you remember Corn Silk from your teenage years? I know I do—hard to believe it's been around that long (myself included). Throughout its existence, Corn Silk has been synonymous with not having to worry about looking like an oil slick by midday. Corn Silk powder was supposed to be the oil-absorbing powder to end all powders. I recall buying it at several different junctures years ago, hoping it would work miracles on my sludge-laden skin. Sad to say, it didn't work wonders back then and it still can't today. In fact, there is very little about ☹ **Corn Silk Shineless Loose Powder** *($3.99)* and ☹ **Corn Silk Shineless Pressed Powder** *($3.99)* that I can recommend. The packaging doesn't allow you to see the colors at all, and most of them are slightly peach or pink (but still sheer), plus the darker shades and all of the loose powders have a subtle shine (who knows what they were thinking with that twist? powder is supposed to eliminate shine, not add to it). Although the powders are now mercifully fragrance free and they do have a dry, soft texture and apply very sheer, that isn't enough to make up for the initial drawbacks.

Corn Silk, which is now owned and distributed by the Sally Hansen Company, has added some ancillary products as a spin-off to its original powders. All of these products are also fragrance-free and replete with lots of oil-busting claims. For information about Corn Silk, call (800) 954-5080 or visit them on the Web at www. planetrx.com

☺ **Corn Silk Liquid Powder Concealer** *($4.29)* is a tube concealer with a wand application. It has a light, minimally creamy texture and dries quickly into place,

The Reviews C

leaving a soft matte finish. It comes in four shades, appropriate for light skin tones only. Due to the powdery finish, it can appear a bit chalky if you're too heavy-handed with your application or have any dry skin.

☺ **Powder Finish Cover Stick** *($4.29)* is a concealer in a lipstick tube that has a rather thick, somewhat heavy application. The four colors are good, but the opaque coverage does not look natural. For heavy coverage this may be an option.

☺ **Liquid Makeup** *($4.96)* has an incredibly limited number of shades, and clearly Corn Silk thinks only fair to light-skinned women have problems with oiliness. For those women, this can be an option for a decent matte-finish foundation that offers light to medium coverage and a fairly powdered finish. It blends well but you must be quick or this dries into place and is difficult to soften. Avoid Creamy Natural, Fair Beige, and Natural Beige; these shades are too pink or peach for most skin tones.

☺ **Zero Shine Powder Makeup** *($7.23)* is a powder-based foundation with a soft, matte, dry finish. The zero shine won't last all day, but it can make it through till lunch. The colors are only appropriate for very white skin.

☺ **Zero Shine Powderstick Makeup** *($6.99)* is a decently smooth stick foundation that comes in four OK colors and applies sheer and light. However, anyone with oily skin will cringe at the amount of waxes in here, which can exacerbate breakouts and do nothing to help with shine control in the least. Still, for a stick foundation, it does have a soft, matte finish and decent colors, and can be an option for someone with normal to slightly dry or slightly oily skin.

## Cover Girl (Makeup Only)

Every now and then, cosmetics companies do an about-face, with the results being nothing short of outstanding. Cover Girl is such a line and is no longer one you need to avoid, as it has introduced a far more elegant, sophisticated array of products (at least far more than before). From my perspective, this merits a name change from Cover Girl to Cover Woman!

Cover Girl has been putting on a whole new look and it's an impressive face-lift. As this book goes to press, Cover Girl is in the process of a major overhaul of its entire line, eliminating most (though not all) of the overly fragranced (meaning malodorous) foundations, blushes, eyeshadows, and pressed powders. Even more significant is its elimination of all of the poor foundation textures, chalky powders, and flaky eyeshadows. It's out with the old and in with the new, featuring some great options and some of the best prices you will find at the drugstore. Before I get too carried away, I should state that some of the powders still have a wafting, sweet fragrance and are, at best, overpowering. Yet points like this are now the exception to the rule and are forgivable due to the fine tuning and positive changes afoot.

Cover Girl's Web site and its consumer relations number are both helpful if you have any questions or concerns. Since many products were discontinued, you may be wondering what new (and pleasantly improved) item has replaced what's gone. It is clear that Cover Girl is starting the millennium with the best intentions and an eagerness to provide not only superior products but also superior service. For more information about Cover Girl, call (800) 543-1745 or visit the interactive Web site at www.covergirl.com.

FOUNDATION: Cover Girl would win even higher marks if it would only pattern itself after sister company Olay and provide adequate testers for all of its products. While some stores do sell mini samples of certain formulas, those are few and far between. For now, and even though the colors have gotten remarkably better, without testers the chance of buying the wrong color is fairly high.

☹ **Clean Makeup Sheer Stick Foundation** *($7.49)* is another option for stick foundation, only there are just six shades to choose from. These are decent options but this formula has a creamy feel and slightly greasy finish that would not please those with any oily areas. For those with normal to dry skin who are looking for a creamy, sheer coverage makeup, it may be worth a test drive but this product serves little purpose and isn't really worth considering. Avoid Honey, it can be too peach, though the colors are so sheer it probably doesn't matter.

☺ **Fresh Look Clear Up Tinted Acne Treatment Cream** *($5.49 for 0.65 ounce)* is a very good 10% benzoyl peroxide in a non-irritating, matte-finish gel base. It is also supposed to be a slightly tinted concealer, but it does a poor job of concealing anything. What it does a very good job of is disinfecting and that is an important step in the treatment of breakouts. However, 10% is quite strong and not the best place to start for all skin types. It would be far better to start with a lower concentration of this active ingredient and move up gradually if your acne is resistant to the lower levels.

☺ **Fresh Look Makeup Oil-Free SPF 15 for Combination to Oily Skin** *($7.79)* has an incredibly reasonable price, the SPF 15 is titanium dioxide–based, the finish is nicely matte (though not as matte as Revlon's ColorStay Lite SPF 15), and there is a huge assortment of colors to choose from, 16 in all. Wow! It really is a great new formula with a smooth, even application and no noticeable fragrance. What a difference from the old Cover Girl! There are shades for very light skin tones, but nothing suitable for darker skin tones. These colors are too peach, pink, or rose for most skin tones: Natural Ivory, Creamy Beige, Warm Beige, Natural Beige, Medium Light, Tawny, Toasted Almond, and Soft Sable.

☺ **CG Smoothers All Day Hydrating Makeup** *($7.29)* actually has great colors (16 in all)—what a shame the color on the container doesn't even vaguely resemble the color inside. For example, the color swatch for Ivory looks like a rather deep beige, but on the skin it's actually an extremely light, almost whitish beige! The talc content gives this sheer-to-medium coverage foundation a soft matte, slightly powdery finish, which is anything but hydrating. It would work well for someone with normal to oily or combination skin.

☺ **CG Smoothers Tinted Moisturizer** *($7.29)* has a name that says it all. These are exceptionally sheer moisturizers that impart the smallest amount of color to the skin. The three shades aren't bad, but this is appropriate only for dry skin because it contains both mineral oil and lanolin oil, which are both too emollient for any other skin type. Perhaps Cover Girl will go one step further and add sunscreen to this dry-skin formula to further its appeal, because until it does, you would still need a sunscreen underneath, unnecessarily doubling up moisturizers on the face.

☹ **Clean Makeup** *($5.69)* is one of the original Cover Girl foundations that hasn't yet been discontinued, but hopefully that's just a matter of time because it contains clove, menthol, camphor, and eucalyptus, which are extremely irritating for skin, plus the colors are largely unusable for any skin tone and the fragrance is intrusive.

☺ **Clean Makeup Fragrance Free** *($5.69)* mercifully deletes the sickly sweet scent from the one above, as well as the irritating extracts. Unfortunately, almost all of the 15 shades (with the exceptions of Ivory and Classic Ivory) are just too peach, pink, or rose for most skin tones.

☹ **Simply Powder Foundation** *($7.29)* goes on thick and heavy, and easily cakes on the skin. It's a lot more than powder, it's a messy layer over the skin and way below my new expectations for Cover Girl.

☺ **Ultimate Finish Liquid Powder Makeup** *($7.29)* features a nice smooth texture, although the aluminum starch (second ingredient) is a skin irritant and the isopropyl myristate in here can aggravate breakouts. It may be OK for normal skin types not prone to blemishes. Drier skins will find it just exaggerates every dry skin cell. The 16 shades are a mixed bag; half of them are too peach, pink, or rose for most skin tones. Avoid Natural Ivory, Creamy Natural, Classic Beige, Medium Light, Warm Beige, Creamy Beige, Natural Beige, and Toasted Almond.

☺ **Continuous Wear Makeup** *($7.39)* has 15 mostly excellent shades (including colors for darker skin tones) that blend on smoothly and would work well for someone with normal to dry skin seeking sheer to light coverage. Unfortunately, since the container is opaque, it is next to impossible to identify your possible color—a serious shortcoming I hope will be corrected at some point.

CONCEALER: ☺ **CG Smoothers Concealer** *($5.59)* is a standard, lipstick-style concealer that doesn't go on as greasy as it appears and provides good coverage with minimal creasing. However, the six shades are on the peach side, and this is opaque enough for that to be a problem for some skin tones.

☺ **Invisible Concealer** *($3.99)* is a surprisingly excellent, affordable concealer.

The six colors are great for lighter to medium skin tones, and it applies smoothly and evenly without creasing! This is one to try.

**POWDER:** ☺ CG Smoothers Fresh Look Pressed Powder Combination to Oily Skin *($5.59)*, ☹ CG Smoothers Fresh Look Pressed Powder Normal to Dry Skin *($5.59)*, and ☹ Clean Pressed Powder Normal Skin *($3.99 in regular or fragrance-free)* are all talc-based powders that have a similar sheer, smooth, almost invisible finish despite the different names and formulations. The colors are all decent, with only a few having slightly pink or peach tones, but so slight it's barely worth mentioning. What is most disappointing is that the powders are packaged in such a way that it is very hard to see the color. Some stores do have an enclosed powder display (usually for the CG Smoothers powders), and this is a welcome bit of assistance. Though I rarely comment on a product's smell, the scents for the versions for normal to dry and normal skin are so pungent I just had to say something. In contrast, the Fresh version has minimal fragrance.

☹ **Professional Loose Powder** *($5.19)* comes in six mostly well-conceived shades, but that is cancelled out by the pointless inclusion of eucalyptus, camphor, and menthol—three potent irritants—and the sickly sweet fragrance.

☺ **BLUSH: Instant Cheekbones** *($4.99)* has three colors in one compact—a blush tone, a contour color, and a shiny highlighter. The colors for these and for the single blush version, **Cheekers** *($2.99)*, haven't been updated for some time, but that may be forthcoming given the sweeping changes at Cover Girl. In the meantime, these are all rather pastel and intense. That may be OK for darker skin tones, but anyone looking for subtle colors will be left out of the running. Most of the colors are slightly shiny, making these an option for normal to dry skin, as most oilier skin types should forgo artificial shine at all costs. Caution: if you are fragrance sensitive, you may want to consider other options, because the smell radiating from these could knock you off your feet.

☺ **CG Smoothers Cheek Glaze** *($5.99)* is a rather unusual twist-up gel blush that applies a very sheer, translucent veil of color. Don't let the perceived depth of these colors fool you! These will work best for normal to very dry skin that wants the slightest hint of color and a moist, slightly sticky finish. **Classic Color Blush** *($4.99)* is a larger-sized single powder blush that comes in four shades that are vivid but blend on sheer. These are fairly powdery, and the color intensity is too soft for darker skin tones.

☺ **EYESHADOW: Professional Eye Enhancers** *($4.69 "4 kit"; $4.29 "3 kit"; $2.79 "1 kit")* are labeled as matte or "perle," but most are very shiny to slightly shiny. Some of the matte shades are indeed matte (but be careful) and are worth checking out. Although in the past I downgraded these for their texture and cling, that seems to have changed and these are no longer textures to shy away from. Some of the 3-kit and 4-kit compacts have practical color combinations, so you can really use all the shades!

EYE AND BROW SHAPER: ☺ CG Smoothers Gel Eye Color *($5.59)* are chubby pencils that go on somewhat wet, which means they glide on easily, and then the color dries to a matte finish that doesn't budge or smear all day. By the way, though I love the way these pencils go on, trying to keep a point on the pencil isn't easy, and that makes it difficult to create a thin, controlled line. **Perfect Blend Eye Pencil** *($3.99)* is a fairly standard pencil that goes on slightly more dry than most others and has decent staying power. There are 11 shades to choose from, all with a sponge tip to ease blending. **Liquid Pencil Felt Tip Eyeliner** *($5.29)* is an excellent, gel-based liquid liner that applies easily and stays on without fading or chipping off. It is also very easy to wash off, so if you're a fan of this type of eyeliner, this is a strong contender. **Perfect Point Plus** *($4.49)* is an automatic eye pencil that glides on easily without being greasy and maintains a consistent, sharp point.

☺ CG Smoothers **Natural Brow and Lash Mascara** *($2.59)* is an acceptably priced, extremely standard clear brow gel that leaves a minimal sticky feel. This brush isn't ideal, but it works—just take care that you evenly coat the brows, because any clumps will dry and flake off, an unpleasant side effect of this particular gel formula. **Brow and Eye Makers** *($2.79)* feature two short pencils that are the same color. It seems you're supposed to use one for eyes and one for brows, but the dry, waxy texture of these makes them best suited for brow pencil, and then only if you insist on using pencil over powder.

☺ LIPSTICK AND LIP PENCIL: Cover Girl has streamlined its lipstick collection, and continues to offer impressive textures and a pleasing array of muted and bright colors. **CG Smoothers Hydrating Lipstick** *($7.19)* claims to provide just as much moisture for your lips as lip balm, but the fact is that most creamy, slightly greasy lipsticks (like this one) will do just that. This lipstick wears well and has enough stain to keep the color around for part of the day, which would be a better basis for a catchy claim. **Continuous Color Self-Renewing Lipstick** *($4.49)* is available in Cremes, Shimmers, and Sheers. All of these are accurately named and have dropped the silly claim that all you have to do is press your lips together to renew the color, which can be attributed to almost any lipstick. These all have a smooth, slightly greasy texture. The Sheers are more fleeting, but the Cremes and Shimmers (which aren't too shiny) have enough stain to go the distance, at least until lunch! **LipSlicks Lip Gloss** *($3.29)* is a basic, emollient gloss with some very shiny shades in packaging that makes getting it on the lips very tricky for anyone with thin lips. **Triple Lipstick SPF 15** *($5.89)* is one of the few lipsticks that offer UVA protection with an in-part titanium dioxide base. This is a creamy, semi-opaque formula with a slightly greasy finish and minimal stain. **CG Smoothers Lip Liner** *($5.59)* is as standard a lip liner as they come, in a nice though limited range of colors. These do need sharpening, and will work as well as any other pencil.

MASCARA: ☹ **Professional Advanced Mascara Curved Brush** *($4.69)* builds OK length and thickness, though I find the curved brush incredibly awkward to use. **Professional Advanced Mascara Straight Brush** *($4.69)* has an easier-to-wield wand than the curved version but this builds lashes unevenly, creating a choppy, brittle appearance.

☺ **Super Thick Lash** *($4.69)* is a great mascara, building long, thick lashes with only a slight tendency to clump. If you don't like the occasional clumpiness common to thickening mascaras, stay away from this one. **Natural Lash Darkener** *($4.69)* is advertised as making the lashes naturally darker with no apparent length or thickness and that is exactly the performance you can expect, plus it doesn't clump or smear in the least.

☺ **Professional Waterproof Mascara** *($2.61)* is a great improvement over Cover Girl's discontinued **Marathon Waterproof Mascara.** This formula applies easily and effortlessly builds nice length and some thickness. Best of all, it really does hold up when wet!

☹ **Remarkable Washable Waterproof Mascara** *($4.69)*—washable/waterproof, isn't that an oxymoron? Nonetheless, this applies evenly and builds good length and thickness. It isn't as waterproof as others; it withstands only a little water (such as a light rain) but does not hold up underwater, so swimmers and others will have to look elsewhere. As a plus, this does come off easily without taking your lashes with it!

☹ BRUSHES: Displayed under the heading "Makeup Masters," the small assortment of brushes is as masterful as signing your name in crayon. The **Large Blush Brush** *($4.59)* and **Medium Blush Brush** *($4.59)* are merely OK, with the bristles being too soft and too sparse for much control. The **Powder Brush** *($5.49)* has a flat-cut top, which tends to work against the natural contours of the face and makes it easy to overpowder.

# *Darphin*

I don't know quite how to present this shockingly flawed, inferior, and overpriced line. Not only are the prices unwarranted for what you get, the formulations are some of the most dated, mundane concoctions I've encountered in a long time. For those who think that buying a line with a French accent is somehow going to net them better skin, I can almost guarantee that the purchase of a group of Darphin products will just bring them problems. Several of the products contain a range of irritating ingredients, including alcohol, camphor, lemon, and menthol. The AHA products do not contain AHA. The basic thickening agents and water-binding agents are not unique in the least. And the (missing) icing on the cake is that there are no sunscreens recommended for part of a daily skin-care routine. I imagine that there may be some emotionally pleasant sensation that accompanies the purchase of these products. Perhaps the act of actually purchasing a $175 moisturizer or a $50 cleanser feels good but, regrettably, none of that will help your skin. If you're going to spend this kind of money for skin care, though it is anyone's guess why you would, I'd suggest you look to lines that are at least well-formulated, with state-of-the-art water-binding agents, sunscreens, AHA or BHA products, topical disinfectants, and antioxidants.

Darphin's makeup selection seems to be little more than an afterthought. The company's brochure states that its makeup line "was created for women who demand only the finest ingredients and the latest technology in makeup." In reality, even those women who have no expectations from their makeup will walk away either in sticker-shock at the prices or puzzled by such an ordinary, run-of-the-mill group of products making extraordinary, absurd promises. There is nothing here that cannot be found countless times over (and many times better) in almost every other makeup line reviewed in this book. For more information about Darphin, call (888) 611-3003 or visit the Web site at www.darphin.net.

# Darphin Skin Care

☹ **Purifying Cleansing Milk** *($48 for 6.7 ounces)* contains menthol and camphor and is absolutely not recommended.

☹ **Purifying Toner** *($48 for 6.7 ounces)* lists the second ingredient as alcohol, and it also contains witch hazel and camphor, all of which can irritate and inflame skin.

☺ $$$ **Oil Free Exfoliating Foam Gel** *($40 for 4.2 ounces)* is a shockingly standard, detergent-based scrub that uses polyethylene (ground-up plastic) as the abrasive. This would work, but for the money it is just embarrassing to even consider it as an option.

☹ **Intensive Purifying Complex** *($85 for 1 ounce)* has alcohol as the second ingredient, and the fragrant oils are high up on the ingredient listing, making this anything but purifying, though it can be intensely drying and irritating. The tiny amount of tea tree oil in this product is not enough for it to be effective as a disinfectant.

☹ **Aromatic Purifying Balm** *($100 for 1 ounce)* contains several problematic plant extracts that can be skin irritants, and is not recommended. It does contain tea tree oil but the amount is not enough to be effective as a topical disinfectant.

☹ **Desincrustant Lotion** *($40 for 1.7 ounces)* lists the third ingredient as sulfur, and that's followed by lemon and arnica extract. As if that weren't enough, this lotion also contains menthol and camphor. All of these are extremely irritating and problematic for skin and this product is absolutely not recommended.

☺ $$$ **Purifying Aromatic Clay Mask** *($45 for 1.7 ounces)*. The soothing agent is negated by the presence of several irritating plant extracts. Other than that, this is

The Reviews D

an OK mask for normal to oily skin, though the thickening agents in here can be problematic for someone with blemish-prone skin.

☹ **Cleansing Aromatic Emulsion** *($40 for 4.2 ounces)* contains sodium lauryl sulfate relatively high on the ingredient list, which makes it a potential skin irritant for all skin types. Other than that, this is a confused product with mineral oil as the second ingredient (which can leave a greasy film on the face) and detergent-cleansing agents (which can dry the skin). It also contains some plant extracts that can be skin irritants and other plant extracts that can be irritating.

☹ **Vitalskin Aromatic Cleansing Milk** *($40 for 6.7 ounces)* contains arnica high up on the ingredient list, which can be a potent skin irritant and should not be used over abraded skin.

☹ **Camomile Aromatic Care** *($59 for 0.5 ounce)* would be a good blend of plant oils but it also contains several fragrant plant oils that can be skin irritants, including lavender, cypress, and bergamot. If you like the idea of the standard plant oils in this product for your skin—sweet almond oil, jojoba oil, and hazelnut oil—using those straight out of the bottle from the health food store would be far better than putting this fragrant, overpriced concoction on your skin.

☺ **$$$ Aromatic Balancing Day Cream** *($75 for 0.7 ounce)* is a good, though exceptionally standard moisturizer that could be easily replaced with just about any moisturizer from Clinique or L'Oreal (except those lines have better-formulated products).

☺ **$$$ Aromatic Soothing Cream** *($60 for 1.7 ounces)*. The amount of "good" ingredients is barely present and the fragrant oils in here are all serious potential irritants.

☺ **$$$ Rose Aromatic Care** *($69 for 0.5 ounce)*. The plant oils in here are very basic and good for dry skin, so forgo the fragrance, which can be a problem for skin, and just use the same oils from your cupboard, namely hazelnut, almond, and sunflower.

☺ **$$$ Arovita Creme Aromatique with Fruit Acids** *($115 for 1.7 ounces)*. The pineapple and grape extract in here are unrelated to AHAs, and the imperceptible amount of those and the vitamin E is almost laughable. This is a good moisturizer for dry skin but given the price, shockingly lackluster and common.

☺ **$$$ Arovita Eye and Lip Contour Gel** *($65 for 1 ounce)* is a good emollient, though light-feeling moisturizer for normal to dry skin.

☹ **Stimulskin Cream** *($175 for 1.7 ounces)* lists the second ingredient as lemon, which is a significant skin irritant in this amount. Several of the plant extracts are anti-irritants but there are also several other plant extracts here that are fairly irritating. It does contain about 1% lactic acid (AHA) but that is not anywhere close to being enough for exfoliation purposes.

☺ **$$$ Stimulskin Complex** *($295 for ten doses—total 1 ounce)*. Several of the plant extracts are anti-irritants but several others in here are fairly irritating. This is indeed a good lightweight moisturizer for normal to slightly dry skin, but there isn't one aspect of this formulation that makes it worth even a fraction of the price (which is $4,720 for 16 ounces).

☺ **$$$ Clear White Clarifying Milk** *($50 for 6.7 ounces)* is an ordinary wipe-off cleanser; it doesn't get any more standard and boring than this. The only thing outstanding about it is the price, which is more nauseating than anything else. Neutrogena's Extra Gentle Cleanser ($7.29 for 6.7 ounces) is almost identical and won't hurt your skin, while Darphin's contains plant extracts that can be anti-irritants as well as plant extracts that can irritate the skin.

☺ **$$$ Clear White Clarifying Essential Cream with Fruit Acids** *($95 for 1.7 ounces)* contains little that is beneficial for skin lightening in a very standard moisturizing base. While there is research showing vitamin C (magnesium ascorbyl phosphate) and mulberry extract may have some effectiveness for skin lightening (though not better than hydroquinone), the amount of mulberry and vitamin C in here is not enough to have any effect on skin. The lemon and pineapple extracts in here are also scant, plus they are unrelated to AHAs.

☺ **$$$ Clear White Clarifying Complex Intense** *($110 for 1 ounce)*. Several of the plant extracts are anti-irritants but there are others here that are fairly irritating. The same comments about skin lightening for the Essential Cream above apply for this one.

☺ **$$$ Clear White Clarifying Toner** *($50 for 6.7 ounces)*. This very basic toner would be good for most skin types, but while several of the plant extracts may be anti-irritants there are also several that are fairly irritating. The same comments about the skin-lightening properties of the Essential Cream above apply for this one.

☺ **$$$ Clear White Clarifying Mask** *($65 for 1.7 ounces)* includes zinc oxide as the second ingredient, so this emollient mask will go on looking white, but that won't change melanin production in skin. The same comments about the skin-lightening properties for the Essential Cream above apply here. This version does contain lactic acid, but only about 0.1%, which is eons away from having any effect on skin exfoliation.

☺ **$$$ Intralderm** *($40 for 2.7 ounces)*. The plant extracts in here can primarily be skin irritants, but aside from that this is just a good, lightweight moisturizer for normal to dry skin.

☺ **$$$ Reducing Cream** *($75 for 1.7 ounces)*. The wheat starch in here will give a matte feel to skin, but the effect is fleeting and it can be a cause of breakouts for blemish-prone skin.

☹ **Firming Vitaserum 70** *($125 for 1 ounce)* contains arnica and ginseng, both irritating plant extracts, in a very ordinary serum base of water, water-binding agents, preservatives, and fragrance. This is a huge "why bother?" unless you are interested in potential skin problems at the going price of $125 for 1 ounce.

☺ **$$$ Vitaserum Eye Contour 40** *($55 for 0.5 ounce)*. The potential for irritation from the salts in here is of concern, but other than that this is so astonishingly ordinary and do-nothing a formulation it is just mind-numbing.

☺ $$$ **Ecran Soleil SPF 30** *($50 for 1.7 ounces)* is a good in-part titanium dioxide–based sunscreen. It is almost identical to formulations at the drugstore from Bain de Soleil to Olay.

☺ **Soleil Filtrant SPF 25** *($48 for 5 ounces)* is similar to the Ecran version above and the same comments apply.

☺ $$$ **Vital Protection Day Fluid SPF 15** *($75 for 1 ounce)* is similar to the Ecran version above and the same comments apply.

☺ **Soleil Douceur** *($48 for 5 ounces)*. The soothing agents in this product are cancelled out by the presence of plant extracts that can be skin irritants. Aside from that, this is a good, though standard moisturizer for normal to dry skin.

☹ $$$ **Fibrogene Intensive Eye Contour** *($55 for 0.5 ounce)*. Though some of the plant extracts in here are soothing agents, there are also those that are potential skin irritants. This is an uninteresting, tonerlike moisturizer for normal skin.

☹ $$$ **Fibrogene Mask** *($65 for 1 ounce)* is a standard clay mask that also contains thickeners, plant extracts, preservatives, and fragrance. Though some of the plant extracts in here are soothing agents, there are also those that are potential skin irritants. Other than that, this is an uninteresting mask for normal to oily skin.

☹ $$$ **Intral Mask** *($50 for 1.7 ounces)*. Some of the plant extracts in here are soothing agents but others are potential skin irritants. This is a good, though ordinary mask for someone with normal to dry skin.

☹ $$$ **Mild Aroma Peeling** *($45 for 1.7 ounces)*, when rubbed over skin, will create exfoliation. That can feel good, but it can also be somewhat irritating. Basically this is just wax and some fragrance.

☹ $$$ **Nebulskin Aromatic Spray** *($29 for 3 ounces)*. This standard toner would be far better without the irritating plant extracts, but it would be suitable for most skin types.

☹ $$$ **Soothing Eye Contour Mask** *($68 for 1 ounce)* would be an OK light-weight moisturizer for normal to dry skin but it won't change any aspect of skin.

☹ $$$ **Vitalbalm Lip Care** *($20 for 0.12 ounce)* is a good but ordinary lip balm. This is all right, but not very emollient, and so incredibly *not* worth the price!

## *Darphin Makeup*

☺ $$$ <u>FOUNDATION:</u> **Teint de Rose Foundation** *($45)* has a moist, liquidy texture and is sheer enough to remind you of a tinted moisturizer, not foundation. For those with normal to dry skin with money to spare, this dewy-finish makeup is an option. The six shades offer choices for lighter skins only; darker skin toness would do well to avoid Sublime and Gold, both of which are too peachy.

☹ <u>CONCEALER:</u> **Concealer Pencil** *($30)* is a thick pencil that is greasy and hard to blend without pulling the skin. Plus the colors are, in a word, appalling with nary a natural skin tone in the bunch.

☹ <u>POWDER:</u> **Pastel Loose Powder** *($40)* is talc-based and very finely textured powder, yet of the two shades, one is sparkly and the other is too peach for most skin tones. **Harmonie Compact Powder** *($35)* is also talc-based and has a soft texture with noticeable shine. The colors are exceedingly unnatural and not worth considering for any skin tone.

<u>EYESHADOW:</u> ☹ **Aquarelle Eye Shadows** *($25)* are sold as singles and apply incredibly sheer. The colors are a hodgepodge of shiny vivids and a range of matte brown shades. The brown shades have a thicker, dry texture that are not the easiest to blend as they tend to grab and stick to skin.

☺ $$$ <u>EYE AND BROW SHAPER:</u> The **Eye Pencil** *($20)* and **Brow Pencil** *($20)* are ludicrously overpriced and both have standard textures and applications like pencils from L'Oreal to Revlon for a quarter of the price.

<u>LIPSTICK AND LIP PENCIL:</u> ☺ $$$ **Perfect Lipsticks** *($22)* make a big deal out of using the same plant wax (candelilla) and plant oils (castor) found in hundreds of other lipsticks. These are nothing more than greasy, semi-opaque lipsticks dressed up in opulent packaging. **Lip Pencil** *($20)* is a standard pencil with a smooth texture and slightly dry finish. There is a brush at one end to help with blending, but that extra touch doesn't justify the high price.

☹ $$$ **Perfect Gloss** *($20)* is a very thick, very sticky gloss that is very expensive for something so very basic.

☺ $$$ <u>MASCARA:</u> The **Mascara** *($20)* applies quickly, building lots and lots of length with minimal effort. Thickness is sketchy, but for those who just need lengthening mascara, this is definitely an option.

☺ $$$ <u>BRUSHES:</u> There are three **Brushes** *($30 and $50)* that are soft and workable, but at this price level they should be exceptional and they're not.

# DDF (Skin Care Only)

DDF is an acronym for Doctor's Dermatologic Formula. Is there any doubt what this line is supposed to represent to the consumer? Even more to the point, this line is one of the many headed up by Dr. Howard Sobel, a real, live, credential-packed dermatologist and plastic surgeon. According to Sobel, "Having an active full-time dermatology practice in Manhattan keeps me on top of skin care issues. I care about the quality and effectiveness of the products I use in my practice and dispense to my patients." As great as that sounds, there is no way these formulations substantiate the notion that this doctor is "on top of skin care issues." Most of the sunscreen formulations do not contain UVA-protecting ingredients, the cleansers contain ingredients that would be unsafe to get in the eye, many of the products contain fragrance (all potential skin irritants and sensitizers), several products contain alcohol and menthol (which are unnecessary skin irritants), and the claims about getting rid of wrinkles are completely without substantiation.

Yet there will be lots of consumers who will believe these products are superior because they carry a physician's endorsement. Regrettably that isn't the case for this line, which has nothing medical or otherwise professional about it. Highlighting the concern about just how serious the issue of doctors selling skin-care products is (and how prevalent), an article in the August 1999 issue of the *Tufts University Health & Nutrition Letter* stated that the "American Medical Association has issued guidelines advising physicians not to sell health-related products for profit. When a doctor stands to gain from something a patient buys, it creates a conflict of interest." The American College of Physicians–American Society of Internal Medicine issued ethical guidelines for physicians selling products, which were in turn reported in the *Annals of Internal Medicine* for December 7, 1999. The paper stated that sales of cosmetics and vitamins by physicians are "ethically suspect."

What is most distressing to me is that so-called dermatological lines like this one sell expensive sunscreens that are no different (and if anything worse) than sunscreens you would find at the drugstore or elsewhere for far less. Further, and according to the *Archives of Dermatology*, the problem with expensive sunscreens is that "… sunscreen users are only applying 50 percent of the recommended amount, so they are only receiving 50 percent of the SPF protection." How likely are you to apply the correct, liberal amount of sunscreen when 1 ounce costs over $20 or $25? And perhaps just as shocking is that a line represented by dermatologist would use fragrance when that is such a known source of skin irritation and dermatitis.

The strength of this line is that there are indeed some well-formulated topical disinfectants, AHA exfoliants, skin-lightening products, and moisturizers using some very good water-binding agents and antioxidants. And not all of the prices are hard to swallow. If you pick and choose there are some great products here to consider, but be wary and proceed with caution.

For more information about DDF, call (800) HDS-SKIN or visit the Web site at www.ddfskin.com.

⊗ **10% Glycolic Cleansing Pads** *($25 for 60 pads)* no doubt contain 10% glycolic acid, but they also contain alcohol and menthol, which are unnecessarily irritating and problematic for skin. This should not get in the eyes, and splashing the face makes that a potential risk.

⊗ **Acne Exfoliating Cleanser** *($26 for 4 ounces)* contains sulfur and resorcinol, which are topical disinfectants that are rarely used because they tend to be extremely irritating and sensitizing for skin. This should not get in the eyes and splashing the face makes that a potential risk.

☹ **Glycolic Exfoliating Wash 7%** *($31.25 for 8.45 ounces)* is a standard, detergent-based water-soluble cleanser that contains glycolic acid. The effectiveness of the glycolic acid would be rinsed away, but what might get left behind is the irritation of the mint oil in here. This should not get in the eyes and splashing the face makes that a potential risk.

☹ **Medicated Skin Cleanser 5% Benzoyl Peroxide** *($21 for 8.4 ounces)* is a standard, detergent-based cleanser that uses sodium C14-16 olefin sulfate as the cleansing agent, which makes it too irritating and potentially sensitizing for all skin types. The benzoyl peroxide is a good topical disinfectant, but in a cleanser its benefits would be washed down the drain. This should not get in the eyes and splashing the face makes that a potential risk.

☹ **Medicated Skin Cleanser 10% Benzoyl Peroxide & Tea Tree Oil** *($24 for 8.45 ounces)* is similar to the 5% version above and the same comments apply.

☺ **$$$ Non-Drying Gentle Cleanser** *($30 for 8.45 ounces)* is an exceptionally standard, detergent-based cleanser that would be good for most skin types except dry skin. The price is outrageous given what's in this ordinary formulation. It does contain coloring agents.

☹ **$$$ Salicylic Wash 2%** *($32.50 for 8.45 ounces)* is a standard, detergent-based water-soluble cleanser that contains salicylic acid (BHA). The effectiveness of the BHA would be rinsed away here, but other than that this is good for most skin types except dry skin. It is exceedingly overpriced for this standard formula. This should not get in the eyes and splashing the face makes that a potential risk.

☺ **$$$ Sensitive Skin Cleansing Gel** *($27.50 for 8.45 ounces)* is an exceptionally standard detergent-based cleanser that would be good for most skin types except dry skin. The price is outrageous given this ordinary formulation. It does contain coloring agents.

☺ **$$$ Wash off Cleanser** *($30 for 8.45 ounces)* is an exceptionally standard, detergent-based water-soluble cleanser that would be good for most skin types except dry skin. The price is outrageous given this ordinary formulation, and it does contain coloring agents. This version also contains lemon oil, which can be a skin irritant, though it is primarily in here as fragrance.

☺ **Bergamot, Herbal, Strawberry, or Coconut Face and Body Polish** *(each one is $22 for 8.45 ounces)* all use almond meal and polyethylene (ground-up plastic) as a scrub in a standard, detergent-based water-soluble cleanser. It would work, though the fragrance in here is completely ill conceived in a supposedly dermatological line of skin-care products.

☺ **Pumice Acne Scrub 2¹/₂%** *($25 for 8.5 ounces)* thankfully doesn't really contain pumice; rather, it uses polyethylene (ground-up plastic), which is far easier on skin, in a standard, detergent-based water-soluble cleanser. Benzoyl peroxide is an effective topical disinfectant, but it would be rinsed away before it had much of a chance to make a difference.

☻ **Aloe Toning Complex** *($20 for 8.45 ounces)* lists the third ingredient as witch hazel. That contains a large concentration of alcohol, making this potentially drying and irritating for skin.

☻ **Glycolic Toner 5%** *($22 for 8.45 ounces)* contains alcohol and menthol, which makes it too irritating for all skin types.

☻ **Glycolic Toner 10%** *($32.50 for 8.45 ounces)* contains alcohol and menthol, which makes it too irritating for all skin types.

☺ **$$$ Marine Balancing Spray** *($42 for 4.4 ounces)*. Algae has water-binding and antioxidant properties for skin (derived from seaweed and pond scum), but not anything unique or special among lots of other plant extracts or antioxidants.

☺ **$$$ Bioactive Nourishing Serum** *($52 for 1 ounce)*. You would be far better off using plain jojoba oil (the main oil in this product) to avoid the list of fragrant plant extracts here that can all be potential skin irritants. The water-binding agents are nice and the plant extracts can be good anti-irritants, but that isn't worth $52 for 1 ounce given the amount of them in here.

☻ **EPF Moisturizer C3 SPF 15** *($70 for 1.8 ounces)* does not contain the UVA-protecting ingredients titanium dioxide, zinc oxide, or avobenzone, and is absolutely not recommended.

☺ **$$$ EPF Environmental Protection Serum C3** *($60 for 1 ounce)*. If you are looking for a topical vitamin C product, this would be one to consider, as it definitely contains the more stable form and a good amount of it. This can be helpful for reducing irritation and melanin production.

☻ **Glycolic Gel 10%** *($32.50 for 2 ounces)* lists alcohol as the second ingredient, which makes this too irritating and drying for all skin types.

☺ **Glycolic Moisturizer 10%** *($32.50 for 2 ounces)* is a good 10% AHA exfoliant in a very standard moisturizing base. There are teeny amounts of good antioxidants in here but that doesn't help the exfoliation and it minimally helps skin.

☺ **$$$ Nourishing Eye Cream** *($35 for 1 ounce)* is a good moisturizer for normal to dry skin.

☺ **$$$ Retinol Eye Renewal** *($49.50 for 0.5 ounce)* does contain retinol; however the glass packaging guarantees it will break down and be ineffective in days. Because retinol is so unstable, it requires opaque and preferably airtight packaging. L'Oreal, Lancome, Alpha Hydrox, and Neutrogena all have retinol products that meet these fundamental criteria. Aside from that, this is a good moisturizer for normal to dry skin. It does contain fragrance.

☺ $$$ **Retinol Energizing Moisturizer** *($85 for 2 ounces)* is similar to the Eye Renewal version above and the same comments apply.

☺ $$$ **Retinol Energizing Serum with Protein Complex** *($85 for 2 ounces)* is similar to the Eye Renewal version above and the same comments apply. This one also contains BHA, but the pH is not low enough for it to be effective as an exfoliant.

☺ $$$ **Soothing Eye Gel** *($35 for 1 ounce)* is a very good lightweight moisturizer for normal to slightly dry skin.

☺ **Ultra Lite Oil Free Moisturizing Dew** *($26.25 for 2 ounces)* is a good moisturizer for someone with normal to dry skin, though it is not oil-free, and the thickening agents in here are not the best for someone looking to avoid pore-clogging ingredients.

☺ $$$ **Vitamin K Cream** *($45 for 1 ounce)*. The only research establishing vitamin K as being effective for reducing the presence of capillaries on the surface of skin was done by the company that manufactures the ingredient, and by the patent holder. Not only that, the study merely looked at 28 women who applied this vitamin K cream and who then, a few weeks later, reported on how they liked it. That isn't a scientific study by any standard; it isn't double-blind, nor were the results measured by any known protocols. This is a good moisturizer for normal to dry skin, and that's it. It does contain scant amounts of vitamin C and kojic acid, which could have potential for affecting skin color, but not in this amount.

☺ $$$ **Erase Eye Gel** *($37.50 for 0.5 ounce)*. For what this can do, please refer to the comments about vitamin K, kojic acid, and the vitamin C content of the Vitamin K cream above.

☹ $$$ **Infusia Vitamin K Kit** *($23.95 for four sheets and activator mist)*. The film former (hairspray) lining the patches in this product doesn't help skin, though it does keep the patches in place. There is no benefit to sleeping in these bandages. The claim that the product can penetrate 20 layers is meaningless; cellular layers are microscopic and that amount is completely insignificant for skin. The plant extracts can be anti-irritants. The activator mist is mostly water with trace amounts of vitamins. See the Vitamin K Cream above for the comments about the vitamin K in here.

☹ $$$ **Infusia Blemish Patches** *($19.95 for 16 patches and activator mist)*. See the comments for the Infusia Kit above for the effect of the these patches. This product contains a small amount of BHA and azelaic acid. While those two ingredients can absolutely be helpful for skin, you would be far better off buying these separately and applying them without these patch contrivances. The plant extracts in here can be skin irritants, as can the film former of polyvinyl alcohol.

☹ $$$ **Infusia Nose Pore Patches** *($19.95 for 16 patches and activator mist)* is similar to the Blemish version above and the same comments apply.

☹ **Moisturizing Photo-Age Sunscreen SPF 30** *($21 for 4 ounces)* does not contain the UVA-protecting ingredients titanium dioxide, zinc oxide, or avobenzone, and is absolutely not recommended.

☺ **Organic Sunblock SPF 30** *($21 for 4 ounces)* is a very good titanium dioxide–based sunscreen for someone with normal to dry skin.

☹ **Sport Proof SPF 30** *($21 for 4 ounces)* does not contain the UVA-protecting ingredients titanium dioxide, zinc oxide, or avobenzone, and is absolutely not recommended.

☹ **Sun Mist SPF 30** *($21 for 4 ounces)* does not contain the UVA-protecting ingredients titanium dioxide, zinc oxide, or avobenzone, and is absolutely not recommended.

☺ **2.5% Benzoyl Peroxide Gel** *($13 for 2 ounces)* is a very good, 2.5% benzoyl peroxide topical disinfectant for those with blemish-prone skin.

☺ **Benzoyl Peroxide Gel 5% with Tea Tree Oil** *($16.50 for 2 ounces)* doesn't contain enough tea tree oil for it to be effective as a topical disinfectant. Other than that, it is still an option as a 5% benzoyl peroxide topical disinfectant for blemish-prone skin.

☺ **10% Benzoyl Peroxide and 3% Sulfur Gel** *($17.50 for 2 ounces)* adds sulfur to benzoyl peroxide, and while that may help very stubborn acne problems, the risk of irritation and inflammation is probably not worth the risk.

☺ **$$$ Clay Mint Mask** *($24 for 4 ounces)* does contain mint, which is an unnecessary skin irritant for all skin types. Other than that, this is a standard clay mask that can help absorb excess oil like most clay masks can.

☺ **$$$ Detoxification Mask** *($22.50 for 2 ounces)* is just clay, and that won't detox anything, although it is a good absorbent for use on oily skin.

☺ **$$$ Fade Gel 4** *($42.50 for 1 ounce)* is a very good, 1% hydroquinone-based skin lightener that also contains AHA, kojic acid, and azelaic acid. All of those are great options for inhibiting melanin production.

☹ **Fade Cream SPF 30** *($27.50 for 2 ounces)* does not contain the UVA-protecting ingredients titanium dioxide, zinc oxide, or avobenzone, and is absolutely not recommended.

☺ **Holistic Skin Lightener** *($37.50 for 2 ounces)* is an option for skin lightening if you are looking to use a well-formulated glycolic acid product that doesn't use hydroquinone. However, while this product does contain azelaic acid, mulberry extract, and kojic acid, which have been shown to be effective for inhibiting melanin production, the amount of these in here makes them only minimally (if at all) effective for that purpose. It contains ascorbyl palmitate, a form of vitamin C, but the research about vitamin C being effective for skin lightening is for magnesium ascorbyl palmitate, not ascorbyl palmitate.

☹ **Sulfur Therapeutic Mask** *($25 for 4 ounces)* does use sulfur, which can be a topical disinfectant but also a potent skin irritant. This version also contains alcohol and eucalyptus, adding irritation and no benefit to this basic clay mask.

☹ **$$$ Surface Peel Cream** *($23.75 for 2 ounces)* contains a minute amount of papain, which as an enzyme could have some exfoliating properties, but not at this amount. Basically this is just wax that you rub over the skin that will roll off dead skin cells. That can make skin feel softer but the effect can also be somewhat irritating.

☺ **$$$ Aloe Cort Cream** *($23.75 for 2 ounces)*. After using some of the products in this line you would need an anti-inflammatory product like this. However, this basic hydrocortisone cream is identical in effectiveness to Lanacort and Cortaid at the drugstore for less than $5 per ounce. The continuous use of hydrocortisone over time can actually cause skin damage by thinning the skin and breaking down the skin's support structure. If you are aware of this very serious shortcoming and plan only occasional use, it can be effective for reducing skin irritation, but there is no reason to use this one rather than the drugstore versions.

## *Decleor Paris (Skin Care Only)*

Perhaps now that Shiseido has purchased Decleor Paris, it will now be called Decleor Japan. That's unlikely as part of Shiseido's interest in this European high-end skin-care line is the image it carries. What Shiseido may have overlooked is that Decleor is almost all image by virtue of the fact that its products are some of the most standard, basic formulations around. None of the products in the line are nearly as impressive or as current as, say, some of the products from Estee Lauder, L'Oreal/Lancome, Alpha Hydrox, Neutrogena, Eucerin, or Avon. What can I say about a line whose average product costs about $50 and whose typical recommended skin-care routine ranges from $250 to $400 (and that doesn't include sunscreen)? What I really want to know is how women can be so misled into believing that exceptionally expensive lines have something to offer that other lines don't. Do they think that these elegant European lines have a roomful of elite scientists using special formulas that will finally erase those wrinkles and bumps that every other product they purchased promised to eliminate but evidently didn't? They don't, though that must be the dream. Basically, I've found nothing special or exclusive about the products offered by Decleor, except for the prices.

If you are one of those women who feel better spending excessive amounts of money on skin care, there are other better-formulated lines to consider with state-of-the-art formulations. It's not that this is a bad line, it is just a regular one with some plant extracts added to make it look exotic. Do be aware that this line consists of an incredibly redundant multitude of moisturizers, a pathetic display of sun protection, mediocre AHA products, no BHA product, and problematic cleansers. Of course, Decleor's brochure tries hard to convince you that every product it sells will bring a wrinkle-free nirvana to your face, but these formulations fall far short of the ad copy, and in more ways than one. For more information about Decleor, call (888) 414-4471 or visit the Web site at www.decleor.com.

☺ $$$ **Cleansing and Make-up Remover Cream** *($26 for 8.4 ounces)* is a fairly standard cold cream–style makeup remover that can leave a somewhat greasy film on the skin, but it may be an option for someone with dry skin.

☺ $$$ **Cleansing Lotion for the Eyes** *($18 for 4.2 ounces)*. This very standard eye-makeup remover is exceptionally ordinary. It also contains oak root extract high up on the ingredient list, and that can be an irritant for skin.

☺ $$$ **Cleansing Oil for the Face and Eyes** *($31 for 8.4 ounces)* is a lot of money for almond oil that you could easily pull out of the cupboard. It will remove makeup, but you'll have to wipe it off. This is an overpriced option for someone with dry skin.

☺ $$$ **Gentle Facial Cleanser** *($24 for 5 ounces)* is a mineral oil–based cleanser that also contains detergent cleansing agents. It also contains other plant oils and emollients, making it an option for someone with dry skin, though it can leave a greasy film on the skin.

☹ **Regulating Cleansing Gel** *($22 for 5 ounces)* is a water-soluble cleanser that uses sodium C14-16 olefin sulfate as the detergent cleansing agent. This ingredient is extremely irritating and drying for all skin types.

☺ **Velvet Cleansing Milk** *($24 for 8.4 ounces)* is a cold cream–like cleanser with basic thickening agents and plant oil. It needs to be wiped off and is embarrassingly overpriced for what you get. The linden extract in here *may* have some anti-inflammatory properties but it can also be a skin irritant.

☺ $$$ **Whitening Cleanser** *($33 for 8.4 ounces)* is a cold cream–like cleanser that contains a scant amount of mulberry extract. That does have some value in preventing melanin production, though there is only one study demonstrating this, and it used the pure concentration (not the minimal amount present in this product), and the study showed mulberry extract to be minimally effective when compared to hydroquinone and kojic acid.

☺ $$$ **Whitening Toner** *($33 for 8.4 ounces)* does contain mulberry extract, but see the comments for this ingredient in the above review for the Whitening Cleanser. The grapefruit extract in here can be a skin irritant.

☹ **Whitening Day Cream SPF 12** *($45 for 1.69 ounces)* doesn't contain the UVA-protecting ingredients titanium dioxide, zinc oxide, or avobenzone, and is not recommended. It does contain mulberry extract and the comments for this ingredient in the Whitening Cleanser above apply here.

☺ $$$ **Whitening Day Emulsion** *($38 for 1.69 ounces)* is an exceedingly average moisturizer containing mostly thickeners, silicone, plant oils, plant extracts, slip agents, and preservatives. It does contain mulberry extract, and the comments for this ingredient in the Whitening Cleanser above apply here.

☺ $$$ **Whitening Night Cream** *($51 for 1.7 ounces)* is similar to the Day Emulsion above, only more emollient, but the same basic comments apply.

☹ **Whitening Aromessence** *($70 for 0.5 ounce)* contains nothing that can lighten skin or inhibit melanin. This is more like putting perfume on your face than anything else, which is not helpful for skin in the least. Several of the fragrant oils in here can be irritants.

☹ **Whitening Powder Complex** *($70 for three 3-ounce vials)* is basically a serum lotion you mix with a powder of ascorbic acid. Ascorbic acid is not considered a stable form of vitamin C and the mulberry extract in the serum part of this product is too scant to have an effect on skin lightening.

☹ **Regulating Tonic Lotion for Combination and Oily Skins** *($30 for 13.5 ounces)* contains several irritating ingredients that are a problem for most skin types, including orris root, witch hazel, zinc sulfate, and chlorhexidine. All of these are known for their sensitizing potential. They may have some antibacterial property for skin, but the irritation would negate that benefit.

☺ $$$ **Soothing Cleansing Water** *($33 for 8.4 ounces)* is a good toner for someone with normal to dry skin but the fragrant oils and some of the plant extracts can be skin irritants.

☺ $$$ **Exfoliating Face Gel** *($26 for 1.7 ounces)*. The apricot kernels will exfoliate and this does rinse off, but it is incredibly overpriced for this standard formulation.

☹ **Face Peel for All Skin Types** *($31 for 1.69 ounces)*. The second ingredient is paraffin, which can clog pores. It also contains lemon oil and lavender oil, which can be skin sensitizers. The silicate in here can exfoliate the skin, but why stick in all these other ingredients that can cause problems?

☺ $$$ **Contour Firming Serum for the Eyes for All Skin Types** *($36 for 0.5 ounce)* is a rather standard, lightweight moisturizer that could be good for normal to slightly dry skin.

☹ **Day Alpha Hydrating Cream with Plant Extracts and Alpha-Hydroxy Acids, SPF 12, for All Skin Types** *($42 for 1.69 ounces)*. For the money you wouldn't want to short change yourself with anything other than an SPF 15, though this does contains part titanium dioxide as one of the active ingredients. The label claims to have a 6% concentration of AHAs but that isn't possible given the ingredient listing (or your face would be unhappy with the other ingredients that come before and would be in amounts that can hurt skin). At best there is about a 3% concentration, plus the pH is about 5, which makes it ineffective for exfoliation.

☺ $$$ **Day Hydrating Cream** *($56 for 1.69 ounces)* doesn't contain a sunscreen, which makes it a very poor daytime moisturizer, though it can be good for dry skin at night.

☹ $$$ **Essential Harmony** *($58 for 1.7 ounces)* is primarily hazelnut oil, which can indeed be emollient for skin, but given the abundance of fragrant oils in here that can be potential skin irritants, you would be far better off just using plain hazelnut oil that you buy from the health food store and skip the problematic ingredients in here altogether.

☹ $$$ **Eternance Cream for Mature Skins** *($53 for 1.69 ounces)* is a very ordinary, dated moisturizing formula. It would be good for someone with dry skin, but for the money there are more interesting and unique formulas out there. The ginseng in here can be a skin irritant.

☹ **Eye Contour Gel for All Skin Types** *($27 for 0.5 ounce)*. This standard gel formulation contains orris root, sweet clover, and rose water, all of which can be skin irritants. This gel is more a problem for skin than a help.

☹ $$$ **Firming Neck Gel with Plant Extract for Mature Skins** *($48 for 1.69 ounces)*. This minimally moisturizing gel has some algae, which can have antioxidant properties, but it also contains *Centella asiatica* that can be a skin irritant. This won't firm skin regardless of your age.

☹ $$$ **Hydra Matte Regulating Fluid** *($29 for 1.7 ounces)* has a minimal matte effect on skin that doesn't last very long. The amount of tea tree oil isn't enough to be effect as a disinfectant, but the orris root in here can be a skin irritant.

☹ $$$ **Instant Beauty Booster for All Skin Types** *($42 for 1.69 ounces)* would be an OK, lightweight moisturizer for someone with normal to slightly dry skin. Expecting anything in the way of instant beauty is great marketing, but this product won't do it.

☺ $$$ **Moisturizing Face Cream with Plant Extracts and Essential Wax for Normal Skins** *($50 for 1.69 ounces)* is a good lightweight, though overpriced, moisturizer for someone with normal to dry skin. The idea of essential waxes is an interesting slant, but I prefer mine in candles; that way they won't have a chance of clogging pores.

☹ $$$ **Moisturizing Face Cream for Dry Skins** *($50 for 1.69 ounces)* would be a good, though exceptionally standard moisturizer for someone with dry skin.

☹ $$$ **Soothing Anti Redness Day Cream** *($61 for 1.69 ounces)*. Some of the plants and oils in here can be skin sensitizers while others are anti-irritants, which sort of cancel each other out. The claim about reducing redness is bogus, and without a sunscreen this is useless as a daytime moisturizer.

☹ $$$ **Soothing Anti-Redness Serum** *($69 for 1 ounce)* is a good lightweight moisturizer for someone with dry skin, but several of the plant oils here are fragrant and can cause skin irritation.

☹ $$$ **Soothing Night Cream for Normal Skins** *($35 for 1.69 ounces)* would be a good though standard moisturizer for someone with normal to dry skin.

☹ $$$ **Stimulating Concentrate for Mature Skins** *($70 for 0.5 ounce)* is a group of very standard grocery store–type oils and fragrant oils. The fragrant oils—musk, clove, and cinnamon—can all be potential irritants, while the grocery-store oils are just fine for the skin.

☹ **$$$ Timecare Cream (Fruit Acids) for Mature Skins** (*$70 for 1.69 ounces*). Nothing in this cream will have any effect on aging skin, and there are no fruit acids (meaning AHAs) here, just plant extracts, which have nothing to do with effective exfoliation. Several of the plant oils in here are fragrant and can cause skin irritation. The linden extract in here *may* have some anti-inflammatory properties but it can also be a skin irritant.

☺ **$$$ Timecare Serum (Fruit Acids) for Mature Skins** (*$72 for 1 ounce*) makes the same claims as the cream above, but the formulations are completely different! This lightweight moisturizer does not contain fruit acids (or AHAs) and cannot change mature skin in any way. Several of the plant oils in here are fragrant and can cause skin irritation. It's a good lightweight moisturizer for normal to slightly dry skin.

☺ **$$$ Timecare Mask** (*$34 for 1.69 ounces*) is fine for a mask, but the miracles it's supposed to accomplish, from toning skin to erasing years off the face, don't hold water.

☺ **$$$ Vitalite Nourishing and Firming Face Cream** (*$56 for 1.69 ounces*) would be a very good moisturizer for someone with dry skin, but it isn't nourishing because you can't feed the skin from the outside in.

☹ **$$$ Vitarome Cream for Dry Skins** (*$39 for 1 ounce*) is a very good emollient (and standard) moisturizer for someone with dry skin, although it contains several fragrant oils that can cause skin irritation.

☺ **$$$ Contour Mask for Eyes and Lips All Skin Types** (*$31 for 1 ounce*) is a standard mask that places a layer of hairstyling-type ingredients over the face. It can't "contour" anything, but your skin will feel temporarily smoother when you take it off.

☺ **$$$ Moisturizing Creamy Face Mask for All Skin Types** (*$32 for 1.69 ounces*) contains a bunch of moisturizing ingredients, similar to those found in all the Decleor moisturizers, along with a film former. It is definitely creamy, and it could be a good mask, but the claims in the brochure have nothing to do with reality.

☹ **Regulating Face Mask for Combination Skins** (*$26 for 1.69 ounces*) is a standard clay mask that also contains lemon and camphor, which are unnecessary skin irritants and don't regulate anything.

☹ **Regulating Gel for Combination Skins** (*$27 for 1.69 ounces*) contains way too many irritating ingredients for any skin type. This won't improve imperfections, but it can cause them. This product contains alcohol, orris extract, lemon oil, and bitter orange oil, all highly sensitizing ingredients.

☹ **Regulating Peel Off Mask** (*$26 for 2.5 ounces*) is primarily water, polyvinyl alcohol (film former/plasticizing agent), and alcohol. The alcohol in here is too irritating, and peeling a layer of plastic off the face might make it feel temporarily smoother but it doesn't help skin in the long run.

☹ **S.O.S Regulating Tinted Gel** *($26 for 0.5 ounce)*. The amount of tea tree oil in here isn't enough to be a disinfectant, the color of this tint doesn't look like skin, the alcohol and orris root can be irritating, and the rice starch can trigger breakouts. You will need an S.O.S. after using this gel.

☹ **T-Zone Regulating Gel** *($29 for 1 ounce)*. The amount of tea tree oil isn't enough to be a disinfectant and the alcohol may be an irritant (though there is only a small amount in here). The film formers can leave a matte feel on the face but they minimally control oil; however there is nothing in here that will help blemish-prone skin.

☹ **High Protection Sun Cream Water Resistant SPF 15** *($26 for 4.2 ounces)* doesn't contain the UVA-protecting ingredients titanium dioxide, zinc oxide, or avobenzone, and is absolutely not recommended.

☹ **Moderate Protection Sun Cream Water Resistant SPF 15** *($26 for 4.2 ounces)* doesn't contain the UVA-protecting ingredients titanium dioxide, zinc oxide, or avobenzone, and is absolutely not recommended.

☹ **Kidsun Cream SPF 15** *($22 for 2.5 ounces)* doesn't contain the UVA-protecting ingredients titanium dioxide, zinc oxide, or avobenzone, and is absolutely not recommended.

☹ **Sea and Mountain Sun Protection Cream SPF 20** *($21 for 2.5 ounces)* doesn't contain the UVA-protecting ingredients titanium dioxide, zinc oxide, or avobenzone, and is absolutely not recommended.

☹ **Self Tanning Cream SPF 4** *($21 for 4.2 ounces)* can't protect skin from UVA rays, and the SPF is so low as to encourage the risk of skin cancer and wrinkles. This product is absolutely not recommended. It does contain dihydroxyacetone, which is the active ingredient in all self tanners, but the other aspects of this products are not worth the trouble.

☹ **Sensitive Zone Stick SPF 15** *($15 for 0.26 ounce)* doesn't contain the UVA-protecting ingredients titanium dioxide, zinc oxide, or avobenzone, and is absolutely not recommended.

☹ **Satin Bronzing Gel SPF 2** *($26 for 4.2 ounces)* has an offensively low SPF and doesn't contain the UVA-protecting ingredients titanium dioxide, zinc oxide, or avobenzone, and is absolutely not recommended. How ironic that this gel makes claims that it can fight free-radical damage.

☹ **Bronzing Emulsion SPF 4** *($26 for 4.2 ounces)* has an offensively low SPF and doesn't contain the UVA-protecting ingredients titanium dioxide, zinc oxide, or avobenzone, and is absolutely not recommended.

☹ **Sun Protection Cream SPF 8** *($26 for 1.69 ounces)* has an offensively low

SPF and doesn't contain the UVA-protecting ingredients titanium dioxide, zinc oxide, or avobenzone, and is absolutely not recommended.

☹ **Tan Accelerator** *($17 for 2.5 ounces)* is as unethical a skin-care product as I can imagine. It is one thing to sell creams that don't protect skin from sun damage; it is another thing to sell a product that encourages women to tan. Why doesn't this line hand out cigarettes too?

☺ **$$$ After Sun Face Mask** *($22 for 2.5 ounces)* is a good emollient mask, but there is nothing in here beneficial for the sun damage you will get from using the sunscreens from this line.

☺ **$$$ Aromaessence Solaire Defense** *($58 for 0.5 ounce)*. The absurdity of this product is that you are spending a lot of money for primarily sunflower seed oil, rice bran oil, and wheat germ oil, easily replaceable at any grocery store for a fraction of the amount, minus the irritating fragrance.

☺ **$$$ Natural Face Oil Neroli for Normal and Sensitive Skins** *($55 for 0.5 ounce)* is plant oil (mostly hazelnut and avocado), with some wax thrown in. That's good for dry skin, but the orange oil makes it a problem for sensitive skin.

☹ **Natural Face Oil Ylang Ylang for Combination Skins** *($55 for 0.5 ounce)* contains a group of oils that are primarily fragrant, feel greasy on the skin, and are known sensitizers.

☺ **$$$ Natural Face Oil Angelique with 100% for Dry Skins** *($55 for 0.5 ounce)* contains a group of oils that can be found on the grocery shelf plus a handful of fragrant oils. The basic oils are great for dry skin, but it would be much cheaper to buy and mix them together yourself, and that way you won't be slathering your face with fragrant oils, which can cause negative reactions.

☺ **$$$ Eye and Lip Precious Contour Balm for Mature Skins** *($34 for 0.5 ounce)* would be a good, but amazingly average moisturizer for someone with dry skin.

☺ **$$$ Aromatic Nutrivital Balm** *($54 for 1 ounce)*. You might as well just consider using the plant oils (primarily hazelnut oil that you can get at the grocery store) and forgo the thickening agents and fragrance in this balm.

☺ **$$$ Aromatic Timecare Balm** *($54 for 1 ounce)* is almost identical to the Nutrivital version above and the same comments apply.

☺ **$$$ Aromatic Harmony Balm for Sensitive Skins** *($52 for 1 ounce)*. This would be good for someone with dry skin, but the fragrant oils can cause problems for sensitive skin.

☺ **$$$ Essential Face Balm for Combination Skins** *($57 for 1 ounce)* has nothing essential in it, but it does contain plant oils and carnauba wax. Some of the oils are fragrant and can irritate the skin, while the wax can clog pores, and so this is inappropriate for oily or blemish-prone skin.

☺ **Prolagene Gel for Face and Body for All Skin Types** *($26 for 1.69 ounces)* has a very fancy name for a stunningly bland product. It contains mostly water, slip agent, thickener, fragrant oil, coloring agent, and preservatives. There is little this gel can provide for the skin, though it probably won't hurt anyone either.

# Derma Wand

This is the first "anti-aging machine" I've seen that comes with a warning. It clearly states, "Do not use Derma Wand on skin which is prone to excessive amounts of broken capillaries or on skin which is prone to rosacea." As forthright and valid as that warning is, that includes about 75% of the female American population. Almost all Caucasian women are prone to broken, surfaced capillaries. It doesn't take much to hurt delicate capillaries and produce a red, spiraling network across the face. And rosacea probably occurs in about 15% of the Caucasian population. That excludes a lot of women from using the Derma Wand, and we haven't even begun to discuss the claims.

The Derma Wand emits an electrical charge that supposedly generates some amount of ozone—that is, supercharged oxygen. It works sort of like a miniature stroke of lightning, and the user feels a slight sting, like a rubber-band snap, which isn't surprising given the electricity being generated. The zapping and the ozone production are supposed to help with the penetration of anti-aging creams and lotions. Naturally that assumes the anti-aging creams and lotions work in the first place, and will work even better if they penetrate the skin. Neither is the case, and anyway, oxygen can't help creams penetrate better, because the skin can't handle more oxygen than is already in the air. Even if it could, the possibility of damage from the electrical charge isn't worth it. The Derma Wand is also supposed to zap zits, because pure oxygen can kill the bacteria causing the blemish. The theory is sound, but skin cells are also destroyed by pure oxygen, and how the wand gets around this dilemma isn't explained. For more information about the Derma Wand, call (800) 704-1209.

# Dermablend

Dermablend is a small line of products designed to help women who may want to cover up some major skin problems. For those women who want to hide hyperpigmentation, vitiligo, port wine stains, or other skin imperfections, Dermablend's offer is hard to refuse. The question is how well these products work and whether they are good for the skin. The **Cover Creme Foundation** *($23; 15 shades)*, **Leg and Body Cover** *($14.50; 11 shades)*, **Quick Fix** *($15, cover stick; 7 shades)*, **$$$ Compact Cover Creme** *($16; 12 shades)*, **$$$ Setting Loose Powder** *($17; 1 shade)*, and **$$$ Setting Pressed Powder** *($17; 3 shades)* are supposed to provide complete, opaque coverage that can hide any kind of scarring or birthmarks (no matter how severe), or scarring on the legs. These are not lightweight products that magically place a camouflaging film over the face and legs. Not surprisingly, each product has an unusually thick texture that can blend out to thin but opaque coverage. This is heavy-duty stuff.

Most of the colors are actually quite good and natural. If you spread an even layer of any of the creamier cover products over your face or legs you can be assured of a good deal of coverage which, depending on the depth of the discoloration, will hide your problem from view. The deeper the discoloration, the less likely you will be able to conceal it. The question is, do you really want that much coverage? What you get in place of the discoloration is a noticeable layer of foundation. Even if this is spread as thinly as possible, it still has a heavy texture. Plus, the sheerer you try to make it, the less coverage you get. There is no way that these products can look totally natural, but they can cover.

The Leg and Body Cover can be a problem to use because even though it is waterproof and won't come off in the rain, it will rub off, and there's nothing you can do to prevent that. The Setting Powder, a white talc powder that looks very pasty on the skin, should not be used at all. Almost any neutral loose or pressed powder would work instead.

It's difficult for me to recommend this product line, yet I know that many women have strong feelings about their facial discolorations. I may think the heavy look of the foundation is no better than the discoloration itself, but the problem isn't on my face. Since emotions are strong when it comes to issues like this, testing the products yourself is the only way to make a decision, which is why I've left out face rating symbols for the makeup products mentioned above.

Dermablend also has a small ancillary group of skin-care products, reviewed below, that have few benefits and many shortcomings. For more information about Dermablend, call (773) 483-4100 or visit the Web site at www. sheen.com.

## *Dermablend Skin Care*

⊗ **Facial Cleanser** *($12.50 for 6.3 ounces)* is a standard, detergent-based water-soluble cleanser that could work well for someone with normal to oily skin, but the lemon, lime, grapefruit, and orange oils in here make this an irritation waiting to happen. It does contain coloring agents.

⊗ **Remover** *($14.50 for 6.3 ounces)* lists the second ingredient as tea-lauryl sulfate, and its potential to cause irritation and sensitizing reactions is a problem.

⊗ **Facial Toner, Normal to Dry** *($15.50 for 8.75 ounces)* contains witch hazel and is potentially too drying and irritating for most skin types. That's a shame, because overall the other water-binding agents and anti-irritants are quite good. This does contain retinol, but the packaging does not assure that it will remain intact.

⊗ **Facial Toner, Normal to Oily** *($15.50 for 8.75 ounces)* is almost identical to the version above for Dry skin and the same comments apply.

☹ **Maximum Moisturizer, SPF 15, PABA-Free** *($22.50 for 2 ounces)* doesn't contain titanium dioxide, zinc oxide, or avobenzone to protect skin from UVA damage, and is not recommended.

☹ **$$$ Wrinkle Fix Line Smoother for Lips and Eyes** *($14.50 for 0.12 ounce)* is little more than a lip gloss—it would be hard to get more greasy and ordinary than this. I would never recommend this for the eye area.

☺ **Advanced Fade Creme with Sunscreen and AHA** *($18.25 for 1.7 ounces)* doesn't contain titanium dioxide, zinc oxide, or avobenzone to protect skin from UVA damage and doesn't list an SPF number, so it is not recommended for sun protection. However, as a 1% hydroquinone-based skin-lightening product to fade brown spots or patching, it is very good for someone with normal to dry skin. It does contain fragrance.

☺ **Chromatone Plus Fade Creme with Sunscreen** *($15 for 3.75 ounces)* doesn't contain titanium dioxide, zinc oxide, or avobenzone to protect skin from UVA damage and doesn't list an SPF number, so it is not recommended for sun protection. However, as a 2% hydroquinone-based skin-lightening product to fade brown spots or patching it is very good for someone with normal to dry skin. It does contain fragrance.

## Dermalogica (Skin Care Only)

Image is a major factor in most women's decisions about buying products. The right image can convey the value of a company's products through an appeal to the emotions. A beautiful model, a charismatic actress, or a distinctive brochure and packaging can be all the impetus necessary to persuade unwary consumers to make a purchase. What other consideration is there for buying a cosmetic product—particularly a skin-care product? If a cream promises to firm the skin or protect it from environmental damage, we have very little to go on other than the impression we get from the advertising and the packaging (and, of course, the salesperson).

With that in mind, I have always been most intrigued by cosmetics lines that choose to create a scientific image instead of a glamorous one. Dermalogica has honed its image to a T. The name implies a relationship to dermatology, which sounds as if you are getting serious skin care. The subtitle on Dermalogica's products is even more commanding: "A Skin Care System Researched and Developed by the International Dermal Institute." But what is the International Dermal Institute? Are there any dermatologists there? Apparently not: the International Dermal Institute is a school for facialists who want an education beyond what is required for their cosmetology license, and the classes are taught by facialists. (If you're going to get a facial, although I would not suggest you spend your hard-earned money on one, it is best to go to someone who has training from somewhere other than just a cosmetology licensing school. In that regard, the International Dermal Institute provides a good, albeit expensive, service.)

Does the professional atmosphere of the school associated with Dermalogica mean better products? The proof is in the pudding, and this pudding is just Jell-O, not chocolate mousse. The company's literature expounds at length on the ingredients the products *don't* contain, such as mineral oil (because it's greasy and sits on the skin, although the same could be said of many of the plant oils and water-binding agents that the products do contain). But some of the products contain petrolatum, from which mineral oil is derived, so even if mineral oil were a culprit in skin-care products (it isn't), this line's claim that it doesn't contain any is misleading.

Dermalogica also wants us to know that its products don't contain isopropyl myristate, lanolin, or coal tar–based dyes, because, as the brochure explains, they can cause breakouts. That is true, but Dermalogica's products do contain ceresin, beeswax, forms of acrylate, and other ingredients that can potentially clog pores; they also use drying and irritating cleansing agents, as well as extremely sensitizing plant extracts that cause well-known problems Dermalogica doesn't want us to know about.

Another misleading statement is the claim that the products don't contain formaldehyde, a preservative that can cause problems for the skin. In fact, many of the products contain diazolidinyl urea, a preservative that can release formaldehyde. The products also claim to be fragrance-free, but many of the plant extracts and oils used in the products indeed provide fragrance. Fragrance, regardless of its origin, can be irritating to the skin. I could go on, but I'll let the products and their ingredient lists speak for themselves. For more information about Dermalogica, call (800) 831-5150 or visit the Web site at www.dermalogica.com.

☺ $$$ **Treatment Foundation** *($29)*. Dermalogica considers its foundations as part of its skin care treatments. The two foundations aren't treatments of any kind despite the "skin care merges with makeup" claims. This one has a lightweight, moist texture and sheer, minimally matte finish. The eight shades are OK, but these darker colors are too rose, ash, or orange for anyone to consider: Intensities 3, 4, and 5.

☹ **Color Corrector** *($15)* is identical in formula to the foundation above but has only two shades, a pure white one and a reddish bronze tone to "correct" skin color or customize the Treatment Foundation. It's an extra step you can easily skip if you had one good neutral foundation color.

☹ **Anti-Bac Skin Wash** *($34 for 16 ounces)* is an extremely drying detergent cleanser, and between the sodium C14-15 olefin sulfate, mint, menthol, and camphor it contains, this product is too irritating for words.

☺ **Essential Cleansing Solution** *($34 for 16 ounces)*. This cold cream–type wipe-off makeup remover would work for someone with very dry skin but the fragrant water can be a skin irritant. It can leave a greasy film on the skin.

☹ **Dermal Clay Cleanser** *($34 for 16 ounces)* contains menthol, mint, lemon, and arnica, all of which are too irritating for all skin types.

☺ **Special Cleansing Gel** *($34 for 16 ounces)* is a standard, detergent-based water-soluble cleanser that can be OK for someone with oily or combination skin. It contains a balm mint, which can be irritating for some skin types.

☺ **$$$ Soothing Eye Makeup Remover** *($15 for 2 ounces)* is a standard, detergent-based eye-makeup remover that would work as well as any. At least this one doesn't contain fragrance of any kind.

☹ **$$$ Gentle Cream Exfoliant** *($27.50 for 2.5 ounces)* contains several potentially irritating ingredients, including sulfur and lemon. The abrasive in here is seashells, and that is anything but gentle.

☺ **$$$ Skin Prep Scrub** *($22 for 2.5 ounces)* is a detergent-based water-soluble cleanser that uses cornmeal as the scrub. It would probably be better to just use cornmeal from the grocery store if you want a cornmeal scrub, then at least you wouldn't be applying some of the irritating plant extracts in here, including arnica and ivy.

☹ **Multi-Active Toner** *($21.50 for 8 ounces)* contains mint and lavender, which are too irritating for all skin types.

☺ **Active Moist** *($38.50 for 3.5 ounces)*. If it weren't for the potentially irritating plant extracts in this one, it could have been a good emollient moisturizer for someone with dry skin.

☹ **Active Firming Booster** *($41 for 1 ounce)* contains too many irritating plant extracts for all skin types, including lemon, arnica, pine, pellitory, and orange. This won't firm anything but it could cause a little inflammation.

☹ **Gentle Soothing Booster** *($41 for 1 ounce)*. Raspberry juice can be irritating for some skin types and may cause allergic reactions. Besides, there is no benefit in putting raspberries on the skin, especially not at $41 an ounce! This is one of the most do-nothing ingredient listings I've seen in some time.

☺ **$$$ Intensive Eye Repair** *($35 for 0.5 ounce)* is a good emollient moisturizer for dry skin, but it won't repair anything. It does contain some good emollients, water-binding agents, antioxidants, and vitamins, but if things did get repaired you wouldn't need to buy this product again, right? One word of warning: there is a small amount of arnica in here that can cause irritation especially around the eyes for some sensitive skin types. It does contain fragrance.

☺ **$$$ Total Eye Care SPF 15** *($33 for 0.75 ounce)* is a good lightweight moisturizer for normal to dry skin with a titanium dioxide–based SPF 15. It also contains lactic acid, though the product doesn't have a low enough pH for it to work as an exfoliant.

☺ **Intensive Moisture Balance** *($31 for 1.75 ounces)* is similar to the product above only somewhat less emollient. It would be good for someone with normal to dry skin. It does contain wild yam extract; for more explanation about why this extract has no effect on skin, please refer to the Appendix Dictionary.

☺ $$$ **Intensive Moisture Concentrate** *($45 for 1 ounce)*, like many moisturizers, uses a film former as the main ingredient. This places an imperceptible layer of plastic over the skin that helps the skin temporarily look smoother. It is just a good lightweight moisturizer for slightly dry skin. It does contain fragrance.

☺ $$$ **Specific Skin Concentrate** *($45 for 1 ounce)* is similar to the Intensive Moisture above, and the same review applies. This one does contain some potentially irritating plant extracts but the amount is probably too small to be a problem for most skin types.

☺ **Skin Smoothing Cream** *($42 for 3.5 ounces)* is a good emollient moisturizer for someone with dry skin. It contains all the appropriate emollients, plant oils, vitamins, and water-binding agents. It also contains some irritating plant extracts, but not very much of them, so it probably won't be a problem for most skin types.

☹ $$$ **MultiVitamin Power Concentrate** *($42.50 for 45 capsules)*. The plant oils in here are citrus and can be potential irritants. The form of vitamin C is ascorbic acid and that is considered not to be the best option for vitamin C as it can be too irritating (the stability is not an issue because it comes in capsule form). The vitamin A in here is the least active form, namely retinyl palmitate. If you're looking for a vitamin-type moisturizer, there are far better ones to consider than this.

☹ **Oil Control Lotion** *($27 for 1.7 ounces)*. This salicylic acid lotion also contains mint, camphor, and menthol, which won't control oil in the least, but will cause redness, dryness, and irritation.

☹ $$$ **Special Clearing Booster** *($37 for 1 ounce)* is a fairly expensive 5% benzoyl peroxide–based product. There are much cheaper benzoyl peroxides available at the drugstore, and I would recommend starting with a 2.5% benzoyl peroxide for breakouts before jumping to a 5% version, which can be far more irritating.

☹ **Skin Renewal Booster** *($41 for 1 ounce)* is a 10% AHA and 0.5% BHA product that also contains sulfur and salicylic acid. The pH of this product isn't low enough for the AHA or BHA to be effective exfoliants, and the sulfur is unnecessarily irritating.

☹ **Solar Shield SPF 15 (stick)** *($9.50 for 0.28 ounce)* doesn't contain avobenzone, zinc oxide, or titanium dioxide for UVA protection, and is not recommended.

☹ **Sunswipes SPF 15** *($28 per carton)* don't contain avobenzone, zinc oxide, or titanium dioxide for UVA protection, and are not recommended.

☹ **Full Spectrum Block, SPF 15** *($23 for 4 ounces)* doesn't contain avobenzone, zinc oxide, or titanium dioxide for UVA protection, and is not recommended.

☺ $$$ **Protective Self-Tan SPF 15** *($24 for 4 ounces)* doesn't contain avobenzone, zinc oxide, or titanium dioxide, and is not recommended for outdoor use; but as a self tanner it should work just fine.

☺ **Solar Defense Booster SPF 30** *($30 for 1 ounce)* does contain avobenzone, so this one has good UVA protection! However for some reason, this line is big on mint and lemon in its products, which just isn't the best for skin. This one even has lavender oil, a known photosensitizer (meaning sun exposure can trigger a reaction). What's that doing in a sunscreen?

☺ **Ultra Sensitive Bodyblock SPF 15** *($22 for 4 ounces)* is a pure titanium dioxide–based sunscreen but, like many other products in this line, it contains mint, lemon, grapefruit, and lavender, which have no place in a product for sensitive skin.

☺ **Ultra Sensitive Face Block SPF 25** *($22 for 1.75 ounces)* is similar to the one above and the same concerns apply.

☹ **Pigment Relief SPF 15** *($45 for 1.7 ounces)* doesn't contain avobenzone, zinc oxide, or titanium dioxide for UVA protection, and is not recommended. The mulberry extract in here has minimal to no effect on inhibiting melanin production.

☺ **$$$ Intensive Moisture Masque** *($32.50 for 2 ounces)* would be a good moisturizing mask for someone with dry skin, although a good emollient moisturizer left on the skin a little thicker and a little longer than usual can have the same effect. This does contain fragrance.

☺ **$$$ Skin Hydrating Masque** *($28.50 for 2.5 ounces)* contains vitamin K, which has no effect on surfaced capillaries, and the form of vitamin C in here (ascorbic acid) is considered to be unstable and potentially irritating.

☺ **$$$ Skin Refining Masque** *($27.50 for 2.5 ounces)* is a standard clay mask that contains little else besides clay. It would be a good mask to absorb oil though it does contain a small amount of irritating plant extracts.

☺ **$$$ MultiVitamin Power Recovery Masque** *($35 for 2.5 ounces)* is a standard peel-off mask. This won't change a wrinkle on your face but this can be a good mask for normal to dry skin. It contains mostly plant water, glycerin, film former, slip agent, thickeners, vitamins, plant oils, silicone, plant extracts, and preservatives. While most of the plant extracts in here are good anti-irritants it also contains lemon, which can be an irritant.

☹ **Skin Purifying Wipes** *($25 for 36 towelettes)* contain camphor and mint, and all I can say is ouch!

# DHC USA (Skin Care Only)

DHC is a Japanese cosmetics company that was launched in the United States several years ago. According to its brochure, the highlight of this line is a single bar of soap. The brochure states, "For more than 15 years women in Japan have relied on this clear, pure, gentle bar of soap." Do Shiseido, Fancl, or several other behemoth cosmetics companies in Japan know about this? Clearly this soap is not the raging success DHC would like you to believe because DHC is far from the largest cosmetics company in Japan. What is probably not surprising is that this soap is not unique in the least: it is a standard, tallow-based bar soap. Tallow can cause breakouts and the cleansing agents can be drying. Plus, if this was the be-all and end-all for soap, what are all the other cleansers in this line for?

The strong points for this line are that most of the products do not contain coloring agents, and the formulations are rather basic and straightforward, which is best for the way skin utilizes good water-binding agents and emollient oils. While DHC boasts that it doesn't use fragrance, that simply is not the case across the board. Some of these products absolutely contain fragrance in the form of fragrant extracts, and there are a handful of other irritating ingredients to look out for too, including alcohol, lemon, and ginseng (though this line does have far less use of these than many other lines). There are lots of good moisturizers to consider. You can ignore the claims about firming and getting rid of wrinkles; these products can't live up to those claims any more then any other cosmetics company's products can. While the latest fad ingredients are here—from vitamin C (the good one) and retinol (though not in packaging that will keep it stable)—they also want you to believe that olive oil will keep your skin young. Now, that's as wishful and unsubstantiated a claim as it comes.

By the way, DHC is great about sending samples of all its products, so you might want to take advantage of that. For more information about DHC USA, call 1-800-DHC-CARE or visit the Web site at www.dhccare.com.

☹ **Mild Soap** *($12 for 3.1 ounces)* is a standard, tallow-based bar soap made of lard and lye, just like any other soap. It does have an attractive appearance, but the lard can clog pores and the cleansing agents can be too drying for most skin types.

☺ **$$$ Deep Cleansing Oil** *($22 for 6.7 ounces)* actually doesn't contain much oil at all. This is just an emollient, wipe-off cleanser with a tiny bit of vitamin E for effect and rosemary oil for scent. The recommendation is to use this product with another cleanser in the line, and you would have to do that to get this stuff off the face.

☺ **Facial Wash for Oilier Skin** *($18 for 6.7 ounces)* is a standard, detergent-based water-soluble cleanser. This standard formulation is an option for normal to oily skin, though the cleansing agents can be somewhat drying and irritating for some skin types. It does contain fragrance.

☺ **Gentle Cleansing Foam for Normal Skin** *($14 for 4.9 ounces)* is a fairly alkaline cleanser that uses myristic acid and potassium hydroxide as the cleansing agents, and that can be too drying for most skin types. The little bit of olive oil in here won't undo the dryness of the cleansing agents.

☺ **Mild Cleansing Cream for Drier Skin** *($14 for 4.9 ounces)* is an exceptionally standard, mineral oil–based wipe-off cleanser. This is just pricey cold cream with lots of ordinary thickening agents and it doesn't rinse off the face, but it can be an option for someone with normal to dry skin.

☺ **Oil-Free Makeup Remover** *($15 for 3.3 ounces)* is a very standard, typical, detergent-based makeup remover that can work as well as any.

☹ **Facial Scrub** *($14 for 4.9 ounces)* uses apricot seeds as the exfoliant, along with some thickeners and fairly drying detergent cleansing agents, and that makes this a standard, OK exfoliant for someone with normal to oily skin.

☺ **Balancing Lotion for Normal Skin** *($12 for 6 ounces)* is a good, irritant-free toner that contains mostly water, glycerin, water-binding agents, AHA, and preservatives. There isn't enough AHA in here for it to act as anything other than a water-binding agent. That's not bad, just maybe not what you were expecting. One of the water-binding agents in here is placental protein; it's just a good water-binding agent, but I have to say that one always makes me uncomfortable—the skin can't tell the difference between sources of proteins, so why use placenta? It's just offensive.

☺ **Soothing Lotion for Drier Skin** *($12 for 6 ounces)* is similar to the Balancing Lotion above and the same comments apply. At least this one doesn't contain placenta.

☹ **Clean Finish Lotion for Oilier Skin** *($12 for 6 ounces)* is mostly alcohol, along with ginseng, sage, and resorcinol, and that makes it extremely irritating and sensitizing for all skin types.

☺ **Renewing AHA Cream** *($34 for 1.5 ounces)* contains 10% lactic acid (AHA), although the pH of this product is not low enough to make it very good for exfoliation. This is a standard (but good) moisturizing base.

☺ **AntioxC** *($32 for 1.4 ounces)*. The vitamin C in here is magnesium ascorbyl phosphate and that is considered to be a good, stable, and effective form, but it won't change a wrinkle, nor is it better than other antioxidants. The teeny amount of algae and kudzu vine in here have no impact on skin. This is a good, lightweight moisturizer for someone with normal to slightly dry skin.

☺ **$$$ Concentrated Eye Cream** *($29 for 0.7 ounce)* is a good lightweight moisturizer for someone with normal to slightly dry skin. The teeny amount of royal jelly can have emollient properties, but it is not an antiwrinkle cure, while the rosemary and ginseng extract in here can be skin irritants.

☺ **Dual Defense SPF 25** *($24 for 3.5 ounces)* is a good, partly titanium dioxide–based sunscreen for someone with dry skin. What is most disappointing about this line are all the moisturizers claiming to fight wrinkles, yet there's only one sunscreen, and it isn't for everyone as the copy claims, because someone with normal to oily skin would not be happy with this product that contains olive oil and rice oil.

☺ **Hydrating Nighttime Moisture** *($28 for 1 ounce)* is a very good, lightweight moisturizer for someone with slightly dry skin.

☺ **Light Moisture for Normal to Oilier Skin** *($24 for 3.3 ounces)* lists the second ingredient as olive oil, and some of the water-binding agents, like collagen, which is good for dry skin, aren't the best for oily skin. This is a good moisturizer for normal to dry skin; just don't use it over oily areas. It also contains retinol, but the clear packaging allows for decomposition of this highly unstable ingredient.

☺ **Oil-Free Hydrator for Oilier Skin** *($22 for 3.3 ounces)* could be a good, very lightweight moisturizer for slightly dry skin.

☺ **Rich Moisture for Normal to Drier Skin** *($24 for 3.3 ounces)* is a good emollient moisturizer for dry skin. The ginseng in here can be a skin irritant, though the amount is probably too scant to be of real concern. The minuscule amount of royal jelly can be an emollient but it serves no great purpose for skin care.

☺ **Extra Nighttime Moisture** *($30 for 1.5 ounces)* is similar to the Rich Moisturizer above and the same basic comments apply. This version does contain a minuscule amount of retinol but the clear packaging will cause this little amount to decompose quickly.

☺ **$$$ Wrinkle Relief** *($28 for 0.7 ounce)*. The teeny amount of royal jelly in here has little benefit for skin. In the long run, you would get just as much benefit by using pure virgin olive oil from your cupboard instead of this version. It does contain ginseng, which can be a skin irritant.

☺ **$$$ Collagen Eye Stick** *($29 for 0.12 ounce)* is a very emollient, clear, lip gloss–type moisturizer for the eyes. It is very emollient and good for very dry skin, but don't expect the collagen to do anything special; it's just a water-binding agent, nothing more. It can't help shore up your own collagen. If only it were that easy, given how long collagen has been around as a skin-care ingredient, none of us would have wrinkles.

☹ **Soothing Eye Gel** *($24 for 0 .7 ounce)* would just be a pretty do-nothing eye gel except this one contains orange peel and lemon, which can irritate the skin around the eyes.

☹ **$$$ Nourishing Mist** *($35 for 6 ounces)*. The price for this is a bit shocking. It can be a good, ordinary toner, but there isn't much reason to spray this on yourself. It's supposed to help with jet lag but I wouldn't use this over melatonin.

☺ **Pure Squalane** *($25 for 1 ounce)* is indeed pure squalane, a plant oil or shark oil (there is no way to know the source). There are lots of oils in the world you can use for far less cost than this one that would work well on dry skin. It is a good moisturizing ingredient, but no more so than safflower or sunflower oil from the grocery store.

☺ **Skin Conditioning Oil** *($30 for 1 ounce)* is just olive oil and some fragrance oils of lavender and rosemary. You don't need the fragrance, so all that counts is the olive oil. You can find much better olive oil than this at your grocery store for a lot less money and forgo the potentially skin-irritating fragrances.

☺ $$$ **Advanced Collagen Treatment** (*$40 for 1 ounce*) definitely contains collagen, but other than being a good moisturizer, this won't do anything else for skin. The collagen won't penetrate or affect the collagen in your skin in any way, shape, or form. It also contains minute amounts of algae and royal jelly, and while they can have some minor emollient and antioxidant properties, in this amount the effect is nonexistent.

☺ $$$ **Olive Virgin Oil** (*$36 for 1 ounce*). At first I thought this was a joke, but it isn't. This is pure virgin olive oil. Even if virgin olive oil was a great skin care ingredient, why would you bother buying this from a cosmetic company for such an absurd amount of money as opposed to getting the exact same thing from a grocery store for a fraction of this price? Olive oil is a good moisturizing oil but that's about it.

☹ $$$ **Hydrating Facial Mask** (*$16 for 3.5 ounces*) is a standard clay mask with some film former that allows this to peel off the skin. It is exceptionally ordinary, but can help absorb oil. There is a small amount of water-binding agents in this mask, but the clay eliminates their impact on skin.

☹ $$$ **Deep Cleansing Facial Mask** (*$24 for 2.1 ounces*) is a standard clay mask that is similar to the Hydrating Mask above, and the same basic comments apply.

☹ $$$ **Firming Kelp Facial Mask** (*$30 for 0.6 ounce liquid and 3.5 ounces gel*) comes in steps. Step 1 is a toner that you place on the skin before you apply the mask, which is Step 2. The toner is just water and some water-binding agents. The DNA in here won't affect your own DNA, and you wouldn't want it to! The mask is mostly film former (hairspray), so you peel this one off. That can help skin feel smooth and soft, just as any peel-off mask does.

☺ $$$ **Lip Conditioner** (*$11 for 0.12 ounce*) is a very emollient, good lip balm for dry lips. It contains mostly lanolin, thickeners, plant oils, and preservatives.

# Diane Young

Diane Young is a New York City facialist and aesthetician whose appearances on QVC have made her line of products an infomercial curiosity. Her credentials as a skin-care expert seem to have garnered her some amount of attention in fashion magazines, and the name of her salon, the Diane Young Anti-Aging Salon, is a name that definitely gets attention. Her product line is a host of products promising nothing less than returned youth. Young's Coneflower (echinacea) Neckline Firmer is supposed to be "clinically proven to decrease lines up to 36% in 4 weeks and to increase skin firmness up to 21% in 4 weeks." Wow, another unpublished skin-care study with miraculous promises; what a shock. It isn't any wonder that this has caught the attention of consumers.

Young's niche in the world of skin care is her use of plants that are relatively unique. An extract called mahimba, from the Asian neem tree, has some antibacterial value in pure form. Another is *long xu cai*, a very exotic name for algae, as well as clematis, a flowering plant some 400 varieties of which are known to exist. There are also the standard plants used in any product line that wants you to think natural thoughts, including cucumber, chamomile, aloe, and horsetail. What any of that can do for the skin is more folklore than established knowledge, but there is no way around it—plants look good on a label. Keep in mind that even if a plant does have known beneficial properties, that information is derived from research done using a pure concentration in a tincture form or a specific individual "tea" product. I have seen few studies establishing that once a plant is added to a cosmetic—in minute amounts, mixed with 10 to 50 other ingredients, and preserved and packaged in a range of containers (most plant concentrates require dark packaging to maintain stability)—it retains any of its original properties. There are exceptions but they are few and far between. What you are relying on with the addition of all these plants is the hope that they will have an effect, and what you get is merely the feel-good emotional reaction from thinking you are putting something "natural" on your skin.

There are some very nicely formulated moisturizers in this small product grouping, and aside from the prices and some fairly extravagant claims, it isn't a line to be dismissed outright, but the lack of a sunscreen is disturbing. This reflects a total lack of knowledge about skin and doesn't provide the consumer with the real foundation for any anti-aging skin-care routine. The anti-aging claims for this line are a figment of the imagination and nothing more.

For more information about Diane Young products, visit www.dianeyoung.com, or call the Anti-Aging salon at (212) 753-1200, or QVC at (800) 455-6685.

☺ $$$ **Age Lift Intensive Hydration** *($42.50 for 1.3 ounces)* is a good moisturizer for normal to dry skin, but don't count on the algae or an extract from the neem tree to help to change even one line on your face.

☺ $$$ **Years Younger Serum** *($45.50 for 1 ounce)* is a good lightweight moisturizer for normal to slightly dry skin. The name is enticing but don't bet on the results.

☹ $$$ **De-Puffing Eye Gel** *($29.75 for Age Eraser Eye Kit)*. The host of plant extracts in this formula can't depuff the eye area. This is a good, extremely lightweight gel that doesn't work very well as a moisturizer. Cucumber extract (the second ingredient), along with bladderwrack, calendula, and chamomile, has been used in these kinds of products before, and I still get hundreds of letters a month from women saying, "I've tried everything to reduce the puffiness under my eyes and nothing works" and do I know of anything that can help? I still don't, at least not in the way of a skin-care product.

☺ $$$ **Coneflower Neckline Firmer** *($34.25 for 1 ounce)*. Echinacea can be a problem for allergy-prone individuals but if that's not a concern for you this is a good, emollient, gel-like moisturizer for normal to dry skin. There are no ingredients in here unique to this product and there is nothing in here that can firm skin.

☺ $$$ **Coneflower Lipline Firmer** *($41 for 0.5 ounce)* is to be rubbed over skin for exfoliation. It's nice, but please forgive me if I mention that my line, as well as BeautiControl and Mary Kay, have identical versions for a fraction of the cost.

☺ $$$ **Moisture Lift Eye Mask** *($29.75 for Age Eraser Eye Kit)* won't erase anything but it is a good moisturizer for normal to dry skin. All of the interesting ingredients are present in tiny amounts (well after the pH balancer).

☺ $$$ **Immediate Appeal Gel Exfoliant** *($38.50 for 0.5 ounce)*. This blue gel can be rubbed over the skin, and that rolls off dead skin cells. That can make skin feel soft, but the ingredients in this product don't amount to much and the price is hardly appealing for what you get.

☺ $$$ **Immediate Eye Appeal** *($42.75 for 0.5 ounce)* has the same basic review as the Immediate Appeal Gel Exfoliant above.

☹ $$$ **Young Glow! Pearl Tone Underbase** *($35 for 0.5 ounce)* is supposed to be worn under makeup but on top of your moisturizer. Talk about adding layers, and still no sunscreen in sight. This is a light moisturizer that adds a bit of shine to the skin. There are lots of products that can do that; but does anyone really need one more product to add shine and another layer of stuff over their face?

# Doctor's Dermatologic Formula (See DDF)

# Dove (Skin Care Only)

For more information about Dove products, call (800) 451-6679 or visit www.dovespa.com.

☹ **Beauty Bar** *($1.99 for two 4.75-ounce bars)* is a standard, tallow-based bar cleanser that contains some emollients to cut the irritation and dryness caused by the detergent cleansing agents. It is still quite drying, and although it is technically not soap, the tallow in here can potentially clog pores. It is probably just fine for most skin types from the neck down, but not from the neck up.

☹ **Beauty Bar (Unscented)** *($1.99 for two 4.75-ounce bars)* is similar to the bar above, and the same review applies.

☹ **Sensitive Skin Beauty Bar New Milder Formula** *($1.99 for two 4.25-ounce bars)* is similar to the bar above and I don't really see any difference that makes it new or more mild.

# Dr. Hauschka Skin Care

Dr. Rudolf Hauschka is no longer around, although the cosmetics company bearing his name definitely is. I had a good deal of trouble finding out anything about the doctor's work, and what little is available is in German, but rather than reviewing the man, I'll concentrate on the products, which is what really counts. What I find particularly intriguing about Dr. Hauschka Skin Care is that the products are some of the most atypical I've seen. Sold primarily at health food stores, the products are a standout for their price alone. A cleansing cream at $15.95 for less than two ounces is literally one of the most expensive around.

If plants are your thing, these formulations, according to the ingredient listing, are some of the most "pure" around (but not 100%; there are animal-derived ingredients in some of them). However, I should state that the products don't appear to contain what the labels reflect. Their consistency leads me to believe that they contain other ingredients not represented on the label, but I have no proof one way or the other and will go by the ingredient listing as fact, as I do for all the products I review.

In looking at the brochures for Dr. Hauschka Skin Care, it's hard to ignore the religious fervor. Some skin-care lines market their products as all-natural, others as all-science combined with nature, and then there are those rare lines that claim to be about a spiritual experience. Dr. Hauschka is as much about skin care as it is about spirituality. The product brochures read more like doctrine than a skin-care manual. "Your skin . . . connects you to the kingdom around you—the earth, the planets, and the stars." The company mission statement is a "holistic concept of health and the four-fold nature of the human being. . . . A person's health is the dynamic interworking and balance between the physical body, the life force, the soul, and the 'I.' " The statement goes on, and it turns out the company's religious bent is based on anthroposophy, a modern religious sect derived from theosophy (a mixture of Buddhism and Brahmanism) that claims to develop knowledge and realization of spiritual reality. What does that have to do with skin care? As you might imagine, it isn't easy to get a straight answer—after all, spirituality through skin care isn't an easy concept to grasp—but the main idea is that the products are supposed to support your natural rhythms. I guess supporting natural rhythms doesn't come cheap.

What about the effectiveness of the products in this line? That depends on your point of view. These products are loaded with fragrant oils and plant extracts that have little place in skin care and a good deal of irritation and inflammation potential on skin. However, there are also plenty of benign nut and vegetable oils here that can be quite good for dry skin. Aside from the fragrant-oil issue, take note of the handful of irritating ingredients that show up in these products, including witch hazel, silver, and alcohol. But then, for the purists looking into this line, there's the handful of synthetics that show up, including cetaryl alcohol, lanolin alcohol, and Vaseline. I don't think those are a problem in the least, but for a line that has such a natural perspective, they seem incredibly out of place. They also make the company's claim about no synthetics completely untrue. I am also skeptical about the disclosure of the ingredients on the products because there is no listing of preservatives on the label. If that is truly the case the risk of contamination after just a couple of weeks of use is fairly significant, especially considering all the plant extracts. The company insists the ingredient labels are accurate; if its claim is true, I'd be concerned about keeping the products around for more than a few weeks at best.

Another problem with these products is that the ingredients are virtually identical product to product to product, with very few exceptions. What makes that strange are the claims that range from getting rid of acne to firming skin—all from the same ingredients. And one more point: the sun-protecting products in this line with SPF 8 and SPF 15 are recommended as being able to provide sun protection "against burning while permitting some tanning." Didn't anyone at Dr. Hauschka Skin Care hear about the very well-publicized fact that there is no such thing as a good tan? The logic of providing this kind of misleading information while recommending holistic skin care is so full of holes it makes me cringe.

For more information about Dr. Hauschka, call (800) 247-9907 or visit the Web site at www.drhauschka.de (please note that this Web site is in German).

☺ $$$ **Cleansing Cream** *($15.95 for 1.7 ounces)* would be an OK scrub for someone with normal to dry skin.

☻ **Cleansing Milk** *($22.95 for 5.1 ounces)*. The alcohol in here (the second ingredient) makes it inappropriate for most skin types. For "a gentle cleanser," that much alcohol just doesn't make sense.

☻ **Facial Toner** *($22.95 for 3.4 ounces)* contains mostly water, alcohol, and witch hazel, and is an irritation waiting to happen. The ingredients just don't warrant the cost.

☻ **Clarifying Toner** *($22.95 for 3.4 ounces)* has similar ingredients to the toner above and the same comments apply.

☻ **Rhythmic Night Conditioner** *($22.95 for ten ampoules)* contains mostly water, rose oil, witch hazel, royal jelly, and silver. Silver can be a skin irritant, as can the rose oil and witch hazel. If silver has some benefit for skin, I can't find any documentation establishing what it can do, especially in the amounts used in this product. As for the royal jelly, it keeps showing up in products, but the claims for this ingredient have never been substantiated either.

☻ **Rhythmic Conditioner Sensitive** *($22.95 for ten 0.34-ounce ampoules)* doesn't have as much rose oil or witch hazel as the one above, but they are still in there, and instead of the silver this one contains copper oxide. This still sounds fairly irritating, though the borage oil can be soothing and emollient.

☺ **Moisturizing Day Cream** *($34.50 for 3.4 ounces)*. Without sunscreen, this moisturizer is absolutely not recommended for daytime. It contains mostly water, plant extracts, plant oils, alcohol, witch hazel, thickeners, and fragrance. The alcohol and witch hazel are a problem in a moisturizer but the plant oils in here could make up for that.

☺ **Rose Day Cream** *($21.95 for 1.1 ounces)* is a far better moisturizer than the one above and, while overpriced, would be great for dry skin. However, without a sunscreen, it is only acceptable for nightwear.

☺ **Quince Day Cream** *($24.95 for 1 ounce)* contains mostly water, plant oils, fragrant plant extracts, emollients, thickeners, and fragrance. This is a good emollient moisturizer for dry skin. The quince seed has skin constricting properties, which makes it a potential skin irritant, but there is only a tiny amount in here so it probably has little to no impact on skin.

☺ **Normalizing Day Oil** *($23.50 for 1 ounce)* contains mostly water, plant oils, plant extract, and fragrance. These are oils that can be found in a kitchen cabinet (almond, wheat germ, peanut, and jojoba) and are just fine for dry skin. What is strange is that this product is recommended "for oily, impure skins . . . [to] remove signs of blemishes and large pores." I can't imagine anything less helpful for oily skin or blemishes than more oil.

☺ **Toned Day Cream** *($23.50 for 1.1 ounces)* contains mostly water, plant oils, plant extracts, thickeners, and fragrance. This is a good moisturizer for dry skin.

☹ **Translucent Bronze Concentrate** *($23.50 for 1 ounce)* is supposed to soften the appearance of small red blood vessels, but with alcohol as the third ingredient, I strongly doubt that claim. Alcohol can cause surface capillaries to look worse.

☺ $$$ **Eye Contour Day Cream** *($22.95 for 0.33 ounce)* is a good emollient moisturizer for dry skin but the price is completely unwarranted.

☹ **Eye Solace** *($18.50 for 1.7 ounces)* contains too much alcohol to be used around the eye area.

☹ **Rhythmic Night Conditioner for All Skin Conditions** *($22.95 for ten ampoules)*. The trace amount of silver in here can potentially be a skin irritant and has no benefit for skin. As for the rose oil, it may smell nice, but it can be a skin irritant too.

☹ **Rhythmic Conditioner, Sensitive for Sensitive Skin** *($22.95 for ten ampoules)* is more like putting eau de cologne on the skin than anything else.

☺ $$$ **Cleansing Clay Mask** *($24.95 for 3.06 ounces)* is a relatively pure clay mask, but clay doesn't do much for skin and the witch hazel can be a skin irritant.

☹ **Rejuvenating Mask** *($29.95 for 1.1 ounces)* is similar to most of the moisturizers in this line, and contains mostly water, plant extracts, alcohol, glycerin, plant oils, and thickeners. If it weren't for the alcohol, this would be a great moisturizer for dry skin.

☺ $$$ **Moisturizing Mask** *($33.95 for 1.1 ounces)* is similar to the Rejuvenating Mask minus the alcohol, plus this one contains Vaseline and lanolin. It would be great for dry skin.

☹ **Facial Steam Bath** *($24.50 for 3.4 ounces)* is supposed to be used with steam heat. Repeated use of steam heat can cause surface capillaries, increase the severity of rosacea, and damage skin. As much as I love soaking in a Jacuzzi, I don't fool myself into thinking it's helping my skin.

☹ **Sunscreen Lotion SPF 8** *($15.95 for 3.4 ounces)* has too low an SPF to be recommended.

☺ **Sunscreen Lotion SPF 15** *($15.95 for 3.4 ounces)* is a very good titanium dioxide–based sunscreen that would be good for someone with dry skin. It can leave a white cast on the skin.

☺ **Sunscreen Lotion SPF 20** *($17.95 for 3.4 ounces)* is similar to the one above only with a higher SPF.

☺ **Sunscreen Cream for Children SPF 22** *($19.95 for 3.4 ounces)* doesn't contain anything different to make it better for children, but it is a good titanium dioxide–based sunscreen.

☺ **After Sun Lotion** *($14.25 for 3.4 ounces)* is a good moisturizer for dry skin, though the amount of alcohol in here can be problematic for some skin types.

☺ **$$$ Lip Balm** *($9.50 for 0.15 ounce)* is a good emollient balm for dry lips, and contains many of the same ingredients as most of the moisturizers in this line.

☺ **$$$ Lip Care Stick** *($7.50 for 0.16 ounce)* is similar to the one above except in stick form.

## Dr. Mary Lupo (Skin Care Only)

Dr. Lupo is a dermatologist with an impressive list of credentials who has created her own skin-care line. There are some interesting AHA products but also a handful of overblown claims. Her sunscreens claim to have UVA protection, but one clearly doesn't contain any UVA-protecting ingredients, and her Conditioning Cleanser uses sodium lauryl sulfate (SLS), known for being one of the most irritating detergent cleansing ingredients around. Surely as a dermatologist, Lupo should know about these issues, and I always find it disappointing to see a line from a medical professional that ignores such fundamentals.

Still, there are some good AHA products in here, particularly lightweight ones. They're pricey for what you get, but they are well-formulated. For more information about Dr. Mary Lupo, call (800) 419-2002 or visit the Web site at www.drmary lupo.com.

☺ **$$$ Conditioning Cleanser** *($22 for 6 ounces)* is an OK, water-soluble cleanser, but the standard detergent cleansing agents are fairly drying and one of them is sodium lauryl sulfate, which can be a skin irritant. There probably aren't large quantities of these in here, but I am always concerned when I see them listed in a product designated as "conditioning" or moisturizing.

☺ $$$ **Gentle Purifying Cleanser** *($22 for 7 ounces)* is a fairly standard, detergent-based water-soluble cleanser that is in many respects quite good for most skin types, except dry skin. It does contain fragrance.

☺ **AHA Renewel Gel I** *($25 for 3.5 ounces)* is a good 8% gel AHA product containing lactic acid. It contains no other irritants and should work well to exfoliate the skin without clogging pores. Given the extremely limited selection of AHA liquids or gels that contain no irritants, this one is pretty good.

☺ **AHA Renewal Gel II** *($25 for 3.5 ounces)* is similar to the one above, and the same review applies.

☺ **AHA Renewal Lotion I** *($25 for 3.5 ounces)* is an 8% AHA lotion in a standard moisturizing base. This is pretty pricey and is just as effective as Alpha Hydrox at the drugstore for far less.

☺ **AHA Renewal Lotion II** *($25 for 3.5 ounces)* is similar to the one above, and the same review applies.

☹ **Daily Age Management Moisturizer, SPF 15** *($23 for 2 ounces)* does not contain avobenzone, titanium dioxide, or zinc oxide for UVA protection, and is not recommended.

☺ **Daily Age Management Oil Free Moisturizer SPF 15** *($23 for 2 ounces)* is a titanium dioxide–based sunscreen with a great SPF. It is a good sunscreen that goes on light, but it would be best for someone with normal to slightly dry skin.

☺ **Full Spectrum Sunscreen UVA/UVB SPF 27** *($17.50 for 3 ounces)* is a good in-part avobenzone-based sunscreen that would work well for someone with normal to slightly dry skin. This very standard formulation holds no advantage over Neutrogena's avobenzone-based sunscreen at a fraction of the price.

☺ $$$ **Intensive Target Moisturizer** *($38.50 for 1 ounce)*. If you want to spend this kind of money on a fairly standard moisturizer with vitamin E, it's up to you, but this is overpriced for a simple product.

☺ $$$ **Vivifying Serum C** *($39.95 for 1 ounce)* uses the stable version (magnesium ascorbyl palmitate) of vitamin C, so if you want vitamin C in a lightweight gel, this one is definitely an option. This product also contains human leukocyte extract (white blood cell extract). White blood cells are the colorless cells in blood that help protect the body from infection and disease. However, there is no research showing that applying white blood cells topically can have any effect on skin whatsoever.

# eb5 (Skin Care Only)

Pharmacist Robert Heldfond is the creator of this line that has been around for as long as I can remember, and little has changed since I first reviewed it more than 15 years ago. Heldfond still wants you to be believe that as a pharmacist he spent years developing his eb5 cream. It is almost embarrassing for anyone to admit that it took years to create what is little more than Vaseline and thickening agents. But what would you expect from a man who still refers to melanin discolorations on skin as "liver spots," which is a completely inaccurate and archaic term (but then, so are these products). Heldfond insists that you need to use no other product than his eb5 to care for your skin. But this line has no sunscreen, which is a guarantee of inevitable continuing skin damage and wrinkling, and the formulations here would leave your skin in the lurch if you were wanting the advantages of any current research on antioxidants, AHAs, elegant water-binding agents, and on and on.

Another quirky assertion from Heldfond is that "only a pharmacist, and one who is schooled in compounding as I was, could produce such an amazing discovery. Back in pharmacy school, I first learned from a renowned professor the art of trituration, maceration, and percolation which no other cosmetics companies have been able to duplicate." If you believe that one, I have a bridge in New York I can sell you for very cheap! First, pharmacists aren't trained in compounding cosmetics or skin-care products in the least. Second, trituration simply means to grind a substance into a powder; maceration means to make something soft by steeping it in a liquid; and percolation, well that's coffee: to pass a substance through a filter. And Heldfond is the only one to know how to do any of that to create a moisturizer? Look out, Estee Lauder! The truth is, these products are so far from state-of-the-art it is laughable.

The bottom line: These are some of the most unimpressive skin-care products around and it's a bit shocking that they are still in production and still so amazingly overpriced. For more information about eb5, call (800) 683-2325 or visit the Web site at www.eb5.com.

☺ **Cleansing Formula** (*$15 for 6 ounces*) is a fairly gentle, though extremely standard, water-soluble cleanser that contains a small amount of detergent cleansing agents, and would be best for someone with normal to dry skin, though it doesn't do a very good job of taking off makeup. It does contain fragrance.

☹ **Toning Formula** (*$15 for 8 ounces*) contains a few too many irritating ingredients to recommend, including arnica (which is not recommended to ever be used on abraded skin) and witch hazel. The teeny amount of lactic acid in here is only effective as a water-binding agent.

☺ **Women's Facial Cream** (*$35 for 4 ounces*). This very ordinary moisturizer would be good for someone with dry skin. The vitamins are nice for antioxidants but not special or unique in skin-care products.

☺ **Men's Facial Cream** (*$35 for 4 ounces*) is almost identical to the Women's version above only this one has a slightly lighter feel, which would work well for women too. There is nothing in this product that would be particularly helpful for men.

☺ **$$$ Eye Gel Formula** (*$18 for 0.5 ounce*) is a good, though fairly greasy, moisturizer for someone with normal to dry skin.

☺ **Age Spot Formula** *($25 for 6 ounces)* is a standard 2% hydroquinone fade cream. It also contains fruit extracts, but these are not the kind of AHAs that can exfoliate the skin and help lighten brown spots, plus the sunscreen in here is not adequate and it doesn't contain any reliable UVA protection.

## Ecco Bella

Ecco Bella means *Behold Beauty* in Italian and it's a lovely thought. It is one of the many smaller lines usually sold in health food stores whose claims of "all natural," "organic," and "pure" seem so saintly and correct that it almost feels wrong be critical of their products. Yet these products do have shortcomings you need to be aware of. What's typical of this line, as well as every other "natural" line from Aveda through Zia, is the way it casts suspicion on many ingredients that are perfectly harmless and safe to use. Ingredients such as talc and mineral oil have gotten bad raps from companies like these largely due to anecdotal or unrelated data as opposed to real evidence of any potential harm or risk. Meanwhile, the products use ingredients such as plant extracts, essential oils, and a garden's worth of herbs (organically grown, mind you), all deemed the perfect solution. Yet scientific research continues to show that plant extracts and oils (especially fragrant ones), in their countless species and forms, can be problematic for the skin and are not automatically beneficial just as they grow from the ground.

Furthermore, when you're dealing with a mass-produced and distributed product, it's doubtful that the finished product has retained any of the benefits these plants are alleged to have, if there were benefits to be gained from their use in the first place. The Ecco Bella brochure states that when its products are used daily, " … fine lines will be reduced as well as breakouts and dryness. Oily skin will become more balanced." If only that were true! But vinegar, some coconut oil–based detergent cleansing agents, fragrant oils, and emollient oils can't do that. There are some great sunscreens in this line and some very emollient moisturizers, and that's wonderful, but they won't change a wrinkle or alter your skin in any way. Plus, if you have normal to oily skin, these products pose more problems than they help to solve.

The makeup collection has some items that are worth a look—the eyeshadows and blushes have excellent textures and a smooth application—but the rest of the makeup goes from standard to stunningly no-frills basic. Bottom line: there are some products to consider here if you can overlook the egregious hype, and the prices are comparatively good. For more information, call (973) 696-7766 or visit the Web site at www.eccobella.com.

## Ecco Bella Skin Care

☺ **Purifying Cleanser for Normal to Oily Skin** *($11.50 for 6.5 ounces)* is a standard, detergent-based water-soluble cleanser that would work well for oily skin

The Reviews E

types, though the cleansing agent may be too drying for more normal skin types. It does contain fragrant oils. The small amount of plant extracts in here can be anti-irritants and have a tiny amount of anti-bacterial properties.

☺ **Soft and Soothing Cleanser for Normal to Dry Skin** *($11.50 for 6.5 ounces)* is almost identical to the Purifying Cleanser above only this version contains oatmeal (a soothing agent), a different fragrance, and a small amount of plant oil. That makes it minimally better for normal to dry skin, so it would actually be best for someone with normal to oily skin.

☹ **Purifying Toner for Normal to Oily Skin** *($11.50 for 6.5 ounces)*. Vinegar (acetic acid) can have antibacterial properties, but it is part alcohol, which makes it drying and irritating for skin. Vinegar is supposed to have a pH similar to skin, which is nice, but nowadays most all skin-care products are the pH of skin (around 5.5).

☹ **Soft and Soothing Toner for Normal to Dry Skin** *($11.50 for 6.5 ounces)* is almost identical to the version above and the same comments apply.

☺ **$$$ Moisture-to-Go Spray On** *($15.50 for 2 ounces)* is actually a very good toner for all skin types but best for normal to dry skin. The plant extracts are here in minuscule quantities; some are potential skin irritants, while others are potential anti-irritants.

☺ **Skin Survival Day Cream SPF 15** *($21.50 for 2 ounces)* is a very good titanium dioxide–based sunscreen for normal to dry skin.

☺ **Skin Survival Night Cream** *($21.50 for 2 ounces)* is a very good emollient moisturizer for normal to dry skin. The plant extracts are here in minuscule amounts; some are potential skin irritants, while others are potential anti-irritants.

☺ **Daily Exfoliant with 8% AHA and BHA** *($17.50 for 2 ounces)* has a pH of about 4.5, which makes it barely passable as an exfoliant. It does contain lactic acid but only about 5%, along with about 1% BHA. However, the lemon and passion fruit acids are not effective as exfoliants. It also contains clay, which gives it more of a matte finish. It's an option, but a pH of 3 to 3.5 would be far better if you are looking for effective exfoliation.

# Ecco Bella Makeup

☹ **FOUNDATION:** **Natural Foundation SPF 15** *($16.95)* does contain titanium dioxide (it's the second ingredient) but this is not listed as an active ingredient, so the SPF, though probably true, should not be relied on exclusively. Unfortunately, this formulation has a pasty texture and a slightly chalky finish, which mars what would otherwise be a good foundation. The eight colors are OK but the pump-bottle applicator isn't the best for economical usage. Overall there are more bad points that outweigh the good ones, making this hard to recommend.

☻ <u>CONCEALER:</u> **Natural Cover-Up** *($8.95)* is about as far from natural looking as can be. This lipstick-style concealer has a thick, greasy, hard-to-blend texture, and the two colors are just terrible.

☺ **BLUSH: Matte Blush** *($8.95)* is aptly named—these do have a soft matte finish and a very smooth application. The color selection is small but has much potential, especially for darker skin tones. Lighter skins may find this is too pigmented for their skin tone.

☺ <u>EYESHADOW:</u> **Matte Eyeshadow** *($8.95)* has a texture almost identical to the Matte Blush and applies equally well. It's slightly powdery, but clings nicely to the skin. The only drawback is the inclusion of blues, greens, and bright purples among some lovely earth-toned neutrals.

☺ <u>EYE AND BROW SHAPER:</u> **Soft Eyeliner** *($8.95)* has a soft texture and goes on very sheer, with a slightly waxy aftereffect. These are very standard, though it would take some effort to get a definite line to show up on the skin.

<u>LIPSTICK AND LIP PENCIL:</u> ☺ **Natural Lipstick** *($8.95)* is a really basic lipstick with a greasy texture and a semitransparent, glossy finish. The colors are nice but there are much more creamy, smoothly textured lipsticks to consider over this one. **Long Lasting Lip Crayons** *($7.95)* are thick lip pencils with the standard two-in-one claim. These need to be sharpened and have a soft, creamy texture and a finish that is neither too greasy nor too glossy. The colors are very sheer with little to no intensity, so the long-lasting claim is erroneous.

☺ **Lipliner Pencil** *($8.95)* is just a standard pencil that has a soft, slightly dry texture and some amount of stain—much more than the lipsticks or lip crayons do.

☻ <u>MASCARA:</u> **Natural Mascara** *($8.95)* is a boring mascara that initially hints at its lengthening potential yet after several strokes just remains a do-nothing mascara. Wait, it does do something—it makes the lashes feel very dry. The mirror on the side of the tube is a nice touch, but not enough to save this mascara from being relegated to the "why bother?" pile.

# *Elizabeth Arden*

Elizabeth Arden was a pioneer in the beauty industry. At the turn of the last century, Arden began her legacy when she opened her first salon, with the now familiar red door. Over the next several years, she introduced new products and services to women unaccustomed to such choices, and almost single-handedly made it acceptable for modern women to wear makeup. And while Arden understood and met these beauty needs, she was also adept at self-promotion and packaging, helping to solidify the idea that what holds the product should be as beautiful as the woman who uses it. She was the front-runner in the cosmetics industry for quite some time,

until another young go-getter by the name of Estee Lauder began her own empire—
one that would eventually lead to the Elizabeth Arden line being almost an afterthought
in the mind of many consumers.

Although Arden will probably never reach the same level of success that Lauder
has, it is nice to see that Arden's makeup image has improved and that the products
have become far more up-to-date. Even its ads, with supermodel Amber Valetta as
the link to today's woman, have taken on a refreshingly casual air. Now, aside from
the marketing struggles, Arden has an attractive collection of foundations, wearable
blush and eyeshadow colors, and some remarkable mascaras. Another plus is its updated tester units, which are readily accessible, with the colors divided into appropriate
groups for relatively easy selection.

When it comes to skin care, Arden is a strange mix of uniqueness and utter disappointment. The worst aspect of this line is that none of the SPF skin-care products
have UVA-protecting ingredients. To make all the claims about repairing and healing
skin, without a good sunscreen in sight, just seems so misleading. What is impressive
about the line is Arden's patented use of ceramides. Ceramides were at the forefront of
what we now know to be significant options for dealing with skin. That won't change
a wrinkle, but they do help the skin behave and look better. What a shame this interesting nuance of skin care gets lost among some absurd sunscreen products.

For more information about Elizabeth Arden, call (212) 261-1000 or visit the
Web site at www.elizabetharden.com.

## Elizabeth Arden Skin Care

☺ $$$ **Millennium Hydrating Cleanser** *($25.50 for 4.4 ounces)* is a standard
mineral oil–based wipe off cleanser that also contains a small amount of detergent
cleansing agent. It can leave a greasy film on the skin but can be an option for some-
one with dry skin. It does contain fragrance.

☹ **Millennium Revitalizing Tonic** *($24.50 for 5 ounces)* contains mostly alcohol
and some amount of menthol, and that is too irritating and drying for all skin types.

☺ $$$ **Millennium Day Renewal Emulsion** *($54.50 for 2.6 ounces)*. This very
rich (though exceedingly emollient) moisturizer is an option for dry skin.

☺ $$$ **Millennium Eye Renewal Cream** *($39.50 for 0.5 ounce)* is a very rich,
thick, ordinary moisturizer. It will indeed take care of dry skin but it is incredibly
overpriced.

☺ $$$ **Millennium Night Renewal Creme** *($82 for 1.7 ounces)* is similar to the
Day Renewal Emulsion above and the same basic comments apply (the only real
difference is consistency, with this one being less thick).

☺ $$$ **Millennium Energist** *($60 for 1.7 ounces)* is far better than the other

Millennium moisturizers, if you're going to spend the money. The antioxidants, plant oils, and water-binding agents are quite good.

☺ $$$ **Modern Skin Care 2-in-1 Cleanser** *($17.50 for 4.2 ounces)* is a very good, detergent-based water-soluble cleanser for someone with normal to oily skin and the only thing modern about it is that it isn't the greasy mess of the Millennium cleanser. It doesn't do anything to "minimize the appearance of pores," and it can be drying for some skin types despite what the brochure claims. It claims to contain antioxidants, but they aren't evident in the ingredient list. Even if the plant extracts in here are supposed to do that job, the effect would be washed down the drain, though some of the plant extracts in here are fragrant and can be skin irritants.

☹ **Modern Skin Care One Great Soap** *($12.50 for 5.3 ounces)* has the ingredients that keep bar cleansers in their bar form, which can clog pores, and the cleansing agents are too drying for most all skin types.

☹ **Modern Skin Care Daily Moisture SPF 15** *($32.50 for 1.7 ounces)* doesn't contain zinc oxide, titanium dioxide, or avobenzone for UVA protection, and is not recommended.

☹ **Modern Skin Care Oil Free Sunblock SPF 15** *($33.50 for 4.2 ounces)* doesn't contain zinc oxide, titanium dioxide, or avobenzone for UVA protection, and is not recommended.

☺ $$$ **Modern Skin Care Illuminating Complex** *($42.50 for 1 ounce)*. How illuminating is this lightweight lotion? Not very. The form of salicylic acid (a salt as opposed to an acid) used in this product is not effective for exfoliating the skin. Skin Illuminating Complex is a good lightweight moisturizer for normal to dry skin, very standard and not illuminating.

☹ **Modern Skin Care Clear the Way Mask** *($19.50 for 3.5 ounces)* is a peel-off mask that contains peppermint and menthol. The irritation, with minimal to no benefit for skin, makes this more of a problem than anything else.

☺ **Visible Difference Deep Cleansing Lotion** *($18.50 for 6.7 ounces)* doesn't clean deeply in the least. It is a standard, cold cream–type cleanser that needs to be wiped off and can leave a film on the skin. It can be an option for normal to dry skin.

☹ **Visible Difference Oil Control Refining Cleanser** *($19.50 for 6.8 ounces)* contains standard detergent cleansing agents, but with a few irritating additions that are hard on skin, such as lemon and sodium lauryl sulfate.

☹ **Visible Difference Oil Control Clarifying Toner** *($18.50 for 6.8 ounces)* contains alcohol, witch hazel, and lemon. Ouch!

☹ **Visible Difference Refining Toner** *($15 for 6.7 ounces)* contains mostly water, witch hazel, alcohol, glycerin, and preservative. The alcohol and witch hazel make it too irritating for most skin types.

☺ $$$ **Visible Difference Eyecare Concentrate** *($30 for 0.5 ounce)* is an ordinary but good moisturizer for dry skin.

☺ $$$ **Visible Difference Perpetual Moisture** *($38 for 1 ounce)* is a very good moisturizer for normal to dry skin.

☹ **Visible Difference Eight Hour Lip Protectant Stick SPF 15** *($12.50 for 0.13 ounce)* doesn't contain avobenzone, zinc oxide, or titanium dioxide for UVA protection, and is not recommended.

☺ **Visible Difference Eight Hour Cream** *($20 for 4 ounces)* is one of the original products in the Arden skin-care arsenal. The teeny amount of salicylic acid and the high pH make it completely ineffective for exfoliation. This is just a good, very old-fashioned, heavy emollient moisturizer for dry skin.

☺ $$$ **Visible Difference Refining Moisturizer Creme Complex** *($47.50 for 2.5 ounces)* is a somewhat heavy, though ordinary, moisturizer for someone with very dry skin.

☺ $$$ **Visible Difference Refining Moisture Lotion** *($28.50 for 1.35 ounces)* is similar to the Creme Complex above and the same basic comments apply.

☹ **Visible Difference Matte Moisture Lotion** *($32.50 for 1.7 ounces)* contains a form of BHA that is not effective for exfoliation—the pH is just too high for it to work in removing skin cells.

☺ **Visible Difference Pore Fix-C** *($12.50 for ten strips)* are pore strips that are almost identical to the Biore strips, with the same warnings and concerns. This version comes with a minuscule amount of vitamin C. The form of vitamin C is ascorbic acid, considered to be more of an irritant than a help for skin.

☺ $$$ **Ceramide Purifying Cream Cleanser** *($19.50 for 4.2 ounces)* is a fairly emollient, standard, cold-cream cleanser that needs to be wiped off. It doesn't purify anything and it can leave a greasy feel on skin, though this can be an option for someone with dry skin.

☹ **Ceramide Purifying Toner** *($18.50 for 6.7 ounces)* is an alcohol-based toner. Alcohol doesn't purify the skin, but it can cause irritation.

☺ $$$ **Ceramide Advanced Time Complex Capsules** *($55 for 0.97 ounce, includes 60 capsules)* are the most popular product Arden sells, yet these tiny gelatin capsules contain some fairly ordinary stuff: silicones, plant oil, water-binding agent (including ceramide), and vitamins. This is a good lightweight, soothing moisturizer for the face, but that's about it. What is particularly nice about this product is the absence of preservatives; due to the encapsulation, there is no need for them.

☺ $$$ **Ceramide Eyes Time Complex Capsules** *($37.50 for 0.35 ounce, includes 60 capsules)* is similar to the Advanced version above only this one contains witch hazel, which can be a skin irritant. Ceramide is a very good water-binding agent, but it won't change a wrinkle or alter skin in any way.

☺ **$$$ Ceramide Firm Lift Intensive Lotion for Face and Throat** *($45 for 1 ounce)* is a good moisturizer for someone with normal to dry skin, but there is nothing startling or particularly interesting about this product. If you already own one of Arden's Ceramide products, there is no reason to add this to your arsenal.

☺ **$$$ Ceramide Night Intensive Repair Creme** *($45 for 1 ounce)* is a good moisturizer for normal to dry skin, but there is nothing about this that will repair skin. The second ingredient is a neutralized form of salicylic acid (BHA), which means the product won't exfoliate the skin.

☺ **$$$ Ceramide Time Complex Moisture Cream** *($45 for 1.7 ounces)* is a good moisturizer for someone with normal to dry skin.

☹ **Ceramide Time Complex Moisture Cream SPF 15** *($45 for 1.7 ounces)* doesn't contain avobenzone, zinc oxide, or titanium dioxide for UVA protection, and is not recommended.

☹ **Ceramide Herbal Botanical Supplement** *($59 for 60 0.59-ounce capsules).* The herbal extracts in these tiny capsules are clever additions with enough buzz to sound convincing to many consumers, but they add nothing to Arden's original ceramide formulations; some of them are anti-irritants and others potentially irritating, while in this amount mulberry has no skin-lightening effect.

☹ **$$$ Ceramide Eye Wish SPF 10** *($39 for 0.5 ounce).* The only wish I have for Arden is for it to have an SPF 15 with UVA protection. Unfortunately, that isn't the case here, and there doesn't seem to be anything I can do about it.

☹ **$$$ Good Morning Skin Serum** *($29.50 for 0.5 ounce)* is a silicone-based, lotion-like moisturizer for dry skin. This can feel silky soft on skin, similar to Cinique Stop Signs ($32.50 for 1 ounce), which is less expensive and better-formulated with state-of-the-art water-binding agents. The plant extracts in here, for the most part, are good anti-irritants. Do not start the morning off with this product unless you are willing to put an effective sunscreen of some kind over it.

☹ **$$$ Good Night's Sleep** *($35 for 1.7 ounces).* The plant extracts in here are mostly fragrant and potentially irritating to skin. This is a good moisturizer but it is fairly ordinary and there are far better ways for your skin to get a good night's sleep.

☹ **All Gone Eye and Lip Makeup Remover** *($16 for 3.4 ounces)* is a silicone-based, wipe-off cleanser that also contains a small amount of detergent cleansing agents. It will work as well as any makeup remover.

# *Elizabeth Arden Makeup*

**FOUNDATION:** Arden still has a bit of work to do in getting its foundations with sunscreen up to par (SPF 15 is the minimum, with reliable UVA protection), but the textures and shade selections are impressive. ☺ **$$$ Flawless Finish Mousse Makeup** *($28)* is a foundation that comes in a metal can that uses a propellant to distribute an airy, bubbly, flesh-toned foam that blends on better than you might expect, though it can waste some product until you get used to it. The coverage is sheer and the texture has enough slip to allow for adequate blending. This dries to a soft matte finish and should work well for normal to slightly oily or dry skin. There are some great colors for very light skin tones, but avoid these shades: Melba (peach), Summer and Bronze (orange), and Natural (slightly ash).

☺ $$$ **Flawless Finish Hydro-Light Foundation SPF 10** *($30)* is a creamy foundation that comes in a jar. The application is soft, with sheer to light coverage and a satin finish that would be good for normal to dry skin. The SPF is pure titanium dioxide, which is great, but SPF 15 would be perfect. Still, this is one to consider if you have normal to very dry skin. All of these colors are too pink, orange, or peach to recommend: Vanilla, Buff, Honey, Bronze II, and Cameo.

☺ $$$ **Flawless Finish Complete Control Matte Makeup SPF 10** *($28)* also offers a pure titanium dioxide–based sunscreen, but again, SPF 15 is the goal. This has a smooth, light texture and a soft matte finish with medium coverage. It would be fine for normal to slightly oily skin that isn't prone to breakouts, and the only colors to avoid are Fawn, Bisque, Cream (all too pink), and Bronze II (orange).

☹ $$$ **Flawless Finish Sponge-On Creme Makeup** *($28)* is a fairly thick and somewhat greasy cream-type compact makeup, making it only an option for someone with dry skin. This one starts out very thick and provides medium to full coverage with a creamy, opaque finish. It blends well enough, but most women do not need this much full-face coverage, and the fragrance is quite strong. All of these colors are too pink, orange, or peach to recommend: Honey, Mocha II, Toasty Beige, Warm Beige, Toasty Rose, and Bronzed Beige.

☺ $$$ **Flawless Finish Smartwear Makeup SPF 15** *($28)* is the only Arden foundation with a high enough SPF, but this one has no UVA protection! Whose "smart" idea was this, given all the other foundations that have titanium dioxide? Although this is unreliable for sun protection, it is a very light-textured foundation with sheer to light coverage and a gorgeous satin-matte finish. The amount of emollients in here would not make someone with oily skin too happy, but normal to slightly dry skin will find this works beautifully. These colors are too pink or orange to recommend: Cameo, Buff, Honey, Bisque, and Bronze II.

☺ $$$ **Flawless Finish Dual Perfection Makeup** *($28)* is a pressed powder meant to be used wet or dry as a foundation, though wet can be really choppy and streaky. It is a standard, talc-based powder that has a silky feel. This type of foundation works best for someone with normal to slightly dry or slightly oily skin. Most of the colors are excellent. The only ones that may be a problem are Cream and Cameo, which may be too peach for most skin tones.

☺ **CONCEALER:** **Concealing Cream** *($14)* has a thick, greasy texture and although it covers well, don't expect much longevity from it but do expect creasing. **Perfect Covering Concealer** *($14)* is an improvement over the cream reviewed above, but this is still creamy enough to crease. There are some colors to consider and the coverage is great, but test this one out at the counter and wear it for a few hours before you purchase it. **$$$ Visible Difference Eye-Fix Primer** *($15.50 for 0.25 ounce)* is supposed to be a sheer cream for the eyelid to prevent makeup creasing, and it's basically talc and wax. Forget the wax, and just use your foundation with powder over it, which would work as well if not better than this product.

☹ <u>POWDER:</u> **Flawless Finish Loose Powder** *($24)* has a soft feel and a very dry texture that shows up easily on the skin. All of the shades have a slight amount of shine, which on top of the dry finish isn't flattering for daytime wear. Avoid Medium 1, which is strongly orange. **Flawless Finish Pressed Powder** *($23)* has a slightly less dry texture than the one above and it is matte; however, the application tends to leave a chalky, cakey finish that is too apparent to make this an option.

☺ **$$$** <u>BLUSH:</u> **Cheekcolor** *($20)* features a velvety-smooth texture and a soft, sheer finish that is a pleasure to apply. There are some beautiful, primarily warm-toned matte shades and almost as many shiny options. What's helpful here is that the blushes are divided into three color families that correspond well with the eye and lip colors.

☺ <u>EYESHADOW:</u> The lovely selection of **Eyeshadow Singles** *($10)* are divided into four color groups, from neutrals and browns to plums and purples. This is a welcome separation that makes coordinating colors a breeze. The shadows all have a wonderful satin-matte finish and a texture similar to Arden's blushes: like velvet. These go from sheer to moderate in intensity, and there are enough matte shades to keep me from griping about the presence of several very shiny colors!

☺ <u>EYE AND BROW SHAPER:</u> **Smoky Eyes Powder Pencil** *($15)* has a powdery texture and a finish that is meant to be smudged, but the point of this pencil is so soft, it is difficult to get an even application and it tends to smear instead. **Smooth Lining Eye Pencil** *($14)* is a creamier pencil that goes on well and offers some deep colors, but the finish of this also makes it prone to smearing. For a soft look, these do blend out well, but watch out. **$$$ Dual Perfection Brow Shaper and Eyeliner** *($16)* has a dry, grainy texture and is meant to be used wet, but the colors are shiny and that just doesn't fly for the brow and the eye. **$$$ Eye Defining Liquid Liner** *($16.50)* has a good formula but a bad brush—it is too long and loose to make using this type of eyeliner worthwhile.

☺ <u>LIPSTICK AND LIP PENCIL:</u> **$$$ Exceptional Lipstick** *($16.50)* is a great name for just a standard, creamy lipstick. These all tend to have a slight to strong glossy finish and enough stain to allow for longer wear. The color range is what's really exceptional! **Lip Definer** *($13.50)* is an automatic pencil (always a plus!) that goes on smoothly and has a creamy consistency. It's fine but not worth the price when there are so many less expensive pencils at the drugstore. **Lip Talkers** *($12.50)* is Arden's attempt at a pencil/lipstick. Of all these chubby lipstick pencils, available from Maybelline Lip Express to Prescriptives Matte Lip Crayon, I think Arden's is great. It is more matte than most, and has a slight stain, so it has great staying power; actually, it's a bit difficult to get off. Give this one a try next time you are at the cosmetics counters.

☺ $$$ **Lip Lip Hooray Lipstick SPF 15** *($16.50)* is a lipstick with a twist. It contains zinc citrate, an ingredient meant to fight bad breath. Zinc citrate works to control bad breath by neutralizing sulfur compounds in the mouth. It's an interesting concept but not all that practical, given that applying zinc citrate to the lips doesn't mean it gets to the mouth or stomach, where the bad breath is generated. Actually, if the notion is to lick the lipstick and get the zinc citrate that way, that's a problem because eating lipstick is hardly healthy. The other problem with this lipstick is that it contains mint and menthol, which can be irritating to the lips. I suspect those are in here to give women a cooling sensation on the lips to create the sensation of fresh breath. That's a false reading at best. This is a good creamy lipstick, but fighting bad breath is best left to other methods. **Crystal Clear Lip Gloss** *($12.50)* is a very thick, sticky gloss that is flavored with spearmint, which tastes nice but can be irritating for the lips. $$$ **Visible Difference Lip Fix Creme** *($17.50)* is supposed to prevent lipstick from feathering. It works well for some lipsticks, but I don't care for the squeeze-tube applicator. It goes on like a moisturizer and must dry before you put on your lipstick. It is less than convenient for touch-ups during the day. I prefer anti-feathering products that come in lipstick or lip-liner forms so there's no waiting between applications and you don't need to remove what you have on to reapply.

☺ $$$ <u>MASCARA:</u> Arden's mascaras are still as good as they were when last reviewed, although it is surprising that, given the nature of the cosmetics industry, Arden has not launched any new mascaras in the past two years. **Defining Mascara** *($16.50)* is great for lengthening the lashes with minimal clumping. If thickness isn't your major goal, it's worth a try. **Two-Brush Mascara Regular** and **Waterproof** *($16.50)* are similar in application to the one above, except this one is double-ended to allow for a standard mascara application and then a lash-separating step. You won't notice much difference, but you will go through your mascara a lot faster—which is great for Arden, not for you! The waterproof version does hold up wonderfully under water. **Natural Volume Mascara** *($16.50)* is excellent; this also applies well and builds noticeable length and some thickness with minimal clumping—and it lasts. If the higher price doesn't bother you, go for it but there are less expensive options that are just as good as this one.

☺ $$$ <u>BRUSHES:</u> There is now a small but good assortment of **brushes** *($20 to $40)* to be found at most Arden counters. There are five to choose from, and you will find the **Face Brush** *($40)* is dense and soft but not too full or floppy, and the **Blush Brush** *($35)* has a great shape and is also dense yet soft. The **Eye Brushes 1, 2, and 3** *($20 to $35)* are fine but overpriced for what you get, although each brush comes with its own case, which is great for traveling.

## *English Ideas*
## *Lip Last (Makeup Only)*

The promise of an all-day lipstick has kept women searching and believing that the next lipstick they buy will really make it through lunch (or even just until midmorning). With its Lip Last, English Ideas is hoping you'll accept the notion that it has the answer for your lips. Well, don't hold your breath; you'll find you need almost as many touch-ups with Lip Last as you would without. English Ideas is a full line of makeup products and its stated goal is to "bring new technology to the cosmetic marketplace." Yet there isn't much new technology here. As always, there are some products to consider, plus enough gimmicky items to placate any full-fledged makeup shopper. And you'll be able to experiment to your heart's content with its well-organized tester units. What is both impressive and perplexing are the number of items (foundations, eyeshadow, concealer, lipsticks) displaying both reliable and unreliable SPF protection. If you can get this idea right for your foundations and eyeshadows, why not your lipsticks?

For more information about Lip Last and English Ideas, call 1-800-LIP-LAST or visit the Web site at www.englishideas.com.

☺ $$$ <u>FOUNDATION:</u> **Perfect Powder SPF 15 Pressed Powder Foundation** *($28)* is a very sheer, slightly shiny, talc-free powder foundation with titanium dioxide as the active sunscreen. There are eight shades available, with options for darker skin tones, and the texture is dry but smooth. Keep in mind that it takes a liberal coverage of sunscreen to get the SPF on the label, so a sheer-finish application won't protect you from sun damage. **Perfect Liquid SPF 15 Foundation** *($30)* comes in a pump bottle and also has titanium dioxide as its active agent. This has a slick, smooth application and dries quickly to an opaque, matte finish, which would be great for very oily skins. Four of the six shades are too peach or pink for most skin tones, but the two winning shades are LF4 and LF5 (for medium to dark skin tones). **Perfect Primer** *($28)* is a thick, viscous silicone primer that has an incredibly slippery texture (that's the nature of silicones) and leaves a soft, slick feel on the skin. This can make the skin look smoother, but the end result is not something everyone will appreciate.

☺ <u>EYESHADOW:</u> **Colour Eyeshadow SPF 15** *($15)* uses zinc oxide as its sunscreen and although that is a reliable ingredient for protection, it lends a dry, chalky texture to these powder eyeshadows. They blend decently and are pigment-rich, but the trade-off for these mostly shiny shadows is undesirable. $$$ **Eye Perfection Color Corrector SPF 15 Eyelid Foundation** *($35)* features three powdery colors in one compact: flesh tone, pale yellow, and mint green. The SPF is zinc oxide–based and has the same texture issues as the Colour Eyeshadows above, only this product tends to flake off easily.

EYE AND BROW SHAPER: ☺ **Kolour Liner** *($12)* is a completely standard, creamy pencil with a slightly powdery finish that can easily smear. $$$ **Brow Hi-Lites** *($22)* is an absurdly overpriced brow gel whose colors all have a strong metallic tint and a sticky texture. If you've ever dreamed of shiny copper or golden brows and can handle the price tag, these are for you. $$$ **Brow Last Brow Sealant** *($18)* is nothing more (literally) that alcohol and cellulose (a thickening agent), and even with two brushes it is not worth the high-end price tag.

☺ **Brow Enhance** *($15)* is a standard pencil with an unusually pleasant texture that applies easily and evenly without streaking or looking heavy. If you prefer pencil to powder for brows, this is an option.

☹ **Liner Last Eye Liner Sealant** *($18)* wouldn't be necessary if the eye pencil was better, but in any event this is nothing but alcohol with thickeners and a hairspray-type fixative, and that is too potentially irritating for the eye area. **Eye Potion Eye Lifting Treatment** *($18)* is a very pale pink, iridescent color that is applied with a wand to give a visual "lift" to the eye area. It is quite drying and the witch hazel in here isn't best for the eye area. Plus, shiny pink isn't the best lifting shade for everyone.

☺ LIPSTICK AND LIP PENCIL: **Kolour Creme SPF 15 Lipstick** *($15)* is a very creamy, opaque lipstick with an unreliable sunscreen and a slightly glossy finish. The color range is impressive, with some excellent reds to choose from. **Lip Works Lip Balm SPF 18** *($9)* is just a very sheer gloss that leaves your lips out to dry when it comes to UVA-protecting ingredients. The five options each have a "theme" (such as tea tree oil or grapefruit extract—which serve no purpose for lips other than to risk irritation, though the amounts in here are so minuscule they probably aren't a problem). The Concealer shades of Lip Works Lip Balm is reputed to hide cold sores, which is far beyond the reach of this product (and most any concealer, for that matter). $$$ **Lip Hi-Lites** *($22.50)* are applied with a sponge tip and have a slightly greasy feel and an ultra-shiny finish. For the money, any iridescent drugstore gloss from Revlon StreetWear to Maybelline would work just as well if not better. **Lip Enhance** *($15)* bills itself as lip liner and foundation in one, but is really just a standard, pink-toned pencil with an overly thick texture. **Kolour Crayon** *($12)* is a standard lip pencil that is a distinct improvement over the Lip Enhance's texture. These apply smoothly and offer a slight powder finish and have an impressive stain.

☺ $$$ **Lip Last Lipstick Sealant** *($17.50)* is supposed to be a "patented breakthrough" meant to solve the problem of keeping lipstick on the lips. While some aspect of the formula or name may be patented, efficacy is not patented (by the way, you can't patent efficacy for *any* product or ingredients). All this very tiny bottle contains is a film-forming ingredient (like hairspray) that burns when you apply it to the lips—there is even a warning on the bottle. If you apply an even layer, you definitely get a great covering over your lips that creates a matte seal and that can prevent feathering and bleeding, though not any better that most ultra-matte lipsticks (Revlon ColorStay comes to mind). This does last for a good length of time but tends to roll and chip off the lips, taking your lipstick with it. Your lipstick will still stay on, but only slightly longer than usual. It is tricky to apply, and the burning can be a problem. There are better ways to keep lipstick from bleeding or feathering than this pricey little liquid.

☹ **Professional Lip Brush** *($20)* has a decent brush, but the overly long, inconvenient handle does not come with a cap—meaning that once this is used, traces of lipstick will be all over whatever the brush touches if it is not kept clean. **Lip Refine** *($32 for 0.5 ounce)* is a lotion that contains AHAs and is supposed to exfoliate the lips. I would be concerned about AHAs on the lips because of the delicate nature of the skin in that area, but this product doesn't have a low enough pH to create any exfoliation. Even if it did, there are far less expensive and far more effective AHA products available.

☺ **Lip Makeup Remover** *($10)* uses plant oil to cut through Lip Last. It works, but any oil would do the same thing. Of course, this product makes much ado about not containing mineral oil– or petroleum-based ingredients, as if they were somehow bad for skin; they aren't. In fact, because mineral oil doesn't go rancid like plant oils, it is better for the skin in many ways.

☹ $$$ <u>MASCARA:</u> **Mega Mascara All Weather Mascara** *($24)* is woefully overpriced, and the very curved and wavy brush is awkward for applying mascara. How you're supposed to get an even mascara application out of this is a mystery. **Mega Primer** *($16)* is a standard, white coating of mascara that is completely unnecessary given the prevalence of superior mascaras that can get long lashes without the help of an additional product.

☹ **Duo Lash Treatment Mascara** *($28)* is a double-sided mascara with one end being the Mega Primer reviewed above and the other a standard mascara that will eventually lengthen lashes with no clumping. The primer makes no discernible difference, and, for the money, this can't compare to L'Oreal's Le Grande Curl, Maybelline's Vol'um Express Mascaras, or any Lancome mascara for far less.

## *Epicuren (Skin Care Only)*

I don't know how to describe how truly unbelievable I found the claims espoused by Epicuren. They rank up there with some of the worst (though, to my chagrin, I have to admit that the companies that are on my "overblown offenders" list is getting longer and longer by the day). Epicuren's marketing nonsense (though an expletive I can't use would have been far better than the word "nonsense") is just infuriating because I'm certain there are lots of consumers who will want to believe what this company professes. First, let's take the natural air out of this overinflated balloon of claims. Epicuren claims that its products are hypoallergenic, non-comedogenic, and absolutely free of chemical preservatives or fragrances. According to the FDA, "hypoallergenic" and "noncomedogenic" are not regulated terms, and cosmetics companies can use them however they like. There are plenty of ingredients in these products that can trigger skin reactions, and these products absolutely contain fragrance. *All* ingredients are chemicals, and fragrant oils and fragrant extracts are chemicals with preservatives to keep them stable.

Epicuren's claims about natural versus chemical are meaningless, and their products contain plenty of synthetic ingredients—didn't the marketing people read their own ingredient listings? Further, many of these products contain quite chemical ingredients that range from sodium lauryl sulfate to triethanolamine, tetrasodium EDTA, butylene glycol, benzoyl peroxide, cetyl alcohol, diazolidinyl urea, sodium C14-16 olefin sulfate, artificial coloring agents, propylparaben, and on and on. The notion of natural is ludicrous.

While some of the unnatural ingredients on the Epicuren label are easy to spot, others are disguised with names like P.C.M.X., something that turns out to be chloroxylenol, a preservative. That's not bad, but it is definitely not natural, though the name helps keep up the facade Epicuren is trying to create.

Epicuren's collection of other erroneous or misleading information is extensive. It states that "glycolic acid without prescription was approved by the FDA in mid-1990." That's not true in the least. Glycolic acid in strengths under 20% has always been available over the counter and never needed a prescription. Epicuren also claims that its "...5% or 10% [glycolic acid] solutions will not make your skin sensitive to the sun like Retin-A does." This flies in the face of recent research published by the FDA that indicates just the opposite. Products with effective AHAs that do their job of exfoliating built-up sun-damaged skin indeed make the skin more sun-sensitive. While Epicuren carries on at length about how its glycolic acid products are far better and more gentle than Retin-A, it also warns that "if you experience a mild stinging effect [from the Glycolic Polymer Solution], this is normal and will subside with usage. However, if the stinging persists, rinse off after an hour until your tolerance increases." The exact same thing can be said of Retin-A. And lots of people do not get used to AHAs or Retin-A.

You have to sit down for this next one! On the one hand, Epicuren states that its zinc-oxide sunscreen "is truly a new millennium product; especially, in the wake of all the medical publications such as the *New England Journal of Medicine*, etc. on the dangers caused [by] using chemical sunscreen ingredients that irritate the skin, such as octyl methoxycinnamate, benzophenone-3, benzophenone-4 and octyl dimethyl and PABA." Not only have there been no such published studies in that journal, it has published just the opposite information: the *New England Journal of Medicine*, October 14, 1993, vol. 329, no. 16, states, "On balance, then, the possible [and unproven] adverse consequences of sunscreen use are dwarfed by their established benefits." What is even more incredible than this erroneous, potentially harmful information is that Epicuren didn't notice that some of its own sunscreens include some of the very ingredients it criticizes, including octyl methoxycinnamate and benzophenone-3, and at levels ranging from 5% to 7.5%.

I won't even get started on the prices for these products. For more information on Epicuren, call (800) 235-1217 or visit the Web site at www.epicuren.com.

☺ $$$ **Herbal Cleanser** (*$48 for 4 ounces*) is a standard, detergent-based cleanser (which isn't natural in the least) that would work well for normal to oily skin. If you think the price brings you the benefit of the plants and vitamins present in the tiniest amounts in this product, remember that in a cleanser they would all just be rinsed down the drain before they could somehow affect the skin.

☹ **Citrus Herbal Cleanser** (*$41 for 4 ounces*) uses lemon oil (and it does smell like lemon oil) and that can be irritating to the eyes. Even if I thought its claim that this product contains "natural surfactants" was true, surfactants are potentially drying.

☹ **Gelle Cleanser** (*$17 for 4 ounces*) uses sodium C14-16 olefin sulfate as one of the main cleansers, which can make it irritating for most skin types.

☺ $$$ **Apricot Cream Cleanser** (*$31 for 4 ounces*) is a good emollient cleanser for dry skin, though it does need to be wiped off and can leave a slight greasy feel on the skin.

☺ $$$ **Facial Scrub** (*$34 for 4 ounces*) is supposed to be "a surgical scrub." Run for your life if your doctor is scrubbing with finely ground apricot and walnut shells, which is what this product contains, along with thickeners, fragrance, and preservatives. It is a decent scrub but there is no reason to use this over other far less expensive scrubs or just plain baking soda for that matter. One more point: Epicuren claims this one is all-natural too, but it contains propylene glycol and propylparaben among other very synthetic ingredients.

☺ $$$ **Fine Herbal Scrub** (*$37 for 4 ounces*) is almost identical to the one above only with a smaller content of shells. The same basic comments apply.

☺ $$$ **Citrus Herbal Extra Fine Cleansing Scrub** (*$37 for 4 ounces*) is similar to the two versions above and the same comments apply.

☺ $$$ **Benzoyl Peroxide Scrub** (*$27 for 4 ounces*). According to Epicuren, "benzoyl peroxide has been medically proven over the past 10 years to be the most effective way to diminish acne through cleansing." While benzoyl peroxide is a good disinfectant for breakouts, there is no research indicating it is the most effective, and definitely not when it is in a cleanser. Despite its first comment, Epicuren's further explanation contradicts its original claim that "Benzoyl Peroxide Scrub is not a preventative measure for acne but rather a treatment for active eruptions and acne clusters." Odd, that's not what it said at first. Nevertheless, benzoyl peroxide is indeed preventive because it kills the bacteria in the pore that are part of what triggers a breakout. In a cleanser, the benzoyl peroxide would be rinsed away before it had much chance to have an effect. This product also contains pumice, which can be very irritating for most skin types.

☹ **$$$ Medicated Acne Cleanser** (*$32 for 4 ounces*) uses sodium lauryl sulfate as the main cleansing agent, which makes it problematic for most skin types. The 1% benzoyl peroxide in here is indeed a good disinfectant for breakouts, but in a cleanser it would be rinsed down the drain before it had much of a chance to be effective.

☺ **$$$ Medicated Acne Gel** (*$49 for 4 ounces*) contains 10% benzoyl peroxide, a concentration that makes it effective for disinfecting the bacteria in skin that can cause acne. The gimmick in this product is that it is supposed to contain 5% asymmetric oxygen, something that is supposed to "make it the most effective acne treatment known." It is true that oxygen can kill bacteria but the notion that this can penetrate skin and help is at best minimally possible.

☹ **$$$ Live Enzyme Conditioner** (*$22 for 2 ounces*) is supposed to invigorate and break down the skin's surface. This product claims to contain an enzyme, but it doesn't state which one. While enzymes in general can have exfoliating properties, enzymes are notoriously unstable in products, and if this one is live, a contention I truly doubt, then it would be even more unstable than most.

☹ **$$$ Enzyme Protein Mist** (*$20 for 4 ounces*) contains the same "live enzyme" as the other enzyme products in this line; this one is even recommended for the hair. Well, let's hope that it can't do what enzymes do, which is exfoliate the surface of skin, because if it can do that, it would also exfoliate the structure of the hair (hair is merely dead skin, almost identical to the skin's surface layer). It can't do much for the skin so I wouldn't worry about what it would do to the hair.

☹ **$$$ Live Enzyme Concentrate** (*$56 for 1 ounce*). I guess if you need one enzyme product, two must be better. But if one of the live enzyme products in this group does work, you don't need more—after all, there is only so much skin you can break down. Instead Epicuren wants you to apply this, then apply the Enzyme Gel Plus and a moisturizer. Supposedly this concentrate was originally developed for treatment of burns. Unbelievable! Does burned skin really need to be further broken down and peeled?

☹ **$$$ Live Enzyme Gel Plus** (*$68 for 2 ounces*) is similar to the other enzyme products but with supposedly more enzyme. The same basic comments apply.

☹ **Glycolic Polymer Solution 5% or 10% Gel or Lotion** *($20 for 2 ounces).* Epicuren recommends you use its AHA products with its Enzyme products. How much skin does Epicuren think we have to exfoliate? But not to worry; according to the ingredient listing the 10% version does not contain that much AHA and the pH of 5.5 to 6 is too high for it to be effective as an exfoliant. The 5% version does seem to contain that amount, but again the pH is too high for it to exfoliate effectively.

☺ **Apricot Facial Emulsion** *($26 for 2 ounces)* is a good facial cream for normal to dry skin. It can also be custom blended with "your favorite aromatherapy" including peppermint, orange, and grapefruit. When it comes to skin care, your skin would be far better off if you just lit a fragrant candle instead of putting the fragrance all over your face.

☺ **$$$ Ultra Rose Treat Emulsion** *($42 for 2 ounces)* is almost identical to the Apricot version above and the same comments apply.

☺ **Evening Emulsion** *($32 for 2 ounces)* is similar to the Rose and Apricot versions above and the same comments apply.

☺ **$$$ Acidophilus Facial Skin Cream** *($60 for 4 ounces)* contains the tiniest amount of acidophilus you can imagine. If you want acidophilus, there are yogurts or supplements that are a far better source. What benefit acidophilus can have for skin is not substantiated anywhere, but even if it did have a positive effect it wouldn't in this quantity (internally acidophilus helps to give the body healthy bacteria if you are taking antibiotics).

☺ **Aloe Vera Gel** *($14 for 4 ounces)* contains aloe vera gel, and that's not the same as pure aloe, despite what the marketing claims imply, because a gel form is already far diluted from the actual aloe plant. That doesn't make it bad, but it is definitely not preferred to the aloe vera gel you can buy at your health food store. This version is supposedly infused with asymmetric oxygen, but if it really could deliver this to the skin, it would trigger free-radical damage.

☺ **$$$ Eye Cream** *($56 for 0.5 ounce)* is a good emollient moisturizer for normal to dry skin.

☺ **$$$ Retinol Concentrate** *($48 for 0.5 ounce)* is basically a good moisturizer for normal to dry skin, with antioxidants and plant oil. Even though I find the research suggesting that what retinol does is related to the effects of Retin-A or Renova completely inconclusive, many products showcase it, and this version is not preferred over others that range from Alpha Hydrox to L'Oreal. The reason for this is that the way it's packaged (in a non-airtight, non-opaque container) makes me strongly doubt the claim that it is stabilized.

☺ **$$$ CXc Stabilized Vitamin C Topical** *($36 for 0.5 ounce)* is supposed to contain a 15% concentration of ascorbyl glucosamine, but so does the Retinol version above (or close to it). So why would you bother with this one and miss the theoretical miracle of retinol?

☹ **$$$ Botanical Elixir Serum** *($48 for 1 ounce)* claims to contain "33 highly beneficial botanical substances." That's a lot of plants to put on one face. There is no way to tackle the claims surrounding each of the substances appearing in this lotion, but the amount of each is minuscule, and a few are relatively irritating to skin, including arnica, lemon, and the fragrant oils. However, those who are seeking carrot extract, green tea, *Ginkgo biloba,* celery extract, broccoli extract, and lemon extract, to name a few, need look no further.

☺ **$$$ Colostrum Serum** *($80 for 2 ounces).* I guess if you want more than just the miracles of Epicuren's vitamin C, enzyme, AHA, retinol, or fragrant-oil rejuvenation products, then this is as good as any. Colostrum is a fluid secreted in animal and human breast milk at the start of milk production. The source of colostrum used in cosmetics or supplements is animal. While there is absolutely no question that human colostrum transfers many important active immunological compounds to a newborn, that is where the benefits start and stop, at least for skin care. When it comes to topical or oral application of colostrum, there have been no in vivo studies monitoring its effect on human skin.

☺ **$$$ Essential Rose Oil** *($48 for 0.5 ounce)* is one way to put perfume on your face if you want to do that, though this can be irritating and sensitizing to the skin. This product also contains other fragrant oils that are also problematic for skin. This oil is great for smelling but not for the skin.

☹ **Conditioning Lip Balm SPF 15** *($8 for 0.25 ounce)* does not contain adequate UVA protection and is not recommended.

☹ **Enzyme Protein Sunscreen** *($18 for 4 ounces)* does not contain UVA-protecting ingredients and is not recommended.

☹ **Enzyme Protein Sunscreen Extra Moisturizing Spray SPF 20** *($18 for 4 ounces)* does not contain UVA-protecting ingredients and is not recommended.

☺ **$$$ Zinc Oxide Sunblock Sunscreen SPF 20** *($58 for 4 ounces)* is a very good, exceptionally overpriced sunscreen. Despite Epicuren's glorification of pure zinc oxide, Neutrogena's SPF 15 and SPF 30 products, both with pure titanium dioxide for one-sixth the price, are excellent and as gentle as this one, and give the same protection, plus Neutrogena's won't burn your wallet.

☹ **$$$ Bulgaricum Powder** *($60 for 4.5 ounces)* is a very fancy way to sell yogurt for the skin. You're supposed to mix the *Lactobacillus bulgaricus* powder in this product with Epicuren's Pure Aloe, and you get something that is supposed to detoxify and oxygenate skin. However, in general skin doesn't like oxygen—oxygen triggers free-radical damage, ergo the need for antioxidants. Even if oxygen in this form could somehow benefit skin, how that bit of extra oxygen is better than what the air provides (21% of air is oxygen) is a mystery. If you like yogurt for skin, there are far cheaper versions than this, like pure yogurt from a health food store.

☺ $$$ **Skin Rejuvenation Therapy (SRT) Facial Emulsion with added Anti-oxidants** (available in **SRT #1: Bulgarian Rose Otto, Jasmine, Neroli, Lavender, and Vetiver;** or **SRT #2: Melisse, Clarysage, Myrrh, and Frankincense**) *($60 for 1 ounce).* According to the Epicuren brochure, "This is the ultimate treatment for cell rejuvenation to help reverse the signs of aging." But if this is the ultimate then what are the all other vitamin, enzyme, AHA, herbal, and colostrum products for? The fragrance in the SRT product can be irritating for skin, but other than that it can be a good moisturizer for normal to dry skin. Just don't expect one wrinkle to change, because it won't. This also contains the same enzyme ingredient as the ones above, but again I suspect it isn't effective to exfoliate skin.

☺ $$$ **Pro-Collagen III** *($30 for 0.33 ounce)* supposedly "selectively amplifies the biosynthesis of Collagen III in human skin. ... The phenomenal results are typically visible within 48 hours." If that were possible, how would the skin know when to stop making collagen? Would your skin just plump up forever? Nonetheless, this is merely a good moisturizer for normal to dry skin with some good water-binding agents and vitamins, but there is absolutely nothing special in this product that would even begin to warrant such exaggerated claims.

**(Unrated) Progesterone Cream** *($63 for 4 ounces)* contains wild yam, but wild yam does not contain anything else that would act like progesterone when absorbed through skin. According to *The PDR Family Guide to Natural Medicines & Healing Therapies,* as well as Dr. John R. Lee, who is the originator of the theory about using topically applied progesterone, "[while wild yam] is used in the production of artificial progesterone it will not yield the hormone in the absence of a chemical conversion process that the body can't supply." However, this product does contain progesterone USP, the kind of ingredient recommended by Lee (though there is no information about the amount of that ingredient this product contains ). Please see the section in Chapter Two of this book on "Battling Hormones: Is Progesterone in Skin-Care Products the Answer?" for information regarding products making claims about their progesterone content. And please note that Dr. Lee does recommend far less expensive progesterone creams than this one.

# Erno Laszlo

Erno Laszlo's continued following is beyond me. I made a bet years ago, when the products first came out in upper-end department stores, that this line wouldn't last. I believed women would never pay $14 (that was the price in the first edition of this book), then $23 (second edition), and now an astounding $25 (fifth edition) for a bar of soap. I was wrong. It is still around and it still has a following.

According to the company's brochure, Dr. Erno Laszlo, an (alleged) Hungarian dermatologist, was "the first to combine the exact science of his profession with the art of cosmetology" using "precisely diagnosed treatments dispensed with a doctor's touch." Great copy, except that Erno Laszlo was never licensed to practice medicine in this country, and some say he was never even a medical doctor in Eastern Europe.

In his time, Laszlo's claim to fame was prescribing skin-care regimens for wealthy women who could afford to "succumb to the 'Laszlo Ritual' of daily skincare." His ritual included washing with old-fashioned bar soap (he had women with dry skin cover their face in oil before using the soap), then splashing the face 30 times with a basin full of the soapy rinse water, then splashing the face 30 times with scalding hot water. When that was done, his patients would finish by soaking their skin with apple cider vinegar. Dr. Laszlo proclaimed that nothing cleaned better than hot water and soap, but because soap's alkaline content destroyed the skin's pH level, apple cider vinegar was needed to restore it.

One of the problems with tried-and-true skin-care routines is that new research, more often than not, negates what we once thought to be true. After all, the good doctor couldn't have known about sun damage or the need for exfoliation, or that hot water can hurt skin and cause surfaced capillaries. He clearly didn't know that soap is too irritating and that irritation is a problem for skin. Plus, alkaline substances (that's what soap is) on skin are extremely drying, and studies have demonstrated that they can increase bacteria content in skin and hurt the skin's healing process. With gentle cleansing, you leave the pH of the skin alone, and there is no reason to worry about bringing it back to the right pH.

Aside from a potpourri of plant extracts (some irritating, others soothing), a rather unique plant oil used in some of the Laszlo products is chaulmoogra oil (which is supposed to be the "*doctor's* discovery" but that is clearly not the case. Chaulmoogra oil was utilized in the 1800s internally to treat leprosy, and rather successfully at the time. However, topically, it is an emollient that can cause skin irritation.

In 1966 Laszlo sold the right to use his name and retail his products to Chesebrough-Pond's. Now, some 30 years after Laszlo's death (and a slew of other owners), are these products in line with Laszlo's original skin-care theories? For the most part, the skin-care routines still include using bar soap and all of that soapy/hot water splashing, but the rest of the regimen is just loosely based on the "doctor's" concepts. All but one of the toners is alcohol-based, just like many other toners on the market. The line's makeup offerings are still small compared with its mammoth skin-care collection, but nevertheless have expanded. Yet there is still nothing spectacular enough to warrant such high and mighty prices. A few of the foundations have some excellent textures and colors, but that's about it. For more information on Erno Laszlo, call (800) 865-3222 or visit the Web site at www.ernolaszlo.com.

# Erno Laszlo Skin Care

☹ **Active pHelityl Cleansing Lotion** *($28 for 6.8 ounces)* is a relatively standard, detergent-based water-soluble cleanser that also contains some emollient, which can make it better for normal to dry skin. It also contains some fairly irritating plant extracts that are supposed to sound like AHAs but they are unrelated to that kind of effect on the skin. It also contains lemongrass, pine needle, and arnica, which just add to the irritation.

☺ **$$$ Active pHelityl Oil Pre-Cleansing Oil for Dry to Slightly Oily Skin** *($30 for 6.8 ounces)* is supposed to be used before you use the soaps below, to protect the skin and help remove makeup. But your skin wouldn't need protection if you weren't using such a drying product to wash your face. This contains mostly mineral oil, plant oil, fragrance, and preservatives. Given this is mostly mineral oil, skip the fragrance and just use plain mineral oil for far less; that's what the doctor did.

☹ **Active pHelityl Soap for Dry and Slightly Dry Skin** *($23 for 6 ounces)* is a standard, tallow-based bar of soap, with the same ingredients found in all soaps. This one does contain some plant oil, but that won't help the dryness caused by the other ingredients. This is a lot of money for a very ordinary bar of soap.

☹ **HydrapHel Cleansing Bar for Extremely Dry Skin** *($24 for 6 ounces)* doesn't contain any tallow, but it has all the other detergent cleansing agents that can cause dry skin. This is a standard bar cleanser with a tiny amount of emollients, and it's not the best for any skin type, and especially not dry skin.

☹ **HydrapHel Cleansing Milk for Extremely Dry Skin** *($28 for 6.8 ounces)* contains several potentially irritating plant extracts, including lemongrass, pine needle, arnica, and kiwi. They can be a problem for any skin type but especially for dry skin. Other than that, this is just a cold cream–type cleanser that needs to be wiped off and can leave a greasy film on the skin.

☺ **$$$ HydrapHel Cleansing Treatment Liquid Cleanser for Extremely Dry Skin** *($25 for 4.3 ounces)* is little more than an expensive, standard cold cream, and not very different from just using mineral oil or Vaseline by itself. It can be an option for dry skin, but it can leave a greasy film.

☹ **Sea Mud Soap for Normal, Slightly Oily, and Oily Skin** *($23 for 6 ounces)* contains the standard soap ingredients of tallow and sodium cocoate, with a little sea mud thrown in. It's still soap, and the mud makes it more drying and leaves a slight film on the skin. Also, tallow can cause breakouts.

☹ **Special Skin Soap for Oily and Extremely Oily Skin** *($23 for 6 ounces)* contains the standard soap ingredients of tallow and sodium cocoate, along with the detergent cleanser sodium lauryl sulfate, which is very drying and irritating. This is a fairly drying, average bar soap, and the tallow can cause breakouts.

The Reviews E

☹ **Sea Mud Cleanser** *($28 for 6.8 ounces)* contains fairly drying detergent cleansing agents as well as some fairly irritating plant extracts, including arnica, pine needle, and arnica. There is sea mud in here but that just adds to the dryness. There are far more gentle ways to effectively clean the face than this.

☹ **Multi-pHase Eye Makeup Remover for All Skin Types** *($25 for 4 ounces)* is basically just silicone and plant extracts. The plant extracts include some that can cause inflammation and irritation and that should not be used repeatedly on skin.

☺ **$$$ pHelitone Gentle Eye Makeup Remover** *($18 for 3 ounces)* is far more gentle than most all of the above cleansers; there are no irritating plant extracts or drying cleansing agents. This is just a basic makeup remover that uses a more gentle detergent cleansing agent and some slip agents, with no fragrance and coloring agents. If they could figure this out for a "gentle" product, why not be gentle with everyone's skin?

☹ **Conditioning Preparation for Oily to Extremely Oily Skin** *($26 for 6.8 ounces)* is almost pure alcohol, and very irritating to the skin; plus, resorcinol is a serious skin irritant, and one the FDA disallowed in 1992 for products making claims to treat acne.

☹ **Heavy Controlling Lotion PM Oil Control for Slightly Oily to Extremely Oily Skin** *($28 for 6.8 ounces)* won't control anything, and the alcohol makes it too drying and irritating for all skin types.

☺ **$$$ HydrapHel Skin Supplement Freshener for Extremely Dry and Dry Skin** *($30 for 6.8 ounces)*. At least this one doesn't contain any alcohol; it's about time. This would be a good nonirritating toner for most skin types.

☹ **Light Controlling Lotion Toner for Slightly Dry to Oily Skin** *($26 for 6.8 ounces)*. The alcohol is too irritating for all skin types.

☹ **Regular Controlling Lotion PM Oil Control for Slightly Dry and Normal Skin** *($28 for 6.8 ounces)* is an alcohol-based toner that also contains some talc and baking soda. The alcohol is too irritating and drying for all skin types but is particularly inexcusable in a product for dry skin.

☹ **AHA Revitalizing Complex** *($95 for 1.5 ounces)* contains about 3% to 4% AHAs and BHA combined, but the pH is too high for it to be an effective exfoliant, not to mention that there are far more effective and less expensive AHA or BHA versions available, and I am also not one to recommend both together; use AHA for sun-damaged skin and BHA for blemish-prone skin.

☺ **Active pHelityl Cream PM Moisturizer for Slightly Dry Skin** *($32 for 2 ounces)* is a standard, emollient, Vaseline-based moisturizer. You're paying a lot of money for what amounts to not much more than Vaseline.

☺ **$$$ Antioxidant Complex for Eyes, Lightening, Firming, Protective Eye Treatment for All Skin Types** *($65 for 1 ounce)*. Tannic acid can be a skin irritant. And though this product does contain mulberry extract and magnesium ascorbyl phosphate (a stable form of vitamin C) that can have melanin-inhibiting effect on skin, the amounts are minuscule and not enough to have any effect.

☺ **$$$ Antioxidant Concentrate for Eyes, Intensive Therapy for the Eye Area** *($48 for 0.5 ounce)* is a very good emollient moisturizer. It does contain a tiny amount of witch hazel but not enough to have an effect on the skin.

☹ **$$$ Antioxidant Mattifying Complex** *($45 for 2 ounces)*. The witch hazel can be an irritant but the film formers can leave a matte feeling, though it won't last long. This is more of a lightweight moisturizer for normal to oily skin than something that will provide many oil-absorbing properties.

☹ **Antioxidant Moisture Complex SPF 15 Oil-Free Moisturizer for All Skin Types** *($55 for 2 ounces)* doesn't contain avobenzone, zinc oxide, or titanium dioxide, and is not recommended.

☺ **$$$ Antioxidant Moisture Complex Cream for Extremely Dry to Normal Skin** *($65 for 2 ounces)*. This is a very good emollient moisturizer for someone with dry skin.

☹ **Daily Moisture Protection Lotion SPF 15 AM Moisturizer with Sunscreen for All Skin Types** *($45 for 2.5 ounces)* doesn't contain avobenzone, zinc oxide, or titanium dioxide, and is not recommended.

☹ **$$$ HydrapHel Complex PM Moisturizer for Extremely Dry and Dry Skin** *($55 for 2 ounces)* is a good, though very ordinary moisturizer for dry skin.

☺ **$$$ HydrapHel Emulsion AM Moisturizer for Extremely Dry and Dry Skin** *($45 for 2 ounces)* is a good emollient moisturizer that still requires a good sunscreen if you are going to be wearing it during the day.

☹ **Moisture-Firming Throat Cream for All Skin Types** *($23 for 2 ounces)* would be a good emollient moisturizer for dry skin, but it contains some fairly irritating plant extracts, including ginseng and arnica.

☹ **$$$ pHelitone Replenishing Eye Cream for All Skin Types** *($42 for 0.5 ounce)*. Pricey for a jar of Vaseline-based moisturizer, with little else, don't you think?

☹ **$$$ pHelityl Cream PM Moisturizer for Normal Skin** *($55 for 2 ounces)* is an exceptionally ordinary emollient moisturizer for normal to dry skin.

☹ **pHelityl Lotion AM Moisturizer for Slightly Dry to Slightly Oily Skin** *($45 for 3 ounces)* is good, lightweight, and emollient for someone with dry skin, but overpriced for a very ordinary mineral oil–based moisturizer. Plus, no one with even slightly oily skin is going to be happy with this much oil in a product of any kind, and without sunscreen it is useless for daytime.

☹ **$$$ R.E.M. Intensive Night Therapy for Normal to Extremely Oily Skin** *($85 for 2 ounces)*, with its emollients and waxes such as caprylic/capric triglyceride, beeswax, ozokerite, and plant oils, is a serious problem for oily skin. Actually, all this product ends up being is a very good moisturizer for normal to dry skin.

☺ $$$ **Total Skin Revitalizer Facial Hydration Enhancer for All Skin Types** (*$54 for 1 ounce*) is a lightweight, emollient moisturizer. It won't revitalize the skin, but it will keep normal to dry skin moist, just like any other moisturizer.

☺ $$$ **Total Skin Revitalizer for Eyes Hydration Enhancer for the Eye Area** (*$45 for 0.5 ounce*). This is a good emollient moisturizer for the eyes (although there is a tiny amount of witch hazel and ivy in here, it's probably not enough to be irritating).

☺ $$$ **Retinol Reparative Therapy** (*$85 for 1 ounce*) is another retinol product, but if you compare the cost and the formulation, L'Oreal's, Neutrogena's, and Alpha Hydrox's are just as good for one-eighth the price and in more airtight packaging (which keeps the retinol stable).

☹ $$$ **Hydra-Therapy Skin Vitality Treatment, Two Phase Moisture Mask for All Skin Types** (*$36 for four applications of each phase*) is a two-part system that is so amazingly ordinary it is almost embarrassing. You mix an ordinary liquid with a simple powder that is mostly salt, apply it to your face, let it set, and then rinse. It contains ordinary ingredients, but an absurdly expensive price tag.

☺ $$$ **pHelitone Firming Eye Gel Mask for All Skin Types** (*$30 for 0.5 ounce*) is an absurdly standard, lightweight gel for minimally dry skin. It does contain a small amount of witch hazel but probably not enough to be a problem.

☹ **Beta Wash** (*$32 for 6.8 ounces*) uses sodium C14-16 olefin sulfate and sodium lauryl sulfate as the main cleansing agents, which would be irritating enough for any skin type, but then this product throws more fuel on the fire with the inclusion of camphor, menthol, and peppermint. This is an irritation waiting to happen.

☹ $$$ **Beta Complex Acne Treatment** (*$65 for 2 ounces*) is a good, irritant-free BHA exfoliant, but the price is almost mind-boggling, especially as the pH is too high for this to be an effective exfoliant. There are far less expensive versions around with the appropriate pH that work. This one is a waste of time for the skin.

☹ **Beta Target Blemish Treatment** (*$18 for 0.5 ounce*) contains too much alcohol, eucalyptus, peppermint, menthol, and camphor for any skin type; this is an irritation waiting to happen.

☹ **Beta Mask** (*$36*) contains too much alcohol, eucalyptus, peppermint, menthol, and camphor for any skin type; this is an irritation waiting to happen.

☹ **Sea Mud Mask** (*$32 for 4 ounces*) is basically a standard clay mask, but it also contains alcohol and peppermint, which makes it too irritating for all skin types.

☹ **Oil-Free Sunblock SPF 25 for All Skin Types** (*$22 for 4.3 ounces*) doesn't contain avobenzone, zinc oxide, or titanium dioxide, and is not recommended.

☺ **Self-Tanning Lotion SPF 8** (*$22 for 4.2 ounces*) doesn't contain avobenzone, zinc oxide, or titanium dioxide, and is not recommended as a sunscreen, but it works fine as a self tanner.

☹ **Sun Control Mist SPF 15** *($22 for 3.5 ounces)* doesn't contain avobenzone, zinc oxide, or titanium dioxide, and is not recommended.

## Erno Laszlo Makeup

FOUNDATION: There are some very good foundations here, including some with reliable sun protection. The shades cater to those with very light to medium skins—darker skins will be forced to search elsewhere. As an aside, the "pH" in the "multi-pHase" names refers to the line's notions about adjusting the skin's pH level and the "multitude of benefits" supposedly bestowed on anyone who wears a Laszlo foundation. Most skin-care and makeup products these days are in alignment with the skin's own pH so this claim is not of special benefit.

☹ **Multi-pHase Active Tint SPF 15** *($22)* is an extremely sheer, tinted moisturizer whose four colors are dated, at best. There is no UVA protection, and according to the company, this product is, thankfully, on the way out.

☺ **$$$ Multi-pHase Dual Option Foundation SPF 8** *($32)* is a standard powder foundation that can be used wet or dry. It has a dry, soft texture and even, matte finish with reliable sun protection (zinc oxide and titanium dioxide), although with an SPF number that is too small to bank on. Of the eight shades, six are great options and two should be avoided: Rose Bisque and Fawn are too rose for most skin tones.

☺ **$$$ Multi-pHase Light Diffusing Foundation SPF 15** *($30)* has a smooth, slightly thick texture that blends out to a natural matte finish with light to medium coverage. The SPF is part titanium dioxide, and of the 14 colors, only Tawny and Rose Beige are best avoided. By the way, this doesn't diffuse light or change the appearance of wrinkles—it's just a good foundation for normal to slightly dry skin. I am not wild about the pump bottle, which tends to deliver more foundation than you need to use with no way to get it back in the bottle.

☺ **$$$ Multi-pHase Oil Free Foundation SPF 15** *($30)* has an in-part titanium dioxide–based sunscreen and comes in a pump-applicator bottle, which can waste product. This one has a slightly drier finish than the Light Diffusing version above and would be best for normal to slightly oily skins needing light to moderate coverage. Of the 14 shades, be wary of Bisque, Linen, and Tawny, which are too pink or rose for most skin tones.

☹ **MultipHase Perfecting Foundation SPF 8** *($32)* has a too-low SPF with no UVA protection and is a poor choice for stick foundation. It does have a creamy texture but the finish is slightly heavy and it can look caked, especially with these 12 shades, which are pretty close to terrible—only Biscotti and Shell may be worth considering by some lighter skin tones.

☹ **Regular Normalizer Shake-It Foundation** *($32)* is a thin, liquidy foundation that is mostly alcohol and talc, and although it does dry to a sheer, matte finish, the alcohol makes it too drying and irritating for anyone.

☹ <u>CONCEALER:</u> **pHelitone Concealer** *($27)* has a creamy-smooth texture and finish but comes in three unimpressive colors, and at this price they should be perfectly neutral. **Multi-pHase Firming Concealer** *($27)* is very concentrated and provides full coverage and a dry finish that can look heavy if blending isn't spot-perfect. The formula tends to separate in the tube and the four colors are a mixed bag of "just passable" and "no way."

☺ $$$ <u>POWDER:</u> **Multi-pHase Finishing Powder** *($35)* is a prism of shades in one compact that end up creating one shiny color on the face. They are available as a flesh-toned color (the Finishing Powder), a **Highlighter** *($32)*, or a **Bronzer** *($35)*, and all share the same comments. If overpriced shine motivates you, here you go.

☺ $$$ **Controlling Face Powder Loose** *($28)* and **Duo-pHase Face Powder Loose** *($28)* are both standard, talc-based powders with a dry, very silky texture and a satin finish. The Duo pHase is recommended for normal to dry skin, but there isn't much difference between the two and the colors are identical.

☺ $$$ **Controlling Face Powder Pressed** *($25)* and **Duo-pHase Pressed Powder** *($25)* are also standard and talc-based, and with the exception of the pressed format, the same comments for the loose versions apply here too.

☺ $$$ <u>BLUSH:</u> **Multi-pHase Blusher** *($35)* is available in one compact that has a prismatic arrangement of colors that apply as a single rosy tone on the skin. It's matte, which is nice, but nothing special or worth this amount of money for what amounts to a standard blush with no color options.

☺ <u>EYESHADOW:</u> $$$ **Multi-pHase Eyeshadow Multi-Wear** *($32)* has a very long name for what comes down to just eyeshadow trios with a powder eyeliner included. At least one part of each set is shiny, and it's usually the eyeliner part. So after you've applied three matte shadows, your lash line will glisten and glitter and look distracting. If you're into that concept, Sand and Taupe are the best ones to consider. $$$ **Multi-pHase Cream Eye Sheer** *($22)* is a cream eyeshadow that blends on thick and choppy and stays creamy, which means it will crease and crease throughout the day. **Multi-pHase Eye Pencil** *($14)* is just a standard pencil with nothing that deserves any type of "multi" prefix to describe what's just a pencil.

☺ <u>LIPSTICK AND LIP PENCIL:</u> $$$ **Multi-pHase Lipstick** *($17)* is a very creamy lipstick with a glossy finish and a noticeable stain, which means it'll last longer than usual. The 25 shades are attractive. $$$ **Multi-pHase Sensual Lip Color** *($18)* makes such sweeping statements as "won't bleed, feather or crack," yet its greasy, opaque texture and slick feel belie each claim, except for the cracking part. $$$ **Multi-pHase Lip Sheer SPF 15** *($17)* does not have suitable UVA protection and remains a standard sheer and very glossy lipstick. **Multi-pHase Lip Pencil** *($14)* is standard and has a creamy texture that glides well. The color selection, though small, is workable.

☹ **Multi-pHase Lip Perfector** *($25)* is supposed to keep lipstick from bleeding, but if anything it can make matters worse than if you didn't use it.

☺ **$$$ MASCARA: Multi-pHase Mascara** *($19)* is a good mascara, but not a great one. It does build decent length and thickness, but nothing special or indicative of this price.

☹ **Multi-pHase Advanced Mascara** *($19)* isn't advanced in the least. It doesn't lengthen very well, tends to go on unevenly, and makes lashes look sparse.

# *Estee Lauder*

What sets the venerable Estee Lauder company apart from its rivals is that it owns most of the cosmetics lines it competes with. Lauder's formidable reach includes Clinique, Origins, Prescriptives, M.A.C., Bobbi Brown, Stila, Aveda, Jane (a drugstore line aimed at teenagers), Tommy Hilfiger, and La Mer (with La Mer being the cosmetics line to boast one of the most expensive skin-care products being sold, at $1,000 for a 16-ounce container). That sort of takes the notion of cosmetic secrets and throws it to the wind, doesn't it? Would Estee Lauder keep so-called secrets away from its own companies?

Of course, Estee Lauder is still the grande dame of makeup lines, with a loyal following and a plethora, if not endless redundancy, of products. Ask any of the salespeople who work for this seasoned cosmetics company and they will tell you the products sell themselves. A few years ago, Night Repair and Eyezone were jumping off the shelves; then Estee Lauder's AHA product, Fruition (discontinued in favor of the far better formulation Fruition Extra), caught fire; and now Diminish and Spotlight (vitamin A and skin-lightening products) are the flavor du jour. It only takes a cursory look at the stable of Estee Lauder products, from the line itself to its protégés, to notice that there is an overwhelming number of antiwrinkle products to choose from (over 300 in all). But the question to ask is this: If just one or two of its products could live up to its claims to get rid of wrinkles, why would you need an additional 250 products claiming to do the same thing? The Estee Lauder lineup boasts some wonderful moisturizers, but also absurd prices for pretty standard products that can't live up to their more glorious claims.

Estee Lauder has an absolutely huge assemblage of makeup, with a particular emphasis on foundations. Bridging the gap from its skin care, Estee Lauder's makeup products are primarily aimed at the wrinkle-concerned baby boomer with copy that reads "firms the skin"; the phrase "time-released moisture" shows up in product after product. Beneath the hype and the Hurley (Elizabeth, that is), Estee Lauder's products remain relatively standard and only mildly unique. It excels in presenting an incredible range of lipstick shades and textures, as well as offering some remarkable foundations with sun protection, and velvety powders. The weak points lie more in the blandness of the rest of the makeup—at these prices and with Estee Lauder's reputation, you should expect an above-average product, distinctive enough to stand apart from the rest in its particular category. Instead, many of the blushes and eyeshadows are nice, but ordinary, too, without the satiny-smooth finish of other lines or the matte color options offered by most every other line. The mascaras are just ordinary, without the impressive lengthening and thickening performance of Lancome mascaras and many others. That isn't bad, but after a while it starts to become apparent that Estee Lauder's competitors (including the companies it owns and doesn't own) are doing a better job of formulating products with exemplary textures and superior performance. That should make Estee Lauder envious, but maybe that's why it went on its buying spree over the past couple of years.

The counter displays for Estee Lauder's makeup are slightly more accessible than they have been in the past. However, even at some of the open-sell, spacious counters the sales pressure can be intense and the salespeople do tend to stay close by. Still, if you know what you need and are prepared to be skeptical, your experience at the Estee Lauder counters should be pleasurable. For more information about Estee Lauder, call (212) 572-4200 or visit the Web site at www.esteelauder.com.

# *Estee Lauder Skin Care*

☺ **$$$ Perfectly Clean Foaming Gel Cleanser, Normal/Oily and Oily Skin** (*$16.50 for 4.2 ounces*) is an exceptionally standard, detergent-based water-soluble cleanser with a tiny amount of BHA. It is best for normal to oily skin types, because the cleansing agents can be a bit drying in this formulation. The pH is too high for the BHA to be effective as an exfoliant.

☺ **$$$ Perfectly Clean Foaming Lotion Cleanser, Normal/Dry and Dry Skin** (*$16.50 for 4.2 ounces*). The oil does help cut the drying effect of the cleansing agents, and this one would be suitable for normal to dry skin.

☹ **Perfectly Clean Solid Cleanser Normal to Dry** (*$16.50 for 4.2 ounces*) is a pricey bar cleanser that is almost identical to Cetaphil Bar Cleanser at five times the price. This contains fragrance and coloring agents. It can be drying, and the ingredients that keep the bar form solid can clog pores.

☹ **Rich Results Hydrating Cleanser** (*$18.50 for 4.2 ounces*) is similar to the Re-nutriv Creme Cleanser below, only this version contains menthol, coriander, and sage, which can all be skin irritants.

☺ **$$$ Splash Away Foaming Cleanser** (*$18.50 for 3.4 ounces*) is a fairly drying, detergent-based water-soluble cleanser. Keep it away from your eyes, because it can sting if you get even a little in them.

☺ $$$ **Tender Creme Cleanser** *($26 for 8 ounces)* is a cleanser that needs to be wiped off with a tissue or a washcloth. It tends to leave a slightly greasy film and does not take off makeup all that well. The tiny amount of vitamins in this product have no benefit for skin. It does contain fragrance. For the money, Neutrogena's Extra Gentle Cleanser is almost identical for a third the price.

☺ **Soft Clean Rinse Off Cleanser** *($16.50 for 6.7 ounces)* contains minimal detergent cleansing agents, which make it extremely gentle but also less effective for cleaning skin. It could be good for dry skin types.

☺ $$$ **Gentle Eye Makeup Remover** *($13.50 for 3.4 ounces)* is an exceptionally standard, detergent cleanser–based eye-makeup remover and it works the same as most, though this one does not contain fragrance.

☺ $$$ **Lip and Eye Makeup Remover for Long Wear Formulas** *($14.50 for 3.4 ounces)* would work well but is just a standard makeup remover.

☺ **Take It Away Makeup Remover** *($18 for 6.7 ounces)* is a fairly standard, wipe-off makeup remover that would work for most skin types.

☹ **Deep Sweep Skin Refiner** *($18.50 for 3.4 ounces)* is basically alcohol, synthetic scrub (ground-up plastic), and slip agents. It also contains menthol, which just adds to the irritation and dryness from the alcohol.

☺ $$$ **Gentle Action Skin Polisher** *($18.50 for 3.4 ounces)* is supposed to be a water-soluble scrub, but it doesn't rinse off well. Although the scrubbing effect is fairly mild, the other ingredients are emollient and rather standard thickeners that can clog pores. This could be good for someone with dry skin.

☺ $$$ **So Polished Exfoliating Scrub** *($19.50 for 1.7 ounces)* is an abrasive scrub that can be rough for most skin types, and is not preferred over using plain baking soda with a gentle cleanser.

☹ **Clear Finish Purifying Toner N/D** *($25 for 13.5 ounces)*. This extremely standard toner contains menthol, which can be a skin irritant for most skin types.

☹ **Clean Finish Purifying Toner N/O** *($25 for 13.5 ounces)* is similar to the version above for N/D skin, only this one adds grapefruit to the menthol irritation factor.

☺ $$$ **Re-nutriv Extremely Delicate Skin Cleanser** *($32.50 for 7.5 ounces)*. Why use this very greasy product when Pond's Cold Cream is essentially the same thing for a fraction of the price? This can be an option for very dry skin, but the teeny amount of royal jelly and vitamin A in here have no effect.

☺ $$$ **Re-nutriv Moisture-Rich Creme Cleanser** *($27.50 for 3.4 ounces)* is similar to the one above only slightly less greasy. The same basic review applies.

☺ $$$ **Re-nutriv Gentle Skin Toner** *($30 for 6.7 ounces)* is an alcohol-free toner whose second ingredient is cetrimonium chloride, a cleansing agent and disinfectant. It isn't bad for the skin, it just isn't all that gentle. There probably isn't much in this product, but this also contains arnica, which is a problem when used repeatedly on skin.

☺ **$$$ Re-nutriv Creme** *($75 for 1.75 ounces)* is a very emollient, though ordinary, moisturizer for extremely dry skin.

☺ **$$$ Re-nutriv Firming Eye Creme** *($47.50 for 0.5 ounce)*. This won't firm the eye area, and the fancy water-binding agents (amino acids and collagen) cannot get rid of wrinkles, but it is a very good emollient moisturizer for dry skin.

☺ **$$$ Re-nutriv Firming Throat Creme** *($53 for 1.7 ounces)* is similar to the one above, but there is nothing about this formulation that makes it better for the throat versus the face. It does contain fragrance.

☺ **$$$ Re-nutriv Intensive Firming Plus** *($95 for 1.7 ounces)* is a very overpriced, basic moisturizer for dry skin. It does contain a small amount of AHAs but the pH is too high for it to be effective as an exfoliant.

☺ **$$$ Re-nutriv Intensive Lifting Creme** *($150 for 1.7 ounces)*. While this is a good moisturizer with good water-binding agents, antioxidants, and anti-irritants, there is nothing in here that will lift skin anywhere, and the price is nothing less than obscene given the ingredient list. Estee Lauder charges a lot less for other moisturizers that have a similar ingredient listing.

☺ **$$$ Re-nutriv Replenishing Creme** *($78 for 1.7 ounces)* is similar to the moisturizer above, only not as greasy, and the same review applies.

☺ **$$$ Re-nutriv Lightweight Creme** *($75 for 1.75 ounces)* is almost identical to the creme above, but slightly lighter in weight. The company suggests using this for normal to oily skin, but ingredients like plant oils, lanolin oil, and thick waxes make that recommendation absurd and the price painful.

☺ **$$$ Resilience Creme** *($60 for 1.7 ounces)* is a good, but extremely ordinary, moisturizer for someone with normal to dry skin. The fish elastin in here won't help firm a fish's skin any more than it will yours.

☺ **$$$ Resilience Lotion** *($60 for 1.7 ounces)* is similar to the product above, only in lotion form, and the same review applies.

☺ **$$$ Resilience Lift Eye Creme** *($42.50 for 0.5 ounce)* is without a doubt a very good moisturizer for normal to dry skin, with several state-of-the-art water-binding agents and emollients like Vaseline and shea butter. But it won't lift the skin anywhere and there is nothing about it that makes this better for the eye area than the face. There are minute amounts of plankton, caffeine, and barley in here, among other extracts. If these ingredients are the answer for wrinkles, then are all the other Estee Lauder products lying? Or does everything get rid of wrinkles? Must be, because there is no uniformity among these products.

☺ **$$$ Resilience Eye Creme** *($42.50 for 0.5 ounce)* is similar to the Lift Eye Creme above only somewhat less emollient. The same basic comments apply.

☺ **$$$ New Resilience Lift SPF 15 Face and Throat Cream** *($45 for 1 ounce)* and **New Resilience Lift SPF 15 Face and Throat Lotion** *($45 for 1 ounce)* are two good sunscreens with part titanium dioxide to help provide UVA protection. But no one is spending this much money on these two products just for sun protection. Clearly, women are hoping that the word "lift" has serious implications and that these can make a difference in the appearance of skin. They can't. They are standard sunscreens in good moisturizing bases; the miracle ingredients of fish elastin and cartilage are just not going to do what you're hoping for. Other than that, these are both good for normal to dry skin, with the cream being better for drier skin and the lotion better for normal to dry skin. The lotion is not recommended for oily skin.

☺ $$$ **Verite Light Lotion Cleanser** *($22.50 for 6.7 ounces)* is an OK wipe-off cleanser that can leave a slightly greasy film. It can be an option for someone with dry skin.

☺ $$$ **Verite Soft Foam Cleanser** *($22.50 for 4.2 ounces)* is the only product in the entire Verite grouping with a fairly irritating ingredient that is totally inappropriate for someone with sensitive skin, and taking care of sensitive skin is supposed to be the hallmark of the Verite line.

☺ **Verite Soothing Spray Toner** *($22.50 for 6.7 ounces)* is a very good nonirritating toner for all skin types. It does contain fragrance.

☺ $$$ **Verite Calming Fluid** *($60 for 1.7 ounces)* won't calm anything, but it is a very good moisturizer for someone with normal to dry skin.

☺ $$$ **Verite Moisture Relief Creme** *($50 for 1.75 ounces)* is a very good moisturizer for someone with dry skin.

☺ **Estoderme Creme** *($25 for 4 ounces)* is a very emollient, rich, almost greasy moisturizer for someone with very dry skin.

☺ **Estoderme Emulsion** *($25 for 4 ounces)* is a good moisturizer for dry skin.

☺ $$$ **100% Time Release Moisturizer Creme** *($35 for 1.7 ounces)* is a good moisturizer for someone with normal to dry skin, but it is one of the more ordinary offerings in the Estee Lauder lineup.

☺ $$$ **100% Time Release Moisture Lotion** *($35 for 1.7 ounces)* is similar to the cream version above and the same basic comments apply.

☺ **Clear Difference Oil-Control Hydrator for Oily Normal/Oily and Blemish-Prone Skin** *($27 for 1.7 ounces)* is a good lightweight moisturizer that also contains BHA, but this won't control oil. The pH of this product is about 4, but it would need a pH of 3 to 3.5 to make it a more effective exfoliant.

☹ **Equalizer Oil-Free HydroGel** *($27.50 for 1.7 ounces)* is basically alcohol and silicone. The alcohol can be drying and irritating.

☺ $$$ **Advanced Night Repair Protective Recovery Complex** *($70 for 1.7 ounces)* is a good moisturizer that also contains a small amount of sunscreen, which doesn't make sense in a product that's meant to be used at night, and can be a skin irritant.

The Reviews E

This product won't repair anything and contains nothing that warrants the price tag, but it is a good lightweight moisturizer for dry skin.

☺ $$$ **Time Zone Eyes Ultra-Hydrating Complex** *($40 for 0.5 ounce)* is a lightweight moisturizer for normal to dry skin. Seaweed and fish collagen won't hydrate the skin, but the water-binding agents are nice. Some of the film formers in here can be irritating for some skin types.

☺ $$$ **Time Zone Moisture Recharging Complex** *($55 for 1.7 ounces)* is similar to the one above, only with more emollients. It would be good for dry skin.

☺ $$$ **Eyezone Repair Gel** *($35 for 0.5 ounce)*. I was told it would last six months because you use so little, but you would have to use almost none for a half-ounce to last that long. The tiny amount of algae and even smaller amount of vitamin A in here won't do anything for skin, but this is an OK, ordinary moisturizer for slightly dry skin.

☺ $$$ **Fruition Extra Multi-Action Complex** *($70 for 1.7 ounces)*. The original Fruition was discontinued, and the Extra is now the only version available. The original was supposed to be an exfoliating AHA product, but it didn't contain enough of the stuff to have any effect; basically it was just a good lightweight moisturizer. Fruition Extra adds salicylic acid to the mix, though only about a 1% concentration of AHA, so this is mostly a BHA product now. It does work well as an exfoliant but is incredibly overpriced for what you get, which is a good, lightweight moisturizing base with silicones, film formers, water-binding agents, vitamins, fragrance, coloring agents, and preservatives.

☺ $$$ **Idealist** *($42.50 for 1 ounce)* is a new product from Estee Lauder, and the spin on it is that it's a non-retinol and non-AHA wrinkle remover; it claims to be the best option around for skin. If that's the case, does that mean Estee Lauder's Fruition Extra (with AHA) and Diminish (with retinol) are now history, along with all the other AHA, BHA, and retinol products the other Estee Lauder–owned lines sell? That would never happen, of course, despite Estee Lauder's claim that Idealist is now the answer for your less-than-youthful visage. The two standout ingredients, according to Estee Lauder "...are acetyl glucosamine and sodium lactobionate." For some reason, if these two ingredients can do that, the only company that knows about it is Estee Lauder.

What we know about N-acetyl glucosamine is that it's an amino acid sugar, the primary constituent of mucopolysaccharides and hyaluronic acid, and is found in all parts of the skin. It has value as a water-binding agent, and is effective (in large concentrations) for wound healing. There is research (*Cellular-Molecular-Life-Science*, 53(2), February 1997, pages 131–40) showing that chitins (also known as chitosan—which is comprised of acetyl glucosamine) can help in the complex process of wound healing. However, that is a few generations removed from acetyl glucosamine being included in a skin-care product. Besides, you have to wonder what any of that has to do with exfoliation, especially in the tiny concentration this product contains. And please understand that wound healing isn't related to wrinkles because wrinkles aren't wounds. What about the sodium lactobionate? It seems to be used in solutions as a preservative, but I wasn't able to find any research confirming Estee Lauder's contentions for it. It's a mystery.

It is a good, lightweight moisturizer for normal to dry skin—the silicone will leave a silky feel on the skin—and it does have plenty of anti-irritants and antioxidants. Whether or not the acetyl glucosamine and sodium lactobionate do something different is yet to be seen.

☺ **$$$ Future Perfect Micro-Targeted Skin Gel** *($45 for 1.75 ounces)* is a good lightweight emollient moisturizer for normal to dry skin. The name of this gel is better than what you get; it sounds as if you can place it over a wrinkle, zero in, and, poof, get rid of it. Not even remotely possible.

☺ **$$$ Age Controlling Creme** *($60 for 1.7 ounces)* is a very good emollient moisturizer for someone with very dry skin, but why this product is for "age control" is anyone's guess.

☺ **Spotlight Skin Tone Perfector** *($30 for 1.7 ounces)* is a standard, silicone-based moisturizer. By the way, Estee Lauder describes the mica and titanium dioxide in a press release previewed in *The Rose Sheet* for November 29, 1999, as follows: "microprism technology enhances the skin's radiance with interference particles that break down the light on the skin." What a great description for ingredients that add shine and a white color and do so in thousands of products! This product is meant to improve skin color thanks to the presence of plant extracts that include mulberry root and licorice extracts. There is some research that indicates these ingredients in pure form can inhibit melanin formation, but not in the tiny amount present in this product.

☺ **$$$ Uncircle** *($37.50 for 0.5 ounce)*. There is nothing in here that will have any more effect on circles than would any other moisturizer in this line. Vaseline and film former is not what I or anyone else would call an exotic or excitingly new formulation, and fish cartilage can't affect anything around the eye.

☹ **Unline Total Eye Care** *($35 for 0.5 ounce)*. I wonder if this means Estee Lauder's other eye products don't work? Otherwise, why else would there need to be so many lotions making the same claims? There are many aspects of this that make for a good moisturizer. However, while the mint and wintergreen oil might provide a cooling sensation, they are also irritants and a problem for the eye area.

☺ **$$$ Skin Perfecting Creme Firming Nourisher** *($35 for 1.75 ounces)* is a lightweight emollient moisturizer for dry skin. One word of warning: this product does contain arnica extract, which can be a serious skin irritant with repeated use.

☺ **Skin Perfecting Lotion Lightweight Moisturizer** *($27.50 for 1.7 ounces)* is lightweight but boring. There is no SPF rating on the label although a sunscreen agent is listed, and that means there is no way to know how much protection this product provides. Do not count on it for use during the day. The Creme version above is far better formulated with more interesting water-binding agents and less fragrance.

☺ $$$ **Nutritious Bio Protein** *($45 for 1.7 ounces)* is a good moisturizer, but despite the clever name you can't feed the skin from the outside in.

☺ $$$ **Diminish Retinol Treatment** *($47.50 for 1 ounce)* came on the scene with a fanfare of claims about getting rid of lines, evening-out skin tone, improving skin texture, and on and on, much like the claims around several of the other products in this line. It definitely contains retinol, but only about 0.1% or 0.2%. Other than that, the rest of the ingredients are standard, lightweight moisturizing ingredients. If you are interested in retinol, Avon Anew Retinol Recovery Complex P.M. Treatment ($17.50 for 1 ounce); Alpha Hydrox Retinol Night ResQ Anti-Wrinkle Firming Complex ($11.99 for 1.05 ounces), or L'Oreal Line Eraser Pure Retinol Concentrate ($12.49 for 1 ounce) all have better versions, because their packaging is more reliable for keeping retinol stable (it's otherwise very sensitive to air and light).

☺ **Swiss Performing Extract Moisturizer** *($37.50 for 3.2 ounces)* is a very emollient, very good moisturizer for someone with dry skin.

☺ **Enriched Under-Makeup Creme** *($25 for 4 ounces)* is definitely rich, but also boring. This is a very emollient and basic moisturizer for someone with very dry skin.

☺ $$$ **Day Wear Super Anti-Oxidant Complex SPF 15** *($37.50 for 1.7 ounces)*. The antioxidants are not exactly at the top of the ingredient list, nor are they any more special than those in hundreds of other products, so none of that is all that super. What is good about this day cream is that it contains an SPF 15 sunscreen that is part titanium dioxide, one of the better ways to protect against sun damage. In that regard, this product is right on, as are most of Estee Lauder's sunscreens, but there is no reason to spend this kind of money on an otherwise standard sunscreen.

☺ **Go Bronze Tinted Self Tanner for Face** *($18.50 for 1.7 ounces)*, like all other self tanners, uses the active ingredient dihydroxyacetone to turn the skin brown. The advantage to the tint is so you can see where you've applied it, to help achieve a more even tan.

☺ **Self-Action Super Tan, Medium** *($25 for 4.25 ounces)*; **Self-Action Super Tan for Face, Medium/Dark** *($18.50 for 1.5 ounces)*; **Self-Action Super Tan Spray, Medium/Dark** *($25 for 4.2 ounces)*; **Self-Action Tanning Creme, Dark** *($17.50 for 4.2 ounces)*; **Self-Action Tanning Creme, Medium** *($17.50 for 4.2 ounces)*; and **Self-Action Tanning Creme, Very Dark** *($17.50 for 4.2 ounces)*, like all other self tanners, all use the active ingredient dihydroxyacetone to turn the skin brown. These work as well as any and the only real difference is your personal preference for application.

☺ **Sun Block for Face SPF 15** *($18.50 for 1.7 ounces)* is a good, in-part titanium dioxide–based sunscreen in a good emollient base for someone with normal to dry skin.

☺ **Sun Block for Face SPF 30** *($19.50 for 1.7 ounces)* is similar to the one above and the same review applies.

☹ **Counter-Blemish Lotion** *($12 for 0.45 ounce)* contains alcohol as the first ingredient, along with other potentially irritating plant extracts of cinnamon and ginger.

☺ $$$ **So Clean Deep Pore Mask** *($19.50 for 3.4 ounces)* is a standard clay mask. This would work as well as any and doesn't contain any irritants.

☺ $$$ **So Moist Hydrating Mask** *($19.50 for 3.4 ounces)* is indeed hydrating but no more so than any other moisturizer in the Estee Lauder family.

☺ $$$ **Stress Relief Eye Mask** *($27.50 for ten 0.4-ounce packets)* is a somewhat sticky mask that doesn't feel great on the skin, though it is a good lightweight moisturizer. Still, there is nothing in here that will relieve skin of anything.

☺ $$$ **Triple Creme Hydrating Mask** *($27.50 for 2.5 ounces)* contains good moisturizing ingredients, so it would feel good on dry skin, but not more so than any other moisturizer in the Estee Lauder lineup.

## *Estee Lauder Makeup*

**FOUNDATION:** Estee Lauder's foundations offer something for everyone in terms of texture and formulation. However, over half of the formulas are without the recommended UVA-protecting ingredients, and while many have an SPF 15 or higher there are still those that don't. Perhaps most disappointing is the nonexistent selection of shades for darker skin tones. Fair to medium skin tones will be overwhelmed with options, but take great care in finding the right shade, as Estee Lauder still likes to sneak in the occasional rosy pink and orange colors.

☺ $$$ **Impeccable Protective Compact Makeup SPF 20** *($27.50)* has been reformulated and is not nearly as greasy as it was before, which is great, but how sad that this new formula dropped the prior sunscreen formulation, which included UVA-protecting ingredients, leaving this version incomplete. The texture is now more in line with Estee Lauder's Minute Makeup, only this is slightly creamier and offers heavier coverage. For normal to dry skin willing to wear an adequate sunscreen underneath, this could work well, but there are better options out there. Of the 14 shades, these can be too pink, coppery, or ash for most skin tones: Vanilla, True Beige, Golden Tawny, and Ginger.

☹ **Bare Skin SPF 10 Sport Makeup** *($27.50)* is supposed to be for "active outdoor life." Well, you may have fun outdoors but if you wear this makeup you will be left with out adequate protection. SPF 10 is not adequate for spending casual (or any) amount of time in the sun. By all standards (including those of the American Academy of Dermatology, the FDA, and the Skin Cancer Institute), SPF 15 is minimum. To make matters worse, this product doesn't even contain UVA protection. It is a decent, sheer tint with a soft matte finish for minimal makeup application, and could be good for normal to dry skin; if you're willing to wear a sunscreen underneath this, the six shades are an option.

☺ $$$ **Minute Makeup SPF 15** *($27.50)* is one of the better stick foundations on the market. This has a light, creamy texture that applies smoothly and dries to a soft, powder finish. But don't let the name fool you—it takes as long to apply as any other makeup. Consider this one if you have normal to dry skin. One word of warning: Estee Lauder claims it is non-acnegenic. I disagree. Several ingredients in here could trigger breakouts, not the least of which is the active sunscreen ingredient, titanium dioxide, which is great for UVA protection but problematic for acne-prone skin. Of the 12 shades, the only suspect colors are Amber and Suede (both slightly orange).

☺ **Maximum Coverage with Non-Chemical SPF 15** *($25)* goes on creamy and smooth and does tend to "stick" to the skin, which can feel uncomfortable. It doesn't provide as much coverage as the name implies (this isn't Dermablend), but it does cover well. In the limited assortment of colors to choose from, most are great. There are two color-correcting shades of green and yellow, but just ignore those and also consider avoiding Cool Beige (too rose), Rich Ginger (copper), and Sun Beige (very rose).

☺ $$$ **Lucidity Light-Diffusing Makeup SPF 8** *($27.50)* claims it gives the face "a soft, air-brushed effect," but this is just a standard moisturizing foundation with a smooth texture and medium coverage. The SPF is not only too low for daily protection, it does not contain UVA-protecting ingredients. Look into this one if you have normal to dry skin. It's an option but there is nothing about this product that will impart "magazine cover model" looking skin. Of the 14 shades the following can be too peach or pink for most skin tones: Outdoor Beige, Natural Beige, Golden Sands, Golden Caramel, Vanilla Beige, and Porcelain.

☺ $$$ **Enlighten Skin-Enhancing Makeup with SPF 10** *($27.50)* is a superior foundation with titanium dioxide as the sunscreen agent; what a shame it only has an SPF 10, which leaves the skin in need of more sun protection. The application is smooth and sheer, leaving a beautiful, slightly matte finish. It is best for someone with normal to combination or slightly dry skin. The color selection isn't the best, with some strange tones of pink, peach, and yellow, though the shade range includes options for very light but not for very dark skin tones. These colors are too pink or copper for most skin tones: Neutral Beige, Gentle Ivory, Outdoor Beige, Vanilla Beige, and Fresh Cocoa.

☺ $$$ **Futurist Age-Resisting Makeup SPF 15** *($32.50)* leaves out the most important anti-aging weapon anyone can have: a sunscreen with UVA-protecting ingredients! How disappointing that a foundation with such a wonderful texture and luminous finish has this as its major flaw. If you have normal to dry skin and are prepared to wear a sunscreen underneath, you will get a great foundation, but be careful of the following colors, all of which can be too rose, orange, or copper for most skin tones: Fawn, Pale Almond, Tender Cream, Cool Sand, Golden Petal, Cameo, Bare Beige, and Mahogany.

☺ $$$ **Compact Finish Double Performance Makeup** *($27.50)* is a standard powder foundation with an excellent soft, silky finish; it works well alone or with foundation. You are supposed to be able to use it wet or dry, but the wet never works well with these kinds of powders. All the salespeople I spoke to warned about streaking, which is what can easily happen no matter how deft you are at blending. Still, there are some impressive shades to choose from, and all are just beautiful. The only colors to consider carefully are Ivory Beige (may be too pink) and Ivory (can be too peach).

☹ $$$ **Double Wear Makeup SPF 10** *($27.50)* is great! At least when it comes to a terrific matte texture that doesn't move. Someone with normal to oily skin will be impressed with the application and the way it holds up over a long day, though it can provide too much coverage—this is pretty thick stuff—and, as is true for all ultra-matte foundations, it's hard to get off. Of course the SPF should be a 15 even though it does have a pure titanium dioxide base. Without it, for someone with normal to oily skin, that means another sunscreen underneath, which can add an oily or layered feel on the skin. For a long-lasting foundation I would start with Revlon's ColorStay Lite SPF 15 first, with its lighter coverage and far better SPF at half the price. Of the 12 shades here, six can be too peach, pink, or rose for most skin tones: Pebble, Tawny, Dusk, Bronze, Spice, and Soft Tan.

☻ **Double Matte Oil Control Makeup SPF 15** *($27.50)* was launched after the winning Double Wear Makeup, and one would think the reliable SPF would carry over, since this foundation has a similar theme. Well, the SPF is higher *but* this one doesn't contain UVA protection! In addition to this, the texture of this is thick, the colors are almost all poor (most are strongly yellow or rose), and the finish is slightly chalky, making this a poor choice. Oilier skins looking for sun protection would do well to consider Revlon's Color Stay Lite SPF 15 instead.

☺ $$$ <u>CONCEALER:</u> **Double Wear Stay in Place Concealer SPF 10** *($16)* has a pure titanium dioxide sunscreen base and six workable colors (although Dark can be too copper), but some of the colors can lean slightly toward the peach side, so be careful. This provides intense coverage and you must be exact in your blending, as this dries very quickly to a matte finish that won't budge. For dark circles, it is preferred to Estee Lauder's **Smoothing Creme Concealer SPF 8** *($16)*. The Smoothing Creme comes in a squeeze tube, so be cautious of squeezing out too much. However, it does have a pleasant, creamy texture and a natural finish that allows for semi-opaque coverage and minimal chance of creasing. The SPF, though pure titanium dioxide, is too low to rely on for daily protection. The five colors are all worthy of consideration, but there is nothing for very light or dark skin tones. **Double Wear Concealer SPF 10** *($16.50)* is a good addition to Estee Lauder's ultra-matte Double Wear Foundation SPF 10. The tiny bottle with a standard wand applicator is nice, and it goes on in a creamy sweep and then dries to a slightly powder finish with good opaque coverage. A more matte finish without the powder effect might have worked better with the foundation, but the coverage is what probably counts for those looking to eliminate dark circles under the eye, and the six shades are impressive, especially the lighter shades that would work great for very light to medium skin tones. Avoid the shade Dark, it can be too coppery for most skin tones. Be careful though—the powder finish does tend to accentuate lines.

☺ $$$ **Uncircle Concealer SPF 20** *($16)* is a thick concealer in a pot that offers an excellent physical sunscreen but despite this and the three very good colors, it can crease into lines, so test it carefully before making the investment.

☹ **Automatic Creme Concealer** *($13.50)* comes in only two colors and a mauve tint. The mauve is completely unnecessary and the other shades are too rosy-peach to recommend.

**POWDER:** ☺ $$$ **Enlighten Skin Enhancing Powder** *($20)* is a standard, talc-based powder, available as a pressed powder only. It has a light, dry texture and applies extremely sheer. It is sold with a brush rather than a puff and that makes sense, given the concept of this "no powder" powder, whose six shades are all excellent. **Lucidity Translucent Loose Powder** *($26)* and **Lucidity Translucent Pressed Powder** *($20)* are also standard, talc-based powders. Both of these have great color selections and a wonderful soft, silky finish. Lucidity is supposed to change the way light focuses on your face. It doesn't. Though it feels nice and smooth, it doesn't look any different from dozens and dozens of other powders. **Double-Matte Oil-Free Loose Powder** *($18.50)* and **Double-Matte Oil-Free Pressed Powder** *($20)* are both standard, talc-based powders. They both have a great texture, with a dry, slightly chalky finish, which can be a problem for some skin tones, but someone with very oily skin will appreciate how well these absorb. All the colors are good options.

☹ $$$ **Instant Sun All-Over Bronzing Duo** *($25)* is a dual-sided powder bronzer that applies unevenly and is quite shiny. Funny, I don't recall any kind of tan glittering so much.

☺ $$$ <u>BLUSH:</u> **Blush All Day** *($20)* is a powder blush with a slightly too-dry texture that can make blending on a smooth sweep of color a challenge. All of the colors are soft and sheer (a few have a slight shine); there are no shades deep enough for darker skin tones. **Minute Blush Creme Stick for Cheeks** *($25)* has a light, creamy, slippery texture that dries to a sheer, minimal powder finish. The six colors are gorgeous, with a couple of options for deeper skin tones (Russet and Spice). This type of product works best for normal to dry skin types.

☺ <u>EYESHADOW:</u> **Two-in-One Eyeshadow** *($12 singles, $20 duos, and $35 for quads)* comes in a soft, attractive range of single colors that all have some amount of shine, some definitely more so than others. They have a smooth, soft application (don't count on intensity from these), but focus your concentration on the matte shades only. One nice feature of these colors is that they can be applied wet and they do this nicely. That provides for a slightly more opaque coverage but also adds an interesting smoothness you should check out. The **Quads** feature three shadows and two thin stripes of darker shadow for lining, and most of them are well coordinated with workable shades that really do go well together.

☹ **$$$ Futurist Full Treatment Eye Makeup** *($25)* is a collection of creamy eyeshadows that apply very sheer and blend out to a soft matte finish. The treatment part is attributed to the moisturizing capabilities of this rather standard formula, but that is exactly what will be this eyeshadow's undoing, leading to creasing and a crepey look on the eyelids.

<u>EYE AND BROW SHAPER:</u> ☺ **Eye Defining Pencil** *($14)* is a basic pencil that needs sharpening and has a creamy texture that glides on. These claim to be a "non-smudge" formula, but this is creamy enough that it can definitely smudge by midday. **$$$ Two-in-One Eyeliner/Brow Color** *($25)* goes on wet or dry. It comes in one compact with two colors: Brown and Black. While it does work to fill in brows or line the eye, the color selection is rather limited and most any matte eyeshadow can perform the identical function.

☺ **$$$ Automatic Pencil for Eyes** *($22.50; $8 for a refill)* is a standard, twist-up pencil in an elegant container. It is among the more pricey pencils on the market, but the refills are a bargain and then you have the sexy container, if you're into that kind of thing. Some of the colors are too shiny and fairly greasy, so be careful; this can smear under the eye. **Brow Gel** *($13.50)* is a fairly standard brow groomer with a good brush and minimal sticky after-feel.

☹ **Liquid Eyeliner** *($13.50)* comes in two shades and features a thin brush that applies an even line. As nice as that is, this tends to dry so slowly as to seriously try your patience and risk smearing. **Natural Brow Filler** *($13)* is a one-color fat eyebrow pencil that isn't by any means a one-size-fits-all product. The fat tip makes it hard to control the color through the brow, and the color isn't in the least natural, so it isn't for everyone. **Automatic Pencil for Brows** *($22.50; $8 for a refill)* is similar to the Automatic Pencil Liner for Eyes, only this one has a slightly drier finish. It comes in a pretty container, but penciling is not the best option for a natural-looking brow, and this isn't an improvement over far less expensive versions.

☺ <u>LIPSTICK AND LIP PENCIL:</u> **$$$ Futurist Full Treatment Lipstick SPF 15** *($16)* does not provide adequate UVA protection and remains a standard, creamy lipstick with a slightly greasy finish and moderate coverage. These do have a slight stain, but are prone to feathering. **$$$ True Lipstick** *($16)* comes in **Satin** or **Matte**. Both have a slick feel and are opaque. The Satins have a glossy finish whereas the Mattes (which are not matte in the least) have a creamy finish. There is enough stain here to let these colors go the distance, at least until lunch! **All Day Lipstick** *($13.50)* is extremely creamy, bordering on greasy, with medium coverage and no stain to speak of. A better choice for a name might have been "Gone Before Lunch Lipstick." **Go Pout Lip Color** *($15)* makes claims that it adds dimension and fullness to the lower lips and shadows the contour of the upper lips. Quite a feat for a standard lipstick, and it looks convincing in the ads; however, all this adds up to is a good creamy lipstick with a fair amount of iridescence. That can affect the way light is reflected off the lips (or anywhere else), just not in the way Estee Lauder wants you to think it does. **Lip Blush SPF 15** *($15)* does not have adequate UVA protection, so count on this being nothing more than a very standard, sheer, glossy lipstick. **High Shine Lip Lacquer SPF 15** *($15)* also does not have reliable UVA-protecting ingredients, making this just a somewhat sticky, semi-opaque "wet" gloss. **Lip Defining Pencil** *($14)* is a standard pencil with a creamy feel and enough stain to help lip color cling a little longer. Before investing in these, take a look at Clinique's pencils, which are virtually identical but less expensive. **$$$ Automatic Pencil for Lips** *($22.50; $8 for a refill)* is a standard, twist-up lip liner, but the tip of these comes out of a wider than normal opening, which makes it too thick to be capable of drawing a thin line outline around the mouth. **$$$ Futurist Lipstick SPF 15** *($16)* is a rather standard, creamy lipstick that has enough of a greasy feel to make those with bleeding-lipstick problems cringe a bit. The SPF 15 sounds impressive but alas—without UVA protection there is no reason to consider this as part of your or anyone else's future plans.

<u>MASCARA:</u> ☺ **$$$ More Than Mascara** *($16.50)* is just mascara, plain and simple. Perhaps Estee Lauder wants you to think that the "More" part comes from the nice length and decent thickness you get from using this, but there are *more* mascaras out there that can do just that for less! **Individualist Lash Building Mascara** *($16.50)* is a good choice if you need a reliable mascara that with some effort will build perceptible length and thickness; it tends not to clump or smear. **Futurist Mascara** *($16.50)* is a distinct improvement over the other Estee Lauder mascaras, building nice length and thickness with no clumps or smudges. If that is somehow futuristic, then Estee Lauder has been living in the past! **Lash Luxe** *($25)*. What a shame you can't wear the container, because it is beautiful. This is a decent mascara that builds decent length (though it does take some work to get there), but no thickness. It is an understatement to suggest that there are far less expensive mascaras that out-perform this one.

☹ **Pure Velvet Dramatic Volume Mascara** *($16.50)*. If length, thickness, and volume are your goals, this mascara may send you over the edge trying to achieve them. **Luscious Creme Mascara** *($14.50)* can build some thickness and length, but is prone to clumping and can smear by the end of the day. It may work for some, but there are far better choices available for reliable mascara.

☺ **Lash Primer Plus** *($15)* is sold as an undercoat for lashes or "pre-mascara." It is an unwarranted step, given the plethora of superlative mascaras industry-wide. A truly excellent mascara should not need the help of an additional product.

☺ **BRUSHES:** Although not up to par with brushes from many other lines, including those from the Estee Lauder family of companies such as M.A.C., Bobbi Brown, and Stila, Estee Lauder's **Brushes** *($4.50 to $20)* do have some potential. Both eyeshadow brushes are nice options (though almost too small for some eye shapes); the **Concealing Brush** *($12.50)* is one to consider, as well as the **Blush Brush** *($18.50)*. The rest are below average in terms of density and shape, even though the price is definitely reasonable.

# Eucerin (Skin Care Only)

For more information about Eucerin call Beirsdorf Inc. at (800) 227-4703 or visit the Web site at www.eucerin.com.

☹ **Cleansing Bar Dry Skin Therapy** *($3.88 for 3 ounces)* is a detergent-based bar cleanser. While it is still milder than others, the ingredients that keep the bar in its form can clog pores and the cleansing agents are fairly drying.

☺ **Gentle Hydrating Cleanser** *($7.99 for 8 ounces)* isn't hydrating, though it is a very good, very standard, detergent-based water-soluble cleanser for normal to slightly dry or slightly oily skin. It is fragrance and color-agent free.

☺ **Original Moisturizing Creme** *($4.19 for 2 ounces)* is an extremely heavy moisturizer. It would be best for someone with extremely dry, parched skin, but there are more elegant formulas than this one available.

☺ **Original Moisturizing Lotion** *($10 for 8 ounces)* is basically just thickeners and mineral oil, which makes it a mediocre but OK moisturizer for very dry skin.

☺ **Tri-Lipid Replenishing Lotion** *($7.49 for 8 ounces)* is a good, though very standard moisturizer for normal to dry skin.

☺ **Advanced Sun Defense SPF 15** *($7.99 for 6 ounces)* this is a very good in-part avobenzone-based sunscreen. It has an ordinary moisturizing base that would work well for someone with normal to dry skin.

☺ **Facial Moisturizing Lotion, SPF 25** *($8 for 4 ounces)* is a very good in-part titanium dioxide– and zinc oxide–based sunscreen in a fairly emollient base for someone with normal to dry skin.

The Reviews E

☹ Face Renewal Alpha Hydroxy Moisturizing Treatment SPF 15 *($6.99 for 4 ounces)* does not contain the UVA-protecting ingredients of titanium dioxide, zinc oxide, or avobenzone, so it is not recommended.

☺ Plus Alpha Hydroxy Moisturizing Lotion *($7.49 for 6 ounces)* uses urea as the ingredient to exfoliate skin, and that's a possibility. This would work for exfoliation but there are more elegant formulations to consider than this one.

☺ Plus Alpha Hydroxy Moisturizing Creme *($7.49 for 6 ounces)* is similar to the lotion above, and the same review applies.

☺ Q10 Anti-Wrinkle Sensitive Skin Creme *($7.79 for 1.7 ounces)* does contain coenzyme Q10, and while that's a good antioxidant, there is no evidence that it has any effect on wrinkles. This is good, emollient moisturizer for someone with normal to dry skin but that's about it.

## Exuviance by Neostrata (Skin Care Only)

The politics that take place in the cosmetics industry are sometimes mind-boggling. From an outsider's point of view, it may seem a bit boring, but from the inside, where I spend some amount of time, it is a fascinating saga of egos, money, and skin-care hopes and dreams. Exuviance has some of that drama in its history. Exuviance was created by Dr. Eugene Van Scott and Dr. Ruey Yu. These two researchers owned the original use patent for glycolic acid (AHA) in relation to its use for diminishing wrinkles. As far as Scott, Yu, and their attorneys were concerned, that meant anyone who used glycolic acid in their products for wrinkles should be paying the two doctors a licensing fee. The ensuing court case never got very far, which must have been quite frustrating, because from Yu's and Scott's perspective, their research and patent was gaining profits for everyone but them. (I should point out that Avon and a handful of other companies did pay licensing fees for their use of glycolic acid.) To add fuel to the fire, Yu and Scott's own line of AHA products, Neostrata, never found much of an audience in the world of dermatology where they were exclusively marketed. The more popular lines of M.D. Formulations, Dr. Obagi, Murad, and many others, showed up far more often in doctor's offices than Neostrata ever did.

Either in frustration or to better compete, Scott and Yu have repackaged themselves in Exuviance, a line of AHA products with supposedly more hypoallergenic, sensitive-skin formulations. Separate from the drama and politics, how do these products rate? Well, I would hardly call these formulations "hypoallergenic," because they contain fragrance, coloring agents, and preservatives, three of the more typical sources of allergy responses from cosmetics (aside from plant extracts), while their cleansers use tea-lauryl sulfate. When it comes to AHA products, this line is AHA overkill. You only need one good AHA product, yet this line uses it in almost every item it sells.

The products also claim they contain a polyhydroxyacid called gluconolactone. However, according to an article in the July 1998 issue of *Cosmetic Dermatology*, the skin can't tell the difference between effective AHAs, and the chance of this one staying on the surface of skin longer did not prove out. So it ends up being as good as any. Nonetheless, when it comes to AHAs these are definitely well-formulated. They are all between 6% to 8% concentrations and have an effective pH of 3.5. Scott and Yu feel strongly that their new blend of AHAs, called polyhydroxy acids (a blend of different hydroxy acids), work better than just plain glycolic acid but I'm skeptical about that. The research doesn't support the claim, as skin can't tell what is exfoliating it, only if an exfoliant is effective.

There is reason to consider these products, and especially for those of you in search of an effective AHA and sunscreen formulation, this line excels. But do be careful; I think Scott and Yu got carried away with their own creation and couldn't imagine a product of theirs without their AHA in it. For more information about Exuviance by Neostrata, call (800) 225-9411 or visit the Web site at www. neostrata.com.

☺ **Gentle Cleansing Creme, Sensitive Formula** *($18 for 8 ounces)* contains a tiny amount of AHA, thankfully not enough to affect the eyes, but this isn't a very effective cleanser unless you use it with a washcloth. It ends up being a cold cream–type cleanser that can leave a film on the face.

☺ **Purifying Cleansing Gel** *($18 for 8 ounces)* is a standard (but good) detergent-based water-soluble cleanser for normal to oily skin. It does contain about 4% AHA but the pH isn't low enough to make it effective as an exfoliant.

☹ **Moisture Balance Toner** *($17.50 for 8 ounces)* contains alcohol as the second ingredient, and that makes it unacceptable for any aspect of skin care!

☺ **Soothing Toning Lotion Sensitive Formula** *($17.50 for 8 ounces)* is a disappointing formulation that is mostly water, glycerin, and preservatives. The amount of AHA in this product isn't even 2% so it has no exfoliating properties.

☺ **Essential Multi-Defense Day Creme SPF 15** *($25 for 1.75 ounces)* is a definite, though very expensive, option if you are looking for an effective 8% AHA product with a decent sunscreen. It is a good in-part titanium dioxide–based sunscreen. The moisturizing base is just a list of thickeners with some silicone; it's nothing very interesting, but would be good for someone with normal to slightly dry skin.

☺ **Essential Multi-Defense Day Fluid SPF 15** *($22.50 for 2 ounces)* is almost identical to the one above, only in lotion form.

☺ **Fundamental Multi-Protective Day Creme SPF 15 Sensitive Formula** *($25 for 1.75 ounces)*, aside from containing slightly less AHA than the others, is still similar to the ones above, and the same review applies.

☺ **Fundamental Multi-Protective Day Fluid SPF 15 Sensitive Formula** *($22.50 for 2 ounces)* is similar to the one above, and the same review applies.

☺ **Evening Restorative Complex** *($27.50 for 1.75 ounces)* is a very average, though good moisturizer with about a 6% concentration of AHA.

☺ **$$$ Hydrating Lift Eye Complex** *($22.50 for 0.5 ounce)* isn't very different from the Evening Restorative above; for all intents and purposes they both work well for normal to dry skin and are decent AHA concentrations for exfoliation.

☹ **Blemish Treatment Gel** *($13.50 for 0.5 ounce)* lists alcohol as the first ingredient, which makes this product too irritating for all skin types.

☹ **Skin Lightener Gel** *($16.50 for 1.6 ounces)* would be a good 2% hydroquinone and AHA skin-lightening product if it wasn't for the alcohol it contains, which is unnecessarily irritating.

☹ **Rejuvenating Treatment Masque** *($16.50 for 2.5 ounces)* is basically alcohol and film former. This is an irritation waiting to happen.

☹ **Essential Multi-Protective Lip Balm, SPF 15** *($8.50 for 0.14 ounce)* doesn't contain avobenzone, zinc oxide, or titanium dioxide, and is not recommended.

## FACE Stockholm

This boutique line of makeup has personality and style. The two Swedish owners, mother and daughter Gum Nowak and Martina Arfwidson, have a passion for what they do and have created an interesting niche in the cosmetics world for women who want makeup to be fun and casual. With little attitude and a large number of color choices, this line indeed offers some interesting products to choose from, even though, in the long run, there's nothing really exceptional. It's hard to tell the difference between this line and M.A.C., Bobbi Brown, or Stila, to name a few.

The skin care here is lackluster, with major problems to be found, especially with the sunscreens and with the presence of irritating ingredients. The prices are another factor: they are unreasonable for what you get. For more information about FACE Stockholm, call (888) 334-FACE or visit the Web site at www.face stockholm.com.

## FACE Stockholm Skin Care

☹ **Aloe Vera Cleansing Cream** *($18 for 4 ounces)* is an emollient, wipe-off, cold cream–style makeup remover that can leave a greasy film on the skin. Wiping off makeup can tug at the skin and encourage wrinkles.

☹ **Aloe Vera Cleansing Lotion Normal to Dry, Sensitive Skin** *($12 for 4 ounces)* is similar to the one above, and the same comments apply.

☺ **Foaming Facial Cleanser Normal to Oily Skin** *($12 for 4 ounces)* is a standard, detergent-based water-soluble cleanser that works quite well both in removing makeup and not drying out the skin.

☹ **$$$ Apricot Gel Scrub Normal to Oily** *($16 for 2 ounces)* is an exceptionally overpriced scrub of gel, thickening agents, and ground-up apricot seeds. Baking soda mixed with Cetaphil Gentle Skin Cleanser would work far better and be vastly less expensive.

☹ **Eye Makeup Remover** *($8 for 2 ounces)* is a standard, detergent-based makeup remover, but this one uses sodium lauryl sulfate, an exceptionally irritating one.

☹ **Aloe Vera Toner All Skin Types** *($12 for 4 ounces)* contains witch hazel, which is a completely unnecessary irritant for the skin.

☹ **Blue Astringent Oily and Problem Skin** *($12 for 4 ounces)* contains alcohol and camphor and that can cause lots of problems for any skin type.

☹ **Botanical Toner Normal to Oily Skin** *($12 for 4 ounces)* contains witch hazel and eucalyptus, which are both irritants that can cause problems for the skin.

☹ **Vegetable Toner All Skin Types** *($12 for 4 ounces)* contains water and plant extracts. That wouldn't necessarily be a problem, though it also wouldn't be helpful, except this toner also contains lemon oil, which is a skin irritant and not recommended.

☺ **Aloe Vera Moisture Cream All Skin Types** *($24 for 2 ounces)* is a very good emollient moisturizer for dry skin. It wouldn't work for all skin types; this one contains lots of ingredients including plant oil and lanolin, that would be a problem for oily, combination, or blemish-prone skin types.

☺ **Aloe Vera Facial Lotion All Skin Types** *($14 for 4 ounces)* is an extremely emollient moisturizer that contains mostly water, plant oils, lanolin, thickeners, vitamin E, and preservatives. It would be very good for someone with dry skin. Much like the product above, this one is not suited for all skin types.

☺ **Orchid Oil Moisturizer All Skin Types** *($24 for 2 ounces)* is similar to the one above, and the same comments apply.

☺ **Vitamin Cream All Skin** *($24 for 2 ounces)* is similar to the one above, and the same comments apply. It does contain vitamins but not enough to matter.

☹ **SPF 15 Moisture Cream All Skin Types** *($24 for 2 ounces)* doesn't contain avobenzone, zinc oxide, or titanium dioxide, and is not recommended.

☺ **Aloe Vera Gel All Skin** *($12 for 4 ounces)* is just fine except for a few plant extracts thrown in that could be skin sensitizers, although for aloe vera you would be better going to the health food store and getting the pure stuff.

☹ **AHA Cream Dry to Mature Skin** *($26 for 2 ounces)* contains lemon and grapefruit as the second and third ingredients. Neither of these are AHAs; all they do is irritate the skin and that's not good for any skin type.

☹ **AHA Face Lotion Normal to Oily** *($14 for 4 ounces)* is similar to the one above, and the same review applies.

☺ **AHA Eye Cream All Skin Types** *($24 for 1 ounce)* is a good moisturizer for normal to dry skin but that's about it. At least with this one, there's no lemon and grapefruit. There is about a 2% concentration of lactic acid, but that isn't enough for it to work as an exfoliant.

☺ **Sage and Aloe Mask All Skin Types** *($18 for 2 ounces)* is just a bunch of thickeners and emollients; it would be good for dry skin (not for all skin types as the name implies). Someone with oily or blemish-prone skin would not appreciate the lanolin oil and plant oils this mask contains.

## FACE Stockholm Makeup

**FOUNDATION:** ☺ **Liquid Foundation** *($21)* is a good but rather ordinary foundation with an even, light-to-medium application and a handful of great colors. It would work well for someone with normal to dry skin. The only colors to avoid are Sno, which can be too pink, and Sommar, which can be too peach.

☺ **Matte Foundation** *($21)* has a soft matte finish, and is lighter-textured than it used to be, but the matte effect doesn't last long, so that makes it best for someone with normal to slightly dry or slightly oily skin. The colors to avoid are Sno, which is slightly pink, as well as Yellow, Mint, and Lilac. The last three are color correctors and they just add a layer of makeup that doesn't correct anything.

☺ **Powder Foundation** *($24)* has excellent shades (15 in all) and a wonderfully soft, dry finish. These are better used as powders than foundation and are definitely preferred over the regular Pressed Powders in this line that are all shiny. The only shades to avoid are July and November, which are both fairly peach.

☹ **$$$ Tinted Moisturizer** *($29)* is very overpriced for such a basic formula, and it doesn't even offer any sun protection. The one color available is limiting, to say the least.

☹ **$$$ Picture Perfect Foundation** *($26)* comes in a jar and is a very thick, emollient formula that is meant for full coverage. The texture is so greasy that the product's directions explain the need to use powder to get any longevity from the makeup, and you would need to powder and repowder, and then repowder all day long. The 13 shades have some worthwhile colors, but this formula has enough drawbacks to pass it up entirely, including a far from natural looking and a far too heavy application for most skin types.

☹ **CONCEALER:** **Corrective Concealer** *($16)* doesn't correct, it just places strange shades of yellow, pink, and blue on the face. **Concealer Wand** *($12)* is a tube applicator concealer that has an extremely poor range of colors; all of them are either too pink, peach, ash, or green to recommend. **Concealer Stick** *($12)* is a standard, lipstick-style concealer; most of the colors are poor—only Light Amber, Amber, and Dark Amber look like skin tone—plus this one tends to crease.

<u>POWDER:</u> ☹ $$$ **Pressed Powder** *($18)* is talc-based and has some great colors and a dry, smooth texture but all of the shades are shiny. Doesn't that negate the reason for using a pressed powder? Unless you're looking for shine, this is one to avoid.

☺ **Galaxy** *($14)* is just loose glitter, large flecks of it, kind of like what you buy at an arts and crafts store. It is fairly messy to apply because it doesn't cling well, but for shine, this is as shiny as it gets.

☺ $$$ **Loose Powder** *($18)* is also talc-based and has some great neutral shades with a very dry, soft finish. There are some shiny shades and strange colors that are best overlooked unless the mood strikes you, but they're not to be taken seriously. **Bronzer** *($18)* is a standard, pressed-powder bronzer that comes in a small but good variety of colors. These omit the iridescence, but the oils do leave a sheen on the skin.

<u>BLUSH:</u> ☺ **Blush** *($13)* are standard, single-tin blushes that have a great soft texture. The large color selection has some excellent options, although these are strongly reminiscent of many other lines and nothing unique or special.

☹ $$$ **Creme Blush-On** *($16)* is standard cream blush that has an old-fashioned, slightly greasy texture, so be cautious unless you have dry skin. It goes on more sheer than the color in the pot would lead you to think. In the long run this can't compete with the more current cream-to-powder blush textures that have a more even and less slippery application and appearance.

☺ <u>EYESHADOW:</u> **Pearl Shadow** and **Matte Shadow** *($13)* are nicely identified; the matte shades are excellent and there are a lot of them.

☹ $$$ **Eye Dust** *($16)* are tins of extremely shiny powder. They are messy to use and hard to control but they do create shine all over and work as well as any. **Face Highlighters** *($16)* are tins of greasy, iridescent color that can be used anyplace you want to add shine. They work best for evening only. **Trinity Eye, Lip, Cheek** *($16)* are pots of creamy, rather slick eyeshadows that are also meant to work for blush or lip color. They're loaded with shimmer and make the skin, lips, or eyes look greasy and iridescent.

☺ <u>EYE AND BROW SHAPER:</u> **Eye and Brow Pencils** *($10)* are all grouped together and they are extremely standard, soft-finish pencils in a wide range of colors. **Cake Eyeliner** *($11)* is a standard cake eyeliner to be used wet that creates a dramatic line along the lashes. **Brow Fix** *($12)* comes in two shades, clear and a medium brown. They work well to make brows look fuller and keep them in place, but the color choice is dismal. $$$ **Brow Shadow** *($16)* is a group of matte eyeshadows that match brow color rather nicely. This is a great way to apply brow color.

☹ **Liquid Eyeliner** *($12)* is hard to apply evenly and tends to go on choppy. The brush is too long and soft to rely on for effective control.

The Reviews F

☺ <u>**LIPSTICK AND LIP PENCIL:**</u> **Lipstick** *($15)* has a vast range of colors that are nicely creamy and opaque. **Matte Lipstick** *($15)* has a great, soft, matte finish and a smaller color selection than the regular lipstick, but it's still a large assortment with great neutral shades. **Lipgloss** *($12)* is just a tube lip gloss with a great range of colors. **Pot Lipgloss** *($12)* is a slightly sticky but very glossy pot of gloss with an exceptionally vivid application of color. **Lip Liner Pencil** *($10)* is a modestly priced, standard creamy lip pencil that comes in some great colors.

☺ <u>**MASCARA:**</u> **Mascara Regular** *($12)* is a decent mascara that builds some amount of length and thickness, but it takes awhile. The more interesting aspect for the mascara is the color selection; lavender, silver, and eggplant are, to say the least, unique and a kick for a noticeably strange look.

☺ <u>**BRUSHES:**</u> The large range of brushes offered in the FACE Stockholm line come in a good price range *($10 to $30)*. The eyeshadow brush selection is excellent and there are many reasons to check these out, especially for size options. However, the larger face brushes tend to be stiff and coarse and are not as dense as I would prefer for easy application.

# *Fashion Fair*

It has always struck me as somewhat sad and ironic that women of color, who on average buy cosmetics at three times the rate of other ethnic groups, have such a limited number of options. One would think a cosmetics line like Fashion Fair would be a welcome oasis in a desert of limited choices, but in fact the opposite is true. Although Fashion Fair distinctly prides itself as a line for women of color, many of its products' textures and color choices leave much to be desired and can't hold a candle to other lines such as M.A.C. and Prescriptives that have recognized the oversights for women of color and successfully corrected them. There are also much better lines specifically devoted to African-American women, particularly Iman (available at J.C. Penney) and Black Opal (a small but good drugstore line that is also available at some Sears stores). This line hasn't changed much at all since I last reviewed it, and that's a shame, as it is in need of some updating. There are some plausible choices to be found here, but they are few and far between. The poor state many of its counters are in (its tester units are poorly organized, outdated, and generally a mess) leads me to believe that African-American women have already spoken loud and clear by opting to ignore this line until it provides them with what they can presently get elsewhere.

One area of utter disappointment is the skin-care products. They are mostly greasy cold cream–like cleansers, water-soluble cleansers with strongly irritating cleansing agents, alcohol-based toners, and greasy moisturizers. Layering greasy moisturizers on darker skin tones can cause a buildup of dead skin cells, making skin look dull and uneven. Almost all of the toners are exceedingly drying and irritating, which is another cause of dull, uneven skin tones and breakouts. An even more glaring defect is the lack of sunscreens or AHA products. Surely by now Fashion Fair knows that darker skin tones also run the risk of sun damage, and that a major cause of ashen discolorations on dark skin tones is damage caused by the sun. For more information about Fashion Fair, call (312) 322-9444 or visit the Web site at www.fashionfair.com.

# Fashion Fair Skin Care

☺ **Botanical Cleansing Gel** *($12 for 6.7 ounces)* is a good (but standard) detergent-based water-soluble cleanser for someone with normal to oily skin. It does contain fragrance but the couple of minuscule plant extracts in here hardly make this botanical.

☺ **Cleansing Creme with Aloe Vera** *($14.25 for 4 ounces)* is a standard, mineral oil–based wipe-off cleanser that can leave a greasy film, though it can be an option for someone with dry skin.

☺ **Deep Cleansing Lotion Balanced for All Skin Types** *($15 for 8 ounces)* is a fairly greasy cleanser that needs to be wiped off. It contains several ingredients that could cause breakouts, including lanolin and isopropyl palmitate. Calling this suitable for all skin types is absurd, though for someone with very dry skin it is an option.

☹ **Facial Shampoo Original Formula for Normal or Oily Skin** *($11 for 3 ounces)* is a standard, detergent-based water-soluble cleanser that uses sodium lauryl sulfate as the main cleansing agent. It can be very drying and irritating for all skin types.

☺ **Gentle Facial Shampoo Mild for Dry Sensitive Skin** *($10 for 2.1 ounces)* is definitely gentler than the shampoo above and could be very good for someone with normal to oily skin.

☺ **$$$ Eye Makeup Remover** *($8.50 for 2 ounces)* is a standard, silicone- and detergent-based eye-makeup remover. It works as well as any and this one doesn't contain fragrance.

☹ **Gentle Facial Polisher for All Skin Types** *($13.25 for 3 ounces)* is a detergent cleanser that also contains synthetic scrub particles. It does contain menthol, which can be irritating for many skin types.

☺ **Botanical Skin Purifier I for Normal to Oily Skin** *($11.50 for 6.7 ounces)* won't purify anything; it is just about as ordinary a toner as you can get, and the lemongrass in here can be a skin irritant.

☺ **Botanical Skin Purifier II for Normal to Dry Skin** *($11.50 for 6.7 ounces)* can't balance skin, but it is an OK toner for the skin type indicated.

☹ **Deep Pore Astringent Regular for Normal to Oily Skin** *($13.25 for 8 ounces)* is primarily alcohol and fragrance, and that makes it too drying and irritating for all skin types.

The Reviews F

☹ **Skin Freshener I Normal to Oily Skin** (*$11.50 for 6 ounces*) contains mostly alcohol, which is very drying, not to mention irritating.

☹ **Skin Freshener II Dry or Sensitive Skin** (*$11.50 for 6 ounces*) has basically the same ingredients as Skin Freshener I and can be just as drying. Alcohol isn't appropriate for any skin type, but even less so for someone with dry or sensitive skin.

☹ **Toning Lotion Mild for Dry Sensitive Skin** (*$13.25 for 8 ounces*) is an alcohol-based toner; alcohol isn't good for even the hardiest skin type, much less dry, sensitive skin.

☺ **Dry Skin Emollient for Excessively Dry Skin** (*$21 for 2 ounces*) is a good but extremely basic and rather greasy moisturizer for someone with very dry skin.

☺ **$$$ Eye Cream** (*$20 for 0.5 ounce*) is a somewhat thick, emollient moisturizer that would be a good moisturizer for dry skin.

☹ **Hidden Beauty Skin Enhancing Creme** (*$24.50 for 1.9 ounces*) is supposed to be a blend of antioxidant vitamins and beta hydroxy acid. The amount of vitamins is minuscule and the willow bark in here is only distantly related to BHA and does not work as an exfoliant.

☺ **Moisturizing Creme with Aloe Vera for Dry Skin** (*$18.50 for 4 ounces*) is a very emollient moisturizer that would work well on very dry skin, but not because of the aloe.

☺ **Moisture Lotion for All Day Beauty** (*$14.75 for 4 ounces*) is a standard emollient moisturizer for someone with dry skin, but rather unimpressive, and without sunscreen it is not good for all-day protection.

☺ **Moisturizing Lotion for Normal to Oily Skin** (*$18.50 for 4 ounces*) is a very standard moisturizer, but what are Vaseline and lanolin doing in a product for oily skin!

☹ **Oil-Free Moisturizer** (*$19.50 for 4 ounces*) is indeed an oil-free moisturizer, but it also contains isopropyl myristate and isopropyl palmitate high up on the ingredient list, and both of those thickening agents are well known for causing blackheads and breakouts.

☹ **Oil-Control Lotion** (*$15 for 3 ounces*) contains mostly alcohol and some minerals that have some ability to absorb oil. The alcohol causes more problems than the minerals can help.

☺ **Special Beauty Creme with Collagen** (*$19.50 for 2 ounces*) is a good ordinary moisturizer for someone with very dry skin. Collagen is a good water-binding agent, but it doesn't affect the collagen in your skin one little bit.

☹ **Deep Pore Cleansing Masque for Normal to Oily Skin** (*$15.25 for 2 ounces*). There are far better mask formulations available than this one.

☺ **Vantex Skin Bleaching Creme with Sunscreens** (*$14 for 2 ounces*) doesn't contain enough sunscreen to protect skin from any amount of sun damage, but it is a good 2% hydroquinone product in a slightly moisturizing base. You would still need a reliable sunscreen in order for this product to be effective.

## Fashion Fair Makeup

FOUNDATION: ☹ **Oil-Free Perfect Finish Souffle** *($21)* goes on thick and creamy but dries to a matte medium finish. It can be tricky to blend, but the color selection and coverage are excellent for someone with normal to oily skin (it may look somewhat pasty on normal to dry skin). The only colors to avoid are Copper Glo, Brown Blaze Glo, and Bronze Glo.

☺ **Oil-Free Liquid** *($17.50)* is a good matte foundation for someone with oily skin who wants heavier coverage. This blends on decently, but don't expect a sheer application. These colors, which are all too orange for most skin tones, should be avoided: Honey, Amber, Copper, Tan, and Tender Brown.

☺ **Liquid Sheer Foundation** *($12.50)* does provide a light, sheer coverage. This is a more emollient foundation that would work well for dry skin. The color range has been whittled down to a few good shades, and those are: Tender Brown, Warm Caramel, Brae Bronze, and Ebony Brown. These shades are too orange or peach to recommend: Tawny, Honey Amber, Copper Tan, and Copper Blaze.

☹ **Oil-Free Perfect Finish Creme to Powder Makeup** *($20)* has a somewhat greasy finish though the colors are quite good. This can be too creamy for someone with oily skin and too powdery for someone with dry skin, so only those with mostly normal skin would find this workable.

☹ **Perfect Finish Creme Makeup** *($16.50)* is appropriate for normal to dry skin only, as this goes on creamy and stays that way. The coverage is sheer to medium, as this foundation blends out fairly well. The pigment in darker foundations tends to interact with the skin's surface oil and can turn orange, and that seems to be the case here. These colors are strongly orange and should be avoided: Tawny Glo, Brown Blaze Glo, Bronze Glo, Copper Glo, and Amber Glo.

CONCEALER: ☹ **Cover Tone Concealing Creme Fragrance-Free** *($15)* is for use under the eyes or over blemishes and scars. It has a very dry, thick consistency and provides fairly heavy coverage with a slightly sticky finish. If you need a lot of coverage this is an option; if not, this product is not the least bit natural looking. All of the colors are very good.

☹ **Fragrance-Free Coverstick** *($10)* has a drier consistency for oily skin. It can be difficult to blend, and the two colors, Medium and Dark, are too peach or orange for most skin tones. The regular **Coverstick** *($10)* has fragrance and a much creamier formula. It does blend sheer, but can slip into lines around the eye. Most of the colors are either too peach or orange. The only neutral color is Very Light, but the application still leaves much to be desired.

☺ **POWDER:** $$$ Loose Powder *($15.50)* is a standard, talc-based powder that has a nice texture and good colors, but it is shiny. The **TransGlo Pressed Powder and Loose Powder** *($13)* follow suit and are also shiny, although the colors are great. Both of these powders contain mineral oil, which isn't bad but also not great for oil control. Luckily, the $$$ **Oil Control Loose Powder** *($17)* and the **Oil Control Pressed Powder** *($13)* are oil free, but they still have a slight shine (which negates eliminating shine from the face) and most of the colors are too peach. Walnut is the only one to consider in both formats. **Fragrance-Free Pressed Powder** *($13)* is a standard talc powder and has a smooth, slightly dry texture and some good colors. The shine is there too, but not enough to be as obvious as the others. Perhaps these would be OK for evening wear, but they certainly won't reduce the shine of a foundation.

☺ **BLUSH: Beauty Blush Fragrance and Fragrance-Free** *($13)* comes in an interesting variety of colors, both fragranced and fragrance-free. They go on dry but smooth and include both vivid and subtle shades, but be careful: many of the colors are also quite shiny.

☹ **EYESHADOW: Ultimate Eyes** *($15)*, **Eye Shadow Collection Quads** *($14.50)*, **Trios** *($13.50)*, and **Touches of Color** *($13.50)* are all extremely shiny. They are a poor option for women of any color. The two shades of brown that aren't shiny each come packaged in a set of four colors, and the other three shades are shiny. I do not recommend any of the Fashion Fair eyeshadows except possibly for evening wear.

☹ **EYE AND BROW SHAPER: Eye Liner Pencils** *($10)* are creamy pencils with a sponge tip on one end so you can smudge them before they do this on their own. **Liquid Liner** *($12)* has three very shiny shades and the brush is hard to control so application tends to be uneven and splatters. **Brow Pencil** ($7) has a very dry, heavy texture with colors that are just OK, but a matte powder eyeshadow is a far better choice than this. **Brush-On Brow** *($11)* has two shades of matte powders that are rather waxy and apply too heavily to look natural.

☺ **LIPSTICK AND LIP PENCIL:** There are three types of lipsticks available, **Cremes, Frosts,** and **Forever Matte** *($12.50)*. The Cremes have a slightly greasy consistency with a nice selection of opaque colors, and the Frosts are identical in texture to the Cremes except they are very iridescent. Forever Matte isn't really matte; it's actually quite creamy with a nice stain for longer wear and a shiny finish. **Automatic Lip Colors** *($11.50)* is just lip gloss with a wand applicator and a nice, non-sticky feel. **Lip Liner Pencils** *($8.50)* are standard, creamy pencils with a small but good selection of colors. They go on as well as most other pencils.

☹ **MASCARA:** Fashion Fair's **Mascara** *($11)* is billed as a treatment mascara with proteins, panthenol, and collagen. None of these ingredients have any effect on the lashes, and certainly not in the amounts used in this product. To top that off, this is one of the worst mascaras I have tested, providing absolutely no length and no thickness, and it smears easily.

# Flori Roberts

Flori Roberts is a cosmetics line that seems to be satisfied staying exactly the same, never improving and reformulating its products as style and improved formulation changes come along. I could almost feel the tumbleweeds roll by as I revisited this stagnating line. Maybe Flori Roberts should just raise the white flag and surrender to the excellent choices for women of color all around, from Iman (usually right next to Flori Roberts at J.C. Penney) to Trish McEvoy and Black Opal, among the many lines that have successfully given women of color wonderful, workable choices and reliable products. For now, Flori Roberts seems content to offer African-American women poor foundation colors; shiny, dry blushes; and eyeshadow color combinations that were popular (who knows why?) back when everyone was wondering, "Who shot J. R?"

Women of color require stronger colors (which tend to cause grainy texture), but that doesn't mean the blushes can't be silky-smooth and have stronger pigment at the same time; many other lines have accomplished this feat. And darker skin tones do not require shiny eyeshadows. If the blushes can be matte, surely the eyeshadows can be too.

This line leaves much to be desired in the skin-care arena as well. It has more than its share of greasy moisturizers and drying toners (containing lots of irritating ingredients), which can create problems that weren't there before for darker skin tones. Irritation on darker skin tones can make skin look flaky and ashen. None of that is good. This line needs an overhaul, but it doesn't look like it's coming anytime soon. For more information about Flori Roberts call (800) 621-6043. As this book went to press, Flori Roberts' Web site, www.floriroberts.com, was under construction.

# Flori Roberts Skin Care

☹ My Everything Double O Soap Gold, for Normal to Oily Skin *($13 for 4 ounces)* is a standard bar soap with many ingredients, such as peppermint oil, eucalyptus oil, and camphor, that are very irritating and drying.

☹ My Everything Treatment Foaming Cleanser *($12 for 6 ounces)* is a standard, detergent-based water-soluble cleanser that can be a bit confusing for some skin types. The cleansing ingredients are on the drying side, but then there are plant oils that can compensate yet also be a problem for oily skin. This one also contains peppermint oil, an unnecessary irritant.

☺ My Everything Foaming Gel Cleanser *($15 for 6 ounces)* is a gentle, detergent-based water-soluble cleanser that contains a small percentage of lactic acid (an AHA). In a cleanser, this small amount of AHA isn't a problem; the lactic acid is more a moisturizing agent than an exfoliant. It does contain fragrance.

☺ **Optima Gel Cleanser Gold Oil-Free** *($15 for 6 ounces)* is a fairly good water-soluble cleanser that should work well for someone with normal to oily skin.

☺ **My Everything Treatment Exfoliating Facial Scrub and Primer** *($12.50 for 4 ounces)* would be an OK and relatively gentle exfoliant, but it can be tricky to rinse off.

☹ **My Everything Gentle Eye Makeup Remover** *($9 for 3 ounces)* isn't gentle. Putting peppermint, sage, and rosemary, which are strong irritants, especially for the eye area, in an eye-makeup remover is a cruel joke.

☹ **Double O Complex Gold for Normal to Oily Skin** *($12.50 for 8 ounces)* contains alcohol and a host of irritating ingredients, such as peppermint oil, eucalyptus oil, clove oil, and camphor. This toner does nothing for the skin other than irritate and dry it, a problem for all skin types and all skin colors.

☹ **My Everything Treatment Skin Balancing Astringent/Toner** *($12 for 6 ounces)* contains mostly water, witch hazel, slip agent, lactic acid, anti-irritant, and preservatives. This is about a 5% AHA product. The witch hazel and orange oil in here make it more irritating than necessary, and this toner is not suitable for most skin types.

☹ **Optima Refining Lotion Gold Oil-Free** *($14.50 for 6 ounces)*. Witch hazel contains a good amount of alcohol, which makes it irritating and drying when used repeatedly.

☺ **Hydrophilic Moisture Complex Gold** *($20 for 2 ounces)* is an OK, very boring moisturizer for normal to dry skin, but as an exfoliant it doesn't even rate.

☺ **My Everything Creme** *($25 for 3.25 ounces)* would be a good emollient moisturizer for someone with dry skin who isn't prone to breakouts.

☺ **My Everything Treatment Advanced Formula Creme, Alpha-Melanix with Sunscreen** *($28.50 for 3.25 ounces)* doesn't contain enough sunscreen to protect skin from sun damage, nor does it contain any UVA protection, and it is not recommended as a sunscreen. It is just a very ordinary moisturizer with mostly thickeners and silicones.

☹ **My Everything Treatment Eye Treatment Complex** *($18.50 for 1 ounce)* is just a bunch of thickeners; what a terribly formulated, overpriced, do-nothing moisturizer.

☹ **My Everything Treatment Oil Free Moisturizer** *($9.99 for 2.6 ounces)* is a do-nothing product that won't help any skin type. The sunscreen isn't rated and it doesn't have UVA protection, so that part is also disappointing.

☺ **My Everything Treatment Oil Control Serum Normal to Oily Skin** *($14 for 1 ounce)* is a good (though simple) lightweight gel moisturizer for normal to slightly dry skin. It contains mostly water, aloe, slip agents, water-binding agents, and preservatives.

☹ My Everything Treatment Revitalized Protection Moisturizer, Alpha-Melanix with Sunscreen *($16.50 for 4 ounces)* doesn't contain enough sunscreen to protect skin from sun damage, nor does it contain any UVA protection, and it is not recommended. Plus, the AHA in here is less than 1%, which makes it ineffective for exfoliation.

☺ My Everything Treatment Advanced Chromatone Plus with Alpha-Melanix Fade Cream with Sunscreen *($14.50 for 1.7 ounces)* is a standard 2% hydroquinone fade cream in an emollient base. Hydroquinone can be an effective melanin inhibitor. This also contains a tiny amount of lactic acid, but not enough to exfoliate the skin or help the hydroquinone perform more effectively by improving cell turnover, and the sunscreen in here is useless for any kind of reliable protection.

## *Flori Roberts Makeup*

<u>FOUNDATION:</u> ☹ **Touche Satin Foundation** *($15)* is a cream-to-powder compact makeup that is decidedly creamy. It does blend on well, offering medium to full coverage, but the colors are just awful. The only possible considerations may be Walnut, Mahogany, or Mocha. The rest are too peach, pink, or red to even try on.

☺ **Maximum Matte Souffle Oil-Free Makeup** *($20)* is the most salvageable of Roberts's foundation formulas. Although this appears to be quite thick, the texture isn't too bad and the coverage ends up on the light to medium side. This can blend on choppy, so use caution. All of the colors are winners, although Sienna is slightly orange. This would be a great option for normal to oily skins.

☺ **Hydrophilic Oil-Free Foundation** *($21)* is a liquid foundation that offers sheer to light coverage and a slightly sticky matte finish. This can be an option for normal to oily skins, but the colors are pitiful. The only possibilities (and these are for lighter skin tones), are Golden A and Chroma A (slightly peach). The rest are some of the worst foundation colors you're likely to see.

☹ **Hydrophilic Demi-Compact** *($18.50)* is another creamy foundation with medium to full coverage that would be OK for normal to dry skin if the colors weren't so bad. Every shade is either too peach, orange, or red to recommend.

<u>CONCEALER:</u> ☺ **Concealer Pencil** *($10)* is a pencil, and that's not the best way to use concealer. Who needs one more thing to sharpen? Plus, as is true for this version, pencils tend to have a heavy, greasy texture and opaque coverage that is destined to crease and cake. If you are a fan of this type of product, and can somehow make it look good, you may want to consider Fair (for medium skin tones) and Bronze (medium to deep).

☹ <u>POWDER:</u> **Chromatic Loose Powder** *($17.50)* has a smooth, soft texture and a lovely dry finish but guess what? All of the colors are too peach or pink for most any skin tone. **Pressed Powder** *($13)* also has a beautiful texture and finish, but the colors—I mean, really! **Compact Face Powder With Oil Control** *($15)* has a nice, dry texture and will assuredly absorb excess oil (that's what any good powder should do), but here we go again with the colors: all are too peach to recommend.

☺ <u>**BLUSH:**</u> **Radiance Blush** *($13)* has a large assortment of colors, all with slight to glaring shine. Even without the shine, the grainy, dry texture of these leaves much to be desired. For the most part, these colors are only an option for women with deep ebony skin tones. **More Than Blush** *($14.50)* is an ultra-shiny liquid that comes in one shade, intended for use with or without blush for a bronze tone, but no one needs this much glitter on the face.

☹ <u>**EYESHADOW:**</u> **Signature Eyeshadow Trios** *($14.50)* have some of the most unusual and shiny color combinations you are ever likely to see in the world of makeup. No one needs this much shine and definitely not as the only option.

☺ <u>**EYE AND BROW SHAPER:**</u> **Eye Contour Pencils** *($8.50)* are fairly standard, but a bit drier than most on the market. This makes them a little harder to apply, but they also don't smear as fast. **Matte Brows** *($10.50)* is a powder shadow meant for use on the brows. It comes in two colors, Brown and Black, and is a great option for shaping eyebrows.

☺ <u>**LIPSTICK AND LIP PENCIL:**</u> Flori Roberts excels in this arena, and the availability of testers can be sketchy, but if you know what you need you should be fine. **Lipstick** *($10)* is just to the greasy side of creamy and comes in a nice range of colors. **Matte Lipstick** *($10.50)* is hardly anyone's definition of matte, but it is a good creamy lipstick with opaque coverage. **Liquid Lip Gloss** *($10.50)* is a wand applicator–type, standard gloss with a light, non-sticky texture. **Lip Polish** *($10)* offers two shades of ultra-shiny, sticky gloss in a pot. **Lip Contour Pencil** *($8.50)* is completely ordinary in every respect except that it is drier and more waxy than most.

☺ <u>**MASCARA:**</u> **Lash Set 2000 Mascara** *($12)*. When I looked at the box, it was dated 1996, prompting me to wonder how long it had been sitting there. I would warn you not to buy any dated products that are more than a year or two old at the most. Dates notwithstanding, this is a nice mascara that thickens quickly but may clump due to the creaminess of the formula.

## Forever Spring (Skin Care Only)

Actress Connie Stevens promotes this line as the reason she looks so wonderful. Well, she does look great, but that has absolutely nothing to do with these products. These are just very basic skin-care products with ingredients similar to a hundred others on the market, and that means they have good and bad points. The good points are some reliable moisturizers; the bad points are irritating plant extracts and poorly formulated sunscreens. I also admit to having a rough time with the name of the company. Any cosmetics-company name that implies that you will stay forever young from buying a set of skin-care products, whether it's Sudden Youth, Instant Youth, Instant Lift, or Forever Spring, is selling a marketing gimmick and not a reality in any way, shape, or form.

The big problem in this line is the ☹ **Time Machine** *($120).* This is by far one of the bigger wastes of money I've seen in the world of cosmetics. It is supposed to exercise facial muscles through topical stimulation. Facial muscles, just like body muscles, cannot be built up through artificial exercise; if they could, why would a bodybuilder ever bother to lift weights? Even if this machine did work, the muscles would simply bulge, not lift skin (you'd look like many an older bodybuilder, with muscles *and* sagging skin). In addition, this machine can create damage by breaking delicate surface capillaries. It is supposed to increase circulation, but there are better ways to increase circulation than with voltage. Running up and down your stairs for 20 minutes will not only increase your circulation but also help your heart and build energy. For more information about Forever Spring call (800) 523-4334 or visit the Web site at www.foreverspring.com.

☹ **AHA Cleansing Pads** *($26.95 for 50 pads)* contains mostly witch hazel, which can be a skin irritant. It also contains AHA and BHA, and the pH of 4 is passable for making this effective for exfoliation. The mix of additional irritating plant extracts is problematic for skin. In the long run, there are far more gentle and effective AHA and BHA products to consider than this one.

☺ **Collagen Facial Cleanser** *($14.25 for 4 ounces)* is a fairly standard, greasy, wipe-off cleanser that is not water soluble. The directions say to wipe up, never down, but regardless of whether you pull the skin up or down, you're still causing it to stretch, and that causes sagging. For someone with very dry skin this is an option. It does contain fragrance.

☹ **Ginseng & Vitamin C Cleansing Gel** *($21.50 for 6 ounces)* contains several ingredients that can irritate the eyes and skin, including grapefruit and tangerine. Those serve no purpose for skin other than to cause irritation.

☹ **Honey Almond Apricot Scuffer** *($13.25 for 4 ounces)* is a detergent-based water-soluble cleanser that uses sodium lauryl sulfate as the main cleansing agent, which is extremely drying and irritating, and is not recommended for any skin type.

☺ **Ambrosia Skin Refresher** *($14.50 for 4 ounces)* is a good basic toner. It would work well for most skin types.

☹ **Ginseng & Vitamin C Balancing & Toning Lotion** *($12.50 for 6 ounces)* lists the main ingredients as pink grapefruit and tangerine extracts, which make it potentially irritating and drying for all skin types, plus it also contains ginseng and witch hazel, and that adds to the irritation potential.

☺ **Retrieve Alpha & Beta Hydroxy Combination for the Face** *($26.95 for 1* *ounce*) doesn't have a pH that's low enough for it to be an effective exfoliant, but it can be a good moisturizer for someone with dry skin. It does contain AHA, BHA, and urea. The urea is not here in enough of a concentration to be effective as an exfoliant.

☺ **Bio Eye and Throat Intensive Lubrication Complex** (*$15 for 1 ounce*) would be a good emollient moisturizer for someone with dry skin.

☺ **Collagen Skin Quencher** (*$22.75 for 4 ounces*) is a good, very lightweight moisturizer for someone with slightly dry skin, but the collagen and elastin can't do anything for the collagen in your skin. This moisturizer is supposed to be used with the Time Machine.

☺ **Collagen Spray** (*$4.95 for 2 ounces*) is an OK toner. This is more like spraying water on the face than anything else. The amount of collagen water in here is negligible and it can't affect the collagen in your skin.

☺ **Fibro Eye Soother** (*$14 for 0.5 ounce*) is almost all water and silicone. These can feel good, but it isn't worth the price tag for this tiny amount.

☺ **Ginseng Facial Feed** (*$21.25 for 4 ounces*) is a very good emollient moisturizer for dry skin. The ginseng can be a skin irritant.

☺ **Ginseng and Vitamin C Intensive Complex with Vitamins E, A, C, and Lipolic Acid** (*$31.50 for 2 ounces*) is a good emollient moisturizer for dry skin and all the vitamins you could want.

☺ **Hy-Persome Facial Lotion** (*$24.50 for 2 ounces*) is a good though unimpressive moisturizer for someone with normal to dry skin.

☺ $$$ **Hy-Persome Eye Emollience** (*$19.50 for 0.5 ounce*) is similar to the one above though definitely more emollient for dry skin.

☹ **Lift and Taut Spring Skin Serum** (*$26.95 for 1 ounce*) contains mostly arnica extract, which is a potent skin irritant and makes this product a problem for all skin types.

☺ $$$ **Mandarin Liposome Oxygen Booster** (*$24.95 for 0.5 ounce*) lists liposomes as an ingredient, which is strange, because liposomes are a delivery system (a way of formulating a product), not an ingredient. In any case, this product can't deliver oxygen into the skin, because it doesn't contain any, unless you consider water a source of oxygen, but then all products contain that. The mandarin extract and fragrance in here can be skin irritants.

☺ **Petal Soft Eye Cream** (*$14 for 0.5 ounce*) would be a very good emollient moisturizer for someone with dry skin.

☺ **Super Rich Emollience** (*$24.50 for 4 ounces*) would be a very good emollient moisturizer for someone with very dry skin.

☹ **Super Rich Emollience Outdoor Protection SPF 15** (*$24.95 for 4 ounces*) doesn't contain avobenzone, titanium dioxide, or zinc oxide, and is not recommended.

☺ **Forever Summer Self Tanning Lotion, Super Rich Emollience** (*$23.50 for 4* *ounces)*, like all self tanners, uses dihydroxyacetone to turn the skin brown. This one works as well as any.

☹ **Acne Blemish Relief** *($17.50 for 1 ounce)* is a mishmash of ingredients that can add up to problems, not help. The clay and BHA aren't bad, but several of the plant extracts are irritants, including arnica, lemon, orange, kiwi, clove, and cypress. It also contains sulfur, another potent irritant. This is redness and flaking just waiting to happen.

☺ $$$ **Baby Soft Facial Clay** *($15 for 4 ounces)* is a standard clay mask. If you want a clay mask, this would be fine, and it can make the skin feel soft, but "baby soft" is stretching things a bit.

☹ **Ginseng Firming Peel-Off Facial Masque with Multi-Fruit AHAs** *($18 for 4 ounces)* is mostly plastic and alcohol with a tiny amount of AHAs. There is no reason to put this combination of ingredients on your skin.

## *Freeman Cosmetics (Skin Care Only)*

For more information about Freeman products (owned by the Dial Corporation), call (800) FREEMAN or visit the Web site at www.freemancosmetics.com.

☺ **Skin + Vitamin C Complex Cleanser and Toner** *($5.99 for 8 ounces)* is a standard, detergent-based cleanser that also contains a good deal of witch hazel, which can be a skin irritant. It can work for some skin types, but I suspect this will be fairly irritating. It does contain fragrance and coloring agents. The amount of vitamin C in here (as all these Vitamin C products) is infinitesimally small.

☹ **Skin + Vitamin C Complex Moisturizer SPF 15** *($6.99 for 2.5 ounces)* doesn't contain avobenzone, zinc oxide, or titanium dioxide, and is not recommended.

☺ **Skin + Vitamin C Complex Eye Cream** *($7.99 for 0.5 ounce)* is a good emollient moisturizer for dry skin. The amount of vitamin C in here (and all the Vitamin C products in this line) is infinitesimally small.

☺ **Skin + Vitamin C Complex Night Repair** *($7.99 for 2 ounces)* won't repair anything, but it is a good moisturizer for dry skin. The amount of vitamin C in here (and all the Vitamin C products in this line) is infinitesimally small.

☹ **Skin + Vitamin C Complex Pore Masque and Clarifier** *($5.99 for 2.5 ounces)* is mainly alcohol and plastic, and there is never a reason to put these kinds of ingredients on your skin. I know it's fun to peel masks of this kind off the skin, but that just isn't good for the skin.

☺ **Blueberry & Lavender Facial Gel Cleanser** *($2.85 for 6 ounces)* is a standard, detergent-based water-soluble cleanser that would be good for someone with normal to oily skin. The small amount of blueberry and lavender here are probably not a risk for irritation, but these do not help skin in any way. This does contain fragrance and coloring agents.

The Reviews F

☺ **Pineapple & Watermelon Alpha & Beta Hydroxy Skin Renewal Facial Wash** *($3.29 for 8 ounces)* is a standard, detergent-based water-soluble cleanser that would be good for someone with normal to oily skin. The small amount of pineapple and watermelon in here can be skin irritants. The plant extracts in here are not AHAs, though this product does contain BHA, but the pH is not low enough for it to be effective as an exfoliant.

☹ **Cucumber & Ginseng Oil-Free Deep Pore Cleanser** *($3.49 for 5.3 ounces)* contains peppermint, menthol, and camphor, which can't deep-clean though they can deeply irritate and inflame skin.

☺ **Apricot & Sea Kelp Facial Scrub** *($3.50 for 6 ounces)* is a walnut shell–based scrub. The plant oil makes this product good only for someone with dry skin. It can leave a greasy film.

☺ **Peach Tree & Coconut Blemish Control Medicated Facial Scrub** *($3.69 for 5.3 ounces)* is almost identical to the Apricot version above and the same basic comments apply. This version does contain a tiny amount of BHA, but the pH isn't low enough for it to be effective as an exfoliant and the plant oil in here won't make someone with oily skin very happy.

☺ **Raspberry & Almond Face & Body Scrub** *($3.50 for 6 ounces)* uses synthetic scrub particles (ground-up plastic) in a detergent cleanser base. It will exfoliate the skin and can work for someone with normal to dry skin. It does contain fragrance and coloring agents.

☺ **Apple Pear & Aloe Alpha-Beta Hydroxy Skin Repair Lotion** *($3.29 for 5.3 ounces)* is an OK, but very ordinary moisturizer that contains mostly water, thickeners, slip agent, glycerin, plant extracts, fragrance, and preservatives. The plant extracts in here are not AHAs. It does contain BHA though the pH is not low enough for it to be effective as an exfoliant.

☺ **Raspberry & Sugar Cane Alpha Hydroxy Lotion** *($2.88 for 18 ounces)* is an emollient, though very ordinary moisturizer that contains mostly water, plant oil, slip agent, thickeners, plant extracts, fragrance, preservatives, and fragrance. But the plant extracts are not AHAs.

☺ **Apricot & Vitamin E Ultra Nourishing Lotion** *($2.88 for 18 ounces)* is a good emollient moisturizer for dry skin.

☺ **French Vanilla & Shea Butter Ultra Moisturizing Lotion** *($2.97 for 18 ounces)* is an emollient, though very ordinary moisturizer.

☺ **Avocado & Oatmeal Mineral Mud Mask** *($2.85 for 6 ounces)* is a standard clay mask with a small amount of oil, which can prevent it from being too drying. If you want to use a clay mask, this is a good one for an exceptionally reasonable price.

☹ **Cucumber & Ginseng Peel-Off Masque** *($2.85 for 6 ounces)* is mainly alcohol and film former, which places a layer of plastic over the skin you can peel off. This is an irritation waiting to happen.

☹ Peach Tree & Pear Blemish Control Medicated Gel Masque *($3.49 for 6 ounces)* is similar to the Cucumber version above and the same comments apply. There is nothing in this product that can help prevent breakouts.

☹ Tangerine & Guava Alpha-Beta Hydroxy Peel-Off Masque *($2.82 for 6 ounces)* is similar to the Cucumber version above and the same comments apply.

☹ Sunflower & Aloe Perfect Moisturizer SPF 6 *($2.85 for 4.6 ounces)* is hardly "perfect." Its SPF rating is only 6, which is not adequate to protect against sun damage, and it doesn't contain avobenzone, zinc oxide, or titanium dioxide, and is not recommended.

# Galderma (See Cetaphil)

# Gale Hayman of Beverly Hills

Gale Hayman's claim to fame was her status as co-founder of Giorgio in Beverly Hills. After a divorce concluded her ownership, she started this line of skin-care and makeup products bearing her own name. Selling primarily at Sears and through the Home Shopping Network, her line is a long distance from the elan of her company's namesake town. Actually, the products are a long distance from anything current, and the makeup collection may remind you more of Beverly Hills circa 1981. The tester unit is actually referred to as The Glamour Center, and the packaging has a kitsch leopard-skin print. Basically, nothing has changed here since this line was reviewed years ago (and there weren't any changes from the edition before that). The beauty "palette," according to Hayman, is based on the color of a woman's eyes, which unlike her skin or hair never changes. Perhaps Hayman is unaware of colored contact lenses or the very fact that basing an entire makeup wardrobe on just your eye color is about as sensible as choosing your clothing wardrobe based on your shoe size. Besides, most of the colors here, especially for the eyes, are ultra-bright and difficult to blend together. If you're nostalgic for makeup colors that faded when Reagan won a second term, look no further than Gale Hayman of Beverly Hills.

Hayman's brochure for her skin-care products is completely implausible. It states "the impression you get in Beverly Hills is obvious. From the very glamorous to the trend-setting elite, the women of Beverly Hills boast a quality found nowhere else in the world. It's an ageless appearance, a beauty that transcends time." Clearly, with its product name attached to a highbrow town, the impression you're supposed to get is that Hayman's products have in some way contributed to this lean and "ageless" look. That's almost funny. What isn't so funny is that despite all of the hyperbole about these products, there's not one sunscreen in the group. So much for ageless beauty. You're supposed to believe that the elastin, amniotic fluid, and DNA in these products can help restore skin. If it were only that easy! In regard to the ladies of Beverly Hills I can assure you—having spent a good deal of time in that town—that the glamorous and even not so glamorous have all seen a plastic surgeon and most every inch of their anatomy from head to toe has either been lifted, suctioned, cut and pasted, or resurfaced more times than you can count. Their beauty has nothing to do with this line of products or any other product line for that matter.

For more information about Gale Hayman of Beverly Hills, now under ownership of Color Me Beautiful, call (800) FOR-GALE or visit the uneventful Web site at www.galehayman.com

# Gale Hayman Skin Care

☺ **Total Eye Make-up & Facial Cleanser** (*$18.50 for 6.76 ounces*) is a detergent-based, wipe-off makeup remover. This will work to remove makeup. However, the trivial amount of amniotic fluid in here has no effect on skin and is an offensive ingredient in skin-care products.

☺ **Total Skin Toner Freshener & Firmer** (*$18 for 6.76 ounces*) is virtually identical to the Cleanser above only minus the amniotic fluid. The same basic review applies. The teeny amount of collagen and elastin in here are nothing more than water-binding agents; they won't affect the collagen in your skin.

☺ **$$$ Eyelift Gel** (*$25 for 0.5 ounce*) is just water, film former, plant extracts, thickeners, preservatives, and coloring agents. This is an OK, completely ordinary, lightweight moisturizer, though several of the plant extracts can be skin irritants. Nothing in here can lift or change skin.

☺ **$$$ Line Lift** (*$27.50 for 0.7 ounce*) contains water, DNA, elastin, plant oils, and preservatives. DNA and elastin can't change skin, period. This can be a good lightweight moisturizer for normal to dry skin, but that's it.

☺ **$$$ Youth Lift** (*$45 for 1 ounce*) is almost identical to the one above; the same comments apply.

☹ **$$$ Youth Lift Firming Night Treatment** (*$55 for 1 ounce*) contains mostly water, plant oil, egg yolk, thickeners, water-binding agents, and preservatives. This is a good, extremely standard moisturizer for dry skin.

☺ **Youth Lift Total Moisturizer** (*$35 for 2 ounces*) is similar to the one above and the same review applies.

☺ **Alpha Hydroxy Cream with Multi Vitamin Complex** (*$20 for 1 ounce*) contains plant extracts that aren't AHAs, and the pH of this product is too high for them to be effective exfoliants even if they were real AHAs. This is just a good, though very ordinary moisturizer for normal to dry skin.

☹ **DHEA 14 Super Moisturizing Cream** (*$47.50 for 2 ounces*) is just a basic moisturizer with a small amount of DHEA, one of the myriad anti-aging supplements being sold in health food stores. According to *HealthNews*, a newsletter from the publishers of *The New England Journal of Medicine,* although there is a small body of research showing that oral intake of DHEA may be helpful, for many reasons it may have more risks than positives. It is, most likely, a potent "steroid hormone called dehydroepiandrosterone, a chemical cousin of testosterone and estrogen. … Since DHEA is converted into testosterone, some women who take it grow body or facial hair and, if they are under age 50 or so, can stop menstruating. DHEA has also been shown to decrease levels of HDL ('good') cholesterol in women, and could increase the risk of heart disease." There is no research showing that DHEA has any effect when used topically.

☺ $$$ **5-Minute Pore Cleanser Exfoliating Mask** *($22 for 2 ounces)* is a clay mask with almond pieces and synthetic scrub particles. Leaving scrub particles sitting on the skin isn't the best way to exfoliate skin, but it won't necessarily hurt either.

☺ $$$ **Lip-Lift** *($16 for 0.04 ounce)* is just a good mineral oil–based lip balm.

# Gale Hayman Makeup

<u>FOUNDATION:</u> ☹ **Light Coverage Treatment Makeup** *($15)* makes much ado about using "Vitamin F.A.C.E." (the initials stand for vitamins F, A, C, and E). They're barely present in here at all, and though they may be good antioxidants they are hardly unique. This does have a light, even texture that provides sheer coverage, but half of the ten shades are too peach, pink, or orange to recommend. Avoid Porcelain, Beige, Medium Beige, Dark, and Bronze.

☹ <u>CONCEALER:</u> **Treatment Concealer Cream** *($12.50)* isn't much of a treatment, and the three colors are just too peach or pink for any skin tone.

☺ $$$ <u>POWDER:</u> **Semi-Translucent Face Powder** *($17)* is a talc-based, standard pressed powder that has a soft, smooth, dry texture. Sun Bronze is part of this group but is just a shiny bronze shade, and since when is a tan iridescent? The remaining colors are very nice.

☺ $$$ <u>BLUSH:</u> **Color Control Blusher** *($17)* has a dry, grainy texture with some amount of shine. There are both soft and vivid colors, and the latter tend to grab on the skin and are hard to blend.

<u>EYESHADOW AND EYE/BROW SHAPER:</u> ☹ **MonoChrome Shadow Liner** *($16)* has colors that are all extremely shiny (even those labeled as matte), and have an uneven, choppy application. **Primer for Eyes and Lips** *($12.50)* comes in a pot and has a cream-to-powder texture that dries to a pale pink, matte finish. It can crease on the eyelid and feels too dry over the lips, and that can prime the face for some problems.

The Reviews G

☺ **Glamour Definer Pencil for Eyes** *($7.50)* is a standard pencil that needs to be sharpened and is prone to smudging, which doesn't sound very glamorous to me.

☺ **$$$ Automatic Brow Definer** *($16)* comes in only two shades, which isn't much choice, but this is still a good, albeit standard, dry-finish brow pencil.

☺ <u>LIPSTICK AND LIP PENCIL:</u> **Treatment Lip Color** *($10)* is a good creamy lipstick with a slightly glossy finish. **Treatment Lip Glaze** *($13)* is billed as a lip gloss that doesn't bleed into the lines around the mouth. Don't believe that for a second; one application and it'll be up into those lines before you know it—but it's still a good lip gloss. **Glamour Definer Pencil for Lips** *($7.50)* is a standard lip pencil that has replaced this line's former Automatic Lip Definer, which is a shame because this is as ordinary as they come and now you have to sharpen it.

☹ <u>MASCARA:</u> **Dramatic Lash Mascara** *($10)* is just an OK mascara; it does build some length and thickness, but I wouldn't call it dramatic or worth the extra price.

# Garden Botanika

Despite Garden Botanika's Chapter 11 woes (filed in April 2000) and the closure of more than half of its locations (at one point Garden Botanika had over 252 stores open; it will now be down to 91 stores according to an article in the cosmetics industry insider newsletter *The Rose Sheet*, February 7, 2000), it is still attempting to keep things current with the addition of skin-care products meeting the consumer's demand for vitamin C and retinol.

Garden Botanika is like The Body Shop but with a Northwest flair (it is, after all, a Seattle-area company). The prices are extremely reasonable, and the packaging a little more upbeat than its competition. Between the prices and the consumer demand for "natural" products (regardless of how senseless that demand is), you're likely to find enough plants and aromatherapy here to satisfy.

As far as products go, Garden Botanika has made some impressive headway in the makeup field, usually not the strong suit of natural cosmetics lines of this type (though The Body Shop has leapt ahead in that area too). There are some great colors here, but most of them are best for Caucasian and Asian women, and not for women of darker skin colors. The color groupings are impressively arranged on a standup wood podium. Regrettably, the display is inconvenient to use, with no shelf space for purses, hands, arms, or note-taking. The colors are divided in two sectors: one half of the dais holds pink and rose tones and the other half yellow and peach tones, and that's very functional for those who want to be careful about choosing the right colors.

For more information about Garden Botanika, call (800) 968-7842 or visit the Web site at www.gardenbotanika.com.

# Garden Botanika Skin Care

☹ **Skin Correcting Cleansing Bar** *($4 for 4.2 ounces)* is a standard bar cleanser that contains ingredients that can be quite drying and may clog pores. It does contain a disinfectant, but disinfectants work only when left on the skin, and you would not want to keep this cleanser on your face for even a second.

☺ **Skin Correcting Deep Cleansing Face Wash** *($10 for 8 ounces)* is a standard, detergent-based water-soluble cleanser that could work well for someone with normal to oily skin. It does have a host of plant extracts, but none of these are helpful for blemishes. While some can be skin irritants, the amounts are so small they probably won't be of any effect one way or the other.

☺ **Skin Correcting Purifying Toning Lotion** *($10.50 for 8 ounces)* does contain the real thing, salicylic acid for exfoliation, and it is listed as the active ingredient with a pH of 3! It comes in a simple slip-agent base with a host of plant extracts. What counts is the BHA, and this is a very good lightweight one to consider.

☺ **Skin Correcting Essential Moisture Lotion** *($12.50 for 1.75 ounces)* is a standard, rather ordinary moisturizer. Unless you have dry skin, this is a truly unnecessary step. If you do have dry skin and want to try it, it is an option, but only over dry areas. The host of plant extracts in this lotion can be a problem for some skin types.

☹ **Skin Correcting Intensive Blemish Treatment** *($8.50 for 0.5 ounce)* lists the second ingredient as alcohol, which makes it irritating and drying, not correcting.

☺ **Skin Correcting Activated Charcoal Mask** *($11 for 3.4 ounces)* is a standard clay mask that also contains some charcoal and plant extracts. The plant extracts are a mix of potential irritants and anti-irritants. The charcoal in here is in too small an amount to have much benefit for skin, although charcoal has great absorption and disinfecting properties.

☹ **Skin Renewing Gentle Foaming Cleanser, with Alpha Hydroxy Acid** *($11 for 8 ounces)* is a standard, detergent-based cleanser. However, the cleansing agent is TEA-sodium lauryl sulfate, which can be very drying and potentially irritating for most skin types, and the plant extracts in here can be irritating as well.

☹ **Skin Renewing Cleansing Bar** *($4 for 4.2 ounces)* is a standard bar cleanser that can be drying for all skin types, and the ingredients that keep the bar in its form can clog pores.

☺ **Skin Renewing Clarifying Toning Lotion** *($10.50 for 8 ounces)* is basically just water and glycerin with a bunch of plant and fruit extracts thrown in. Some of the plant extracts are anti-irritants while others can be irritating. The plant extracts make claims about being AHAs but they cannot perform in that capacity.

☹ **Skin Renewing Moisture Replenisher SPF 8** *($15 for 1.75 ounces)* has only minimal sun protection, and with all the good SPF 15s around, why bother with such inadequate daily protection?

☹ **Skin Renewing Balancing Creme, SPF 8** *($15 for 1.75 ounces)* has only minimal sun protection, and with all the good SPF 15s around, why bother?

☺ **Skin Renewing Night Serum with Vitamin C** *($15 for 1 ounce)* contains mostly water, thickener, slip agent, plant extracts, silicone, glycerin, ascorbic acid, and preservatives. If you are looking for a vitamin C product, the research indicates that the ascorbic acid in here is not the best option because it is unstable and can be irritating. The amount in here is so tiny as to have almost no effect even if it was a decent option for an antioxidant. Other than that, this is a good though ordinary lightweight moisturizer for normal to slightly dry skin.

☺ **Skin Renewing Retinol Skin Smoother** *($15 for 1 ounce)*. Because retinol is such an unstable ingredient, the way it's packaged is of vital concern. This container allows sunlight and air exposure, which means the retinol will not be stable for very long if at all after it's opened.

☺ $$$ **Skin Renewing Vitamin C Treatment** *($25 for 1 ounce)* is a silicone-based serum that uses ascorbic acid as its form of vitamin C. If you are going to use a vitamin C product, ascorbic acid is not the one to try, as it is not considered a stable form and the risk of irritation with this variation is not great for skin. Other than that it would probably feel good as a lightweight moisturizer for normal to dry skin, and it does contain a handful of other antioxidants (in very tiny amounts)—it's just not one of the versions to consider as a vitamin C product.

☺ **Skin Renewing Triple C Moisture Infusion** *($25 for 1.7 ounces)* is similar to the Treatment version above and the same comments apply.

☹ **Skin Renewing Vitamin C Peel Off Mask** *($10 for 3.4 ounces)* is a polyvinyl-based mask (polyvinyl is basically hairspray, and it's what creates the plastic-like layer over the face) that contains far too many irritating ingredients to be a consideration for any skin type, including alcohol, orange, lemon peel, tangerine, lime, and grapefruit extracts.

☺ **Skin Renewing Shadow Stopper** *($12.50 for 0.5 ounce)* is a decent moisturizer for dry skin, though it does contain some irritating plant extracts as well as some soothing ones, which makes no sense. The teeny amount of vitamin K in here (or vitamin K in any amount) cannot change dark circles.

☺ **Skin Renewing Clarifying Facial Mask** *($11 for 2 ounces)* is a standard clay mask that is almost identical the Skin Correcting version above, minus the charcoal; the same basic comments apply.

☺ **Chamomile Cleansing Milk** *($10 for 8 ounces)* is a plant oil–based, standard wipe-off cleanser. It will take off makeup and can be an option for someone with dry skin, but it can leave a greasy feel on the skin.

☺ **English Violet Cleansing Milk** *($10 for 8 ounces)* is similar to the one above and the same comments apply.

☺ **Linden Flower Cleansing Milk** *($10 for 8 ounces)* is similar to the one above and the same comments apply.

☺ **Citrus Cleansing Gel** *($11 for 5 ounces)* is a standard, detergent-based water-soluble cleanser. It also contains a minute quantity of orange oil, but the small amount is in here primarily for fragrance and probably won't be a problem for irritation. It does contain coloring agents.

☺ **Cucumber Cleansing Gel** *($10 for 8 ounces)* is a standard, detergent-based water-soluble cleanser that can be good for someone with normal to oily skin or slightly dry skin. It does contain fragrance and coloring agents.

☹ **Oatmeal & Glycerine Cleansing Bar** *($3 for 4 ounces)* is fairly alkaline, which is drying for all skin types, and the ingredients that keep the bar in its form can clog pores.

☺ **Gentle Eye Makeup Remover** *($6.50 for 4 ounces)* is a very standard detergent cleanser makeup remover. It will do the job and does contain fragrance.

☺ **Jojoba Scrub** *($9.50 for 2 ounces)* is a gentle scrub that could work well for someone with normal to dry skin, but some of these ingredients could clog pores.

☺ **Elder Flower Toning Lotion** *($9.50 for 8 ounces)* is just glycerin and fragrance; it's OK for someone with normal to dry skin, but it's mostly a do-nothing formulation.

☺ **Honey and Rosewater Toning Lotion** *($9.50 for 8 ounces)* is similar to the one above and the same comments apply.

☹ **Witch Hazel & Thyme Toning Lotion** *($9.50 for 8 ounces)* contains witch hazel, which is irritating enough, but this one also contains camphor and is not recommended.

☺ **AHA Skin Renewing Treatment for the Face** *($25 for 3.4 ounces)* is mostly a good emollient moisturizer for dry skin, because the plant extracts in here are not AHAs and cannot perform in that capacity.

☺ **Angelica Moisture Creme** *($10.50 for 2 ounces)* contains mostly water, plant extracts, thickeners, and preservatives. This is a very ordinary moisturizer that has little benefit for skin of any type.

☺ **Ivy and Yarrow Moisture Creme** *($10.50 for 2 ounces)* is a good moisturizer for dry skin. Ivy and yarrow can be irritants but there aren't enough of them in here to have an effect.

☺ **$$$ Daily Vitamin C Treatment** *($15 for 0.5 ounce)* does contain vitamin C, but it uses ascorbic acid, which is considered to be one of the more irritating and unstable forms.

☹ **The Great Perfector** *($15 for 2 ounces)* contains several irritating plant extracts, including eucalyptus, clove, orange, and cedar, and is not recommended.

☹ **Night Normalizing Gel** *($11 for 2 ounces)* contains too many potentially irritating ingredients, including lemon, to be recommended.

☹ **Oil-Absorbing Moisture Gel** *($10.50 for 2 ounces)* is similar to the Normalizing Gel above and the same comments apply.

☹ **Soothing Herbal Eye Gel** *($9.50 for 1 ounce)* is just plant water, thickener, preservatives, and coloring agent. The plant extracts in here are mixed bag of some that are irritants (ivy and hypericum) and those that are anti-irritants. This is problematic for skin.

☺ **Nourishing Eye Creme** *($10.50 for 1 ounce)* is a good, though very ordinary moisturizer for dry skin.

☺ **Nutrient Night Creme** *($12 for 2 ounces)* is a good moisturizer for normal to dry skin.

☺ **Vitalizing Night Creme** *($12 for 2 ounces)* is a good moisturizer for someone with dry skin, but it's very basic. The tiny amount of retinol in here would not be stable in the type of container it comes packaged in.

☺ **Skin Balancing Moisture Cream** *($10.50 for 2 ounces)*. This can't balance skin, it is merely an ordinary moisturizer for slightly dry skin that contains potentially irritating plant extracts including arnica and ivy.

☺ **Calendula Moisture Cream** *($10.50 for 2 ounces)* is a good moisturizer for dry skin.

☺ **Chamomile Moisture Mask** *($9.50 for 2 ounces)* is just waxes, plant oils, and fragrant oils. It is moisturizing, but the fragrant oils in here are overwhelming and can be skin irritants.

☺ **Desert Mud Mask** *($9.50 for 2 ounces)* is a standard clay mask that contains merely clay and preservatives. It doesn't get much simpler than that and it is a good option for someone with oily skin.

☺ **Soothing Botanical Gel Mask** *($9.50 for 2 ounces)* is a very standard mix of thickening agents and plant extracts (some that are irritants and others that are anti-irritants). It may feel refreshing but it won't do much for skin.

## Garden Botanika Makeup

<u>FOUNDATION:</u> ☺ **Moisturizing Foundation SPF 8** *($11)* is a liquid foundation with a very nice, soft application. Most of the 12 colors are fine, particularly Linen, Vanilla, and Honey, but Alabaster is too pink, Willow is too peach, and Sand and Flax can turn peach. The SPF 8 isn't the best (it should be at least SPF 15), although it does contain titanium dioxide. **Oil-Free Foundation SPF 8** *($11)* isn't all that different from the Moisturizing Foundation above; they have a similar texture and finish. This is not the best for someone with oily or combination skin but it can

be suitable for someone with normal to dry skin. However, the same concerns about SPF and color choice apply here.

☺ **Natural Color Powder Plus** *($12.50)* is a pressed powder–style foundation that has a rich, soft texture in a small but good selection of six colors. It can be used alone or over foundation. It does have a small amount of oil, so it may not be preferable for someone with normal to oily skin. The only two colors to watch out for are Sand Dollar and Sesame, which may be slightly too pink for some skin tones.

☹ **CONCEALER: Color Corrector Stick** *($8)* and **Color Corrector Creme** *($8)* are shades of yellow and green that are an unnecessary extra layer of makeup. Too many layers of makeup can feel thick and heavy on the skin. If the foundation color is right (meaning neutral with no overtones of peach, pink, rose, or ash), and the consistency is smooth and even, there is no need for this step. **Cream Concealer** *($8)* comes in a wand applicator, but the colors are fairly peach and not the best to consider for any skin tone.

**POWDER:** ☺ **Pressed Powder** *($10)* comes in three good shades with a dry, soft finish.

☹ **Translucent Loose Powder** *($10)* has a very dry, choppy finish, and all the shades are shiny, which negates the effect of dusting down shine with a powder.

☺ **BLUSH: Natural Color Blush** *($9.50)* comes in some great, neutral, earth-toned, matte shades. There are only a handful of shiny colors to steer clear of. **Face Shimmer** *($9.50)* is very iridescent. The shine is overkill, but then everyone seems to need shine these days, so why not this line?

**EYESHADOW:** ☺ **Natural Color Eyeshadow** *($8.50)* has a small but workable group of matte eyeshadows. It also has its share of shiny shades but they are easily avoidable. Check out Birch, Papyrus, Dogwood, Logan Berry, and Smoky Quartz. **Shadow Primer** *($8.50)* has a cream-to-powder finish that can be helpful to keep eyeshadows on if you are using a moisturizing foundation; if you are using a more matte-finish foundation, this wouldn't be necessary. **Shadow Liner** *($8.50)* is a dark powder eyeshadow that can be used wet or dry for eyelining or extra drama.

☺ **Eye Crayon** *($7.50)* is a standard chubby pencil with a creamy texture and a fair amount of shine.

☺ **EYE AND BROW SHAPER: Brow Gel** *($8)* comes in one shade, Clear. It works fine but is clearly limited. **Natural Color Eye Pencil** *($6.50)* is just a standard, slightly dry-finish pencil in a small but good range of colors.

**LIPSTICK AND LIP PENCIL:** ☺ **Sheer Lip Crayon** and **Matte Lip Crayon** *($7.50)* are just a sheer gloss and a matte lipstick in the shape of fat pencils. These require sharpening, which makes them inconvenient to use. **Lip Shimmers** and **Lip Shines** *($15 for a set of six colors)* are a stack of six pots of shiny glosses (that's the

Shimmers) or non-shiny glosses (the Shines). They are fun to use if you are into gloss, and the price is almost too lip-smacking to pass up. **Lip Polish** *($6.50)* is just a standard gloss in a tube, but a rather good one considering the consistency and price. **Natural Color Lipstick** *($8.50)* is an excellent group of creamy lipsticks with good opaque coverage. **Natural Color Lip Pencil** *($6.50)* is a standard, slightly dry-finish pencil in a small but good range of colors. **Natural Color Sheer Lipstick** *($8.50)* is identical to Natural Color Lipstick except it is not opaque.

☺ **Lip Primer** *($8)* is an option only if lipstick tends to turn color on you. It lays down a neutral beige tone that you then apply lipstick over. It doesn't stop lipstick from feathering.

<u>MASCARA:</u> ☺ **Mascara** *($8)* is just an OK mascara. It doesn't build much length and definitely no thickness, and the tube can get pretty gloppy and messy.

☹ **Lash Primer** *($8)* is an extra step that shouldn't be necessary. If a company makes a good mascara, that should be all it takes to make beautiful long, thick lashes.

<u>BRUSHES:</u> ☺ This isn't the best assortment of brushes, but there are some that are definitely worth consideration. The **Dome Brush** *($15)*, **Shadow Brush** *($6)*, **Fluff Brush** *($5)*, **Lip Brush** *($5)*, and **Angle Brush** *($5)* are all excellent, with great shapes and soft bristles, and are nicely packed to hold powder well.

☺ However, the **Blush Brush** *($7)* is too small, the **Shadow Contour** *($6)* is too floppy to control, the **Blender** *($6)* is too big for the eyes yet too small for the face, and the **Powder Brush** *($10)* is too loose and sloppy for even application.

# *Givenchy*

The name Givenchy rolls off the tongue like an infusion of French wine and haute couture fashion. Yet as eloquent and refined as it sounds, when it comes to cosmetics, image doesn't equal substance and it turns out the Givenchy products have more accent than quality. Skin care is the most disappointing aspect of this line, although the packaging is some of the most elegant in the industry. What a shame packaging won't help your skin. Ordinary formulations abound, and despite the presence of some exotic-sounding ingredients, these are mostly waxy bases with few to no current formulations. As fascinating as it may sound to have some ginseng, coltsfoot, or hawthorn extract, or placental enzymes and thymus peptides, which show up repeatedly in scant amounts, your skin would be far happier with more interesting water-binding agents, antioxidants, and anti-irritants than the standard concoctions this line is filled with. And not one of the sunscreens has any UVA-protecting ingredients. Placenta and thymus—is anyone intrigued by these types of ingredients anymore?

Givenchy's small makeup collection is about as far removed from its haute couture as an eight-track cassette is from compact discs. This is one of the few lines that unabashedly still offers an appalling amount of pink, rose, or peach-toned hues in all of its foundations. The eyeshadows and blushes are gorgeous to look at, but good luck using the strange color combinations and shine with any sense of order or placement. If you hold a special place in your heart for Givenchy, consider purchasing what it does best: fashion and fragrance. Opting for Givenchy's makeup is simply saying "yes" to high style over real substance.

Please note that several of the Givenchy products contain coltsfoot extract. According to *The PDR Family Guide to Natural Medicines & Healing Therapies*, coltsfoot has potential carcinogenic activity from its pyrrolizidine alkaloid content and is not recommended for repeated use.

For more information on Givenchy products, call (212) 931-2600 or visit the Web site at www.givenchy.com.

# *Givenchy Skin Care*

☺ $$$ **Cleansing Foam** *($22 for 4.2 ounces)* is a standard, detergent-based water-soluble cleanser that uses cleansing agents (myristic acid and potassium hydroxide) that are considered more drying and irritating than most.

☹ **Gentle Cleansing Gel** *($28 for 4.2 ounces)* is a very standard, detergent-based cleanser that includes a form of tallow that can irritate and clog pores. There are far more elegant cleanser formulations out there for a fraction of this price.

☹ **Gentle Cleansing Milk** *($28 for 6.7 ounces)* is an extremely confused cleanser and isn't gentle. It contains mineral oil, which can leave a greasy film on the skin, and it uses sodium lauryl sulfate as the cleansing agent, an ingredient notorious for being one of the more irritating cosmetic ingredients.

☺ $$$ **Regulating Cleansing Gel, Purifying Care for Radiant Skin Combination and Oily Skins** *($20 for 4.5 ounces)* is a standard, detergent-based water-soluble cleanser that would work well for someone with normal to oily skin. It does contain fragrance and coloring agents.

☺ $$$ **Gentle Eye and Lip Makeup Remover Gel** *($15 for 1.3 ounces)* is a standard, detergent-based makeup remover with a handful of plant extracts thrown in for effect; some of these can be irritants (coltsfoot and bladderwrack) and others anti-irritants (scullcap).

☺ $$$ **Gentle Eye and Lip Makeup Remover** *($15 for 1.3 ounces)* is similar to the Gel version above only this is in a liquidy lotion form.

☺ $$$ **Make-off Emulsion** *($22 for 6.7 ounces)* is merely a mineral oil–based, wipe-off cleanser that includes slip agents, fragrance, and preservatives. It will take off makeup and can leave a greasy film on the skin. This is virtually identical to using plain mineral oil, which is available for about $2 for 16 ounces.

☺ **$$$ Gentle Exfoliating Massage** *($27 for 1.7 ounces)* is a standard, synthetic-based scrub (ground-up plastic is the abrasive) mixed in with thickening agents and mineral oil. It can be an option for dry skin but can leave a film on the skin.

☹ **Bain des Soin Toner for Combination/Oily Skin** *($22 for 6.7 ounces)* lists the second ingredient as alcohol, which would be drying and irritating enough for any skin type, but this one also has camphor, menthol, and coltsfoot, and is absolutely not recommended.

☺ **Bain des Soin Toner for Dry/Sensitive/Tired Skin** *($22 for 6.7 ounces)* would work for normal to dry skin, but it is exceptionally ordinary, and sensitive skin does not need fragrance or coltsfoot extract.

☺ **Bain des Soin Toner for Normal/Dry Skin** *($22 for 6.7 ounces)* is almost identical to the Sensitive version above and the same comments apply.

☹ **Balancing Mist** *($30 for 5 ounces)*. The menthol and some of the plant extracts are skin irritants and the DNA and placenta are just useless for skin, though I imagine they make a great impression.

☺ **$$$ Gentle Toning Lotion** *($28 for 6.7 ounces)* is a standard, irritant-free, glycerin-based toner, with some silicone and a few water-binding agents. It would be good for someone with dry skin.

☹ **Regulating Mist** *($30 for 5 ounces)* contains urea, which can exfoliate skin, but the witch hazel and some of the plant extracts can be skin irritants.

☺ **$$$ Double Sequence Eye Contour Firming Balm** *($75 for 60 doses)* is a two-step process that comes in medical-looking vials. As therapeutic as this appears to be, the ingredients are less than remarkable. This is a combination that may make for a good moisturizer but it won't firm anything. Dose 1 contains several thickening agents, water-binding agents, emollients, preservatives, and plant extracts. Dose 2 is almost identical. There are minuscule amounts of vitamins, some interesting water-binding agents, and an anti-irritant, but not anything unusual or special for skin, along with several plant extracts that can be skin irritants. Plus, both Dose types contain aluminum starch high up on the ingredient list, which can be drying and irritating for dry skin.

☺ **$$$ Lifting Double Sequence** *($100 for 0.5 ounce total, 30 treatments)* is a lighter-weight version of the Eye Balm above. These two Doses are good moisturizing formulations with some interesting water-binding agents, but this is by far more image than substance. You are actually spending $3,200 for a pound of this stuff, and all you are getting is a moisturizer for normal to slightly dry skin. For this kind of money you would have enough for a great face-lift in less than a year or two.

☺ **$$$ Firm Profile** *($55 for 1.7 ounces)* contains mostly water, thickeners, silicone, preservatives, fragrance, film former, plant extracts, water-binding agents, and coloring agents. This is a shockingly standard moisturizer for someone with normal to dry skin.

☺ $$$ **Fundamental Care** *($69 for 1.7 ounces)* contains a tiny amount of lactic acid, but nowhere near enough to be considered an exfoliant. It is just a good, though very ordinary moisturizer for normal to slightly dry skin. The plant extracts can be skin irritants.

☹ **Hydra Tricellia Creme SPF 15** *($45 for 1.7 ounces)* does not contain the UVA-protecting ingredients avobenzone, zinc oxide, or titanium dioxide, and is not recommended.

☹ **Hydra-Tricellia SPF 15 Tri-Activating Hydration Lotion, Oil-Free** *($58 for 2.5 ounces)* does not contain the UVA-protecting ingredients avobenzone, zinc oxide, or titanium dioxide, and is not recommended.

☹ **Matte Regulating Day Care** *($38 for 1.7 ounces)* is indeed matte: the second ingredient is aluminum starch (octenylsuccinate), a thickening agent that has some absorbing properties (like alum), but it is more likely to absorb the moisture in this product than the oil on your skin, plus it can be an irritant. This also contains witch hazel, silicones, and thickening agents.

☺ $$$ **Nutritive Care** *($54 for 1.7 ounces)* is a standard, mineral oil–based moisturizer that contains thickening agents and a tiny amount of water-binding agents. It's fine for dry skin, but absurdly overpriced for what you get.

☺ $$$ **Protective Day Care** *($43 for 1.7 ounces)* does not include sunscreen, so this only counts for evening care. It is a standard, mineral oil–based moisturizer with thickening agents and a tiny amount of water-binding agents. This is so standard as to be almost embarrassing.

☹ **Relaxing Complex** *($44 for 1.7 ounces)* contains nothing relaxing, although it does contain alcohol, which can dry and irritate skin.

☺ $$$ **Hydra-Tricellia Mask** *($40 for 2.8 ounces)* contains mostly emollients, minuscule amounts of some good water-binding agents, and clay. It does contain a tiny amount of alcohol but probably not enough to be a problem. This could be a good mask for someone with normal to slightly dry skin, but this is mostly a "why bother," because there are far better moisturizers in the world to consider than this one. The plant extracts in here can be skin irritants.

☺ $$$ **Hydrating Cream Mask** *($40 for 1.7 ounces)* is similar to the Tricellia version above and the same comments apply.

☹ **Regulating Purifying Mask** *($38 for 2.8 ounces)* is a standard clay mask that also contains a lot of alcohol and witch hazel, which makes it too irritating and drying for any skin type.

☺ $$$ **Whitening Concentrate** *($48 for 1 ounce)* is a hydroquinone-based skin-lightening product. When used with sunscreen, this can be an effective way to improve the appearance of sun-damaged skin discolorations. (This formula does have sunscreen ingredients, but no UVA-protecting ingredients, and no SPF is listed.)

# Givenchy Makeup

**FOUNDATION:** ☹ **Teint Transparent Powder Foundation SPF 15** *($42)* is a standard wet/dry powder foundation whose texture and color selection leave much to be desired. If peach- to orange-toned powder is what you're looking for, you've found it—and with a reliable SPF to boot.

☺ $$$ **Teint Minimal Foundation SPF 10** *($35)* has a disappointing SPF of 10 (15 is the standard) with no UVA-protecting ingredients of titanium dioxide, zinc oxide, or avobenzone. It offers borderline skin tone colors, save for Voile Champagne and Voile Ivoire, and is otherwise a basic tinted moisturizer with sheer to light coverage and a natural matte finish.

☹ **Teint Estompe Concealing Matte Foundation** *($42)* makes such lofty claims and is overpriced for what you get. Please do not believe for one minute that any foundation is capable of "controlling skin's moisture levels in all climates, while absorbing sebum and controlling perspiration while tightening the skin." I was tempted to read further to see if it could also keep my blood pressure in check, but decided to test the colors instead. No surprises here—all of the eight shades are too pink, rose, peach, or copper to recommend.

☺ $$$ **Teint Couture Moisturizing Foundation** *($42)* has a smooth, light, creamy texture and a satin finish. It is a decent but (overpriced) option for normal to very dry skin needing medium coverage. Of the seven shades, only two are acceptable: Ocre #12 and Safran #17. The rest are too peach, rose, or orange to recommend.

☹ **Touche Multiple Face and Body Makeup** *($30)* is a twist-up highlighter stick that has a creamy, somewhat greasy texture and soft, sheer colors that would work for any part of the face, but on the body it's up to you. The creamy application tends to stay that way on the skin and leaves a fairly strong shine, which can easily be transferred to clothing.

☹ **Teint Ecran SPF 15** *($42)* is a compact foundation that appears to be cream-to-powder but ends up far more powdery than creamy. The SPF is pure titanium dioxide, and that's the only outstanding feature this foundation has to offer. The texture of this thick powder tends to apply a heavy layer that looks dry and cakey on the skin, which is a shame because the colors aren't half bad.

☹ **CONCEALER: Perfect Corrector** *($23)* is perfectly suited to anyone who has truly pink or orange skin and wishes to make it more prominent. Sarcasm aside, this would be an option if the colors weren't so poor.

☺ $$$ **POWDER: Powder Prism** *($40)* features four tones of powder in one compact. The idea is to use them individually or in combination to achieve a softly powdered finish. The texture is smooth and slightly dry but the color combinations—from very pale pastels to ivory with coral, are makeup accidents waiting to happen (you would not want to dust these tones over your skin and change a flesh tone look to an unnatural one). **Serial Colors Powder Prism** *($40)* is identical to the one above, only here you have 16 tiny squares of powder, lightly infused with sparkly particles. The same comments apply, although this one does apply slightly more sheerly.

☺ $$$ <u>BLUSH:</u> **Blush Prism** *($36)* is stunning to look at, reminiscent of a gem with a satiny-soft texture. It's also best left at that, as all of these colors are too shiny and they can be difficult to use.

☹ <u>EYESHADOW:</u> **Eyeshadow Prism Duos** *($30)* is a small group of eyeshadow duos, each with one shiny shade and most with contrasting colors. Between these and the other Prisms in this line, you risk making your face look like a kaleidoscope of colors. **Eyeshadow Prism** *($38)* is a five-color eyeshadow compact. Each block of color is so tiny that you can easily miss the separation. The center color is intensely shiny and the other colors don't work together. This is a compact that is prettier to look at it than it is to use.

<u>EYE AND BROW SHAPER:</u> ☹ **Eye Liner Pencil** *($20)*. Despite the exaggerated claims for these overpriced, exceptionally standard pencils, the cream-to-powder texture smudges easily, and there's a sponge tip provided to help start the mess. **Eye Brow Pencil** *($20)*. The only difference between this brow pencil and almost every other brow pencil being sold is that this one tends to ball up on the skin as you blend, and who needs that?

☺ $$$ **Perfect Liquid Eyeliner** *($24)* is actually about as close to perfect as this type of eyeliner can get. The brush is thin and easy to control; it applies well, dries quickly, and then stays put! What a shame the cost is so absurd for what you get.

<u>LIPSTICK AND LIP PENCIL:</u> ☺ $$$ **Rouge a Levres** *($20)* is also known as "Givenchy Lipstick," but a rose by any name is still just a standard creamy, moist lipstick. **Rouge Couture Long Lasting** *($21)* is a very good creamy lipstick with opaque coverage and a satin-matte finish. The long-lasting claim is debatable, but at this price it should be almost permanent! **Couture Glossy Lipstick** *($21)* is merely a greasy lipstick with a high-gloss finish and minimal staying power. **Rouge Miroir Lipstick SPF 8** *($21)* comes in a tube that has a space-aged, aerodynamic look. There is even a built-in mirror for quick touch-ups, which will be necessary given the consistency of this particular formula. Truly a work of form over function. As a postscript, the SPF offers no UVA protection. **Lip Pencil** *($20)* is a standard pencil with a somewhat greasy finish, so don't count on much wear or stain. One end is a lip brush, which is a nice convenience, but lots of less expensive pencils have the same advantage, and I mean lots less expensive.

☺ $$$ <u>MASCARA:</u> The **Mascara** *($19)* is quite good. It builds fairly long, thick lashes with little effort. It also doesn't clump or smear. However, there are lots of mascaras for one-fourth the price that match or surpass this mascara's performance.

## Glymed Plus (Skin Care Only)

Glymed Plus is one of many skin-care lines being sold by dermatologists and spas. Of course there is nothing particularly medical about these products. As far as spa lines are concerned, I've yet to see anything particularly special about any of them. Glymed claims its products are naturally manufactured (who doesn't?), but they aren't, though I imagine you could argue that there's no such thing as "unnatural" manufactured cosmetics. The ingredients in these products aren't any more natural than those in any other cosmetics line, and include plenty of synthetics and a share of plant-extract ingredients. There are some good AHA moisturizers in this line, but its Acne Management line contains several unnecessary irritants, and similar and more gentle formulations with the same active ingredients are available for far less at the drugstore. Oxy Radical Anti-Oxidant Therapy can't fight oxidative skin damage, but theoretically it works the same as hundreds of other products containing antioxidants. A definite plus here are some well-formulated sunscreens; only the price makes me reluctant to recommend them wholeheartedly.

For more information about Glymed Plus, call (800) 676-9667 or visit the Web site at www.glymedplus.com.

☺ $$$ **Gentle Facial Wash** *($29 for 8 ounces)* isn't all that gentle, but it is a good, albeit exceptionally overpriced, detergent-based water-soluble cleanser that would work well for normal to oily skin. It does contain about 2% to 3% AHA, which isn't much, but the pH isn't high enough for it to be effective as an exfoliant anyway.

☹ $$$ **Oxy Radical High Purification Skin Cleanser** *($29 for 8 ounces)* has a singularly lavish name for a singularly ordinary creamy cleanser for dry skin. It needs to be wiped off with a washcloth or it can leave an emollient film on the skin. It does contain a minuscule amount of plant extracts and some antioxidants such as superoxide dismutase. But in the amount used here, their value is at best limited, and no matter what the amount, there is no research showing their benefit for skin—plus in a cleanser they would be wiped away. For the money and formula, you would be far better off with Neutrogena's Extra Gentle Cleanser for a third the cost.

☺ $$$ **Serious Action Skin Wash** *($28.60 for 8 ounces)* is a standard, detergent-based water-soluble cleanser that contains 2.5% benzoyl peroxide. That can be great for blemish-prone skin, but in a wash the benefit would be mostly washed down the drain. If you do want a benzoyl peroxide wash this is as good as any, but for the price, and given that the effective ingredient would just be rinsed away, you would be far better off with a benzoyl peroxide topical that is left on the skin.

☺ $$$ **Serious Action Exfoliant Scrub** (*$28.60 for 8 ounces*) is similar to the Skin Wash above, with similar issues, only this version contains scrub particles.

☹ **Serious Action Skin Astringent No. 5** (*$26.95 for 8 ounces*) contains alcohol and menthol, which are problematic ingredients for irritation and have no positive effect on skin.

☹ **Serious Action Skin Astringent No. 10** (*$28.05 for 8 ounces*) does contain BHA and tea tree oil, and that could be helpful for breakouts, but this version also contains menthol and arnica, which are unnecessarily irritating to skin with no benefit whatsoever for healing skin.

☹ **AHA Accelerator** (*$60.50 for 4 ounces*). It goes without saying that there are less expensive AHA products available. Besides, although this version does have a good concentration of AHA and a pH that makes it effective as an exfoliant, it also contains lemon, citrus, and balm mint oils, which add no benefit and can be too irritating for most skin types.

☹ **Facial Hydrator** (*$47.75 for 4 ounces*) has alcohol as the second ingredient, and that is too irritating for most skin types. It also contains lemon, citrus, and balm mint oils, which add irritation without bringing any benefit for the skin.

☹ **Serious Action Skin Gel** (*$58.85 for 4 ounces*) is aimed at controlling breakouts, but this is a lot of money for some fairly irritating ingredients, including alcohol (second on the ingredient list), camphor oil, and eucalyptus oil. There are far better products for breakouts than this, not to mention for far less money.

☺ $$$ **Treatment Cream** (*$69.55 for 2 ounces*) is a very good emollient, glycolic acid–based AHA moisturizer with about 7% AHA and a pH of 3.5, which makes it an effective exfoliant for dry skin. To suggest that there are less-expensive versions that would work as well is unnecessary, right?

☺ $$$ **Vital-A Protein Binding Trans-Dermal Retinyl Cream** (*$36.25 for 1.5 ounces*) does contain retinyl palmitate, a form of retinol, but it isn't retinol anymore than retinol is tretinoin (tretinoin is the active ingredient in Retin-A and Renova that retinol is likened to—or at least that's what all the hype about retinol is aimed at when it's described as working similarly to Retin-A and Renova). While I am skeptical about the effectiveness of retinol, there is some minimal research showing that it there is some token comparison between the two. However, there is no research demonstrating retinyl palmitate to be of much help for skin over any other vitamin-related ingredient. This also contains lactic acid (about 7%) but the pH is too high for it to be effective as an exfoliant. Otherwise, it is a good basic moisturizer for dry skin.

☺ $$$ **Oxy Radical Daily Skin Repair Cream** (*$68.25 for 2 ounces*) is a very good moisturizer for dry skin, with plenty of the latest buzz ingredients that have little proof of efficacy but that theoretically are worth considering. What is a joke is the inclusion of RNA and DNA, genetic material that, thankfully, is useless on the surface of skin.

☺ $$$ **Oxy Radical Daily Cell Repair Serum** *($68.25 for 0.5 ounce)* is similar to the Repair Cream above only in lotion form. This version works better for normal to slightly dry skin. It also contains salicylic acid (BHA, at about a 0.1% concentration), but the pH is too high for it to be effective as an exfoliant.

☺ $$$ **Eye and Lip Renewal Complex** *($36.75 for 0.75 ounce)* contains mostly water, thickeners, silicone, plant oil, AHA (about 3%), vitamins, water-binding agents, plant extracts, fragrant oils, film former, and preservatives. The amount of AHA isn't enough for it to be effective as an exfoliant, and that's good, because it would be a problem for the lips, which can be irritated far more easily than other skin. It's a good moisturizer for normal to slightly dry skin but there is nothing about it that makes it especially suited to the eyes or lips.

☺ $$$ **Oxy Radical Photo-Age Protection Cream 35** *($42.75 for 2 ounces)* is a part titanium dioxide–based sunscreen that would work well for normal to dry skin, but the cost makes it unlikely anyone will use this liberally, which is essential to obtain the SPF number on the label.

☺ **Photo-Age Environmental Protection Gel SPF 20** *($47.25 for 7 ounces)* is a very good, titanium dioxide–based sunscreen. It works well but it can leave a white film on the skin. The gel feel is a great option for some skin types that like gels and want titanium dioxide–based sun protection to prevent irritation to skin and eyes. Only the price is a problem, because concern about the cost can affect how liberally you are likely to apply it.

☹ **Photo-Age Protection Cream SPF 15** *($27.50 for 2 ounces)* doesn't contain UVA-protecting ingredients and is not recommended.

☹ **Alpha-Hydrox Exfoliant Masque** *($39.40 for 4 ounces)* is a waxy mask that contains mostly paraffin and scrub particles. The wax does help roll off skin, but it can be pore clogging for some skin types, and the scrub particles can be rough on dry skin. It also contains small amounts of AHA and BHA, but they aren't effective as exfoliants because the pH is too high for these to work. However, that's good news, because a scrub is meant to be washed off and AHAs and BHA are meant to be left on to have an effect.

☹ **Oxy Radical Skin Repair Fruit Enzyme Masque** *($41.80 for 2 ounces)*. Because papain tends to be an unstable enzyme, this product is minimally effective as an exfoliant. It also contains fractional amounts of some marketing buzzword ingredients—such as Dead Sea salts, live yeast, and RNA and DNA—but the amounts are too tiny to add up to any consideration for skin, and there is no evidence that they are helpful for any skin type in any amount.

☹ **Serious Action Masque** *($39.50 for 4 ounces)* is a standard clay mask that also contains eucalyptus and camphor, which makes it unnecessarily irritating for all skin types.

☺ **Derma Pigment Bleaching Fluid** *($33.60 for 2 ounces)* is a good, 2% concentration hydroquinone-based moisturizer. It contains mostly water, slip agents, aloe, thickeners, and preservatives. Less-expensive versions of skin-lightening products like this are available of course, but this is definitely an option to consider.

☺ **Derma Pigment Skin Brightener** *($33.60 for 2 ounces)* contains mostly water, AHA (about 8%), glycerin, plant oil, aloe, vitamins, more thickeners, and preservatives. This is a good glycolic acid–based moisturizer for normal to slightly dry skin. However, while AHAs do help surface texture, they do not affect the production of melanin, which can help improve skin discolorations.

☺ **Living Cell Clarifier** *($33.60 for 2 ounces)* contains live yeast cells, sort of like bread dough. There is no known benefit for using this on skin, but it won't hurt either. There are other plant extracts in here too, and vitamins, but nothing different from those that most of the moisturizers in this line contain.

☺ **Serious Action Skin Medication No. 5** *($26.95 for 4 ounces)* is a good 5% benzoyl-peroxide gel that also contains a teeny amount of tea tree oil. It is a very good option for blemish-prone skin, but keep in mind that this one is virtually identical to PersaGel at the drugstore.

☺ **Serious Skin Medication No. 10** *($26.40 for 4 ounces)* is similar to the No. 5 version above, only this one contains 10% benzoyl peroxide.

☹ **Serious Skin Peeling Lotion** *($28.05 for 2 ounces)* contains sulfur, salicylic acid, resorcinol, and alcohol, so I would absolutely call this serious, and potentially seriously irritating too. There are far better ways to exfoliate skin and disinfect it at the same time without the use of sulfur, resorcinol, and alcohol.

# *Guerlain*

If any cosmetics company can be considered sensual, luxurious, and elitist, Guerlain is it. Before even taking quality into consideration, it is hard to ignore the lavish gold packaging, intricate designs, and the monumental price tags that accompany everything from eyeliner to powder. As an example, a refillable powder compact sells for $140 and a lipstick compact is $80! The containers are exquisitely bedecked with faux jewels, and if it were chic to powder your nose and apply lipstick in public, you'd be the talk of the party. But therein lies the problem with overzealous packaging: it is essentially a waste, because no one but you and your makeup bag will see it. All that really counts when it comes to makeup is how it looks on your face. Though it may be a sight to behold, if the product inside is only a blush and the lipstick only a lipstick, there is no real reason to lust after a container.

Guerlain's skin-care products contain ordinary cosmetic ingredients, without any of the unique antioxidants, water-binding agents, or emollients that show up in less-expensive lines from Clinique to L'Oreal. Actually, if you are looking to spend money on skin care, there are many other pricey lines with far better formulations than this. What is most inexcusable is the line's blatant lack of sunscreen options. There are dozens and dozens of moisturizers in this line, and no reliable sunscreen as part of the daily routine! That is unconscionable from a skin-care point of view. Repetitive formulations are the hallmark of the Guerlain line, despite specialty claims for each product grouping.

In terms of the color line, the strong points are the blushes and foundations, while the weaknesses are the shiny eyeshadows and pressed powder. What are worth considering, if you can overlook the exorbitant prices, are the blush and lipsticks. To be fair, I should add that Guerlain is not the most expensive product line at the cosmetics counters, although it's definitely up there, with several products costing over $100. Yet, if you read the ingredient listings, you would understand that what you were really buying is a Hostess Twinkie and not Crème de Caramel. In the end, don't worry if you can't afford this line; your skin won't be left out in the cold without it. For more information about Guerlain, call (800) 882-8820 or visit the Web site at www.guerlain.com.

# Guerlain Skin Care

☺ $$$ **Issima Blue Voyage Ready to Go Cleanser** *($27 for 0.8 ounce)* is a standard, wipe-off makeup remover, and I mean really standard. It contains mostly water, slip agents, detergent cleansing agent, preservatives, and fragrance. It works as well as any liquid makeup remover.

☹ **Issima Blue Voyage Recovery Creme SPF 15** *($72)* doesn't contain the UVA-protecting ingredients of titanium dioxide, zinc oxide, or avobenzone, and is not recommended.

☺ $$$ **Issima Blue Voyage In-Flight Serum** *($72)* adds up to a good, though very standard moisturizer for normal to dry skin for a bizarre amount of money. If only you could read this ingredient listing you would be as shocked as I am.

☺ $$$ **Issima Foaming Milky Cleanser** *($49 for 6.8 ounces)* is a very standard, mineral oil–based, cold cream–style, wipe-off cleanser. It can leave a greasy film on the skin but may be an option for someone with dry skin. The ordinary ingredient listing for this one is shocking given the price.

☺ $$$ **Issima Moisturizing Cleansing Milk** *($32.50 for 6.8 ounces)* is similar to the Foaming version above and the same basic comments apply.

☺ $$$ **Issima Smoothing Gentle Exfoliator Radiance** *($37 for 2.5 ounces)* is a plant oil–based cleanser with gentle detergent cleansing agents. That very basic combination doesn't add much to exfoliation and the teeny amounts of lemon and papaya in here don't either.

☺ $$$ **Issima Fresh Purifying Toner** *($32.50 for 6.8 ounces)* is a good, but exceedingly mundane toner. The minuscule amount of mushroom extract and retinyl palmitate in here have no effect on skin.

☺ $$$ **Issima Radiant Moisturizing Toner** *($32.50 for 6.8 ounces)* is similar to the Purifying version above and the same basic, disappointing comments apply.

☹ **Issima Mythic Creme SPF 10** *($50 for 0.5 ounce)* does make mythic claims about protection and hydrating skin, but they're the only thing mythic about this product. The SPF 10 is seriously wanting, and the lack of UVA-protecting ingredients makes this product a big no-no.

☹ **Issima Hydramythic Fluid SPF 15** *($58 for 1 ounce)* doesn't contain the UVA-protecting ingredients titanium dioxide, zinc oxide, or avobenzone, and is not recommended.

☺ $$$ **Issima Intensive Protective Emulsion** *($89 for 1.7 ounces)* is a good moisturizer for someone with dry skin, but the price could make you feel worse than any amount of flaky skin ever could.

☺ $$$ **Issima Intensive Protective Emulsion** *($89 for 1.7 ounces)*. This very basic, humdrum formulation would be good for someone with normal to dry skin. The plant extracts in here are a mixed bag of anti-irritants and irritants; what a waste.

☺ $$$ **Issima Intensive Revitalizing Creme** *($125 for 1.7 ounces)* is similar to the Protective Emulsion above only in cream form, and the same basic comments apply.

☺ $$$ **Issima Midnight Secret Late Night Special Treatment** *($89 for 1 ounce)* is a good, extremely ordinary moisturizer for normal to dry skin, but nothing more. The secret must be that there's nothing interesting inside the bottle.

☺ $$$ **Issima Success Day Smoothing Anti-Wrinkle Day Care** *($125 for 1.7 ounces)* does not carry an SPF but does have sunscreen ingredients, though they are not UVA-protecting ones. This is a good moisturizer for normal to dry skin. The plant extracts in here are minimally present, and while some can have antioxidant properties, others can be irritants.

☺ $$$ **Issima Success Lift** *($95 for 0.5 ounce)* lists its sixth ingredient as aluminum starch (octenylsuccinate), which can be a skin irritant and absorbent, and for dry skin that doesn't make any sense. It is primarily just thickeners and slip agents, and exceedingly mundane and overpriced. The teeny amount of plant extracts in here will not lift skin anywhere.

☺ $$$ **Issima Success Night Firming Anti-Wrinkle Night Care** *($145 for 1.7 ounces)* contains mostly water, slip agent, thickeners, glycerin, silicone, fragrance, preservatives, vitamins, and water-binding agents. This is a good though markedly standard moisturizer for normal to dry skin.

☺ $$$ **Issima Serenissime Restructuring Treatment with Active Genesium** *($175 for 1 ounce)* ends up costing $2,800 a pound for extremely standard ingredients and something called "genesium," which supposedly can tackle all the things that cause the skin to age. However, there is no such thing as "genesium"—it is just a marketing term. The ingredients here are the same ones in product after product in this line. Further, Serenissime does not contain a sunscreen, and without a sunscreen it can't handle the number-one cause of *aged*-looking skin, and that's sun damage. It does have some good water-binding ingredients and some antioxidants, but they are overwhelmed by the waxy thickening agents and mineral oil, which you can find in a hundred other products. Even the interesting ingredients come well after the fragrance and preservatives, meaning they are barely present.

☺ $$$ **Issima Super Aquaserum** (*$125 for 1.7 ounces*) is about a 2% AHA product, which means it doesn't contain enough AHAs to exfoliate, although the AHAs are good water-binding agents. The urea in here can be an exfoliant, but not at this tiny amount, though it can be a water-binding agent. I can't even comment about the prices anymore—they are too preposterous to believe and completely unwarranted.

☹ **Issima Creme Camphrea, Anti-Blemish Care** (*$25 for 0.56 ounce*). Mineral oil and beeswax for blemish care? They've got to be kidding. On top of that it also contains camphor. Irritation and grease, now there's an original combination. Don't put this on blemish-prone skin.

☺ $$$ **Issima Eyeserum/Eye Contour Treatment** (*$68 for 0.5 ounce*) contains water, slip agent, thickeners, vitamin E, water-binding agent, preservatives, vitamins, and plant extracts. This standard formulation for normal to dry skin contains several plant extracts that can be irritants and others that are anti-irritants. The other ingredients are completely ordinary and average.

☺ $$$ **Issima Intenserum Beauty Treatment** (*$175 for ten 0.08-ounce ampoules*) is, to say the least, inanely overpriced. For $3,300 per pound, you get mostly water, slip agents, thickeners, silicone, vitamin E, fragrance, water-binding agents, and preservatives. It isn't worth it. To be fair, it is a good lightweight moisturizer for someone with normal to dry skin, but these ingredients do not warrant a price tag that's even one-tenth of this one.

☹ **Issima Matiday Oil-Control Hydrating Fluid** (*$52 for 1 ounce*) contains orris root and zinc sulfate, which are irritating; mineral oil, which is greasy; and aluminum starch (octenylsuccinate), which can absorb oil but is just standard and can be overly drying.

☹ **Issimat T-Zone Matifying Secret** (*$40 for 0.5 ounce*) lists the second ingredient as alcohol, and some of the same problems for the Matiday above apply here as well.

☺ $$$ **Issima Revitalizing Moisturizing Mask** (*$65 for 2.5 ounces*) is moisturizing but hardly revitalizing. This product contains a host of thickening ingredients, minimal vitamins, and water-binding agents. That's not bad, just not worth $65. This would be a good mask for someone with dry skin.

☺ **$$$ Issima Neck Firming Creme** *($89 for 1.7 ounces).* The preservative is way too high on this ingredient listing, indicating this stuff is 99% wax! It makes no sense why this should be for the neck as opposed to any other part of the body, because even at this steep price, the formulation doesn't differ from the other Guerlain products.

# Guerlain Makeup

**FOUNDATION:** Guerlain has enough foundations to appeal to a broad range of needs and preferences. What's lacking here are light, smooth textures and realistic colors. There are some shades to consider, but at these prices, they should be the best around, and these don't come close to anything but mediocre.

☺ **$$$ Issima Foundation** *($55)* has a very thick, emollient texture that can blend out easily enough to a sheer, dewy finish. This is only appropriate for drier skins, and of the seven shades, two (#4 and #7) are not recommended due to peachy-rose overtones.

☺ **$$$ Perfect Light Foundation SPF 8** *($45)* does not list any active sunscreen ingredients but does contain titanium dioxide high up on the list. Don't rely on it for secure sun protection until Guerlain learns what the FDA requirements for sunscreen labeling are. This does have a smooth, light texture and light to medium coverage that dries to a soft matte finish. The 11 shades are not the best, as many of them have a slight pink or peach tone, but may work for some skin tones. The ones to avoid are Beige Tendre, Beige Dore, and Dore Soleil.

☹ **Issima Anti-Aging Creme Foundation SPF 12** *($48)* does not offer reliable UVA protection, the SPF is disappointing, and the other ingredients aren't going to change a wrinkle, so there goes the anti-aging claim. It is an emollient foundation with a soft texture and moist finish, providing sheer to light coverage, yet all of the shades are just too peach, pink, or rose for most skin tones.

☹ **Sophistik SPF 18** *($32)* gets high marks for an excellent, partially titanium dioxide–based sunscreen but falls woefully short on texture (thick and greasy) and colors. Of the nine shades, two are shiny (dubbed **Enhancers**) and the remaining colors, with the exception of #3, are varying degrees of pink, peach, or ash.

☺ **$$$ TwinSet Compact Foundation SPF 15** *($50)* is a compact foundation available in either **Powder** or **Cream-to-powder** textures. Both have reliable, all titanium dioxide–based sunscreen, and can provide sheer to light coverage. The Cream-to-powder tends to stay creamy, but of the six shades, three are far removed from real skin tones: Rose 23, Apricot 33, and Dore 45. The Powder is quite standard but nice and the colors are more realistic; where they lose credibility is the inclusion of shine in each one!

☹ <u>CONCEALER:</u> **Corrective Concealer SPF 12** *($26)* has titanium dioxide as its active UVA-protecting ingredient, but this is one creamy concealer that tends to slip and crease in spite of your best preventive efforts. **Protective Base for Eyelids** *($25)* is the type of product that only seems to show up in high-end lines like Guerlain. It goes on creamy and then dries to a powder finish, which is fine; what's not fine are the colors: one is pink, the other is shiny bronze. They are sheer, but that only serves to interfere, not help, with your other eyeshadow colors.

<u>POWDER:</u> ☺ $$$ **Meteorites Voyage Compact Powder** *($145; $45 for refill)* is a rainbow of pastel and muted colors in a breathtaking compact accompanied by a price that should leave you all choked up. **Meteorites Finishing Powders** *($42).* You have to sit down for this one! This is supposed to be "powder pearls for the face … sent down from heaven." Flowery language aside, these are multicolored powder beads that all have a slight to moderately intense shine. There are much less expensive ways to gleam yourself up than this, and you'll have no trouble finding facsimiles of this product at The Body Shop, the drugstore, or less expensive cosmetics counters.

☹ **Voilettes Loose Powder** *($43)* comes in four colors, all with a pink cast and a wafting violet fragrance, and they're shiny as well.

☺ $$$ **Compact Powder for the Face** *($50)* is a standard, talc-based powder that has a soft, dry texture and comes in a small but good choice of colors, but the price will give you sticker shock when you realize that everyone from L'Oreal to Clinique has pressed-powder options than are equal to if not better than this one.

☹ **Terracotta Bronzing Powder** *($32 for women's; $47 for men's)* is a bit confused. In the "women's line," there are three believable, tan-looking colors although the shine these have negates the real look (real tanning does not yield iridescence), while the Men's Bronzer is perfectly matte and priced higher. So women's tans are supposed to shine but not men's? Go figure. These may be worth the splurge if the shine was absent, but until then there are much better options for bronzer, such as Bobbi Brown and even Bonne Bell! **Terracotta Refreshing Tinted Gel SPF 8** *($32)* features no active ingredient for sun protection and is just a very, very shiny bronzing gel available in three tints. **Terracotta Stick Bronzer** *($32.50)* has a cooling, wet feel and is quite sheer but blindingly shiny. If you prefer bronzing sticks, check out the ones from Bobbi Brown, which are attractively matte.

☺ $$$ <u>BLUSH:</u> **Mozais Powder Blusher** *($19)* has a great silky-soft texture and a sheer finish. The ten shades are mostly winners, with several matte options available.

☹ $$$ <u>EYESHADOW:</u> **Mozais Eyeshadow** *($16)* can be combined with the blush color and two eyeshadows of your choice in one compact. You may want to avoid this convenience, since almost all of these eyeshadows are very shiny, with a powdery texture and sheer application that imparts little color or effect.

☹ $$$ <u>EYE AND BROW SHAPER:</u> **Mozais Eyebrow Shaper** *($16)* is identical to the eyeshadows and is not identified on the tester unit as being specific to the brows. Keep in mind that even the natural brown and taupe colors here have at least a slight shine and are quite powdery (meaning they can flake off during application and will look completely unnatural on the brows). **Eyeliner** *($25)* is a standard liquid liner available in matte or metallic finishes. It dries quickly and stays put, but the brush is not the best for a smooth application. **Mozais Eyeliner** *($16)* has a greasy texture and choppy application, and at this price it should be stellar.

LIPSTICK AND LIP PENCIL: ☺ $$$ **KissKiss Haute Tenue Lipstick** *($23)* has a wonderfully smooth texture and a full-coverage, satin-matte finish. **KissKiss Douceur Lipstick SPF 10** *($19.50)* has no UVA-protecting agents and is just a standard, creamy lipstick with 18 shades to choose from. **Lipshine SPF 8** *($23)* is also without adequate UVA protection and the price is staggering for what amounts to generic, slightly greasy gloss.

☹ **Lipliner Pencil** *($19)* is totally commonplace and has a greasy, slightly slick texture that can be unappealing.

☺ $$$ MASCARA: **Super-Cils Beauty Treatment Mascara** *($21)* takes forever to build any length and even then it never makes much difference. The container is handsome, but that won't do a thing for your lashes. It's not really a bad mascara, just a boring one. **Super-Cils Waterproof Mascara** *($21)* has the same drawbacks as the one above, which isn't great, but this is waterproof and takes some effort to remove.

# Guinot (Skin Care Only)

What's in a name? If it's French, usually a high price tag and the promise of "European" skin care. Of course, in Europe the women praise American know-how when it comes to skin care—but I guess the grass is always greener in someone else's lawn. As it turns out, French products are no different from American products. All the gimmicky plant extracts and vitamins, standard thickening agents, basic detergent cleansing agents, preservatives, slip agents, emollients, lightweight silicone moisturizing gels, and problematic ingredients are virtually identical, but the claims have a French accent.

Guinot is a long-established salon/spa line of skin-care products with a reputation for being an elegant, elite, serious, and intricately designed way to take care of skin. The price tag definitely makes them elite, and the packaging can be described as elegant, but in terms of formulation, these products are rather ho-hum, with some downright inferior formulations. Many of them seem old-fashioned.

Despite the extravagant-sounding product names, this line seems unusually overpriced for what you get, and in need of revamping. I could go on at length about the claims, which range from "remodels your silhouette" to "blackheads disappear," "transforms the appearance of oily skin," "diffuses the water needed to keep skin moist all day," and (this one's my favorite) "dynamizes the complexion, smoothing away signs of fatigue." It would take another entire book to do justice to this kind of obtuse profundity. That's not to say there aren't some good products mixed in here, but they just can't do what the claims may lead you to believe. Guinot's name turns out to be the most impressive part of this skin-care line, which means its elite, serious image is just that: image. Guinot's customer service number is (800) 444-6621 or you can visit the Web site at www.guinotusa.com.

☺ $$$ **Moisture Rich Cleansing Milk** *($22.50 for 6.7 ounces)* is a standard mineral oil– and plant oil–based wipe-off cleanser that can leave a greasy film on the skin, though it can be an option for someone with dry skin. It does contain fragrance and coloring agents.

☺ $$$ **Refreshing Cleansing Milk** *($22.50 for 6.7 ounces)* is virtually identical to the Moisture Rich above and the same comments apply.

☹ **Purifying Cleansing Gel** *($22.50 for 6.7 ounces)* is a relatively standard detergent-based water-soluble cleanser that would be an option for someone with normal to oily skin, but this one contains sulfur, which makes it extremely alkaline and problematic for irritation and can encourage breakouts.

☹ $$$ **Wash-Off Cleansing Cream** *($28.50 for 5 ounces)* is almost identical to Neutrogena's Extra Gentle Cleanser ($6.06 for 6.7 ounces). It doesn't remove makeup very well and can leave a slightly greasy film on the skin, but it can be an option for someone with dry skin.

☺ $$$ **Gentle Eye Cleansing Gel** *($19.50 for 4.2 ounces)* is a standard detergent-based makeup remover that would work as well as any. This does contain fragrance and coloring agents.

☹ **Purifying Toning Lotion** *($22.50 for 6.7 ounces)* lists the third ingredient as sulfur, which makes this extremely alkaline and means it can encourage bacteria growth in skin and cause irritation. This is not recommended.

☺ $$$ **Moisture-Rich Toning Lotion** *($22.50 for 6.7 ounces)* is a rather standard toner. The plant extract in here is cornflower, which can have antibacterial properties but that is not helpful in the least for dry skin. The urea can be an exfoliant but probably not at this tiny an amount. There are far more interesting toners around than this one.

☺ $$$ **Gentle Face Exfoliating Cream** *($36 for 1.7 ounces)* isn't the best way to exfoliate skin as it is hard to rinse off and can leave a greasy film on skin. It does contain fragrance.

☺ $$$ **Huile Fine Nutri Comfort** *($40 for 1 ounce)* contains mostly fragrant oils, which may be comforting to smell but can be irritating for skin.

☺ $$$ **Longue Vie Cellulaire, Vital Face Care** *($67 for 1.6 ounces).* It isn't possible to make a more ordinary moisturizer for normal to dry skin than this one. There isn't one interesting ingredient except for microscopic amounts of water-binding agents so far at the end of the ingredient listing, they may as well not be there at all.

☺ $$$ **Skin Revitalizing Concentrate** *($52 for 1 ounce)* is an OK moisturizer for normal to slightly dry skin, but it is one of the more ho-hum, do-nothing formulations around.

☹ **Anti-Fatigue Eye Gel** *($29.50 for 0.5 ounce)*. The plant extracts in here are a mix of irritants (ivy) and anti-irritants (cucumber), which makes it a boring and potentially problematic gel.

☺ $$$ **Desensitizing Serum** *($40 for 1.69 ounces)* is a good moisturizer for dry skin, but rather basic and uninteresting. The teeny amount of vitamin C in here is barely detectable.

☺ $$$ **Intense Protection Cream** *($35 for 1.7 ounces)*. There is nothing intense about this product other than it is intensely boring. It is just water, thickeners, fragrance, and preservatives. What a waste.

☺ $$$ **Radiance Renewal Cream** *($52 for 1.7 ounces)* is similar to the Protection Cream above and the same comments apply. It has a few more bells and whistles (a form of vitamin A, vitamin E, and water-binding agents) but they are in such microscopic amounts as to be useless for skin.

☺ $$$ **Renewing Care with Gentle Fruit Acids Radiance Revealer Mask** *($31 for 1.7 ounces)* contains mulberry, black currant, and raspberry extracts, which are supposed to be "fruit acids" –they aren't and for the most part have no benefit for skin other than potential irritation.

☹ **Eye Lifting Crème** *($34 for 0.5 ounce)*. What is aluminum starch octenylsuccinate doing in a moisturizer? This embarrassing formulation isn't even a good moisturizer. The interesting ingredients are in microscopic amounts and have no impact on skin.

☺ $$$ **Anti-Wrinkle Cream for the Eyes** *($34 for 0.5 ounce)* is a good but exceptionally ordinary moisturizer for dry skin.

☺ $$$ **Firming Neck Cream** *($40 for one ounce)*. Not only won't this firm skin but it is just an average moisturizer for dry skin.

☺ $$$ **Lifting Day Cream** *($48.50 for 1.6 ounces)*. This ordinary lanolin-based moisturizer for dry skin contains a miniscule amount of water-binding agents that have no impact on skin and ginseng, which can be a skin irritant. It is only minimally passable as a moisturizer for dry skin.

☺ $$$ **Anti-Redness Treatment** *($28 for 1 ounce)* there is nothing in here that can reduce redness. The plant extracts are good anti-irritants but they would mostly be reducing the irritation from the fragrance in here, not helping skin.

☹ **Anti-Wrinkle Rich Night Cream** *($48.50 for 1.5 ounces)* could be an option for dry skin but it contains sulfur, which makes this too potentially irritating for skin.

☹ **Youth Replenishing Skin Cream** *($70 for 1.6 ounces)* is a confused product. Using absorbents with emollients in one formula means it would be too drying for dry skin and too emollient for oily skin, and combination skin would still end up getting ingredients over areas that don't need it.

☺ $$$ **Hydrazone Moisturizing Cream Dehydrated Skin** *($67 for 1.6 ounces)*. Like most of the Guinot moisturizers this is just water, wax, preservatives, and fragrance. The minute amount of vitamin A in here is almost nonexistent.

☺ $$$ **Liftosome Lifting Cream** *($72 for 1.6 ounces)* is a just a very ordinary moisturizer for dry skin that contains the same boring ingredients as most Guinot products. This does contain one decent water-binding agent, but that doesn't warrant the price tag for this otherwise run-of-the-mill product.

☹ **Pure Balance Cream** *($29 for 1.7 ounces)* is supposed to reduce the size of pores and disinfect skin. It can't. If anything, this product contains thickening agents that can cause problems for oily or blemish-prone skin. The teeny amount of zinc in here has no effect.

☹ **Pure Balance Concealer** *($22 for 0.5 ounce)* is a strange color and doesn't conceal anything though some of the ingredients can clog pores.

☺ $$$ **Pure Balance Serum** *($36.50 for 1.7 ounces)* can minimally make skin feel smoother but it has a tacky feel and won't hold oil back for very long. It does contain fragrance.

☺ $$$ **Instant Relaxing Anti-Wrinkle Mask** *($31 for 1.7 ounces)*. The only wrinkle this will remove are the ones from your wallet. The spleen extract in this mask has no effect on skin, and the miniscule amount of collagen cannot affect the collagen in your skin.

☺ $$$ **Pure Balance Mask** *($26.50 for 2.1 ounces)* is mostly chalk and clay. That will indeed absorb oil and would be an option for oily skin types only this product contains alcohol and camphor, which can be skin irritants.

☺ $$$ **Soothing Gel Mask** *($32 for 1.7 ounces)* is a standard clay mask with some emollients. It is an OK option for a mask but there is nothing soothing about it. If anything, the aluminum starch (octenylsuccinate) in here can be a skin irritant.

☺ $$$ **Instant Eye Mask** *($31 for 1 ounce)* is a do-nothing product that offers no benefit for skin.

# Hard Candy (Makeup Only)

Hard Candy is a modern-day success story. Founder Dineh Mohajer was a premed student in Southern California who had an eye for fashion. Frustrated that she couldn't find a blue pastel nail polish that matched her blue sandals (don't you just hate that?), she decided to create her own at home. So, after adding blue dye to a standard white nail polish, she found herself back on campus getting an extraordinary amount of attention from the female students, who flipped over the color. Shortly after trademarking the name "Hard Candy" in 1995, Mohajer stepped into the ultra-trendy Fred Segal boutique and presented her new colors (four in all), which were snatched up immediately. From there the line exploded to a broad range of flashy, glittery, brash colors and products.

In May 1999, Hard Candy was purchased by Sephora, which features the line in many of its stores. Interestingly, Hard Candy's chief competitor, Urban Decay, was also purchased by Sephora and the two rivals are now under the same umbrella, with big plans for expansion.

While the story of Hard Candy is intriguing, its products and displays are strictly image. This is a color line that relishes the chance to provide sparkly, glittery *everything,* from polish to pencils. Yet as eye-catching as this line appears, the formulations are either exceptionally standard or leave much to be desired, which proves the old adage, "all that glitters is not gold."

As always, the final decision to "shine on" is up to you. For more information on Hard Candy, call Sephora at (415) 392-1545, or visit the Hard Candy Web site at www.hardcandy.com.

☹ **FOUNDATION:** There is only one foundation-type product in the lineup, called **Hint Tint SPF 15** *($28)*. This does not include UVA-protecting ingredients so it is absolutely not recommended for sun protection. Second, this is really closer to a foundation than a tinted moisturizer, and two of the three colors are terrible—which makes this a great big "why bother?"

☹ **BLUSH: Cream Blush/Highlighter** *($28)* comes in a compact with one-half cream blush and the other a cream-to-powder highlighter. The blush part has a heavy, thick texture that blends on sticky but sheer, while the highlighter is too shiny for anything but an evening look.

☹ **EYESHADOW:** The **Eyeshadow Quartets** *($35)* are absurdly overpriced and have an opaque, dry, powdery texture. The color combinations are mostly unworkable and all of the shades are either subtle or eye-glaringly shiny. **Heavenly Hi-Lites/ Heavenly Lo-Lites** *($15)* are cream eyeshadow sticks with a slightly dry texture and sheer, ultra-shiny colors that are difficult to blend.

**EYE AND BROW SHAPER:** ☺ $$$ Here comes the glitter: **Eye Glider** *($16)* is just a standard automatic pencil with a creamy application and shiny colors. **Glitter Eye Pencil** *($17)* has a smooth, powdery texture and glides well, but be prepared for the glitter to fly everywhere.

☹ **Super Sonic Pencil** *($18)* is a standard chunky pencil with a waxy, sticky texture that is truly awful, with or without the flecks of glitter. **Sonic Glitter Stick** *($18)* is worse than the one above, with a grainy, greasy, and sticky texture that feels terrible on the skin.

☺ **$$$ Brow Pencil** *($16)* is worth a look if the price doesn't bother you. The texture of this one is light and powdery, with a good sheer application that builds nicely. It is almost a shock that all of the colors are matte. **$$$ Training Brow Compact** *($28)* is cute but overpriced for what you get: two shades of matte eyeshadow in a compact with an itty-bitty pair of tweezers and a minuscule brow brush. There are scads of inexpensive matte brow colors and far better tweezers to use that negate the need for this kit.

☺ **Training Brow Gel** *($14)* is exceedingly standard and absolutely not worth the price tag. Use hairspray on an old toothbrush instead and treat yourself to a nice lunch out!

☺ **$$$ LIPSTICK AND LIP PENCIL: Super Good Lipstick** *($16)* is more like "super standard." This is a creamy lipstick with a finish that borders on greasy. **Caffeine Lipstick** *($16)* is supposedly enriched with caffeine for a quick lift every time you lick your lips. However, upon closer inspection of the ingredient list, caffeine was nowhere to be found! Please ignore this gimmick so they're not encouraged to take it further! Plus, the notion of encouraging consumers to lick their lips and consume lipstick to get a hit of caffeine is not good for anyone's health. **Glitter Dip Lipstick** *($16)* is a creamy lipstick speckled with chunks of glitter. It's showy—what more can I say? **Lip Sync Quartet** *($35)* is like the eyeshadow quartets above, meaning poor quality and very overpriced. What does $35 get you? Three sheer lip colors and one sticky gloss, all packaged in a compact with a mini brush. Completely not worth it in every way, and not recommended.

☺ **Lip Gloss** *($12)*, **Lip Gloss Ring** *($12)*, **Super Shine Lip Gloss** *($12)*, and **Sonic Lip Gloss** *($12)* are basic, shiny lip glosses with varying degrees of glitter and stickiness. If you're really into gloss you may appreciate this attention to nuance, but shine is shine and after awhile it just all looks too trendy to be taken seriously. Isn't shine, like, so five minutes ago? **Digital Lip Pencil** *($12)* is the glittery counterpart to the Glitter Dip Lipstick, and all I can say is, why? Someone tell me why! **Lip Pencil** *($12)* is completely standard, needs sharpening, and the color choices are poor.

☺ **MASCARA:** If performance doesn't matter as much to you as color, you'll feel right at home among this average **Mascara** *($15)* that proudly showcases blue, pink, green, and copper shades to cake up your lashes. The **Glitter Mascara** *($15)* is so shiny and flaky, even a Las Vegas showgirl would pass it up.

☺ **SPECIALTY PRODUCTS:** As the backbone of this line's business, the **Nail Polish** *($12)* features a wild assortment of colors and textures, from the chip-prone glittery shades to the palest pastels. These are quite ordinary except for the colors and if one of these somehow fits in to your wardrobe or color scheme, why not?

# *Hope Aesthetics*

Hope Aesthetics is a line of skin-care products marketed to cancer patients, and it claims to address the special needs of women who are in the midst of cancer treatments. What is most intriguing about this line is that a woman who survived breast cancer created it. Let me state from the beginning that this is a hard line for me to review. I am incredibly sympathetic to the fight against breast cancer and the toll it can take. I have mentioned before that my older sister had breast cancer, and her struggle for physical health and emotional well-being was all-consuming. Vincene Parinello, the creator of Hope Aesthetics, lived through a bilateral mastectomy and chemotherapy. After all she went through, she felt the effects of the battle were showing up on her skin. According to her story, she investigated all kinds of skin-care products and was appalled to find that many were toxic. So she decided to create her own. She feels that her ". . . line is the healthiest thing you can use on your skin, cancer or no cancer." I wish I could say the same for it, but I can't.

Her products just aren't the miracles she claims they are, and there is nothing about the formulations that makes them special or unique for women struggling with cancer. Parinello claims she has support for her statements from in-depth testing that generated astonishing results. If I only had a dime for every cosmetics company that makes claims about its astounding studies, I would be a wealthy woman by now. Parinello says "in a four month double blind study on 200 subjects as well as a successful test market study on over 300 women, the preventive [skin-care] system, which stabilizes free radicals and protects the lipids from damage when used in higher levels, enhanced the collagen synthesis process." Even if her product line improved the appearance of skin, there is no way you can demonstrate that free radicals have been stabilized in skin. There is no way to see it without cutting out a good chunk of skin and even then that wouldn't give you any information for what happens throughout the day to skin. Further, her product line simply could not accomplish this long-term, given it doesn't have an effective sunscreen among the product options.

She also states that "over 500 women have successfully used Hope Aesthetics with no adverse reactions or sensitivities." While I'm sure there are lots of women who can use these products, overall, given the preservative base used, the fragrances, and other potentially irritating ingredients, statistically there are going to be reactions. That's not bad; I just strongly doubt her claims. What is really distressing, given the audience this line is trying to reach, is that the prices are just galling.

There are other statements Parinello makes about her products' contents that just aren't based in reality. For example, Hope Aesthetics products are supposed to be formulated with pharmaceutical-grade essential oils, yet there are no such things as pharmaceutical-grade essential oils. And there are some other infuriating statements associated with this line; for example, that the product line "is free of harmful chemicals and all petroleum derivatives, which deprive the skin of oxygen." I thought the whole purpose of antioxidants was to keep air off the face, which Vaseline and mineral oil do quite nicely. But keeping air off the face is not the same thing as suffocation; and mineral oil and Vaseline do not suffocate skin and are actually decent moisturizing ingredients. As far as "chemicals" are concerned, the products in this pure and botanical line do contain plenty of ingredients that have nothing to do with plants. That doesn't make them bad for the skin, it just makes this another line pretending to be something it isn't.

For more information on Hope Aesthetics, call (800) 266-4799 or visit the Web site at www.hopeskincare.com. I should mention that at the time I first reviewed Hope Aesthetics in my newsletter, its Web site provided ingredient listings. They have since taken that feature off and replaced it with hype about the showcase ingredients that are supposed to impress you (all the natural-sounding ones without any information about order of inclusion or what else the product contains). This happened exactly one week after my story ran.

☺ $$$ Tea Elle Sea Foaming Cleanser for Normal/Combination Skin ($28.50 for 6 ounces). The cleansing agent, sucrose cocoate, derived from coconut acid, can be a skin irritant.

☺ $$$ Purifying Cleanser for T-Zone/Oily Skin ($28.50 for 6 ounces) contains the same cleansing agent as the Tea Elle above as well as sodium laureth sulfate, a detergent-based water-soluble cleansing agent. It would be an option for normal to oily skin, but it contains salicylic acid and glycolic acid, ingredients that would be best not to accidentally splash in the eyes.

☹ Gentle Lotion Cleanser for Dry/Sensitive Skin ($28.50 for 6 ounces) contains bitter orange extract, which would be a problem for sensitive skin. Other than that, this is just wax and water and preservatives, which are not great at cleaning skin if you wear makeup.

☹ Hope Glycolic Facial Toner for Combination, Sun Damaged and Oily Skin ($27.50 for 6 ounces) does contain glycolic acid, lactic acid, and salicylic acid, but the product's pH is over 5, too high a number to allow it to be effective as an exfoliant. This product also contains balm mint, which can be a skin irritant.

☹ Hope Botanical Facial Toner for Normal/Dry Skin ($27.50 for 6 ounces) would be a decent toner with soothing agents and water-binding agents, but it also contains balm mint, which can be a skin irritant.

☺ BHW Hydrating Antioxidant Complex for All Skin Types ($35 for 2 ounces) would be a good moisturizer for dry skin, but since it doesn't contain sunscreen, I disagree with the recommendation to apply it twice a day.

☺ $$$ Protective Eye Gel for All Skin Types ($40 for 0.5 ounce) contains mostly plant oils, about 5% AHAs, vitamin A, impressive water-binding agents, and preservatives. If you aren't allergic to the rose hips oil in this product, it could be a very good moisturizer for normal to dry skin.

☺ $$$ **Triplice Antioxidant Creme for Normal to Dry Skin** *($50 for 2 ounces)* lives up to its claim about antioxidants and would be a good moisturizer for normal to dry skin. It also contains about a 7% concentration of AHA, and the pH would make this a good emollient exfoliant.

☹ **Bellissima Regenerating Creme for All Skin Types** *($50 for 2 ounces )* contains far too many potentially irritating ingredients, including lavender oil, citrus acids, grapefruit oil, and lime oil, to make it appropriate for any skin type.

☹ **Serum Di la Hope for All Skin Types (Except Oily Skin)** *($50 for 1 ounce)* contains mostly grape seed oil and plant extracts. You would be far better off just going to your health food store and buying grape seed oil, because several of the plant extracts in here, including tangerine, lemon, and lime, can be a problem for most skin types.

☺ $$$ **Angel's Kiss Creme Di la Hope for Dry Skin** *($45 for 1 ounce)* is a very good moisturizer for dry skin.

☹ **Beta Hydroxy Blemish Buster** *($26 for 1 ounce)* is made with 2% BHA, which would be great, except that the product contains other irritating ingredients such as witch hazel and camphor.

# Hydron (Skin Care Only)

Hydron is sold on QVC, and it is simply captivating to watch the host of the show swear by it while enthusiastic callers echo the sentiment. The presentation is *very* convincing, but before you pick up your phone and order, you need more information than just what the company wants you to know.

The Best Defense Collection by Hydron supposedly can restore your skin's natural moisture balance by creating a water-insoluble film over the surface of your skin. According to the company, "Hydron is a polymer, which is an extremely high-molecular-weight compound." What Hydron really is, is polyhydroxyethylmethacrylate. That makes it basically a film former, like most of the other acrylates that show up in skin-care products. The other aspect of Hydron is that, like any polymer, it is too large to penetrate the skin, so it sits on top and covers the surface. That water-insoluble film also has water-binding properties, which are nice and can benefit dry skin, but the film is hardly miraculous or rare or the only way to keep water in the skin, and it's not unique in terms of function compared to other film-forming agents used in lots and lots of skin-care products.

Hydron's advertising gimmick is to compare skin to rawhide, demonstrating what happens to rawhide if you put water versus other types of ingredients on it.

Skin cannot be compared to rawhide (nor to a dead leaf, contrary to a Pond's demonstration years ago on a dried-up oak leaf). First, skin is constantly being produced and shed (it is mostly a living organ of the body); rawhide, on the other hand, is completely dead. Further, the causes of wrinkling have nothing to do with dry skin. *Dry skin and wrinkles are not associated.* The Hydron ad demonstrates that oil does not provide water (moisture) to the skin, and although that is true, it is not exactly shocking news. However, it does take oil or other water-binding agents to *keep* water in the skin. For dry skin, the issue is getting water to the skin and keeping it there. That process can be as simple as spraying the face with water before you use a moisturizer. (You don't need to spray expensive toners on your face; water will do, and the moisturizer will trap the water underneath.)

Although Hydron claims to be a unique water-delivery system, it is by no means the only one. It uses liposomes, which were developed by Lancome/L'Oreal more than 15 years ago. One more point: all of the ingredients listed on Hydron's products are completely standard. That doesn't make them bad, but they're not the skin sensations they claim to be. For more information about Hydron, call (800) 4-HYDRON or visit the Web sites at www.iqvc.com or www.hydron.com.

☹ **Best Defense Gentle Cleansing Creme** *($16.50 for 6 ounces)* is supposedly a rinseable cleanser that contains mostly thickeners and a detergent cleansing agent. It can be a good cleanser for someone with normal to dry skin, but it can leave a film on the skin.

☺ **Best Defense Antibacterial Facial Cleansing Gel** *($9.97 for 4 ounces)* is a standard, detergent-based water-soluble cleanser that uses a small amount of triclosan as the antibacterial agent. Triclosan is primarily used in products claiming to kill germs on the hands. There is little evidence that it is helpful for reducing bacterial or viral infections. This cleanser would still work well for someone with normal to oily skin.

☺ $$$ **Best Defense Gentle Eye Make Up Remover** *($17 for 4 ounces)* is just water, silicone, and a detergent cleansing agent. It will take off eye makeup.

☺ $$$ **Best Defense Micro-Exfoliating Creme** *($16.75 for 3.6 ounces)* can be a good standard scrub for someone with dry skin.

☺ **Best Defense Botanical Toner** *($14.50 for 6.5 ounces)*. The plant extracts in here can have anti-irritant benefit. This product does contain fragrance and coloring agents.

☹ **Best Defense Tri-Activating Skin Clarifier** *($37.75 for 1 ounce)* is Hydron's version of an AHA product, but the ingredient list just says it contains plant extracts such as lemon and sugarcane, and that's not the same thing as an AHA (such as lactic or glycolic acid). It sounds natural, but if you want to be certain you're getting an effective AHA product, look for glycolic or lactic acid on the ingredient list, not a plant extract.

☹ **Oil Balancing Toner** *($16 for 6.5 ounces)* has alcohol as the second ingredient, which makes this too drying and irritating for all skin types.

☺ **Best Defense All Over Moisturizer** *($13.25 for 8 ounces)*. This very basic moisturizer would be OK for someone with normal to dry skin but it is more of a "why bother?" than anything else.

☺ $$$ **Best Defense Facial Moisturizer Oil-Free with SPF 15** *($29 for 2 ounces)* is a good, in-part avobenzone-based sunscreen for normal to oily skin. It does contain some good antioxidants and water-binding agents. The tiny bit of lanolin in here is not enough to be a problem for someone with normal to oily skin.

☺ $$$ **Oil Balancing Serum** *($19.75 for 0.45 ounce)* contains three absorbent powders that include nylon-6, silica, and magnesium aluminum silicate. That will absorb oil nicely but it doesn't balance anything, and definitely not any better than an oil-absorbing powder. It does contain some good water-binding agents but a few irritating plant extracts as well. This is an option to consider but be cautious about lightweight lotion's limitations.

☺ $$$ **Best Defense Fragile Eye Moisturizer** *($26 for 0.5 ounce)* is a good emollient moisturizer that can be used all over the face, not just around the eyes.

☺ $$$ **Best Defense Line Smoothing Complex** *($37.75 for 0.5 ounce)* is a good lightweight moisturizer for normal to slightly dry or oily skin.

☺ **Best Defense Moisture Balance Restorative Overnight Liposome Complex** *($36 for 2 ounces)* would be a good emollient moisturizer for someone with dry skin.

☺ **Hydronamins Moisturizing Vitamin Therapy Day Creme SPF 15** *($29.75 for 1.9 ounces)* is a good, in-part avobenzone-based sunscreen for normal to dry skin. The minimal amount of vitamins in here have no real impact on skin, though the water-binding agents are a rather good addition.

☺ **Hydronamins Moisturizing Vitamin Therapy Night Creme** *($36.75 for 2 ounces)* is a good moisturizer for normal to dry skin but the amount of vitamins in here can have no real impact on skin.

☹ **Best Defense Self-Adjusting Tinted Moisturizer** *($24.50 for 2 ounces)* doesn't contain avobenzone, titanium dioxide, or zinc oxide, and is not recommended.

☹ **Best Defense Sportscreen SPF 15** *($15 for two 3-ounce tubes)* doesn't contain avobenzone, titanium dioxide, or zinc oxide, and is not recommended.

☹ **Best Defense Sportscreen SPF 30** *($15 for two 3-ounce tubes)* doesn't contain avobenzone, titanium dioxide, or zinc oxide, and is not recommended.

☹ **Best Defense Sunless Tanning Creme SPF 8** *($17.50 for 4 ounces)* has a dismal SPF 8, and it doesn't contain the UVA-protecting ingredients of titanium dioxide, zinc oxide, or avobenzone. As just a self tanner, it uses the same active ingredient to turn skin brown as all self tanners do.

☹ **Best Defense Five-Minute Revitalizing Masque** *($24 for 2.65 ounces)* is a standard clay mask that also contains plant extracts, glycerin, thickeners, silicone, and preservatives. The plant extracts include eucalyptus, balm mint, pine needle, sage, and thyme, all potential skin irritants. The mask also contains some water-binding agents and a detergent cleansing agent. The water-binding agents are nice, but the detergent cleansing agent is sodium lauryl sulfate, which can be a skin irritant. This product has too many potential problems to be of any benefit for skin.

☹ **Best Defense Menthol Ice** *($15 for 4 ounces)* contains both menthol and alcohol, both drying and irritating; that may be OK for sore muscles, but keep this one off the face or abraded skin.

☹ **Best Defense Tender Lip Care** *($15.75 for two 0.5-ounce tubes)* doesn't contain avobenzone, titanium dioxide, or zinc oxide, and is not recommended.

# *IGIA*

There probably isn't a woman in the United States right now who hasn't seen the ads for this line. In one form or another, whether they are for the IGIA Hair Removal System, the IGIA Sun System Facial Tanner, the IGIA Clear Blemish Remover, or the IGIA Epil-Stop, IGIA ads seem to have perfected the art of convincingly selling miracle, useless beauty products. These products are widely advertised in fashion magazines and mail order catalogs throughout the United States and Canada. Let's start with the IGIA Sun System, because this product speaks to the ethics of this company more than the other three, which, though useless, at least aren't harmful.

☹ **Sun System Facial Tanner** *($149)* claims to let you "[do] in minutes what usually takes hours to acquire. Compact, easy to use, and safe. Comes with a convenient 30-minute timer so there's no need to worry about burning. You control the amount of color you receive, while its four UV lamps help you get that even tan. Stop wasting money on unhealthy tanning salons and get better results in the privacy of your own home with the IGIA Sun System." According to the FDA, the FCC (Federal Communications Commission), the American Academy of Dermatology, and the Skin Cancer Foundation, suntanning machines are nothing more than skin-cancer machines, and should be made illegal. They radiate the most damaging effects of the sun only inches away from your body and, worse, they are available day after day, month after month, in areas of the country where you would not normally see the sun on a daily basis, radiating body parts that are usually covered. Not only do they put users at serious risk for skin cancer, but in all likelihood they age the skin faster than normal sun exposure would because of the proximity of the radiating light source. This is a senseless machine to make readily available to an unsuspecting public that believes something is safe when the contrary is true. There is no such thing as a safe tan generated by any kind of UV exposure, indoors or out. This machine alone casts a great shadow over IGIA. In fact, trust is the one thing this kind of company is *not* radiating.

☹ **Epil-Stop Hair Removal Cream** *($29.95 for 4 ounces)*. The Food and Drug Administration issued a recall on September 13, 1997, for this product, manufactured by International Chemical Corporation, Amherst, New York. Previously, on September 4, 1997, the California Poison Control Office had issued a press release warning that Epil-Stop "is adulterated in that it has high pH levels which may cause skin irritation and burning." Check out the FDA home page at www.FDA.gov for more information.

IGIA Epil-Stop products were advertised on television, in magazines, and over the Internet, with claims about removing hair and stopping hair growth naturally and painlessly. If only all that were true, my midweek leg stubble would be a thing of the past. It isn't. Epil-Stop is a horrendous example of marketing claim abuse, which isn't surprising, at least not to this cosmetics watchdog. It turns out that Epil-Stop works like any other drugstore depilatory: by dissolving hair with a high-pH ingredient base. Unlike other drugstore products, however, Epil-Stop took the pH to a higher level, eating away not only the hair but the skin as well.

☹ **IGIA's Hair Removal System** *($119)* is supposed to be a "painless home electrolysis system that helps keep hair from growing back! Unlike common [tweezing] and depilatory devices that can cause skin irritation, this system uses mild radio frequency pulses that [are] absolutely safe and delivered through the tweezers to remove hair without touching the skin." Well, that much is true. This overpriced machine delivers low-wattage radio waves through the hair shaft. Does that kill off a hair follicle? There is no research indicating that these machines do anything but tweeze the hair. The low voltage may make these machines ineffective, but they are also extremely low risk. In comparison to the other IGIA products, this one is the safest in the bunch. Keep in mind that these kinds of self-electrolysis machines have been advertised for years and years. I remember them from when I was a kid. The chances of operating these successfully yourself are at best slim. You probably would end up just tweezing instead of zapping the hair because getting the device to work right is extremely tricky and incredibly time-consuming. Given the time it takes for a hair to grow back, it could take months before you knew if it was really working. What a waste.

☹ **IGIA Clear Blemish Remover** *($99)*, while more benign than the Sun System, is a shocking waste of money. Here's the marketing language used in the brochure: "The IGIA Clear Blemish Remover uses a non-invasive process [a dull, metal-tipped, plastic wand] that produces negative ions to destroy bacteria and remove unattractive blemishes within seconds. Once the bacteria [are] destroyed the natural healing process can occur through the pores. The IGIA Clear Blemish Remover works best on small raised spots and typical skin problems such as pimples, blemishes, black-heads, ingrown hairs, and mild acne." The brochure carries on further, saying "this is the safe, painless way to remove unsightly skin spots and let your natural beauty shine through. Includes one bottle of cleanser and one moisturizer lotion, and comes in an attractive, slim, white plastic case." The idea that ions (which are nothing more than a group of atoms with a positive, negative, or neutral electric charge) can penetrate a pore and kill blemish-causing bacteria is preposterous. Even if ions could do that, bacteria are only part of the reason a blemish occurs. This expensive little implement doesn't address hormonal issues, the pore lining, oil production, or the use of skin-care products that can clog pores and cause breakouts. All it will remove is money from your wallet.

What about the two skin-care products packaged with the machine? The ☹ **Cleansing Lotion** contains mostly alcohol, water, witch hazel, glycerin, and menthol. If your skin isn't red and irritated before you use this product, it will be after, or worse. The ☹ **Deep Moisturizing** product contains mostly water, mineral oil, sesame oil, slip agents, thickeners, lanolin, Vaseline, preservatives, and coloring agents. Are they serious? Sesame oil and lanolin are notorious for clogging pores, and Vaseline and mineral oil leave a greasy feel on the skin. This rather dated formulation may be good for someone with seriously dry skin, but it is the worst imaginable for someone struggling with breakouts.

For more information, call (800) 716-8667 or visit the Web site at www.igia.com.

# *Iman*

Only a handful of women are known by their first name alone, including Madonna, Cher, Ann-Margaret, and, of course, the exquisite, regal Iman. As her story goes, she was hand-picked as a teen from the streets of Nairobi, Kenya, to become a model. From that point on Iman broke the fashion color line, along with model Beverly Johnson, gracing the covers of fashion magazines and runways that had previously deemed black women unacceptable as cover models.

After "retiring" in 1989 Iman became active in food and aid relief for her war-torn, impoverished homeland, and has fought for the rights of Ethiopian women regarding the horror of female circumcision. Clearly Iman is no ordinary woman.

Venturing into the world of makeup seems a natural for this elegant, savvy aristocrat. And in some areas, Iman has achieved breakthroughs for women of color that other cosmetics lines could learn from. Regrettably, her line loses considerable ground with its skin-care products, called Liquid Assets. Whoever put these products together for her doesn't seem to have had a plan, or to have realized that different skin types exist. The cleansers are disappointing, the toners are mediocre, the AHA products are limited, and the oil-free products are too emollient and may cause breakouts. Additionally, not one of the daytime moisturizers contains sunscreen, even though women of color are also subject to sun damage. In fact, sun damage is often responsible for darker skin tones becoming ashen, and lighter-skinned women of color run a risk of skin cancer. Like most of the skin-care lines glutting the cosmetics market right now, these products have the requisite plant extracts. But don't get too excited if you're a consumer who thinks plant extracts are what good skin care is all about; most of the green stuff comes after the preservatives, which means there isn't much.

Iman's line excels when it comes to her color collection. Most of the blush, eyeshadow, and lip colors are stunning, with a majority of matte neutral shades in a wide variety of tones that don't include blues, greens, or purples. These products are appropriate for a wide range of skin colors, from Asian to Latin and all shades of African-American skin; even lighter skin tones looking for more pigmented shades would be happy with the selection. There are a few shortsighted areas, such as limited concealer colors, and the lack of a good foundation for drier skins, and while the tester unit is nicely organized, you need a salesperson's assistance to try anything, but these are more nitpicky than real complaints.

Not to be outdone by some of the trendier, artistry lines, Iman has launched I-Iman Cosmetics, because, according to her, women "…want some color, some couture, some flash … you don't want to be safe all the time!" While not everyone is likely to agree with that, there is nothing wrong with the occasional flash of color, if worn appropriately (meaning *not* for your next job interview).

I-Iman cosmetics is available exclusively at select Sephora stores, and on Sephora's Web site, www.sephora.com. For more information about Iman cosmetics, visit her Web site at www.i-iman.com.

## *Iman Skin Care*

☹ **Perfect Response Oil-Free Cleanser, for Acne Prone, Very Oily Skin** *($15 for 4 ounces)* includes sodium C14-16 olefin sulfate as the primary detergent cleansing agent, plus peppermint extract and lemon extract, and all of those are exceedingly irritating. This product is not recommended for any skin type.

☹ **Perfect Response Gentle Toner, for Acne Prone, Very Oily Skin** *($15 for 6 ounces)* contains a small amount of salicylic acid (BHA), but it also contains witch hazel, citrus, yarrow, and nettle, all potential skin irritants. The pH of this product also isn't low enough for the BHA to be effective as an exfoliant.

☹ **Perfect Response Oil-Free Hydrating Gel, for Acne Prone, Very Oily Skin** *($18 for 1.7 ounces)* contains water-binding agents, vitamins, and slip agents. It also contains several irritating ingredients, including alcohol and sulfur. The sulfur can be a disinfectant but it is also a skin irritant; the alcohol is just irritating.

☹ **Perfect Response Blemish Gel, for Acne Prone, Very Oily Skin** (*$12 for 0.5 ounce*) would be a great 5% benzoyl peroxide gel to disinfect blemishes, except that it also contains peppermint and lemon, which are unnecessary irritants that can make acne-prone skin redder and tend to break out more.

☹ **Perfect Response Clay Masque, for Acne Prone, Very Oily Skin** (*$12 for 4 ounces*) is an OK clay mask with 2% salicylic acid and a small amount of charcoal. It doesn't have a low enough pH for the BHA to be an exfoliant but the clay mask can absorb oil. It also contains a small amount of peppermint and lemon, which are unnecessary skin irritants.

☹ **Perfection Even-Tone Fade Cream** (*$20 for 2.1 ounces*) is a standard 2% hydroquinone product (which does inhibit melanin production when used with an effective sunscreen) in a good emollient base for normal to dry skin. It also contains a tiny amount of lemon and grapefruit, but probably not in enough concentration to be a problem for most skin types.

☹ **Perfect Response Even-Tone Fade Gel with AHA** (*$20 for 1.7 ounces*) contains several skin-irritating plant extracts and ingredients, including spearmint, sodium sulfite, sodium methabisulfite, and styrene. It also doesn't contain any effective melanin-inhibiting ingredients.

☹ **Cleansing Bar with Grapefruit Normal/Oily Skin Formula** (*$8.50 for 3.5 ounces*) is a standard detergent-based cleansing bar that contains tallow along with some plants and grapefruit. The grapefruit supposedly makes it good for oily skin types, although there isn't much in this bar. (If there were, it would be a skin irritant. Ever get grapefruit juice on an open cut? Ouch.) Also, tallow can cause breakouts.

☹ **Cleansing Bar with Rose Petal** (*$8.50 for 3.5 ounces*) is almost identical to the Cleansing Bar with Grapefruit (including the grapefruit), and the same review applies.

☺ **Liquid Assets Gentle Cleansing Lotion** (*$13 for 3 ounces*) is a standard, detergent-based water-soluble cleanser that would work well for most skin types. It does contain a small amount of plant extracts that can be skin irritants but probably not enough to be of concern for most skin types.

☹ **Eye Makeup Remover with Aloe Vera** (*$10 for 3 ounces*) would be a good, standard eye-makeup remover, but it also contains lemon and grapefruit, which can definitely be irritating for the eye area.

☹ **Liquid Assets Skin Refresher Lotion** (*$12.50 for 3 ounces*). The orange oil and menthol are skin irritants and not refreshing for skin in the least.

☺ **$$$ Instant Replay AHA Perfecting Lotion** (*$35 for 1 ounce*) has about a 4% concentration of AHA in a good pH. It isn't going to perfect anything and it contains grapefruit and lemon, which can be skin irritants, but for a very mild AHA exfoliant it is an option.

☺ **$$$ Time Control Renewal Complex** *($29.50 for 1 ounce)* contains only about 3% to 4% AHA in a pH that's too high to make this an effective exfoliant. However, it is a good lightweight moisturizer for normal to dry skin.

☹ **$$$ Time Control Sloughing Gel** *($18 for 2.8 ounces)* is a standard synthetic scrub that uses ground-up plastic as the abrasive in a standard detergent cleansing agent base. It is an option for someone with normal to oily skin.

☻ **Time Control Peeling Masque with AHA** *($18 for 2.8 ounces)* has polyvinyl alcohol (plastic) and alcohol as the first two ingredients, while the amount of AHA is less than 2%, adding up to a useless, irritating mask.

☻ **All Day Moisture Complex, SPF 15** *($16.50 for 3 ounces)* doesn't contain avobenzone, titanium dioxide, or zinc oxide, and is not recommended.

☻ **Oil-Free Hydrating Lotion, SPF 15, for Acne Prone, Very Oily Skin** *($20 for 1.7 ounces)* doesn't contain avobenzone, titanium dioxide, or zinc oxide, and is not recommended.

☺ **Eye Firming Cream with Cucumber** *($15 for 0.5 ounce)* won't firm anything, but it is a good, ordinary emollient moisturizer for someone with normal to dry skin.

☻ **Night Time Complex Oil-Free Moisturizer** *($20 for 1.8 ounces)* contains several thickening agents (isopropyl myristate and shea butter) that can cause problems for someone with oily skin. It also contains lemon and grapefruit, which can be skin irritants.

☻ **Oil-Free Advanced Moisture Complex** *($16.50 for 3 ounces)* contains isopropyl myristate (fourth on the ingredient list) and shea butter, which are great for dry skin but are both known to cause breakouts. Neither are great for oily to combination skin despite the claim about being oil-free.

☻ **Under Cover Agent Oil-Control Lotion** *($16 for 1 ounce)* is a liquid version of Phillips' Milk of Magnesia that uses magnesium aluminum silicate instead of magnesium carbonate to absorb oil. It would do the trick, but it also contains balm mint and camphor, which are skin irritants.

☺ **PM Renewal Cream** *($20 for 1.8 ounces)* is a good, but exceedingly ordinary, emollient moisturizer for someone with dry skin. Like most of the products in this line, this one also contains grapefruit and lemon, which can be skin irritants, but the amount in here is so small it probably won't have an effect on skin.

☻ **Oil Free SPF 8 Moisturizer** *($16.50 for 3 ounces)* has a dismal SPF and doesn't contain avobenzone, titanium dioxide, or zinc oxide, and is not recommended.

☻ **Sun Defense Lip & Eye Stick, SPF 15** *($15 for 0.14 ounce)* doesn't contain avobenzone, titanium dioxide, or zinc oxide, and is not recommended.

☻ **Sun Defense Lotion, SPF 25** *($20 for 4 ounces)* doesn't contain avobenzone, titanium dioxide, or zinc oxide, and is not recommended.

# Iman Makeup

☺ <u>FOUNDATION:</u> **Second to None Cream to Powder Foundation SPF 8** *($18.50)* has a beautiful texture, a smooth application, and a powdery finish. This type of foundation would work well for normal to slightly dry or slightly oily skin types (the cream part can be too greasy for oily skin types and the powder part too drying for those with dry skin). The coverage is light to medium and there are only a few colors to avoid—Sand 5 (too peach), Earth 3 (slightly red), Clay 1 (too ash), and Clay 4 (red)— but all of the other colors are exquisite. **Second to None Oil-Free Makeup SPF 8** *($16.50)* does not list the active sunscreen ingredient, so the SPF is unreliable (and an SPF 8 is too low to be considered anyway). This is still a good foundation for normal to slightly oily skins, with sheer to light coverage and a soft matte finish. This formula dries quickly, so deft blending is essential. The only colors to consider avoiding are Clay 2 and 5, and Sand 1 and 5, as they can be too ash or orange.

☹ <u>CONCEALER:</u> Iman's **Concealer** *($12)* formula has changed from a thick, dry formula to a lightweight, fairly greasy formula. I wish I could say this was an improvement, but aside from the more natural-looking coverage from the original, this tends to stay "wet" and will assuredly crease into any lines around the eyes. This is a shame because the three colors available (no shades for dark skin tones) are superb.

<u>POWDER:</u> ☺ $$$ Both the **Luxury Loose Powder** *($17.50)* and the **Luxury Pressed Powder** *($18)* are standard, talc-based powder with a wonderfully soft, silky texture and a good selection of sheer matte shades that are appropriate for medium to very dark skin tones. The only color to avoid is Clay Medium, which is very orange.

☹ **Sheer Finish Bronzing Powder** *($16)* comes in three gorgeous bronze tones but all of them are very iridescent. These may work for a nighttime walk on the beach but in daylight it will look like you ran into some glitter.

☺ <u>BLUSH:</u> **Luxury Blushing Powder** *($15)* comes in a spectacular array of colors, is a pleasure to apply, and has great staying potential. However, the texture can be too dry for someone with dry skin.

☺ <u>EYESHADOW:</u> **Luxury Eyeshadow** *($10)* has the same slightly dry texture as the blush. There is a nice selection of rich, matte shades to choose from, as well as some obviously shiny colors to sidestep. These colors are beautiful: Plum, Chili, Oak, Onyx, Vanilla, Almond, Cedarchip, and Mahogany.

<u>EYE AND BROW SHAPER:</u> ☺ **Perfect Eye Pencil** *($8.50)* is indeed perfect if you prefer a creamy pencil with a slight powder finish that could easily smudge. **Luxury Liquid Eyeliner** *($12)* claims it is smudge resistant, when it is not in the least. This has a nice, fine-tipped brush and applies evenly but takes way too long to dry, and once it does it can smudge and chip!

☺ **Perfect Eyebrow Pencil** *($12.50)* is standard but nice. This goes on well, and should stay around for a while. There is a brush at the end of the pencil for softening the color.

**LIPSTICK AND LIP PENCIL:** ☺ **Luxury Moisturizing Lipstick** *($12)* calls itself a cream-matte lipstick, which is somewhat misleading. This is really just a nice, creamy, opaque lipstick that leaves a slight stain for longer wear. The color range is gorgeous, and there are some nice sheer shades that are labeled as such but have the same base formula as the rest. **Luxury Lip Gloss** *($10)* is indeed quite luxurious. The texture is smooth and non-sticky, so for gloss aficionados, this is a find! The color selection is small but workable.

☺ **Perfect Lip Pencil** *($11)* is similar to the eye pencil and the same comments apply. These are probably too creamy to prevent lipstick from feathering. **Dual-Tone Lipstick** *($11.50)* is a standard creamy lipstick that has a light and a dark half in colors such as silver and black. These really have no purpose, although the claim is that it helps "adjust the intensity of your lipstick." Save your money and blot with a tissue instead, or just choose a different color.

☹ **MASCARA: Perfect Mascara** *($12)* isn't perfect in the least, unless your definition of perfection is to build no length and absolutely no thickness for your lashes.

# *Jafra*

Regardless of what in-home line of products you choose to try out, each makeup/skin-care demonstration begins the same way. An array of products is set in front of you, and a presentation placard of information is placed next to the salesperson or, to use the preferred term, beauty consultant. You are then taken through a rather fun, hands-on demonstration of products and uses after your skin type has been assessed. Of course, skin typing is almost always hit-or-miss, but I'll get to that in a minute. The skin-care routine generally involves a minimum of six products and, more often than not, "if you really want great skin," an average of seven products, although that rarely includes an adequate sunscreen. Once your face is clean and loaded up with several moisturizers, including an exfoliator, "firming" gel, protective cream, and eye lotion, the makeup application begins.

Jafra's routine is no exception, although this just as accurately describes the techniques of Mary Kay, Shaklee, Amway, and all the others. Like its peers, Jafra offers some products that are great, some that are good, some that are bad, and some that are really bad.

What is unique to Jafra is the way its salespeople determine skin type. They have a cute little machine called a Skin Programmer. It supposedly measures the moisture level of the skin by assessing its electrical conductivity. You hold a metal cylinder in one hand while the salesperson holds a plastic handle with a metal tip on your face.

You don't feel a thing, but a very small electrical charge is generated. How long it takes that electrical charge to complete its circuit—from your cheek or chin to your hand—rates a number. The theory is that the less water (moisture) you have in your skin, the slower the electrical charge; the more water in your skin, the faster the electrical charge. Unfortunately, it only *sounds* good. It doesn't really tell you much about the true condition of your skin. There is so much room for error it's almost a joke. The way your skin registers an electrical current will be different depending on the time of day, what skin-care products you have on, and even the weather. My skin was rated as normal to dry. I explained that I've never had dry skin in my life. I was told that my skin may look oily, but it is only compensating for the dry skin underneath.

That would be fine if oil production worked that way, but it doesn't: oil production is regulated by hormones, not some biological homeostasis. If that weren't so, women with dry skin would automatically have oily skin too, since their oil glands would react to the state of dryness, but, as anyone with dry skin would tell you, that is clearly not the case. You would do much better to follow the skin-type suggestions in Jafra's brochures, which are standard, and ignore the output of the Skin Programmer.

Jafra's color collection has a few fairly interesting selections. It is a rather straightforward line, with all the basics and some good options for a wide range of skin tones. The color line is divided into Warm, Cool, and Neutral, which is helpful, except that some of the Neutrals tend to be warm rather than truly neutral. For more information about Jafra, call (800) 551-2345 or visit the Web site at www.jafra.com.

# Jafra Skin Care

☺ **Cleansing Gel** *($12.50 for 4.2 ounces)* is a good, though very standard, water-soluble detergent-based cleanser for someone with normal to oily skin. It does contain a small amount of chamomile oil, probably more for fragrance than as an emollient oil.

☹ **Cleansing Lotion for Dry to Normal Skin** *($12.50 for 8.4 ounces)* is an oil-based cleanser that needs to be wiped off and can leave skin feeling greasy. It can be an option for someone with normal to dry skin. It does contain a small amount of chamomile oil, probably more for fragrance than as an emollient oil.

☻ **Cleansing Cream for Dry Skin** *($12.50 for 4.2 ounces)* is a thicker version of the Dry to Normal version above; the same review applies, but even more so. While the greasy film may not be a problem for dry skin, wiping off makeup is.

☻ **Cleansing Lotion for Normal to Oily Skin** *($12.50 for 8.4 ounces)* is meant to be wiped off with a washcloth, and that's essential, because it won't come off with simple splashing, as any self-respecting water-soluble cleanser should, especially one for oily skin. This cleanser leaves skin feeling somewhat greasy, which is not great for someone with oily skin.

☺ **Replenishing Cream Cleanser** *($14 for 4.4 ounces)* is a wipe-off cleanser that can leave a somewhat greasy film on the skin. It can still be an option for someone with normal to dry skin. It does contain lemon extract but too small an amount to have an impact on skin.

☹ **$$$ Original Formula Cleansing Cream** *($14 for 3 ounces)* is cold cream, and it is thick, heavy and greasy. It contains mostly mineral oil, wax, lanolin, plant oil, and preservative. It can leave a greasy film on the skin but it is an option for very dry skin.

☺ **Purifying Gel Cleanser** *($14 for 4.4 ounces)* won't purify anything. It is a standard detergent-based water-soluble cleanser that also contains a small amount of salicylic acid, though the pH is too high for it to be an effective exfoliant. It does contain a tiny amount eucalyptus and juniper, which can be skin irritants, though the amount is so small, they probably won't negatively affect skin.

☺ **Balancing Foam Cleanser** *($14 for 4.2 ounces)* is almost identical to the Purifying version and the same basic comments apply.

☹ **Soothing Results Cleansing Lotion** *($12.50 for 8.4 ounces)* is a wipe-off makeup remover that contains lemon peel, which isn't soothing for the skin, but can be an irritant. This can leave a greasy film on the skin.

☺ **$$$ Dual-Action Eye Makeup Remover** *($9 for 2 ounces)* is a silicone-based eye-makeup remover that also contains plant oils. It can leave a slightly greasy film on the skin but it will take off eye makeup.

☺ **Gentle Exfoliating Scrub for All Skin Types** *($12.50 for 2.5 ounces)* isn't all that gentle and it can be slightly greasy. It contains standard synthetic scrub particles, plus several plant oils and other emollient thickeners that make it very hard to rinse off. It also contains several plant extracts that can be skin irritants including balm mint, sage, nettle, coltsfoot, and rosemary.

☹ **Original Formula Skin Freshner** *($14 for 8.4 ounces)* contains mostly water and alcohol as well as menthol, which makes it too irritating for all skin types.

☺ **Skin Freshener for Dry Skin** *($13 for 8.4 ounces)* is a very good toner for someone with normal to dry skin. It does contain a tiny amount of ammonium alum, which can be an irritant, but the amount is so small it won't be a problem for most skin types. This does contain fragrance.

☺ **Skin Freshener for Dry to Normal Skin** *($13 for 8.4 ounces)*. The witch hazel, sandalwood oil, and rose oil this product contains can all be skin irritants.

☹ **Skin Freshener for Normal to Oily Skin** *($13 for 8.4 ounces)* contains a lot of alcohol, which can dry and irritate the skin (causing it to become more oily). It also contains plant oils, the last thing someone with oily skin would want on her face.

☹ **Skin Freshener for Oily Skin** *($13 for 8.4 ounces)* contains a lot of alcohol and plant extracts that can all be potent skin irritants for all skin types. It also contains lemon extract and menthol, which only add fuel to the fire.

☺ **Soothing Results Calming Toner for Sensitive Skin** *($13 for 8.4 ounces)* is a good toner for normal to dry skin. It contains mostly water, water-binding agents, plant extracts, fragrance, and preservatives.

☹ **Stimulating Tonic Spritzer** *($15 for 6.7 ounces)* is just glycerin and water with some fragrant plant extracts. That can be refreshing, but the plant extracts in here can be a problem for the skin.

☹ **Rediscover Alpha Hydroxy Complex** *($31 for 1 ounce)* contains several fruit extracts, but sugarcane extract and apple extract are not related to AHAs. This moisturizer cannot exfoliate skin and that is the only real purpose of a well-formulated AHA product. It contains lavender and coriander oil, which are potential skin irritants.

☺ **$$$ Advanced Time Protector Daily Defense Cream, SPF 15** *($38 for 1.7 ounces)* is a very good in-part zinc oxide–based sunscreen. It is also in a very good moisturizing base for someone with normal to dry skin.

☹ **Day Cream Moisturizer for Dry to Normal Skin SPF 6** *($15 for 1.7 ounces)* SPF 6 is inadequate for daily protection from sun damage and it doesn't contain UVA-protecting ingredients of titanium dioxide, zinc oxide, or avobenzone. This is absolutely not recommended.

☹ **Day Lotion for Normal to Oily Skin SPF 6** *($15 for 4.2 ounces)* has similar issues to the Dry to Normal Skin version above and the same comments apply.

☹ **Day Lotion for Oily Skin SPF 6** *($15 for 4.2 ounces)* has similar issues to the Dry to Normal Skin version above and the same comments apply.

☹ **Lipid Intense Hydrator SPF 12** *($23 for 1.7 ounces)*. SPF 15 would be far better, though this is a good in-part zinc oxide–based sunscreen. This isn't intense but it is a good moisturizer for normal to dry skin.

☹ **Moisture Response Hydrator SPF 12** *($19 for 1.7 ounces)* is similar to the Lipid Intense Hydrator above and the same basic comments apply.

☹ **Moisture Manager Hydrator SPF 12** *($16 for 1.7 ounces)*. SPF 15 would be far better, though this is a good in-part zinc oxide–based sunscreen. The rather boring moisturizing base is mostly water and thickeners, making it a mediocre product all around.

☹ **Oil Control Hydrator SPF 12** *($16 for 1.7 ounces)* is similar to the Moisture Manager above and the same basic comments apply.

☺ **$$$ Elasticity Recovery Hydrogel** *($35 for 1 ounce)*. There is nothing in here that will help elasticity in skin but it is a good lightweight moisturizer for normal to slightly dry skin.

☹ **Extra Care Cream** *($8 for 0.5 ounce)* is a very emollient, very greasy, and mundane moisturizer for someone with very dry skin.

☹ **Royal Moisture Cream** *($16 for 1.7 ounces)* is almost identical to the Extra Care above and the same comments apply.

☺ **Night Cream for Dry Skin** (*$15 for 1.7 ounces*) is a very good moisturizer for someone with normal to dry skin.

☺ **Night Cream Moisturizer for Dry to Normal Skin** (*$15 for 1.7 ounces*). Someone with normal skin will probably find this too emollient, but it is a very good moisturizer for someone with dry skin.

☺ **Night Cream for Normal to Oily Skin** (*$15 for 1.7 ounces*). Women with oily skin could find themselves with clogged pores and more oil than they started out with, but it could be a good moisturizer for normal to dry skin types.

☺ **Night Lotion** (*$15 for 4.2 ounces*) is a very good moisturizer for someone with normal to dry skin.

☺ **Overnight Replenisher** (*$25 for 1.7 ounces*) is a good moisturizer for normal to dry skin. This isn't the most exciting of the moisturizers to be found in this group but it is still well-formulated.

☺ **$$$ Time Corrector Firming Moisture Cream** (*$38 for 1.7 ounces*) won't correct one minute on your face, or firm anything, but it is a good moisturizer for dry skin.

☹ **$$$ Royal Jelly Moisture Balm Lotion, Original Formula** (*$60 for 1 ounce*). You may be wondering why this otherwise standard moisturizer sells for $60 an ounce. Jafra touts royal jelly as a miracle ingredient. The salesperson told me it could heal burns, get rid of scars, and erase wrinkles. It sure sounds like a miracle. Is it? Well, bee larvae who get fed *fresh* royal jelly turn into queen bees. But if you try to sneak *stored* royal jelly into them, they don't turn into queens. As natural and interesting as that all sounds, there is still no evidence that royal jelly has any miracle benefit for the skin, though it can be a topical disinfectant. The other moisturizers in the Jafra line up are far more interesting than this one or the others with royal jelly that follow.

☺ **$$$ Royal Jelly Milk Balm Moisture Lotion Dry and Normal to Dry** (*$60 for 1 ounce*) is a good moisturizer for normal dry skin, but if you are expecting something special from the royal jelly, give it up. This royal jelly gimmick doesn't translate to good skin care. The far more interesting water-binding agents and emollients in this product are what make it worthwhile, not the bee-stuff.

☹ **$$$ Royal Jelly Milk Balm Moisture Lotion, Unscented** (*$60 for 1 ounce*) is a very heavy, ordinary moisturizer. Of course there is some royal jelly, but it's unimportant. This can be an option for very dry skin, but it can clog pores and dull skin.

☺ **Sunblock Cream SPF 15, Advanced UVA/UVB Protection** (*$11.50 for 4.2 ounces*) is a very good in-part avobenzone-based sunscreen that would be appropriate for normal to slightly dry skin. On the ingredient label, avobenzone is listed by its formal chemical name butyl methoxydibenzoylmethane.

☺ **Sunblock Cream SPF 30, Advanced UVA/UVB Protection** (*$12 for 4.2 ounces*) is similar to the Sunblock Cream SPF 15 above, only with longer sun protection. The same basic review applies.

☹ **Sunscreen Cream SPF 8, Advanced UVA/UVB Protection** *($10.50 for 4.2 ounces)*. While this does contain avobenzone for UVA protection, the SPF 8 makes it unreliable for daily sun proteciton.

☹ **Clear Blemish Treatment** *($9.50 for 0.5 ounce)* has a pH of 3, which is great, but it also contains alcohol and that's a problem for healing breakouts.

☹ **Clear Pore Clarifier** *($15 for 1.7 ounces)* has a pH closer to 5, which means it isn't low enough for the BHA (salicylic acid) to have an effect. This product also contains clove oil, which can be a skin irritant.

☺ **Deep Cleansing Mask for Normal to Oily Skin** *($12.50 for 2.5 ounces)* is a fairly standard clay-based mask that also contains a small amount of fragrant plant extracts, silicone, and lots of thickening agents. This would be an OK clay mask for someone with normal to dry skin. The teeny amount of tea tree oil in here isn't enough to be effective as a topical disinfectant.

☹ **Malibu Miracle Mask** *($13.50 for 1.7 ounces)* is about as an unmiraculous a skin-care product as you can get. The only miracle is that Jafra can convince some women that it is a miracle. This contains peppermint and spearmint oil, which makes it potentially irritating for all skin types.

☺ **Refreshing Moisture Mask for Dry and Dry to Normal Skin** *($12.50 for 2.5 ounces)*. Although I'm not one to recommend clay masks for dry skin, this one contains such a small amount of clay that it would be quite a good emollient mask. This does contain fragrant oils.

☺ **Soothing Results Cooling Yogurt and Honey Mask, for Sensitive Skin** *($12.50 for 2.6 ounces)* is a clay mask with several plant oils, thickeners, and water-binding agents. Clay isn't the best thing for sensitive skin, and can be a skin irritant, but this would be a good mask for someone with dry skin.

# Jafra Makeup

**FOUNDATION:** ☹ **Moisturizing Makeup SPF 6** *($12)* does not offer UVA protection, and even if it did, the SPF is embarrassingly low. This does have a very smooth texture that provides medium coverage, but the range of 12 shades are too peach, pink, or rose for most skin tones. The only shade to consider is Cashmere, which may work for some darker skins.

☹ **Oil-Controlling Makeup SPF 6** *($12)* has fewer shades than the one above, and the same problems with overly peach, pink, or rose colors. The texture is great, but that's no consolation for a lack of neutral, flesh-toned shades and a dismal SPF with no UVA protection.

☹ **Always Color Stay On Makeup SPF 10** *($15)* does not list any sunscreen ingredients and after much searching, Jafra's Customer Service relayed that they use non-active sunscreens, which makes no sense, as the FDA stipulations regarding sunscreen labeling are quite strict: all sunscreen ingredients are active ingredients. This remains a lightweight, ultra-matte finish foundation that dries quickly and provides medium, semi-opaque coverage. The 16 shades are disappointing; the only colors to consider are for darker skins, and they include Espresso, Rich Mahogany, and Chestnut.

CONCEALER: ☹ Cream Concealer *($8.75)* comes in stick form, and offers six mediocre colors. The newer dark shades are decidedly more neutral than the lighter tones, which are too peachy-pink to look natural. On top of that, the texture of this makes creasing all too easy. Total Concealer *($9.75)* comes in a tube with a wand, and the three shades aren't much better than those for the Cream Concealer above and are therefore not the best option for most skin tones.

☺ White Soufflé Highlighter *($9)* is a liquid concealer that is indeed white, but it goes on very subtly, requiring just a tiny bit to lighten a shadow under the eye or along the corners of the mouth or nose. It can be used under or over foundation for highlighting without iridescence.

☺ POWDER: Translucent Face Powder *($12)* and Pressed Powder *($12)* are talc-based and have an improved texture that is incredibly soft and smooth. The finish is light and not as dry as most powders, making it a good choice for normal to dry skin. The six colors are good albeit slightly peach so be careful, though the sheer finish can negate that concern. Check this in the daylight to make sure.

☺ BLUSH: Powder Blush *($11)* has a great soft texture that blends on smoothly and evenly without grabbing or streaking. All of the colors are great, but be aware that Bronze, Pink Silk, and Soft Peach all have shine. Beyond that, the colors, though lacking many neutrals, are great. There are some good options for darker skins, such as Terra Cotta, Desert, and Copper.

☺ EYESHADOW: Jafra offers Eyeshadow Duos *($11.50)* and Trios *($11.50)*. This is a line that simply doesn't sell single eyeshadows, and some of the color combinations available are too shiny or strangely contrasting to be able to create a coordinated eye design. However, in spite of the fact that I think buying sets of three shadows is a great way to waste money (you rarely use all the colors), there are a handful of surprisingly neutral, workable groupings. The only matte combinations to consider are Bazaar, Caravan, Neutral Ground, and Mirage. The Duos feature one shiny shade, so those are up to you.

☺ EYE AND BROW SHAPER: Eye and Brow Pencils *($7)* are both standard pencils with a creamy application and dry finish. The colors are fine, but for the Eye Pencils, avoid the gold, green, and blue shades. Liquid Eyeliner *($9.25)* has a very thin, soft brush that tends to make the application spotty and more difficult than usual. Inkwell Eyeliner *($9.25)* is a better choice for liquid liner, and has a brush that is soft but firm enough to get the job done without incident. The only drawback is that this takes some time to dry, and that risks smearing. **Automatic Eye Liner** *($8.50)* is a standard twist-up pencil that applies smoothly but stays creamy, so smudging can be an issue.

LIPSTICK AND LIP PENCIL: ☺ **Classic Long Lasting Moisturizing Lipsticks** *($8)* are basic creamy lipsticks with a slightly glossy finish. The color selection is wonderful. **Always Color Stay-On Lipstick** *($9.50)* is Jafra's version of Revlon's ColorStay lipstick. This one works quite well, with a soft and opaque ultra-matte finish. The best part is that these tend not to flake or peel off like a lot of ultra-matte lipsticks do. **Lip Lacquer** *($7.50)* is a smooth, slightly sticky lip gloss with some strong, opaque colors to choose from. It will last longer than traditional gloss due to the higher pigmentation.

☹ **Time Protector Lipstick SPF 15** *($10.50)* left out reliable UVA protection and that is the only ingredient that could have been realistically tied to the "time-protecting" name. These also claim to be anti-feathering, but the slightly greasy, semi-opaque texture negates that possibility entirely. **Lip Pencil** *($7)* is reasonably priced for a very standard, slightly creamy pencil. **Automatic Lip Pencil** *($8.50)* is a creamy, soft twist-up pencil that glides on but won't help keep lipstick in place for long if you're prone to colors bleeding.

☹ MASCARA: **Optimascara** *($7.75)* does build nice length and some thickness but tends to smear and flake after just a few hours. **Waterproof Mascara** *($7.75)* builds good length and noticeable thickness though it can feel sticky and heavy when applied. Plus, if this gets even slightly wet, you'll see what a joke the waterproof claim is.

☹ BRUSHES: Jafra's brush sets tend to come and go, but they regularly feature the **Deluxe Face Powder Brush** *($11)* which is full but loose and floppy, so powder will fly everywhere, and the **Retractable Blush Brush** *($7)* would be OK in a pinch, but is too small and loose for professional results.

# *Jan Marini Skin Research*

Jan Marini Skin Research, Inc. was founded, of course, by Jan Marini, who originally started out marketing products for M.D. Formulations. Thus it isn't surprising to find that her own line is also aimed at dermatologists and plastic surgeons much the way M.D. Formulations is. Marini's line stands out in direct contrast to many of the other skin-care lines reviewed here, with far more realistic and varied skin-care products. First, there are no spiraling-out-of-control ingredient listings where everything is thrown in except the kitchen sink. But more important, there are some well-formulated products that include sunscreens, an acne formulation, glycolic acid–based alpha hydroxy acid (AHA), beta hydroxy acid (BHA) products, and skin-lightening options. Two additional strong points are that many of the products are fragrance-free, while all are free from coloring agents!

For good or bad, there are also some of the current trendy ingredient offerings, ranging from retinol to vitamin C and growth factors, along with a smattering of exotic plant extracts. It is interesting to note that Marini attributes the research for her "topical form of lipid (fat) soluble Vitamin C that is stable and able to be absorbed as developed in conjunction with physician researcher Nicholas Perricone, M.D." Now that Perricone has his own version of vitamin C products (quite similar to Marini's, by the way, using ascorbyl palmitate and magnesium ascorbyl palmitate), and given that he claims his are the best ever with the highest concentration of the stuff, I wonder if she would now agree with his findings. Does that mean we should all buy Perricone's products? Or do they both get rid of wrinkles and Perricone is wrong about the superiority of his products? The saga of the cosmetics and vitamin C wars continues.

As I discussed earlier in this book, there is no conclusive research about vitamin C eliminating even one wrinkle on the skin, something Perricone concludes in his own writings. I've also discussed at length the limited research (and thus my resulting skepticism) about the value of vitamin A (retinol) cosmetics products on the skin. If you still want in on either vitamin C or vitamin A, this line definitely has some pricey versions to consider. Ironically, the claims made by the world of cosmetics for vitamin C and vitamin A are almost identical. So once again you have to wonder, if vitamin C gets rid of wrinkles, why would you need vitamin A? It never fails to amaze me that women still have wrinkles with all these anti-aging products.

Marini uses "growth factor" in a group of products called "Transformation." The actual ingredient is transforming growth factor (TGF beta-1). TGF beta-1 is a complex protein known to bring about changes in connective tissue. TGF is a human growth factor responsible primarily for wound-healing. It stimulates collagen production, or, a far better description, according to Dr. Bruce A. Mast, M.D., Division of Plastic and Reconstructive Surgery, Department of Surgery, University of Florida, Gainesville, would be that TGF beta-1 "is a proscarring component of healing." Mast explained that in order for a wound to heal, the body has to be able to create scar material, or collagen, for skin. That kind of collagen production is not related to the skin's support structure. Mast's concern in regard to TGF beta-1 in skin-care products is that if it really worked, it could encourage scar formation on skin, and that doesn't improve the appearance of wrinkles.

For the most part, Marini's professional information packet is exceptional, offering a wealth of accurately stated facts about skin care and the effect products have on the skin. The information about vitamin A, vitamin C, and the growth factors is overblown, but it is nevertheless in essence accurate. For example, one of the information sheets for the Marini line explains that "approximately 90% to 95% of what we think is inevitable aging is the result of cumulative sun damage. Most of this damage is programmed into the skin in childhood, but it takes many years to manifest itself." No one argues with this fact. It then goes on to say that most of that damage is reversible by using these products. Wouldn't that be nice! But then it would be true for lots of products out there that contain similar if not identical formulations, not to mention many that are less expensive than these.

For more information about the availability of Jan Marini Skin Research products, call (408) 362-0130 or (800) 347-2223, or visit the Web site at www.jmskin research.com.

☺ **Bioglycolic BioClean Cleanser** *($25 for 8 ounces)* is a standard, detergent-based water-soluble cleanser that would work well for most skin types.

☹ **Bioglycolic Facial Cleanser** *($25 for 8 ounces)* is a standard detergent-based water-soluble cleanser that includes AHA. While AHAs are great for exfoliating, their effectiveness would be rinsed down the drain and problematic if it got into the eyes on the way. Thankfully the pH of this product is too high for it to be effective as an exfoliant and so it doesn't pose much risk.

☹ **Bioglycolic Oily Skin Cleansing Gel** *($25 for 8 ounces)* is similar to the Facial Cleanser above only with a higher concentration of detergent cleansing agents. That may be better for oily skin but the AHA in here is still a problem.

☺ **$$$ Bioglycolic Cream** *($60 for 2 ounces).* This is a well-formulated AHA moisturizer that would be great for normal to dry skin. It does contain sodium hyaluronate, but that is just one of many good water-binding agents for skin and doesn't make this a superlative formulation. If you are looking for AHAs, there are many far less expensive options to consider.

☺ **$$$ Bioglycolic Facial Lotion** *($45 for 2 ounces)* is similar to the cream above only in lotion form. The same basic comments apply.

☺ **$$$ Bioglycolic Facial Lotion SPF 15** *($45 for 2 ounces)* is a good, titanium dioxide–based sunscreen for someone with normal to slightly dry skin. It has about an 8% to 10% AHA content (glycolic acid); however, the pH of 4 to 5 makes it minimally effective for exfoliation. Using an expensive sunscreen can also be problematic. As is true for all sunscreens, a liberal application is essential to receive the SPF number on the label, and expensive ones tend to make users reluctant when it comes to applying sunscreen generously.

☹ **$$$ Bioglycolic Eye Cream** *($33 for 0.5 ounce).* The pH of 4.5 to 5 is too high for this to have an effect as an exfoliant.

☺ **Bioglycolic Even Tone Pigment Lightening Gel** *($35 for 2 ounces)* is a good, hydroquinone-based skin-lightening solution in a lightweight gel formula. It also includes AHA, although the pH is too high for that ingredient to be effective as an exfoliant. A separate, well-formulated AHA product would be of help with this gel because the exfoliation AHAs provide can improve the appearance of skin discolorations. Along with the AHA, a well-formulated sunscreen is essential to get results. This product also contains kojic acid, which has some effect in reducing melanin production, but that information is derived from in vitro studies and not on human skin.

☺ $$$ **Bioglycolic BioClear** *($50 for 1 ounce)* contains about 8% to 10% AHA and about 1% BHA in a fairly basic, lightweight moisturizing formula. It would work well for exfoliation for someone with normal to dry skin. Generally, though, the combination of AHA and BHA isn't the best option. BHA can exfoliate both in the pore and on the surface of skin, so it isn't necessary to have the AHA, which only affects the surface. Given that BHA can cover both territories, using it alone is the best way to start to reduce the risk of irritation. This one contains mostly water, AHA, thickeners, glycerin, water-binding agents, plant extracts, BHA, and preservatives.

☹ **Bioglycolic Acne Gel I** *($35 for 2 ounces)* contains a mixture of AHA and BHA, though either one or the other alone would be better. BHA is preferred for fighting breakouts due to its ability to exfoliate in the pore and on the surface of skin, while AHA works primarily on the surface. Regardless, alcohol is the first ingredient in this product, and that can cause dryness and irritation, making breakouts worse, and while the lavender oil in here has a nice fragrance it's best left off reddened, acne-prone skin.

☹ **Bioglycolic Acne Gel II** *($35 for 2 ounces)* is almost identical to the Acne Gel 1 above and the same comments apply.

☺ **Bioglycolic Sunless Self Tanner** *($25 for 4 ounces)* is a standard, dihydroxyacetone-based self tanner, and although this product contains AHA it is in a high-pH base that makes it ineffective as an exfoliant; that's actually preferred, or you would simply lose the tan you just applied.

☹ **Benzoyl Peroxide Wash 2.5%** *($25 for 4 ounces)* is a cleanser, and because a cleanser is washed away, the effective ingredient, benzoyl peroxide, would be rinsed down the drain. For most all skin types, any of the following three benzoyl peroxide products would be a far better consideration, especially since then there would be no risk of accidentally splashing it in the eye.

☺ $$$ **Benzoyl Peroxide 2.5%** *($25 for 4 ounces)* is a reliable topical disinfectant to use for fighting breakouts, but there are similar if not identical versions available for far less.

☺ $$$ **Benzoyl Peroxide 5%** *($25 for 4 ounces)* is similar to the one above, only in a more potent strength.

☺ $$$ **Benzoyl Peroxide 10%** *($25 for 4 ounces)* is similar to the one above, only in a more potent strength.

☺ $$$ **C-Esta Cleansing Gel** *($25 for 6 ounces)*. If you want vitamin C, this line has enough options to keep you well supplied. This is a standard, detergent-based water-soluble cleanser. For the money, if you want vitamin C on your skin, it would be better to get it in a form that stays on the skin rather than in a cleanser that would rinse down the drain.

☺ $$$ **C-Esta Cream** *($75 for 1 ounce)* now brings you more vitamin C. It is a fine, though overpriced option for vitamin C.

☺ $$$ **C-Esta Eye Contour Cream** *($40 for 0.5 ounce)* is similar to the version above and the same comments apply.

☺ $$$ **C-Esta Eye Repair Concentrate** *($55 for 0.5 ounce)* is similar to the versions above, only in a gel-like lotion form.

☺ $$$ **C-Esta Lips** *($40 for 0.5 ounce)* assumes that none of these other products can be used around the mouth, so now you have one just for the lips. But it's similar to the versions above and the same comments apply. This version does contain fragrance.

☺ $$$ **Factor-A Cream** *($45 for 1 ounce)* is as good an option for vitamin A as any, though there are far less expensive options available.

☹ $$$ **Factor-A Plus Cream** *($45 for 1 ounce)* would have been a good option if you were looking for a combination of vitamin A and AHA, but the pH is too high to make this one an effective exfoliant.

☹ **Factor-A Plus Lotion** *($40 for 1 ounce)* contains alcohol as the second ingredient, which can be a problem for skin.

☺ $$$ **Factor-A Lotion** *($40 for 1 ounce)* is much like the one above minus the AHA and alcohol, and is a good lightweight version of the Plus Lotion, assuming vitamin A is what's needed.

☹ $$$ **Transformation Cream** *($60 for 1 ounce)*. The big-deal ingredient in this product is transforming growth factor (TGF beta-1). As I described above, the claims for what this ingredient can do are at best exaggerated and its effectiveness is not established in skin-care products.

☹ $$$ **Transformation Eye Cream** *($40 for 0.5 ounce)*. Like the above Cream, this version also contains TGF beta-1 and the same comments apply. This one also contains sugarcane extract, but that is not an AHA, nor is the pH here appropriate for exfoliation.

☹ $$$ **Transformation Serum** *($50 for 1 ounce)* is similar to the one above, only this version is lighter in weight and would be better for someone with normal to slightly dry skin.

☺ $$$ **Antioxidant Group Skin Silk Protecting Hydrator** *($40 for 1 ounce)* is a good basic moisturizer for normal to dry skin.

☺ $$$ **Antioxidant Group Recover-E** *($40 for 1 ounce)* is a good moisturizer for dry skin, and vitamin E is a good antioxidant.

☹ **Antioxidant Group Daily Face Protectant SPF 30** *($45 for 2 ounces)* doesn't contain UVA protection and is not recommended. Further, the risk of buying an expensive sunscreen is that you will not use it "liberally" and liberal application is essential for the product to perform up to the SPF number on the label.

☺ **Clean Zyme** *($20 for 4 ounces).* Despite all the fancy words about how papaya (a source of the enzyme papain) works, this is basically just another topical exfoliant much like AHA or BHA. This version is an option for someone with normal to oily skin, though issues of how stable the papaya is are still a concern.

☺ **$$$ Day Zyme** *($40 for 1 ounce)* is similar to the version above only in a slightly thicker form for someone with normal to slightly dry skin.

☺ **$$$ Night Zyme** *($40 for 1 ounce)* is similar to the Day Zyme, only slightly more emollient. It would be an option for someone with normal to dry skin.

☺ **Skin Zyme** *($35 for 2 ounces)* is almost identical to the Night Zyme above and the same comments apply.

# *Jane*

Jane was a little-known cosmetics line aimed at teenagers and sold in drugstores. But the "little-known" status is a thing of the past since Estee Lauder purchased the line in 1997. Jane is still a group of products aimed at teenagers, only the line now has far more money to launch a bevy of new products. Aside from the financial infusion, what remains intact are the brochures accompanying the display for Jane products, with bright young faces bemoaning the beauty problems and needs of adolescence and extolling cute makeup and skin-care solutions.

At first glance this is all harmless fun, but there is an aspect to this kind of marketing directed at teenage girls that is quite disturbing. Most, if not all, of Jane's marketing is aimed at encouraging girls to achieve status and happiness through makeup. For example, Jane's LipKick Liquid Lipstick is explained as follows: "What a rush. 8 all-new, kick @#$$% [kick-ass is the likely translation] colors with those high-energy botanicals Ginseng and Ginkgo. ... Great when you feel down in the mouth." While there is the occasional Jane comment that says, "Feeling good about yourself is sexy," the overwhelming impression is that feeling good takes makeup. This message is problematic and makes me worry about the influence that outlook has on impressionable young girls whose self-esteem at this age is extremely fragile and vulnerable.

While Jane's approach might be directed at teenagers, the simple black packaging, neutral colors, and vivid, creamy lipstick colors seem to be much more in alignment with what adults would be interested in. The prices are more than reasonable, and many of the colors are appropriate for a wide range of skin tones. What is certainly aimed at teenagers are Jane's flavored lip products that taste like vanilla, butterscotch, pineapple, peach, cinnamon, and several others. Flavored lipsticks are clearly aimed at teenage girls too old for Barbie, but not old enough to make adult decisions.

The Reviews J

Now that Estee Lauder's money is fully invested in Jane, the line has launched a group of skin-care products called Good Skin. These products do not veer from the teenage angle, and are about feeling fresh, getting rid of oil, and fighting blemishes every step of the way. Regrettably, this is also about giving teenagers what they think they want instead of what can help. While that makes good marketing sense—it's hard to change a teenager's mind about anything she believes is true—it isn't the best for skin.

For more information about Jane, call (800) 820-JANE or visit the Web site at www.janecosmetics.com.

## Jane Skin Care

☺ **ClenZing Gel, Gentle** *($5.99 for 5 ounces)* is a standard, detergent-based water-soluble cleanser that would work well for normal to oily skin. However, there is nothing gentle about this product. It is highly fragranced too, and that can be problematic for those with sensitive skin.

☺ **ClenZing Gel, Normal** *($5.99 for 5 ounces)* is a standard, detergent-based water-soluble cleanser that would work OK for oily skin. It is highly fragranced and that can be problematic for those with sensitive skin. It also uses TEA-lauryl sulfate as the third ingredient, and that can make it drying for some skin types.

☺ **ClenZing Gel, Oily** *($5.99 for 5 ounces)* is almost identical to the Normal version above, only this one contains clove extract, which can be a skin irritant. This is not the one from this group to choose for any skin type.

☺ **ClenZing To-Go, Stick Cleanser, Gentle** *($5.49 for 2 ounces)* is more of a makeup remover/toner in a stick form. It would work well to remove makeup but can feel slippery on skin that's looking to feel fresh and oil-free.

☹ **ClenZing To-Go, Stick Cleanser, Normal** *($5.49 for 2 ounces)* contains cornstarch, lemon extract, and lots of fragrance. Cornstarch is problem for clogging pores, and in general the Gentle version above is the better choice.

☹ **ClenZing To-Go, Stick Cleanser, Oily** *($5.49 for 2 ounces)*. Cornstarch is problem for clogging pores, and the other ingredients are potentially irritating. Overall, the Gentle version above is the better choice. This version does contain tea tree oil (melaleuca) but not enough to make a difference for breakouts.

☹ **Cloudburst Cleanser, Foaming Face Wash, Gentle** *($6.99 for 4 ounces)* uses sodium C14-16 olefin sulfate as the main detergent cleansing agent (listed as the second ingredient), which makes it potentially too irritating for all skin types.

☹ **Cloudburst Cleanser, Foaming Face Wash, Normal** *($6.99 for 4 ounces)* is similar to the Gentle version above and the same comments apply.

☹ **Cloudburst Cleanser, Foaming Face Wash, Oily** *($6.99 for 4 ounces)* is similar to the Gentle version above and the same comments apply.

☺ **Seeds & Weeds Face Scrub** *($6.99 for 5 ounces)* is a fairly abrasive scrub that would indeed exfoliate skin, but the thickening agents in here can be problematic for those worried about breakouts.

☹ **Automatte Mattifying Toner** *($5.99 for 6 ounces)* lists alcohol as the second ingredient and that makes it too irritating, drying, and reddening for all skin types.

☹ **Be Pure Astringent for Oily Skin** *($5.49 for 6 ounces)* lists alcohol as the second ingredient, and it also contains menthol among other potentially irritating ingredients, and is not recommended.

☺ **Light Energy Oil-Control Moisturizer** *($5.99 for 4 ounces)*. This has a fairly matte finish and is barely (really not) moisturizing at all, which is great for someone with oily skin. The amount of witch hazel in this product isn't enough to be a concern for skin. The BHA is about a 1% concentration but the pH of 4.5 makes it minimally effective as an exfoliant.

☹ **Mudville Cooling Earth Mask** *($6.99 for 4 ounces)* is a standard clay mask that would be an option, except the cooling effect is caused by the menthol it contains and that makes it too irritating and reddening for all skin types.

☹ **Peel Out Acne Treatment Gel Patch** *($5.49 for 0.75 ounce)* has alcohol as the second ingredient, which makes it too irritating, drying, and reddening for all skin types.

☹ **Spot Off Invisible Acne Treatment Gel** *($5.49 for 6 ounces)* has alcohol as the second ingredient, which makes it too irritating, drying, and reddening for all skin types.

# Jane Makeup

<u>FOUNDATION</u>: Jane's foundation formulas do not have any colors suitable for darker skin tones, so this is clearly a line aimed at fairer-skinned youth and definitely not African Americans. ☹ **Oil Free Foundation** *($2.99)* features eight mostly neutral shades and a soft matte finish. What a shame it applies so choppy and tends to just sit on the skin, looking obvious. With some slight adjustments, this could be a wonderful option.

☺ **True to You Sheer Finish Foundation** *($2.99)* has a rather good range of neutral colors and a nice, smooth texture that goes on quite sheer and smooth. It is assuredly an improvement over the one above. There are shades to avoid and testers are usually scarce but occasionally they sell a small sample bottle for less than one dollar, so consider giving this a try if you have normal to slightly dry skin and prefer sheer coverage.

☺ **Lightweight Liquid Powder** *($2.38)* is a cream-to-powder makeup that has a very slick, almost wet feel and a dry, powdery finish. Before you get too excited, keep in mind that, because of the waxes used to hold this product together, oilier skins will see shine in no time and the possibility of breaking out would also be increased. It can also make any dry skin you have look more noticeable. Still, this would be an option for normal skin types seeking a smooth, sheer finish and the price is almost too good not to give it a try! These colors may be too pink, rose, or orange for some skin tones: Beige, Creamy, and Tan.

CONCEALER: ☺ **No Show Concealer** *($2.99)* comes in stick form but has a surprisingly satiny texture and three workable colors. This has a slight tendency to slip into lines around the eyes as the day goes by, although it's not as bad as some and it shouldn't be a problem at all for those who do not have any lines to speak of. **Clueless Two Way Concealer** *($2.99)* is a decent concealer with soft coverage and good staying power, but it does tend to slip into lines under the eyes. The color choices are limited but what's there is neutral enough to work well.

☹ **Write Away Concealer** *($2.99)* is a standard pencil concealer that features two very good colors but a greasy, thick application that will undoubtedly crease and look obvious on the skin.

POWDER: ☹ **Oil-Free Finishing Powder** *($2.38)* is a talc-based pressed powder with a soft, silky-dry texture that applies sheer and even, and a range of colors that are decidedly peach-toned. Lighter skin tones may want to try Colorless or Fair, but should still be cautious.

☺ **Staying Powder Loose Powder** *($2.99)* is a very good, dry-finish, exceedingly standard talc-based powder. This would be best for someone with oily skin, and the colors (four in all) are fine except for Light, which is too orange. **Radiation All-Over Body Glimmer** *($2.38)* is simply loose, iridescent powder in both flesh-toned and vivid shades. If the shine trend continues, this would be a cheap way to keep up with the fad.

☺ BLUSH: **Blushing Cheeks** *($2.99)* all have a soft, smooth texture and go on quite sheer. The color range is impressive, and although there are a few with noticeable shine, the majority are matte. These would be excellent for very light to medium skin tones. **Sweet Cheeks Instant Blush** *($2.99)* is a very good cream-to-powder blush that comes in a small but viable range of colors. The texture is identical to the Lightweight Liquid Powder reviewed above and these all apply sheer and blend surprisingly well, though it does take some effort to keep this looking smooth.

☺ EYESHADOW: **Eye Zing Shadow** *($2.99)* is a collection of powder eyeshadows that have a soft, easy-to-blend texture. Many of the shades are shiny, so choose carefully (if you have lines, these will make them more apparent), and you're bound to be pleased with both performance and price!

☺ EYE AND BROW SHAPER: The fairly standard **Gliding Eye Liner, One Liners for Eyes** (automatic pencils) and **High Brow Pencils** *(all $2.99 each)* all go on well without being greasy, dragging, or looking choppy. They would be an option for anyone, regardless of age. If you prefer using pencils to matte powder eyeshadows, these are as good as any you'll find. **Brow Beaters Tinted Brow Groomer** *($2.99)* is a standard, slightly sticky brow gel with such a small amount of color as to be almost insignificant. For those who need some brow taming with a slight, sheer, brownish color, this is an option to consider. **Express Lines Liquid to Powder Liner** *($2.99)* is a decent option for liquid eyeliner, with a thin, firm brush that lays down an even line. This dries quickly, so precision is key, but for those who have the knack or prefer liquid liner, this is a welcome addition.

LIPSTICK AND LIP PENCIL: ☺ Jane must know that teenagers can't help but buy lipsticks and glosses because the options for lips from this small line of products is astounding. **Lip Huggers Satin Lipstick** *($2.99)* may be too creamy and opaque for teens and too glossy and slippery for adults. The colors are fine, but this is one slippery, glossy lipstick. **Lip Huggers Matte/Shimmer Lipstick** *($2.99)* are not really matte but they are smooth and light with a frosty finish and only a slightly creamy feel. **Barely Lips Sheer Lipstick** *($2.99)* is right up a teen's alley and may work for adults looking for an emollient, glossy lipstick with only a hint of color. **Hip Lips Lipstick** *($2.99)* has a creamy, smooth texture and a fair amount of stain. There are only eight shades, but these are worth a look and the Pez-style dispenser is truly unique and fun. **Quik Stix** *($2.99)* are the traditional chubby lip pencils that seem like a good idea but end up being just a slightly greasy lipstick you have to sharpen. At this price, that may not be such a bad trade-off! **Gloss Overs** *($2.99)* is reasonably priced, very standard, pot lip-gloss—nothing more, nothing less. **One Liners Lip Liners** *($2.99)* are automatic lip pencils that have a smooth texture and a great color selection. **Shaping Sticks** *($2.99)* are standard pencils with a middle-of-the-road texture: not too dry or too greasy. The color selection is worth checking out and at these prices, feel free to experiment. **One for All** *($2.99)* has a creamy application with a somewhat dry finish. It is intended for use on the eyes, cheeks, and lips, but may be too oversized for the shape of most women's lips. Still, if you can get the knack for applying this, it can work well as a multipurpose product.

☺ **MegaBites Flavorful Lip Color** *($2.99)* are standard creamy lipsticks that are all food-flavored. The accompanying taste may seem inviting or repulsive, depending on your mood. **LipKick Energizing Liquid Lipstick** *($2.99)* is an intensely flavored sheer lipstick that you apply with a wand. These are more akin to lip gloss, only with more color. **Lickety Stix Double Gloss** *($2.99)* are two flavored, Chap Stick–style lip balms with a slight tint. If you like the idea of tasty lipsticks, that's one issue; the other is that ingesting any major amount of lipstick is not a good idea and these kinds of products encourage young girls to do just that. **Lip Dips Pot Lipstick** *($2.99)* is similar to the Gloss Overs above but these have an undesirable sticky, goopy texture.

MASCARA: ☺ Flashes Ultra-Rich Mascara *($2.99)* is surprisingly good; it goes on fast, building thick, even lashes with little to no smearing.

☹ Splashes Water-Resistant Mascara *($2.99)* builds just OK length and minimal thickness. It doesn't smear, which is good, but it's unreliable as waterproof mascara.

☺ BRUSHES: Jane's brushes aren't awful, they are just the wrong shape and tend to have a poor consistency. The eyeshadow brushes are too small and thin, while the powder and blush brushes are soft enough but aren't the best sizes and don't have the best density of bristles for proper application.

# Jane Iredale (Makeup Only)

If you haven't heard about "all mineral" makeup yet, you will. Jane Iredale's line of products wants you to believe that "all mineral" makeup is the absolute best option for creating next-to-perfect skin. Iredale wasn't the first kid on the block with this concept. The makeup collection from Jane Iredale is actually reminiscent of a another "all mineral" line of makeup products called Youngblood. It turns out the correlation between the two lines isn't all that surprising because Iredale helped start Youngblood, but eventually severed ties with them and branched out on her own.

Iredale's small color line is advertised as "The Skin Care Makeup." It isn't skin care–like in the least, but it does have some very good products to consider, at least if you prefer the look of a powder foundation instead of traditional liquids, creams, or cream-to-powders. Regrettably, many of the claims surrounding the products, though not always entirely untrue, certainly tempt the line between fact and fiction. For example, Jane Iredale's Web site states that when applying her powder base with SPF 20 "the SPF increases when the product is layered... because of the minute crystals of titanium dioxide and zinc oxide [that] act like tiny mirrors reflecting back the sun's rays." While the part about how titanium dioxide and zinc oxide (as physical/inorganic sunscreens) work is true, once the SPF has been established through FDA testing, a product (or company) cannot make claims of increased protection and would in fact need to be reevaluated and reassigned a different SPF based on those results.

Another less serious claim is that its powder bases, which are quite thick and relatively opaque on the skin, are "...so sheer it actually looks like skin yet gives coverage that traditional makeups can only envy." These powders can be applied sheer, but the very nature of their ingredients results in a heavy-textured product that, like it or not, does look powdery and "made-up" on the skin. That is especially true if you have any dry patches on the skin—these mineral powders, which also claim to "trap moisture," will exacerbate any dryness and can look caked and change color over very oily areas. Actually, they do trap moisture, but they trap it away from the skin, which is the nature of any powdered mineral: they are extremely absorbent and drying.

There are several more dubious claims, but you get the idea. If the concept of a different type of powdered makeup than the traditional talc-based powders you're used to at the cosmetics counters or drugstore appeals to you, then this line presents some fine choices. Just keep in mind that, true to the nature of the cosmetics industry at large, Iredale's line often makes much ado about nothing—not that these products are not worth looking into but, rather, you'll need to be cautious about the inflated benefits of some rather ordinary but nevertheless effective ingredients. And Iredale is not the only game in town, with bare escentuals, Origins, and Youngblood all having good options.

There is only one skin-care product in the Jane Iredale collection and it is a rather controversial one. The toner-like liquid is ⊗ **D2O Mist Spray** *($16 for 1.7 ounces)*, which contains mostly "heavy water" and fragrant extracts. The big deal here is the "heavy water" or $D_2O$, which is deuterium oxide. This is supposed to help set makeup and hydrate skin because heavy water, according to Iredale, "...has a higher resistance to vaporization, which helps it stay on the skin for longer periods of time." I have seen no research that substantiates that claim, though even if that were the case, overhydrating the skin is not necessarily a good thing, as too much water in the skin can actually hurt the skin's healing process (I discuss this issue at length in the introduction of this book under "What Makes a Great Moisturizer"). However, while there is research suggesting that $D_2O$ is not toxic to skin, there is also research indicating that heavy water is quite toxic by interfering with cell production (according to some, it blocks mitosis and prevents cells from being created). It is definitely toxic when ingested. For those reasons alone, whatever benefits this may have, the potential negatives make this a no-no.

For more information about Jane Iredale, call (888) 496-8007 or visit the Web site at www. janeiredale.com.

☺ **$$$ <u>FOUNDATION:</u> Amazing Base SPF 20** *($34)* uses titanium dioxide as its active sunscreen and this same ingredient also contributes to the powder's opacity, cling, and long-wearing capabilities. This loose powder foundation is talc-free (although there is nothing wrong with including talc in cosmetics) and has a very smooth texture and dry finish that tends to get drier in feel and appearance the longer it is worn. It can be used dry or mixed with a moisturizer to approximate a liquid foundation or allow an easier application over drier skins. Either method can be messy (true for any loose powder application), and is a definite drawback. Keep in mind that this provides medium to full coverage and is not as natural-looking as the brochure claims. It has an overall smoother texture and less noticeable shine than Youngblood's or Origin's versions. Jane Iredale's ten shades are mostly neutral but can go on a bit darker than they appear. The only shades to be careful of due to slight peach or rose tones are Amber, Warm Sienna, and Rose Beige. There are no colors in this version for darker skins.

☺ **$$$ Purepressed Base SPF 17** *($32.50)* is a pressed powder version of the Amazing Base and this one is recommended by Jane Iredale for oily skins, as it is more matte and not as thick, so oilier skins will be less likely to experience a heavy, caked look once their oils and the powders mix. The sunscreen is pure titanium dioxide and the same comments made for the Amazing Base apply to this as well. The exception with this is the much broader range of shades, with some excellent options for darker skins called **Global Shades**. These are richly pigmented and as a result do not look as ash or gray on deeper skin tones like many other powders can. Of the 18 shades, the only ones to consider avoiding are Natural, Honey Bronze, and Fawn. Caramel and Autumn can be too yellow for most skins, but may work for some.

☹ <u>**CONCEALER:**</u> **Circle/Delete** *($28)* comes in a pot with two colors; one is lighter and the other is a medium tone. The texture is quite thick and creamy, with a vague waxy odor and opaque coverage. This will definitely crease, and applying one of the mineral powders over this tends to look heavy and obvious. Over and above that, the three duos have colors that are mostly a far cry from real skin tones. **CoverCare** *($19)* is a full coverage, matte finish concealer with a dry texture that can make blending it on evenly difficult. The consistency of this is actually semi-solid, and when squeezed out of the tube (which takes some effort), tends to come out (and fall off) in chunks. If you have the patience to use this and can apply it quickly, it can be an option. It is unlikely this will crease, although any prominent lines around the eyes will be accentuated by the dry, somewhat powdery finish. The three available colors are neutral.

☺ **$$$ <u>BLUSH:</u>** The **Pressed Mineral Powder Blush** *($25)* has a silky texture that goes on well. It isn't tightly pressed, so it is messier than most powder blushes but the color range is impressive for a smaller line, with options for light and dark skins.

☺ **$$$ <u>EYESHADOW:</u> Pressed Mineral Eyeshadows** *($16.50)* are sold as singles and have a silky texture that isn't as powdery as the blush. There are some worthwhile matte shades that go on sheer and blend well; the shiny shades are clearly marked as shimmer or pearlescent, so you can pick and choose accordingly.

☹ <u>**EYE AND BROW SHAPER:**</u> **Eye Pencils** *($8.50)* are creamy, run-of-the-mill pencils that apply well but can easily smudge.

☺ <u>**LIPSTICK AND LIP PENCIL:**</u> **LipColours** *($14)* are standard creamy lipsticks that have a slightly glossy finish and medium coverage. **LipSheres** *($14)* are sheer, glossy lipsticks that have minimal staying power, like most every other sheer lipstick. **Lip Pencils** *($8.50)* have a creamy texture and great colors but are otherwise quite boring and need regular sharpening.

☹ <u>**MASCARA:**</u> Jane Iredale's **Mascara** *($14)* doesn't contain shellac, lacquer, or petroleum—which is fine if you happen to have a sensitivity to any of those standard mascara ingredients. If not, there is no reason to think this is better for sensitive eyes than most other mascaras, and in fact, there isn't much about this that makes it even worth trying. It takes a lot of effort to get length and some thickness, but there are clumps along the way.

☺ **BRUSHES:** The brushes available here are mostly very good, and the ones to consider for their excellent shapes and soft but firm feel are the **Chisel Powder** *($20)*, the **Eye Shader** *($9)*, and **Eye Contour** *($9)*; the **Eye Liner** *($10)* and **Camouflage Oval** *($13.50)* are options as well, and both are synthetic. The **Handi Brush** *($30)*, which is recommended for applying Jane Iredale's powder bases, is cut straight across and applies the powder much like a sponge would, and may be worth a test to see how you like the results. The **Lip Brush** *($14)* is OK but really too small for most lips to use efficiently.

## *Janet Sartin*

To say the least, this is a high-end line that is absurdly overpriced. Yet the products are just standard—alcohol-based astringents, standard AHA products, bar soaps, mineral oil–based cleansers, and mineral oil– and lanolin-based moisturizers—without much of anything interesting. Given the prices, you would at least want the latest water-binding agents, anti-irritants, and sunscreen formulations. Even the packaging is ordinary and clumsy. (At least when you buy Chanel or Dior, the packaging has an elegance all its own, no matter what's in them.) In some ways this line is almost schizophrenic: the astringents and masks are all exceptionally drying and irritating, while the cleansers and moisturizers are rather greasy and emollient. I can't imagine how someone's skin wouldn't be disturbed by most combinations of these products.

One of the more provocative sections in Sartin's brochures are the lists of foods that are said to be best for specific skin types. For example, she suggests that vegetable soup, fish, cooked cereals (grains), and fruit are great, but oily nuts, fried foods, and chocolate can cause problems. This kind of blatant fiction sends skin care for those with oily and acned skin back to the Stone Age. A healthy diet low in fat and without excess sugar is good for the body, but there is no evidence that fatty or sugary foods can affect even one oil gland. In fact, quite the contrary. Dermatologists and researchers searched for decades to find a dietary correlation between food and skin care, and none exists. You may have food allergies that can show up on the skin, but they are more likely to be associated with shellfish, milk, wheat, and some vegetables, such as tomatoes. While I'm on the subject of food, although I advocate drinking lots of water for good overall health, no matter how much you drink it won't pass through to the skin. Excess water is just eliminated; it doesn't travel to skin cells.

For more information about Janet Sartin products, call (800) 321-1779 or visit the Web site at www.sartin.com.

The Reviews J

# *Janet Sartin Skin Care*

☹ **1012 Soap, Specially Formulated Soap for Oily Skin** *($14 for 3.25 ounces)* is basically lard and lye. Lye dries the skin and lard can clog pores. The price is excessive for this ordinary bar of soap.

☹ **Gentle Cleansing Soap, for Normal to Combination Skin** *($14 for 3.6 ounces)* is similar to the soap above and the same review applies.

☹ **Superfatted Soap, Specially Formulated Soap for Dry Skin** *($14 for 3 ounces)* is similar to the 1012 Soap above, except with plant oil, but that won't undo the problems of dryness from the cleansing agents in here.

☹ **Cleansing Oil, Nourishing Cleanser for Normal to Dry Skin** *($27 for 7 ounces)* is a joke, right? How can they charge $27 for mineral oil, peanut oil, and preservatives? Did they think no one would notice? If you are interested, plain mineral oil would work far better without the preservatives.

☹ **Gentle Cleanser, for Normal to Oily Sensitive Skin** *($23 for 7 ounces)* is anything but gentle. It is mostly just water, alcohol, and glycerin, which is incredibly drying and irritating for all skin types.

☺ **$$$ Nourishing Cleanser** *($25 for 6 ounces)* won't nourish one skin cell, but it is a good, gentle, detergent-based water-soluble cleanser with water-binding agents. The amino-acid water-binding agents in here don't hold up well under water or with detergent cleansing agents.

☺ **$$$ Sensitive Skin Cleansing Treatment** *($23 for 7 ounces)* is basically a lightweight toner that uses a standard detergent cleansing agent and glycerin to remove excess makeup. It is OK but incredibly ordinary and overpriced, and you'll need to use a lot of it to clean your face even once.

☺ **$$$ Gentle Eye Makeup Remover** *($17 for 4 ounces)* is a standard, completely ordinary eye-makeup remover that would work as well as any.

☺ **Gentle Eye Makeup Remover Pads** *($17 for 60 pads)* is similar to the remover above only it provides the wipe-off pads. If you want this type of product, Huggies Baby Wipes Refills, Natural Care, Unscented *($5.29 for 160 towelettes)* will do the exact same thing for far less money.

☹ **Papaya Enzyme Scrub** *($25 for 1 ounce)* not only contains alcohol, but a host of irritating plant oils as well. Ouch.

☹ **Clear Astringent, Treatment Cleanser for Normal to Oily Skin** *($23 for 7 ounces)* contains mostly water, alcohol, and glycerin. Alcohol irritates skin, causing redness, dryness, and flaking.

☹ **Controlling Astringent, Pore Refining Lotion for Excessively Oily Skin, Day and Night Treatment** *($28 for 7 ounces)* is almost identical to the Normal to Oily version above and the same comments apply.

☹ **Skin Application Clarifying Lotion, for Excessively Oily and Blemished Skin** *($27 for 7 ounces)* is similar to the two astringents above, but with salicylic acid. Salicylic acid as an exfoliant has some good points, but in an alcohol base it can only cause problems, irritating the skin and causing inflammation and dryness.

☹ **White Astringent, Pore Refining Lotion for Normal to Oily Skin, Night Treatment** *($28 for 7 ounces)* is almost identical to the product above, and the same review applies.

☺ **$$$ Active Skin Replenishing Cream, Super Rich Nourishing Cream** *($39 for 1.85 ounces)* is an incredibly emollient, though ordinary moisturizer that is best for someone with dry skin. What this moisturizer is doing in the middle of all these drying soaps and toners is at best confusing.

☺ **$$$ Continual Action Cream Age Protection with Kalaya Oil** *($45 for 1.7 ounces)* is a very good emollient moisturizer for dry skin and while the kalaya oil (emu oil) is a good oil for skin, it isn't a miraculous ingredient.

☺ **$$$ Eye Care for Sensitive Eyes, Enriched with Kalaya Oil** *($45 for 1 ounce)* is similar to the one above except more emollient, though the same basic review applies.

☺ **$$$ Eye Care Serum, Enriched with Kalaya Oil** *($45 for 1 ounce)* does contain kalaya oil (emu oil), a good emollient, but that's it. Though if you are sold on this ingredient, it is the second one in here. Other than that, this is good emollient moisturizer for dry skin.

☺ **Hydrating Lotion Advanced Skin Conditioning** *($38 for 1.75 ounces)* is a good, though ordinary moisturizer for someone with dry skin. The tiny amount of algae in here can have no impact on the health of skin.

☺ **$$$ Nutri Performance Cream, Soothing Emollient to Help Nourish Dry Skin** *($39 for 1.85 ounces)* is an ordinary but extremely emollient moisturizer for someone with super-dry skin.

☺ **$$$ Nutri Performance Eye Care Cream** *($35 for 0.5 ounce)* is similar to the Performance Cream above and the same basic comments apply. The few more vitamins in here have minimal impact on skin.

☺ **$$$ Superfatted Cream, Rich Nourishing Cream for Dry Skin** *($70 for 4 ounces)* is one of the most overpriced standard formulations around. All this product contains is Vaseline, lanolin, mineral oil, and beeswax! It is great for very dry skin, but the price is just a joke and the effect easily replaced at the drugstore with Aquaphor Healing Ointment *($5.69 for 1.75 ounces)*.

☺ **$$$ Highly Active Collagen Cream** *($44 for 1.85 ounces)* is similar to the Superfatted version above and the same comments apply. The tiny amount of collagen in this product (or any amount of it) has no effect on the collagen in your skin.

☺ **$$$ Revitalizing Cream with Plant Extracts** *($44 for 1.7 ounces)* is a moisturizer that contains three different AHAs, totaling about 5% to 6% AHAs in a moisturizing base of Vaseline, thickeners, silicone, and plant extracts. The plant extracts are so far down the ingredient list they're hard to see, but they are a mixed bag of potential skin irritants and anti-irritants. In many ways this product is extremely similar to Pond's Age Defying Cream, but at four times the price.

☺ $$$ **Revitalizing Lotion with Plant Extracts** *($32 for 1 ounce)* is similar to the one above only in lotion form.

☺ $$$ **Revitalizing Lotion Advance Strength with Plant Extracts** *($35 for 1 ounce)* is similar to the one above, except it contains about 8% AHA and includes glycolic acid; the same basic review applies.

☹ **Daily Firming Neck Cream** *($25 for 1 ounce)* is a good basic moisturizer for normal to dry skin but contains nothing unique or special for the neck. It does contain a mix of plant oils and extracts that may be skin irritants, including ginseng, grapefruit, lime, and lemon.

☺ $$$ **Skin Clarifying Mask with Green Tea** *($25 for 1.7 ounces)* is a standard clay mask. It would work to absorb oil, but the amount of green tea in here is so minuscule as to have no impact on skin.

☺ $$$ **Triple Performance Moisture Mask with Kalaya Oil** *($25 for 1.7 ounces)* is a good emollient mask for dry skin. It contains several emollient ingredients that could trigger breakouts, so this is only appropriate for very dry skin. Emu oil (kalaya) is a good emollient but there is nothing about this oil that provides miraculous properties for the skin.

☹ **Normalizing Mask, for Normal to Oily Skin** *($22 for 2.5 ounces)* is just water, clay, and alcohol. It won't normalize anyone's skin, but it can be extremely irritating.

☺ $$$ **SPF 15 Sunblock Face Cream with Plant Extracts** *($39 for 1.85 ounces)* contains in-part titanium dioxide, plus a host of standard thickening agents. This is an incredibly standard, overpriced sunscreen for someone with normal to dry skin. It would work, but this is easily replaced with any UVA-protecting sunscreen you find at the drugstore.

☺ **Sunblock SPF 15 Waterproof Lotion with Plant Extracts** *($18 for 4 ounces)* is similar to the Face Cream version above, only this one is in lotion form, and the same basic comments apply.

☺ **Sunblock SPF 25 Waterproof Lotion with Plant Extracts** *($18 for 4 ounces)* is similar to the SPF 15 Waterproof version above, only with a higher SPF, the same basic comments apply.

☹ **SPF 15 Oil Free Sunspray** *($18 for 4 ounces)* doesn't contain avobenzone, titanium dioxide, or zinc oxide, and is not recommended.

☹ **SPF 15 Waterproof Sunspray with Plant Extracts** *($18 for 4 ounces)* doesn't contain avobenzone, titanium dioxide, or zinc oxide, and is not recommended.

☺ **$$$ Lip Sartinizer, Lip Balm for Dry and Chapped Lips** *($19 for 0.5 ounce)* is an extremely standard Vaseline- and wax-based balm for the lips. At $19, you are buying little more than Vaseline.

☺ **$$$ Eye Rest Pads** *($16 for 60 pads)* contain aloe, tea, fragrance, and preservatives. Unless you are allergic to the tea or rose water these won't hurt your skin, but they are a waste of your time and money.

## Janet Sartin Makeup

<u>FOUNDATION:</u> ☺ **$$$ Dual Performance Treatment Makeup Extra Coverage** and **Regular Coverage** *($36 and $32)* come in the largest foundation containers I've ever seen, but neither formula qualifies as a "treatment." They are virtually indistinguishable from Clinique's Pore Minimizer foundation, and they have the same problems. Both contain mostly alcohol, which can cause irritation, dryness, and increased redness. There is no reason for any skin type to consider these foundations.

☹ **NutriPerformance Treatment Makeup** *($31)* has a very sheer, soft matte finish with a slight sheen, but it comes in only five shades, which is absurdly limited, and three of those colors are extremely peach or rose. Sand and Beige are the only possibilities. It won't reduce wrinkles, and the second ingredient, isopropyl myristate, is notorious for causing breakouts.

☹ **Blemish Fix** *($10)* is almost identical to the Dual Performance Makeup, and the same review applies. This one also comes in just five colors, and you only get 0.5 ounce. It won't fix any blemishes and may make matters worse.

☺ **$$$ Daily Protection Makeup SPF 10** *($35)* has not only a too-low SPF for daily protection, but offers unreliable UVA protection. This is otherwise just a lightweight makeup suitable for normal to dry skin looking for sheer coverage and willing to wear an adequate sunscreen underneath. The five colors are not the best, but sheer enough to not be much of an issue.

☹ <u>CONCEALER:</u> **NutriCover Eye Cream** *($21)* comes in three shades that are unacceptable for most skin tones, and is unusually greasy, easily creasing into the lines around the eyes.

☺ **$$$ <u>POWDER:</u> Dual Performance Compact Powder** *($24)* is a good standard powder that comes in only three OK shades. Don't expect this one to control oil any better than any other pressed powder. **Face Powder Loose** *($21)* is a good soft powder, but rather messy and inconvenient to use.

☺ **$$$ Bronze Fusion 2 in 1 Bronzing Powder** *($22)* is a multicolored bronzer that perpetuates the sparkly tan look seen in countless other bronzing powders that sell for less than this one.

☺ **$$$ <u>BLUSH:</u>** The standard **Refined Powder Blush** *($19)* comes in a nice array of 12 colors. It has a slightly dry finish, and while in general I prefer blush that feels silky, this one still works. The shades do have a slight bit of shine, but it ends up being barely noticeable on the skin.

☺ **EYESHADOW:** Although the Sartin concept of creating your own eyeshadow compact by selecting the shades you want *($10 per color)* and putting them in a compact you purchase *($2.50 for a duo; $3 for a trio)* is nice, most of the colors are extremely shiny and should be avoided. The only matte colors to consider, and they are rather attractive and go on nicely, are Toast, Dark Brown, Teakwood, Cocoa, Light Gray, Gray, Dark Gray, Sea Gray, Tan, Cashew, Cameo, Golden, and Pumpkin.

☺ **PENCILS:** There are four standard **Eyeliner Pencils** *($12)* and three standard **Lip Liner Pencils** *($12)*. It doesn't get much sparser than this. They are fine but boring. **$$$ Cake Eye Liner** *($16)* is just what the name says, but the colors are all way too obvious. Violet, Royal Blue, Midnight, and Turquoise are all too colorful. Midnight Gray is the only one to consider.

☹ **MASCARA: Extra Performance Mascara** *($15.50)* is one of the all-time worst mascaras I've ever tested. You can apply this one for hours and actually lose length, and it smears and smudges.

☺ **BRUSHES:** If this line has any strengths, it is in its brush selection *($12 to $19)*. These are, for the most part, very good brushes, with a silky feel and a firm but soft bristle density.

# *Jason Natural Cosmetics*

As the name implies, Jason Natural Cosmetics is about—surprise!—natural ingredients. According to its brochure, "We believe consumers must have a reliable natural alternative to chemically synthesized, technical grade products, and to that end we are devoted to developing and manufacturing a wide range of personal care and beauty care products that are truly botanical in origin." Several of the Jason products contain laureth sulfosuccinate, lauramide DEA, cocamidopropyl betaine, and sodium myreth sulfate, among many others, so you have to ask, how natural are those?

This line also wants you to know its information dates back to the ancient Egyptians and that much of their "knowledge of the healing power of herbs and their special effects on the skin was gathered into books during medieval times." Is there really anything from ancient Egypt or medieval Europe that would be of interest to us today? After all, they didn't have sunscreens, they didn't have antibiotics, and they didn't live past 50. While the notion of ancient folklore is romantic, it is nonsense when it comes to the health of your skin.

Jason also states that its products don't contain offensive chemical ingredients like lauryl/laureth sulfates, pore-clogging ingredients, and other known irritants. In its brochure it has a big red stamp saying, "No Lauryl Sulfate or Laureth Sulfates." But that's simply not true: some of these products absolutely contain those cleansing agents! (Not that laureth or lauryl sulfates are dangerous in any way—there is no research substantiating this—but if a company adopts popular misconceptions it should at least stand up to its own distorted claims.) They also contain cornstarch, which can clog pores, and eucalyptus and SD alcohol, which are irritants and can trigger breakouts, not to mention flaky, dry skin.

What is relatively unique to the Jason line is the listing of international units (IU) for some of the vitamins used in its products. That does sound impressive, but given that no one knows how much or how little vitamins (as antioxidants) are needed for skin, the numbers are meaningless and more for marketing than of real help. Several products have an ingredient called MSM showcased on the label. MSM is short for methylsulfonylmethane, an antibacterial agent and degreasing agent. What that is doing in some of these moisturizing creams is unclear.

Still, there are some good and even great products to be found in this line, particularly moisturizers containing all the antioxidants you could ever want. For a line with great prices, that's really impressive. Given the price point, I would consider a closer look. But ignore the claims—even Jason Natural Cosmetics can't keep its own ingredients and claims straight. For more information about Jason Natural Cosmetics, call 1-800-JASON-05 or check out the Web site at www.jason-natural.com.

☺ **Clean Start Refreshing Cleanser for Normal Skin** *($8.49 for 8 ounces)* is a standard, detergent-based water-soluble cleanser that also contains mixed citrus oils, which can be irritating to the eyes and face.

☻ **D-Clog Naturally Balancing Cleanser** *($9.69 for 8 ounces)* contains several ingredients that can be problematic for oily or blemish-prone skin, including witch hazel, cornstarch, flour, and camphor.

☺ **Fresh Face Rehydrating Cleanser** *($9 for 8 ounces)* is a standard, wipe-off cleanser using plant oil. It can leave a greasy film behind on the skin.

☻ **Satin Soap, Natural Tea Tree Oil, Anti-Bacterial Liquid Soap** *($3.99 for 17.5 ounces)* contains triclosan, which can be effective as an antibacterial agent, but there are problems associated with its use in regard to certain bacteria adapting to its application. Separate from that issue, this soap contains eucalyptus, which is too irritating for all skin types.

☺ **Quick Clean Eye Makeup Remover for All Skin Types, Oil Free** *($7.49 for 75 pads)* is a standard, detergent-based eye-makeup remover. At least they left most of the fragrant ingredients out of this one. It would be OK for wiping off makeup, but it is best in the long run never to wipe off eye makeup—or any makeup for that matter.

☺ **Citrus 6-in-1 Facial Wash & Scrub with Ester-C** *($7 for 4.5 ounces)* is supposed to contain AHAs and BHA, but it doesn't, which is good, because it would all just be rinsed away in this cleanser. Aside from that, it is a mild cleanser with a soft scrub that can be good for exfoliation.

☹ **Original Apricot Scrub Facial Wash and Scrub** (*$4.50 for 4.5 ounces*) contains sodium lauryl sulfate, a potent skin irritant, as the third ingredient, and is not recommended.

☹ **Fruit Cooler Refreshing Toner for Normal Skin** (*$8.49 for 8 ounces*) has witch hazel as the second ingredient, and that can be too irritating for most skin types.

☹ **Vegee Tonic Balancing Astringent** (*$9.50 for 8 ounces*) contains witch hazel and alcohol, and is not recommended.

☺ **70% Aloe Vera All Purpose Moisturizing Creme** (*$4.79 for 4 ounces*) would be a very good moisturizer for normal to dry skin. The amount of aloe sounds impressive, at least to those who think aloe is a miraculous ingredient. However, the gel in here is more water than aloe.

☺ **84% Aloe Vera All Purpose Moisturizing Creme** (*$6.49 for 4 ounces*) is similar to the one above and the same comments apply.

☺ **98% Aloe Vera Super Gel** (*$7 for 8 ounces*) is indeed mostly aloe, with some thickening agents and preservatives. The price isn't bad, but for those looking for aloe, pure aloe from the health food store may be of more interest. The spirulina in this product can't moisturize skin.

☺ **Aqua Moist Balancing Moisture Lotion SPF 12** (*$9.50 for 4 ounces*) would be far better with an SPF 15, but it is a part titanium dioxide–based sunscreen that would be good for someone with normal to slightly dry skin. It does contain witch hazel, which can be drying.

☺ **Beta-Gold Rehydrating Freshener** (*$9 for 8 ounces*) is a good lightweight toner for most skin types. It also contains citrus oils, but the amount is tiny and is mostly added as fragrance.

☺ **Hemp Plus Natural EFA Moisturizing Creme** (*$10.50 for 4 ounces*) would be a very good moisturizer for normal to dry skin, but the hemp oil is not any better for skin than any other effective plant oil.

☺ **Natural Cocoa Butter All Purpose Moisturizing Creme** (*$4.49 for 4 ounces*) would be a very good moisturizer for dry skin.

☺ **Oil Free NaPCA Naturally Lite Moisturizing Creme** (*$7.50 for 4 ounces*) contains mostly water, aloe, plant extracts, thickeners, water-binding agents, vitamins, and preservatives. This would be a very good, lightweight moisturizer for normal to slightly oily skin.

☺ **Perfect Solutions Ester-C Moisture Creme, Daily Age Defense** (*$14 for 2 ounces*) is a good moisturizer for dry skin, though there's nothing in here that can defy age. The vitamin C, vitamin A, and other antioxidants in this product are good for skin but they won't change or stop wrinkling.

☺ **Perfect Solutions Ester-C Moisture Lotion, Daily Age Defense** (*$16 for 4 ounces*) would be a very good moisturizer for someone with normal to dry skin.

☹ **Quick Recovery Rehydrating SPF 12 Lotion** *($9 for 4 ounces)* is a good, in part titanium dioxide–based sunscreen, but the SPF 12 is not worth the trouble, especially considering that this line has so many good sunscreens with SPF 15 or greater, so there is no reason to even consider this one.

☺ **Skin-amins Topical Vitamin Therapy Hi-Vitamin A Complex with MSM, 10,000 I.U.** *($9.99 for 2 ounces)*. While this product can be a very good moisturizer for someone with dry skin, the claims about improving acne and age spots are bogus (there are no such things as age spots, these are sun-damage spots, resulting in hypermelanin production, so the term used is very misleading). The ingredients in here are great for dry skin but can be a problem for breakouts, and there are no melanin-inhibiting ingredients in this product. The 10,000 International Units (IU) listed here sound impressive, but why 10,000 IUs? With no information about the amount of any substance the skin needs for antioxidant protection, the number is meaningless.

☺ **Skin-amins Topical Vitamin Therapy Hi-Vitamin B Complex with MSM, 3,000 mg** *($9.99 for 2 ounces)* is similar to the one above, and the same basic review applies.

☺ **Skin-amins Topical Vitamin Therapy Hi-Vitamin C Complex with MSM, 3,000 mg** *($9.99 for 2 ounces)* is similar to the one above, and the same basic review applies.

☺ **Skin-amins Topical Vitamin Therapy Hi-Vitamin D Complex with MSM, 12,000 I.U.** *($7.99 for 2 ounces)* is similar to the one above, and the same basic review applies.

☺ **Skin-amins Topical Vitamin Therapy Hi-Vitamin E Complex with MSM, 10,000 I.U.** *($7.99 for 2 ounces)* is similar to the one above, and the same basic review applies.

☺ **Skin-amins Topical Vitamin Therapy Hi-Vitamin HFK Complex with MSM, 6,000 mg** *($11.99 for 2 ounces)* is similar to the one above, and the same basic review applies.

☺ **Suma Moist Active Creme Concentrate with Live Yeast Cell Extracts** *($12.99 for 2 ounces)*. Yeast can be good as an antioxidant but it isn't a miracle ingredient. Other than that, this is a good moisturizer for dry skin. This product also contains germanium. According to Dr. Andrew Weil (www.drweil.com), "[There is] an FDA import ban aimed at germanium, a trace element used in the production of computer chips, which sometimes is identified as vitamin O. The FDA noted that consumption of germanium has caused kidney injury and death when used chronically by humans, even at dosages suggested on product labels. It has banned germanium imports intended for human consumption on the grounds that these products are either poisonous and deleterious to health or unapproved new drugs." The bottom

The Reviews J

line: there is no evidence that germanium has any positive effect for skin and it can be problematic and therefore should probably be avoided.

☺ **Super Anti-Oxidant Youth Enhancing Tea Time Anti-Aging Moisturizing Creme** *($4.99 for 4 ounces)* is similar to the one above, and the same basic review applies.

☺ **Super E Creme, Super Moisture Creme, 25,000 I.U.** *($7.49 for 4 ounces)* is similar to the one above, and the same review applies.

☺ **Vitamin E All Purpose Moisturizing Creme, 5,000 I.U.** *($9.49 for 4 ounces)* is similar to the one above, and the same review applies.

☺ **Vitamin K Creme Plus with Bioflavonoids and Calendula** *($20 for 2 ounces)* would be a very good moisturizer for normal to dry skin but the claims about vitamin K improving circulation or eliminating surfaced capillaries are unsubstantiated.

☹ **Witch Vera Aloe Gel Cooling Moisturizer** *($5.99 for 8 ounces)* would definitely be cooling, but it would also be irritating, as the first ingredient is witch hazel; therefore this product is not recommended.

**(Unrated) Woman Wise 1,000 mg Progesterone Max Comfort and Balancing Creme** *($18.99 for 2 ounces)*. Please see the section in Chapter Two of this book on "Battling Hormones: Is Progesterone in Skin-Care Products the Answer?" for information regarding products making claims about their progesterone content.

☹ **Woman Wise 10% Wild Yam Balancing and Moisturizing Creme** *($9.99 for 4 ounces)* contains wild yam, but wild yam does not contain progesterone or anything else that would act like progesterone. According to the *The PDR Family Guide to Natural Medicines and Healing Therapies,* wild yam "is used in the production of artificial [synthetic] progesterone but it will not yield the hormone in the absence of a chemical conversion process that the body can't supply." So while it may seem nice that wild yam is natural, it has no benefit for women going through perimenopausal or menopausal skin changes.

☺ **SPF 16 Sun Block** *($9 for 4 ounces)* is a great, part titanium dioxide and zinc oxide sunscreen for normal to dry skin.

☺ **SPF 26 Total Sun Block** *($9.50 for 4 ounces)* is similar to the one above, and the same review applies.

☺ **SPF 36 Family Sun Block** *($10.50 for 4 ounces)* is similar to the one above, and the same review applies.

☺ **SPF 40 Active Sun Block** *($10.75 for 4 ounces)* is similar to the one above, and the same review applies.

☺ **SPF 46 Kids Sun Block** *($11 for 4 ounces)* is similar to the one above, and the same review applies.

☺ **SPF 20 Natural Lip Protection on a String** *($5 for 0.16 ounce)* is a great, part titanium dioxide and zinc oxide sunscreen (there are other sunscreen agents in this formula) for normal to dry skin.

☺ **SPF 26 Sun Block Sport Stick** *($8 for 0.75 ounce)* is a great, part titanium dioxide and zinc oxide sunscreen (there are other sunscreen agents in this formula) for normal to dry skin, but the price is unwarranted unless you only use this on your lips.

☹ **Fresh Papaya-Pineapple Facial Peel & Mask** *($9 for 4.5 ounces)* contains lemon oil, which can be a skin irritant. Other than that, it does contain papain and bromelain, but both are considered fairly unstable for purposes of exfoliation.

☺ **Meditation Masque, Anti-Stress Aromatherapy, Soothing, and Refreshing Masque** *($7.50 for 4 ounces)* is a standard clay mask with thickening agents. For a clay mask, it's just fine.

☺ **T-Zone Ultimate Balancing Clay Oil-Control Aromatherapy Masque** *($9.50 for 4 ounces)* is similar to the one above only this one includes camphor, and that can be too irritating for most skin types.

☹ **Super-C Cleanser Gentle Face Wash** *($9.99 for 6 ounces)* is a standard, detergent-based water-soluble cleanser that isn't all that gentle; this can be fairly drying for most skin types. It also contains witch hazel.

☺ **C-Light Skin Tone Balancer** *($19.99 for 1 ounce)* would be a good moisturizer for someone with normal to dry skin. The pH of this product is too high for the BHA to be an effective exfoliant. Also, this product contains kojic dipalmitate, a melanin inhibitor, and while that may have benefit, it is not as effective as hydroquinone, and all skin-lightening products are useless without the consistent daily use of a good sunscreen.

☹ **$$$ Ultra-C Eye Lift Treatment** *($19.99 for 0.5 ounce)* contains mostly water, glycerin, plant extracts, thickeners, water-binding agents, silicone, preservatives, and fragrance. There is every form of vitamin C imaginable in this product, so if you are looking to cover your vitamin C bases, you might as well consider this one. However, the main form of vitamin C here is ascorbic acid, which can be irritating for most skin types.

☺ **$$$ Hyper-C Serum Anti-Aging Therapy** *($30 for 1 ounce)* contains most every form of vitamin C imaginable in an emollient serum. If you're looking for vitamin C, this is a pricey, though valid option.

☹ **"C" My Lips Protector SPF 15** *($7.99 for 0.47 ounce)* doesn't contain UVA protection and is not recommended. It also contains BHA (though that would be a problem for lips—lips don't need that kind of penetrating exfoliation), yet this product doesn't have a low enough pH for the BHA to be effective.

☹ **Deep-C Orange Peel, Peel off Masque** *($17.50 for 2 ounces)* contains alcohol and witch hazel, which can be too irritating for most skin types.

☹ **New Cell Therapy 7 1/2 Plus Balancing Cleansing Pads with Alpha/Beta Hydroxy Acids** *($9 for 50 pads)* do contain about 4% AHAs (as glycolic acid), but the other forms, sugarcane and sugar maple extract, are not AHAs. It also contains

BHA, but the pH of this product is not low enough for any of these to be effective as exfoliants. Plus, there are several irritating ingredients in here, including witch hazel, lemon extract, and alcohol, and that makes it a problem for all skin types.

☺ **New Cell Therapy 6 Plus Daytime Moisturizing Emulsion with Alpha Hydroxy Acids** *($10 for 2 ounces)* contains about 2% to 3% AHA, which isn't enough for this to work as an exfoliant. Aside from that, this would be a good standard moisturizer for dry skin.

☺ **New Cell Therapy 12-1/2 Plus Moisturizing Oil-Free Gel with Alpha Hydroxy Acids** *($18.99 for 1.1 ounces)* does contain about 8% AHA, but the product's pH isn't low enough for it to be an effective exfoliant. It would be a good moisturizer for someone with normal to slightly dry or slightly oily skin.

☺ **New Cell Therapy 10 Plus Nighttime Creme with Alpha Hydroxy Acids** *($15 for 1 ounce)* contains about 2% to 3% AHA, which isn't enough to be an exfoliant. Aside from that, this would be a good standard moisturizer for dry skin.

☹ **New Cell Therapy 12-1/2 Plus Protective Moisturizer Alpha Hydroxy Acids with SPF 12 1/2 Alpha Hydroxy Acids** *($18.58 for 1.6 ounces)* has an SPF 12. Given that this line has so many excellent sunscreens with SPF 15 or greater, this one is a waste of your time.

☺ **New Cell Therapy 3-1/2 Plus Gentle Eye Gel with Alpha Hydroxy Acids** *($12.99 for 1 ounce)* contains "mixed fruit acids," and that means you don't know what you are getting. With a concentration of less than 2% of lactic acid, there isn't enough to make this effective as an exfoliant anyway. This is a good lightweight moisturizer for slightly dry skin.

☹ **New Cell Therapy 5-1/2 Plus Fast Acne and Blemish Relief with Alpha Hydroxy Acids** *($9 for 1 ounce)* contains both lemon and orange extract high on the ingredient listing, making it too irritating for most all skin types. It doesn't contain AHA (the plant extracts listed here are not the same thing as glycolic or lactic acid).

# J.C. Penney Professionals

J.C. Penney Professionals makeup and skin care falls down in so many areas, my review could easily be summed up in a definitive "Why bother?" For what you get, the skin-care products are strangely overpriced. None of the formulations address any current skin-care research in fields ranging from sunscreens to AHA or BHA, all the formulations are at best described as ordinary, and in addition there is little to no differentiation between skin types. The makeup products are even more of a disappointment. Foundations and powders are either too shiny or some strange shade of peach, pink, or ash. The concealer is in a pencil form, which isn't the best applicator tool, with a texture that is too dry for most skin types. The large range of blushes and eyeshadows have great textures but are almost all too shiny (now really, who needs more shiny eyeshadows?). J.C. Penney Professionals' brushes are impressive though not any cheaper than the brushes found at other cosmetics counters from higher-end department stores. For more information, call (800) 222-6161 or visit the Web site at www.jcpenney.com (as this book went to press, the Web site did not have the J.C. Penney Professionals products available).

# J.C. Penney Professionals Skin Care

☺ **Total Cleanser** *($17 for 8 ounces)* is a standard, ordinary, detergent-based water-soluble cleanser, though the cleansing agent, TEA-cocoyl glutamate, can be too drying for some skin types. The plant extracts in here can be good anti-irritants. It does contain fragrance.

☹ **Total Freshener** *($17 for 8 ounces)* contains both witch hazel, sage, and lemon extract, making it too potentially irritating for all skin types.

☹ **Total Toner** *($17 for 8 ounces)* is virtually identical to the freshener above and the same review applies.

☺ $$$ **Total Eye Cream** *($22.50 for 0.5 ounce)* would be a good moisturizer for normal to dry skin.

☺ **ProVide C Pure Vitamin C Prolipid 131 Botanic Enriched** *($32.50 for 2 ounces).* This is the most amazing name for an otherwise unamazing product. While it is a good moisturizer for dry skin, it turns out it contains hardly any vitamin C. I won't bore you with the pros and cons of vitamin C in a moisturizer.

☺ **Total Moisture Normal to Dry Skin** *($18 for 4 ounces)* is similar to the ProVide above and the same basic comments apply.

☺ **Total Moisture Oil Free** *($18 for 4 ounces)* is similar to the ProVide above and the same basic comments apply.

☺ **Total Night Cream** *($25 for 2 ounces)* is almost identical to the ProVide above and the same basic comments apply.

☺ **Total Clay Moisture Mask** *($17 for 4 ounces)* is a standard clay mask with some plant extracts. There is a small amount of lemon extract, but that probably won't affect the skin if the mask is used intermittently and kept on the face only for brief periods of time (which is how most masks are used).

# J.C. Penney Professionals Makeup

**FOUNDATION:** ☹ **Perfect Foundation** *($20)* is a good foundation, but the colors! They are about as far from perfect as I can imagine. There are lots of shades but almost all of them are unusually peach, orange, or pink for most all skin tones.

The only ones to consider are #0, #1, #2, #4, and #9. The texture is fine for someone with normal to dry skin and the application is smooth and sheer, but with these colors, there are just too many to avoid to make this a real consideration.

☺ **Dual Active Foundation** *($20)* is a pressed powder–type foundation that comes in only four shades. Four shades can only be described as limited. What's more shocking is that all four shades are shiny, and I mean iridescent, sparkling shiny! You can maybe consider this for an evening look, but the finish is powdery and chalky looking, so it can look uneven and caked even in dim light.

**POWDER:** ☺ $$$ **Professional Finish Powder Foundation** *($20)* is a loose powder and all five shades are shiny. That doesn't make for a great finish except for evening wear and then only if sparkling all over is your idea of glamour.

**CONCEALER:** ☹ **Concealing Pencil** *($12.50)* comes in pencil form with five shades. Two are pink and yellow, which are strange colors meant to be color correctors, but that just place an eerie tone over the face. The other colors are OK but tend to be slightly peach. The stick has a dry texture that isn't bad, although it can make wrinkles more evident.

**BLUSH:** ☺ **Powder Blush** *($15)* has a great soft texture and a large selection of colors, but most all of the shades are iridescent and that's too much shine.

**EYESHADOW:** ☺ **Rich Eyeshadow** *($12.50)* isn't rich, but it does have a soft, smooth texture and application; unfortunately, amid this large range of colors there are only five that are matte, all the rest are shiny.

**EYE AND BROW PENCIL:** ☹ **Brow Pencil** *($10)* comes in only three shades with a too-hard, dry finish, making application almost impossible.

☺ **Eye Liner** *($10)* is similar in texture to the Lip Liner, and, like most pencils, is just very standard, ordinary, but good.

**LIPSTICK AND LIP PENCIL:** ☺ **Lipstick** *($12.50)* comes in a nice range of colors and in three textures. However, the descriptions are not what you end up getting. The **Cream Lipstick** is extremely glossy and greasy, the **Matte Lipstick** is exceptionally creamy and not in the least matte, and the **Sheer Lipstick**—well, it is sheer, more of a gloss than anything else. **Lip Liner** *($10)* is a very standard pencil that needs sharpening. It has an impressive color selection and the texture is slightly drier than most, which can help prevent lipstick from moving into the lines around the mouth. **Lip Gloss** *($12.50)* is a standard pot of gloss that comes in nine shades. This is a very thick, greasy gloss that feels quite slick but has decent staying power.

**MASCARA:** ☹ **Mascara** *($12)* is just OK, but doesn't build much length, thickness, or definition. It isn't even worth mentioning, but then I couldn't really leave it out now, could I?

**BRUSHES:** ☺ **Brushes** *($15 to $22)*. If there is any strong point to this line, it is the selection of brushes offered. The textures are soft and the brush density is good.

Most of the shapes are quite workable and are all options for applying color to the face. Perhaps the only brush shape missing is a tiny eyeliner brush.

## *Jergens (Skin Care Only)*

The Andrew Jergens Company created the Biore Strips, those strips of gauze-like paper meant to pull blackheads out of the nose and face. Jergens decided to create an identical version with an accompanying skin-care line under its own brand name. You won't find much of a difference between these, and it is unclear why Jergens would want to compete against itself, but my comments about the Biore Strips apply to the Jergens Pore Strips as well. For more information about Jergens, call (800) 742-8798 or visit the Web site at www.jergens.com.

☺ **Gentle Foaming Face Wash** *($3.89 for 6 ounces)* is a standard but OK, detergent-based water-soluble cleanser. There are tiny scrub particles in this cleanser that feel somewhat scratchy. This can be drying for some skin types, but it is still worth considering. It does contain fragrance.

☺ **Moisturizing Creamy Cleanser** *($1.99 for 6 ounces)* is a gentle cleanser that is water-soluble but doesn't take makeup off very well. It can be an option for someone with dry skin. It does contain fragrance.

☹ **Naturals Soap with Aloe & Lanolin for Normal to Dry Skin** *($1.89 for 9.5 ounces)* is a standard tallow-based bar soap that also contains some lanolin. The lanolin won't undo the drying effect of the soap or prevent the clogged pores tallow can cause.

☹ **Naturals Soap with Vitamin E & Chamomile for Sensitive Skin** *($1.89 for 9.5 ounces)* is almost identical to the soap above, and the same review applies. Nothing about this soap makes it appropriate for sensitive skin.

☺ **Daily Nourishing Cream Alpha & Beta Hydroxy Complex** *($6.59 for 2 ounces)* contains a minimal amount of AHA and a form of salicylic acid that is not effective for exfoliation; further, the pH is too high to make any of this work for cell turnover. Other than that, this is just wax and some silicone and not much of an option for skin care.

☺ **All-Purpose Face Cream** *($2.79 for 6 ounces)* is fairly greasy and thick. It is a waste of time, although it can be an option for someone with dry skin, but only minimally so.

☺ **Aloe Enriched Lotion, for Very Dry Skin** *($2.99 for 6 ounces)* is a good though mundane moisturizer for very dry skin.

☺ **Original Scent Lotion, for Dry Skin** *($2.99 for 6 ounces)* is an exceedingly standard moisturizer with alcohol as the second ingredient. It's probably there as an emulsifier, but my concern is that it could be irritating for the skin in this quantity.

☹ **Protective Moisture Lotion SPF 15 with Vitamin E** *($6.59 for 4 ounces)* doesn't contain avobenzone, zinc oxide, or titanium dioxide in the active ingredients, and is not recommended.

☹ **Replenishing Moisture Lotion Vitamin E Enriched** *($6.59 for 4 ounces)* is a very standard moisturizer. It can be OK for slightly dry skin but this is as boring a formulation as it gets.

☹ **Ultra Healing Cream, for Extra Dry Skin** *($4.99 for 8 ounces)* is a good, basic (though boring) Vaseline-based moisturizer for dry skin. It does contain a tiny amount of AHA but the amount is too small and the pH to high for it to be an exfoliant.

☹ **Ultra Healing Lotion, for Extra Dry Skin** *($2.99 for 6 ounces)* is similar to the Cream version above and the same basic review applies.

☹ **Ultra Healing Lotion, Fragrance Free, for Extra Dry Skin** *($3.49 for 10 ounces)* is similar to the Cream version above and the same review applies.

☹ **Vitamin E Enriched Lotion, for Very Dry Skin** *($2.99 for 6 ounces)* is similar to the Cream version above and the same review applies.

☹ **$$$ Pore Cleansing Strips** *($3.99 for 5 nose strips)* are the Biore strips, repackaged under the Jergens label, so please refer to the Biore Pore Strips review comments.

## Joan Rivers Results (Skin Care Only)

If you shop QVC you know that Joan Rivers sells everything from a Melissa doll (named after Rivers' daughter) to handbags and jewelry. Now add skin care to that grouping. While I think of Joan Rivers as one of the truly funny women on television and have long admired her humor, her entry into the skin-care field seems, well, funny. Could it be that Rivers has forgotten that we all know she has had her share of cosmetic surgeries and that's why her skin looks so smooth, and that these products have nothing to do with the appearance of her tightly readjusted skin? Did anyone at QVC think a sunscreen might be helpful? I guess not. For more information, call (888) 345-5788 or visit the Web site at www.iqvc.com.

☺ **Thoroughly Cleansing Facial Bath** *($20 for 6.7 ounces)* is a good but extremely basic, detergent-based water-soluble cleanser. It would work well for normal to oily skin types but could be too drying for normal to dry skin. The vitamins and plant extracts are present in minuscule amounts and, even if they could have an effect on skin, would be rinsed down the drain.

☹ **$$$ Polished Perfection Exfoliating Scrub** *($19.50 for 4 ounces)* lists the third ingredient as sodium lauryl sulfate, which can be a problem for irritation and dryness. Other than that, this is just a detergent-based water-soluble cleanser with synthetic beads for scrubbing skin. It also contains some plant extracts, vitamins, fragrance, and coloring agents.

☹ **Clean Splash Toner** *($17.25 for 6.7 ounces)*. Witch hazel can be an irritant, which sort of negates the anti-irritant in here.

☺ **Daily Improvement Treatment Formula** (*$33.25 for 1.7 ounces*). The pH of this product is about a 5, which makes it a poor exfoliant and not recommended as a well-formulated AHA product. However, it would be a good moisturizer for normal to slightly dry skin though the amount of vitamins in here is negligible and the formula rather basic and uneventful for the money. I should mention that the third ingredient in this product is strontium nitrate, which is utilized in flares and pyrotechnic devices because it burns with an intense red flame—but what that has to do with skin care, I have not been able to discern (and I've been looking).

☺ **Nightly Improvement Treatment Formula** (*$33.75 for 1.7 ounces*) is similar to the version above and the same comments apply.

☺ **$$$ Constant Nourishment Eye Smoother** (*$31 for 0.5 ounce*) is hardly nourishing but it is a good moisturizer for normal to dry skin.

## Joey New York (Skin Care Only)

So who's Joey? His name is Joey Roer and that is all the Web site for this line wants you to know about the founder. Joey's main claim to fame seems to be a very hip New York location that is described as being "…among America's premiere destinations for world-class therapeutic skin care treatments and beauty enhancement products. All of Joey New York products contain only all-natural quality ingredients." This may indeed be a premier destination, located at 24 West 57th Street, Suite 503, New York, New York, and the products do get a lot of attention in fashion magazines, but none of that explains the primarily problematic formulations this line struggles with. First, these aren't natural in the least. A mere cursory look at the ingredient listing proves that. Plus, the dusting of plant extracts in here are present in such minute amounts as to be barely worth mentioning. Even more significant is that while some of the plants used have anti-irritant properties (licorice and chamomile), many others have an irritating effect on skin (including camphor, peppermint, yarrow, coltsfoot, pine, lemon, grapefruit, and nettle). What a waste. The Pure Pore products have a good amount of salicylic acid (BHA), but not one has an appropriate pH to make it an effective exfoliant and the inclusion of peppermint, camphor, and alcohol in several cause unnecessary inflammation and irritation, which only make matters worse for clogged pores.

There are a few positives in this line to take note of. There is a skin-lightening product with 2% hydroquinone, which makes it an option for inhibiting melanin production; there is a sunscreen that contains zinc oxide as one of the actives and an SPF 30; and there are a couple of well-formulated moisturizers, but that's about it. For the most part, Joey New York has a far better location than it has formulations. For more information, call (800) 563-9691 or visit the Web site at www. joeynewyork.com.

☺ **Pure Pores Cleansing Gel with Vitamin C** *($22 for 8 ounces)* is a standard detergent-based cleanser that also contains plant oils and about a 1% salicylic acid (BHA). The jojoba oil in here can be a problem for oily skin types, and the grapefruit and orange oil can be skin irritants. The pH of this product isn't low enough for the BHA to be effective as an exfoliant, though even if it were, it would just be rinsed down the drain before it could have an effect on skin.

☹ $$$ **Pure Pores Crushed Almond and Honey Scrub** *($28 for 4 ounces)* is just what the name implies, a honey and almond meal scrub that also contains clay, making it slightly difficult to rinse off. It's an option, but it doesn't really get much more standard than this when it comes to a scrub.

☺ $$$ **Pure Pores Oil-Free Moisturizer with Ginseng** *($22 for 2 ounces)* contains several thickening agents high up on the ingredient list that would be problematic for someone with breakouts. Other than that, it is an OK moisturizer for someone with normal to slightly dry skin. It contains fennel and ginseng, which can be skin irritants.

☹ **Pure Pores Blackhead Remover and Pore Minimizer Gel** *($20 for 2 ounces)* contains about 1% BHA but the pH of this product isn't low enough for it to be effective as an exfoliant. It also contains something called "fruit acids" but that isn't the same as AHA, it is a sound-alike that leads you to believe this product contains something it does not. There are a handful of potentially irritating plant extracts, which just adds up to a product with more potential problems than benefits.

☹ **Pure Pores Masque and Blemish Treatment** *($21 for 2 ounces)* contains too much alcohol as well as sulfur and camphor, making this too irritating for all skin types. Sulfur can be a mild disinfectant but the irritation it can cause makes it more of a problem for skin than a help.

☹ **Roll on Blemish Fix** *($18 for 3.3 ounces)* contains too much alcohol as well as camphor, making this too irritating for all skin types.

☹ **Chin Breakout Relief** *($25 for 2 ounces)* contains mostly water and alcohol along with peppermint oil, which makes it too irritating for all skin types.

☹ **Hide and Heal** *($13)*. The salicylic acid in here can't exfoliate because of the high pH and it is no more effective a concealer than any other. This version also contains menthol, camphor, eucalyptus, and peppermint, which, because of the irritation and inflammation they cause, can actually hurt the skin's healing process.

☹ **Milk and Honey Cleanser with Vitamins** *($22 for 8 ounces)* uses sodium lauryl sulfate as the main detergent-cleansing agent, which can be fairly irritating. The teeny amount of milk in here has no impact on skin. This also contains several problematic plant extracts including nettle, yarrow, coltsfoot, horsetail extract, and sage, which are all skin irritants.

☺ **Extra Gentle Eye Makeup Remover** *($16 for 6 ounces)* is an exceptionally standard makeup remover. It is no more gentle than hundreds of other similarily formulated products.

☺ **Gentle Makeup Remover Pads** *($10 for 50 pads)* is identical to the version above, only it comes with presoaked pads.

☹ **One Step Toner and Moisturizer** *($22 for 8 ounces)*. While this does contain about 6% glycolic acid (AHA) in a passable low pH, the plant extracts in here of horsetail, pine, and lemon are too irritating for all skin types and are not moisturizing in the least.

☺ **Vitamin Toner with Ginseng** *($16 for 8 ounces)*. Ginseng is a skin irritant but given most women don't know that, the name of this product sounds healthy and natural. It also contains a good deal of fragrance, making this a real do-nothing toner with potentially more problems than benefits. The vitamin C in here is ascorbic acid, which is considered to be the most irritating and unstable form of vitamin C.

☺ **Green Tea with Multivitamins SPF-30** *($20 for 1 ounce)* is a very good, in-part zinc oxide–based sunscreen for someone with normal to dry skin. The minuscule amount of vitamins in here have no effect on skin and the plant extracts are mix of irritants and anti-irritants, which make them a waste in this product.

☺ **Red Marine Algae Vitamin Enriched Moisturizer** *($20 for 1 ounce)* is a very good emollient moisturizer for normal to dry skin. The plant extracts in here are a mix of irritants and anti-irritants and negate any purpose for skin, good or bad.

☹ **Firm and Tone Eye Cream** *($20 for 0.5 ounce)* contains several problematic ingredients, including arnica, witch hazel, and ivy, for the skin that would be even more of a problem around the eye area.

☺ **$$$ Lift Up Eye Gel** *($20 for 0.5 ounce)* is an OK lightweight moisturizer. The vitamin C in here is ascorbic acid, considered to be one of the more irritating and unstable forms.

☹ **Line Up** *($40 for 1 ounce)* is supposed to prevent wrinkles. This toner-like lotion can't do that in the least though it can irritate the skin. The second ingredient is sodium silicate, a highly alkaline earth mineral that has absorbing properties and can irritate the skin. The fourth ingredient is magnesium aluminum silicate, which also has absorbing properties. None of that is helpful for skin, particularly when it comes to wrinkles. The teeny amount of collagen in here has no effect on the collagen in your skin.

☺ **$$$ Skin Lightener Treatments** *($40 for two 0.5-ounce containers)*. The **Day Skin Lightening Treatment SPF 15** has no UVA-protecting ingredients of titanium dioxide, zinc oxide, or avobenzone and is not recommended. That is disappointing because it does contain 2% hydroquinone, which can inhibit melanin production. The **Night Skin Lightening** portion also contains 2% hydroquinone in a standard Vaseline-based moisturizer that is an option for inhibiting melanin production. It also contains kojic acid, which can inhibit melanin production, but it is a highly unstable skin-care ingredient and probably doesn't have much impact on skin.

☺ **$$$ Calm and Correct** *($38 for 1 ounce)* is supposed to "diminish the appearance of dark circles under the eyes, spider veins on the face and legs, and the redness that results from laser treatments and chemical peels." As if any of those things are related. Not surprisingly, the fish cartilage and seaweed in here can't do any of that. This is a good, though extremely standard lightweight moisturizer for normal to slightly dry skin that contains mostly water, thickeners, water-binding agents, silicone, plant extracts, vitamin E, film former, and preservatives. Vitamin E does not help wound healing, and reducing the appearance of surfaced capillaries on the face is not possible with a cosmetic.

☺ **$$$ Super Duper Lips** *($25 for 2-piece kit)*. It doesn't get much more hyped than this. You're supposed to believe that this "…will instantly and dramatically help to enhance your lips making them fuller, smoother, softer and 'kiss-able' in minutes!" The Lip Gel contains mostly corn syrup, glycerin, honey, and AHA. The slight swelling the AHA causes does not enhance lips and the Super Duper Lipstick Pencil is as standard a lip pencil as it gets. You can give this a test run, but it won't make you want to pucker up.

## Kalo Hair Inhibitor

Getting rid of unwanted body hair is a desire probably second only to wanting more perfect hair on your head. The cosmetics industry has been selling products claiming it can do both for you painlessly and, of course, naturally. **$$$ Kalo Hair Inhibitor** *($39.95 to $59.95 for 4 ounces, depending on the distributor)* wants you to believe it can take care of the former. Let's look at the claims: "Kalo is a soothing, all-natural, herbal-based, aqueous mist that you spray on after shaving, waxing, or sugaring. It was formulated by top Canadian scientists and underwent 5 years of extensive clinical and safety tests. . . . Kalo's proprietary formula works directly in the follicle, neutralizing the key elements necessary for hair to grow, without damaging skin tissue or causing irritation. After each removal session, you will notice that 10–15% of your hair will not grow back. . . . Within 6 months, you should expect 50% of your hair to be permanently eliminated. Best of all, with continued usage, growth can ultimately be ceased completely. Test results show that even in a worst case scenario—a man with a very dense, coarse beard who shaves two or three times a day—the growth will most likely be retarded to the point that this person need shave only two or three times a week."

Where to start? Those extensive Canadian studies are as good a place as any. When the distributors for Kalo sent me their research and documentation for this claim, it turned out to be strictly about irritancy and had absolutely nothing to do with efficacy. Next, there is nothing natural about Kalo in the least. The ingredients include propylene glycol, triethanolamine, propylparaben, methylparaben, diazolidnyl urea, and EDTA. None of those are bad, but the "natural" claim is one of the many misleading ones generated by this company.

The Kalo Web site states, "We cannot disclose what herbs are included as this would give our secret formula away." Perhaps the best way to go about this completely unsubstantiated bombast is with the ingredient list. According to the FDA (and since this product is sold in the United States, Kalo must comply with FDA regulations), legally you must disclose all ingredients in a cosmetic regardless of any purported "secret formula." The only exceptions to this are fragrance, soap, and products developed before 1978. According to Kalo, it has chosen not to comply with the legal mandate to disclose all ingredient listings. It's an odd twist to boast about doing something illegal.

There is also a discrepancy between the ingredients listed on the product itself and on the box. The box includes an ingredient called dithiothreitol that, for some reason, is left off of the container itself. However, dithiothreitol is ultimately significant, which may be why the company is trying to keep it secret. Dithiothreitol is a reducing agent, meaning a depilatory, and in its pure form has quite a list of cautions, including severe skin and eye irritancy (Material Safety Data Sheet—MSDS #C4807). Despite the safety data, there doesn't seem to be enough of it in Kalo to be a problem in the least. But this depilatory agent is hardly a natural hair inhibitor. It is a thiol, just like any depilatory you buy at the drugstore that uses forms of ammonium or sodium thioglycolate.

*But here's the final catch:* Kalo's "effectiveness relies on first physically removing the unwanted hair in a way that removes the hair shaft and bulb without breaking the hair and leaves the follicle open usually accomplished by waxing, sugaring or tweezing." You then apply Kalo and "every time you wax, you can expect that 10 to 15 per cent of the hair will never grow back." Well, duh! If you keep waxing, sugaring, and tweezing you will never know if your hair has grown back. There would never be a way to know what is creating the results. Waxing, sugaring, and tweezing by themselves produce a sense of reduced growth because of the intermittent nature of hair production. Plus, by the time you figured out that the herbs weren't telling the cell to stop forming hair (by the way, it isn't the cells that trigger hair growth but hormones telling the cells what to do), your guarantee would be up and you would have purchased over $500 of this stuff trying to get it to work. And how many men are going to wax, sugar, or tweeze their beard?

Kalo is not the only company making the same spurious claims about its product being a natural hair inhibitor; there are others and every one I've seen is making the same claims and are all using depilatory agents. For more information about

Kalo, call Sunset International Distribution at 800-65-NISIM or visit the Web site at www.nisim.com.

## Karin Herzog Skin Care

It is strange to review a cosmetics line whose primary formulations are based on a major, faulty premise, but Karin Herzog's line of skin-care products is just that. Most all of her skin-care products are based on the notion that oxygen in creams, lotions, and masks can help skin—that is, get rid of wrinkles, cure acne, and heal rosacea and an assortment of other skin ills. Based on this assumption, most all of the Herzog products contain hydrogen peroxide, a source (albeit not a great source) of oxygen. I've discussed many times why the notion of oxygen in skin care is a bogus concept (see "Oxygen for Skin Care" in Chapter 2).

Separate from the oxygen issue, another Herzog claim I find disturbing is that her "products are so pure, and the quality standards so rigorous, that many of the Karin Herzog products require no preservatives." A head of lettuce can be entirely pure and natural too, yet give it a week or two in your refrigerator and it will yield mold and bacteria growth. Not a pretty picture, and extremely bad for skin and eyes. Bacteria, mold, and fungus contamination can invade a cosmetic the second it is formulated. While only a handful of Herzog's products don't list preservatives, I suspect they are there nonetheless or there would be serious problems with using them.

Another substantial marketing focus of the Karin Herzog line is her Vita-A-Kombi products. The vitamin A used is "vitamin A palmitate, a neutral form of vitamin A. Vitamin A has proven to be an important nutrient in the fight against aging skin, in products such as Retin-A, recognized as one of the most effective products to reduce wrinkles and fine lines." Yes, Retin-A has been shown to be significant in altering abnormally produced cell formation caused by sun damage, but that doesn't mean retinyl palmitate—there actually isn't an FDA-approved ingredient called vitamin A palmitate—can do the same thing. In fact, retinyl palmitate is so many levels removed from the active ingredient in Retin-A that even in high concentrations it has no significance for skin other than as a good antioxidant. But it isn't the only antioxidant, and hardly the only one to look for. Ironically, retinyl palmitate doesn't seem to be the primary form of vitamin A that's used in all the Karin Herzog products. For some reason, the other less-showcased products use retinol, which in many ways is the preferred form of vitamin A to consider. It still won't change a wrinkle, but it's an interesting change of direction between the Vit-A-Kombi product and the others in the line; so why bother with Vit-A-Kombi?

I know it may get boring to hear me carry on about sunscreen, but here is yet another "scientifically designed" line talking about its vast research and product superiority yet ignoring the skin's need for sun protection. I find that either lamentably ignorant if a company is truly unaware of this fact (but then why you would trust any of its formulations and research is unfathomable to me), or totally unconscionable if it does know about the need for sunscreen and then doesn't provide one.

A strange side note: a quick and even cursory look at the ingredient label catches the repetitive nature of the formulations; one after the other have almost the same combination of ingredients—water, mineral oil, Vaseline, hydrogen peroxide, thickeners, vitamins, and fragrance. One after the other. If you thought one of these moisturizers was good, there would be absolutely no reason to buy the others; they are all that similar. Buy the way, the Vaseline and mineral oil make these products only suitable for those with dry skin.

One strong, true point of the Karin Herzog line is the truly simple and basic nature of its formulations. There are no long, contrived ingredient listings throwing in every plant that grows to make it appear all natural. If it wasn't for the added fragrance and hydrogen peroxide included in these products, they would be an option for sensitive skin types. For more information about Karin Herzog Skin Care, call (800) 261-7261 or (707) 586-7991 or visit the Web site at www.karinherzog.ch.

☺ $$$ **Cleansing Milk** *($30 for 7.05 ounces)* doesn't clean the skin very well since it needs to be wiped off with a washcloth or Kleenex.

☺ $$$ **Professional Cleansing Cream** *($32 for 1.76 ounces)* is one of the most overpriced cold creams I've ever seen. It can leave a greasy film on the skin and using it is no different from using old-fashioned Pond's Cold Cream, which I wouldn't recommend either. The brochure brags that this product doesn't contain preservatives; it doesn't, but then neither does Vaseline, which is what you are mostly buying in this product.

☻ **Mild Scrub** *($34 for 1.76 ounces)* is scratchy stuff and the mineral oil can leave the skin with a bit of a greasy feel.

☺ $$$ **Vita-A-Kombi 1, Vita-A-Kombi 2, or Vita-A-Kombi 3** *(#1 $50 for 1.94 ounces; #2 $54 for 1.94 ounces; #3 $56 for 1.94 ounces)*. The varying numbers for these products indicate the concentration of oxygen—1% oxygen; 2% oxygen, or 3% oxygen. These standard, mundane moisturizers are hardly worth the money. Though if you do want to believe the hype about hydrogen peroxide, you could just go to the drugstore and buy 3% hydrogen peroxide for 89 cents and have the same thing.

☺ $$$ **Vita-A-Kombi Fruit Acids 1% Oxygen** *($50 for 1.94 ounces)* is similar to the one above only with the addition of AHA. However, the pH of this product and the concentration of AHA—less than 2%—make it a poorly formulated AHA product.

☺ **Day Cream** *($30 for 1.76 ounces)* doesn't have an SPF and only lists octyl methoxycinnamate (a UVB-protecting ingredient) in the regular list of ingredients, so this product should not be used during the day. There is little difference between this product and the Night Cream below.

☺ **Night Cream** *($32 for 1.76 ounces)* is a good, though exceptionally standard, moisturizer. There would be no reason to use this one rather than Eucerin.

☺ **$$$ Eye Cream 0.5% Oxygen** *($48 for 0.6 ounce)*. It's interesting to buy an eye cream that contains the warning "rinse immediately if in contact with eyes." Other than that, this is a good, standard moisturizer for dry skin.

☹ **Oxygen Face Cream 2% Oxygen** *($34 for 1.76 ounces)* contains—yes, more hydrogen peroxide, in water, mineral oil, and thickeners. For some reason this one is recommended for teenagers to control acne. There is nothing in this product capable of doing that and the emollients will only feel greasy on blemish-prone skin.

☺ **$$$ Facial Oil** *($20 for 0.49 ounce)* is mostly emollients and water-binding agents. It is good for dry skin and is one of the only uniquely formulated products in the bunch.

☺ **$$$ Mask** *($38 for 1.76 ounces)* is virtually identical to many of the moisturizers in this line. There is literally no reason to think of it doing anything special or different for the skin.

☺ **Oxygen Body Cream 1% with Fruit Acids** *($34 for 4.3 ounces)*. I guess if your face needs oxygen, your body would too. However, this formula is identical to the face products, and as long as it's cheaper, you might as well use this. It does contain about a 1% concentration of AHA but that isn't enough to serve any function for skin.

☺ **Oxygen Body Cream 3%** *($34 for 4.3 ounces)* is similar to the one above, minus the AHA.

## *Kiehl's (Skin Care Only)*

Kiehl's independent, small-town image went by the wayside in April 2000 when it was purchased by L'Oreal. How did this very expensive, obscure skin-care line become so well known? Especially when you consider that the company doesn't advertise (although it does have a PR firm that handles its press relations, which garnered it a lot of attention in fashion magazines). Kiehl's has definitely gotten value out of its attention-getting media mentions.

The line has been around for quite some time; it has its origins in a family-owned pharmacy. Still, the products hardly warrant excitement or even mild enthusiasm. Most of them are surprisingly ordinary, with a dusting of natural ingredients almost always at the very end of the ingredient list, well past the preservatives. That amounts to little more than a token attempt to make the products appear more natural to consumers who want to believe a plant or vitamin must somehow be better for the skin than something that sounds more chemical. Nevertheless, that token amount is enough to allow Kiehl's to brag about how its products nourish the skin or are more environmentally friendly, even though that may only be true for less than 1 percent of the product's content.

Of course, those who know better understand that vitamins can't nourish the skin, that using nonfat milk and plant extracts means the amount of preservative in a product must be increased to prevent deterioration, and that while plant oils may be moisturizing, they are not wonder ingredients.

The company's most interesting claim is that its products are all made by hand, just the way they were when the original Kiehl's pharmacy began selling cosmetics in 1851. Today, given the wide distribution of Kiehl's products—they are available at Bergdorf Goodman, Neiman Marcus, Barney's, Harrods, and many other stores— that claim is extremely hard to swallow. The person I talked to at Kiehl's said each product is made the way I would make a cake. But I've never baked thousands of cakes at once, or baked one cake that could serve thousands of people. I can't stir 100 pounds of flour and water; how can someone stir 100 pounds of water and waxes? Yes, it is all hand-stirred, she insisted. Even if that were true, which I strongly doubt, what extra benefit is there to hand-stirring a cosmetic anyway? It's just more personal, she said; there's better control. It may *sound* more personal, but the possibility of error or contamination is far greater and the concept itself mistaken.

Regardless of how the products are processed, the bottom line is, can they do what they claim and are they worth the money? In this case, the products consist of totally ordinary ingredients, despite the fact that they are called special or natural. Many ingredients are questionable for sensitive skin types or for oily skin, and in some instances would be irritating for any skin type, and the sunscreen products are mostly a serious problem for reliable sun protection. For more information about Kiehl's, call (800) KIEHLS-1.

☹ **Foaming Non-Detergent Washable Cleanser** *($13.50 for 8 ounces)* is not in the least a nondetergent cleanser: the second ingredient is sodium C14-16 olefin sulfate, a cleansing agent in shampoos that is known for stripping hair color. I would call this a standard detergent facial cleanser that can dry out the skin.

☺ **Gentle Foaming Facial Cleanser for Dry to Normal Skin Types** *($13.50 for 8 ounces)* is a standard, detergent-based water-soluble cleanser that also contains a small amount of plant oils. The plant oils in here can leave a greasy film on the skin, so this would only be appropriate and worth considering for someone with very dry skin.

☹ **Oil-Based Cleanser and Makeup Remover** *($10.50 for 4 ounces)* at least has an honest name. This very greasy cleanser needs to be wiped off like cold cream and can leave a film on the face. The second ingredient is isopropyl myristate, notorious for causing breakouts. The cleanser also contains lanolin oil, which is emollient but can be a problem for sensitive skin types. If you like grease, this product is an option.

☹ **Rare-Earth Oatmeal Milk Facial Cleanser #1 (Mild)** *($17.50 for 8 ounces)* doesn't contain any earth that is remotely rare, just standard kaolin and bentonite, better known as clay. But I guess if you want to charge this kind of money for clay and standard detergent cleansing agents, you have to call it rare. The minuscule amounts of vitamins, nonfat milk, and oat flour are included to boost the natural appearance of a completely unnatural product.

☹ **Rare-Earth Oatmeal Milk Facial Cleanser #2 (Medium Strength)** *($17.50 for 8 ounces)* is very similar to the facial cleanser above, only much more drying.

☹ **Rare-Earth Foaming Cleanser #2 (Medium Strength)** *($17.50 for 8 ounces)* contains both sodium lauryl sulfate and TEA-lauryl sulfate as the main detergent cleansing agents, both of which are extremely drying and irritating. I definitely would not recommend this for the face. The standard natural ingredients are listed well after the preservatives, and they won't make this cleanser any less irritating.

☺ **Ultra Moisturizing Cleansing Cream** *($16.95 for 8 ounces)* is a very ordinary, somewhat greasy wipe-off cleanser that can leave a film on the skin, though it can be an option for very dry skin.

☺ **Washable Cleansing Milk a Moisturizing Cleanser for Dry or Sensitive Skin** *($13.50 for 8 ounces)* is not what I would consider a "washable" cleanser. It contains oils that can leave a greasy film on the skin. Protein, nonfat milk, and other "natural ingredients" are at the very end of the ingredient list, well after the preservatives, so there aren't enough of them to make this product even vaguely milky.

☺ **Milk, Honey, and Almond Scrub** *($18.50 for 6 ounces)* is a standard scrub that uses ground almonds. It also contains talc and flour, which can be hard to rinse off and can be irritating when rubbed into the skin. The nonfat milk, plant oils, and vitamins are at the end of the ingredient list. The oils may leave a greasy residue but this can be an option for dry skin.

☺ **Ultra Moisturizing Buffing Cream with Scrub Particles** *($16.50 for 4 ounces)* is a scrub that uses a synthetic scrub ingredient (ground-up plastic); it also contains thickening agents and oils. It would be suitable for someone with very dry skin.

☹ **Pineapple and Papaya Facial Scrub Made with Real Fruit** *($26.50 for 4 ounces)* does contain pineapple and papaya, but they are potent skin irritants. (Ever get pineapple on abraded skin or in your eyes? It hurts.) This is a standard detergent cleanser with cornmeal as a scrub. You can use plain cornmeal if you want a scrub similar to this for a lot less money and without the irritation from the other ingredients.

☹ **Blue Astringent Herbal Lotion** *($12.50 for 8 ounces)*. Not only is the alcohol in this product drying and irritating, but the aluminum chlorohydrate (yes, the stuff used in antiperspirants) can cause infection of the hair follicle. What were the chemists who made this product thinking?

☺ **$$$ Calendula Herbal Extract Toner Alcohol-Free** *($32.75 for 8 ounces)*.

The plant extracts in here are a mixed bag of irritants (gentian and ivy) and anti-irritants (burdock and calendula). This is hardly worth the confusion to your skin.

☹ **Cucumber Herbal Alcohol-Free Toner for Dry or Sensitive Skin** *($13.95 for 8 ounces)* is alcohol-free, but not irritant-free. It contains balm mint, pine needle, camphor, and sulfonated oils, all of which can be serious irritants. There is nothing about this product appropriate for sensitive skin.

☺ **French Rosewater** *($10.50 for 8 ounces),* as the name implies, is mostly rose water, which is merely fragranced glycerin, not particularly helpful for skin.

☹ **Herbal Toner with Mixed Berries and Extracts** *($19.95 for 8 ounces)* does have berries but it also has peppermint and lemongrass, which can be irritating for skin.

☹ **Rosewater Toner #1** *($12.50 for 8 ounces)* is mostly alcohol with rose fragrance. It can be irritating and drying.

☹ **Tea Tree Oil Toner** *($22.95 for 8 ounces)* contains eucalyptus and grapefruit in the number two and three spots on the ingredient listing, making this a skin irritation waiting to happen. The teeny amount of tea tree oil in this product isn't enough to be an effective disinfectant for blemishes.

☺ **$$$ Anti-Oxidant Skin Preserver** *($55 for 0.5 ounce)* contains mostly thickeners, plant oil, and vitamins. This is a very emollient, though ordinary moisturizer for normal to dry skin. The vitamins are decent antioxidants though they hardly are unique to this product or warrant the price tag.

☺ **Creme d'Elegance Repairateur Superb Tissue Repairateur Creme** *($25.50 for 2 ounces).* Regardless of what language you say it in, this cream will not repair skin. It would be a good moisturizer for someone with very dry skin.

☺ **Original Formula Eye Cream, Ultra Nourishing** *($10.50 for 0.5 ounce)* isn't even vaguely nourishing, but it is a very good, though ordinary, moisturizer for someone with dry skin.

☺ **$$$ Light Nourishing Eye Cream** *($15.95 for 0.5 ounce)* uses a film-forming agent as a way to smooth the skin and keep water in. Other than that, it is a good ordinary moisturizer for normal to dry skin.

☺ **Moisturizing Eye Balm with Pure Vitamins A & E** *($14.50 for 0.5 ounce)* is a good, though standard and somewhat heavy moisturizer for dry skin.

☺ **Panthenol Protein Moisturizing Face Cream** *($22.50 for 4 ounces)* is a good basic moisturizer for someone with dry skin. The really interesting ingredients are listed way after the preservatives and are hardly worth mentioning.

☺ **Sodium PCA Oil-Free Moisturizer** *($22.50 for 4 ounces)* would be a good moisturizer for someone with normal to dry skin. There are thickening agents here that can be a problem for someone with oily skin and the formulation is exceedingly ordinary.

☺ **$$$ Algae Masque for Balancing Skin Types** *($39.95 for 4.5 ounces)* contains nothing that can balance skin and is certainly not suitable for all skin types, particularly not for someone with oily or combination skin. This can be a good peel-off mask for someone with dry skin, but the algae has no magical benefit. It is an antioxidant, but no better than lots and lots of antioxidants that show up in skin-care products.

☹ **All-Day Masque Oily-Acne** *($12.50 for 1 ounce)* contains several plant oils, and that makes it completely inappropriate for someone with oily skin, plus there is nothing in here of benefit to someone with breakouts.

☺ **$$$ Moisturizing Masque** *($35 for 2 ounces)* is indeed moisturizing and good for someone with dry skin. All of the fancy natural-sounding ingredients are at the end of the ingredient list, but even if there were more, they still couldn't repair skin as this mask claims.

☺ **Rare-Earth Facial Cleansing Masque** *($16.50 for 5 ounces)*. There is nothing rare about the clay in here—it is just standard bentonite and kaolin. It also contains cornstarch, which can clog pores, and several plant oils that can be problematic for oily skin. This can be an option for someone with normal to slightly oily skin but be cautious of this mask's limitations.

☹ **Rare-Earth Face Masque (Gently Astringent for Oily-Acne Skin)** *($13.50 for 4 ounces)* is a sulfur-based clay mask. There is nothing gentle about sulfur, though it is a disinfectant. That wouldn't be all that bad, but there are several thickening agents in this mask that can clog pores and cause breakouts.

☺ **Soothing Gel Masque** *($14.95 for 8 ounces)* is just a layer of film former over the skin and some plant extracts. That can feel OK, and peeling off the layer of plastic will make skin feel temporarily smoother, but for the most part it is really just a waste of time.

☹ **Treatment and Concealing Stick for Blemishes** *($14.50 for 0.5 ounce)* contains more ingredients that are problematic for breakouts than you can imagine, including zinc oxide, lanolin oil (can you believe lanolin oil in a product for acne?), isopropyl palmitate, and carnauba wax (that's car wax).

☹ **Superb Total Dermal Protection Face Cream SPF 8** *($22.95 for 2 ounces; $39.99 for 4 ounces)* is blatantly exaggerating when it claims to provide "total dermal protection" with an SPF of only 8, plus it doesn't contain any UVA-protecting ingredients, and is absolutely not recommended.

☹ **Superb Dermal Protection Eye and Throat Cream with SPF 6** *($27.95 for 2 ounces)* is similar to the Total Dermal version above and the same comments apply.

☺ **Ultra Facial Moisturizer** *($11.50 for 2 ounces)*. This dull formulation is minimally useful for normal to dry skin, although the minuscule amounts of vitamins and plant oils are undetectable.

☹ **Ultra Facial Moisturizer SPF 13** *($27 for 4 ounces)* doesn't contain avobenzone, titanium dioxide, or zinc oxide for UVA protection, and is not recommended.

☹ Ultra Protection Moisturizing Face Gel SPF 15 *($29.95 for 1 ounce)* doesn't contain avobenzone, titanium dioxide, or zinc oxide, and is not recommended.

☹ Ultra Moisturizing Eye Stick with SPF 26 and Vitamin E (Matte) #3 *($19.50)* does not contain avobenzone, titanium dioxide, or zinc oxide, and is not recommended.

☹ Ultra Protection Moisturizing Eye Gel SPF 18 *($28.50 for 0.5 ounce)* does not contain avobenzone, titanium dioxide, or zinc oxide, and is not recommended.

☹ Ultra Moisturizing Eye Stick SPF 18 and Vitamin E *($15.95 for 0.5 ounce)* doesn't contain avobenzone, titanium dioxide, or zinc oxide, and is not recommended.

☺ $$$ Ultra Moisturizing Concealing Stick SPF 26 and Vitamin E (Matte) #1 *($19.50 for 4 grams)* is a part titanium dioxide–based sunscreen that also works as a concealer, but not a very good one. This is a fairly greasy concealer that can crease into the lines around the eyes. If you are already using a sunscreen on your face, using another one in your makeup is completely unnecessary.

☹ Ultra Protection Face Cream and Sunscreen SPF 18 PABA-free *($40 for 2 ounces)* doesn't contain avobenzone, titanium dioxide, or zinc oxide, and is not recommended.

☺ Heidegger's All-Sport Water-Resistant Skin Protector SPF 30 *($17.95 for 4 ounces)* is a good in-part titanium dioxide–based sunscreen that would be good for someone with normal to slightly dry skin.

☹ Sun Screen—Tan Creme, "Tan Smart—Not Fast," SPF 15 *($15.95 for 8 ounces)* doesn't contain avobenzone, zinc oxide, or titanium dioxide for UVA protection, and is not recommended; so much for a smart sunscreen. There is no such thing as a safe tan of any kind except from a self tanner.

☺ Sun Shield Sunblock with SPF 15 *($23.50 for 8 ounces)* is a very good, pure titanium dioxide–based sunscreen for someone with dry skin.

☹ Ultra Protection Water-Based Sunscreen Lotion SPF 24 *($44 for 8 ounces)* doesn't contain avobenzone, zinc oxide, or titanium dioxide, and is not recommended.

☹ Water-based Sunscreen Lotion With SPF 16 *($35 for 8 ounces)* doesn't contain avobenzone, zinc oxide, or titanium dioxide, and is not recommended.

☺ Lip Balm #1 *($4.95 for 0.7 ounce)* is a very emollient lip gloss that contains mostly Vaseline, plant oils, lanolin, and preservatives.

# *Kinerase*

Just when I was wondering what the new antiwrinkle bandwagon was going to be for the new millennium, it starts showing up in ads, fashion magazines, and news stories. It even showed up in an article in the Sunday *Parade* magazine for September 15, 1999. If the press releases for the products containing this new ingredient are to be believed, your new expenditures to fight wrinkles starting in the year 2000 are going to be for something called growth factor (GF). But before you run out to spend your money on this new twist in the antiwrinkle game, read the following information closely. The information is complicated, but the story is every bit as interesting as antioxidants.

The latest products making claims about getting rid of wrinkles are **$$$ Kinerase Lotion 53** *($77 for 53 ml)*; **Kinerase Cream 40** *($77 for 40 ml)*; **Kinerase Lotion 112** *($140 for 112 ml)*; and **Kinerase Cream 80** *($140 for 80 ml)*. These products were developed by Senetek PLC (www.senetekplc.com) and are distributed by ICN Pharmaceuticals, Inc. Kinerase contains a plant growth hormone called N6-furfuryladenine.

Note: Kinerase and a product sold by Osmotics called Kinetin (reviewed in the March 1999 issue of *Cosmetics Counter Update)* both contain N6-furfuryladenine. N6-furfuryladenine also goes by the name "Kinetin." Osmotics chose to name its product after the less chemical-sounding name of the ingredient. For the sake of not confusing the Osmotics product Kinetin with the active ingredient N6 furfuryladenine, I will use the longer technical name for this review.

Here's what you have heard or will be hearing about Kinerase (and Kinetin): "A revolutionary skin rejuvenation product . . . available though dermatologists and plastic surgeons. The active ingredient is a natural botanical growth hormone, called N6-furfuryladenine. Kinerase rivals Renova's effectiveness in diminishing fine lines and discoloration, but without any of the side effects. Kinerase also helps improve moisture retention, leaving skin smooth and supple. Imagine not having to put up with the burning, redness, peeling, and sun sensitivity associated with Renova or other Vitamin A creams. . . . Kinerase contains 0.1% N-furfuryladenine compared to only .05% found in Kinetin [the product sold by Osmotics]. All University of California Irvine studies showing the product's effectiveness were performed using .1% N-furfuryladenine."

The notion that Kinerase is in some way special because it is sold through a doctor's office is not true. Doctors sell all kinds of skin-care products and none of them are formulated by any other standards than those that apply to cosmetics regulations. Kinerase is a cosmetic, not a pharmaceutical, and thus is subject to none of the regulations governing medical products.

Further, as I mentioned in the May 1999 issue of my newsletter, *Cosmetics Counter Update,* the physician who conducted the study on Kinetin (though he asked me not to mention him by name) told me in no uncertain terms that while he did do a clinical study with Kinetin, his results were not remotely like those associated with the claims in the Osmotic brochure [and therefore can't substantiate anything about Kinerase] and that he was shocked his name was being connected with the product in any way, shape, or form. After I interviewed this physician and told him how his name and research were being bandied about on the Web site for Osmotics, I noticed that Osmotics eliminated that information and exaggeration from its site (though it is still alluded to, only much less directly).

But that's about Osmotics' exaggerated claims. What about the actual study showing Kinerase to be as effective as Renova?

According to Dr. Jerry L. McCullough, professor of dermatology, University of California, Irvine, who was part of the research team, "The UCI study was a double-blind study, which involved subjective assessments of clinical improvement and safety by both the physician and the subject. This is the protocol design used in the pivotal multicenter clinical trials of Renova, which were reviewed by the FDA and led to FDA approval. The above studies focused on the clinical assessment of safety and efficacy as did the kinetin [Kinerase] studies. The only objective measures of efficacy in the Renova clinical studies were skin replica analysis and histologic evaluation. The studies at UCI involved over 160 subjects in two studies each lasting one year. ... These studies employed objective assessment of the skin-barrier function using measurements of transepidermal water loss (TEWL) in addition to state of the art clinical photography (Canfield Scientific) to document clinical response. I think that the efforts made by Senetek PLC [the company that makes Kinerase] to document the efficacy and safety of this product far exceed those of the numerous anti-aging skin products [that] flood the cosmetics counters and Web pages making unsubstantiated claims."

While on the surface it does appear that Kinerase performs like Renova, it is important to recognize that this study does not indicate any results about cellular effects or changes. This study looked at surface improvements. As I've reported in the past, the studies the FDA accepted about Renova's performance for wrinkles were hardly definitive. TEWL tells you about moisturization, not about wrinkles, and visual assessment may be impressive but it doesn't tell you if other moisturizers with other ingredients would net you the same improvements. The main interest in this product for skin care actually has nothing to do with wrinkles; instead, the active ingredient in Renova, tretinoin, has a wealth of established literature in regard to its effect on improving abnormal skin-cell production caused by sun damage. That makes Renova (or any other drug containing tretinoin) significant. Kinerase has no such data backing up its effects.

Aside from the single study from UC Irvine, companies selling products that contain plant and human growth factors are claiming different issues about cellular production. I tracked down a Dr. Suresh I. S. Rattan, Ph.D., D.Sc., associate professor of biogerontology at the University of Aarhus, Denmark, who happens to be the patent holder for N6-furfuryladenine in relation to how it is used for aging skin. Rattan discovered this plant growth factor in 1988 and obtained the U.S. patent in 1994. That is, Rattan discovered what happens to skin cells in a petri dish when N6-furfuryladenine is added.

Rattan told me, "Normal cells, as they divide and age, go through a progressive accumulation of changes that are irreversible until they reach a stage where they finally die. This in vitro [meaning in a petri dish as opposed to in humans or animals] form of creating cellular aging, which takes place over one year—consider that it takes our cells more than 70 years to age—is a well-known biochemical phenomenon called the Hayflick Phenomenon, named after the researcher who discovered this method of studying cellular aging in a laboratory setting."

All this relates to N6-furfuryladenine and what it does when added to cells aging in a petri dish. Rattan continued, "Normally when we grow cells in culture, as they become older, regardless of sun exposure, they go through over 300 varying changes and alterations. A young cell is plump, round, smooth (and the functions and chemical processes orderly and vigorous). As the cells age, they become irregular, flattened, and large, full of debris—debris meaning they fill up with waste products that they can't get rid of. Further, when you grow normal cells in the lab, they have a limited number of times they multiply and divide—termed a cell's replicative life span. But when I added N6-furfuryladenine to these cultures the cells did not age as fast, the process slowed down dramatically. In the presence of various concentrations of N6-furfuryladenine, cells act younger, longer."

As exciting as this sounds, and Rattan is indeed excited about his research, he also said, "Topically [applied to the surface of skin] no one knows how or if N6-furfuryladenine is being taken up or used by the cell. There are no studies done on the biochemical action on human skin or animal skin. It has only been observed for in vitro systems. On one level, I feel this compound can be a health-preserving molecule. But it would take a lot of money to find out its full potential.

"What will put my mind at rest is knowing what the full up and down side is. We are curious about negative effects; even water is toxic in certain doses. In cell cultures when a concentration of say 250 micromolars of N6-furfuryladenine was used, we got good results, but when we used 500 micromolars of N6-furfuryladenine, the cells started dying."

I asked Rattan if the hoopla in the U.S. media was disappointing to him. "Often cosmetics companies get carried away. I believe this compound has more potential, but we only really know how it acts in culture, not in humans."

But let me get back to the issue of growth factors, which I will definitely be discussing more with you in the future, because the cosmetics industry is going to be making a lot of noise about the growth factors their products contain. What is significant about N6-furfuryladenine is that even though the literature refers to it as a plant growth factor, it is not a "cell divider," and that is a significant distinction. There are biochemical ingredients that cause cells to divide, such as peptidic hormones or cytokines (human growth factors such as epidermal growth factor (EGF) and transforming growth factor-Beta (TGF-beta 1)). According to an article by Dr. Donald R. Owen in the March 1999 issue of *Global Cosmetic Industry*, "The body produces these [cytokines or peptidic hormones] in exquisitely small concentrations at just the right location and time.... Actual growth factors such as [EGF and TGF-beta 1] are [large] configurations which do not penetrate the skin.... They [also] lose their activity within days in water or even as solids at normal temperatures.... [Yet], even after all these complications, the siren's song is too strong. We [the cosmetics chemists] will use them."

While many skin-care ingredients leave me cold in terms of their claims, more often than not, they are not dangerous. However, the risks associated with growth factors, if scientists do learn how to get them stabilized and into skin, are alarming. In skin, you don't need extra cell division. For example, hyper cell division in the upper layers of skin can cause psoriasis.

More important, increasing cell division is a cancer risk. Cancer cells never age, they have an indefinite or an immortal life of hyperactive division, which is what makes them deadly. Dr. Rattan explained, "Numerous studies have looked at cortisone, other plant extracts, and various other growth factors; most all of these affected multiplication, or replicative life span . . . [a risk to healthy cells]. N6-furfuryladenine (kinetin) helped the skin cell act younger. It wasn't that it altered cell division, but it slowed down the changes that take place [in vitro] as cells age."

One more thing Rattan described: "If cells are old they can't become young, you can't make an old cell revert. A fundamental biological precept is, if it's a disease you can reverse it, but if it is a natural biological process you can't reverse the effect. Aging is a biological process not a disease. You can affect its rate of progression but you can't stop it or make it revert back." For more information, call the Senetek Corporation at (707) 226-3900.

## *Kiss My Face (Skin Care Only)*

I love the name of this skin-care line. It evokes a sense of tenderness and affection that is sweet and caring. You may have run into this line in health food stores and the occasional drugstore. It is particularly hard for teens to ignore. Perhaps even more beguiling are the incredibly low prices. I only wish the thoughtful name translated into thoughtful products, but I'm not sure what this company was thinking. Despite the claims about the line not using any unnecessary chemicals, there are plenty of them in these products. Actually, its brochure states that its products contain "no synthetics or chemicals, artificial preservatives or fragrances of any kind. ... All the ingredients coming from renewable resources are environmentally sound. Many of the herbs are grown or harvested by indigenous people, helping preserve their way of life." What kind of renewable resource is cocamide DEA, propylparaben, or sodium lauryl sulfate? While some of its "chemical" ingredients are derived from plant sources, that still doesn't mean you can eat the stuff. Plus, as you all know, the process of creating a cosmetic ingredient and then preserving it has very little to do with nature. Once extracted from the plant and preserved, cosmetic ingredients are also no longer edible and only vaguely related to their natural origins.

And no fragrance? It states further down in the brochure about how aromatic its products are. Well, aromatic ingredients such as rose oil, geranium oil, or bergamot oil are fragrance, as are the myriad plant extracts in here! I'm concerned that the amount of plants in these products serves little purpose for the skin and that it is more allergy-provoking than anything. Further, this line seems to have a penchant for lime, lemon, camphor, eucalyptus, grapefruit, and peppermint. These serve no purpose for skin other than to cause unnecessary irritation, which impedes the skin's healing process.

While the prices are more than reasonable, there are other aspects of this line that leave much to be desired, such as cleansers with sodium lauryl sulfate as the main cleansing ingredient, AHA products with either minimal concentrations or a high pH, blemish products with extremely irritating ingredients, and lots of fragrant, sensitizing plant oils.

For more information about Kiss My Face, call (800) 262-KISS or check the Web site at www.kissmyface.com.

☹ **Fragrance Free Antibacterial Moisture Soap** *($3.99 for 12 ounces)* contains sodium lauryl sulfate as the second ingredient, which means a high risk of irritation for all skin types. It also contains triclosan, an effective antibacterial agent. In order for any antibacterial agent to do its thing, it needs to be left on skin for a period of time (for example, doctors scrub with far more potent antibacterial scrubs for several minutes before they consider themselves germ free). In a cleanser, ingredients like triclosan would be rinsed down the drain before they could have a real effect.

☹ **Hawaiian Heaven Antibacterial Moisture Soap** *($5 for 12 ounces)* is similar to the one above and the same comments apply.

☹ **Pear Antibacterial Moisture Soap** *($3.99 for 12 ounces)* is similar to the one above and the same comments apply.

☹ **Original Moisture Soap** *($3.99 for 12 ounces)* contains sodium lauryl sulfate as the second ingredient, which means a high risk of irritation for all skin types.

☹ **Almond Creme Moisture Soap** *($4.40 for 12 ounces)* is similar to the one above and the same comments apply.

☹ **Peaches & Creme Moisture Soap** *($3.99 for 12 ounces)* is similar to the one above and the same comments apply.

☹ **Summer Melon Moisture Soap** *($3.99 for 12 ounces)* is similar to the one above and the same comments apply.

☹ **Chamomile Olive Soap** *($1.99 for 4 ounces)* has a standard soap base that can be drying for most skin types.

☹ **Pure Olive Oil Soap** *($1.99 for 4 ounces)* is similar to the one above and the same comments apply.

☹ **Olive & Aloe Soap** *($1.99 for 4 ounces)* is similar to the one above and the same comments apply.

☹ **Olive & Herbal Soap** *($1.99 for 4 ounces)* is similar to the one above and the same comments apply.

☹ **Olive & Honey Soap with Calendula** *($1.99 for 4 ounces)* is similar to the one above and the same comments apply.

☹ **Citrus Cleanser** *($6.95 for 4 ounces)* is a standard wipe-off, cold cream–type cleanser with the addition of lime oil, lemon oil, and other plant extracts that are completely unnecessary skin irritants.

☹ **Exfoliating Face Wash** *($8.95 for 4 ounces)* contains oils of lemon, grapefruit, tangerine, lemongrass, orange, and lime. All are irritating, and useless for the skin.

☺ **Gentle Face Cleanser for Normal to Dry** *($10 for 4 ounces)* is a relatively rinseable cleanser with plant oil and detergent cleansing agent. The orange oil in here isn't the best, but it's probably not enough to be a problem for the skin. This could be an option for someone with dry skin.

☹ **Normal/Oily Foaming Facial Cleanser** *($10 for 4 ounces)* contains witch hazel, lime oil, lemon oil, grapefruit oil, orange oil, and tangerine oil, which are too irritating for all skin types.

☹ **Organic Jojoba & Mint Facial Scrub** *($10 for 2 ounces)*. Between the mint, peppermint, eucalyptus, camphor, and bergamot oil, I can't imagine why anyone would want to put this much irritation on skin.

☹ **Scrub Masque** *($7 for 5 ounces)* is basically just almond meal and cornmeal with thickeners, including oatmeal. This is a fairly abrasive scrub and can be a problem for most skin types, especially dry or sensitive skin.

☹ **Aloe & Chamomile Toner for Normal/Dry Skin** *($9 for 4 ounces)* does contain aloe and chamomile but it also contains witch hazel and tea tree oil, which are both out of place in a product for dry skin. Tea tree oil can be a good topical disinfectant and the witch hazel can also be drying and irritating for most skin types but especially dry skin.

☹ **Aloe & Tea Tree Astringent for Normal/Oily Skin** *($9 for 4 ounces)* is similar to the one above only with the addition of camphor to add to the irritation.

☹ **Citrus Essence Astringent for Oily and Combination Skin Types** *($5 for 8 ounces)* contains witch hazel and lemon juice, along with extracts of more citrus fruits. This is a problem waiting to happen.

☺ **Flower Essence Toner** *($5 for 6 ounces)*. I'm concerned about the fragrance extracts in this toner but, aside from that, this would be an option for someone with normal to dry skin. It contains mostly water, glycerin, slip agent, water-binding agent, plant oil, and preservatives.

☺ **Alpha Aloe Oil Free Moisturizer 5% Alpha Hydroxy Acid Fragrance Free** *($9.95 for 16 ounces)* is indeed oil free, but it does contain other ingredients such as isopropyl palmitate and emulsifying wax that can be a problem for oily skin. While this product contains a concoction of AHAs, it would be far better if it only contained lactic and/or glycolic acid (they perform the best for skin). Regardless, the pH of this product isn't low enough to make it an effective exfoliant, though this would be a good moisturizer for dry skin.

☺ **Alpha Aloe Oil Free Moisturizer Vanilla Scent 5% Alpha Hydroxy Acid** *($9.95 for 16 ounces)* is similar to the one above and the same basic review applies, though products with no scent are best for skin.

☹ **Aromatherapeutic Alpha Hydroxy Creme** *($15 for 1 ounce)* contains about 1% of something called natural mixed fruit acids, which isn't the same as an alpha hydroxy acid, and even if you could rely on this amorphous mixture, there isn't enough of it to be effective as an exfoliant. While this could be a good, standard moisturizer for dry skin, the inclusion of lemon oil, lime oil, tangerine oil, orange oil, and grapefruit oil makes it too irritating for most skin types.

☺ **Peaches & Creme Moisturizer 8% Alpha Hydroxy for Face and Neck** *($8.95 for 4 ounces)*. This version of an AHA product uses nicely identified mixed fruit acids. However, it's glycolic acid and lactic acid that are the best versions of AHAs for skin. The others listed here—citric acid, malic acid, and tartaric acid—are just not the best for exfoliation. Plus, the pH of this product is too high for it to be an effective exfoliant anyway. There are fewer irritating plant extracts in here than in most of the products in the Kiss My Face lineup, which makes this a good moisturizer for dry skin but the citrus oils can be a problem.

☹ **Botanical Acne Gel** *($16 for 1.7 ounces)* contains witch hazel, peppermint oil, and camphor oil, which will only make acne worse by making skin redder and more irritated.

☺ **All Day Moisture Creme** *($9 for 4 ounces)* has no sunscreen, so you wouldn't want to use this during the day—but as a standard, exceedingly ordinary moisturizer for dry skin, it's worth a consideration.

☺ **All Night Olive & Aloe Moisture Creme** *($8.95 for 4 ounces)* is an excellent option for dry skin.

☺ **Chinese Botanical Moisturizer** *($9.95 for 16 ounces)* is similar to the one above and the same basic review applies. The plant extracts in here all have Chinese names but they all correlate to regular plant extracts that have some antibacterial, anti-inflammatory, and potentially irritating effects. They are a bizarre mixture seemingly unrelated to a standard moisturizer that appears to be for dry skin.

☺ **Fragrance Free Oil Free Moisturizer with NaPCA** *($5.89 for 16 ounces)* is basically just water, wax, fragrance, preservatives, and a tiny amount of something called NaPCA, which is short for sodium pyrrolidone carboxylic acid. That very unnatural-sounding ingredient is a good water-binding agent, but nothing to get excited about and there's not enough of it here to make this otherwise ordinary, waxy moisturizer worth considering.

☺ **Oil Free with NaPCA Moisturizer with Green Tea and Ginkgo Biloba** *($5.89 for 16 ounces)* is similar to the one above and the same basic review applies. One additional comment: while this product is oil-free, it contains emulsifying wax, which can clog pores. The inclusion of *Gingko biloba* extract can be a problem for reddened skin.

☺ **Fragrance Free Olive & Aloe Moisturizer for Extra Sensitive Skin** *($5.89 for 16 ounces)* contains extracts of chamomile, marigold, sage, yarrow, orange blossoms, lavender, elder flowers, and fennel, and so I would hardly consider this fragrance-free. Other than that, it is a good standard moisturizer for dry skin, containing water, thickeners, plant oils, vitamins, water-binding agent, and preservatives.

☺ **Honey & Calendula Moisturizer for Extra Dry Skin** *($5.89 for 16 ounces)* is almost identical to the Olive & Aloe version above, only with honey and calendula, which aren't useful for dry skin anyway, and the same review applies.

☺ **Olive & Aloe Moisturizer for Sensitive Skin** *($5.89 for 16 ounces)* is a good standard moisturizer for dry skin, but the fragrance in here makes it inappropriate for sensitive skin types.

☺ **Vitamin A & E Moisturizer** *($5.89 for 16 ounces)* is similar to the one above and the same basic review applies.

☺ **Ultra Light Facial Creme** *($10 for 4 ounces)* is a good moisturizer for dry skin.

☺ **Vitamin C & A Ultra Rich Moisturizer** *($15 for 1 ounce)* would be very good for dry skin.

☺ **A, C, & E Eye Opener** *($15 for 0.5 ounce)* is similar to the one above and the same basic review applies.

☹ **Anti-Ox Facial Serum** *($15 for 1 ounce)* contains lime, lemon, and grapefruit oil, and is not recommended.

☹ **Deep Pore Cleansing Masque Normal/Oily Skin** *($10 for 2 ounces)* contains peppermint, grapefruit, clove, lemongrass, and witch hazel. Ouch!

☹ **Ester-C Serum** *($15 for 1 ounce)*. The type of vitamin C in this product isn't indicated on the label, which isn't acceptable by FDA standards; however, what is listed are irritating ingredients such as grapefruit oil and lemon oil.

☺ **Lemongrass Souffle Masque** *($10 for 2 ounces)*. The lemongrass oil may smell nice, but it is as useless for skin as the rose oil in here. Other than that, this is a good standard clay mask with almond oil, which makes it OK for dry skin.

☹ **Organic Botanical Lifting Serum** *($12 for 1 ounce)* contains two ingredients that can be a problem for skin: witch hazel and grapefruit oil. And the other ingredients in this serum won't lift the skin anywhere either.

☹ **Everyday SPF 15 Moisturizer** *($11.95 for 12 ounces)* doesn't contain the UVA-protecting ingredients titanium dioxide, zinc oxide, or avobenzone, and is not recommended.

☺ **Oat Protein Sunblock SPF 18** *($9 for 4 ounces)* is great stuff to consider for dry skin, though it does go on very white and heavy.

☺ **Oat Protein Sunblock SPF 30** *($10 for 4 ounces)* contains part titanium dioxide and would be good for normal to dry skin.

☹ **Spray On Sun Block SPF 30** *($9 for 4 ounces)* does not contain UVA-protecting ingredients, and is not recommended.

☹ **Sunswat SPF 15** *($9 for 4 ounces)* doesn't contain UVA-protecting ingredients, and is not recommended.

☺ **Instant Sunless Tanner** *($10 for 4 ounces)* contains the same active ingredient as all self tanners, and this one is as effective as any, though the concentration is low, meaning it takes several applications to get a tan.

☹ **After Sun Aloe Smoother with Jewelweed and Yucca** *($6 for 4 ounces)* is 95% pure aloe, which is nice and can be soothing; however, it also includes mint oil, which can take the soothing effect and turn it into irritation. You would be far better off with no additives and pure aloe, available from most health food stores.

## *L'Occitane*

With a very lush French accent and an inviting boutique that emanates an atmosphere reminiscent of southern France, L'Occitane also emanates wafting fragrances from the moment you pass its doorway. L'Occitane started out as a fragrance company that moved on to aromatherapy and then ventured into skin care. The staples of the line are shea butter and essential oils. Shea butter is indeed a good emollient for dry skin, but it is not a cornerstone or must-have by any means, and it is a must-not for oily or combination skin types. Essential oils are lovely to inhale but problematic for skin when it comes to a high risk of irritation or an allergic reaction. Several of the moisturizers, though basic, are quite good for dry skin but the sunscreens are appalling, with SPF 8s and 10s the mainstay, accompanied by dangerous information such as "helps to fight harmful rays while allowing a natural suntan to develop." If you are tanning, the harmful rays of the sun are causing serious and most likely irreversible damage. There are options here, but L'Occitane is just another highly fragranced line of skin-care products, extolling their natural contents when they are anything but all-natural. All in all, this line seems to have very little available for what it takes to create healthy skin for a wide range of skin types. For more information, call (888) 623-2880 or visit the Web site at www.loccitane.net.

☺ $$$ **Cold Cream** *($21 for 2.64 ounces)* has a name that's appropros. It can leave a greasy film on the skin and is easily replaced with less-expensive versions at the drugstore with far less fragrance.

☹ **Cold Cream Soap** *($6 for 5.3 ounces)* is a standard bar soap loaded with fragrance and it contains mint, which adds to the irritation of the cleansing agent.

☺ **Extra Gentle Cleansing Milk** *($16 for 8.4 ounces)* is similar to the Cold Cream above only in lotion form. The same basic comments apply.

☺ **Very Mild Cleansing Lotion** *($20 for 8.4 ounces)* is similar to the Cold Cream above only in lotion form. The same basic comments apply. This does contain a good deal of fragrance.

☹ **Gentle Makeup Remover Cream-Gel** *($20 for 8.4 ounces)* is basically fragrant plant water and plant oil with thickening agents. It also contains fairly irritating plant extracts including lemon, eucalyptus, juniper, and orange. This product has more problems than positive aspects, and isn't worth the trouble.

☹ **Purifying Foaming Gel** *($20 for 8.4 ounces)* is a standard, detergent-based water-soluble cleanser that would work well for normal to oily skin, but the problematic plant extracts of lemon, cypress, peppermint, niaouli, and ylang-ylang in here give it more risks than positives.

☺ **Extra Gentle Cleansing Water** *($14 for 8.4 ounces)* is more like applying eau de cologne on the skin than anything else. This would work as a toner but has little positive about it.

☺ **Gentle Eye Makeup Remover** *($15 for 5.1 ounces)* is a standard eye-makeup remover that contains mostly plant water, slip agent, detergent cleansing agents, and preservatives. It would work as well as any.

☹ **Clarifying Toner** *($26 for 2.6 ounces)* is just water, witch hazel, fragrant plant extracts, and preservatives. Witch hazel from the drugstore at least wouldn't contain the fragrance, but in any form witch hazel can be a skin irritant with repeated use.

☹ **Lavender Vinegar** *($15 for 5.1 ounces)* contains alcohol and camphor—ouch! The vinegar, which can also be an irritant, is incidental to the other ingredients.

☺ **Toning Lotion** *($15 for 5.1 ounces)* is just fragranced plant water with a tiny amount of water-binding agents. This is an option, but there are far better formulations to consider for good skin care.

☹ **Intensive Restructuring Day Care SPF 10** *($22 for 1.4 ounces)* has a dismal SPF and no UVA-protecting ingredients, and that makes this one to avoid at all costs.

☹ **Moisturizing Active Care SPF 8** *($20 for 1.4 ounces)* has a dismal SPF and no UVA-protecting ingredients, and that makes this one to avoid at all costs.

☺ **Ultra Moisturizing Daycare SPF 15** *($22 for 2.6 ounces)* is a good, in-part titanium dioxide–based sunscreen for someone with normal to dry skin.

The Reviews L

☺ **100% Pure Shea Butter** *($32.50 for 4.9 ounces)*. This would be a good, pure emollient for dry skin and not one you see every day, and it is even fragrance-free!

☹ **Eye Contour Cream-Gel** *($21 for 0.5 ounce)*. The oils of lemon, eucalyptus, juniper, and mandarin orange make this standard moisturizer fairly problematic for the eye area—or the face for that matter.

☺ **$$$ Firming Serum** *($20 for 0.5 ounce)* is a good lightweight moisturizer for normal to slightly dry skin, but it is not firming in the least.

☺ **Intensive Regenerating Night Care** *($22 for 1.4 ounces)* is a very good, though overly fragranced, moisturizer for normal to dry skin.

☹ **Nourishing Protective Care** *($20 for 1.4 ounces)* lists the third ingredient as alcohol, which makes this too potentially irritating and drying for all skin types, and it is not nourishing in the least.

☹ **Matte Finish Rebalancing Cream-Gel** *($20 for 1.4 ounces)* has peppermint, lemon, and cypress, and that adds up to be potentially irritating for all skin types.

☹ **Clarifying and Exfoliating Face Mask** *($26 for 2.6 ounces)* has peppermint, lemon, and cypress, and that adds up to be potentially irritating for all skin types. The crushed apricot seeds will exfoliate, but there are far more gentle ways to do this than with these irritating unnecessary extras.

☹ **Moisturizing Radiance Face Mask** *($26 for 2.6 ounces)* includes lemon, eucalyptus, juniper, and mandarin orange, and that makes this too potentially irritating for all skin types.

☺ **$$$ Soothing Exfoliating Face Mask** *($26 for 2.6 ounces)* is an extremely standard clay mask that also contains oatmeal. It will exfoliate and is an option for someone with normal to oily skin, but watch out for the fragrance.

☹ **Dry Oil Sun Care Spray SPF 8** *($24 for 8.4 ounces)* has a dismal SPF and no UVA-protecting ingredients, and that makes this one to avoid at all costs.

# L'Oreal

It is fitting that L'Oreal precedes Lancome so closely in an alphabetical listing, because both are owned by the same parent company. As a result, many products present in both lines are essentially indistinguishable, like L'Oreal's Hydra Renewal that is almost ingredient by ingredient the same as Lancome Hydrative. Despite the similarities between Lancome and L'Oreal, there are also glaring differences. Foundation colors for L'Oreal are mediocre to poor (and there's usually not a tester in sight), while Lancome excels in foundation colors and textures. L'Oreal's powders have followed the trend toward heavy shine and shimmer (except for its Feel Naturale and Quick Powder pressed powders) and most of the eyeshadow offerings are noticeably iridescent. Lancome's have far less shimmer though the textures are similar. What you can investigate from L'Oreal "because you're worth it," as they say, are

the many superior mascaras that, dollar for dollar, rival Lancome's most every step of the way. The blush options have increased and are largely impressive, and the lipsticks, though standard, are quite good and reminiscent of, guess who?

When it comes to skin care, though, especially moisturizers, I think you would find more similarities than contrasts between these two sister lines. For more information about L'Oreal, call (800) 322-2036 or visit the Web site at www.lorealparisusa.com.

## L'Oreal Skin Care

☺ **Hydra Fresh Deep Cleanser Foaming Gel for Normal to Oily Skin** *($4.99 for 6.5 ounces)* is a very good, very basic, detergent-based water-soluble cleanser that would work well for someone with normal to oily or slightly dry skin. It does contain fragrance.

☺ **Hydra Fresh Cleanser Foaming Cream for Normal to Dry Skin** *($4.99 for 6.5 ounces)* is a standard, detergent-based cleanser that can be too drying for someone with normal to dry skin, but it is still an option for someone with normal to slightly oily or slightly dry skin. The tiny amount of corn oil in here has minimal impact on skin. It does contain fragrance.

☺ **Shine Control Foaming Face Wash with Pro-Vitamin B5** *($4.99 for 6.5 ounces)* is virtually identical to the Hydra Fresh Foaming cleanser above, minus the plant oil. That is helpful for oily skin, but other than that, this is just a cleanser and it doesn't control shine in the least.

☺ **RevitaClean Cold Cream for Dry or Maturing Skin** *($5.29 for 5 ounces)* is an option for dry skin, but it can leave a greasy feel on the skin. The teensy amount of retinyl palmitate (a form of vitamin A) has no effect for skin.

☺ **RevitaClean Gentle Foaming Cleanser** *($7.29 for 6 ounces)* is a very good, very basic, detergent-based water-soluble cleanser that would work well for someone with normal to oily or slightly dry skin. It does contain fragrance. The teeny amount of vitamin A and peanut oil in here have little to no impact on skin.

☺ **Refreshing Eye Makeup Remover** *($4.99 for 4.2 ounces)* contains mostly water, slip agent, detergent cleansers, preservatives, and fragrance. This is a standard eye-makeup remover and it works as well as any.

☺ **Turning Point Instant Facial Scrub** *($8.99 for 1.7 ounces)* is a basic scrub that uses ground-up plastic (polyethylene) as the abrasive in a fairly emollient base that includes thickeners, silicone, and mineral oil. The form of salicylic acid in here isn't the kind that can exfoliate skin. This would work just fine for someone with normal to dry skin. It does contain fragrance and coloring agents.

☹ **Hydra Fresh Toner** *($4.99 for 8.5 ounces)* is an alcohol-based toner with a small amount of salicylic acid (BHA). There is never a reason to use alcohol on the skin, and the form of BHA in here isn't the kind that can exfoliate skin.

☹ **Shine Control Double-Action Toner Oil Free** *($4.99 for 8.5 ounces)* is an alcohol-based toner and that can be drying and irritating for all skin types.

☹ **Shine Control Oil-Free Toner** *($5.99 for 4 ounces)* is similar to the Double-Action version above and the same comments apply.

☺ **Future E Moisture + A Daily Dose of Pure Vitamin E** *($8.99 for 4 ounces)* is just an OK moisturizer with tiny amounts of vitamin E and BHA (though not the form that makes BHA effective for exfoliation). The fifth ingredient is aluminum starch, which can lend a matte feel but doesn't make for a great moisturizing base. Almost all of the other L'Oreal moisturizers are a better choice than this one or the one below.

☹ **Future E Moisture + A Daily Dose of Pure Vitamin E for Your Skin SPF 15** *($8.99 for 4 ounces)* doesn't contain the UVA-protecting ingredients avobenzone, titanium dioxide, or zinc oxide (an issue it is clear L'Oreal knows something about), and this product is not recommended.

☺ **Line Eraser Pure Retinol Concentrate** *($12.49 for 1 ounce)* is another product joining the others on the retinol bandwagon. This one from L'Oreal is in a rather simple but good moisturizing base and contains about 0.25% retinol, which is the same amount as all retinol products being sold. It is good for someone with normal to dry skin. The packaging is the kind that assures the retinol will be stable.

☹ **Line Eraser Pure Retinol Concentrate SPF 15** *($16.99 for 1.2 ounces)* doesn't contain UVA protection and is not recommended.

☺ **Eye Defense with Liposomes** *($9.99 for 0.5 ounce)* is a good emollient moisturizer for dry skin. The caffeine in here does not "wake up" eyes.

☺ **Overnight Defense** *($11.99 for 1.7 ounces)* is a very good emollient moisturizer for dry skin.

☺ **Wrinkle Defense** *($10.44 for 1.4 ounces)* won't change or fight off a wrinkle but it is a good moisturizer for dry skin.

☺ **Hydra Fresh Super Fresh Moisturizer for Normal to Dry Skin** *($8.99 for 2.5 ounces)* is a good but unimpressive moisturizer for normal to dry skin.

☺ **Hydra Fresh Super Fresh Moisturizer for Normal to Oily Skin** *($8.99 for 2.5 ounces)* is almost identical to the Normal to Dry version above and the same comments apply.

☺ **Hydra Renewal Daily Dry Skin Cream with Pro-Vitamin B5** *($5.99 for 1.7 ounces)*. At least this one left out the alcohol. It is a good, extremely standard, emollient moisturizer for dry skin. There is a tiny amount of vitamin E, but too little to have much effect. The urea can have exfoliating and water-binding properties similar to those of an AHA product.

☺ **Revitalift Anti-Wrinkle Firming Cream with Pro-Retinol A & Par-Elastyl, for Face and Neck** *($9.99 for 1.7 ounces)*. This product does not contain retinol;

rather, it contains retinyl palmitate, which is several generations removed from retinol. There is no ingredient called Par-Elastyl; that is a marketing term L'Oreal created to make a rather basic moisturizing formula sound more exotic.

☺ **Revitalift Eye Anti-Wrinkle and Firming Cream** *($9.99 for 0.5 ounce)* is similar to the one above, and the same review applies.

☺ **Revitalift Oil-Free Anti-Wrinkle + Firming Lotion** *($10.69 for 1.7 ounces)* is just an OK moisturizer with a rather ordinary formulation for normal to slightly dry skin.

## L'Oreal Makeup

<u>FOUNDATION:</u> L'Oreal is one of the few drugstore lines to sometimes make foundation tester units available, but it isn't consistent from store to store and its foundation colors for the most part are shockingly poor.

☺ **Feel Naturale Compact Light Softening One Step Makeup** *($12.29)* is a very good cream-to-powder makeup for someone with dry skin. It has a wonderfully smooth, creamy application; a soft, slightly matte finish; and some excellent colors (though nothing for darker skin tones). However, this is creamy enough to slip into any lines on the face and at the same time powdery enough to exaggerate any flaky, dry skin. Normal to slightly dry skin would fare best with this. Although the label makes the ubiquitous "oil-free" claim, this does have waxes that will nicely aggravate oily skins or those prone to breakouts. Of the 12 shades, the ones to avoid are Golden Beige (can be too peach), Caramel Beige (too golden), Soft Ivory (slightly pink), and Cocoa (too red).

☹ **Feel Naturale Liquid Foundation SPF 15** *($12.29)* has no reliable UVA protection and too much slip and slide to blend on evenly. That may have been forgivable, but the colors are just ghastly, making this one to ignore completely. Note: this is the same foundation formula as L'Oreal's former Feel Perfecte foundation, just with a different name.

☺ **Visible Lift Line Minimizing Makeup SPF 12** *($12.29)* has titanium dioxide as its active sunscreen and is the only L'Oreal foundation that provides adequate UVA protection. What a shame this isn't SPF 15, because it has a light texture and provides soft, sheer coverage with only a slight tendency to settle into imperfections (such as wrinkles). The antiwrinkle claims surrounding this one are dubious. It can help to smooth out skin to some degree, but that's by virtue of its application. By the way, side-by-side comparisons between this foundation and Chanel's Teint Lift Eclat SPF 8 *($50)* yielded favorable responses in favor of the L'Oreal side in terms of which one looked less wrinkled from whomever I asked, proving again that price is irrelevant. There are 12 shades to consider, including options for very light skins. These shades should be avoided by most skin tones: Buff, Golden Beige, Sun Beige, Cocoa, and Cappuccino.

The Reviews L

☹ **Mattique Oil Free Matte Makeup** *($9.99)* has a good, fairly matte texture but it is accompanied by a slightly sticky feel, which someone with oily skin might not like. With the possible exception of Nude Beige, all of the nine colors are too peach or pink to recommend.

☺ **Quick Stick Foundation** *($11.49)* comes in a stunning container and is almost identical in every way to Lancome's Stick Express Teint Idole Foundation *($32.50)*. Both are twist-up stick foundations that have a slight cream-to-powder finish, and both are far less creamy than you might expect from looking at the applicator. The smooth application dries to a solid, unmovable, difficult-to-remove matte base. If matte, full coverage is what you're after, this one would be an option. There are 12 shades to consider, but six are a problem for most skin tones: Soft Ivory, Pale, Nude Beige, Buff, Sand Beige, and Golden Beige are all too pink or peach. There are some good choices for dark skin tones, and as expected, Lancome's version mostly has the superior colors.

☹ **Colour Endure Stay On Makeup** *($12.29)* might indeed stay on, but why would you want it to? The colors in this grouping are almost embarrassing. Of the nine shades, only two are worth considering if you prefer ultra-matte foundation: Sand Beige and Natural Beige. The rest are either too peach, pink, orange, or yellow.

☺ **Translucide Lasting Luminous Makeup SPF 18** *($11.25)* could have been a contender in the battle of drugstore foundations. But with no UVA-protecting ingredients, it can't compete with Neutrogena's SPF 20 version that does have them. L'Oreal's does have a soft matte finish and light to medium coverage, but the nine shades available (with nothing for very light or dark skins) weigh in a bit too heavily on the peach or pink side, although they still may work for some skin tones. These shades should be considered with caution: Soft Ivory, Nude Beige, Golden Beige, Caramel Beige, and Buff.

☺ <u>CONCEALER:</u> **Feel Naturale Concealer** *($7.49)* comes in three fairly neutral shades and has a smooth, flawless finish! It is a great option for sheer to medium coverage. **Hydra Perfecte Concealer SPF 12** *($6.39)* is another good, lightweight, and sheer concealer that provides even coverage. It does have a slight tendency to slip into lines under the eyes. An SPF 15 with reliable UVA protection would have been preferred; this one has neither. **Visible Lift Line Minimizing Concealer** *($9.69)* has a creamy application that dries to a soft matte finish and it doesn't crease into the lines around the eyes. The line-minimizing claim can be put to the test by anyone who knows that wearing foundation and/or concealer in and of itself can make any lines more noticeable, and this one is no exception. The five shades are mostly workable—there's even a shade for very light skin tones, but the deepest shade won't make the cut for darker skin tones. The yellow shade won't reduce redness any better than "natural" skin-toned concealers; all it will do is add a strange, jaundiced cast to the skin.

**POWDER:** ☺ **Visible Lift Line Minimizing Powder** *($12.29)* is a standard, talc-based powder with a silky, very sheer finish. It won't diminish one line on your face, but it nicely sets makeup and could work for all skin types. All but one of the shades is excellent: avoid Colour Lift, a pink tone that no one should be dusting all over their face.

☺ **Quick Powder Sheer Matte Finish** *($9.19)* is also standard and talc-based, with a great silky feel, and would be easy to recommend except the packaging and application directions are just bizarre. The small round package, with the teeniest amount of powder in it, is meant to be rubbed directly on the face—no sponge or brush needed. Yet this is neither a quick nor efficient way to apply powder; you just end up with streaks of powder on your face that still need to be blended over with a sponge or brush!

☻ **Feel Naturale Powder SPF 15** *($11.19)* is a talc-free pressed powder that has a dry, grainy texture and a shiny finish, courtesy of the mica base this powder contains. The SPF is without UVA protection, which makes this powder a real "why bother?"

☺ **Hydra Perfecte Perfecting Loose Powder** *($9.19)* is an iridescent powder that is a contradiction in terms when you stop to consider that the purpose of powdering is to dust down shine and set makeup. However, for a sparkly face, this has a smooth finish and soft shine.

☺ **On the Loose Shimmering Powder** *($5.99)* comes in small pots with an intense though smooth application of shiny powder. For evening, it's an option and will give you the appropriate glittering shine everyone else is wearing.

☺ **BLUSH: Feel Naturale Light Softening Blush** *($10.99)* is a great collection of matte blushes with beautiful colors, textures, and an application that is strikingly similar to Lancome's Blush Subtil. It should suit all skin types very well. **Quick Stick Face and Body Blush** *($12.29)* is an excellent cream-to-powder blush with a smooth, even finish. It does take some deft blending to get it on correctly, but it can provide an exceptionally natural-looking blushed appearance, especially on normal, smooth skin. For fans of stick makeup, this is one to consider—but bear in mind that there are some shiny shades right alongside the non-shiny ones. **Translucide Luminous Gel Blush** *($9.25)* is an interesting option for a sheer-gel tinted blush. It appears to have a shiny finish but blends out exceptionally sheer to almost no color at all. The application is wet-feeling and then dries to a matte powder finish. It would be hard to make a mistake with this one, since the color is so soft, yet it takes patience to blend it on and wait for it to dry, and if you want any noticeable color, it can take a lot of trouble to build up much intensity.

☺ **EYESHADOW: Soft Effects Singles** *($3.69)* have a handful of very good neutral shades that are mostly matte; some of the colors are labeled as "perle" and are easy to avoid, but some of the mattes are deceptively shiny. These are the best mattes: Bark, Sable, Sand, and Raven. I would recommend staying away from the **Duos** *($4.39)* and the **Quads** *($6.29);* they either come in strange color combinations or one or more of the colors is very shiny and ready to exaggerate any lines you may have.

☺ <u>EYE AND BROW SHAPER:</u> **Le Grande Kohl Line and Define Pencil** *($6.69)* is an extra-long standard pencil and very reminiscent of Lancome's Le Crayon Kohl for $16.50. This one from L'Oreal goes on smooth without being greasy and blends well without streaking. Many of the colors have shine, so choose carefully. **Pencil Perfect Automatic Eye Liner** *($6.69)* isn't what I would call perfect; if anything, it tends to go on creamier than most, and that means a greater risk of smearing. As a plus, it doesn't need sharpening. **Lineur Intense** *($6.99)* is traditional liquid liner that goes on like the name says—intense—and stays that way all day without flaking or smearing. **Super Liner** *($6.99)* is a very liquidy liner with a soft pen applicator tip. It is not preferred over the one above as it takes too long to dry and never really seems to set. **Eye Highlighter** *($8.19)* is a very creamy, almost greasy pencil with a sponge tip on the end. Basically, the color selection is a pastel potpourri of shine galore and it's there for a trendy consumer purchase. **Eye Smoker** *($8.19)* is a chubby pencil that goes on creamy, and also features shiny colors. **Brow Colorist** *($8.19)* is a two-sided pencil. One end is your typically standard brow pencil, with some decent color choices, and the other end is a sponge tip that dispenses a shiny white eyeshadow. The cap is outfitted with a brush that is too stiff for comfort, and this whole concept needs to be thought through one more time.

☺ <u>LIPSTICK AND LIP PENCIL:</u> **Colour Riche Gold Hydrating Creme or Perle Lip Colour** *($12.19)* is a fairly creamy, semi-opaque lip color available in both shiny and non-shiny finishes. They're a nice improvement over the former Colour Riche lipsticks, which were more akin to gloss than true lipstick. **Colour Riche Rich Creamy Lipliner** *($5.69)* is a standard twist-up pencil that has a built-in sharpener. The sharpener part isn't necessary given the finer point most twist-up pencils like this one already have. The application is smooth and creamy, and the color range nicely complements the Colour Riche Lipsticks. **Colour Endure Stay On Lip Colour** *($9.19)* is very similar to Revlon's ColorStay, and I'll bet only true aficionados of the latter will be able to tell the difference. They are both matte, go on thick, and stay in place. However, regardless of the claims about not feeling dry there is no emollient feel to this at all. There is a wide assortment of colors, so for fans of ultra-matte lipsticks, this is a boon. **Rouge Virtuale** *($8.79)* is a group of pearl, cream, and matte lipstick shades that seem about as standard as any others in the L'Oreal lipstick library (with the exception of Colour Endure). The Mattes are not matte in the least; in fact, they're rather creamy and have poor staying power. The Creme is more like a gloss, and the Perle is nicely iridescent and sheer. Techno-savvy name notwithstanding, there is really no reason to give these a try. **HydraSoft Deeply Softening Lip Color SPF 12** *($9.99)* doesn't contain UVA protection but it is a very good, standard, glossy lipstick in a slim container. This one has no distinct advantage over dozens of other creamy, sheer lipsticks. **Rouge Pulp** *($7.99)* is standard lip gloss that comes in vivid colors, some of which are opaque. It's got a great name and a feminine package, but that's about it. **Crayon Petite Automatic Lip Liner** *($6.69)* is a standard twist-up lip pencil that is slightly more creamy than most and offers some good colors, including a Clear version. **Rouge Pulp Anti-Feathering Lip Liner** *($7.79)* is an automatic pencil that comes in six very good shades and really is impressive at keeping lipstick in place. This is definitely worth considering.

☺ **Crayon Grande** *($6.69)* is a dual-function, stocky lip pencil that is supposed to be a lipstick and liner in one. It falls short on both counts, as this type of product is hard to sharpen and the formula is too creamy to keep a pointed edge for lining.

☺ <u>MASCARA:</u> **Lash Out Extending Mascara** *($6.69)* is really excellent, but it would be easier to control with a shorter wand. It does build long, thick, non-clumped lashes with no chance of smearing. **Le Grand Curl** *($7.39)* is a great mascara that goes on well without clumping, holds up through the entire day, remains smear-free, and, oh yes, lengthens and thickens with ease. It will lift and curl as you apply it, but that is the nature of any good mascara, and the claims on this one are a bit out of line, but forgivable. **Voluminous Mascara** *($6.69, straight or curved brush)* used to be a poor contender but just keeps on getting better. The latest version, promoting "4 times fuller lashes," is slightly better than the former version, in that it does build a touch more thickness. It builds lots of length and copiously thickens lashes quickly, but the downside is that it can go on heavy and create a very dramatic lash look, which some women may not want or appreciate. Also, the odd colors seen before (Blue, Gold) seem to be gone for good. **Voluminous Waterproof Mascara** *($6.69)* is great in all departments. It builds noticeable length with just a few coats and nicely defines the lashes without clumping. As stated, it is waterproof too! **Le Grand Curl Waterproof Mascara** *($7.39)* applies very easily and lengthens slightly better than the two waterproof versions above, is tenaciously waterproof, and refuses to smear, even if you beg and plead.

☹ **Colour Endure Stay On Mascara** *($7.39)* builds decent length but minimal to no thickness, and it takes a long time to get anywhere. It doesn't smudge or smear, and is water resistant—not waterproof yet still can be stubborn when it is being removed. **Featherlash Mascara** *($6.99)* is billed as "softly sweeping" mascara and ends up being a patchy application of mascara that builds uneven length and minimal thickness. It won't smear and doesn't clump, which is great, but the payoff is not on par with the usual standards set by L'Oreal/Lancome mascaras. **Lash Out Waterproof Mascara** *($6.69)* is just a very mediocre mascara that can take up to 15 coats before you see much length or thickness, and even then not too much, and it can clump slightly. It does hold up underwater, so may be worth the drawbacks for those times when waterproof is required.

## *La Mer*

What can $530 buy you? It can buy you a night out on the town including limo, dinner for two, and a nice dress. Or you can decide to spend it on three pairs of really nice designer shoes. Or another option is a rather elegant designer necklace, earring, and bracelet set. Or if you were someone who is seduced by distorted cosmetics advertising, you could end up wasting your money on four or five skin-care products from the La Mer line, and that wouldn't even include sunscreen, because this overpriced group of products doesn't include one.

The original Creme de la Mer was launched by Estee Lauder as a miracle product for wrinkles based on research from Max Huber, a NASA scientist. How does space technology relate to wrinkles? Well, it doesn't. Huber at one time suffered severe burns in an accident and then, according to the Max Huber Laboratories, it took 12 years and 6,000 experiments to come up with the cream, "which he made through an arcane and lengthy process." That was over 30 years ago. Of course, given that none of this self-experimentation was ever documented, there is no way to know what Huber was using before or what else could have produced whatever results he was so happy about.

It turns out that Creme de la Mer was, and still is, almost exclusively water, thickening agents, and some algae. But this miracle product wasn't enough, at least not for the Estee Lauder company, which was selling a lot of product and understands that, in the world of skin care, if one product sounds good, women will buy other unrelated products with the same name. With the new assortment of La Mer products, Estee Lauder has added a new range of hocus-pocus ingredients to the continuing list of concoctions that were never in Huber's original formula; so much for that mythic story having any real credibility. These supplementary products contain powdered silver, diamond dust, something called declustered water, and a semiprecious stone, tourmaline, that is supposed to have magnetic properties. Wow! It's almost too outlandish to even begin explaining, but I'll do my best. And do keep in mind that if these products were the be-all and end-all for the Estee Lauder company, why is it selling all those other products at the dozen or so other lines it sells just around the counter or next door?

Supposedly, these products are worth the money because some of them contain magnetized tourmaline, colloidal silver, and declustered water. Declustered water is water manufactured to have smaller ions, which supposedly makes the water penetrate the skin better. There is no proof that this synthetic water does what the company claims, but even if the water could penetrate better, is that better for skin? There is definitely research indicating that too much water in the skin can make it plump, but that could also prevent cell turnover and renewal, and inhibit the skin's immune response. Either way, the skin likes taking on water—it plumps to a thousand times its normal size just from taking a bath—and it doesn't need help to do any more, nor would that be good for skin in the long run.

Tourmaline does have unique electrical properties and is used in some machinery to control the direction of light. While that might sound like it can throw light away from the face, it doesn't change the appearance of wrinkles. After all, it would take a great deal of lighting (take it from someone who has been involved with fashion photography makeup) to hide wrinkles, and then you still need to digitally improve the picture and erase the wrinkles. Even if this ingredient could have that effect, in a cleanser the tourmaline would be wiped or rinsed away. The other claim is that this magnetized crystal somehow attracts the iron in blood and helps pull the blood to the surface. I won't get into the argument about the issue of magnets for sport injuries (which, from the research I've seen, is bogus), but for the face, if the tourmaline could provide that benefit, that could cause too much blood flow to tiny capillaries and cause risk of their appearing on the surface of the skin.

As for the colloidal silver, that simply refers to ground-up silver being suspended in solution. Silver can have disinfecting properties, but prolonged contact with it can turn skin grayish-blue and can be irritating to skin. That can't help erase wrinkles, heal skin, or provide any benefit. Silver is better worn as jewelry, though if you are allergic to silver you will be allergic to the silver in this product as well.

The other gimmicky ingredients include fish cartilage, algae (explained in the Creme de la Mer review below), sea minerals (copper, sodium, calcium, quartz), and other forms of algae. While all of these may have some water-binding properties (all except the minerals, which have no benefit for skin care and are barely present in these formulations), the fiction that any of them have an impact on wrinkles is not substantiated in any published scientific study.

For more information about La Mer, call (888) 243-8825 or visit the Web site at www.elcompanies.com.

☺ $$$ **The Cleansing Lotion** (*$65 for 6.7 ounces*). Supposedly, this milky emulsion derives its remarkable cleansing powers from magnetized tourmaline, colloidal silver, and declustered water, but see the comments in the paragraphs above for an explanation about this bravado. What you can most certainly expect is a standard wipe-off cleanser for dry skin that is mostly thickeners, plant oil, preservatives, and fragrance. You would not find it all that different from Neutrogena's Extra Gentle Cleanser (for a fraction of the price). This does contain fragrance and coloring agents.

☺ $$$ **The Cleansing Gel** (*$65 for 6.7 ounces*) is similar to the product above, only this one contains standard detergent cleansing agents found in cleansing gels the world over. It would work well for most skin types—but that price, can that make anyone's skin feel better? See above for more explanation about the claims. This does contain fragrance and coloring agents.

☹ **The Oil Absorbing Tonic** *($60 for 6.7 ounces)* is a toner that contains mostly alcohol, and at any price, much less this amount of money, that's a burn for skin.

☺ $$$ **The Tonic** *($60 for 6.7 ounces)* would be a good, though average toner for most skin types—that is, if the price doesn't get you first. It also has declustered water, colloidal gold, and sea plant extracts. While that keeps with the ocean theme, it doesn't have any benefit for the skin. The gold can be a contact allergen, but probably not in this amount, which is not enough to create a ring for an ant.

☹ $$$ **Creme de la Mer** *($155 for 1.7 ounces)* is the original product created by Max Huber, as described above. As enticing as this dramatic story sounds, the reality is that this very basic cream doesn't contain anything particularly extraordinary or unique, unless you want to believe that seaweed extract (sort of like seaweed tea) can in some way heal burns and scars. Even if it could, burns and scars don't have much to do with wrinkling, and this product is now being sold as a wrinkle cream. According to Susan Brawley, professor of plant biology at the University of Maine, "Seaweed extract isn't a rare, exotic, or expensive ingredient. Seaweed extract is readily available and [is] used in everything from cosmetics to food products and medical applications." Creme de la Mer contains mostly seaweed extract, mineral oil, Vaseline, glycerin, waxlike thickening agents, plant oils, plant seeds, minerals, vitamins, more thickeners, and preservatives. This rather standard moisturizer contains some good antioxidants, which can help heal skin by keeping air off it, but these ingredients are also found in many other moisturizers that cost a *lot* less. According to the cosmetics chemists I've interviewed, it costs pennies, not hundreds of dollars, to stick some seaweed and vitamins in a cosmetic.

☹ $$$ **Moisturizing Lotion** *($135 for 1.7 ounces)* would make a good moisturizer for dry skin, though the price is just bizarre. However, what makes this product not good for skin is the inclusion of lime and eucalyptus, which are potentially irritating and sensitizing for all skin types.

☹ $$$ **Oil Absorbing Lotion** *($135 for 6.7 ounces)* uses a film-forming agent, like most lotions with oil-absorbing claims do. Oh, it still has the algae and water-binding agents, but like the one above, it also includes irritating ingredients that are not helpful for skin.

☺ $$$ **Eye Balm** *($95 for 0.5 ounce)*. The belief about fish cartilage and algae benefits is up to you. But the inclusion of eucalyptus, mint, and powdered almonds is unnecessary and potentially irritating. This could be an emollient moisturizer if the plant extracts don't bother you.

☺ $$$ **The Mist** *($75 for 6.7 ounces)* would be a very good toner for most skin types. A small amount of potentially irritating plant extracts are here, but probably not enough to be a problem for most skin types.

☺ $$$ **Serum de la Mer** *($175 for 1 ounce)*. You would think that for $150 the original Creme de la Mer would be enough, but no, it now takes more, because this product is supposed to prepare your face for the Creme. This is a good lightweight moisturizer for normal to dry skin, but the price, even if fish cartilage was something special, is just unwarranted.

☺ $$$ **Refining Facial** *($75 for 3.4 ounces)* is a relatively standard clay mask. The sea stuff is in here, as is tourmaline and diamond powder. If you feel that scrubbing with microscopic amounts of gem stones (and then rinsing them down the drain) is the way to go, then nothing I can say about this marketing gimmick is going to deter you.

# La Prairie

La Prairie has been at the forefront of expensive antiaging products for more than three decades. Many of the products in this originally Swiss skin-care line are called "cellular treatment." After a while, it all starts sounding silly. Even the mascara is named "Cellular Treatment Intensified Mascara." The concept is incredibly gimmicky, and even if your skin could improve with these products, the prices might cause premature aging. So what do the few women who can safely afford these products get for their money? The prestige of knowing they can afford them, period. High-priced skin-care lines attract women who think that the dollars they spend will buy them something special that most other women can't afford. To some extent, they're right: other women can't afford these. Yet anyone who reads and understands the ingredient lists would find the prices as ludicrous for the contents as they actually are. Many of La Prairie's claims are based on the use of ingredients such as placental protein, flower and herb extracts, marine collagen, and amino acids. There is no research that indicates any of these ingredients can alter one wrinkle, and many less-expensive lines contain the same gimmicks, but that doesn't stop La Prairie from trying to convince you that its versions are worthy of the sky-high price tags.

In retrospect, and despite how marvelous those previous miracle ingredients commanding immense price tags were supposed to be for the skin, that didn't stop La Prairie from joining the vitamin C, AHA, and retinol craze. But if placental extract was supposed to be the fountain of youth, what are these other products and ingredients for? One good bandwagon La Prairie did jump on was providing UVA-protecting ingredients in its suncare products—though selling sunscreens at $125 an ounce should be illegal. Given that a generous application is the cornerstone for getting correct sunscreen coverage, this price almost guarantees that you will not be using enough to get the essential protection from sun damage that the skin really needs and that the label indicates.

La Prairie's makeup does have some sumptuous textures and decent colors. A few of its foundations even have reliable UVA ingredients. There is nothing here that is really worth La Prairie's prices. For more information about La Prairie, call (800) 821-5718 or visit the Web site at www.laprairie.com.

## La Prairie Skin Care

☺ $$$ **Purifying Creme Cleanser** *($50 for 6.8 ounces)* is meant to be rinsed off, but it actually requires a washcloth. It leaves a film on the skin. This is merely a very expensive cold cream. It does contain fragrance.

☺ $$$ **Foam Cleanser** *($50 for 4 ounces)* is a standard, detergent-based water-soluble cleanser that is about as ordinary as they come. It does contain some Vaseline and silicone to cut the drying effect of the rather strong cleansing agents, as well as some anti-irritants, but those are nothing special either, and it would just be better if this product didn't contain such drying detergent cleansing agents. It does contain fragrance.

☺ $$$ **Cellular Eye Make-Up Remover** *($40 for 4.2 ounces)* is a silicone-based, wipe-off cleanser that contains some plant extracts (some that can be irritants and others that can be anti-irritants). That's nice, but I wonder if the executives for these companies laugh about the women who believe they're getting something special when they spend this kind of money for such an ordinary product. It does contain fragrance.

☺ $$$ **Essential Exfoliator** *($50 for 7 ounces)* This is a good scrub for dry skin, but it doesn't rinse off very well and, to say the least, is overpriced for what you get.

☹ **Cellular Purifying Lotion** *($55 for 8.2 ounces)* is a standard alcohol-based toner with a small amount of placental protein thrown in, but that can't compensate for the irritation and dryness caused by the alcohol. Besides, at best, protein extracted from the placenta does what all proteins do for the skin: it acts as a good water-binding agent; the skin can't tell where the protein came from.

☺ $$$ **Cellular Refining Lotion** *($55 for 8.2 ounces)* would be a good toner for most skin types. The plant extracts in here are a mixture of anti-irritants and irritants, but they are present in such tiny amounts that they probably have no effect on skin. The tiny amount of urea in here works as a water-binding agent and not an exfoliant.

☺ $$$ **Age Management Balancer** *($65 for 8.4 ounces)*. This is a good, irritant-free toner, but hardly worth the price tag. There is nothing in here that will manage age.

☹ **Age Management Cream Natural with SPF 8** *($125 for 1.7 ounces)* isn't a natural for this kind of money, and you don't even get an SPF 15! This is an embarrassing product and offensive in defining itself as a skin protector, especially with the other far better, though exceedingly overpriced, SPF 15 sunscreens La Prairie now has with avobenzone.

☹ **Age Management Intensified Emulsion with SPF 8** *($100 for 1.7 ounces)* is similar to the one above and the same review applies.

☺ $$$ **Age Management Eye Repair** *($100 for 0.5 ounce)*. This huge ingredient list is like throwing in everything and the kitchen sink, with good emollients, good water-binding agents, good anti-oxidants, and some good plant extracts. It would work fine for normal to dry skin. The 3% of AHAs is not enough to have exfoliating properties, plus the pH is too high for it to work even if the minimum of 5% was included.

☺ $$$ **Age Management Intensified Serum** *($140 for 1 ounce)* contains about 8% AHAs, which is fine for an exfoliant, though the pH is too high for it to be truly effective. Aside from that, it is a good lightweight moisturizer for normal to dry skin. The plant extracts in here are a mixture of irritants and anti-irritants but the amounts of these are not enough to have much effect on skin.

☹ **Age Management Serum** *($125 for 1 ounce)* is similar to the Intensified Serum above, only this one contains arnica, which should not be used regularly on skin.

☺ $$$ **Age Management Line Inhibitor** *($100 for 0.5 ounce)* is similar to the Age Management Intensified Serum above, and the same review applies.

☺ $$$ **Age Management Night Cream** *($125 for 1 ounce)*. The pH is too high for the AHA in here to be effective as an exfoliant. It would be good for someone with dry skin. While there are a lot of interesting ingredients, there's mostly just a dusting of each.

☹ **Age Management Retexturizing Booster** *($150 for 1 ounce)* contains mostly alcohol, which is too drying and irritating for any skin type, and is not recommended.

☹ $$$ **Age Management Stimulus Complex PM (Delicate)** *($150 for 1 ounce)*. Unbelievable—a completely standard moisturizer for someone with dry skin. If you're going to spend this kind of money, there are other products in this line that have more interesting formulations than this.

☹ $$$ **Age Management Stimulus Complex PM (Normal)** *($150 for 1 ounce)* is almost identical to the one above, and the same review applies.

☺ $$$ **Age Management Stimulus Complex SPF 25** *($150 for 1 ounce)*. How liberally is anyone going to apply this insanely expensive standard moisturizer? The trace elements of the fancy-sounding ingredients are so far at the end of the ingredient listing you aren't even getting a few cents worth of the stuff. But even if you were, there are far less expensive products with those fad ingredients, ranging from L'Oreal to Nivea, and those products contain more of the CoQ10 and retinol to boot.

☺ $$$ **Cellular Brightening System Day Emulsion with SPF 15** *($125 for 1 ounce)* is a good sunscreen with titanium dioxide for an absurd amount of money. And for skin lightening, it is essential to correctly and religiously wear a sunscreen. This product does contain magnesium ascorbyl phosphate, a form of vitamin C that can have some skin-lightening effect, but the research shows that for it to work it takes a 10% concentration and this product contains less than 2%. It's a good moisturizing base, but there are far better ways to deal with skin discolorations than this one.

☹ **Cellular Brightening Systeme Intensive Essence** *($100 for 0.5 ounce)* lists the third ingredient as alcohol, which makes this lotion too potentially irritating for all skin types, and that won't help brighten anything (except for already red skin).

☹ **Cellular Brightening Systeme Soothing Lotion** *($65 for 4.2 ounces)* is similar to the Intensive Essence above and the same comments apply. This product does contain zinc oxide and barium sulfite, which will leave a white cast on the skin, but that won't lighten anything, and the barium sulfite can be a skin irritant. Calling this soothing is a joke, right?

☺ $$$ **Cellular Brightening Systeme Night Treatment** *($125 for 1 ounce)*. The vitamin C in here is magnesium ascorbyl palmitate in about a 4% concentration, which makes it minimally effective at inhibiting melanin production. Other than that, this is a good emollient moisturizer for normal to dry skin. The plant extracts in here are a mixture of irritants and anti-irritants, but the amount is so minimal as to have no real impact on skin either way.

☺ $$$ **Cellular Balancing Complex** *($65 for 1.7 ounces)* is a good (though standard) lightweight moisturizer for normal to dry skin. If you're going to waste money on skin-care products, La Prairie has better formulations than this boring one.

☺ $$$ **Cellular Day Creme** *($100 for 1 ounce)* is a lot of money for a product that is mostly thickeners and Vaseline, but I think La Prairie was hoping you wouldn't notice. Plus, without a sunscreen it is a definite no-no for daytime. It would be good for dry skin but doesn't compare to some of the other more interesting products in this line.

☺ $$$ **Cellular Defense Shield Eye Cream, SPF 15** *($100 for 0.5 ounce)* is a good titanium dioxide–based sunscreen with lots of good emollients, anti-oxidants, water-binding agents, and vitamins. The base is a good emollient moisturizer for normal to dry skin; if used correctly, this wouldn't last two weeks. The plant extracts in here are a mixture of irritants (pinus bark and ginseng) and anti-irritants (licorice and yarrow), but the teeny amounts of these make them insignificant. The vitamin K in here has no effect on skin.

☹ **Cellular Defense Shield with SPF 15** *($95 for five 0.22-ounce vials)* has an impressive hook, similar to Avon's Anew Formula C Treatment Capsules. The crux of the matter for this product is not the sun protection, but what vitamin C can do for the skin. Like Avon's Anew, the vitamin C for this product is encapsulated, or, as the La Prairie brochure explains, hermetically sealed. A powdered form of vitamin C is kept separate from the SPF 15 moisturizer. You mix the first of the five tiny vials with a bit of the vitamin C, and so on, and, voilà, you have a stable antioxidant with SPF 15. The vitamin C in here is ascorbic acid, considered to be the most irritating form of vitamin C and the least effective as an antioxidant or lightening agent for skin, but after all, this doesn't include UVA-protecting ingredients. What a waste.

☹ **Cellular Defense Shield Vitamin C Cream** *($125 for 1 ounce)* lists alcohol as the fourth ingredient, while the vitamin C in here is ascorbic acid, considered to be the most irritating form of the vitamin and the least effective as an antioxidant or lightening agent for skin. If you're looking for vitamin C, this is not the product to even remotely consider.

☺ **$$$ Cellular Eye Contour Creme** *($80 for 0.5 ounce)* weighs in at $2,560 per pound, yet it is nothing more than a Vaseline-based moisturizer. It is a good emollient moisturizer for someone with dry skin, but is basically ordinary, with most of the interesting ingredients coming well after the preservatives. It does contain fragrance.

☹ **Cellular Lipo-Sculpting Systeme Eye Gel** *($125 for 0.5 ounce)* has alcohol as the fourth ingredient, which makes this potentially drying and irritating for all skin types. The handful of plant extracts are strange mix of anti-irritants and potentially irritating ones. There are some good water-binding agents and antioxidants, but there are better ways to get these on the skin than this.

☺ **$$$ Cellular Lipo-Sculpting Systeme Face Serum** *($125 for 1 ounce)*. There is nothing in here that will sculpt the face. The plant extracts are a mixture of skin irritants (caffeine—high up on the ingredient listing—and pine) and anti-irritants (algae and chamomile). The lactobacillus in here is a good bacteria used to ferment beer but has no known benefit for skin. I can't even begin to make a decision on this concoction, it just makes no sense.

☺ **$$$ Cellular Night Cream** *($105 for 1 ounce)* is a rather emollient, though standard moisturizer for dry skin. This rather boring Vaseline-based moisturizer would be good for someone with dry skin.

☺ **$$$ Cellular Neck Cream** *($105 for 1 ounce)*. There is nothing in here special for the neck, in fact it is quite similar to the Night Cream above, and the same comments apply.

☺ **$$$ Cellular Skin Conditioner** *($70 for 4 ounces)* is similar to the Night Cream above, minus the Vaseline, but the same basic comments apply.

☺ **$$$ Cellular Wrinkle Cream** *($105 for 1 ounce)*. If this is a wrinkle cream, what are all these other products for? It is similar to the Night Cream above and the same basic comments apply.

☺ **$$$ Cellular Time Release Moisture Lotion SPF 15** *($125 for 1.7 ounces)* is a good, in-part avobenzone-based sunscreen that contains almost everything but the kitchen sink when it comes to trendy cosmetic ingredients, but only minuscule amounts of each one. It does add up to a good lightweight moisturizer for normal to dry skin with reliable sun protection, but the hodgepodge of plant extracts can't provide any benefit (some are irritants, others anti-irritants). The mulberry in here for skin lightening is in such a tiny amount as to be useless, and the water-binding agents and antioxidants, while nice, are not unique to this product.

☺ $$$ Cellular Time Release Moisturizer-Intensive ($125 for 1 ounce) is a good moisturizer for normal to dry skin, but this is a lot of money for castor oil. The water-binding agents are good but not unique to this formulation and the horsetail and ginseng in here can be skin irritants.

☹ Cellular Purifying Systeme Cleansing Gelle ($60 for 5 ounces) uses TEA-lauryl sulfate as the main cleansing agent, which makes it potentially too irritating for all skin types. It contains a mix of plant extracts that can be anti-irritants and some that can cause irritation. There is also a tiny amount of AHAs in here but not enough and not with the right pH to be effective as an exfoliant.

☺ $$$ Essential Purifying Gel Cleanser ($50 for 7.3 ounces) is a shockingly run-of-the-mill, detergent-based water-soluble cleanser. Some of the herb extracts can be potentially irritating, but they are at the end of the ingredient list, in too minuscule an amount to matter. This cleanser does rinse off, and can be good for someone with normal to dry skin, but the price is a joke, right?

☹ Cellular Purifying Systeme Dual Phase Toner ($65 for 8.4 ounces) is a standard, alcohol-based toner with a small amount of plant extracts and AHAs added. The irritation and dryness from the alcohol are a problem for all skin types.

☺ $$$ Cellular Purifying Systeme Hydrating Fluid SPF 15 ($100 for 1.7 ounces) is an avobenzone-based SPF 15 for $100! I'm just speechless. And there are women who are going to buy this, and probably under-use it (sunscreen requires liberal application and no one is going to apply this overpriced sunscreen liberally) and then not even get the SPF protection on the label. While the plant extracts may add some soothing benefits and the neem extract some antimicrobial activity, there are others that are irritants, including pine, cypress, and horsetail. The water-binding agents are nice, but again the amounts are very small, at least for the amount of money you're spending.

☺ $$$ Cellular Purifying Systeme Hydro Repair ($125 for 1 ounce) is a good 8% AHA and about 0.5% BHA exfoliant in a good but lightweight moisturizing base for someone with normal to dry skin. The plant extracts can offer some anti-irritant properties but others can be irritants. For an AHA product, there are versions just as effective from Neutrogena to M.D. Formulations for far less.

☹ Cellular Purifying Systeme Normalizing Serum ($150 for 1 ounce) lists its fourth ingredient as alcohol, and that won't normalize anything, at least not at this price, which is truly abnormal for what you get.

☺ $$$ **Cellular Cycle Ampoules for the Face** *($275 for seven 0.1-ounce treatments)* is a two-part self-mixed treatment that contains the most ordinary assembly of ingredients you could imagine, and it prices out to about $5,700 a pound! They can't be serious. This isn't even as interesting as a lot of other La Prairie products.

☺ $$$ **Cellular Balancing Mask** *($110 for six 0.12-ounce ampoules)* is a two-part mask that you mix together. Minuscule amounts of aloe vera and baking soda are not going to balance anyone's skin, and the other ingredients aren't as interesting as many others in the La Prairie products.

☺ $$$ **Cellular Moisture Mask** *($65 for 1 ounce)* is a good mask for someone with dry skin.

☺ $$$ **Cellular Purifying Systeme Cleansing Gelle** *($60 for 5 ounces)* is a standard, detergent-based water-soluble cleanser. What a joke—only women who can't decipher an ingredient label won't be laughing. The main cleansing agent is TEA-lauryl sulfate, one that can be irritating for some skin types. This does contain a teeny amount of AHA, but not enough to be an exfoliant, not to mention that the pH isn't effective for that purpose either.

☹ **Cellular Purifying Systeme Blemish Control** *($65 for 0.5 ounce)*. Are you sitting down? Well, at least I am. This BHA product contains alcohol, which is problematic enough for blemish-prone skin, but what is really shocking is that this offers no advantage over PersaGel, Neutrogena, or Paula's Choice BHA products, and in fact La Prairie's version is more irritating than those others! Plus several other plant extracts in here are potentially irritating. There are some good water-binding agents too, but in such teeny amounts they don't amount too much. This also contains neem extract, which has pesticide and antimicrobial activity, as well as horsetail extract, which has been used anecdotally for wound-healing but can also cause dermatitis reactions. While their wound healing and antimicrobial activity may also affect blemishes, there is no research to show that.

☺ $$$ **Cellular Purifying Systeme Regulating Mask** *($100 for 2.6 ounces)* is a standard clay mask with a huge ingredient listing. The tiny quantity of AHAs in here are insufficient to act as exfoliants, the plant extracts are a mixture of irritants and anti-irritants, and the water-binding agents are nice but useless in a clay (absorbing) mask. It's a good basic mask, but for the money, a true "why bother?" product.

☹ **Cellular Purifying Clay Mask** *($65 for 1 ounce)* is a standard clay mask that contains plant oils and plant extracts. Clay can be drying, but the emollients can make up for that. This mask does contain menthol, which can be a skin irritant, as can the ginseng and horsetail in this one.

☺ $$$ **Essence of Skin Caviar Cellular Eye Complex with Caviar Extract** *($85* *for 0.5 ounce)* is a good lightweight moisturizer for someone with dry skin. It does contain 0.04% caviar, which amounts to half an egg—now, isn't that exciting? The notion that this is an instant face-lift in one minute doesn't hold water. Some of the plant extracts in here can be irritants (horsetail and ginseng) while others can be anti-irritants (algae).

☺ $$$ **Skin Caviar Cellular Face Complex with Caviar Extract** *($85 for 1 ounce)* is similar to the one above only it is silicone-based and with a dusting of vitamins. The silicone gives this one a silkier feel on the skin but the same basic review for the Eye Complex applies here.

☹ **Skin Caviar** *($100 for 2 ounces)* is mostly silicone, some water, alcohol, and otherwise has similar ingredients to the ones above. Why not skip the alcohol, which can be drying and a skin irritant?

☹ **Skin Caviar Firming Mask** *($125 for two-piece set)* includes two parts. The Serum part is a blend of standard plant oils (like those from your kitchen cupboard) and fragrant oils, which are best not used on the skin. The Firming Complex part is mostly alcohol, which adds up to irritation and dryness regardless of the other sprinkling of ingredients.

☺ $$$ **Skin Caviar Luxe Cream** *($300 for 1.7 ounces).* If you were going to spend an unseemly amount of money to get a great skin-care product, choosing this incredibly mundane formulation would not be the way to do it. The plant extracts in here are a waste, with some being incredibly irritating (ginseng, horsetail, arnica, and sage), and others anti-irritants, while there's not enough of the mulberry root to have an effect on skin lightening. The water-binding agents are nice but so close to the end of the listing to be only a mere dusting. The vitamins are good antioxidants, but not unique, as they show up in an endless array of products. And for the minuscule amount of caviar in here, you're better off shopping at the grocery store and having it on toast than on your skin.

☺ $$$ **Suisse De-Sensitizing Systeme Cleansing Emulsion** *($65 for 5 ounces)* is more of a ridiculously priced cold cream than anything else. It needs to be wiped off and it can leave a slight film on the skin, but can still be an option for dry skin. The plant extracts in here can be anti-irritants, though some (rose and perilla) can be skin irritants.

☺ $$$ **Suisse De-Sensitizing Systeme Soothing Mist** *($65 for 4 ounces)* would be an OK toner for some skin types. The balm mint, horsetail, ginseng, and rose extracts in this one can be skin irritants, while other plants here are anti-irritants. What a waste.

☺ $$$ **Suisse De-Sensitizing Systeme Nurturing Cream** *($125 for 1.7 ounces)* has balm mint and arnica as two of the main plant extracts, both of which are potential skin irritants and skin sensitizers—very strange things to include in a product for sensitive skin. Other than that this absurdly overpriced moisturizer contains mostly plant water, thickeners, glycerin, silicone (are you bored yet?), plant oil, more thickeners, slip agents, water-binding agents, vitamins, even more thickeners, preservatives, and fragrant plant oil.

☺ $$$ **Suisse De-Sensitizing Systeme Barrier Shield SPF 15** *($100 for 1 ounce)* is a very good sunscreen that contains only titanium dioxide and zinc oxide as active ingredients, which indeed makes it fine for sensitive skin, but the price is shocking for this unbelievably basic group of ingredients. Not to mention that the plant extracts in here can be skin irritants! Neutrogena has far better titanium dioxide–based sunscreens for a fraction of the price.

☺ $$$ **Suisse De-Sensitizing Systeme Age Management Retexturizing Booster** *($150 for 1 ounce)* isn't part of La Prairie's sensitive line, it's just a new AHA and BHA product, and a very overpriced one at that. It's an irritating one too: alcohol is the third ingredient. That's a shame, because except for the surrealistically distorted price, the pH is actually around 3.5, which makes it effective for exfoliation, plus it does have some good water-binding agents and antioxidants.

☹ **Suisse De-Sensitizing Systeme Nurturing Cream** *($125 for 1.7 ounces)* shows the main ingredient to be arnica, which is not recommended for regular use on skin due to the potential for irritation and inflammation. It also contains balm mint high up on the ingredient listing, which adds to the problem. There is little else of interest in this un-nurturing moisturizer.

☺ $$$ **Suisse De-Sensitizing Systeme Exfoliating Enzyme Mask** *($100 for 1.7 ounces)* contains mostly fragrant plant water, glycerin, slip agent, water-binding agents, plant extracts, plant oil, thickeners, fragrant oils, and preservatives. The purported enzymes in this product are papaya extract and pineapple extract, but these aren't enzymes, they're just irritating plant extracts. Enzymes like papain or bromelain can exfoliate skin, but they're not the same as these extracts. And several of the other plant extracts in here can be skin irritants too.

☺ $$$ **Soleil Suisse Cellular Anti-Wrinkle Sun Cream SPF 30** *($100 for 1.7 ounces)* is a titanium dioxide–based sunscreen that would be good for someone with dry skin. It is a basic moisturizer with a sprinkling of plant extracts (some that can be irritants), water-binding agents, and vitamins. That's good, but if you aren't using this product liberally, all of that is useless because you won't be getting adequate protection. All sunscreens must be applied liberally.

☺ $$$ **Soleil Suisse Cellular Anti Wrinkle Sun Block SPF 50** *($125 for 1.7 ounces)* is similar to the SPF 30 above. However, while an SPF 40 sounds like you are getting "more" protection, all you are really getting is more *hours* of protection and there just isn't that much sunlight in a day. Not to mention you still have to reapply if you are perspiring or swimming. An SPF 50 does protect from 98% of the sun's rays, but that's identical to what an SPF 30 does.

☹ **Soleil Suisse Cellular Self Tan for the Body Spray Auto-Bronzant SPF 15** *($75 for 5 ounces)* contains, like all self tanners, the active ingredient dihydroxyacetone. It will turn skin brown exactly the same way a $6 self tanner will. However, the sunscreen here doesn't include the UVA-protecting ingredients titanium dioxide, zinc oxide, or avobenzone, and this is not recommended.

☹ **Soleil Suisse Self Tanner for Face SPF 15** *($75 for 1.7 ounces)* has the same review as the one above.

# La Prairie Makeup

<u>FOUNDATION:</u> ☹ **Perfecting Primer** *($55)* is a shiny, semi-opaque white liquid that leaves an obvious whitish cast on the skin. If you think giving your face a white, shiny cast will "perfect" your look, this is for you, but hopefully most will recognize what a waste this is.

☺ **$$$ Cellular Treatment Foundation Satin SPF 15** *($60)* has a good, partially titanium dioxide–based sunscreen and a lightweight but slick texture that can provide sheer to light coverage with a satin finish. This is best for normal to dry skin. Of the nine shades (with nothing for darker skins), five are best avoided: 1.0, 3.2, 3.5, 4.0, and 4.5.

☹ **Cellular Treatment Foundation Naturel SPF 8** *($60)* has a dismally low SPF (though it is part titanium dioxide) in a creamy-textured, satin-finish foundation that is capable of light to medium coverage, but all eight shades are too peach, pink, or rose to recommend.

☺ **$$$ Cellular Treatment Foundation Flawless SPF 8** *($75)* is outrageously priced, especially with no effective UVA-protecting ingredients and an embarrassing SPF for any claim about fighting wrinkles. If you're somehow still intrigued, this has a creamy texture and provides medium to full coverage. It can look heavy on the skin, but dry skin will appreciate the feel. Of the eight shades, these are too pink, peach, or rose for most skin tones: #100, #500, #600, and #800.

☺ **$$$ Cellular Treatment Powder Finish SPF 10** *($60)* is a wet/dry powder foundation that has a wonderfully smooth texture and a gorgeous silky finish. It would work best for normal to slightly dry or slightly oily skin types. What a shame the price is so ridiculous, as this also has a decent titanium dioxide sunscreen and four of the six shades are great (there are no options for darker skins). Avoid Rose Beige (too rose) and Soliel Beige (too peach).

☺ **$$$ Cellular Treatment Creme Finish SPF 15** *($70)* has a great, all-titanium-dioxide sunscreen, a creamy-smooth texture that blends beautifully, and some neutral colors (except Shade 2 and Shade 5). In spite of this, the price should stop most women dead in their tracks, especially since there is nothing in here that will aid in the uphill battle against wrinkles. It's just a nice (very, very overpriced) foundation and is easily replaced by lots of other good foundations with sunscreen from Neutrogena to Olay.

☹ <u>CONCEALER:</u> **Professional Cover Creme SPF 15** *($40)* has a reliable, titanium dioxide–based SPF, which is great, but it also has a creamy (bordering on greasy) texture with an opaque, slightly greasy finish that can easily crease into lines. The colors are good, but not that good, given the expense. **Cellular Treatment Concealer** *($30)* has a lower price point than the one above, a drier texture, and colors that are decidedly *not* neutral.

<u>POWDER:</u> ☹ **Cellular Treatment Loose Powder** *($40)* claims that it leaves a matte finish, but La Prairie may want to revisit that claim given that this one has a noticeably shiny finish and ends up being anything but matte.

☺ $$$ **Cellular Treatment Pressed Powder** *($36)* is just a regular pressed powder with a nice silky feel. It does not look dry or too matte on the skin, meaning normal to dry skin will appreciate this finish the most. The three shades are slightly peachy-pink.

☺ $$$ <u>BLUSH:</u> **Cellular Treatment Blush** *($37.50)* has an even, smooth texture that applies and builds well. The colors look vivid, but apply sheer, and only Vin is too shiny to recommend. **Creme Lumere Stick** *($35)* is a cream blush with two shades that are sheer but shiny. It is nothing exceptional, and shiny cheeks, especially on someone fighting wrinkles, look strange.

☹ <u>EYESHADOW:</u> **Cellular Treatment Eye Color** *($32)* are a group of single eyeshadows with fairly nice textures and minimal to heavy shine. Why these are labeled as being a treatment makes no sense as there are not enough ingredients in here that can treat the eye area, and the shine only makes wrinkles look more pronounced. **Ensemble de Coleur** *($50)* is a kit of two eyeshadow colors and a powder eyeliner. The shadows claim to have a matte finish, but they are undoubtedly shiny, with a good, smooth texture. The eyeliner part is very dry, and works best with a wet (damp) brush.

☺ $$$ <u>EYE AND BROW SHAPER:</u> **Eye Pencil** *($25)* and **Brow Pencil** *($25)* are standard pencils that are dressed up in elaborate packaging. Please don't be fooled: the packaging doesn't affect performance, and why waste your money for something so ordinary?

<u>LIPSTICK AND LIP PENCIL:</u> ☺ $$$ **Cellular Treatment Lip Color Sheer** *($27)* is, as the name implies, more glossy tint than lipstick. **Cellular Treatment Lip Color Moisturizing** *($27)* has a greasy, wet finish and will bleed into lines almost faster than you can apply it. **Cellular Treatment Lip Color Matte** *($27)* isn't matte in the least but it isn't nearly as greasy as the others and has enough pigment to keep it around for a while. **Cellular Treatment Lip Color Lasting** *($27)* is just a creamy, opaque lipstick with a greasy finish and no stain to speak of, which negates the "long lasting" claim. The **Lip Pencils** *($25)* are in the same boat as the eye and brow pencils, and it's best to let them just sail on by.

☺ $$$ **Cellular Treatment Lip Enhancer** *($40)* is a slightly shiny lipstick that leaves me red-faced. For $40, this actually claims it "redefines the lip outline and extends wear" and "prevents feathering and bleeding." Puh-leeze! If that is even partially true, may lightning strike me down right now. See? I'm still here!

☺ $$$ <u>MASCARA:</u> **Cellular Treatment Intensified Mascara** *($25),* at this price, should be amazing. It isn't, but it is a good mascara that makes the lashes long, thick, and soft, and doesn't smudge.

☺ $$$ <u>BRUSHES:</u> La Prairie has added a few token **Brushes** *($28 to $65; $250 for collection).* They are nicely shaped and look elegant but still don't compare to the fine offerings from Trish McEvoy or Prescriptives, for example.

# Lac-Hydrin (Skin Care Only)

These were the original AHA products sold anywhere! They have been in drugstores for years, and much of what we know about how AHAs behave is a result of these formulations. Lac-Hydrin Five (stands for 5% lactic acid) and Lac-Hydrin Twelve (this one is prescription-only and represents 12% lactic acid) are in bases that have the correct pH to be effective exfoliants. These aren't elegant formulations, but they are some of the best AHA exfoliants available. For more information about Lac-Hydrin, call Westwood Squibb Pharmaceutical at (800) 333-0950.

☺ **Lac-Hydrin Five Lotion** *($10.99 for 8 ounces)* and **Lac-Hydrin 12 Lotion** *($34.98 for 7.6 ounces)* are both good AHA products containing lactic acid in a standard Vaseline-based moisturizer. Either of these are appropriate for someone with dry skin. Lac-Hydrin Five contains 5% AHA and is available over the counter, and the Lac-Hydrin is a 12% AHA product available for some reason by prescription only. Both are fragrance-free.

# Lancome

This very French line maintains a more casual air when compared to the other French lines sold at department stores such as Yves St. Laurent, Orlane, Givenchy, Guerlain, or Chanel, whose elitist airs are so thick you can cut them with a knife. Over the years, Lancome has done a noteworthy job of making sure its products and image radiate a contemporary elegance. Owned by L'Oreal, one of the top five cosmetics companies in the world, Lancome has the advertising dollars to keep its "high-end" line in place in consumer's minds as one of the standards for beauty products. In tandem with the air of European style Lancome exudes, its products have always been aimed at baby boomers and anyone else concerned with the "ravages of time." This has even been reflected within its color line, where several new products have been launched with names such as Teint Optim' Age and in an overabundance of claims that range from "progressively firms the skin" to "soft-focus finish" and "skin illuminating." Paradoxically, Lancome has also been racing fast and furiously to establish itself as a trend line, launching new color collections with some decidedly strange or frivolous concepts such as red glitter eyeshadow, among other vivid colors. My concern is that women will delve into these trends in an effort to stay current but only end up with disappointing products or vividly garish features.

Looking at Lancome's customary lineup of colors, it's clear it continues to offer excellent foundations, great blush and lip colors and textures, and superlative mascaras. There are many superb colors for a wide range of skin tones, from light to dark (including several suitable for darker skin tones). And although there is a lot more to wade through in terms of selection, many of the counters are well equipped to allow for women to experiment on their own.

Two warnings about Lancome. First, its color units, though readily accessible, have no rhyme or reason in their organization. Very few products are grouped by color tones or families and that can make coordinating selections difficult. The other issue is more serious. Some of the Lancome sun-protecting products (particularly its foundations) do not contain UVA-protecting ingredients. Yet it is absolutely self-evident that Lancome has a complete knowledge of the issues surrounding UVA protection in sunscreen formulations. Its new sun-care line has been reformulated to include avobenzone, and L'Oreal (which owns Lancome) uses its own patented UVA ingredient, called Mexoryl SX™, outside of the United States. Given that knowledge, why Lancome (and L'Oreal) would continue to make any sunscreen products without UVA protection is just shocking.

Aside from sun protection, Lancome's skin care is a vast group of products. Some of these have all the latest bells and whistles, but in the world of interesting water-binding agents and antioxidants they fall far short—so in this area the Estee Lauder people, to name one company, are far ahead of Lancome. It is interesting to note that Lancome is rarely the company to set trends, but whatever the next skin-care fad may be, Lancome is there just a few months behind with its version, whether it be products with vitamin C, vitamin A, or a group of anti-acne products (and particularly if Estee Lauder has added it to its line). Perhaps most interesting to the consumer is that because Lancome is owned by L'Oreal, I often find that virtually identical products are first launched at the L'Oreal shelves and then turn up at the Lancome counter a month or two later. In terms of quality both L'Oreal and Lancome have some very good skin-care products—however, their fragrance wafts from many of the products and that is a concern for many skin types.

One more comment: On its Web site Lancome states quite clearly that all skin types need moisturizers. When you're selling dozens of them I imagine you would want everyone to use one. But it is absolutely not true that every skin needs a moisturizer, though every skin type needs an effective sunscreen, something Lancome is only now getting straight in the United States.

For more information about Lancome, call (800) LANCOME or visit the Web site at www.lancome.com.

# Lancome Skin Care

☺ $$$ **Ablutia Fraicheur Purifying Foam Cleanser** *($21.50 for 6.4 ounces)* is a very standard, detergent-based water-soluble cleanser that can be drying for some skin types but is appropriate for someone with normal to oily skin. It does contain fragrance and coloring agents as well as fragrance.

☺ **Clarifiance Oil-Free Gel Cleanser** *($21.50 for 6.8 ounces)* is a very good, very standard, detergent-based water-soluble cleanser that would work well for most skin types except dry skin. It does contain fragrance.

☺ **Galatee Douceur Milky Creme Cleanser** *($37.50 for 13.5 ounces)* is supposed to be a splash- or tissue-off cleanser for all skin types. It is a standard, mineral oil–based wipe-off cleanser that can leave a greasy film on the skin. It may be good for extremely dry skin, though it needs to be wiped off to get both the makeup and the cleanser off. It does contain fragrance.

☹ **Gel Eclat Cleansing Gel** *($18.50 for 4.4 ounces)* uses sodium C14-16 olefin sulfate as the main cleansing agent, which makes it potentially drying and irritating for all skin types.

☹ $$$ **Pur Controle Cleanser for Oily and Normal to Oily Skin** *($18 for 4.1 ounces)* is a very drying detergent cleanser that contains several cleansing agents known for their harsh effect on the skin, including potassium hydroxide, rather high up on the ingredient list. It could be an option for very oily skin but the irritation is not the best for any skin type. It does contain fragrance.

☹ $$$ **Pur Douceur Cleanser** *($18.50 for 4 ounces)* is similar to the Pur Controle above and the same comments apply. It does contain fragrance.

☹ $$$ **Bi-Facil Double-Action Eye Makeup Remover** *($18.50 for 4 ounces)* is a silicone-based wipe-off cleanser, nothing more. The price is steep for this very basic eye-makeup remover. It does contain fragrance.

☹ $$$ **Effacile Gentle Eye Makeup Remover** *($17.50 for 4 ounces)* is a detergent-based eye-makeup remover that isn't all that gentle, but it will take off eye makeup. It does contain fragrance.

☹ $$$ **Eau de Bienfait Cleanser Water with Vitamins for Face and Eyes** *($23.50 for 6.8 ounces)* is similar to the Effacile above, only this one throws in a few teeny amounts of vitamins that have no real effect on skin. This will take off makeup.

☺ $$$ **Exfoliance, Delicate Exfoliating Gel** *($21 for 3.5 ounces)* is a reformulation, and it is a good one. The original contained tallow, which has now been re-placed with other, somewhat less problematic thickening agents. It would work well as fairly gentle scrub for someone with normal to dry skin. It contains about 0.1% to 0.5% salicylic acid (BHA), but the pH is too high, and the amount really too small for it to have any benefit for exfoliation.

☹ **Clarifiance Alcohol-Free Natural Astringent** *($18.50 for 6.8 ounces)* contains menthol, which is an irritant, but so is the potassium alum here, which has skin-constricting properties that may be helpful when used occasionally but with regular application can cause inflammation and irritation, and that hurts skin.

☹ **Tonique Controle Toner for Oily and Normal to Oily Skin** *($18.50 for 6.8 ounces)* is basically just alcohol, and that is too irritating and drying for all skin types.

☺ **Tonique Douceur Non-Alcoholic Freshener for Dry/Sensitive Skin** *($27.50 for 13.5 ounces)* is indeed alcohol-free. This is a very average, do-nothing toner, and way too pricey for such a mundane formulation.

☺ **$$$ Tonique Eclat** *($18.50 for 6.8 ounces)* is an OK, irritant-free toner with glycerin, fragrance, and preservatives. It contain plant extracts that are supposed to sound like AHAs but they cannot perform the same function or provide any benefit for skin.

☹ **Vitabolic Clarifier Radiance Boosting Tonic** *($27.50 for 3.4 ounces)* is basi-cally just alcohol, along with some potentially irritating plant extracts that just boost the risk of skin irritation and dryness.

☺ **$$$ Vitabolic Dark Eye Circle Treatment** *($42.50 for 0.5 ounce)* is another addition to the world of vitamins. And just like the first Vitabolic this one uses ascorbic acid as its form of vitamin C, and that's not the version the research has talked about. If anything, the information I've seen indicates ascorbic acid is one of the more irritating, unstable forms of vitamin C. This is not an improvement over the original, and there is nothing about it that's better for the eye area. In fact, you just get less product for about the same amount of money. It isn't even a very good moisturizer. Avon's version is far more interesting, even with the same form of vitamin C.

☺ **$$$ Vitabolic Deep Radiance Booster** *($45 for 1 ounce)* is almost identical to the Dark Circle version above and the same basic comments apply.

☺ **$$$ Vitabolic Oil Free** *($49 for 1 ounce)*, except for the addition of a film-forming ingredient, is almost identical to the Dark Circle version above, and the same basic comments apply.

☺ **$$$ Bienfait Total Fluide SPF 15** *($55 for 3.4 ounces)* has been reformulated and it now includes avobenzone as part of the active ingredients, which means it can protect from UVA sun damage. So why the neutral face rating? Now that so many products contain UVA-protecting ingredients you can be more picky about what you choose, and this formulation includes alcohol as the third ingredient. That can be drying and irritating for most skin types. Not to mention that the price is completely unwarranted. There is nothing in this product that Neutrogena's or my sunscreens with avobenzone or titanium dioxide don't do better for far less. And why didn't Lancome include UVA-protecting ingredients in the first version that made such wonderful claims but was clearly poorly formulated?

☹ **Bienfait Total Creme SPF 15** *($35 for 1.7 ounces)* got left out when Lancome reformulated the Bienfait Total Fluide above to include UVA-protecting ingredients; why they didn't add them to this one is a mystery. This version is not recommended.

☺ **$$$ Vinefit Complete Energizing Lotion SPF 15** *($37.50 for 1 ounce)*. The best part of this overpriced sunscreen is the sunscreen, which is an appropriate SPF 15 titanium dioxide. Other than grape seed oil and grape extract, there is absolutely nothing in this product that it makes it preferred over Neutrogena's Sensitive Skin UVA/UVB Block SPF 17 (8.99 for 4 ounces). The notion that grapes are one of the best sources of antioxidants when it comes to food is absolutely not the fact for skin-care products. However, if you want grapes and a decent sunscreen you may want to consider this product.

☺ **Hydra Controle Hydrating & Matifying Long-Lasting Treatment Oil-Free Fresh Gel** *($30 for 1.7 ounces)* has minimal ability to keep a matte feel on skin but it is worth a test drive next time you're at a Lancome counter. The tiny amount of papaya and pineapple extract in here have no impact on skin.

☹ **Hydra Controle Mat** *($57 for 1.7 ounces)* includes three forms of alcohol (the irritating kind), film formers, silicone, clay, and thickeners. Clay can absorb oil and the film formers provide a matte feel on the skin, but this has more potential problems than benefits.

☺ **$$$ Hydrative Continuous Hydrating Resource** *($42.50 for 1.75 ounces)* is a good emollient (though very basic) moisturizer for dry skin. It does contain urea, which can have exfoliating properties for skin. For some strange reason this product contains Aspartame (NutraSweet) but I know you're not supposed to eat this stuff.

☺ **$$$ HydraZen** *($42.50 for 1.7 ounces)* is supposed to be relaxation in a jar, or at least that's what the name and ad copy suggest. It's "stress relief for your skin" and contains something called "Acticalm." Even if stress were an issue for skin and you could apply something to the face to make it calmer, according to HydraZen that would only take a moisturizer, because that's all this product is. The only unique thing about HydraZen is the name. If mind over matter works, then you will feel calmer, but it probably isn't from applying this good, but rather ordinary, ho-hum moisturizer for dry skin.

☺ **$$$ Niosome + Perfected Age Treatment** *($60 for 2.5 ounces)* is a good, basic moisturizer for dry skin. There are some antioxidants in it, but in such negligible amounts that they don't count for much. The minuscule amount of lactoferrin in here is a protein usually derived from milk (particularly breast milk) but that can also be found in saliva. It can have antiviral, antibacterial, and anti-inflammatory effects on skin but in this amount, the skin would never notice. This one also contains a teeny amount of lactoperoxidase, an enzyme derived from milk that has antibacterial properties for skin, also in an amount that isn't effective for much of anything.

☺ **Nutribel Nourishing Hydrating Emulsion** *($38 for 2.5 ounces)* is a good, very emollient moisturizer. It would work for dry skin, but there are far more elegant formulations to consider for the money.

☺ **$$$ Nutriforce Double Nutrition Fortifying Nourishing Creme** *($40 for 1.7 ounces)* is a good basic (but ordinary) moisturizer for someone with dry skin.

☺ **Nutrix Soothing Treatment Creme** *($32 for 1.9 ounces)* is a lot of money for mineral oil and Vaseline, but it would be good for someone with very dry skin. Lubriderm to Eucerin, however, offer similar formulas for far less money.

☹ **$$$ Primordiale Intense** *($72.50 for 1.7 ounces).* There is simply nothing intense about this moisturizer for dry skin except the price. And Lancome has far better moisturizers than this one. It does contain a teeny amount of bilberry extract, which is alleged to lighten skin discolorations, but the research about this ingredient having that kind of effect on skin is minimal. The teeny amount of plant extracts in here has no AHA properties.

☺ **$$$ Primordiale Lip** *($29 for 0.5 ounce)* is an emollient, clear, somewhat glossy lipstick, period.

☺ **$$$ Primordiale Nuit** *($75 for 2.5 ounces)* is a good, exceedingly ordinary, emollient moisturizer for someone with dry skin.

☺ **$$$ Primordiale Yeux Visibly Revitalizing Eye Treatment** *($42.50 for 0.5 ounce)* is similar to the Primordial Nuit above only less emollient. It does contain caffeine, but that can be a skin irritant, and it won't wake up the eyes in any manner.

☺ **$$$ Progres Counter des Yeux Eye Creme** *($37.50 for 1.5 ounces)* is a thick, heavy eye cream. This is a good, very basic emollient moisturizer for dry skin around the eyes or anywhere on the face.

☺ **$$$ Renergie Double Performance Treatment** *($72.50 for 2.5 ounces)* is a good, boring, emollient moisturizer for dry skin.

☹ **$$$ Renergie Emulsion Oil-Free Lotion** *($57.50 for 1.7 ounces).* In many respects, this is a very ordinary moisturizer that might be OK for someone with normal to slightly dry skin, but at best this is a "why bother?".

☹ **$$$ Renergie Yeux** *($40 for 0.5 ounce)* is similar to the Renergie Emulsion above and the same basic comments apply. The caffeine in this one can be a skin irritant and will not wake up the eye as its inclusion seems to imply.

☺ **Trans-Hydrix Multi-Action Hydrating Creme** *($36.50 for 1.9 ounces)* is a good standard, boring moisturizer for dry skin.

☺ **$$$ Complexion Expert** *($45 for 1 ounce)* has a basic formulation that makes this moisturizer very similar to other moisturizers from both L'Oreal and Lancome; what makes this one different is the inclusion of kojic acid. Kojic acid has some reported value for preventing melanin production, though not as effectively as hydroquinone. Kojic acid is also considered to be more irritating than hydroquinone though kojic acid does have antioxidant properties.

☺ **$$$ ReSurface** *($52.50 for 1 ounce)* is Lancome's addition to the retinol bandwagon, only L'Oreal beat Lancome to the punch a few months earlier with its Line Eraser Pure Retinol ($12.89 for 1 ounce). These products are virtually the same, with the same retinol, the same small amount used, and the same lightweight lotion formulation. If you're thinking of retinol, despite the meager evidence that there is any reason to use it, why would you choose the Lancome version over the L'Oreal version? Just to be clear for those taken by the retinol craze, be aware that L'Oreal does have two products that sound like they contain retinol but don't. RevitaLift Face & Neck with Pro-Retinol-*A* ($13.49 for 1.7 ounces) and RevitaLift Eye with Pro-Retinol-A ($13.49 for 0.5 ounce). These both contain retinyl palmitate, but retinyl palmitate is about as far removed from retinol as retinol is from tretinoin (that's the truly active ingredient in Renova and Retin-A that retinol is hyped as being similar to), so we are talking really far.

☺ **$$$ Touche Optim' Age** *($22.50 for 0.52 ounce)* is nothing more than wax, silicone, and film former, basically. This slippery, waxy cream is meant to be patted over wrinkles to make them look less noticeable and can be used either over or under makeup or alone. Its application is sort of like spackle but more sheer. It definitely leaves a visible film over the skin, but does it make the lines on the face go away? From my experience (I used it on only half my face over and then later under the Teint Optim' Age foundation), I found some areas definitely looked smoother, like my forehead and eye area, while the laugh lines and crows feet looked no different, except for the film left by the film-forming ingredients. This is one you should test for yourself. It is a curious product that is interesting to experience, but be sure to wear it for the day and check the results in daylight before giving in to the temptation of spending a lot of money on a very small amount of product. By the way, M.A.C. has an identical version for about half the price, called Matte Creme Matifiance *($16.50 for 0.75 ounce)*.

☺ **$$$ Empreinte de Beaute Deep Cleansing Clay Masque** *($21 for 2.5 ounces)* is a basic clay mask. It does contain camphor, and that can be a skin irritant.

☹ **Extra Controle Anti-Imperfections Acne Treatment Matifying Solution** *($30 for 1 ounce)* is a BHA product in an alcohol base. Alcohol can increase breakouts from the irritation it causes as well as dry out the skin and cause redness; also, the pH of this product negates the effectiveness of the BHA.

☹ **Spot Controle Acne Treatment** *($15 for 0.5 ounce)* contains a good amount of alcohol and about 1% BHA. The alcohol won't spot control anything, though it can cause redness, dryness, and irritation, and the pH is too high for the BHA to be effective as an exfoliant.

☹ **Masque Controle, Peel-Off Purifying Mask** *($22.50 for 2.5 ounces)* is an alcohol- and film former–based mask; the alcohol is irritating, and peeling plastic off the face doesn't do much for skin.

☺ **$$$ T. Controle Oil-Free Powder Gel Instant T-Zone Matifier** *($22.50 for 1 ounce)* is an interesting product made of silicone and film former, period; there is no powder in here. It will put a silky film over the skin, but don't count on this to help your oily skin, because there is nothing in this product that can hold back oil. It is a decent lightweight silicone moisturizer but that's about it. Definitely test before you even consider this misleading product. If anything, it will make someone with oily skin feel more oily!

☺ **SPF 15 Face and Body Lotion with Pure Vitamin E** *($21 for 5 ounces)* is a very good, avobenzone-based sunscreen for someone with normal to dry or slightly oily skin. The price is high, but not terrible.

☺ **SPF 25 Face and Body Lotion with Pure Vitamin E** *($21 for 5 ounces)* is similar to the one above and the same review applies.

☺ **SPF 15 Water-Light Spray** *($21 for 5 ounces)* is a very good avobenzone-based sunscreen that is mostly slip agents, film former, and plant oil. It should work well for someone with normal to slightly dry skin.

☺ **High Protection SPF 30 Face Creme with Pure Vitamin E** *($23 for 1.7 ounces)* is similar to the ones above, but there is nothing unique in here that warrants the smaller amount for the same price.

☺ **UV Expert SPF 15 Sunscreen, Daily UVA/UVB Protection Water-Lite Fluide** *($30 for 1 ounce)* is a sunscreen whose name describes itself, except to say that the UVA/UVB protection comes from avobenzone. That's really all there is to say, except that the amount you get isn't worth the price, as the other avobenzone-based sunscreens in this line above are the same for far less. This is about as arbitrary an example of cosmetics pricing as I've ever seen.

☺ **$$$ Soleil Expert Sun Care SPF 30 High Protection Sun Stick** *($19.50 for 0.26 ounce)* is an avobenzone-based sunscreen, and the amount and price are ludicrous given that what you get is a basic sunscreen with avobenzone and there are far less expensive versions from many lines. The price for this is almost $100 an ounce.

☺ **Soleil Ultra Eye Protection SPF 40** *($23 for 1.2 ounces)* is a good but extremely overpriced sunscreen that includes titanium dioxide and zinc oxide as part of the active sunscreen ingredients. This combination is not unique to Lancome and the use of an SPF 40 sounds like you are getting "more" protection, but all you would be getting is longer protection and there just isn't that much sunlight. Nothing about this makes it preferred for the eye area; if anything, the talc and other active ingredients (octyl methoxycinnamate and oxybenzone) can be irritating if they get in the eye.

☺ **After Sun Tan Prolonger Refreshing Gel** *($25 for 5 ounces)* is a bit of a confusing product; it is basically a self tanner (it contains dihydroxyacetone like all self tanners do), but the marketing makes it sound like a soothing product for sun-damaged skin. It isn't; the chemical that makes skin turn brown isn't a soothing agent in the least.

☺ $$$ **Stick Nutrix Levres, Lip Balm** *($16.50 for 0.13 ounce)* is a very emollient but standard lip balm. It's good for dry lips, but very overpriced, given its similarity to products at one-third the price.

## Lancome Makeup

**FOUNDATION:** Lancome's foundation types are almost overwhelming, with more on the way. Each new foundation purports to have benefits that are always tied to the latest buzzwords and "hot" ingredients, but these are nothing more than marketing incantations and have nothing to do with good skin care or how the products perform. Nevertheless, when you look at color choice, application, and color selection, Lancome's foundations are some of the best available.

☺ $$$ **Photogenic Makeup SPF 15** *($32.50)* is awfully similar to L'Oreal's Translucide Foundation SPF 18 *($11.25)*—both lack UVA-blocking ingredients (they don't contain titanium dioxide, zinc oxide, or avobenzone, and Lancome of all lines knows better than to leave this important sunscreen element out). But both do have a light, fluid texture that blends to a soft, natural finish with light to medium coverage. As usual, Lancome's 17 shades are mostly wonderful whereas L'Oreal's lean too much toward the peachy-pink side to work for most skin tones. If Lancome would just add some UVA protection to this version it would be a great recommendation for normal to slightly dry or slightly oily skins. If you're willing to wear sun protection underneath this as it stands now, there are some superior colors to consider for both light and dark skins (but no very dark skins). These shades are too pink, peach, or copper for most skin tones: Ivoire 2, Bisque 4, Bisque 8, and Suede 0, 4, and 6.

☺ $$$ **Dual Finish** *($30)* is a wet/dry powder foundation that offers a soft matte finish and a beautiful selection of colors. The application, especially when used dry, is smooth and even, although this type of foundation is best for normal skin; dry skin may find this too dry and oilier skin will find it too cakey after it is applied. Wet application is not recommended as this type of product tends to go on choppy and streak. The only color to be wary of is Matte Miel Fonce IV, which may turn orange on some skin tones.

☺ $$$ **MaquiLibre SPF 15** *($32.50)* is a lightweight, sheer-coverage foundation with no UVA-protecting ingredients. What a shame, because this would be one to consider for a soft, natural finish. It's still worth a look, but not for reliable sun protection. Avoid Beige Rose III and Rose Clair II, which are very pink.

☺ $$$ **Maquicontrole** ($32.50) is Lancome's original ultra-matte foundation (launched over 15 years ago, well ahead of its time) and it's an exceptional oil-free foundation that offers medium to full coverage and a true matte finish. It has incredible staying power and a solid matte finish. This is definitely one for oily skins to consider, but avoid these shades: Rose Clair II, Beige Natural III, Beige Bisque III (all too pink), Sable III, and Bronze IV (too orange or ash).

☺ $$$ **Tient Idole** *($32.50)* is an ultra-matte foundation Lancome has recently introduced that has somewhat less coverage than its Maquicontrole. This one offers the same finish and budgeproof wear as all the others (see Almay's Amazing Lasting, Maybelline's Great Wear, and Revlon's ColorStay foundations for excellent, less-expensive options). Teint Idole has medium coverage with an opaque finish. It dries very quickly, so blending must be precise the first time through. All of the colors are wonderful except Porcelaine (slightly pink), Beige Sable III (pink), and Amande Bronze (orange).

☺ $$$ **Stick Express Teint Idole Foundation** *($32.50)* is a twist-up stick foundation that has a cream-to-powder finish but is far less creamy than you might suspect from looking at the applicator. The smooth application dries to a solid powder base, providing excellent medium to heavy coverage. But be forewarned: once you blend this one out, which you must do quickly, it really stays put. In fact you may find it hard to remove! The 12 shades available are for the most part terrific—the only one to watch out for is Clair I, which can be too pink for most skin tones.

☹ $$$ **Tient Idole Hydra Compact** *($35 with compact; $25 refill)* is Lancome's revision of its problematic Cool Finish Foundation (which was similar to Vincent Longo's popular Water Canvas foundation). Sadly, this version doesn't come close to the strengths of the previous one. Although the claim is "30% water," that means nothing except that it is 70% something else! That something would be the thickening agents, plant oils, and silicones that give this foundation a nice creamy finish and opaque appearance—and a far more heavy feel than the original. It can be an option for someone with normal to dry skin, but the colors aren't up to par with Lancome's other foundations, so if you decide to try this, choose carefully and avoid Bisque 6 (too peach), Suede 0 (very orange), and Suede 10 (too red). I do wish Lancome had worked out the kinks in its Cool Finish, because it had some strong points that the Hydra Compact doesn't come close to having.

☺ $$$ **Teint Optim' Age SPF 15** *($32.50)* contains no UVA-protecting ingredients, which is very disappointing. If sun protection isn't your goal, this one does have a wonderful, silky-smooth feel and blends on superbly, offering sheer to light coverage with a soft matte finish. It is best for normal to dry skin. The claims about "age minimizing" are bogus—there is nothing in here to support that and it won't make one wrinkle on your face look less noticeable—but it is still an excellent foundation. Be careful with the following shades: Porcelaine D'Ivoire (slight yellow), Porcelaine I, and Beige Bisque III (may turn slightly pink).

☺ $$$ **Maquivelours** *($32.50)* is an emollient, natural-finish formula that is best for normal to dry or very dry skin looking for medium coverage. Of the ten shades, the ones to avoid are Rose Clair II, Beige Rose III (both too pink); Beige Bisque III, and Beige Sable III (too orange).

☹ $$$ **Imanance Tinted Cream SPF 15** *($33)* is a part titanium dioxide–based SPF 15 tinted moisturizer. The coverage is sheer and the emolliency of this makes it suitable for normal to dry skin only. The only useful skin-tone color is Bisque; the three remaining shades are all quite orange or red.

☹ $$$ **Palette Mix** *($28.50)* is a compact with three different flesh-toned shades that you mix together to get just the right color for your skin, to be used alone or over or under foundation. Although this cream-to-powder formula has a superbly smooth finish, most women will have difficulty combining colors like this on their face. It isn't a bad idea, just more trouble and more time-consuming than a makeup application should be.

**CONCEALERS:** ☺ $$$ **Effacernes** *($19.50)* comes in a squeeze tube, which is not my favorite type as it is easy to squeeze out too much, which wastes product. It doesn't crease and provides light to medium coverage. This does offer a smooth, creamy finish with four workable shades. Lancome claims it is waterproof, but the ingredients and real-world testing confirmed otherwise. **Maquicomplet** *($19.50)* is an exceptional concealer that offers great, natural matte coverage and stays put without creasing! Of the six shades available, the only one to ignore is Correcteur (very yellow) and possibly Beige III (slightly pink).

☹ **Face Perfecting Pencil** *($15)* is a chubby pencil concealer that has an opaque, slightly greasy application. This can cover well but does tend to crease . . . and crease. This started out as five shades and has now been whittled down to one; no surprise there, as this is an inconvenient way to use concealer. **Palette Pro** *($28.50)* offers three different compacts, each with varying shades of orange, mauve, yellow, and mint green. Each compact contains one concealer and three color-correcting shades of green, yellow, and mauve. Color correctors are minimally useful on the face and generally cause more problems than they help, leaving a strange tint on the skin that mixes poorly with foundation. Any of Lancome's wonderfully neutral or yellow-based foundations will provide enough color correction for anyone's face. The concealing cream in the Palette Pro Kit comes in three excellent shades, but it is just a concealer that creases minimally. It would be very good for someone with dry skin, but, regrettably, it isn't sold separately.

☺ **$$$ Aquatique** and **Ombre Perfecteur** *($19 and $20)* are billed as "eye foundations." You're supposed to believe you need a separate product (beyond foundation or concealer) to even out the skin tone on the eyelid and prevent eyeshadows from creasing. These two products offer an opaque, thick formula that most certainly can crease, and what's worse is that the color for both is strongly peach, not exactly the color all women need or want.

☺ **$$$ Touche Optimage** *($22.50)* isn't so much a concealer (it has no color) as it is a sort of spackle for wrinkles. It has a smooth finish and a waxy, gel texture that can fill in lines to some extent, but not as much as the ads imply. This may be an option, but test it out first.

POWDERS: ☺ **$$$ Poudre Majeur Loose** *($32.50)* and **Poudre Majeur Pressed Powder** *($28.50)* are talc-free powders with a soft, silky, dry finish. The colors available are fine, although there are only a handful to choose from.

☹ **Poudre Bronzee** *($28.50)* is perhaps one of the worst bronzing powders I've seen. I guess Lancome thinks because suntanned skin is always so shiny the loads of glitter in here will imitate it; that wouldn't be so bad but add to that the incredibly dry and chalky texture and this is one to avoid. **Powder Pro Complexion Perfecting Powder** *($20)* is a selection of three separate shades of color-correcting powders. Not only is this unnecessary, but these also have a shiny finish, making a strange color on the skin even that much more obvious. I never recommend color correctors, but if you do choose to do this step, only use correctors that go under the makeup. Dusting mauve, green, or yellow powder on top of foundation would give the foundation a strange hue, especially out in daylight. The Pearl shade of powder can add a nice halo of shine over the face, neck, and shoulders, but shine is appropriate for nighttime only, right?

☺ **$$$ Poudre Blanc Neige** *($28.50)* is a standard pressed powder with a smooth, silky finish and a truly soft shine. For a subtle amount of shine, which is a welcome change of pace from the glitter in most products, this is an option. Ignore the strange shades of peach, yellow, pink, and bronze—the sheer application makes the colors inconsequential.

☹ **Poudre Liberte** *($25 for powder insert; $10 for compact)* is a talc-based loose powder with a light, airy texture and beautiful finish that has an intriguing concept and terrible execution. The idea was to create a "take along" loose powder in a pressed-powder style compact. The effect would be to achieve the lightness of a loose powder with none of the usual messiness. The compact has a large air bubble on the bottom that, when pressed, pushes up a small amount of powder over a sifter screen and onto the waiting puff. It is then ready to apply, *à la* pressed powder. However, this ends up being worse than taking along loose powder, as *any* pressure on the bubble (from jostling around in your purse, for example) will cause powder to be dispensed up into the puff. Then, when you open the compact for a "quick" touch-up, loose powder spills everywhere. Or if you press the bubble to firmly you can get a shot of powder up in the air and all over your counter or you. The seven colors are just fine, but who needs this much of a mess applying powder?

☺ $$$ <u>BLUSH</u> **Pommette** *($24)* is a wonderfully silky cream-to-powder blush with a beautiful selection of colors and a sheer finish. This is one of the better cream blushes and is best for normal to dry skin. There are two shiny colors, Perle and Lame, which are easily identified and avoided if need be. **Blush Subtil** *($24)* is a talc-free powder blush that comes in an excellent range of colors and has a soft, sheer finish. Darker skin tones take note: there are some great options here. Of course, there are some shiny colors but these are also easily identified.

☺ $$$ **Couleur Flash Blush Stick** *($27.50)* is a twist-up cream-to-powder blush that is nearly identical in texture, finish, and application to L'Oreal's QuickStick Face and Body Blush ($12.29). Both have a creamy slip that quickly dries to a soft, sheer powder finish and would be an option for normal to slightly dry skin. The color selection for Lancome's is smaller than usual and, save for the shiny Desert Gold, are all beautiful.

<u>EYESHADOW:</u> ☺ $$$ **Maquiriche Eye Color Duo** *($10 per tin/$5 per compact; $25 for duo with compact)* are Lancome's powder eyeshadow selections, and you get to create your own compact by selecting the eyeshadow colors of your choice. There are some great matte shades but more and more shiny, shimmery shades to be wary of. The latest additions are strange tones of red, blue, and violet that are attention getters but clearly not for everyone (actually who these are selling to is an interesting question). The texture is fairly smooth, and these blend on more sheer than many others, possibly due to the fact that they are quite powdery (watch out for powder flaking onto the cheek areas with these!).

☺ $$$ **Eye Colour in Two** *($18.50)* is a two-in-one pencil with a cream-to-powder shadow on one end and eyeliner on the other. Cute idea, but all of the shadow colors are shiny and can easily crease, while the eyeliner end is quite dry and tends to drag and pull the skin, making this a wash. **L'Ombre Style Duo** *($24 for pen with two colors)* is a unique concept: this is a dual-ended pen with each end holding a sponge-tip applicator that is "fed" with color from the base. However, several shades that are labeled matte have obvious shine. For a simple eye design this could work—but it's not for everyone. **Eternal Eyes** *($16.50)* is a cream-to-powder shadow with a wand applicator. There are easier ways to apply shadow than this, and blending is difficult. Still, some women prefer this type of product and these are worth a look. They are not waterproof, as claimed, but do hold up well throughout the day, though they are also rather shiny.

☺ $$$ <u>EYE AND BROW SHAPER:</u> **Le Crayon Kohl** *($16.50)* is a standard eye pencil in a nice range of colors. This one is longer than most, so it may seem clumsy at first. These are no better than others for far less money (particularly those from L'Oreal). **Le Crayon Poudre for the Brows** *($17.50)* is a standard brow pencil with a good brush at one end for softening and blending the color. It goes on easily, though slightly creamy, and the colors are matte and soft. **Modele Sourcils Brow Groomer** *($17.50)* is a brow gel with both a clear shade and three tints. The brush is quite full, so it may be difficult to apply. The colors, though limited, are otherwise great and this type of product is an excellent way to make brows look fuller. **Brow Artiste** *($28)* offers two matte-finish, powder-type brow colors in a compact. While most women only need one brow color and mixing takes time, these are still a viable option and have a nice dry texture and matte finish.

(Unrated) $$$ **Artliner** *($24.50)*. As this book went to press, Artliner was being reformulated. It was an excellent (albeit overpriced) liquid eyeliner. I will report on the changes in an issue of my newsletter.

☹ **Maquiglace Lumineuse** *($18.50)* is similar to the former Artliner liquid eyeliner, with two shades and a floppy, thin brush. The salesperson steered me away from this, commenting that it is very difficult to apply evenly. She was right, plus the two shades are intensely shiny. **Le Stylo Waterproof** *($17.50)* is a twist-up eye pencil with mostly shiny colors that all tend to smudge. That's not too bad for a soft look, but otherwise skip it. Plus, it isn't any more waterproof than any other standard pencil.

☺ $$$ <u>LIPSTICK AND LIP PENCIL:</u> For the most part, the textures are true to the names and the shades are gorgeous, but there are now a growing number of trendy shades (silver, gold, lime green) available that you would never have expected to see at a Lancome counter. **Rouge Absolu Matte** *($18.50)* is supposed to be long lasting, but it isn't, at least not any more so than any other creamy, opaque lipstick. Despite the fact that some colors in this group are called matte, they are all creamy. **Rouge Absolu Hydrating Long Lasting LipColor** *($18.50)* is mostly a creamy lipstick with a slightly glossy finish. That might make it more hydrating, but definitely not longer lasting. **Rouge Idole** *($18.50)* is a very good ultra-matte lipstick with an excellent color range. L'Oreal's Colour Endure *($9.19)* is virtually identical to this, so you may want to start there for half the price. All ultra-matte lipsticks can be drying on the lips. **Rouge Sensation** *($18.50)* is a very greasy lipstick that is noticeably more sheer than the other formulas. Again, these are great colors (over 50 shades!) but this one could easily bleed and feather into lines and won't last. **Rouge Magnetic** *($18.50)* supposedly has a "new technology" with fewer waxy ingredients to allow for "comfortable wear." It ends up being just a good creamy, slightly glossy lipstick that doesn't hold up all that well. What it does have over other lipsticks is that it doesn't deposit as much wax on the lips. That feels great and relatively lightweight, but it also doesn't keep the color on as well. **Le Crayon** *($17.50)* is a standard automatic lip pencil with good colors and a smooth application. This may be too creamy to prevent feathering and it is definitely overpriced. **Le Lipstique** *($19)* is a standard pencil with a blending brush at the other end. That's a nice idea, but not worth the price. This does have some good staying power, leaving a slight stain on the lips, and it has a drier texture than the Le Crayon version, and that can reasonably help prevent feathering. **Lip Brio** *($20)* is just standard lip gloss in a tube. Anyone willing to shell out this kind of money for gloss would surely not be reading this book. The packaging is unique, but given you can't wear the tube, this is no different from many other glosses at a fraction of this price.

☺ **Lip Perfecting Pencil** *($15)* is a chubby pencil available in three shades. It's meant to be used as a lip primer or a color by itself. When I inquired as to why this was necessary, the makeup artist at the counter commented that she never uses it and that it's a "why bother?" type of product. My thoughts exactly. **Liplights SPF 15** *($15)* is a thick pot gloss with nine very iridescent colors and a sticky texture. The sunscreen offers no UVA protection. **$$$ Colour in Two** *($18.50)* is a two-sided chubby lip pencil that can be used as a liner or a lipstick. Both sides of the pencil have a similar shade, only one is matte and the other shiny. That's a nice option, but sharpening is difficult, and given that it requires sharpening almost every time you apply it, you'll use the product up faster than any lipstick you may buy.

☺ **$$$ MASCARA:** Here is where Lancome has a well-deserved (and enviable) reputation: its mascaras are some of the best around. There are nine to choose from, and they do get repetitive, so bear with me. **Definicils** *($19)* is Lancome's top seller, and it is easy to see why: this is an excellent lengthening mascara that builds nice thickness with minimal to no chance of clumping. **Immencils** *($19)* is a good thickening mascara, as is **Intencils** *($19)*. The latter builds extremely thick, full lashes but does have a slight tendency to clump. **Extencils** *($19)* is as good as any of the Lancome mascaras, though it won't curl your lashes as claimed. Despite my review, if you are just dying of curiosity to find out if a mascara can replace your eyelash curler, then check out Le Grand Curl *($5.99)* by L'Oreal, Lancome's owner—it has the same claims and the same formulation for far less money.

☺ **$$$ Aquacils** *($19)* is a good waterproof mascara that holds up well through tears and rain. **Eternicils** *($19)* is also waterproof and makes the claim "won't flake, fade or smudge." While that's true, it's also difficult to remove, as are all waterproof mascaras, and it's not recommended for daily use.

☺ **$$$ Forticils** *($15.50)* is still lingering here. This is a lash conditioner that is supposed to be applied before mascara. This will not condition the lashes at all but will add an extra layer, which may help, but if you need this product, it just means you bought an inferior mascara to start with. **Tendercils** *($19)* is Lancome's weakest mascara. Building any length or shred of thickness takes lots of effort and there is nothing in this formulation that makes it any better for sensitive eyes (as the name implies). **Magnificils** *($19)* can't compete with Definicils. I'm shocked to find myself saying this, but this is one Lancome mascara you can pass up. Just to be clear, it's not a bad mascara, it's just not a great mascara.

☹ $$$ <u>BRUSHES:</u> Lancome offers a decent assortment of brushes with a gorgeous feel and softness, though they are truly overpriced for what you get. While the bristles may feel great, the shapes and sizes of the brushes are not the best for most face shapes and are awkward to work with. When you're considering spending $25 and up on an eyeshadow brush, it should be perfect. For the money you would be far better off shopping at Bobbi Brown, Trish McEvoy, or Stila for brushes.

# Laura Mercier

Over the last couple of years, Laura Mercier has become a much more familiar name not only to beauty aficionados but also to the cosmetics consumer at large. If you've flipped through almost any fashion magazine recently, it is hard to overlook her handiwork in editorials or on the cover. She is a formidable makeup artist who has successfully shown us what she is capable of. What sets her makeup line apart from the rest is her trademark "flawless face." Mercier believes that perfecting the complexion is the most important step to makeup application, and her line presents some incredible options for doing just that. Much like her competitors, Mercier has continued to expand her product offerings, segueing from a soft, neutral palette to a blitz of shine and shimmer. All of these artistry lines, from Mercier's to Nars, are viewed by both the industry and consumers as the trendsetters. Each season, we look to them for guidelines on what to change, what to keep, and how to apply and wear the next new look. It all gets very tedious after a while, and I believe a far more sane option is just focusing on the products and techniques you need to enhance and work with your own beauty. As trends come and go, with each new one presenting makeup possibilities, you can choose to adopt just the ones that work best for you.

You will discover that Mercier's makeup, particularly her foundations, is in many ways a step above the rest. The tester unit is very user-friendly and the counter staffs I've come across really have their act together, merging makeup skill with an obvious affection for the line's namesake. Mercier herself regularly visits her counters for special appearances, and my guess is that sitting in her chair would be an experience you wouldn't soon forget.

In 1999, Mercier launched her skin-care line. These overpriced products are fairly standard and almost boring, without options for a range of skin types, and with no topical exfoliants, but the sunscreens are nicely formulated with avobenzone and all the products are fragrance-free. The only aspect of this group worth discussing is that all of the products include emu oil. This large bird native to New Zealand is supposed to have magic properties for the skin. Ah, the poor emu. There are no magic properties hidden in emu oil, but there are studies indicating that the pure oil is a good moisturizing ingredient that mimics the human skin's own oil production. That's nice for dry skin. There are also some animal-model studies indicating that it has some good anti-inflammatory properties, specifically concerning arthritis and skin irritation. All of that is great and there is reason to consider a *pure* form of emu oil (which is actually quite tricky to process and relatively unstable) if you have dry, irritated skin. What has not been researched in regard to emu oil is how it benefits skin in the fractional amounts like those included in skin-care products. While the oil has some nice emollient properties, so do many plant oils. Overall, the oil's anti-irritant properties are fine but probably minimal when present in the amounts used in mass-market skin-care products.

For more information about Laura Mercier, call (888)-MERCIER or visit the Web site at www.lauramercier.com.

## Laura Mercier Skin Care

☺ $$$ **One Step Cleanser** (*$35 for 8 ounces*) is an extremely standard, detergent-based water-soluble cleanser that would work as well as any for most skin types except extremely dry skin. It does contain coloring agents, but there's no apparent fragrance.

☺ $$$ **Firming Eye Cream** (*$32 for 0.5 ounce*) is a very good moisturizer for normal to dry skin but there is nothing firming about it or special for the eye area.

☺ $$$ **Mega Moisturizer Cream with SPF 15** (*$38 for 2 ounces*) is a good, avobenzone-based sunscreen for normal to dry skin. However, the price is out of line for what you get.

☺ $$$ **Moisturizer Cream with SPF 15** (*$38 for 2 ounces*) is almost identical to the version above and the same comments apply.

## Laura Mercier Makeup

**FOUNDATION:** ☺ $$$ **Oil-Free Foundation** (*$38*) is a superlative foundation for normal to slightly oily skin. The texture is very smooth and it blends out to a seamless, soft matte finish with medium coverage. There are 13 shades, with options for very light but not very dark skin tones. The only ones to consider avoiding are Shell Beige (slightly pink) and Summer Beige (slightly orange).

☺ $$$ **Moisturizing Foundation** (*$38*) would be suitable for normal to dry skin seeking medium coverage. The texture is exquisitely light and creamy, leaving a beautiful, natural finish. All six colors are excellent, although there is nothing for darker skin tones.

☺ **$$$ Foundation Stick to Go** *($35)* presents yet another twist-up stick option. Thankfully, Mercier's formula is sheer and light, with a cream-to-powder texture that meshes well with the skin instead of sitting on top of it. All five shades are superb, but there are no options for very light or dark skin tones. As you know, this type of foundation works best on normal to slightly oily skin not prone to breakouts.

☹ **$$$ Tinted Moisturizer SPF 15** *($38)* has no reliable UVA protection but is still a decently creamy, very sheer moisturizer that blends on effortlessly. Of the five shades, be careful with Almond and Tan—both can be too coppery for most skin tones.

☹ **$$$ Foundation Primer** *($27)* is a very thin, lightweight, clear gel of silicone and film former. It's supposed to contain light-reflecting ingredients that protect the skin, but it doesn't (unless you consider the emollient shine from the finish protecting). It can be a good, simple, matte-finish moisturizer for someone with slightly oily skin, but without sunscreen it can't protect from anything and the skin doesn't need protection from Mercier's foundations—or anyone else's for that matter.

☹ **$$$ CONCEALER: Secret Camouflage** *($26)* is a two-sided compact concealer with a thick, dry texture and truly opaque, camouflage coverage. All of the duos have yellow to beige or peach to copper colors that can work if they are mixed in the right proportions, but why would you want to do that (and use two separate brushes for the task, as is recommended at the Mercier counter) when there are so many excellent one-step concealers available? Secret Camouflage is meant as a cover-up for facial blemishes or birthmarks, and if all else has failed, it can be an option. SC4, 5, and 6 are too peach or copper to recommend. For the eye area, there is **Secret Concealer** *($18),* which is far more user-friendly than the Camouflage concealer. It comes in three great shades in a small pot and has a very creamy-smooth texture. It covers well but it does tend to crease on and off during the day. Give this a test run before you decide to make a purchase.

☺ **$$$ POWDER: Loose Setting Powder** *($30)* has an out-of-this-world silky texture that blends beautifully over the skin and leaves a satiny-smooth, dry finish. All of the shades are workable and have a subtle yellow undertone. Only Stardust is too shiny to recommend, although it could work for a glistening evening look. Caution: the cornstarch in here could cause irritation or breakouts for those who are sensitive to it. **Pressed Setting Powder** *($28)* has many of the same qualities as the loose powder, minus the cornstarch. The texture is smooth and dry and all of the colors are very good.

☹ **$$$ Bronzing Powder** *($28)* produces a great soft tan color but the amount of shine in here is too distracting to look natural.

**BLUSH:** ☹ **$$$ Cheek Color** *($19)* is a small group of sheer blush colors that have a smooth texture and are all slightly shiny. The shine is tolerable, but there are more than enough matte options elsewhere to consider first.

☺ $$$ **Cheek Color Stick to Go** *($25)* is a swivel-up blush stick with a creamy-soft texture and three great, sheer colors. It actually blends quite well and, though overpriced, is an option for those who prefer this type of product.

☺ $$$ **EYESHADOW: Eye Colour** *($17)* has an adequate assortment of both matte and shiny shades. The texture is slightly dry and the colors tend to go on softer than you might expect.

☹ $$$ **Creme Eye Colour to Go** *($19)* applies with a wand applicator and has a very slick texture that can make blending a challenge. All four shades are extremely shiny and have a creamy, slippery finish.

☹ $$$ **EYE AND BROW SHAPER: Eye Pencil** *($16)* and **Brow Pencil** *($16)* are both utterly standard and not worth more than a fraction of this price. Mercier apparently developed "an exact texture" for these, but there isn't a difference between these and any other pencil being sold.

☺ $$$ **LIPSTICK AND LIP PENCIL: Lip Colour** *($17)* claims it "fills in ridges and lines," which is something this fairly greasy lipstick simply cannot do. It is just a standard lipstick with an excellent range of colors and a slight stain. **Lip Shimmer and Lip Metallics** *($17)* are both slightly greasy and moderately to boldly iridescent. **Lip Sheer** *($17)* is exactly that, a sheer lip color with a glossy finish and great colors that all have a slight stain. **Lip Pencil** *($16)* is also overpriced, with a standard creamy texture and dry finish. The choices are slim, compared to the vast number of lipsticks.

☹ $$$ **Lip Gloss** *($18)* is outrageously expensive for what amounts to a standard, very sticky gloss.

☻ **MASCARA: Mascara** *($16)* is still a poorly formulated mascara that adds minimal length and tends to spike and clump the lashes no matter how you wield the wand.

☺ $$$ **BRUSHES:** Mercier has done her homework when it comes to **Brushes** *($20 to $52; $150 and $250 for half or full sets with portfolio)*. You will find that most of these are masterfully shaped and dense enough to hold and deposit color evenly on the skin. Every brush is available with a long or short handle, which is an attractive option. The best ones among this collection of either natural or synthetic hairs are the **Powder Brush** *($52)*, **Camouflage Powder** *($28)*, which is more appropriate for eyeshadows, and the **Cheek Colour Brush** *($42)*; all of the **Eyeshadow Brushes** *($24 to $29)* are worth a closer look. The rest are too small, pointed, or stiff to recommend.

# Le Mirador (Skin Care Only)

Le Mirador was created by the American owner of the Le Mirador Resort and Spa in Geneva, Switzerland. These products were supposedly the winners of the first (and, by the way, only) International Skin Care Competition. Not surprisingly, we are never given the results of that competition. Aren't you curious who else was in the running? I'd love to know who came in second or third, or even tenth place. Plus, how was the winner determined? Did a group of women end up looking 10, 20, or 30 years younger, or were there some other determining factors? And who judged those results? None of this information is available anywhere in the world—strange for a competition, don't you think? Usually contestants are part of the news. As it turns out, the competition was created, funded, and overseen by the owner of Le Mirador. There was no scientific process or protocol involved, and the winner was an arbitrary decision of the owners, not some independent, unbiased group of judges as the infomercial for these products claims. While the misinformation regarding these products is disturbing, that doesn't mean there aren't some interesting products in this line to consider. Just ignore the ad, and consider whether or not these products suit your skin type. For more information about Le Mirador, call (800) 345-1515 or visit www.iqvc.com.

☺ **Dual Action Facial Cleanser** *($19 for 6 ounces)* is a standard, detergent-based water-soluble cleanser for most skin types. It contains a small amount of AHAs, but the pH isn't low enough for them to work as an exfoliant. There are hosts of vitamins in tiny amounts, but even if they did have an effect on the skin, they would be rinsed down the drain before they had a chance. This does contain fragrant plant extracts.

☺ **Anti-Oxidant Night Cream with AHA and Pycnogenol** *($24.53 for 2 ounces)* is a very good emollient moisturizer for someone with dry skin, and it definitely contains antioxidants, including pycnogenol. That's all fine and good, but pycnogenol is no more impressive than lots of other antioxidants being used in cosmetic lotions these days. The product also doesn't contain enough AHA to have an effect as an exfoliant. One word of warning: this product contains a host of irritating plant extracts, including spearmint, clove, cinnamon, coltsfoot, sage, horsetail, dandelion, ivy, and witch hazel. While there isn't much of each in this formulation, the total has me concerned about irritations and inflammation for all skin types.

☹ **$$$ Firming Complex** *($30 for 0.9 ounce)*. While this does contain some very good water-binding agents and plant oils in a silicone base that feels soft on skin, the fragrant oils, include ylang-ylang, patchouli, anise, and peppermint, make this potentially irritating for all skin types.

☹ **$$$ Performage Age-Defying Renewal Complex** *($38 for 1.5 ounces)* does contain some very good water-binding agents and soothing plant extracts, but it also contains some fairly irritating plant extracts that can be a problem for all skin types, including lime, sandalwood, spearmint, menthol, and horsetail. It does contain a protein derived from silk, and though that sounds nice, protein has the same effect on skin—which is as a good water-binding agent and emollient—regardless of the source.

☹ **$$$ Revitalizing Eye Cream** *($22 for 0.5 ounce)* is a lightweight moisturizer.

This is a lot of money for a fairly ordinary eye product. It would be good for normal to dry skin but there are far better formulations from dozens of other than lines than this one.

☺ **Triple Action Revitalizing Moisturizer SPF 15** *($21.71 for 2 ounces)* is a good, in-part avobenzone-based moisturizer that would work well for normal to dry skin. It is fairly standard, but good; however there is nothing in here that will repair skin or provide unique moisturizing properties.

☺ **Advanced Formula Sunscreen Protection SPF 15** *($14.50 for 6 ounces)* is a very good, basic, avobenzone-based sunscreen that would work well for normal to dry skin. It does contain fragrant plant extracts. This formula isn't advanced in the least and is actually rather boring in the moisturizing part of the formulation, with minimal water-binding agents and antioxidants.

☺ **Firming Eye Mask with Honey** *($16 for 1 ounce)* won't firm anything, but it is a very good moisturizer with water-binding agents, vitamins, and thickeners. It does contain some plant extracts that can be irritating and others that can be anti-irritants so they sort of negate each other; what a waste.

☺ $$$ **Glowing Skin Facial with Milk Protein** *($15 for 3 ounces)* uses marble powder and ground-up plastic as the abrasives, which can be somewhat rough on skin, but it does the job of a scrub. The rest of the ingredients are primarily thickening agents, though they can rinse rather easily. It does contain fragrance.

## Lip Ink (Makeup Only)

☺ $$$ **Lip Ink** guarantees indelible lip color, or as close to it as you can get anywhere in the cosmetics world. It lasts 50 percent longer than any other lipstick, according to their ads. Well, hold on to your lips, because this product delivers, maybe not as well as the claims profess, but it is impressive. Despite the name, it's not ink, just a very strong, semipermanent lip stain that doesn't rub or easily wear off. Mine lasted a full day and a half—through meals, a shower, bedtime, and past the next morning—but readers of my newsletter have complained that it didn't last quite that long for them, ranging anywhere from a few hours to not much better than any other lipstick.

Lip Ink is a quick-drying liquid lip-color that feels very wet when applied, and after it dries—and you must let it dry—it feels like nothing on the lips. What is left behind are fully colored, dyed lips!

Unfortunately, Lip Ink doesn't add a drop of moisture, so if you have dry, cracked lips, using Lip Ink will give you fully colored, dyed, dry, cracked lips. To that end, the ☺ $$$ **Lip Ink Starter Kit** *($45)* includes **Lip Ink Shine**, which is just an emollient lip gloss, to keep the lips from drying out. Surprisingly, that gloss doesn't compromise the staying power of the lip color, but it will rub off on anyone you are snuggling up to! By the way, Lip Ink claims that Lip Ink Shine contains light reflectors to reduce signs of aging. Any gloss can provide a dewy, moist surface that looks smoother; they make theirs sound unique, and it isn't.

I know this all sounds great, but I have a few warnings about this product. First and foremost, it isn't that easy to use. Here are some excerpts from the instructions that come with the kit: "Always start with clean, dry lips. Then, before applying Lip Ink Color, massage a small amount of Lip Ink Shine into the lips until the shine disappears. [This isn't really necessary if your lips aren't dry, and it can make the color bleed.] Shake the vial three times against the palm of your hand before using. When open, always keep the vial vertical and remove the applicator slowly. [If you don't, it will spill or splatter and make a mess.] Apply with long, smooth strokes in one direction only, not back and forth. Allow 20 seconds between layers for drying. Keep your lips apart and do not blot or pucker your lips during this time. After each application you will feel a refreshing mint-like tingle on your lips. [It felt like burning, not tingling, to me, and caused my lips to feel swollen and irritated.] After the third layer is dry, apply a small amount of Lip Ink Shine to your lips. Once every two weeks, take a paper towel and wipe the Lip Ink applicator tip free of any oil, wax, or food particles that may have accumulated." Like I said, this product definitely takes work! And you have to be careful about applying it perfectly or your mistakes will be semipermanent.

Lip Ink also insists that you are not to combine its product with any other lipstick products because they are not compatible. I did not find that to be true in the least. If anything, I found that it helped provide a lasting base, and I could experiment with other colors over it. Of course, those colors came off, but the Lip Ink did last.

I was also disturbed by a few of Lip Ink's claims, such as its being hypoallergenic, which is a completely meaningless, unregulated term, especially given the burning sensation they warn about (but play down by calling it "tingling"). It also claims its products are "93% formulated from natural herbs and botanicals" but they aren't in the least: these products have a preponderance of synthetic ingredients and dyes, including everything from aluminum lakes (a synthetic dye) to alcohol (lots of alcohol), propylene glycol, phenoxyethanol, and on and on.

The Lip Ink Kit contains two **Lip Ink Colors** *($15 each);* one **Lip Ink Shine** *($15);* one **Lip Ink Off Vial** *($5),* for carrying a transportable version of the lip color remover; one **Lip Ink Off Refill Bottle** *($10);* and one **Purse Carrying Case** *($15).* If you're a fan of the liquid lip stains from Lip Ink (which for many people really do stay put for most of the day and part of the night), then you may be interested in Lip Ink's ☺ **Eye Liner** *($15)* and ☺ **Brow Liner** *($15).* Even with many of the same pros and cons of the Lip Ink Lip Color, Lip Ink's eye products are still fascinating. They are very waterproof and they stay and stay and stay and stay. Because your eyes are less inclined to come in contact with liquids and food, unlike your mouth, the liner and brow color could probably stay on for days. However, there are problems with the application that makes these products tricky to use. Supposedly, the Brow and Eye Liner were reformulated to be better suited for the eye area than lips, but you can't tell that from the ingredient listing. The first ingredient is alcohol, and among the extracts are peppermint and arnica, which explains why it burns and why Lip Ink includes a warning about not using this over broken skin. The other issue is the liquid, runny consistency of the product itself. You will want to practice on your hand before you consider using this on your eyes. It can be hard to get the watery finish to go on dark enough or thin enough, so it tends to spread and is hard to control. You need to wait a minute or so for it to dry, and don't blink or you can end up with liner or brow color where you don't want it. Lip Ink products do eventually wear off and can be removed with most any makeup remover. For more information on Lip Ink, call (310) 796-0595 or (800) 496-9616 or visit the Web site at www. lipink.com.

## *Lip Last (See English Ideas)*

## *Liz Earle Naturally Active Skin Care*

The name Liz Earle may not sound familiar, but her appearances on QVC are creating quite a stir, at least for those women who are writing me to ask, "Do those products work?" Every time a new infomercial airs, I get hundreds of immediate requests to review those products and to determine whether or not the products are "really worth it." You all know that it is astounding to me that women wonder who is really telling the truth about any product being advertised by the cosmetics industry, but even more so in the world of infomercials. Given the large number of celebrities or made-for-infomercial-celebrities endorsing cosmetics, that alone should give one pause. What about all the other TV lines? Is Connie Selleca (Selleca Solutions) telling the truth? What about Joan Rivers (Results)? Linda Evans (Rejuvenique)? Kathie Lee Gifford (Natural Advantage Anti-Aging System and the since defunct Mon Amie, and from 1993 the Timeless Essence Night Recovery Cream—Gifford has been very free with her endorsements)? Marilyn Miglin (her own line); Adrien Arpel (Signature Club A); Diane Young; Victoria Principal (Principal Secret); Stacey Schieffelin (Models Prefer)—need I go on? The never-ending question, "Are any of these really worth the money?" is easily answered by saying no, at least not the way the products are represented in the ads and commercials. So what about Earle's products already?

Liz Earle is a former beauty editor. From this experience, and working with a skin-care product manufacturer, she has arrived at these products bearing her name. There isn't much else to discuss except the products, which are fairly basic and, with no sunscreen, a real disgrace. So much for the notion that being a beauty editor means you know anything about skin care. If you're going to bother looking at a new group of products, you may as well switch channels now. For more information about Liz Earle, visit the Web site at www.lizearle.com or www.iqvc.com.

**Please note:** All of these products were included in a package that sells for $39 for a total of 4.6 ounces worth of product content.

☹ **Cleanse & Polish** *(1 ounce)* has a wafting smell of eucalyptus that penetrated through the box I received. That can irritate the eyes and skin. Other than that, this is more of a cold cream and can leave a slightly greasy film on the skin.

☺ **$$$ Instant Boost Skin Tonic** *(1.7 ounces)* would be a good toner for normal to dry skin, if you can get past the fragrance.

☺ **$$$ Daily Eye Repair** *(0.2 ounce)* does contain a teeny amount of AHA but not enough for exfoliating purposes. If you are looking for a vitamin E cream, this is one to consider; just remember that although it is a good antioxidant the vitamin does not repair skin. It would be a good moisturizer for normal to dry skin.

☺ **$$$ Skin Repair for Dry/Sensitive Skin** *(0.5 ounce)* is a very good moisturizer for normal to dry skin, though the fragrance makes it inappropriate for sensitive skin types.

☺ **$$$ Skin Repair for Normal/Combination Skin** *(0.5 ounce)* is almost identical to the version above and the same comments apply. This moisturizer is too emollient for combination skin types.

☹ **Smoothing Line Serum** *(0.2 ounce)* does contain a form of menthol that can be a potential skin irritant.

☹ **Brightening Treatment** *(0.5 ounce)* contains camphor; that won't brighten skin, but it can cause redness and irritation.

# *Lorac*

In an effort to make her line stand out, Carol Shaw has capitalized on the natural angle with many of her products. And while "infusions of parsley, lemon and cucumber" might sound like a veritable salad for your eyes, they have little if anything to do with the performance of a blush or an eyeshadow. The lipsticks supposedly are the first "moisture matte" on the market, but not only is this a stretch, it's untrue. A lipstick cannot be both moisturizing and matte, and Shaw's are simply a standard creamy lipstick with a good amount of stain. While there are certainly some good products to be found here (though the skin-care products are dismal, with only six options, which means women with oily skin and women with very dry skin would be using the same products), the lack of varied color options when compared to Lorac's competitors, and these include M.A.C., Bobbi Brown, Stila, Trish McEvoy, NARS, Vincent Longo, and on and on, make this a line you could easily overlook and not feel like you've missed out on looking like an "A-list star"! For more information about Lorac, call (800) 845-0705 or visit www.eve.com.

# Lorac Skin Care

☺ **Oil-Free Face Wash** *($20 for 8 ounces)* is a very basic, detergent-based water-soluble cleanser that can work for most skin types, except for someone with dry skin.

☹ **Oil-Free Makeup Remover** *($15 for 4 ounces)* is a fairly standard eye-makeup remover that will indeed take off eye makeup.

☺ **Oil Makeup Remover** *($17 for 6.5 ounces)* is just as standard detergent-based makeup remover that is as mundane as it gets. It will work as well as any.

☹ **Alcohol-Free Toner** *($18 for 4 ounces)* contains menthol, which makes it too irritating for all skin types.

☺ **Moisturizer** *($37.50 for 2 ounces)*. This remarkably ordinary and almost boring moisturizer would be good for someone with normal to dry skin, but for this money it should contain something unique or state-of-the-art.

☺ **$$$ Vitamin E Stick** *($16 for 0.15 ounce)* contains almost no vitamin E to speak of. It is just a basic, greasy, clear lipstick that contains mostly castor oil, waxes, and Vaseline. It's good for dry lips but there is nothing even vaguely unique in here.

# Lorac Makeup

**FOUNDATION:** ☹ **$$$** There are two liquid foundations in this line, the **Oil-Free Makeup** *($30)* and the **Satin Makeup** *($35)*. Both have a similar texture and offer sheer to light coverage and a soft, natural finish. What's disappointing are the colors. Of the ten shades of Oil-Free Makeup, only a handful are neutral (S1, S2) The other shades are varying degrees of orange and deep yellow. The Satin Makeup offers slightly better colors and a touch more coverage, but stay away from M6, M7, and M8, which are obviously orange.

☺ **$$$ Translucent Cream Makeup** *($35)* is a creamy compact makeup that stays moist on the skin and offers sheer to almost no coverage. For normal to dry skins, this is an option and the five shades are fairly good; only CM5 is too peach for most skin tones.

**CONCEALER:** There is one type of regular concealer, the ☹ **Coverup** *($14)*. It comes in a pot and offers great emollient coverage, but also tends to crease almost immediately and keeps on creasing. If creasing isn't a concern for you, there are a few good shades to consider, but just as many to avoid so be careful. Also available is a **$$$ Neutralizer** *($28)*, which is meant to be used on any blue or red discolorations. The color is a greenish-yellow, and ends up looking odd on skin.

**POWDER:** The ☺ **$$$ Loose Powder** *($28)* has a very dry texture, smooth finish, and some workable colors. Of the five shades, avoid P3 and P5, which are too golden orange. **Perfect Powder** *($32 with compact; $24 refill)* is a pressed powder with minimal to light coverage. It makes a big deal about being talc-free, which is strange since its other powder is mostly talc. What this does contain is mica, a shiny mineral pigment that negates the purpose of powder, which is to reduce shine. Still, all four shades are fairly neutral and offer a light finish. If shine is what you want, this is as good an option as any. **Translucent Touch Up Powder** *($32)* is a talc-based powder that has a smooth-as-silk texture and three very good colors. This provides a bit more coverage than traditional pressed powder, and blends on easily. If the price wasn't so prohibitive, it would be an excellent option.

☺ **$$$ Bronzer** *($28)* is a pressed powder bronzer with a silky feel and sheer finish, but like so many others of its ilk, it is very shiny which doesn't add up to a natural looking tan.

☺ **BLUSH:** Shaw's powder **Blush** *($14)* offers a small but very good palette of colors to choose from. Plum, Rose, Peach, and Earth are particularly great. Avoid Desire, unless the goal is extreme shimmer on your cheeks. The texture and application are beautiful. The **Lip/Cheek Tint** *($13.50)* is a pot of color that goes on somewhat greasy and then dries to a smooth, slightly dry finish. There are three shades and all are better suited for lips due to their high concentration of pigment and the difficulty in blending this type of product over skin.

☺ **$$$ EYESHADOW:** All of the **Eyeshadows** *($16)* offer a soft finish and smooth application. Compared to M.A.C., these are not nearly as pigmented, so building intensity may take some effort. However, for a softer look, there are some great matte shades and a horde of shiny shades to ignore. Like most shadows, they can be used wet or dry and several of these shades would make excellent eyeliner or brow colors.

☺ **EYE & BROW SHAPER:** There are two **Eye Pencils** *($12)*, which is, to the say least, very limited, but for pencils these are just fine. (Using powder eyeshadow is a better option.)

☺ **LIPSTICK AND LIP PENCIL:** The **$$$ Lipstick** *($17.50)* is a standard opaque lipstick with a creamy, slightly greasy feel and a shiny finish. These are not even close to being matte, but they do stick around a little longer due to the stain. There is a large, very good selection of colors. **$$$ Sheer Lipstick** *($17.50)* is the exact same formula as the other lipstick, but with less pigment. The colors are fine, but nothing exceptional. **Lip Gloss** *($15)* is a standard greasy pot gloss that is highly fragrant. It would work as well as any other gloss, and this is less sticky than most. **Lip Pencil** *($12)* is just a standard pencil with a great color selection (far more impressive than the selection of eye pencils).

☺ **$$$ MASCARA:** The mascara, **Lorac Lashes** *($17)*, goes on well and lengthens beautifully, with minimal to no clumping. It offers very little in terms of thickness, but for a natural lash look, it is an option.

☺ **BRUSHES:** Another strong point of this line is the excellent assortment of **Brushes** *($12 to $35)*. The eyeshadow brushes are very workable and nicely shaped, and the **Coverup Brush** *($23)* works well for more detailed concealer or blending jobs if this kind of brush is of interest to you. Avoid the **Powder** and **Eye Contour** brushes, both of which are floppy and hard to control.

## Lord & Berry (Makeup Only)

Along the sales aisle of your local drugstore are a handful of small cosmetics lines specializing in a modest array of inexpensive color items. Lines such as Wet 'n' Wild, Jane, Bonne Bell, and Prestige are easy to miss but worth hunting down for some exceptional products that deserve attention—not only for saving you money but also as an aid to creating beautiful makeup elegance. Lord & Berry is a line that I kept overlooking and I admit that was a mistake. While this isn't an exciting line, it does offer some excellent, inexpensive options you may wish to consider for lipsticks, lip pencils, and eyeliners. The only significant negative, and this is true for many drugstore lines, is the lack of testers for any of the products. In fact, oftentimes the actual color of the product is hidden from sight and the color swatch provided is a poor facsimile of what you actually are getting. However, at these prices, you can afford to make a mistake or two! For more information on Lord & Berry, call (201) 998-8890, ext. 2260.

☹ <u>CONCEALER:</u> **Conceal It** *($3.99)* is a thick pencil concealer with a poor texture and colors that are just too peach or pink to recommend.

☺ <u>EYESHADOW:</u> **Eyeshadow Supreme** *($3.99)* is a creamy eyeshadow in pencil form. It dries to a soft powder finish, but all of the colors are mildly to intensely shiny. Still, it can hold its own with others like it sold at much higher prices.

<u>EYE AND BROW SHAPER:</u> ☺ **Powder Liner** *($3.99)* is an eye pencil that gives a surprisingly soft, powdery finish that can be an attractive look for lining. What a shame you can't see the colors of these pencils, or test them yourself! There is a smudge tip at one end for softening the line, but some women may not want to play guessing games with the colors. **Luxury Liner** *($3.99)* is not the *Titanic* of eyeliners but is just a good automatic (no sharpening!) pencil that works well and has a much softer application than the Line 'N Shade reviewed below. **Ink Well** *($3.99)* is a basic liquid liner that goes on solid, dries with a matte finish, and doesn't chip or peel all day. **Liquid Liner** *($4.99)* is a felt-tip pen liner that is capable of creating a thin or thick line, though thinner takes a bit more patience. It dries quickly, but if you're not careful it will smudge slightly.

☹ **Smudgeproof Liner** *($3.99)* has a great, soft application. It goes on almost wet and smoothly, then dries to a solid, almost sticky finish—but that doesn't keep it from smearing.

☺ **Line 'N Shade Waterproof Eye Liner** *($3.99)* isn't any more waterproof than other pencils. In fact, this one has a fairly greasy, opaque application that goes on easily but can slide into lines if used along the lower lashes.

LIPSTICK: ☺ **Ultimate Matte Lipstick** *($3.99)* isn't what I would consider ultimate but it is a rather good lipstick in pencil form. It is supposed to be a cream-to-powder formula, but it applies like any other lipstick pencil. I would rather not have to sharpen my lipsticks, but some women undoubtedly enjoy the two-in-one benefit enough to tolerate this drawback. **Intense Lipstick** *($3.99)* is a noteworthy, opaque cream lipstick with a small but feasible color selection. This glides on and feels great, isn't greasy, and should last beyond the morning coffee break! **Satin Intense Lipstick** *($3.99)* isn't all that intense but is nevertheless an excellent cream lipstick with considerable staying power. **Sheer Lipstick** *($3.99)* is accurately described. This is just greasy, lightly tinted lip color, and is as good as any in this category. **Soft Shine Lipstick** *($3.99)* is another lipstick in pencil form, this time with all of the colors being iridescent. The formula is standard and nicely creamy, and if you're wild about chubby pencils, this would be a good place to turn. **Brilliance Lip Gloss** *($3.99)* is a standard but very emollient lip gloss that can compete with those that sell at four and five times this amount. **Kiss Proof Lip Liner** *($2.99)* has as much staying power as any lip pencil, but it conveniently twists up and has a great, smooth texture. **Waterproof Ultimate Matte Lip Liner** *($2.99)* isn't any more waterproof than any other pencil. It remains a good, standard pencil you have to sharpen.

MASCARA: ☹ **Dramateyes Thickening Mascara** *($3.99)* easily clumps, builds minimal length, and is just a poor mascara on all counts. **Dramateyes Lengthening Mascara** *($3.99)* doesn't clump as badly as the Thickening version, but it also doesn't build much length or define lashes in the least.

# *Lubriderm (Skin Care Only)*

For more information about Lubriderm, call (800) 223-0182, or visit the Web site at www.skinhelp.com.

☹ **Body Bar** *($2.79 for 4 ounces)* is a standard, detergent-based cleansing bar that contains tallow. Tallow can cause breakouts and allergic reactions, and the detergent cleansing agent can be quite drying. The bar also contains some Vaseline and mineral oil to soften the blow, but they aren't much help in the long run.

☹ **Loofa Bar** *($2.79 for 4 ounces)* is similar to the bar above, only with scrub particles, and the same review applies.

☺ **Moisturizing Lotion Normal to Dry Skin Fragrance Free** *($6.59 for 10 ounces)* is a very good, emollient (though boring) moisturizer for someone with dry skin.

☺ **Moisturizing Lotion Dry Skin Care Lotion Original Fragrance** *($6.59 for 10 ounces)* is identical to the lotion above only with fragrance, and the same review applies.

☺ **Skin Therapy Moisturizing Lotion for Normal to Dry Skin** *($6.99 for 16 ounces)* is a very good, though ordinary, moisturizer for very dry skin.

☺ **Skin Therapy Moisturizing Lotion Fragrance-Free, for Normal to Dry Skin** *($6.99 for 16 ounces)* is similar to the one above, only fragrance-free.

☺ **Advanced Therapy Gel Cream for Rough, Dry Skin** *($5.23 for 7.5 ounces)* is similar to the one above, and the same review applies.

☺ **Seriously Sensitive Lotion for Extra Sensitive Skin** *($6.59 for 10 ounces)*. Nothing about this product makes it better for someone with sensitive skin. It is a good, ordinary, emollient moisturizer for someone with dry skin.

☺ **Seriously Sensitive Lotion for Extra Sensitive Dry Skin** *($6.59 for 10 ounces)* is almost identical to the lotion above, and the same review applies.

☹ **Daily UV Lotion with Sunscreen Moisturizer & Sun Protection SPF 15** *($5.68 for 10 ounces)* doesn't contain avobenzone, titanium dioxide, or zinc oxide for UVA protection, and is not recommended.

## Lush (Skin Care Only)

Originating in Canada, and with a handful of boutiques in other parts of the world, Lush is a concept store trying to go one better than The Body Shop. Natural is a major theme here (but heavily laced with essential oils, like most of the products these "natural boutiques" feature; so if you have allergies or a sensitive nose, the fragrance will knock you over), with "cruelty-free" and "all-handmade" following it up. The unique angle you'll find is that Lush sells skin care the way your health food store may let you shop for bulk groceries. You can scoop the stuff up yourself from bins and tubs or buy prepackaged items. While all those points seem clever enough, they don't hold water.

There is no benefit to scooping cosmetics out of a bin, and besides, I would be very concerned about bacterial contamination.

The cruelty-free comment is a dubious one as well, in the same way it is for all companies—because the basic ingredients in these products have at some point all been tested on animals (which is why we know they are safe). As for natural—OK, you already knew this one—with ingredients like sodium lauryl sulfate, TEA-lauryl sulfate, propylene glycol, and lauramide DEA, these products are loaded with very unnatural stuff. Actually, what is a bit startling is finding that this company included ingredients that many "natural" companies have abandoned (or are trying to), namely, the few I just mentioned.

I feel badly that the claims this company makes are so disingenuous and artificial because the names of the products are just adorable: Sympathy for Skin, Skin Drink, Angels on Bare Skin, and Draught of Immortality are my absolute favorites. But cute names and concepts may or may not be the best for your skin, and Lush products end up having more problems than cute answers for skin.

For more information about Lush, visit the Web site at www.lushcanada.com or call (888) 733-LUSH. (**Please note:** All prices here are in Canadian dollars.)

☹ **Honey Lumps** (*$4.20 for 200 grams*), **Fizzy o'Therapy** (*$3.20 for 95 grams*), **Butterball** (*$3.20 for 95 grams*), **Bon Bain Bonnard** (*$4.94 for 200 grams*), **Tisty Tosty** (*$4.95 for 100 grams*), **Summer Blues** (*$4.20 for 200 grams*), **Slammer** (*$4.20 for 200 grams*), **Green Man** (*$4.95 for 200 grams*), **Waving not Drowning** (*$3.20 for 95 grams*), and **Double Extra Lucky** (*$4.20 for 200 grams*) are all Lush's **Bath Ballistics:** "lumps of water softening bicarbonate of soda which fizzes and releases beautiful fragrances throughout the bathroom. … Each one is created with a different combination of fragrances. … Run the bath and add a Bath Ballistic just before or after you get in." As lovely as that sounds, you would be far better off just taking good old-fashioned baking soda (a huge box isn't even $2 in Canada or in the States) and adding that to the bath. The problem with these bombs is that they are highly fragranced, and I mean *highly*, with ingredients that are a high risk for skin irritation, especially for female genitalia. One of these bombs has ginger powder and mustard, clove, and cinnamon. And you're supposed to soak in this! Unbelievable. Another has orange oil and rose oil. While that smells nice, you're better off not sitting in it. Slammer has lemon oil, and Double Extra Lucky has tangerine oil and cardamom. As I said, if you like the scent, buy the pure oil, buy a heat diffuser, light a candle, and let the aroma waft through the bathroom while you sit in an unscented, skin-healthy tub of water with just some pure baking soda or Epsom salts added to soften skin.

☹ **Floating Island** (*$6.50 for 95 grams*), **Dreamtime** (*$3.95 for 30 grams*), **Elixir** (*$3.95 for 35 grams*); **Ceridwen's Cauldron** (*$7.50 for 100 grams*); **13 Rabbit** (*$3.95 for 30 grams*); **Phoenix** (*$7.95 for 30 grams*); **Aqua Mirabilis** (*$3.95 for 50 grams*); and **Creamy Candy Bath** (*$3.95 for 50 grams*). These are Lush's **Bath Melts**, which are creamy, emollient lumps that melt in a hot bath and release their fragrant oils. The emollients are nice enough—cocoa butter and almond oil—but again, much like the Ballistics above, you would be better off with just the almond oil (you can buy that at any grocery store for $2) and skip soaking in fragrances such as sandalwood oil, lemon oil, clove oil, cinnamon, and grapefruit oil.

☹ **Crush** (*$15.50 for 250 grams*) is a bath foam that not only contains potentially skin-irritating plant oil, but also sodium lauryl sulfate, which is a potential skin irritant. It also contains sodium lauryl ether sulfate, orange peel decoction, orange juice, orange oil, lemon oil, perfume, and preservatives.

☹ **Skinny Dip** (*$15.50 for 250 grams*) is similar to the one above, and the same review applies.

☹ **Flying Saucers** (*$15.50 for 250 grams*) is similar to the two above, and the same review applies.

☹ **Bathos** *($15.50 for 250 grams)* is similar to those above, and the same review applies.

☹ **Back for Breakfast** *($15.50 for 250 grams)* is similar to those above, and the same review applies.

☹ **Gumbo Express Smoothie** *($14.95 for 250 grams)* is a bath wash containing sodium lauryl sulfate as well as soap, with plant oils and fragrance. The sesame oil and apricot oil would be fine but the sodium lauryl sulfate and fragrant oils are all skin irritants.

☹ **Scrumptious Smoothie** *($14.95 for 250 grams)* is similar to the one above only with lime and lemon oil, which makes it even more irritating for skin.

☹ **Creamed Almond & Coconut Smoothie** *($14.95 for 250 grams)* is similar to those above, and the same basic review applies.

☹ **Lush Lime Smoothie** *($14.95 for 250 grams)* is similar to those above and the same concerns apply.

☹ **Dreaming of Summer** *($15.95 for 240 grams)* is a bath oil that contains mostly almond oil, sunflower oil, grape seed oil, jojoba oil, and fragrant oils, including orange and lemongrass. The fragrant oils can all be irritants. Your skin would be better off with just the plant oils minus the fragrance.

☹ **Dust to Dust** *($8.50 for 100 grams)*, **Silky Underwear** *($8.50 for 100 grams)*, **T for Toes** *($8.50 for 100 grams)*, **Allelujah** *($8.50 for 100 grams)*, and **Olygist** *($8.50 for 100 grams)* are talc-free dusting powders that contain mostly cornstarch, clay, and magnesium carbonate. They are highly absorbent and better for the neck down than talc any day. However, these are all highly fragranced and so present the same risk problems as the fragrances in all the other Lush products.

☹ **Skin Drink for Dry Skin** *($19.50 for 55 grams)* is a moisturizer for the face. The emollients in here are great, but the rose water, fragrance, and avocado are all potential irritants that should be avoided.

☹ **Imperialis for All Skin Types** *($19.50 for 50 grams)*. The amount of emollients in this product makes it unsuitable for any skin type but dry skin, and the amount of fragrance is a problem waiting to happen.

☺ **Celestial for Sensitive Skin** *($19.50 for 50 grams)*. Finally a product in the Lush lineup with minimal fragrance! Though it still contains vanilla water and orchid extract, I imagine that it contains the least amount of all the products they sell. But while this may be the least for Lush, it isn't little enough to make this emollient moisturizer good for sensitive skin.

☹ **Angelicum for Oily Skin** *($19.50 for 50 grams)* contains a lot, and I mean a lot, of plant oils, lavender water, preservatives, fragrance, and pine oil. This is so inappropriate for oily skin! And what is the pine oil for—is someone polishing furniture with this stuff?

☺ **Spring Cleanser for All Skin Types** *($15.95 for 250 grams)* can leave a greasy film on the skin and is hardly suitable for all skin types.

☺ **Draught of Immortality for Young and Slightly Oily Skins** *($19.95 for 250 grams)* is supposed to be a moisturizer and cleanser in one, but why someone with oily skin would need that is anyone's guess. It's a wipe-off cleanser that can leave a greasy film on the skin.

☺ **Fresh Farmacy** *($7.95 for 100 grams)* is a bar cleanser with calamine powder and fragrant oils. The soap can be drying and calamine can be a skin irritant.

☺ **Angels on Bare Skin** *($8.95 for 100 grams)* is a scrub containing ground-up almonds and clay, with some fragrance. It's not bad, but it isn't as effective as plain baking soda or cornmeal (if you're are looking to scrub your face with food).

☹ **Angel Water** *($12.95 for 250 grams)* is a toner that contains fragrant water and preservatives. This serves no purpose for skin, and there are no soothing agents, anti-irritants, or water-binding agents in this product. It may be great for angels, but angels don't have to worry about their skin.

☹ **Tea Tree Water** *($12.95 for 250 grams)* contains mostly tea tree water and grapefruit. Tea tree oil can be a disinfectant, but tea tree water is too diluted to be effective, and grapefruit is just a skin irritant and has no helpful skin properties.

☹ **Eau-Roma Water** *($12.95 for 250 grams)* is a toner that contains fragrant water and preservatives. This serves no purpose for skin other than to be a potential irritant.

☹ **Sympathy for Skin** *($18.50 for 250 grams)*. The basic moisturizing formula is great, but the amount of fragrance isn't sympathy, it's more like a condolence for possible skin problems.

☹ **Trichomania** *($6.50 for 100 grams)*, **Gentle Lentil** *($6.50 for 100 grams)*, **Chamomile Lawn** *($6.50 for 100 grams)*, and **Very Berry** *($6.50 for 100 grams)* are Lush's bar-form shampoos. They use standard soap ingredients along with sodium lauryl sulfate. The bar ingredients can make hair feel thick and limp, while the soap and sodium lauryl sulfate are very drying for scalp and hair, not to mention being skin irritants.

# M.A.C.

Once the new kid on the block as a start-up cosmetics company with edge and attitude, M.A.C. is now a serious contender in the prestigious world of department-store cosmetics. In fact, M.A.C.'s rampant success clearly paved the way for every other artistry line that took the "imitation is the sincerest form of flattery" concept to dizzying new heights. But this Toronto-based company, now under the ownership of Estee Lauder, is well funded and is launching new products that keep it nicely up to date with its more elegant neighbors at the high-end cosmetics counters. And, in many respects, M.A.C. continues to set precedents that leave many other lines scrambling to catch up. The name of the company (which stands for Makeup Art Cosmetics) more often than not is quite accurate. M.A.C. claims many professional makeup artists use its products, and in my experience that is true. Most professional makeup artists prefer neutral-toned foundations and matte eyeshadows and blushes (despite the current iridescent craze), and this line has a generous offering of each. In fact, the color selection for everything from lipsticks to pencils is exceptional. Also, most of the makeup brushes are beautiful, full, and soft, as well as properly sized to fit the contours of the face and eyes. For the most part, you will find this line a pleasure to shop, and M.A.C.'s salespeople are usually well trained as makeup artists and are a pleasure to deal with. The user-friendly tester units are divided by product type, but not consistently by texture or finish. It is easy to get overwhelmed by the choices, but once you get acclimated, making sense of it all is not too difficult.

One of the clear signs that Estee Lauder is now at the helm of M.A.C. is its new selection of skin-care products (Estee Lauder did this for Jane products as well). There are no surprises here with no unusual or gimmicky ingredients or claims. The standard plant extracts are included (chamomile and cucumber) with no potentially irritating or sensitizing ones, which is great news! Of particular interest is that the moisturizers use some very good water-binding agents and plant oils, which make the products particularly good for dry skin. What is a real drawback is the lack of any treatment products such as a skin lightening product, AHA, or topical disinfectant for breakouts. But most likely these are only the new launch products with lots more on the way.

A stand-up-and-notice feature of the M.A.C. line is its recycling program. If you bring in six empty M.A.C. plastic packages (no glass, pencils, or brushes), you will get a free lipstick of your choice. This is a great marketing strategy that's good for the company, the consumer, and the environment! For more information about M.A.C., call (800) 387-6707 or visit the Web site at www.maccosmetics.com.

## M.A.C. Skin Care

☺ **Cold Cream Cleanser** *($15 for 4 ounces)* is an accurate name for this standard, wipe-off cleanser that can leave a greasy film on the skin. It can be an option for dry skin though Neutrogena's Extra Gentle Cleanser ($6.06 for 6.7 ounces) is virutally identical for far less. It does contain fragrance.

☺ **Everyday Lotion Cleanser** *($15 for 5 ounces)* is virtually identically to Neutrogena's Extra Gentle Cleanser ($6.06 for 6.7 ounces). Both are indeed gentle, and both don't remove makeup very well and can leave a slightly greasy film on the skin, but can be an option for someone with dry skin. You did notice that the Neutrogena one is less than half the price, right?

☺ **Green Gel Cleanser** *($15 for 5 ounces)* is a standard detergent-based water-soluble cleanser that can be an option for someone with normal to oily skin, though the third ingredient is TEA-lauryl sulfate, which can be an irritant for some skin types. It does contain fragrance.

☺ **$$$ Wipes** *($12.50 for 45 sheets)* is basically silicone with some thickening agents soaked on disposable sheets. It will wipe off makeup, but for the money, this isn't all that different or more effective than baby wipes, which you can get fragrance-free, unlike this version that contains fragrance.

☺ **$$$ Scrub Mask** *($16.50 for 3.6 ounces)*. This very standard clay mask is an option for exfoliating but the menthol in here is an unnecessary, risky skin irritant.

☺ **EZR Day/Night Emulsion** *($28 for 1 ounce)*. The interesting ingredients are so far at the end of the ingredient listing as to be barely detectable. And what is a sunscreen agent doing in a product meant to be worn at night? There is more sunscreen in here than any of the water-binding agents or antioxidants. This isn't a bad moisturizer, just not as impressive as many, many others.

☺ **$$$ Fast Response Eye Cream** *($25 for 0.5 ounce)* is a silicone-based moisturizer rather similar to another Estee Lauder product from Clinique called Stop Signs ($32.50 for 1 ounce), which ends up being cheaper than this version. This is a good moisturizer for dry skin. Caffeine's tannin content constricts skin, and that can make it look temporarily smoother, though it can also cause irritation; it does not in any way make eyes look more awake.

☺ **Oil Control Lotion** *($22 for 1.7 ounces)*. The salicylic acid in here cannot control oil, nor can any other ingredient in here. This is just a good BHA product with some good water-binding agents for normal to dry skin that can also help exfoliate skin.

☺ **Studio Moisture Fix** *($22 for 1.7 ounces)* is a very good moisturizer for dry skin.

☺ **Strobe Cream** *($25 for 1.7 ounces)* is a good, though not particularly exciting, moisturizer for dry skin. The plant extracts in here are decent anti-irritants, there just isn't much in here and the same is true for the vitamins. The AHA is less than 2%, which makes it ineffective for exfoliating.

# M.A.C. Makeup

**FOUNDATION:** M.A.C.'s foundations are divided into five color groups, and, according to the company, this is how they break down: The N's have a pink/beige undertone, the C's have a golden yellow to olive undertone, the NC's are olive with pink undertones, the W's are the ones that have the most pink (but many of them are neutral), and the NW's are warmer colors with a pink/beige undertone. In spite of M.A.C.'s attempt to categorize its vast selection of shades, the colors mostly fall on the neutral side, with only minor differences between the groups. It's best to just try to zero in on finding your color and not take the labeling system so seriously, and there are options for almost every skin tone.

☹ **Hyper Real Foundation** *($24)* is supposed to create "synthetic skin texture" by manipulating light rays to beautifully reflect light off the face. Let's get real here: this is a sheer, neutral-colored range of eight foundation shades with a good deal of iridescent pink shine. Yes, a pink, sparkly undertone that shows clearly through the foundation. Perhaps M.A.C. thought plain iridescence would convince women there was a great light manipulation occurring? There are also additional shades of pale, shiny Violet, Green, Gold, and Bronze that are adept at creating a soft shimmer effect wherever you put them.

☺ **Studio Finish Satin Foundation SPF 8** *($19.50)* does not provide UVA protection and the sunscreen level would be too low even if it did. This is still an excellent fluid foundation for normal to dry skin. It leaves a moist, satin finish and provides sheer to light coverage. The 23 shades nicely represent most skin tones, although very dark skins may still have some challenges. These shades are too pink, peach, copper, or ash for most skin tones: NC45, NW20, NW25, NW35, NW45, NW50, W15, W30, and W60.

☺ **Studio Finish Matte Foundation SPF 8** *($19.50)* does not provide UVA protection and the sunscreen level would be too low even if it did. It comes in a long tube that makes controlling the amount you use a bit tricky. The feel is a great, smooth texture with lots of slip, and it dries to a minimal matte finish that is similar to the Satin foundation above. The 24 shades are quite wonderful, providing light to medium coverage, but these colors should be tested with caution: NW25, NW30, NW40, NW45, NC50, NC60, and W30.

☺ **EPT Day Emulsion** *($24)* is a very light-textured, sheer foundation that leaves a soft, minimal matte finish. In terms of coverage, this is more akin to a tinted moisturizer than foundation, and would be a suitable option for normal to slightly dry or slightly oily skins. Of the 12 shades, the lighter colors are beautifully neutral, but the medium to darker colors are too pink, peach, rose, or ash for most skin tones. Avoid N5, N6, N7, and C5.

☺ **StudioFix Powder Plus Foundation** *($21)* has an exceptionally silky texture that applies and blends like a dream. This can be used wet or dry, though wet application runs the risk of streaking, as is true with any powder foundation. Dry application provides light to medium-full coverage. Most all of the more than 24 colors are impressive for a broad range of skin tones, but these shades are best avoided by most skin tones: C50, NW25, NW30, NC50, W15 (almost pure white), W25, W40, and C6.

☺ **Matte Creme Matifiance** *($16.50)* competes nicely with and is more reasonably priced than Prescriptives' Invisible Line Smoother *($35)*. It's a thick liquid that has a matte-cream texture reminiscent of a soft spackle. It can definitely give the appearance of a smoother skin, but the effect is temporary, lasting only a few hours depending on what you wear over it and how much you move your face. Still, it's worth a test run to see if it works for you.

☺ **CONCEALER:** **Concealer SPF 15** *($11.50)* comes in a pot and goes on rather heavy and thick, but provides excellent coverage and stays on all day without much slippage. For those who prefer a more sheer application, M.A.C. recommends mixing this with a bit of foundation or moisturizer to soften the effect. The SPF is pure titanium dioxide, and that's great.

**POWDER:** ☺ $$$ **Studio Finish Face Powder** *($17)* is a very soft, talc-based powder that comes in a tub (the additional shaker-bottle has been discontinued, thankfully) and has an excellent texture and finish. The 20 shades present almost too many options, and there are some red-, rose-, and orange-toned powders to check carefully to ensure a match. Also, the deeper colors tend to "grab" on the skin, which makes a mismatch that much more obvious. $$$ **Pressed Powder Compact** *($18.50)* also has talc-based powder, with a silky-smooth texture and a sheer finish. There are 18 shades to consider, and only these colors are too rose, peach, or ash for most skin tones: NC45, NW35, NW45, and W60. **Blot Powder** *($14.50)* comes in only three colors (all fine), has a drier texture than the one above, and gives a translucent finish.

☺ **Bronzing Powder** *($15)* comes in pressed form, and the three great tan shades are marred by lots of shine. If you prefer an iridescent, sun-kissed look, these are perfect.

☹ $$$ **Iridescent Powder** *($18)* comes in a tub and is exactly named. There are two shades, one pale white and the other a bronze/gold, and both do well in terms of providing high shine.

**BLUSH:** ☺ **Powder Blush** $$$ *($16)* is a fairly standard powder blush that comes packaged in see-through containers with a new stay-on flip top (Estee Lauder did away with the classic M.A.C. two-piece screw-on top). These are a bit on the dry, grainy side but the impressive range of colors goes on true and lasts well. **Cream Color Base** *($14)* is just a very nice cream-based range of colors that can be used on the eyes, cheeks or lips. The color range presents options largely in favor of cheeks or eyes, and these tend to work best as a basic cream blush. Used as eyeshadow, the effect can be intriguing but it's also short-lived, as these tend to readily fade and crease on the eyelids. There are extremely shiny, intense shades as well as soft, minimally shiny colors to choose from.

☹ **Paints** *($15)* are tiny metal roll-up tubes that dispense a thick but light textured cream that lays on intense shine. These can be used alone or mixed with other products, but the heavy shine harks back to the disco glory days of Studio 54!

☺ **EYESHADOWS:** The **Eye Shadows** *($12 small; $14 large)* have a large neutral matte selection and are, for the most part, a pleasure to work with. Be aware that

The Reviews M

many of the colors go on darker or stronger than you might think, which can make achieving a softly blended look a bit tricky. For those with a yen for experimentation, you'll find a plethora of bold colors to play with, most with lots and lots of shine. As a whole, the color range nicely accommodates all skin tones.

☺ <u>EYE AND BROW SHAPER:</u> The **Eye Pencils** *($11.50)* and **Brow Pencils** *($12)* are utterly standard and comparable to most every other pencil out there. For lining the eyes, M.A.C.'s eyeshadows are more than up to the task. **Creme Liner** *($11)* is an ultra-dramatic liner that comes in a pot. It is best used with a damp brush, and once it sets, it stays on quite well. There are basic colors and more than a few metallic or iridescent shades for your consideration. **Liquid Liner** *($15)* is fairly standard and straightforward, applying nicely with a decent brush and drying quickly without flaking or smearing. **Brow Set** *($11)* is just a basic brow gel that can double as a clear mascara. It's not too sticky and works well for either purpose.

☺ <u>LIPSTICK AND LIP PENCIL:</u> M.A.C.'s **Lipsticks** *($13.50)* are mostly excellent, and the range of colors is remarkable. The **Mattes** are true mattes, and are wonderful for a rich, opaque look that does not bleed, though this can feel drying for those not used to a matte lipstick. The **Satins** are great and nicely creamy without being too thick. The finish is creamy—opaque without being too greasy or glossy. The **Sheers** and **Tones** both go on softly and provide a hint of heightened color; the Sheers are noticeably more glossy than the Tones. The **Glazes** are nearly identical to the Sheers, only with iridescence, and the **Frosts** are identical to the Satin lipsticks, except they're frosted. **LipGlass** *($10)* is very thick, tenacious gloss whose heavy texture is not for everyone. For a slightly lighter option, there's **LipGlass (coloured)** *($11.50),* which comes in a range of soft or vivid hues and is easy to work with using the wand applicator. It's still heavier in texture than many other glosses, which may or may not be your preference. **Lip Pencils** *($11)* have a superior color selection; that's the only thing that separates these standard pencils from the ones found in almost every other line.

☺ <u>MASCARA:</u> **Mascara S** *($12)* and **Mascara N** *($12)* are almost indistinguishable. Both build similar decent length and thickness without clumping, though they have a slight tendency to smear as the day goes by. **Mascara X** *($12)* is billed as M.A.C.'s most dramatic mascara, and it does provide more oomph than the other two, yet it's just average in the lengthening and thickening departments and takes some effort to get the best results. It's an option.

☺ $$$ <u>BRUSHES:</u> As stated in earlier editions of this book, M.A.C. has one of the best selections of brushes you'll find anywhere *(28 different brushes, ranging from $5 to $62.50).* The big brushes are a little pricey, but they last forever if you take care of them. Though there are indeed good, inexpensive brushes to be found, if you're going to splurge, this is one area where the extra expense won't be wasted. Be sure to check out M.A.C.'s variety of eyeshadow brushes, particularly the #275 **Medium Angled Shading Brush** (formerly #142), an excellent, versatile eyeshadow brush. The only brushes to really avoid are the #201 Sponge Tip Brush, which comes free in most eyeshadow kits, the #204 Lash Brush, easily duplicated by washing off an old mascara wand, and the #207 Duster, a fantail brush that I'm sure has some function but is truly not imperative for daily makeup application.

# *M.A.C. Professional Studio Makeup*

Aside from the familiar line of makeup products M.A.C. has at department stores across the country, M.A.C. also has several free-standing boutique cosmetic stores in a handful of cities in Canada and the United States that carry everything found at the department-store M.A.C. counters and a few extras that are interesting to check out. For a full exposure to everything M.A.C. has to offer, these stores are definitely worth a visit.

☺ **$$$ Face and Body Foundation** *($28.50)* comes in a 4-ounce bottle and is very liquidy and sheer. It takes some patience to blend this on, as it tends to slide around a lot before drying. This can be layered for more coverage (as can most foundations) and is reasonably waterproof. For body makeup it can be a problem, as it can come off onto clothes and is not a great choice for anything that may need to be fully concealed. There are 18 shades, and most are neutral and workable. The deeper shades can be sketchy; most of them have a slight peach to red cast that won't work for many skin tones.

☺ **Sheer Coverage Foundation SPF 15** *($19)* is a compact foundation with a creamy, emollient texture. It does not dry to a powder finish but, rather, stays moist on the skin and is best for normal to very dry skin seeking sheer to medium coverage. The SPF is all titanium dioxide, and the range of 29 shades is one of the largest selections of foundations you will find. These colors are too pink, peach, orange, red, copper, or ash for most skin tones: NC55, NC65, NW30, NW40, NW50, W10, W40, W45, C35, C50, and C70.

☺ **Full Coverage Foundation SPF 15** *($23)* is virtually identical to M.A.C.'s main line Concealer, only you get more of it in this packaging. The SPF is all titanium dioxide, so sun protection is not an issue. The question is whether or not this type of heavy-duty, opaque coverage is necessary for the entire face. The formula is wax- and oil-based, an automatic drawback for anyone prone to breakouts. The application can be manipulated to look somewhat natural, but will still feel heavy and creamy. For a concealer, it works quite well and the range of 33 shades is extensive to say the least. There are colors for very light to very dark skins, but the following shades are too pink, peach, orange, red, copper, or ash for most skin tones: NC15, NC45, NC50, NW30, NW35, NW45, NW50, W10, W30, W40, W45, and C50.

☺ **$$$ Face Powder** *($22)* is identical to the Studio Finish Loose Powder, except this is a much larger amount of product with a smaller color selection. The same comments as above apply.

☺ **$$$ Pigment** *($18)* are small jars of very shiny loose powder, available in almost every color imaginable. However, there is little benefit in using this product over similar versions from Revlon StreetWear and L'Oreal for a third the price.

☺ **Tint** *($10)* is a collection of liquid color-correctors and highlighters (gold, white, bronze) that can be used alone for a soft shine or mixed into a foundation or with any other color product. The color-correcting tints only place a noticeable layer on the skin that looks strange, and the rest are merely another way to incorporate shine into your makeup routine.

☺ **Glitter** *($10)* are small jars of loose glitter particles that represent a messy, extreme method of shining yourself up.

☺ **Lipmix** *($9.50 per tube; $18 for compact)* is a collection of mostly iridescent, intensely pigmented colors that can be used alone or mixed with an existing lipstick to customize a shade. It's an intriguing option, and I wish there were more practical shades to experiment with, but as it stands now, many of the colors are odd and easily passed up in favor of M.A.C.'s brilliant assortment of lipsticks. Caution: these products can stain, and it takes some effort to remove them from skin and lips; on the plus side, that can be construed as a benefit for the lips!

## Marcelle (Canada Only)

This reasonably priced drugstore line has some very good products that perform well and look great. The packaging is simple, and some of the products are fragrance-free, which is a definite strong point. However, while many of the products don't include fragrance, lots do. Ingredients like lavender are more recognizable as fragrant additives, but there are others you won't recognize, such as floralozone and hedione. The claim that these products are hypoallergenic isn't accurate in the least. There is no way any company can know what your skin may be allergic to, and fragrance is not the only culprit that can cause allergic reactions. Many of these products contain ingredients that have a rather high potential for irritation or a sensitizing reaction, or can cause breakouts, such as witch hazel, several sunscreen ingredients, plant extracts, menthol, alcohol, a form of tallow, sodium lauryl sulfate, and isopropyl myristate.

Sad to say, the makeup pales in comparison to the skin care. The foundations have an incredibly poor color selection, the eyeshadows all have some amount of shine, many of the blushes do too, and the pressed powders are fairly peach or pink. However, the lipsticks and pencils are worth investigating. For more information call (800) 387-7710, ext. 355. **Note:** All prices listed for Marcelle products are in Canadian dollars.

# Marcelle Skin Care

☹ **Aquarelle Aqua-Pure Cleansing Bar Oil-Free** *($5.38 for 125 grams)* is a standard bar soap that can be quite drying for almost all skin types. It contains tallow, which can cause breakouts, and menthol, which can cause irritation.

☹ **Hydractive Hydra-Pure Cleansing Bar for Dehydrated/Normal to Dry Skin** *($6.38 for 125 grams)* is similar to the Cleansing Bar above and the same comments apply, though this version does not contain menthol.

☹ **Soap** *($3.75 for 100 grams)* is similar to the Cleansing Bar above and the same review applies, though this version does not contain menthol.

☺ **Aquarelle Oil-Free Purifying Cleansing Gel for Oily Skin** *($11.95 for 170 ml)* is a good, standard detergent cleanser for most skin types. It won't purify anything, but it can clean the skin without irritation or dryness, and it won't irritate the eyes.

☺ **Cleansing Cream** *($7.98 for 240 ml)* is a mineral oil–based detergent cleanser that can leave a greasy film on the skin, though it can be an option for someone with dry skin. Calling this product hypoallergenic is stretching the facts; it contains sodium lauryl sulfate, an ingredient well known for being a skin sensitizer. There isn't much of it in this product, but using that ingredient at all is suspect in a cleanser that claims to be hypoallergenic.

☺ **Cleansing Milk for Dry to Normal Skin** *($11.25 for 240 ml)* is similar to the Cream version above only in lotion form. The same basic comments apply.

☺ **Cleansing Milk Combination Skin** *($11.25 for 240 ml)* is a standard, detergent-based water-soluble cleanser. It contains a tiny amount of lactic acid that probably isn't enough to be a problem for the skin or eyes, but there are several waxes in here that could clog pores, which would make it a problem for combination skin. This can still work well for normal to dry skin.

☺ **Cleansing Milk Oily Skin** *($11.25 for 240 ml)* is similar to the Combination Skin version above and the same comments apply.

☺ **Gentle Foaming Wash All Skin Types** *($10.50 for 170 ml)* isn't all that gentle, but it is a good, standard, detergent-based water-soluble cleanser that can be drying for most skin types. It does contain a small amount of sodium lauryl sulfate, but not enough to be a problem for most skin types.

☺ **Hydractive Water Rinseable Cleansing Lotion for Dehydrated/Normal to Dry Skin** *($11.95 for 180 ml)* is a wipe-off cleanser that isn't all that rinseable, and it isn't very good at removing makeup either. It could be an option for someone with dry skin.

☹ **2 in 1 Face and Eye Cleanser** *($11.25 for 170 ml)* is a wipe-off eye-makeup remover that is minimally effective at removing makeup. It does contain some plant extracts of which some are potential anti-irritants while others are potential irritants.

☺ **Creamy Eye Make-Up Remover** *($6.99 for 50 ml)* is basically just mineral oil, some thickeners and slip agents, and Vaseline. It will wipe off makeup and leave a greasy film on the skin, but this isn't much different from the mineral oil–based face cleansers above.

☺ **Gentle Eye Make-up Remover—Sensitive Eyes** *($9.98 for 120 ml)* is a good, standard makeup remover that can leave a greasy film behind on the skin but it does work as well as any.

☺ **Eye Make-Up Remover Pads** *($8.50 for 60 pads)* are mineral oil–soaked pads. This is a way to get waterproof makeup off, but it is only minimally different from buying a bottle of mineral oil and using some cotton pads.

☺ **Eye Make-Up Remover Lotion Oil-Free** *($8.50 for 120 ml)* works as well as any makeup remover does.

☹ **Scrub Wash for All Skin Types** *($10.95 for 100 ml)* is a clay cleanser that also contains witch hazel, alcohol, and menthol, and that makes it too potentially irritating for all skin types.

☹ **Aquarelle Oil Normalizing Toner Alcohol-Free for Oily Skin** *($9.98 for 240 ml)*. Technically, it is alcohol-free, but the witch hazel contains a good amount of alcohol and is potentially a skin irritant.

☺ **Hydractive Reviving Toner, Dehydrated and Normal to Dry Skin** *($11.25 for 180 ml)* would be a very good nonirritating toner for most skin types.

☹ **Skin Freshener, Combination Skin** *($10.95 for 240 ml)* is mostly just alcohol and glycerin along with a small amount of menthol, and that makes it potentially too irritating and drying for any skin type.

☹ **Skin Freshener, Normal to Dry Skin** *($10.95 for 240 ml)* is similar to the product above, and the same review applies. This product also contains aluminum chlorohydrate, a key ingredient in underarm deodorant, which can cause breakouts and allergic reactions.

☹ **Skin Toner, Combination Skin** *($10.95 for 240 ml)* is similar to the Skin Freshener for Combination Skin above, and the same review applies.

☹ **Skin Toner for Oily Skin** *($8.98 for 240 ml)* is similar to the Skin Freshener for Combination Skin above, only it contains even more alcohol and the same review applies.

☺ **Alpha-Radiance Cream Normal to Dry and Sensitive Skin** *($15.95 for 60 ml)* doesn't contain more than 3% AHAs, and that isn't enough to make it effective as an exfoliant. Other than that it is just a fairly ordinary moisturizer for normal to dry skin. The fragrance in here is definitely not appropriate for sensitive skin.

☺ **Alpha-Radiance Lotion, Combination to Oily and Sensitive Skin** *($15.95 for 120 ml)* is almost identical to the Normal to Dry version above and the same comments apply.

☺ **Aquarelle Aqua-Matte Hydrating Fluid** *($14.95 for 120 ml)* contains farnesol and farnesyl acetate rather high up on the ingredient listings. These are components of plants and used in cosmetics primarily for fragrance. There is research demonstrating farnesol's effect in reducing pancreatic cancer in mice, but there is no evidence that this translates to a positive effect on skin. This can be an option for normal to slightly dry skin, but it doesn't feel all that matte on skin and won't hold back oil in any way.

☺ **Hydractive Eye Contour Gel** *($11.95 for 15 ml)* is a good lightweight moisturizer for normal to slightly dry skin. There is nothing in here that is unique for the eye area.

☺ **Hydractive Hydra-Repair Night Treatment for All Skin Types** *($17.95 for 60 ml)* is a good emollient moisturizer for someone with dry skin, but there is nothing in here that will repair skin.

☹ **Hydractive Hydra-Replenishing Cream** *($15.75 for 40 ml)* is a very ordinary, boring moisturizer for dry skin. The Night Treatment above is a far better and more interesting formulation for dry skin.

☹ **Moisture Cream** *($12.98 for 60 ml)* is an exceptionally mundane moisturizer for dry skin. The tiny amount of lactic acid (AHA) in here is not enough to have exfoliating properties.

☹ **Moisture Lotion** *($14.75 for 120 ml)* is similar to the Moisture Cream version above and the same basic comments apply.

☹ **Night Cream** *($10.75 for 40 ml)* is almost identical to the Moisture Lotion above, and the same basic review applies.

☺ **Eye Care Cream, Ultra-Light** *($7.68 for 15 ml)* is a good moisturizer for someone with normal to dry skin.

☹ **Eye Cream Ultra Rich** *($8.75 for 15 ml )* is about as close to Vaseline as you can get, which makes it greasy and good for very dry skin but not worth using over just plain Vaseline.

☹ **Dry Skin Lubricating Cream** *($9.95 for 120 ml)* is almost identical to the Eye Cream Ultra above and the same comments apply.

☺ **Moisture Cream Eye with Gingko Biloba SPF 15** *($12.50 for 15 ml)* contains titanium dioxide and zinc oxide as the sunscreen ingredients, which makes this a great sunscreen. Other than that, the base is incredibly ordinary and there is nothing in here that makes this preferred for the eye area; in fact, there are several ingredients that would be problematic. The tiny amount of *Gingko biloba* in here is a mere dusting and has no impact on skin.

☺ **Anti-Wrinkle Cream with Collagen & Elastin** *($15.25 for 40 ml)* is a good emollient moisturizer for normal to dry skin. The collagen and elastin in here are good moisturizing ingredients but they have absolutely no effect on the collagen and elastin in your skin.

☹ **Multi-Defense Cream Daily Moisturizer SPF 15** *($15.25 for 60 ml)* doesn't contain the UVA-protecting ingredients avobenzone, zinc oxide, or titanium dioxide among the active ingredients, and is not recommended.

☹ **Oil-Free Multi-Defense Lotion Daily Moisturizer SPF 15** *($13.48 for 120 ml)* doesn't contain the UVA-protecting ingredients avobenzone, zinc oxide, or titanium dioxide among the active ingredients, and is not recommended.

☺ **Clay Mask** *($10.95 for 100 ml)* is a standard clay mask, but the witch hazel can be a skin irritant.

☺ **Gentle Purifying Mask** *($10.95 for 50 ml)* is a standard clay mask that also contains some plant oil and water-binding agents to help reduce the drying effect of the clay. This can be good for someone with normal to dry skin. The plant extracts in here are a mixed bag, with some being anti-irritants (matricaria) and others being irritants (sage).

☺ **Time Release Hydrating Mask** *($10.95 for 50 ml)* is a clay mask with several water-binding agents, thickeners, and preservatives. This includes a tiny amount of fruit extracts, and although they sound like they are AHAs, they are not. This product also contains menthol, which can be a skin irritant, and that's too bad, because the moisturizing ingredients here are good ones.

☺ **Protective Block No Chemical Sunscreen Cream SPF 25** *($12.95 for 50 ml)* is an excellent sunscreen that contains both titanium dioxide and zinc oxide as the active ingredients in a very standard moisturizing base that would be OK for someone with normal to slightly dry skin.

☺ **Protective Block No Chemical Sunscreen Lotion SPF 25** *($12.95 for 120 ml)* is almost identical to the Cream SPF 25 version above and the same comments apply.

☺ **Protective Block No Chemical Sunscreen Spray SPF 15** *($12.95 for 120 ml)* is similar to the Lotion SPF 25 version above and the same comments apply.

☹ **Sun Block Cream, SPF 15** *($6.78 for 90 ml)* doesn't contain the UVA-protecting ingredients avobenzone, zinc oxide, or titanium dioxide among the active ingredients, and is not recommended.

☹ **Sun Block Cream, SPF 20** *($7.95 for 90 ml)* doesn't contain the UVA-protecting ingredients avobenzone, zinc oxide, or titanium dioxide among the active ingredients, and is not recommended.

☹ **Sun Block Lotion SPF 15** *($6.78 for 120 ml)* doesn't contain the UVA-protecting ingredients avobenzone, zinc oxide, or titanium dioxide among the active ingredients, and is not recommended.

☹ **Sunblock Lotion, SPF 20** *($7.95 for 120 ml)* doesn't contain the UVA-protecting ingredients avobenzone, zinc oxide, or titanium dioxide among the active ingredients, and is not recommended.

☺ **Self-Tanning Lotion with Alpha-Hydroxy Acid Moisturizing Formula for**

Face *($11.25 for 50 ml)* is a standard, dihydroxyacetone-based self tanner that would work as well as any. It contains about 2% to 3% AHA, which isn't enough for it to be effective as an exfoliant, plus the pH is too high for that purpose as well.

☺ **Self-Tanning Spray with Erythrulose** *($13.95 for 120 ml)* uses erythrulose, which is chemically similar to the self-tanning agent dihydroxyacetone used in most self tanners. Depending on your skin color, there can be a difference in the color erythrulose produces. However, dihydroxyacetone completely changes the color of skin within two to six hours, while erythrulose needs about two to three days for the skin to show a color change.

☺ **After Sun Lotion, All Skin Types** *($8.50 for 120 ml)* is a good, extremely mundane moisturizer for dry skin.

☹ **Sheer Tint Moisturizer SPF 15** *($11.95 for 120 ml)* doesn't contain the UVA-protecting ingredients avobenzone, zinc oxide, or titanium dioxide among the active ingredients, and is not recommended.

## Marcelle Makeup

<u>FOUNDATION:</u> ☹ **Aquarelle Oil-Free Makeup** *($9.50)* is very similar to Clinique's discontinued Pore Minimizer Makeup, in that it is mostly alcohol, water, talc, and pigment. The consistency makes application difficult, the four colors are embarrassingly poor, and the alcohol is drying and irritating for all skin types. **Moisture Rich Foundation for Dry/Normal Skin** *($9.50)* would be a good foundation for the stated skin type if the colors weren't so pink and peach. **Matte Finish Oil-Free Foundation** *($9.50)* has a suitably matte finish but, once again, the available colors disappoint. **Sheer Tint Moisturizer SPF 15** *($11.95)* comes without reliable UVA protection and of the three shades, only Creme Beige resembles any known skin tone.

☺ **True Radiance Oil-Free Liquid Makeup SPF 15** *($9.95)* is also without UVA protection but does have an even, light texture that blends well and provides light to medium coverage. There are six shades to consider and they are best for light to medium skin tones. Avoid Tan Beige and Golden Beige, both are too rose for most skin tones.

☺ **Dual Cream Powder Makeup** *($11.95)* is briefly creamy but dries very quickly to a sheer matte finish. Don't count on this for much shine control, but it will go further than most cream-to-powders do for oily skins. This is still best for normal skins, and of the six shades the only one to avoid is Soft Beige.

☺ **Satin Glow Face and Body Shimmer** *($9.25)* is just a shimmery golden bronzer that is one more product to consider if you're keen on gleaming up.

☹ <u>CONCEALER:</u> **Cover Up Stick** *($7.75)* is a standard, lipstick-style concealer with three terrible colors that I cannot recommend for any skin tone. **Concealer Crayon** *($7.75)* is a fat pencil that comes in three OK shades: Light, Beige Cameo, and Dark (which isn't all that dark). The texture is workable, but be prepared to deal with creasing if you have any lines around the eye area.

☹ <u>POWDER:</u> **Pressed Powder** *($9.95)*, **Face Powder Loose** *($9.95)*, and **Silky Finish Powder** *($8.75)* are almost all too pink or peach to recommend. The only passable shade for each is Translucent. **Pressed Bronzing Powder** *($9.95)* comes in only two shades, and both are too peach or red for most skin tones.

☺ <u>BLUSH:</u> **Velvety Powder Blush** *($7.25)* has a very soft, smooth finish and there are some matte options to consider, but the application is too sheer and light for darker skin tones. **Cream Blusher** *($9.25)* is a standard cream blush whose texture is assuredly creamy and leaves a dewy finish on the skin. If you have normal to dry skin and the knack for blending these on right, you'll find some good color choices here, but watch out for the iridescent ones.

☺ <u>EYESHADOW:</u> **Eyeshadow Singles** *($6.25)* now have a handful of matte options along with an assembly of shiny colors to embrace or ignore, depending on your tastes. Both types apply softly and evenly, and neutral colors outweigh the vivid hues.

<u>EYE AND BROW SHAPER:</u> ☺ **Kohl Eye Liner** *($7.25)* is similar to many other pencils on the market, though this one has a slightly drier texture than most. **Waterproof Eyeliner** *($7.25)* is a standard eye pencil that goes on creamy and soft; it does stay on well when wet, but so do most eye pencils. **Accent Eyebrow Crayon** *($7.25)* is a standard brow pencil with a great, smooth application, good colors, and a dry finish. There is a brush on one end to soften the color, and if you prefer brow pencil to powder, this is one to try.

☹ **Powder Eye Liner** *($7.25)* is not all that powdery; it's really just a pencil that goes on somewhat choppy and then tends to roll off.

☺ <u>LIPSTICK AND LIP PENCIL:</u> Marcelle has a good but limited selection of lipsticks. **Hydra Rouge Lipstick** *($7.95)* has a smooth texture, applies evenly, and leaves a slightly glossy finish. **Rouge Impeccable Lip Color** *($7.25)* has a great, creamy, soft-matte application. **Sheer Lip Color** *($7.25)* is exactly that, with a small color selection and standard glossy finish. **Lipsheen Liquid Lip Gloss** *($8.25)* is tube lip gloss that has a pleasant texture and works as well as any other gloss. **Lip Definition Crayon** *($5.75)* is a standard pencil with a nice range of colors. **Waterproof Lip Definition Pencil** *($4.49)* is almost identical to the one above and is as waterproof as any standard pencil can be.

<u>MASCARA:</u> ☹ **Superlash Mascara** *($9.25)* won't take your lashes up, up, and away and in fact it takes a long time to build even slight definition. For a lightweight lash look, it's fine. **Ultimate Lash Mascara** *($9.25)* does build length and thickness but also tends to clump and makes lashes look stiff and unnatural. **WaveLength Waterproof Mascara** *($9.49)* goes on a bit too thick and heavy, sticking the lashes together in the process. It can easily smear while applying but once dry it is extremely waterproof.

☺ **Lash Extreme Lengthening Mascara** *($6.49)* takes some effort to do very little. It doesn't clump or smear but there is nothing extreme about its performance.

# Marilyn Miglin (Skin Care Only)

Marilyn Miglin found her niche in the world of television home shopping with her skin-care products and promises of younger-looking skin. The line Miglin showcases frequently is her Perfect Balance P.D.S. (P.D.S. stands for patented delivery system), accompanied by the Iolight Facial Enhancer. I only wish the products were even half as miraculous as the brochure descriptions. Alas, they aren't even minimally as effective as the copy makes them sound.

A patented delivery system sounds interesting, but lots and lots of different cosmetics companies, from Estee Lauder to L'Oreal, offer lots and lots of patented delivery systems (L'Oreal owns several hundred). A delivery system is the way a product delivers its ingredients to the skin. Almost any mixture of ingredients placed on the skin uses a delivery system, and you can patent any myriad of combinations for this, so it doesn't tell you anything about performance or effect. Liposomes, for example, are a good delivery system but not a miracle for skin.

Miglin's TCN-NA is supposed to be a "metabolic activator" but it is just a bunch of amino acids, and on the surface of skin those are good moisturizing ingredients—they have no effect on the skin's functioning. Oxygen is another Miglin showcase ingredient, but not only isn't there enough oxygen in these products to revive an ant, let alone revitalize the skin, there is no way for the oxygen in this product to get into skin. But even if it could, it would create free-radical damage, because that's what oxygen generates, ergo the need for *anti*oxidants in most skin-care products. What is even sillier is that the source of the oxygen is from oxygenated water. Well, all water is oxygenated (that's what $H_2O$ stands for, two hydrogen molecules and one of oxygen). Only the cosmetics world can make plain water sound like a miraculous ingredient for wrinkles!

What is most stunning, after all the effusiveness about getting youthful skin from the array of products being sold, is that there is no sunscreen in the bunch. Miglin's products aren't bad, just incapable of living up to even a fraction of the claims being professed for them.

For more information, call (800) 284-3900 or (800) 662-1120, or visit the Web site at www.marilynmiglin.com or www.hsn.com.

⊗ **Iolight Facial Enhancer** *($99)* is an infrared light and heat source as well as a vibrating facial massager. Scientifically speaking, when it comes to wavelength frequency, infrared light is just beyond visible light radiation. That means you get heat without light, and that's about it. This little lamp warms up the skin and the massage action vibrates the skin, which can definitely increase blood flow, but it can cause more problems than benefits. Artificially heating up the skin and vibrating it can cause capillaries to surface, so you risk having a network of spider capillaries all over the face.

☹ **$$$ Clean Tone** *($25 for 4 ounces)* is a wipe-off makeup remover that contains a long list of vitamins and water-binding agents. You are still just wiping off makeup and that can be an option for someone with dry skin. This is quite similar in many ways to Neutrogena's Extra Gentle Cleanser for a fraction of the price. The vitamin C in here is ascorbic acid, which is considered to be the least stable and most irritating form of vitamin C.

☹ **Liquid Veil** *($25 for 4 ounces)* is an alcohol-based facial mask that contains a hairstyling agent. It dries into a plastic-like layer over the skin that you then peel off. Both of the main ingredients can dry and irritate the skin. The brochure says, "The tingling tells you it is working." What all the tingling really communicates is irritation and dryness.

☺ **Energy** *($22.50 for 4 ounces)* is a good toner-like moisturizer for someone with normal to dry skin, but don't expect the vitamins to feed your skin. The brochure copy explains that "surface cells get a metabolic boost, taking in nutrients and eliminating waste and toxins." How absurd. Surface skin cells are dead and are incapable of taking in or excreting anything.

☺ **Restore** *($40 for 4 ounces)* is a very good moisturizer for normal to dry skin, although some of the plant extracts in here can be skin irritants.

☺ **Skin Lift** *($25 for 1 ounce)* won't lift skin anywhere, but the large amount of film-forming agents in here can make skin look temporarily smoother. This is a very good moisturizer for someone with normal to dry skin. The vitamin C in here is ascorbic acid, which is considered to be the least stable and most irritating form.

☺ **Perfect Balance Oxygen 600** *($37.50 for 4 ounces)* contains a minuscule amount of oxygenated water (though all water is oxygenated). It would be a good moisturizer for someone with dry skin. This product claims to be super-oxygenating for the skin, amplifying the skin's oxygen intake. Even if it were possible to improve the skin's appearance by delivering oxygen to it, there isn't enough oxygen in here to serve that function. The skin's aging process is very complicated, and there is no single cause of aging that can be bandaged up with a cosmetic. If extra oxygen were the answer, we would all live in oxygen tents and no one would wrinkle. But it isn't just oxygen, or free-radical damage (which requires the presence of oxygen), or the depletion of many other components of the skin's structure. All it takes to stop most of the skin's wrinkling is a sunscreen. Too bad that isn't part of Miglin's skin-care routine.

☹ **Perfect C Cleanser** *($20 for 4 ounces)* is a wipe-off makeup remover that contains a teeny amount of ascorbic acid, which is considered to be the least stable and most irritating form of vitamin C. There is also a tiny quantity of AHAs in here but not enough to have exfoliating properties of any kind. The plant oils in this one, including lemongrass, lime, spearmint, and tangerine, can be skin irritants.

☹ **Perfect C Cleansing Bar** *($20 for three 4.2-ounce bars)* is a standard bar cleanser that can be fairly drying for most all skin types.

☺ **Perfect C Skin Toner** *($20 for 6 ounces)* is a good, relatively irritant-free toner; however, the vitamin C in here, ascorbic acid, can be an irritant.

☹ **Perfect C Firming Creme, Daily Anti-Oxidant Skin Protection** *($30 for 2 ounces)*. The citric acid in here is considered an irritating and unstable form of vita-min C. Several of the plant oils in here are fairly potent skin irritants, including orange, lime, lemon, and spearmint.

☺ **$$$ Perfect C Firming Eye Creme** *($20 for 0.5 ounce)* is a good moisturizer for dry skin. The vitamin C in here has the same problem as the product above but the amount is so tiny it doesn't really matter.

☺ **Perfect C Radiance Skinglo** *($25 for 1 ounce)* contains sparkles, and they're the only thing in this product that make the skin glow. This is mostly just a good, though average moisturizer for normal to dry skin.

☹ **Perfect C Serum, Nightly Free-Radical Neutralizer** *($35 for 0.85 ounce)*. Given all the oxygen claimed for Miglin's other products, I imagine you would need a free radical–fighting product to deal with them. (I'm only kidding.) The ascorbic acid in here, though, is considered a skin irritant and an unstable form of vitamin C, plus this product contains several potentially irritating plant oils including berga-mot, lemon grass, lime, and spearmint.

☺ **$$$ Perfect C Smoothing Stick** *($20 for two 0.1-ounce sticks)* is little more than a clear lipstick. It's a good emollient for dry skin but rather ordinary and heavy.

# Mario Badescu

Fashion magazines have been mentioning Mario Badescu products for some time, and in New York the Badescu salon has been around for more than three de-cades, but only Badescu's recent distribution in Martha Stewart's catalog (and mentions on her show) have made the name of this line more recognizable and mainstream.

Like an old familiar song, these products are supposed to be all-natural skin-care treatments, and are touted by actors and supermodels. I can't confirm whether or not celebrities really use these products, but even if there are some who do, there are lots of celebrities using lots of different products, so that's no way to make a skin-care decision (though for lots of women, it is the only way they decide to do anything).

It probably goes without saying, or at least you won't be surprised when I men-tion, that none of these products are natural in the least. They contain all the same old standard ingredients that show up in almost every product line I've ever reviewed.

The Badescu line does have strong points: there are some well-formulated sunscreens to consider, the price points aren't terribly exorbitant, and there are some very good moisturizers. That's great! The downside is the presence of some really unimpressive cleansers, an irritating blemish product, and poorly formulated AHA products.

Several of the Badescu products contain an ingredient called "seamollient." As exotic as the name sounds, it is just a fancy term for water and algae. Given the Creme de la Mer products that brag about algae and cost an astronomical sum, if you want algae on your skin, you may as well put it there via these products for far less (though why algae has a cult following of any kind for skin care is just beyond me).

An interesting note for those consumers who are becoming more aware of ingredient listings: I'm finding a disturbing trend in the cosmetics industry that is affecting the way ingredient labels are being worded. I suspect that many cosmetics companies are worried about consumers who are now understanding the heretofore indecipherable list of cosmetic ingredients. Companies always added their share of food and vitamins on the ingredient list for marketing purposes, because those were easy names to understand. Plus companies know consumers can't get enough of anything they recognize as natural. As a result of this, cosmetic companies started identifying unnatural-sounding ingredients with wording such as "plant derived" or "from coconut," added parenthetically next to the chemical-sounding name. It looks something like this: "magnesium laureth sulfate (source coconut)." I imagine that does reassure most women, though in truth by the time it reaches the container, the ingredient is no longer even remotely related to coconut.

I'm now concerned about a new bit of deception taking place on ingredient labels, which the Badescu line demonstrates quite nicely. Rather than listing mineral oil or Vaseline in the Cucumber Makeup Remover Cream, for example, the company lists the terms Protol and Protopet. Those are nothing more than trade names for mineral oil and Vaseline, respectively. While there are those consumers who erroneously believe them to be bad for skin, there's nothing wrong with mineral oil and Vaseline. This trend of cloaking ingredients in trade names doesn't help the consumer, though it does help the cosmetics companies make their ordinary products sound more mysterious and natural.

I should mention that the Badescu line is huge—there are over a hundred products. I was only able to obtain a handful of them. For more information about Mario Badescu, call (800) BADESCU or (212) 223-3728; or visit the Web site at www.mario badescu.com.

⊗ **Orange Cleansing Soap** *($12 for 8 ounces)* is a rather simple, standard detergent soap that can be irritating and drying for some skin types. The orange extract can burn the eye area.

⊗ **Enzyme Cleansing Gel** *($12 for 8 ounces)* is a standard, detergent-based water-soluble cleanser that also contains grapefruit and papaya extract, which makes it potentially irritating for most skin types.

☺ **Cucumber Makeup Remover Cream** *($10 for 4 ounces)* is a standard cold cream that contains mostly mineral oil and Vaseline. Pond's Cold Cream is the same thing for far less money, though I wouldn't recommend it either.

☺ **Cucumber Cream Soap** *($10 for 6 ounces)* is a standard, detergent-based water-soluble cleanser that can be OK for some skin types. It would be a problem for someone with dry skin.

☺ **Cleansing Milk with Carnation & Rice Oil** *($10 for 4 ounces)*. You would be far better off using canola oil than this greasy and waxy cold-cream concoction.

☹ **Almond & Honey Non-Abrasive Face Scrub** *($15 for 4 ounces)* uses cornmeal and ground-up almonds as the scrub, and that's hardly nonabrasive.

☺ **Facial Spray with Aloe, Herbs, and Rosewater** *($12 for 8 ounces)* is, as the name says, water, aloe, plant extracts, and fragrance. That's not going to do much of anything for skin. Without water-binding agents or anti-irritants or even an emollient, this is pretty useless.

☺ **Seaweed Cleansing Lotion** *($15 for 8 ounces)* is a standard detergent cleanser with small amounts of witch hazel and thickening agents. It can be OK for someone with normal to oily skin, though the witch hazel can be an irritant.

☹ **Cucumber Cleansing Lotion** *($15 for 8 ounces)*. At best, this is irritating and drying for the skin.

☹ **Keratoplast Cleansing Lotion** *($15 for 8 ounces)*. The lemon peel is too irritating for all skin types. By the way, keratoplast is the trade name for isodecyl salicylate. It isn't BHA, and in this product it ends up being more of an emollient than anything else.

☺ **Elasto-Seamollient Hand Cream with Vitamin E** *($24 for 4 ounces)* is a good, though extremely standard, moisturizer for dry skin. There are far more elegant formulations around, but this one would do the trick.

☺ **$$$ Ceramide Complex with NMF and AHA** *($35 for 1 ounce)*. While this is a good moisturizer for normal to dry skin, it isn't worth the price and doesn't contain AHA (fruit extracts are not alpha hydroxy acids).

☹ **AHA & Ceramide Moisturizer** *($20 for 2 ounces)* is not the kind of AHA formulation I would ever recommend. It doesn't contain lactic acid or glycolic acid and the pH is around 5, which makes it an ineffective exfoliant. The lemon extract in this product can be a skin irritant, and it also contains several ingredients that can clog pores. While it wouldn't be bad for dry skin, why bother?

☺ **$$$ Hyaluronic Eye Cream** *($18 for 0.5 ounce)* is a good, emollient moisturizer for dry skin.

☹ **Hyaluronic Moisturizer SPF 10** *($22 for 2 ounces)* has a foolishly low SPF without UVA protection and is not recommended.

☺ **$$$ Seaweed Nightcream** *($18 for 1 ounce)* is a relatively emollient moisturizer for dry skin. The seaweed is useless, but the thickeners, water-binding agents, and plant oils make this a decent moisturizer.

☹ **Drying Lotion** *($17 for 1 ounce)* is an incredibly accurate name for this product that contains mostly alcohol, calamine, camphor, and sulfur. You can't heal skin by drying it out; that only hinders the skin's healing process. Skin must be intact to heal. Plus these ingredients will only make skin red and risk causing capillaries to surface. Calamine, by the way, contains about 5% zinc oxide (which can clog pores) and a good deal of phenol, which is extremely toxic to skin. In 1992, the FDA actually tried banning calamine altogether, but that didn't happen. Absorbing oil and reducing the swelling of blemishes is not achieved with these ingredients.

☺ **Oil Free Moisturizer SPF 17** *($20 for 2 ounces)* is a sunscreen that contains avobenzone (Parsol 1789) and therefore provides very good sun protection. However, this oil-free product would only be good for someone with normal to dry skin because several of the ingredients, including stearic acid and myristyl lactate, can potentially clog pores.

☺ **Aloe Moisturizer SPF 15** *($35 for 4 ounces)* is similar to the product above and the same review applies, except more so, since this one contains isopropyl myristate.

☹ **Quick Tanning Oil SPF 2** *($8 for 2 ounces)*. There is something incredibly unethical about a cosmetic line selling a product that encourages sun tanning!

☹ **Solargen SPF 4** *($15 for 2 ounces)* has an almost useless SPF and no UVA-protecting ingredients. That someone at the Badescu company thinks this offers anyone sun protection is frightening.

☹ **Solargen SPF 6** *($15 for 2 ounces)* is similar to the one above and the same comments apply.

☹ **Sunscreen Moisturizer SPF 6** *($12 for 8 ounces)* is similar to the one above and the same comments apply.

☹ **Sunscreen Moisturizer SPF 8** *($12 for 8 ounces)* is similar to the one above and the same comments apply.

☹ **Collagen Moisturizer SPF 8** *($20 for 2 ounces)* is similar to the one above and the same comments apply.

☹ **Drying Cream** *($8 for 0.5 ounce)* can definitely dry the skin, because it contains sulfur, a strong irritant and disinfectant, but meanwhile the zinc oxide, beeswax, and palmitate in it can clog pores. Why would anyone make a drying product (assuming that drying will stop breakouts, which it won't) in the form of a cream? This is a very confused product that will confuse almost anyone's skin.

☺ **Azulene Body Soap** *($14 for 16 ounces)* is a good body shampoo but it can also be used for the face. It contains a standard detergent cleansing agent.

☺ $$$ **Strawberry Tonic Mask** *($18 for 2 ounces)* is a standard clay mask. The strawberry serves no purpose (it has no relation to fruit acids or AHAs).

☹ **Azulene Calming Mask** *($18 for 2 ounces)* is a mask that forms a plastic-like layer over the face. It also contains some oil and clay. That wouldn't be a problem for the skin, although it's also not very helpful, but this product also includes wheat starch, which can clog pores, and balsam peru, which can be a skin irritant. This won't calm anything, especially not your skin!

☺ $$$ **Enzyme Revitalizing Mask** *($20 for 2 ounces)* contains mostly papaya and film former. Papaya is a highly unstable exfoliant and somewhat irritating.

☺ **Body Lotion with Alpha-Hydroxy Acid, Cremerol, and Papaya** *($22 for 16 ounces)*. Papaya isn't AHA, so the name of this product is misleading. If you are looking for a good body exfoliant, papaya (assuming this is papain—the active ingredient in papaya) isn't the best way to go; it is considered one of the more unstable enzymes in cosmetic use. Other than that, this is a good emollient moisturizer for dry skin.

# *Mary Kay*

Mary Kay is one of the original home-sales cosmetics companies. Since beginning her firm in 1963, Mary Kay Ash (with her son's help) has built herself quite an empire. There are now more than 300,000 Mary Kay salespeople. As impressive as this all sounds, and it is impressive, the average salesperson's income is more like $5,000 to $10,000 a year. Obviously, the ability to sell does not come naturally to every member of the sales force.

Much of the Mary Kay lineup is a mixed bag of strong and weak points. For example, the foundations have some great textures and color choices, but the SPF 8 is completely behind the times (SPF 15 is minimum), yet they do contain a great UVA-protecting ingredient. The makeup colors are conveniently divided into Cool, Warm, and Neutral but there are lots of pitfalls to watch out for, such as a huge selection of iridescent and, yes, blue eyeshadows; a cream concealer that easily creases into the lines around the eyes; lipsticks that tend toward the greasy side; and a skincare system (including foundation) that often forces you to buy all or none of it, although that usually depends how stalwart a position your line rep takes. The skincare products have only one decent sunscreen and some of the moisturizing formulas are terribly archaic, while some others have current, interesting formulations.

Until recently Skin Revival has been Mary Kay's skin-care essential. To some extent that has been replaced with the launch of TimeWise, two new products being billed as "…the breakthrough you've been waiting for. Now, you can get younger-looking skin every time you cleanse and moisturize your face. [A] revolutionary new skin-care system that delivers… firmer, smoother, younger-looking skin." If these are a revolution for younger-looking skin, why is Mary Kay still selling all those other lotions and potions claiming to make skin look younger? Nonetheless, these two products do not replace nor are they an improvement over other Mary Kay skin-care cleansers and moisturizers. And TimeWise doesn't include a sunscreen, which makes this pair of products time-foolish. Another supposed timesaving feature are the Masking Cleansers, which are supposed to be a two-in-one product, a mask or cleanser. Two of them don't rinse very well and the other one is a problem if you leave it on the skin. These are not innovations or a helpful change in skin care for anyone. For more information about Mary Kay, call (800) 627-9529 or visit the Web site at www.marykay.com.

## *Mary Kay Skin Care*

☺ **$$$ TimeWise 3-in-1 Cleanser** *($18 for 4.5 ounces)* is a standard, wipe-off cleanser (read cold cream) that can leave a greasy film behind on the skin but may be suitable for someone with very dry skin. However, the price is just bizarre for what you get. The tiny amount of vitamin E and vitamin A along with some plant extracts won't change a wrinkle or anything about your face.

☺ **TimeWise Age Fighting Moisturizer** *($20 for 3.3 ounces)*. While there are some good water-binding agents in here, they are in the smallest amount imaginable. This is a good basic moisturizer for someone with normal to dry skin but that's about it.

☺ **Gentle Cleansing Cream Formula 1** *($10 for 6.5 ounces)* is a traditional, greasy cold cream. It might be gentle, but it is also quite heavy, and can leave a greasy film on the skin. It is an option for very dry skin.

☺ **Creamy Cleanser Formula 2** *($10 for 6.5 ounces)* is a mineral oil–based, wipe-off cleanser that can leave a greasy film on the skin. It is less heavy than the Gentle version above but is also little more than using plain mineral oil on the skin. It is an option for someone with dry skin.

☺ **Deep Cleanser Formula 3** *($10 for 6.5 ounces)* is an extremely standard, but good, detergent-based water-soluble cleanser that can be an option for most skin types except dry skin.

☹ **Purifying Bar** *($12 for 4.2 ounces, $10 for refill)* is a standard bar soap that won't purify anything, but it may dry out the skin and clog pores.

☺ **Oil-Free Eye Makeup Remover** *($14 for 3.75 ounces)*. This very simple product will remove eye makeup, the same as most eye makeup removers will.

☹ **Hydrating Freshener Formula 1** *($11 for 6.5 ounces)* contains a small amount of arnica and peppermint, which can irritate the skin. What a shame, because this toner has some good water-binding agents and antioxidants.

☹ **Purifying Freshener Formula 2** *($11 for 6.5 ounces)* contains mostly water and alcohol, which can irritate and dry skin.

☹ **Blemish Control Toner Formula 3** *($11 for 6.5 ounces)* is too irritating to even be considered an option for any skin type.

☺ **Moisture Rich Mask Formula 1** *($12 for 4 ounces)* is a very emollient cream. It contains an insignificant amount of vitamin A. This should feel very good on dry skin.

☺ **Revitalizing Mask Formula 2** *($12 for 4 ounces)* is a standard clay mask that also contains ground-up walnut shells. That can be a good exfoliant, but the waxes in here (carnauba, in particular) can be a problem for blemish-prone skin. It is also hard to rinse off.

☺ **Clarifying Mask Formula 3** *($12 for 4 ounces)* is similar to the Revitalizing Mask above and the same basic comments apply.

☹ **Indulging Soothing Eye Mask** *($15 for 4 ounces)* isn't indulging as much as it is potentially irritating because of the witch hazel.

☺ **Enriched Moisturizer Formula 1** *($16 for 4 ounces)* isn't all that enriched or all that different from the Balancing and Oil-Control ones below. This is an extremely standard, mundane moisturizer for normal to dry skin. The tiny bit of collagen in here can't affect the collagen in your skin.

☺ **Balancing Moisturizer Formula 2** *($16 for 4 ounces)* is a very boring, basic moisturizer for normal to dry skin. This is OK for normal to dry skin but there are far better options for skin than this humdrum choice.

☺ **Oil-Control Lotion Formula 3** *($16 for 4 ounces)* is a lightweight moisturizer. Nothing in this product can control, change, or affect the amount of oil your skin produces. It is just an OK moisturizer for slightly dry skin with a matte finish and that's about it.

☺ **Acne Treatment Gel** *($7 for 1.25 ounces)* contains benzoyl peroxide (5%). This would work fine as a disinfectant for acne.

☹ **Daily Protection Moisturizer with Sunscreen SPF 15** *($16 for 4 ounces)* doesn't contain the UVA protecting ingredients of avobenzone, zinc oxide, or titanium dioxide, and is not recommended.

☺ **Day Solutions SPF 15** *($30 for 1 ounce)* is a good, in-part avobenzone-based sunscreen that would work well for normal to dry skin. While the protection is great, the price is embarrassing, because it's just a sunscreen with very standard ingredients. There is an immensely long list of thickeners, water-binding agents, and plant extracts after the preservative but they hardly amount to a fraction of this product.

☹ **Night Solutions** *($30 for 1 ounce)* has alcohol as the second ingredient, and though this gel-based moisturizer with AHA and BHA has a good concentration of each and a relatively low pH of 3.5 to 4, the alcohol is no solution for any skin type.

☺ **Nighttime Recovery System** *($25 for 2.8 ounces)* is a rather unimpressive lightweight moisturizer for normal to slightly dry skin.

☺ **Advanced Moisture Renewal Treatment Cream** *($19 for 2.5 ounces)* is a good emollient moisturizer for dry skin. It would be an option for dry skin.

☺ **Extra Emollient Night Cream** *($11 for 2.5 ounces)* is a very standard, very emollient moisturizer for very dry skin. It does contain menthol, which can be a skin irritant, though the amount is so small it probably doesn't affect skin in the least.

☺ **Instant Action Eye Cream** *($15 for 0.65 ounce)* is a good moisturizer for dry skin but there is nothing about it special for the eye or that will do anything but moisturize skin.

☹ **Triple-Action Eye Enhancer** *($15 for 0.65 ounce)* claims to have more benefits in one little product than almost any other I've ever seen. According to the company's magazine, it has much more than just triple action; I lost count after six benefits. It has free-radical scavengers, AHAs, and light-diffusing ingredients; it can be used as an eyeshadow base or as an under-eye concealer; it reduces puffiness and increases skin firmness; and, finally, it reduces the appearance of wrinkles. What's in this little miracle? Mostly silicone, film former, clay, several thickeners, and preservatives. There are tiny amounts of vitamins E and A, but they are at the end of the ingredient list and are completely insignificant. Then what about those benefits? Well, there aren't enough AHAs in this product to exfoliate skin (less than 1% lactic acid). It doesn't have light-diffusing properties, unless you consider a little shimmer a camouflage. The film-forming ingredients can form a tight layer over the skin, giving the illusion of smoother skin. This product is a poor under-eye concealer. It would probably work well as an eyeshadow base, although for most women, an eyeshadow base is unnecessary.

☺ $$$ **Triple Action Lip Enhancer** *($15 for 0.5 ounce)* is a very good emollient moisturizer for the lips, but the amount of AHA is minimal and the triple benefit it should have contained but doesn't is sunscreen.

☹ **Skin Revival System** *($40 when purchased together)* is a two-part product consisting of **Skin Revival Cream** or **Skin Revival Cream Oil-Free** *($25 for 1.5 ounces)* and **Skin Revival Serum** *($25 for 1.5 ounces)*. This is Mary Kay's answer to the AHA and BHA craze. The claims are just short of miraculous, yet it is overpriced and neither part contains much AHA (about a 1% concentration). You're supposed to apply the serum, let it dry, then apply the cream, then add an additional moisturizer if you want. That's more complicated than it needs to be. The Skin Revival Serum is mostly alcohol in a gel form that contains about 3% to 4% AHA and about 1% BHA. Those would be an option but the alcohol is completely unnecessary. The Skin Revival Cream is mostly a standard (though emollient) Vaseline-based moisturizer with less than 1% AHA and a form of BHA that doesn't exfoliate. The Skin Revival Cream Oil-Free just leaves out the Vaseline. Don't waste your time with these; there are plenty of products that contain 8% AHAs in a good pH that don't include alcohol and don't require this many steps to get the benefit.

☺ $$$ **Balanced Response Masking Cleanser** *($22 for 5 ounces)* is one of the Masking Cleansers. These are supposed to be a revolution because you can use them either for cleansing or as a facial mask. Washing your face with clay has never made sense to me, but this one can be an option, though for dry skin the clay part may be too drying. The plant extracts are a mix of potential irritants (kiwi) and anti-irritants (burdock).

☺ $$$ **Maximum Moisture Masking Cleanser** *($22 for 5 ounces)* is similar to the Balanced version above only with oat flour instead of clay. The same basic comments apply.

☺ $$$ **Oil Relief Masking Cleanser** *($22 for 5 ounces)* contains several potentially irritating plant extracts and the second ingredient, sodium cocoyl isethionate, is a detergent cleansing agent that should never be left on the face, so the only option is to use this as a cleanser.

☹ **Sun Essentials Ultimate Protection Sunblock SPF 30** *($9.50 for 4.5 ounces)* doesn't contain the UVA-protecting ingredients avobenzone, zinc oxide, or titanium dioxide, and is not recommended.

☹ **Sun Essentials Sensible Protection Sunblock SPF 15** *($9.50 for 4.5 ounces)* doesn't contain the UVA-protecting ingredients avobenzone, zinc oxide, or titanium dioxide, and is not recommended.

☹ **Sun Essentials Intense Protection Sunblock SPF 20** *($9.50 for 4.5 ounces)* doesn't contain the UVA-protecting ingredients avobenzone, zinc oxide, or titanium dioxide, and is not recommended.

☹ **Sun Essentials Lip Protector Sunblock SPF 15** *($6.50 for 0.16 ounce)* doesn't contain the UVA-protecting ingredients avobenzone, zinc oxide, or titanium dioxide, and is not recommended.

## Mary Kay Makeup

☺ **FOUNDATION: Day Radiance Formula I Foundation for Dry Skin SPF 8** *($11 for refill, $8 for compact)* is a thick, creamy foundation that comes in pancake form. It goes on somewhat heavy but can blend out smooth. It can be good for someone with very dry skin. The SPF number is disappointing but it is a titanium dioxide–based sunscreen. These colors are too peach, pink, ash, yellow, or copper for most skin tones: Rose Petal Ivory, Blush Ivory, Delicate Beige, Mocha Bronze, Bittersweet Bronze, Rich Bronze, Toasted Beige, and Cocoa Beige.

☺ **Day Radiance Formula II for Normal to Dry Skin SPF 8** *($11)* has a beautiful texture with a smooth, light finish and is great for someone with normal to dry skin. The SPF number is disappointing, but it is a titanium dioxide–based sunscreen. These colors are too peach, pink, ash, yellow, or copper for most skin tones: Rose Petal Ivory, Soft Ivory, Blush Ivory, Delicate Beige, Dusty Beige, Mocha Bronze, Rich Bronze, Walnut Bronze, Bittersweet Bronze, and Mahogany Bronze.

The Reviews M

☺ **Day Radiance Formula III Oil-Free for Oily and Combination Skin** *($11)* is a lightweight foundation that works great for oily skin types, but it would be better with an SPF like the other foundations. These colors are too peach, pink, ash, yellow, or copper for most skin tones: Delicate Beige, Dusty Beige, Blush Ivory, Rose Petal Ivory, Mocha Bronze, Bittersweet Bronze, Walnut Bronze, and Rich Bronze.

☺ **Cream-to-Powder Foundation** *($11 for refill, $8 for compact)* has a great, smooth, soft finish without feeling greasy or thick. There are only a handful of colors but for the most part they are all excellent; only Bronze 1 and Bronze 2 are too orange for most skin tones.

☹ **CONCEALER: Full Coverage Concealer** *($9.50)* is a tube concealer with a soft, creamy application that provides good, smooth coverage. Unfortunately, it tends to crease and continue creasing long after it's applied. **Full Coverage Neutralizing Concealer** *($9.50)* is a group of lavender, mint, and yellow tints that just add strange colors to the face. These types of products never really help even-out skin tone.

☺ **POWDER: Powder Perfect Loose Powder** *($12.50)* and **Powder Perfect Pressed Powder** *($7.50)* are talc-based powders with a soft, dry consistency. They go on sheer, and three of the four colors are quite good; only Bronze can be too peach for most skin tones.

☹ **BLUSH: Powder Perfect Cheek Color** *($8)* is sold in separate tins that can be placed in a refillable compact. You buy the compact *($7)* separately and fill it with the colors of your choice. In a way, it's very convenient: you don't have to keep paying for a compact. Unfortunately, most all of the blush colors are very shiny; only Nutmeg is a matte shade. What a shame, because these do have a soft, silky-smooth finish. **Creamy Cheek Color** *($6)* is a standard cream blush that comes in two shades. These are OK, but they tend to be greasier and to slide off rather than blend on smoothly.

☹ **EYESHADOW: Powder Perfect Eye Color** *($5 for each eyeshadow, $15 for the compact)* is sold in separate tins that can be placed in a refillable compact. You buy the compact separately and fill it with the colors of your choice. The only negative is that all of the eyeshadows, even the matte ones, have some amount of shine. There is also an incredible range of pastel blues, green, and pinks—an incredibly long-out-of-date eye color selection.

☺ **EYE AND BROW SHAPER:** The **Luxury Eye Pencils** *($9.50)* are standard, twist-up pencils that have a smooth finish and a reasonable price.

☹ The **Luxury Brow Pencils** *($9.50)* have a slightly slick texture, which can make for a shiny brow.

☺ **LIPSTICK AND LIP PENCIL: High Profile Lipstick** *($10)* has a creamy, slightly glossy finish with a good range of colors, though there need to be more neutral tones—the large group of vivid shades is dated. **Luxury Lip Liner** *($9.50)* is a small but good group of standard lip pencils.

☹ <u>MASCARA</u>: **Flawless Mascara** *($8)* and **Conditioning Mascara** *($8)* has different brush sizes but end up applying identically. They build no length or thickness and are a complete disappointment. **Waterproof Mascara** *($8)* doesn't hold up well under water; it tends to chip and peel off after a few dunks. **Endless Performance Mascara** *($8.50)* just doesn't perform up to any standard. It doesn't build any length or thickness. If you wanted a mascara that didn't do anything, this would be one to choose.

## *Max Factor (Makeup Only)*

Max Factor earned his place in the annals of cosmetic history by being *the* makeup artist for movie stars and the rich and famous of the 1920s and beyond. Among his many credits, Max Factor developed innovative makeup colors and textures that were unheard of at the dawn of cinema's Technicolor era. Movie studios and Hollywood's elite relied on his expertise to create all manner of makeup, from the line's still-available Pan Cake Makeup and Erace Secret Cover Up to the very first lip gloss, circa 1930. (I don't recommend pancake foundation for anyone, but it's nice to recognize the roots of the makeup we are all wearing.) Another little-known but monumentally important contribution made by Factor was his Theory of Color Harmony. This theory referred to the art of selecting and blending colors based on a woman's skin tone, eye, and hair color, and you would be hard-pressed to find a cosmetic company who doesn't use some incarnation of this idea to coordinate makeup palettes.

In recent years, Max Factor (owned by Procter & Gamble) has made a token effort to modernize its fading image. There is nothing here that's really new since Factor launched High Definition and Lasting Performance foundations, and that was more than three years ago. Then it tried to piggyback on the success of the film *Titanic* with Tina Earnshaw, the movie's makeup artist (and Factor's spokesperson). Neither has done much to change a line in dire need of a face-lift. There is more to cringe at here than one might expect, including poor foundation colors and textures, shiny blush and eyeshadows (sad but true, although the textures are exemplary), and an overall dark and drab look, as evidenced by Factor's dreary packaging. The pencils and lipsticks are good, but then it's hard to make such products bad. In his heyday, Factor was inventing makeup; nowadays, Factor is years behind the competition and the chance of catching up seems remote. For more information on Max Factor, call (800) 526-8787 or visit the Web site at www.maxfactor.com.

<u>FOUNDATION</u>: ☺ **Seamless Stick Makeup** *($8.89)* may be too little, too late in the growing number of stick foundations on the market. Compared to Factor's other offerings in the foundation category, it is very good. However, this breaks no new ground and pales in comparison to other options from Maybelline to L'Oreal and Olay. The six shades for this one are clearly limiting, as all of them have a subtle to strong peachy tint. The texture is very slick and blends well, drying to a soft,

The Reviews M

natural finish with a bit of a sheen. For those with normal to slightly dry skin who want to give Max Factor a chance, this is an option, but be cautious with your color choice. It is not an option for oily skin (too greasy) or dry skin (the powder part can look pasty). Avoid Sable at all costs: it is too red for almost all skin tones.

☺ **Seamless Makeup** *($8.79)* has a semifluid, smooth texture with a lot of slip. It provides light-to-medium coverage and a soft matte finish. The formula is nothing exceptional and the six shades are all slightly peach to orange, but overall it's not so bad as to be shunned entirely for some fair skin tones. It does not "blend itself," as the brochure states. In fact, its slipperiness demands careful blending to avoid looking streaky or uneven.

☺ **Shimmer Pan Stik** *($7.69)* is basic Pan Stik makeup, in all its thick, waxy glory, infused with loads of pale white or bronze iridescence. It will shine you up, but also has a texture that feels greasy and heavy.

☹ **Pan-Cake Makeup** *($7.69)* and **Pan-Stik Makeup** *($7.69)* are both packaged in sealed plastic wrap that prevents you from viewing the colors (and testers are almost always absent) For that reason alone, these are difficult for me to recommend, but in addition, the textures of both foundations are too heavy, thick, and greasy and almost all of the colors are strongly peach or pink.

☹ **Whipped Creme Makeup** *($7.69)* has the most awful array of foundation colors I have ever seen, making me wonder who is really buying this stuff?

☹ **Lasting Performance Stay Put Makeup** *($8.99)* does stay put and actually has some real-skin colors, but the overly powdered finish makes the skin look grainy and rough and it just feels terrible.

☹ **Powdered Foundation** *($8.99)* works better as a talc-based pressed powder than a foundation. Although the colors are not half bad, this tends to be too powdery and cakey on the skin.

☹ **Silk Perfection Liquid to Powder Makeup** *($7.69)* has a thick, waxy consistency and a dreadful selection of colors, save for Light Champagne.

☹ **CONCEALER: Erace Secret Cover Up** *($4.69)*. Concealer stick was the staple of my first makeup experiences. The coverage with this one was and still is good, with a creamy consistency that doesn't get greasy, but the strong fragrance and turn-for-the-worse color selection makes me glad I've moved on to better cosmetic pastures!

☹ **POWDER: Lasting Performance Loose Powder** *($7.49)* is talc-based powder that has way too much shine, and the one available color is unattractively pink. **Lasting Performance Pressed Powder** *($8.99)*. The texture of this is silky yet strangely waxy powder takes forever to get any on the skin. If you like the most minimal application possible, this is an option, though all of the colors have a slight shine.

**BLUSH:** ☺ **Natural Blush-On** *($6.79)* is a soft, exceedingly smooth blush in a subtle range of pastel and earth tones. Lamentably, all of the shades are shiny, yet if you don't mind shine, this is an option for soft application of color.

☺ **Pan Stik Blush** *($7.69)* is a cream-blush stick that has a lighter texture than traditional Pan Stik Makeup. It comes in three shades, and two are shiny. The texture is cream-to-powder, and they all go on sheer. The one to consider is Bronzer, a believable matte tan shade.

☺ **EYESHADOW: Lasting Color Eyeshadow** *($3.39)* is a small group of single eyeshadows that have a gossamer texture and sheer application. Why did they have to rain on the parade and make every color noticeably shiny? If you want to make wrinkles more obvious, this is a choice, or if you do happen to like shine, but the limited options are disappointing.

☹ **High Definition Eyeshadow Quartet** *($5.79)* has an agreeable texture but is either too shiny and/or too poorly color-coordinated to recommend. **First Coat Eyeshadow Primer** *($6.69)* is a creamy, opaque eyeshadow base that lends a heavy, crease-prone look to the eyes. A lightweight, matte concealer could do double duty here instead.

☺ **EYE AND BROW SHAPER: PenSilks Glide On Eye Pencil** *($5.79)* is an automatic eye pencil that glides on and stays relatively creamy. There is a sponge tip to smudge the line before that happens naturally. **Linemaker Eyeliner** *($5.79)* is the new name for the former Eyeliner Pen. It's a liquid liner that is applied with a felt-tip pen applicator, which works well except for the slightly sticky finish. **Eyebrow and Eyeliner** *($4.69)* are just standard pencils that are a tad too greasy to earn a recommendation. **Stardust Shade and Shine Pencil** *($7.29)* is a small collection of creamy pencils infused with enough iridescence to light a small tunnel. This has limited use but is an option for those in the glitter frame of mind.

☺ **LIPSTICK AND LIP PENCIL:** Except for the noticeably waxy fragrance, Max Factor has some good lipsticks to consider. **Lasting Color Lipstick** *($6.49)* has an extremely creamy finish but it's doubtful you'll find it lasting longer than any other creamy lipstick. **LipSilks** *($7.69)* are standard lip fare with a glossy, sheer application. **High Definition Lip Liner** *($6.19)* is great and one end is a lipstick brush, which is convenient. The only drawback is the small color selection.

☺ **MASCARA: 2000 Calorie Mascara** *($5.79)* goes on easily, doesn't smear, and effectively makes lashes thick and long. As a caution, it does tend to flake if you overdo it, but those who exercise wand-waving restraint will find this one a pleasure. **S-T-R-E-T-C-H Mascara** *($5.79)* isn't as nice as the one above, but is fine for lengthening and some amount of thickness. **Lash Enhancer No. 1 Mascara** *($5.79)* is the latest mascara from Max Factor and although it lengthens and thickens well and applies easily, it isn't noticeably different from what was already here. **2000 Calorie Aqualash Mascara** *($5.79)* builds enough length and thickness to be satisfactory enough for those occasions when reliable waterproof mascara is called for.

The Reviews M

# Maybelline (Makeup Only)

Maybelline is one of the best known and most recognized mass-market makeup lines. Throughout its long history, which began in 1915 when T. L. Wilson founded the company and named it after his sister, Mabel, the company has prided itself on bringing innovative products to cosmetics consumers. Fast forwarding to today's Maybelline shows it is still going strong and has shown a marked improvement in its products since being bought by L'Oreal in early 1996. With improved product selection and modern textures, it is getting harder to tell the difference between L'Oreal and Maybelline. They both specialize in offering a large selection of lipsticks, nail polishes, and mascaras, and their foundations share the same strengths and weaknesses (smooth textures and finishes but poor colors, plus the inclusion of sunscreens, but often without much-needed UVA-protecting ingredients). The pressed powders, mascaras, pencils, and blushes are impressive and inexpensive. With a little caution, there's no reason you can't come away from Maybelline with some great bargains and a beautiful look. For more information, call (800) 944-0730 or visit the Web site at www.maybelline.com.

FOUNDATION: For the most part, there are no testers available for any of Maybelline's foundations, making it difficult to recommend even the ones I liked a lot, which have good textures and color choices. Without being able to test the color first, you can easily end up with the wrong color and with makeup that looks unnatural and mask-like.

☺ True Illusion Makeup SPF 10 ($6.39) was the first major launch that showcased L'Oreal's influence on Maybelline. The bottle closely resembles those for the Lancome foundations, which is also owned by L'Oreal. Yet in spite of the attractive packaging and the smooth, sheer application you get with this foundation, it lacks reliable UVA-protecting ingredients and the SPF 10 is meager for a full day of protection. If you're willing to wear an SPF 15 with UVA-protecting ingredients underneath, this may be an option because the colors are great, the texture impressive for someone with normal to dry skin, and the price—well, it's cheap. There are now 15 shades to choose from, with options for darker skins, and most are suitably neutral. These shades may be too peach or orange for most skin tones: Buff, Beige, Golden, and Cocoa.

☺ True Illusion Liquid to Powder Makeup SPF 10 ($5.99) is not a liquid-to-powder foundation in the least. It is a standard but good cream-to-powder makeup whose SPF is titanium dioxide–based, though because an SPF 15 is basic to healthy skin care, this leaves skin needing more. Still, the colors are mostly excellent, and there are 15 to choose from, including options for darker skin tones (but nothing for very light skin tones). Like all cream-to-powder foundations this works best on someone with normal skin, as these are too emollient for oily skins and the powder finish tends to exaggerate skins that are already dry.

☺ **3 in 1 Express Makeup SPF 15** *($7.44)* is the one to choose if you want a stick foundation that goes on creamy and dries to a soft powder finish with a reliable, all titanium dioxide–based SPF 15. This would work well for normal to slightly oily or slightly dry skin needing sheer to medium coverage. As with most stick foundations, the waxes that keep this in stick form are not great for oily skins prone to breakouts. There are 12 shades to choose from, but the best ones are strictly for light to medium skin tones—all of the darker shades, from Caramel on down, are just too peach or copper for most women of color.

☺ **Great Wear Makeup** *($6.39) is* great! This liquid foundation goes on incredibly smooth and has an ultra-matte finish that would work best for someone with oily skin who prefers medium coverage. As is true for all ultra-matte foundations, blending can be tricky, because once it dries into place it truly doesn't budge. The color range of nine shades is mostly wonderful; be careful of Fair Ivory, which can be too pink, as well as Sand (too peach), Honey, and Natural Beige (both too rosy). What a shame there are no testers, as this is a real find worth checking out if your skin tone is light to medium and your skin type fits the criteria.

☺ **Shine Free Oil Control Makeup** *($3.99)* has been reformulated and now has a very smooth, silicone-based texture that blends easily and dries to a soft matte finish. For normal to slightly oily skin types, this could work well, although the all-day shine control claim won't hold for those with oily skin. The number of shades is limited, but there are some options for light to medium skin tones that prefer light to medium coverage. Avoid Light Ivory/Buff—it is too peach for most skin tones.

**CONCEALER:** ☺ **Great Wear Concealer** *($4.69)* gets the same raves as the Great Wear foundation. This excellent, noncreasing concealer goes on matte but smoothly, without looking dry or heavy. It comes in four superb shades and is best for someone with normal to oily skin. **Undetectable Creme Concealer** *($4.99)* goes on easily and dries to a smooth, matte finish that stays in place and really covers. I wouldn't go so far as to call it undetectable, but it comes in three good shades that don't crease.

☺ **True Illusion Undetectable Concealer SPF 10** *($4.39)* has no UVA-protecting ingredients and the SPF 10 is too low a number for all-day protection, so it is unreliable for sunscreen, but it is a very good concealer with a smooth texture and semi-opaque, natural matte finish. It blends easily and does not crease; however, the bad news is that only one of the three shades looks like skin: Ivory/True Ivory, a great option for light skin tones.

☹ **Shine Free Blemish Control Concealer** *($4.14)* lists salicylic acid as its active ingredient and while that certainly has its place in the battle against blemishes, it takes more that one weapon to win the war. Besides, all three shades for this tube concealer are glaringly peachy-pink, and would only draw attention to what you're trying to hide. **Coverstick** *($4.19)* is packaged so that you cannot see the color, and although most of them are quite good, this has a greasy consistency that will easily crease. **Revitalizing Coverstick** *($4.69)* comes in two reliable shades, but this lipstick-style concealer also creases into lines under the eyes, and that's hardly revitalizing.

POWDER: ☺ **True Illusion Pressed Powder SPF 10** *($5.99)* has a disappointing SPF number but does have a great titanium dioxide–based sunscreen. Do not rely on this for sun protection, but for a soft, silky-feeling powder this excels. This talc-based powder has some lovely colors for very light to medium/dark skin tones, but can go on somewhat chalky. Avoid True Beige, which is too pink for most complexions. **Shine Free Oil Control Translucent Pressed Powder** *($4.89)* won't control shine anymore than most powders can, but it is a wonderfully soft, dry powder that applies smooth and sheer and is indeed oil-free. It's talc-based and comes in three good colors. **Finish Matte Pressed Powder** *($4.39)* is an exceptional talc-based powder with beautiful colors and a silky, even texture. It does contain a tiny bit of mineral oil, but not enough for your skin to notice one way or another.

☹ **Shine Free Oil Control Loose Powder** *($4.89)* comes in two shades, but it is impossible to see them and that makes this talc-based, dry-finish powder hard to recommend. **Moisture Whip Translucent Pressed Powder** *($4.19)* is talc-based, has a slightly peach assortment of colors, but gives a smooth, soft finish.

☺ BLUSH: **Brush/Blush** *($4.09)* is a standard powder blush that comes in an enticing array of colors and has a silky-soft texture that provides a sheer color application with a bit of sheen. There are some sparkly shades to be careful of, but they are in the minority. **Express Blush** *($6.39)* is a nice partner to Maybelline's 3 in 1 Express Makeup. This is a cream blush in stick form that goes on sheer and soft, creating a gentle wash of color for those who prefer creamy blushes with a slight powder-finish. There are eight beautiful shades, of which three have a slight amount of shine. The colors are nicely grouped into warms and cools. This would work for women with normal to slightly dry skin who have the patience to blend this on evenly. **Pure Blush** *($4.74)* has a purely wonderful, velvety-smooth texture and a completely even, professional application. It would be hard to make a mistake with this one, and the twelve pastel to brown-toned shades are all top-notch. The one drawback is the domed shape of the blush, which makes getting it onto a brush a bit tricky—but that's just a technicality. This is worth checking out on texture alone!

EYESHADOW: ☹ **Expert Eyes Eyeshadow Singles** *($2.49)*, **Duos** *($2.94)*, **Trios** *($3.99)*, **Quads** *($3.39)*, and **Octets** *($4.14)* mostly have shiny shades or dreadful color combinations, with a texture that clings unreliably and is just all-around messy. To top that off, these have almost no staying power to speak of. **Great Wear Eyecolor** *($4.49)* come in lipstick-type applicators and go on like a cream, blend relatively easily, and dry to a matte finish. None of them stay on all that well, and it's hard to control your blending with this type of texture and applicator. Still, if you've got the technique down for cream eyeshadows, these are an option—but don't give up your powder eyeshadows yet.

☹ **Cool Effect Cooling Cream Eyecolor** *($3.99)* has no cooling effect whatsoever, but what it does have is opaque, intense shine that can go on as thick as gold lame or just sheer but intensely shiny. For an evening look, it has possibilities, but the mood has to be right. **Cool Effect Cooling Eyeshadow/Liner** *($3.39)* is a chubby eyeshadow pencil that goes on somewhat wet, which means it glides easily, and then dries to a matte finish that doesn't smear or move all day. I only wish the colors were more varied and that you could actually see the color before purchasing it; you have to judge this one by a color swatch on the end of the pencil.

<u>EYE AND BROW SHAPER:</u> ☺ **Expert Eyes Brow and Defining Liner Pencil** *($4.19)* is an automatic pencil that can be sharpened (the sharpener is built into the pencil) to a finer tip than most. Other than that, it's just a standard pencil with a dry texture, which means less smudging. **Smoked Kohl Liner** *($4.49)* is a standard pencil that has a smudge tip at one end, and is as reliable as any. **Ultra-Brow Brush-On Brow Color** *($3.39)* is a great, standard, matte brow-powder that comes packaged with the standard hard brush that needs to be tossed away and replaced with a good soft professional brush. There are two shades, which is, to say the least, limiting, but what's there works if it matches your brow color. **Natural Brows Brow Pencil** *($3.39)* is an affordably priced, very standard brow pencil that can draw on a brow with the best of them. There's a brush on the cap to soften the color, which is helpful.

☹ **Eye Express Easy Eyelining Pen** *($4.19)* does go on easily, and it takes a while to dry. Actually, it never quite set itself the way I was expecting, and stayed tacky to the touch for quite a while. If you accidentally touch it later in the day, it can come off in pieces—so it may be best to pass up this Express. **Expert Eye Twin Brow and Eye Pencil** *($2.49)* is a very greasy pencil dating back to the 1940s. This has to be the way Joan Crawford drew on her severely arched eyebrows. **Lineworks Ultra-Liner Waterproof Liquid Liner** *($4.29)* is just a standard liquid liner that has good staying power underwater, but it tends to peel or smudge if accidentally rubbed.

☺ **Lineworks Liquid Liner Washable** *($4.29)* is a basic liquid liner that dries to a smooth, flat finish. Unfortunately, it applies a bit unevenly, and mistakes are hard to correct. For those who can ace the application, it does wear well during the day. **Lineworks Felt-Tip Eyeliner** *($4.29)* is just like a felt-tip pen, and it delivers a liquid liner that dries to a smooth, matte finish that doesn't budge once it's in place—so applying this is serious and it can be unforgiving. The end result is a dramatic line that doesn't chip or flake during the day. **Expert Eyes Softlining Pencil** *($3.44)* is a standard "sharpen me again" pencil that goes on creamy and stays that way. It smudges and smears easily. **Great Wear Water Proof Eyeliner** *($4.34)* is a standard, twist-up pencil that glides easily over the skin and draws a thick line. The texture is creamy but the tacky finish it has doesn't feel great. This does hold up really well, and resists smudging, but it is no more waterproof than most pencils.

<u>LIPSTICK AND LIP PENCIL:</u> ☺ **Moisture Whip Lipstick** *($4.29)* has a rich, creamy, slightly glossy texture that remains an average lipstick; it's not for those prone to feathering or bleeding. **Great Wear Budge-Proof Lip Color** *($4.74)* has a great range of colors and provides some stiff competition to Revlon's ColorStay Lipsticks. This one doesn't bleed and stays on as well as any other ultra-matte lipstick. **Hydra Time Lipstick** *($4.49)* makes the de rigueur claim of extended wear, yet it doesn't even last as long as most lipsticks. The name is nice, but this is just an emollient lipstick with a small amount of shine and a slight stain. **Great Wear Budge Proof Lip Liner** *($4.74)* works very well and is a good choice for an automatic lip liner.

☺ **Lip Express** *($3.99)* is an oversize (width-wise) lip pencil that is supposed to do double duty as lipstick and lip liner. To some extent that's exactly what it does, just not very well. Like all chubby pencils, this is difficult to sharpen and the color part is so soft, it's impossible to keep a decent tip on the end without perpetual sharpening, which causes you to go through the product much faster than you would with an ordinary lipstick. After all that, the lipstick part is, well, just lipstick. **Lip Polish** *($4.99)* provides a somewhat creamy but also powdery texture that spreads sheer, colored glitter over the lips. It isn't as greasy or messy as some glosses, but it also isn't as smooth—just lots of sparkle.

<u>MASCARA:</u> Maybelline launched the first mass-market Cake Mascara way back in 1915, and has, like L'Oreal and Lancome, become "known" for its reliable mascaras. Some are worthy of attention, but others pale in comparison to those from Maybelline's sister lines.

☺ **Illegal Lengths Mascara** *($4.29)* is an excellent mascara without being too thick or clumpy and it doesn't smear or flake. And yes, it builds lots and lots of length—almost too much! **Volum' Express Mascara** *($3.29; regular or curved brush)* definitely has its strong points, like building long, thick lashes without smearing—but it's not a look all women will covet. If you crave noticeably thick, long lashes and don't mind taking a bit more time with this one, the payoff is great. This has been reformulated and does not apply as heavily as it used to, but it's still best for those who like dramatic, full lashes. **Full N' Soft Mascara** *($6.39)* is a very good mascara. It doesn't build much thickness, but it does quickly build long lashes without clumping or smearing. **Volum' Express Waterproof Mascara** *($3.29)* builds quickly and thickens well, with no clumps. It stays on underwater too! **Illegal Lengths Waterproof Mascara** *($4.29)* definitely lengthens but don't count on getting any thickness from this one. It does stay on well underwater. **Great Lash Waterproof Mascara**

*($2.19)* won't get you much thickness, but you will get decent length without clumping and you can swim for most of the day without a smudge! **Full N' Soft Waterproof Mascara** *($3.99)* builds excellent length and noticeable thickness, and defines and separates lashes beautifully. It is waterproof and removes without much trouble.

☹ **Great Lash Mascara** *($2.19; regular or curved brush)* builds some amount of length, though it takes a good deal of effort to get anywhere. The big drawbacks are that it does not build any thickness and has a tendency to smear. Its continual mention in beauty magazines' "best-of" lists astonishes me, as it does every makeup artist I've ever interviewed. **Lash by Lash Mascara** *($4.29)* should be renamed Hour by Hour Mascara, as this will take that long to build any definition and then go on to smear during the day.

☺ <u>**BRUSHES:**</u> The **Eyeshadow Brush** *($3.99)*, **Blush Brush** *($3.99)*, and **Face Brush** *($6.09)* are extremely soft but firm and work surprisingly well. The **Eye Contour Brush** *($3.69)* is an option for brows or eye lining but is too small for eyeshadow, and the **Retractable Lip Brush** *($4.74)* is a standard lip brush that travels well.

# *M.D. Formulations (Skin Care Only)*

In the area of serious AHA products, M.D. Formulations far surpasses its competition, offering some of the highest-percentage glycolic acid–based AHA products on the market. Not only do most of its products have over 12% AHAs (8% to 10% is the standard percentage in most other good AHA products) and a pH level that makes the AHA effective for exfoliation, but M.D. Formulations also has a line of AHA products, called Forte, with up to 20% glycolic acid. If you're of the opinion that more is better, then look no further. I encourage looking into M.D. Formulations with one caveat: I do not encourage or recommend the use of AHA products with over a 10% concentration on a daily or even semi-regular basis. At this time, there have been no long-term studies that have established the effect of higher concentrations of AHA products on the skin. However, this much irritation of the skin on a daily basis theoretically can be harmful, and could actually cause skin to wrinkle (because repetitive irritation damages skin tissue). This concern has also been echoed in a press release issued by the European Commission's (EU) Scientific Committee on Cosmetic Products dated August 8, 2000. It stated that the EU is "…considering tough new limits on anti-wrinkle creams containing ingredients known as alpha-hydroxy acids, or AHAs. … The EC committee found that the chemicals appear to increase the number of skin cells that are damaged, stimulate reddening, blistering and burning … Dr. Nick Lowe, a dermatologist, says the problem stems from consumer misuse or abuse. 'Improper use, too frequent use and use by those with sensitive skin, this is where you see the damage," he says. While AHAs can play a vital role in making skin feel smoother, overuse can be problematic.

The line has also included some salicylic acid (BHA) in its formulations. From the research I've seen, there is no need to combine these two ingredients in a single product. BHA is better for exfoliation in the pore, and AHAs for sun-damaged skin on the surface. If you don't have clogged pores you don't need the BHA, and if you have both sun-damaged skin and clogged pores, the BHA will do both (exfoliate on the surface of skin and in the pore) quite nicely.

M.D. Formulations makes everything from moisturizers and acne products to shampoos (considered good for dandruff or psoriasis) and foot and nail treatments. If you want to exfoliate skin on any part of your body with an AHA concentration that can really make a difference, you will be impressed by some of these products. However, M.D. Formulations makes several products that are problematic for skin, containing unnecessarily irritating ingredients, and its AHA moisturizers are fairly ordinary and absurdly overpriced for what you get. Other than for their AHA content, these are not elegant or even very interesting formulations, and one face can only take so much exfoliation. Despite those reservations, and the fact that these products are incredibly overpriced, if you pick and choose carefully you stand to find some very good AHA products.

M.D. Formulations was originally sold only to physicians for retail sale, but now, to expand its market while retaining its so-called professional air, it is also sold through salons and spas. For more information, call (800) 55-FORTE or (800) 822-1223, or visit the Web site at www.mdformulations.com.

☺ $$$ **Sensitive Skin Cleanser** (*$28 for 8 ounces*). A skin cleanser for sensitive skin that contains AHA is an oxymoron. And to recommend more than one product with AHA, as this line does (a cleanser, toner, and moisturizer for one face) is a problem for irritation and too much exfoliation. After all, you only have so many skin cells that need to come off the face. However, this cleanser, has a pH of about 4.5, and that makes it ineffective for exfoliating and a much lower risk for causing irritation. Other than that, this is just a standard, detergent-based water-soluble cleanser with thickening agents and preservatives. To suggest that there are cheaper, more gentle ways to clean the skin is an understatement.

☺ **Facial Cleanser Basic** (*$16 for 8 ounces*) is a gentle, water-soluble cleanser for most skin types. But wait before you buy, because this product is pretty much a knock-off of Cetaphil Gentle Skin Cleanser, which is less than half the price of this one.

☺ **Glycare Cleansing Gel for Oily Skin, with 12% Glycolic Compound** (*$25 for 8 ounces*) is a standard, detergent-based water-soluble cleanser for normal to oily skin that contains 12% AHA in an appropriate pH. The effective AHA ingredient would be rinsed away before it had much of a chance to exfoliate, but for a cleanser with a good concentration of AHA that can exfoliate, this is an option, though not an option I recommend.

☺ **Facial Cleanser, with 12% Glycolic Compound** *($25 for 8 ounces)* is similar to the oily skin version above only with a smaller amount of detergent cleansing agents, which does make it an option for normal to dry skin if the goal is a face cleanser with an effective amount of AHA.

☹ **Glycare 5 for Extremely Oily or Acne-Prone Skin** *($40 for 4 ounces)* is an alcohol-based toner with 7% AHAs. I don't recommend using alcohol on anyone's skin, and the alcohol in combination with the AHAs can cause extreme irritation. The product also contains eucalyptus oil, another potent and unnecessary skin irritant.

☹ **Glycare 10 for Extremely Oily or Acne-Prone Skin** *($43.75 for 4 ounces)* is identical to the Glycare 5 except that it contains 14% AHAs. The same warnings about irritation from the alcohol apply.

☹ **Glycare Acne Gel Acne Medication** *($20 for 2 ounces)* would be an option for a combined BHA (1%) and AHA (5%) product if it wasn't for the alcohol content.

☺ **Benzoyl Peroxide 5% for Extremely Oily and Acne-Prone Skin** *($25 for 4 ounces)* is a good benzoyl peroxide topical disinfectant in an extremely lightweight base for someone with problem skin; of course you can buy virtually identical products for less, but this is still a good alternative.

☺ **Benzoyl Peroxide 10% for Extremely Oily and Acne-Prone Skin** *($25 for 4 ounces)* is identical to the toner above except for the proportion of benzoyl peroxide, and the same review applies.

☺ **$$$ Advanced Hydrating Complex Cream Formula** *($40 for 1 ounce)* is a good, though very basic moisturizer for normal to dry skin. Yeast is one of the ingredients, and it can be a good antioxidant, but the amount here is so minuscule that it is barely worth mentioning.

☺ **$$$ Advanced Hydrating Complex Gel Formula** *($40 for 1 ounce)* is more of a toner for normal to slightly dry or slightly oily skin than anything else.

☺ **$$$ Facial Lotion with 12% Glycolic Compound** *($55 for 2 ounces)* is just AHAs with a thickener and preservatives. This is a very good, basic AHA product for most skin types; however, if you have normal to dry skin you will most likely need a moisturizer too (this product contains no emollients, water-binding agents, or antioxidants).

☺ **$$$ Facial Cream with 14% Glycolic Compound** *($75 for 2 ounces)* is similar to the one above, only with slightly more AHA content and a thicker base, but it offers minimal moisturizing benefit for dry skin. This amount of AHA used daily is potentially an unknown, long-term problem for skin.

☺ **$$$ Smoothing Complex with 10% Glycolic Compound** *($35 for 0.5 ounce)* is almost identical to the Facial Cream above except that it has 10% AHA. The same basic comments apply.

☺ **Sensitive Skin Lotion** *($36 for 2 ounces)* has a pH of 4.5 to 5 with a 12%

concentration of AHA, but because the pH is so high (over 4), it is not effective for exfoliating, and that's good news for someone with sensitive skin. But then what does your $36 get you? An amazingly boring moisturizer for normal to slightly dry skin.

☹ $$$ **Sensitive Skin Cream** *($36 for 1 ounce)* is similar to the Lotion above and the same basic comments apply.

☺ $$$ **Vit-A-Plus Night Recovery Complex** *($56.25 for 1 ounce)* is mixture of AHA (8%), BHA (2%), and a tiny amount of vitamin A; it has a pH of 4, which is just borderline for an effective exfoliant. I'm not one to recommend BHA with AHA, but this is an option. I've written about the overblown claims concerning vitamin A (retinol) in Chapter Two of this book, but this product doesn't even contain retinol; instead it contains retinyl palmitate, which is several generations removed and even that more unlikely to have any impact whatsoever on skin. For an exfoliating moisturizer with good water-binding agents, this is an option, though it is overpriced for what you get.

☹ $$$ **Vit-A-Plus Revitalizing Eye Cream** *($61.25 for 0.5 ounce)* includes an 8% AHA content, but the pH of 4.4 makes it a poor choice for exfoliation. The same basic comments about the retinyl palmitate in here apply as for the Night Recovery version above.

☹ $$$ **Vit-A-Plus with Vitamin A** *($35 for 1 ounce)* is a lightweight serum that contains about 10% AHA, although its pH of 4.4 makes it a poor choice for exfoliation. The vitamins in here are good antioxidants, but the retinyl palmitate is not worth your attention for the same reason noted in the Night Recovery version above.

☹ $$$ **Vit-A-Plus2 with Alpha Retinyl Complex** *($62.50 for 0.4 ounce)* contains 20% AHA, although the pH of 4.4 makes it a poor choice for an exfoliant. The vitamins in here are good antioxidants, but the retinyl palmitate in here is not worth your attention for the same reason noted in the Night Recovery version above.

☹ $$$ **Vit-A-Plus Hydra-Firming Masque** *($37.50 for 4 ounces)* is a standard clay mask with AHA and BHA, but the pH of 4.5 makes these ineffective for exfoliation. For a basic clay mask it's an option, but it is really more of a "why bother?" than anything else.

☺ $$$ **Moisture Defense Antioxidant Hydrating Serum** *($42 for 1 ounce)* is a good moisturizer for normal to dry skin and there are good antioxidants in here, but pretty much the same ones that show up in lots of products. However, the urea concentration in this can act as an exfoliant, which isn't bad but can be a problem when used in conjunction with some of the AHA and BHA formulations in this line.

☹ **Skin Bleaching Gel** *($30 for 1.5 ounces)* is a standard 2% hydroquinone product with a 10% AHA content, although the pH of 4.5 makes the AHA ineffective for exfoliation. It also contains vitamin C but not the type (magnesium ascorbyl palmitate) known to help inhibit melanin production. This would be an option nevertheless, but the alcohol content makes it unnecessarily drying and irritating.

☹ Sun Protector, SPF 20 *($30 for 4 ounces)* doesn't contain the UVA-protecting ingredients avobenzone, titanium dioxide, or zinc oxide, and is not recommended.

☺ Total Daily Protector SPF 15 *($15 for 2.5 ounces)* is a good, in-part zinc oxide–based sunscreen in a rather mundane moisturizing base of just thickeners and silicone. There are far less expensive ways to get great sun protection than this one.

☺ Total Protector 30 *($20 for 2.5 ounces)* is similar to the SPF 15 above and the same basic comments apply.

# M.D. Forte

☺ Facial Cleanser I, with 12% Glycolic Compound *($25 for 8 ounces)* is similar to the M.D. Formulations Facial Cleanser with 12% Glycolic Compound above and the same basic review applies.

☺ Facial Cleanser II, 15% Glycolic Compound *($21 for 8 ounces)* is similar to the Facial Cleanser 12% above, only this version has more AHA; the same basic review applies.

☺ Glycare Cleansing Gel with 15% Glycolic Compound *($21 for 8 ounces)* is similar to the Facial Cleanser 12% above, only with more AHAs, but the same review applies.

☹ Glycare I with 15% Glycolic Compound *($18 for 2 ounces)* is an alcohol-based toner with 15% AHAs. I don't recommend using alcohol on anyone's skin, and alcohol in combination with the AHAs can cause extreme irritation. The product also contains eucalyptus oil, another potent and unnecessary skin irritant.

☹ Glycare II with 20% Glycolic Compound *($20 for 2 ounces)* is almost identical to the Glycare I only with more AHAs, but the same warnings about irritation apply. The long-term effects of this much AHA are unknown.

☹ Glycare Perfection Gel, 1% Salicylic Acid in a Base Containing 5% Glycolic Compound *($18 for 1.7 ounces)* does contain an effective amount of AHA and BHA (although this is a combination I don't recommend); however, the real problem is the amount of alcohol in here, which makes it too drying and irritating for all skin types, and that's hardly perfection.

☺ $$$ Facial Cream I with 15% Glycolic Compound *($32 for 1 ounce)* is just AHAs with a thickener and preservatives. This is a very good basic AHA product for most skin types; however, if you have normal to dry skin, you will most likely need a moisturizer too (this product contains no emollients, water-binding agents, or antioxidants).

☺ $$$ Facial Cream II with 20% Glycolic Compound *($35 for 1 ounce)* is similar to the Facial Cream I above only with even more AHAs, and the same review applies. This product is pretty intense and definitely not for everyone. The long-term effects of this much AHA are unknown.

The Reviews M

☺ **$$$ Facial Cream III, 30% Glycolic Compound** *($55 for 1 ounce)* is similar to the Facial Cream II above only with even more AHAs, and the same review applies. This product is pretty intense and definitely not for everyone. The long-term effects of this much AHA are unknown and this much irritation on a daily basis is a definite risk to skin.

☺ **$$$ Facial Lotion I with 15% Glycolic Compound** *($45 for 2 ounces)* is just AHAs with a thickener and preservatives. This is a very good basic AHA product for most skin types; however, if you have normal to dry skin, you will most likely need a moisturizer too (this product contains no emollients, water-binding agents, or antioxidants). This amount of AHA used daily is potentially an unknown, long-term problem for skin.

☹ **$$$ Facial Lotion II with 20% Glycolic Compound** *($47 for 2 ounces)* is similar to the Facial Lotion I 15% above, but with more AHAs, and the same review applies. The long-term effects of this much AHA are unknown.

☹ **$$$ Advanced Hydrating Complex Cream Formula** *($45 for 1.7 ounces)* is identical to the Advanced Hydrating version in the M.D. Formulation line.

☹ **Advanced Hydrating Complex Gel Formula** *($45 for 1.7 ounces)* is a very overpriced, ordinary gel with too much alcohol content and is not recommended.

☹ **$$$ Skin Rejuvenation Eye Cream** *($41 for 0.5 ounce)* has an 8% AHA content, but the pH of 4.4 makes it a poor choice for exfoliation. The matte base is minimally moisturizing and the retinyl palmitate in here is not the same as retinol (and the hype even about retinol is completely overblown).

☺ **$$$ Skin Rejuvenation Lotion I, 10% Glycolic Compound** *($33.50 for 1 ounce)* is an effective 10% AHA exfoliating lotion in a minimally moisturizing base. It contains a tiny amount of antioxidants, but absolutely nothing to warrant the price.

☺ **$$$ Skin Rejuvenation Lotion II, 20% Glycolic Compound** *($51 for 1 ounce)* is almost identical to the Lotion I above and the same basic review applies. The 20% concentration is a concern because the long-term effects of this high a concentration of AHA are unknown.

☹ **$$$ Skin Rejuvenation Hydra-Masque** *($24.50 for 4 ounces)* is a standard clay mask with AHA and BHA, but the pH of 4.5 makes them ineffective for exfoliation. For a basic clay mask it's an option but it is really more of a "why bother?" than anything else.

☹ **Sun Protector, SPF 20** *($17 for 4 ounces)* doesn't contain the UVA-protecting ingredients avobenzone, titanium dioxide, or zinc oxide, and is not recommended.

☺ **Total Daily Protector SPF 15** *($12.50 for 2.5 ounces)* is a good, in-part zinc oxide–based sunscreen in a rather mundane moisturizing base of just thickeners and silicone. There are far less expensive ways to get great sun protection than this one.

☺ **Sun Protector 30** *($18 for 2.5 ounces)* is similar to the SPF 15 above and the same basic comments apply.

☺ **Skin Bleaching Gel with 2% Hydroquinone in a Base Containing 10% Glycolic Compound** *($30 for 1.5 ounces)* is a standard 2% hydroquinone product with a 10% AHA content, though the pH of 4.5 makes the AHA ineffective for exfoliation. It also contains vitamin C but not the type (magnesium ascorbyl palmitate) known to help inhibit melanin production. This would be an option nevertheless, but the alcohol content makes it unnecessarily drying and irritating.

## *Mederma*

Selling products that promise to get rid of scars is getting to be big business. With that kind of popularity, and given how hard it is to get rid of scars (just like it is so difficult to get rid of wrinkles, cellulite, and breakouts), it isn't surprising that a product called ☹ **Mederma** *($24.95 for 1.76 ounces)* is now on the market claiming to get rid of scars, diminish redness, and make skin look smooth and flawless.

How does Mederma do this? I know this is going to be hard to believe, at least it was for me, but Mederma uses onion extract as the scar-changing ingredient. Mederma contains water, thickeners, onion extract, fragrance, and preservative. I asked three different dermatologists if they have ever seen any research showing the effectiveness of onion extract on scarring, and they all asked if I was joking. I'm not joking, this product does contain onions and the customer service representative for Mederma told me that the onion extract "prevents the release of histamines which causes scarring." Even if onions could prevent the release of histamines, histamines have everything to do with allergic reactions but little to nothing to do with scarring. Histamines are produced by the body in response to an allergic reaction. Histamines are sent to fight the allergen that causes the redness, swelling, and itching. While histamines can cause the skin to react, that reaction isn't related to the breakdown of collagen and elastin that causes scarring and the wound healing process the body goes through to produce a scar (a necessary function for the healing of a wound).

Apart from the theory, the March 1999 issue of *Cosmetic Dermatology* published a study about Mederma. The results were as follows: "Treated and placebo [untreated] subjects were compared on all covariants: age, gender, ethnicity, scar age, and use. No significant difference exists between treated and placebo groups for any of these variables. … More placebo patients than treated patients reported improvement with a less noticeable scar [after] 1 week and a less red scar after 1 month." Interestingly, "More treated patients reported improvement with a softer scar after 2 months. There were no differences in improvement for either of the physician-related measures between the two groups." Not exactly the cure for scars Mederma presents. For more information about Mederma, call (888) 925-8989 or visit the Web site at www.merz usa.com.

# Merle Norman

Merle Norman herself began with a background in cosmetics chemistry, and started making her first products in her kitchen before opening up her Studio in 1931. Her famous "Try Before You Buy" philosophy was an industry first, and is still a mainstay feature of the Merle Norman stores. History aside, many of Merle Norman's boutiques are still in dire need of some serious cosmetic surgery, not just a face-lift (all of the stores I visited had a slightly worn, fairly antiquated feel), and the makeup items seem to be stuck in a time warp. Although the pencils and some of the lipsticks have been improved, virtually all of the foundations and concealers have some of the poorest shades imaginable. If you want to check out what I mean by a foundation or concealer being the wrong color or not related to real skin color, these mostly pink, peach, and rose tones are the products to inspect. The display units are still poorly organized and not very user-friendly; in fact, they appear almost haphazard. It would be much better if there were some color or style groupings. As it stands in most stores, the colors have no relation to each other, and are strewn all over.

I admit this all sounds pretty dismal, but with some tweaking this line could really be a contender. The matte blushes and eyeshadows are good, and the color selection is extensive for women of all skin tones and colors; it's just that the color choices are all wrong. Merle Norman needs to take a look at itself through more contemporary, fashionable glasses if it has any hope of joining the rest of the cosmetics world in this new millennium. For more information about Merle Norman, call (800) 348-8889 or visit the Web site at www.merlenorman.com.

**Please Note:** Since the Merle Norman boutiques are privately owned and operated, each one can set prices as they see fit, so the prices listed below may vary from store to store.

# Merle Norman Skin Care

☹ **Luxiva Collagen Cleanser** *($18.50 for 6 ounces)* is just a mineral oil–based wipe off cleanser. The teeny amount of collagen in here has no effect on the collagen in your skin. It does contain fragrance.

☺ $$$ **Luxiva Foaming Cleanser for Dry Skin** *($18 for 4 ounces)* is a detergent-based cleanser that can be effective for most skin types. The plant extracts in here can be anti-irritants. This does contain fragrance and coloring agents.

☹ **Luxiva Foaming Cleanser for Oily Skin** *($18 for 4 ounces)* is almost identical to the Dry Skin version above, only this one contains eucalyptus and lemon, which are drying and irritating problems for all skin types.

☹ **Luxiva Skin Refining Cleanser** *($18.50 for 4 ounces)* won't refine anyone's skin. It has some synthetic scrubbing beads, which are OK for mechanical exfoliation, but it also contains a fair amount of potassium hydroxide, which can be a skin irritant. This product has more problems than benefits.

☺ **Luxiva Dual Action Eye Makeup Remover** *($12.50 for 4 ounces)* is a very standard, but good silicone-based eye makeup remover that also contains detergent-cleansing agents. It does contain fragrance.

☹ **Luxiva AHA Toner** *($14.50 for 6 ounces)* is mostly alcohol and some amount of menthol, which makes it mostly irritating for all skin types.

☺ **Luxiva AHA Toner for Dry Skin** *($14.50 for 6 ounces)* doesn't contain alcohol but the plant extracts in here are not effective forms of AHA.

☹ **Luxiva Collagen Clarifier** *($14.50 for 6 ounces)* this definitely contains collagen, and while collagen is a good water-binding agent, it offers no other benefit for skin. It also contains menthol, which makes it potentially irritating for all skin types.

☺ **Luxiva Preventage Firming Defense Creme for Oily and Normal/Combination Skin Types SPF 15** *($36 for 2 ounces)* is a very good in-part titanium dioxide–based sunscreen in a good moisturizing base for normal to dry skin that includes water-binding agents, anti-irritants, and antioxidants. There is nothing about this product that is appropriate for oily or combination skin types.

☺ **Luxiva Preventage Firming Defense Creme for Dry Skin SPF 15** *($36 for 2 ounces)* is almost identical to the Oily and Normal version above and the same comments apply.

☺ $$$ **Luxiva Preventage Firming Eye Crème SPF 15** *($19.50 for 0.5 ounce)* is similar to the Dry Skin Version above and the same basic comments apply.

☺ $$$ **Luxiva Changing Skin Treatment SPF 15** *($42 for 1 ounce)* is a very good, though very overpriced in-part zinc oxide–based sunscreen for someone with normal to dry skin. It does have its share of interesting water-binding agents but the gimmick here is that it also contains soybean and wild yam extract. Wild yam extract is supposed to contain progesterone to affect menopausal symptoms. According to the *The PDR Family Guide to Natural Medicines & Healing Therapies* and the *American Journal of Obstetrics and Gynecology*, volume 18, 1999, wild yam is used in the production of artificial [synthetic] progesterone but it will not yield the hormone in the absence of a chemical conversion process that the body can't supply, though it can be created in a laboratory. The same issue holds for soybean extract, which is supposed to contain estrogens. While it can effect estrogen levels when eaten, it cannot be converted into estrogen through the skin.

☺ $$$ **Luxiva Energizing Concentrate** *($37.50 for 1 ounce)*. The collagen and yeast in here are good water-binding agents but they offer no other benefit for skin. The ginseng in here can be a skin irritant, though over all this is a good moisturizer for normal to dry skin.

☺ $$$ **Luxiva Fine Line Minimizer** *($42.50 for 1 ounce)* is a good lightweight moisturizer for someone with normal to dry skin. The film former in here can make skin look temporarily smoother but nothing about your skin will be altered one iota.

☺ **Luxiva Triple Action Eye Gel** *($20 for 0.5 ounce)*. The third ingredient is witch hazel, which makes this a potential skin irritant.

☺ **Luxiva Collagen Support** *($21.50 for 2 ounces)* is a good lightweight moisturizer for normal to dry skin. This does contain collagen, which is a good water-binding agent, but it has no effect on the collagen in skin.

☺ **Luxiva Day Creme with HC-12** *($23 for 2 ounces)* is a rather ordinary moisturizer for normal to dry skin. The plant extracts are a mix of some anti-irritants and irritants. Without sunscreen, this is inappropriate for day time.

☺ **Luxiva Night Creme with HC-12** *($38.75 for 2 ounces)* is similar to the Day Creme above and the same comments apply.

☺ **$$$ Luxiva Hydrosome Complex** *($34.50 for 1 ounce)* is a rather ordinary moisturizer for normal to dry skin. The interesting ingredients are in such minuscule amounts they are inconsequential for skin.

☺ **Luxiva Protein Creme** *($39.50 for 4 ounces)* is a very ordinary Vaseline-based moisturizer for dry skin. It does contain a teeny amount of collagen but that doesn't warrant the price or the interest in this product.

☺ **Luxiva Nighttime Recovery Creme** *($38 for 2 ounces)* is a very good moisturizer for normal to dry skin with many state-of-the-art ingredients.

☺ **Luxiva Firming Neck and Chest Creme** *($32.50 for 2 ounces)*. Many of the plants in here can be good anti-irritants but some can be irritants. What a shame. It does contain a tiny amount of salicylic acid but the pH is to high for it to be effective as an exfoliant. Over all this is a good moisturizer for normal to dry skin with nothing that makes it special for neck and chest area.

☹ **Luxiva AHA Intensive Complex** *($32 for 1 ounce)* contains about 7% lactic acid, which would be great except the pH of this lotion is too high for it to be effective as an exfoliant.

☺ **Luxiva Lip Revive** *($15 for 0.5 ounce)* is just a good moisturizer for dry skin. It is supposed to help prevent lipstick from feathering but it does a poor job of this.

☹ **Luxiva Shine Control Hydrator** *($33.50 for 2 ounces)* contains grapefruit, eucalyptus, horsetail, witch hazel, and lemon peel; all of that adds up to irritation and dryness and you will still have oily skin.

☹ **Luxiva Shine Control Lotion** *($16.50 for 1 ounce)* is similar to the Shine Control Hydrator above and the same comments apply.

☹ **Miracol Booster Revitalizing Lotion Concentrate** *($13.50 for 1.25 ounces)* is mostly water, alcohol, a form of milk, and preservatives. If this didn't have a price tag on it I would have thought it a joke. Not only is this drying and irritating for skin, but it is one of the more useless skin-care products in this entire book.

☹ **Miracol Revitalizing Cream** *($14 for 6 ounces)* is mostly water, egg white, fragrance, and preservatives. The question is, why bother?

☹ **Miracol Revitalizing Lotion** *($16.75 for 5.5 ounces)* is similar to the Cream version only in lotion form and a complete waste.

☺ **Cleansing Cream** *($14.50 for 7.5 ounces)* is a mineral oil–based wipe-off cleanser that contains thick waxes and cocoa butter. It's pretty much just cold cream, which can be an option for very dry skin but it can clog pores and feel heavy on skin. It does contain fragrance.

☺ **Cleansing Lotion** *($18 for 14 ounces)* is a mineral oil–based wipe-off cleanser that contains thick waxes and lanolin. It's pretty much just cold cream, which can be an option for very dry skin but it can clog pores and feel heavy on skin. It does contain fragrance.

☹ **Special Cleansing Bar** *($9.50 for 4 ounces)*. There is nothing special about this bar cleanser, except that the third and fourth ingredients are sodium lauryl sulfate and sodium C14-16 olefin sulfate, which are both extremely irritating and drying for all skin types.

☺ **Instant Eye Makeup Remover** *($11 for 3 ounces)* is just a very standard, detergent-based makeup remover. It would work as well as any. It does contain a fragrant plant oil.

☹ **Fresh 'N Fair Skin Freshner** *($14.50 for 5.5 ounces)* lists the second ingredient as alcohol, which makes this too drying and irritating for all skin types.

☹ **Refining Lotion** *($14.50 for 5.5 ounces)* is just water and witch hazel. Even if the witch hazel wasn't a potential skin irritant, this is a do-nothing toner.

☺ **Intensive Moisturizer** *($15 for 1.25 ounces)*. There is nothing intense about this unless you are looking for a heavy, greasy moisturizer for dry skin.

☺ **Moisture Emulsion** *($16.50 for 3 ounces)* is an exceedingly humdrum moisturizer for normal to dry skin.

☺ **Moisture Lotion** *($13 for 3 ounces)* is similar to the Moisture Emulsion above and the same comments apply.

☹ **Protective Veil** *($12 for 3 ounces)* is just water, thickeners, preservatives, and fragrance. What a complete waste of time for your skin.

☺ **Aqua Lube** *($13.50 for 2 ounces)* is a greasy, boring option for dry skin.

☺ **Super Lube** *($14.50 for 2 ounces)* is a greasy, boring option for dry skin.

☹ **Sun Defense Sunscreen for Face and Body, SPF 25** *($16.50 for 4 ounces)* doesn't contain avobenzone, titanium dioxide, or zinc oxide, and is not recommended.

☺ **Sun Free Self Tanning Creme Light** *($13.50 for 4 ounces)*, like all self tanners, contains dihydroxyacetone, the ingredient that turns skin brown. It works as well as any of them.

# *Merle Norman Makeup*

**FOUNDATION:** ☺ **Liquid Makeup SPF 16** *($16.50)* is an extremely light but emollient foundation; however, the SPF offers no UVA-protecting ingredients of avobenzone, zinc oxide, or titanium dioxide and the 24 shades are almost all too peach, pink, orange, or ash to even suggest this as a possibility.

☺ **Luxiva Ultra Powder Foundation** *($21.50)* is a standard talc-based powder foundation that goes on slightly grainy but still has a sheer finish. The texture could easily look cakey if you overdo it. The 16 shades are OK—this is sheer enough so the really bad colors aren't so obvious—but for the money, M.A.C.'s Studio Fix Foundation ($21) has a texture and colors that are light years ahead of this product.

☺ **Luxiva Lasting Foundation** *($24.50)* would be a great option for an ultra-matte foundation that has enough slip to allow more time for blending before it "sets," but the majority of the 19 shades are overwhelmingly pink, peach, rose, or orange. The only colors that look like skin are Palest Ivory, Ivory, and Ecru. Café Beige is OK but may be too red for some skin tones.

☺ **Luxiva Face the Day Crème-to-Powder Makeup SPF 25** *($24.50)* has a slightly grainy but still smooth texture and a solid powder finish. Titanium dioxide is the only active sunscreen agent but once again, the 16 shades are shockingly poor. Only Palest Ivory can be considered neutral and would be an option for light skin tones.

☺ **Luxiva Ultra Foundation with HC-12** *($21.95)* claims it contains a "special treatment complex" with its HC-12, which stands for Hydrating Complex and seems to be a combination of plant oils, water-binding agent, plant extracts, and vitamins. If you have very dry skin, they will help to moisturize but that's about it. This has a creamy texture and sheer finish, so the mostly poor colors aren't as apparent as they are in the other formulas. If you're set on trying a Merle Norman foundation and have dry skin, you may be able to find a worthwhile color among the 20 shades, but this is really stretching the realm of possibilities, which is limited.

☺ **Total Finish Compact Makeup** *($17.25)* is as close to greasepaint as you're likely to find, but even greasepaint isn't *this* greasy. The salesperson confided that everyone calls this the "Tammy Faye Bakker" foundation, and all of the 24 shades are as far from natural skin tone as you can get.

☺ **Powder Base Foundation** *($14.75)* is more creamy, actually greasy, than powdery, and has an almost sticky feel and 26 shades to choose from. It finally blends out smooth and sheer, but with almost no powder feel, so the name is confusing. Plus, it tends to stain the skin, it is that thick.

☺ **Aqua Base Foundation** *($14.75)* is an extremely creamy, rather thick foundation that is supposed to provide matte coverage. It is somewhat matte but can feel more thick and heavy than matte, especially if you don't blend it out carefully. If you want medium coverage with a silky feel and have normal to dry skin, this is the only real foundation option in the Merle Norman lineup, with some of the better skin tones to consider. These colors are too peach, pink, rose, or yellow: Translucent, Bamboo Beige, Fawn Beige, Delicate Beige, Champagne Beige, Porcelain, Taffy Cream, Golden Birch, Bronze Glow, and Gentle Tan.

☹ <u>CONCEALER:</u> **Cover Up** *($11)* can be a decent option for an opaque, soft matte-finish concealer if you can find a reliable skin tone shade among the 14 choices. The majority of them are too pink, peach, or rose and there are a handful of color correctors (yellow, green, lavender) that add a strange cast to the skin. The best options for this one are Warm Light, Olive, and Warm Medium, but make sure you sample this before buying to make sure the color looks even remotely natural. **Retouch Cover Creme** *($11)* has mostly pink and peach shades, and can crease into the lines around the eyes. **Oil-Free Concealing Creme** *($11)* is oil-free but still has a fairly emollient texture. It does go on drier than the Retouch but the colors are just really bad.

<u>POWDER:</u> ☹ **Remarkable Finish Pressed Powder** *($12.50)* and **Remarkable Finish Loose Powder** *($15.50)* are both talc-based powders that go on soft and smooth but the seven colors are mostly too peach or pink to recommend. **Remarkable Finish Pressed Powder Gold Compact** *($24.50)* is identical to the one above, save for an elegant compact and the fact that there is only one shade available, and it is sheer but with a rather noticeably pink-toned finish. **Remarkable Finish Oil Control Pressed Powder** *($13.50)* and **Remarkable Finish Oil Control Loose Powder** *($15.50)* are talc-based powders that are basically indistinguishable from the ones above, and like the others, the colors here are too peach or pink for most skin tones. **Sheer Face Powder** *($16.50)* is one more talc-based powder than is needed for this line; like the Gold Compact above, there is one shade available, and even though it is a sheer application, it can still add a peach tone to skin.

☺ **Highlighting Powder** *($12)* comes in a small pot and is just a very shiny loose powder that can be messy to use but will indeed add lots of sparkles.

☺ <u>BLUSH:</u> **Luxiva Crème Blush** *($13.50)* has a soft, smooth texture and sheer finish. The color range is very good, and if you prefer a traditional cream blush (meaning one that stays creamy) this is a fine option. **Blushing Powder** *($13.50)* has textures that vary a bit, but most of them are soft and blend on easily. There is a vast selection of colors suitable for a wide range of skin tones; most have a small amount of shine, but not enough to be a problem.

<u>EYESHADOW:</u> ☺ **Luxiva Lasting Eyecolor** *($13)* has a silky texture that blends quite well. The color range presents some good choices, but watch out for the satiny shine most of these have. **Crease Resistant Shadow Base** *($9)* is a cream-to-powder concealer for the eyelids and may work for some but won't hold up nearly as well as a matte finish concealer.

☹ **Automatic Shadow Base** *($9)* comes in a compact and is too creamy to even stand a chance at preventing your shadows from fading or creasing. **Shimmerstick Crème Eyeshadow** *($11)* is a cream eyeshadow in pencil form that is intensely shiny, blends out to nothing, and is hard to sharpen.

☺ <u>EYE AND BROW SHAPER:</u> **Automatic Definitive Eye Pencil** *($11)* is a standard twist-up pencil that has a soft, creamy texture and does dry to a transfer-resistant finish with impressive staying power. **Definitive Eyelining Pen** *($11)*, **Automatic Eyeliner** *($7.95)*, and **Waterproof Eyeliner** *($7.95)* are standard liquid liners with stiff applicators. They work for a dramatic look, but shade selection is limited. The waterproof version is quite tenacious, so count on it lasting under most conditions. **Definitive Eye Pencil** *($11)* is a standard pencil that needs sharpening and has a soft texture that smoothes on without being greasy. **Tinted Brow Sealer** *($11)* is a lightweight mascara for the brows that comes in six excellent colors. This works well to softly define and groom the eyebrows, and is not sticky. This is also available in Clear. **Only Natural Brow Powder** *($11)* is a group of matte brow powders that come with a stiff brush. Forget the brush but the powders work well to create a defined brow that doesn't appear artificial or drawn on. **Definitive Brow Pencil** *($11)* is a basic brow pencil with the usual dry finish, it will work as well as any.

<u>LIPSTICK AND LIP PENCIL:</u> ☺ **Lipstick** *($10.50)* is a traditional, creamy, semi-opaque lipstick that has a slight stain to keep the color around longer. Ditto for the **Luxiva Ultra Lipcolor SPF 15** *($12.50)*, which has no UVA-protecting ingredients and offers slightly more coverage than the one above. **Moist Lip Color** *($10.25)* is a very greasy, sticky gloss that comes in a tube and has little to no staying power. **Lip Pencil Plus** *($12.50)* is a fat, two-sided pencil; one end has a matte finish and functions as a lip liner, the other end is creamy with a "lipstick" finish. I find these types of products more gimmicky than useful, and keeping it sharpened can be a pain, but this is a fun product to check out. **Definitive Lip Liner** *($10.50)* has a soft, slightly creamy application that dries to a transfer-resistant finish. It comes in a twist-up container and really does have impressive staying power.

☹ **Luxiva Lasting Lipcolor** *($13.50)* is an ultra-matte lipstick that applies beautifully and sets to a solid matte finish. Regrettably, once this sets it quickly fades and what's left of the color tends to ball up and feel uncomfortable.

<u>MASCARA:</u> ☺ **Creamy Flo-Matic Mascara** *($10)* is an OK mascara. It doesn't clump, but is not the one to choose if you prefer any sort of thickness. **Luxiva Ultra Mascara** *($15)* isn't bad either, just unimpressive for the money. It builds some length and thickness with time, but at this price it should perform far better.

☺ **Waterproof Mascara** *($12.50)* builds average length and enough thickness to qualify for those occasions where waterproof mascara is a must, and this is extremely waterproof!

☹ **Ultra Thick Mascara** *($12)* goes on in a thick, clumpy mess that makes lashes look unnatural with an unattractive, spidery appearance.

**BRUSHES:** Merle Norman's brush selection has some great shapes and sizes but the ☹ **Powder** *($20)* and **Blush Brush** *($15)* bristles are too sparse and stiff to be of much use and don't feel very nice against the skin. **Makeup Artistry Brush Set** *($50)* seems like a bargain, as you get all eight Merle Norman brushes; yet the ones to avoid are the highest priced, and you can just pick and choose from the good ones and still come out ahead in terms of price.

The best brushes to consider in this group are the three ☺ **Eyeshadow Brushes** *($5.50–$6.50)* and the **Concealer Brush** *($6.50),* which is synthetic and is an option for either concealer or eyeshadow.

## MetroGel, MetroLotion, and MetroCream

These three prescription-only drugs are applied topically to treat rosacea. They contain the active ingredient metronidazole, an antimicrobial thought to combat the cause of rosacea. For many people, this is in fact an optimal way to treat rosacea, and it is considered the place to start when putting together an effective skin-care program. MetroCream contains the active ingredient metronidazole in a simple emollient base that is best for someone with dry skin; MetroGel is in a simple, water-based gel formula and is excellent for someone with oily skin; and MetroLotion is great for someone with normal to dry skin. As another option, the active ingredient metronidazole is also found in the prescription-only topical drug Noritate. For more information, call (800) 582-8225 or visit the Web site at www.metrocream.com.

## Models Prefer

I shouldn't be shocked by those of you being seduced by this new line of makeup products on the QVC channel. The line's main representative on QVC, Stacey Schiefferlin, is a beautiful former fashion model who comes on the air presenting her own "before" and "after" photos. Sans makeup, and with her hair done up in curlers (I'm not sure what the rollers are for, but it does add to the dramatic results), she then uses Models Prefer and goes from plain to dazzling by the end of the segment. Now that's powerful marketing, and the phones do ring off the hook. But please keep in mind that popularity is not a reliable gauge for a good product. Pet rocks were popular and so are cigarettes, but that doesn't mean you should join in for popularity's sake alone. And stunning makeup applications showing before-and-afters go way back to the earliest makeup advertising.

The logic for Models Prefer is to "simplify everyday beauty routines . . . [with a] back-to-basics approach using products that produce maximum results with minimal effort, all at an affordable price in neutral colors that will suit anyone." Clearly, all those selling points are debatable; at least I wouldn't agree with any of those claims. These products are by most standards pricey, far more expensive than anything at the drugstore, and some of the items even surpass the prices of M.A.C., Clinique, and Lancome. For example, Models Prefer's two rather standard chubby pencils sell for a startling $19.25 plus $4.22 for shipping and handling. These are almost identical to Sephora's lip, eye, and cheek pencils that cost only $4.50, or to Jane's (Estee Lauder's new drugstore line acquisition) Quik Stix that sell for $2.99.

Besides, there is nothing back-to-basics or special about any of this. The entire line has the same standard makeup products of foundation, concealer, mascara, lipsticks, eyeshadow, blush, and pencils that show up all over the industry.

Another point: for the money, the faux-silver plastic packaging is somewhat cheesy and the amount of product you get is some of the tiniest around. OK, one last point: the concealer not only creases, but also the colors are some of the most bizarre shades I've seen lately. While the rest of the cosmetics industry is changing to neutral skin shades, Models Prefer is trying to sell peach and yellow tones of concealer. That's not back to basics, that's just back to bad.

The skin-care line for Models Prefer has its share of problems. Primarily the set of products is overpriced for what you get, but beyond that the product choice is at best described as limited, and it is aimed at those with normal to dry skin. Then there's the name for the products, Ecogenics. It's supposed to create the image of being ecologically sound, yet the packaging for these products is almost completely wasteful, so you get huge cardboard boxes with cardboard insets wrapped around small containers of product. By anyone's definition, this is ecologically unsound.

For more information about the products, visit QVC's Web site at www.iqvc.com or call (800) 455-8845.

## Models Prefer Skin Care—Ecogenics

*The following products are sold in a set for $76.65; the set includes the cleanser, moisturizer, serum, and the facial bath (with three facial bath packets).*

☹ **Facial Bath** *(three packets)* is supposed to be used as a facial sauna, by adding the contents to a pot of boiling water and then placing your face over that to collect the steam. Steam is damaging to skin for many reasons but primarily it can cause surface capillaries or make them look worse! The packets contain mostly fragrance, as well as sage, peppermint, and spearmint, which makes this potentially irritating for all skin types.

☺ **$$$ Skin Cleanser** *(5.1 ounces)* is a good, though exceptionally standard, detergent-based water-soluble cleanser that would work well for most skin types. It does contain fragrance. The minimal amount of plant extract in here has no impact on skin.

☺ **$$$ Moisturizer** *(1.7 ounces)* is a very good moisturizer for normal to dry skin but there is nothing in here that will change a wrinkle on your face.

☺ **$$$ Skin Serum** *(1 ounce)*. The plant extracts are mix of irritants (pineapple and grapefruit) and anti-irritants (echinacea and hydrocotyl), which is just a waste. This is a good lightweight moisturizer for normal to slightly dry skin.

## Models Prefer Makeup

☺ **Hands-Free Light Diffusing SPF 8 Foundation** *($22)* has an SPF 8, which leaves much to be desired, and it is not recommended. That's truly disappointing because the texture and colors are rather nice though extremely limited (three shades don't cover the range of skin color), and the SPF is part titanium dioxide–based. The hands-free part just means you're supposed to apply the foundation with their standard sponge. What a claim for a basic makeup technique!

☹ **Blend N' Conceal Collection** *($16)* is a compact group of concealers that come in three strange shades of pale pink, yellow-tan, and brown. The dark shade is great but the pink and yellow-tan shades are not recommended for any skin tone and they are definitely not used by any makeup artists I've ever met. Plus the consistency is fairly greasy, and if you have any lines around the eye area, this can easily crease.

☹ **Flawless Neutralizing Powder** *($18.50)* is a yellow powder. Why a jaundice color is supposed to neutralize anything is a mystery. The standard talc base has a smooth finish, but this "universal" color leaves much to be desired.

☺ **Textured Duo-Blush Compact** *($16.25)*. It always seems like a bargain when two types of products come packaged in one container, but in this case you just end up getting one that isn't best for your skin type or application preference, while the amount you get is pathetic, unless you happen to like both colors. The powder blush weighs in at 0.07 ounce and the cream blush part at 0.053 ounce. The average amount you get in most blushes you buy is 0.25 ounce; that's four to five times more than the amount in one of the Models Prefer shades. The compact comes with one shade in a cream and the other a powder. If you have normal to dry skin, a cream texture is fine, but not for oily skin. The colors are fine though limited; you get one shade of rosy pink and one that is a soft peach, and those are the only two options.

☺ **$$$ Bronzer with Spiral Brush and Bag** *($27.50)* has a shaver mechanism on top of it that allows you to grate a layer off of the pressed powder underneath. The powder does have a soft feeling but the mode of application is messy and unnecessary. There is no benefit to taking a pressed powder, turning it into a loose powder, and then applying it.

☺ **$$$ Back to Basics Eyeshadow Trios** *($21)* is a compact of three eyeshadows that are fairly matte and have a silky-soft texture; they go on easily and blend beautifully. The three colors of beige, tan, and copper are great but definitely not for everyone.

☹ **3 Piece Monomatic Eye Collection** *($19.50)* are three eyeshadow "pens" in shiny navy, green, and maroon shades. I do love the applicator for shading the eye very precisely, but the colors are terrible.

☺ **Set of 2 Lip, Eye & Cheek Pencils** *($19.25)* are fat pencils with a very sparkly, somewhat matte finish. There must be a reason for using these, perhaps an evening look, but there are far less expensive versions of this exceptionally standard product.

☺ **Liquid Eyeliner** *($12.50)* is a felt-tip type, penlike liquid eyeliner almost identical to Revlon's Jetliner Intense (for $4.84), only Revlon's has a much smoother application. This goes on choppy but does dry to a solid though shiny finish.

☹ **2 piece Brow and Mascara Set** *($16)* is a clear brow-gel and a mascara. The brow gel is just hairspray in gel form and works well to hold brows in place. That would be fine by itself, but this mascara is one of the worst I've tested in a long time. It builds minimal to no length and takes forever to do that.

☺ **$$$ Mix N' Match Lip Pallet** *($29.25)* is a compact of eight shades of lipstick. These are fairly greasy and sheer though the color selections are rather attractive. The compact is rather small and convenient to carry in your purse. It is a nice a range of colors, but the amount you get of each doesn't add up to even a quarter of the amount of a typical lipstick. This is no bargain by any standard. Supposedly if you follow Schieffelin's *Tricks of the Trade* "you will learn tricks that models use to achieve the perfect shade by mixing different shades together!" Don't all women mix lipsticks together to create a new color? That's a trick?

☺ **$$$ 2 Piece Lip Shaping Liner with Brush** *($16.75)* are standard lip-liners with a brush at one end. These are fine, though the color selection is minimal.

☺ **$$$ Set of 2 All-Over Glamour Sticks** *($27.50)* brings you two shiny, foundation-like sticks, one gold, one silver. It's a bit greasy but the shine is, well, shiny and interesting for an evening look.

☹ **$$$ Set of 2 Eye Brow Pencils** *($16.25)* are two twist-up, standard, slightly greasy, brow pencils, both in the same shade of "gray-brown" or taupe that is supposed "to go with any skin or hair coloring," but doesn't. The notion that one shade of anything can work for everyone is like the myth about one-size fits all pantyhose!

☺ **$$$ Brush Collection** *($34.50)* includes an angle brush, lip brush, sponge brush, eyeliner brush, and a blush/powder brush. The quality isn't as good as in many lines that have single brush selections, like those available from M.A.C. or Hilfiger. Plus, the sponge brush is a waste of money and you can't use one brush for blush and powder or you would be dusting your face all over with residual blush color.

## Moisturel (Skin Care Only)

For more information about Moisturel, call (800) 494-7258 or visit the Web site at www.bms.com.

☺ **Sensitive Skin Cleanser** *($7.76 for 8.75 ounces)* is a good, though extremely basic, detergent-based water-soluble cleanser for normal to dry skin.

☺ **Therapeutic Cream** *($7 for 4 ounces)* is a Vaseline-based moisturizer that also contains silicone, glycerin, and thickeners. This is a good but extremely standard moisturizer for dry skin.

☺ **Therapeutic Lotion** *($8 for 8 ounces)* is similar to the one above, only in lotion form and with less Vaseline; the same basic review applies.

## Mojave Magic (Makeup Only)

Michael Maron has been a makeup artist for many years, and his portfolio of celebrities has clearly impressed lots of QVC shoppers. QVC is where Maron sells his line of cosmetics, called Mojave Magic. I have no intention of discrediting a talented makeup artist, because clearly Maron is a good one, but where Maron really excels is in advertising his own overpriced, completely ordinary products on television. With charisma and enough finesse to charm a makeover wannabe into the next cover girl, Maron extols the multipurpose benefits of Mojave Magic and the "natural minerals" it uses. The fact is, many of the benefits he goes on and on about can be obtained with almost any makeup. For example, any creamy lipstick can also double as a cream blush, and most bronzing powders can be used on the eyes, lips, and—if you're patient—the nails. The "special minerals" used here are nothing more than those good old standbys mica and iron oxides used in most every eyeshadow, blush, or powder you've ever seen, which is about as exotic as any rock in your backyard. Their association to the Mojave Desert is marketing posturing and nothing more.

If you're still intrigued by these very standard products, proceed with caution. For the most part they are overpriced, and virtually everything here can be found in products with much more pleasant textures, finishes, and colors at the drugstore, or from the major lines such as M.A.C. or Clinique, with better quality and for similar if not far lower prices.

The line offers a handful of kits designed to "simplify your life," but look to these only if you can reasonably see yourself using everything they include—otherwise, these are no bargains (although from watching Maron on QVC you would think these were the makeup equivalent of white gold). And for those of you who watch HSN, Maron's products are almost identical to those being sold on that channel by makeup artist Jerome Alexander.

The Reviews M

For more information about Mojave Magic, call QVC at (800) 345-1515 or visit the Web site at www.iqvc.com.

☺ $$$ **The Full Color System** *($49.95)* contains what Mojave Magic considers to be "the most essential, multifunctional products that … give mistake-proof results each and every time." It goes on to suggest that these products work with any skin tone or clothing color as well, leading one to believe that these colors can basically do no wrong. The kit includes ☹ **Multipurpose Powder** *($19.95 alone),* which is simply a pressed-powder blush with two colors, a pink-brown and a red-brown. These are talc-free and have an incredibly dry texture. The powder applies sheer and leaves a slight sheen on the skin, but blending is difficult. This is also recommended as an eyeshadow, but it tends to flake and the colors are not the best around the eye for lighter skin tones. Next is the ☺ **Tinted Lip Conditioner Duo** *($15 alone),* a dual-sided lipstick that is slightly creamy but more glossy than anything else. One half is opaque and the other is sheer and iridescent. Applying this kind of lipstick is awkward, because to get one of the colors you have to use the edge or a lipstick brush—so therefore, no quick, easy application. The "multipurpose" claim with this is that it can be used as a cream blush, but that is hardly unique to just this lipstick; any lipstick can be drawn on the cheek area! ☹ **Maxim-Eyes Duo Mascara** *($17.50 alone)* is a two-sided mascara tube. One half is mascara, which goes on clumpy and thick, sticking the lashes together. The other half is called **Amplifier** and is meant to be a mascara primer and tinted brow-shaper. The wand isn't the best for filling in brows and the taupe-brown shade limits its use to specific eyebrow shades. As a lash primer, it is merely like adding another coat of mascara, which is fine but unnecessary with this kind of product.

☺ The **Lip and Eye Duo Pencil** *($15 alone)* is a dual-sided pencil with one half a standard, deep-brown eyeliner that has a powdery texture and the other end a standard lip pencil in a soft brownish-mauve shade that is slightly creamy. There is only one duo available, which is really no choice at all. In addition to these items, Mojave Magic also includes a pencil sharpener and a retractable powder brush that is functional in a pinch, but the bristles are loose and slightly stiff.

☺ **Perfect Palettes** *($25)* includes an **Eyeshadow Trio** that has a soft, powdery texture (almost too powdery) and colors that apply much sheerer than they look, and all of them have shine. There are three assortments of three shades to choose from and they aren't the best assortment of colors. One is black, white, and gray; another is lavender, pink, and brown, and a third green, beige, and brown. Clearly Maron isn't fond of these shades either, as the model on the cover of his brochure isn't wearing them. The **Lipstick Duo** is a two-sided lipstick with one half a creamy, opaque color and the other a sheer tint. This is supposedly a "three-in-one" product (meaning on the cheeks), but it can be tricky to use that way and the results are not really worth it.

☹ **Hide and Highlight Wand** *($19.50)* is a dual-ended concealer and highlighter.

The concealer has a workable texture but is rose-colored and just doesn't look natural on skin. The highlighter is a convincing flesh tone but is shiny, which serves to draw attention to what you may be trying to hide and otherwise just adds more sparkle to the face. It can be used as a highlighter for evening but be careful about glittering during the day.

☺ **Line and Wrinkle Filler Stick** *($15)* is an automatic concealer that Maron proclaims "is like plastic surgery in a pencil." Perhaps if your plastic surgeon is still in grade school that would make sense, but this remains a slightly creamy, peach-tinted concealer that, like any lighter-toned concealer, can optically make a recessed, dark area (deep wrinkles, laugh lines) look less prominent—but it is no more efficient than any other concealer and this one can crease.

☺ **Luminizing Moisture SPF 20** *($22 for 1.7 ounces)* is a good, in-part avobenzone-based sunscreen for normal to dry skin. But the price is unwarranted for what you get, which is just an effective sunscreen and not very much of it.

☹ **$$$ Lipsicles Collection** *($29)* contains six mini-sized lipsticks and two lip glosses. The lip glosses are just glosses with flavoring, one peppermint and the other kind of like vanilla cookies. The lipsticks are fairly glossy, the colors are nice enough and versatile, but the sizes are indeed small.

☺ **Complexion Perfection System** *($39)* includes the Hide and Highlight Wand reviewed above as well as the **$$$ Weightless Corrective Powder** *($19.50 alone)*, which has a silky, slightly dry texture and is fairly opaque. It is talc-free, and the color, a pale yellow, can be a problem for most skin types and mars an otherwise decent pressed powder. Caution: this is not a lightweight powder, as Maron claims. The kit is rounded out with the soft and reasonably dense **Deluxe Powder Brush**, which would be better suited as a blush brush, as it is really too small for an all-over powder application. Given that the concealer and powder in this system both fall short, it ends up being a lot of money for a good brush.

☺ **$$$ Retractable Lipliner Trio I** *($25)* consists of three very standard, twist-up pencils in rose, peach, and red. These work great, but at $25 this is no bargain and not any different from any pencil you might consider from the drugstore.

☺ **Brush Collection** *($35)* contains seven brushes that are decent for the money. These are workable, relatively soft brushes that are worth consideration for a starting kit. However, for those looking for great brushes, there are shortcomings. The brow brush is extremely tiny and not the most practical, the liner brush is rather hard, and the blush brush is also supposed to double as the powder brush, which is a bad idea (you just end up dusting your entire face with the color of your blush).

# Murad (Skin Care Only)

Like M.D. Formulations, Neostrata, SkinCeuticals, Cellex-C, BioMedic, Dr. Mary Lupo, N.V. Perricone, M.D., and other lines of skin-care products created by or aimed at physicians, the Murad line, from Dr. Howard Murad, wants you to believe that his products are all about science and sound medical advice. They aren't. Although there are some good products here, they are just cosmetics, and there is nothing medicinal about them.

Murad was one of the first doctors to appear on an infomercial selling his own line of skin-care products. At the beginning, Murad's products were all about AHAs and his products were indeed well-formulated in this regard. But Murad had (and still has) its share of products that contain alcohol and other irritating ingredients, ranging from arnica to citrus oils. Some of Murad's products still have SPFs under 15 and some have no UVA-protecting ingredients. He makes much ado about the vitamin C in his products but for the most part the vitamin C is not magnesium ascorbyl palmitate, which is the form considered to be the most stable and the most able to inhibit melanin production.

Where Murad takes a back seat to other doctor-oriented skin-care lines is that every skin type has a routine that calls for a total of at least eight to ten products. By most medical standards that is not only excessive, it is overkill and harmful to skin.

Regardless of whether dermatologists know best about lotions and potions, no scrupulous doctor would, with a clear conscience, sell products using the ludicrous claims made for Murad's products. Any doctor who is willing to sell products such as Murasome Cellular Serum, claiming it neutralizes free-radical damage to stop wrinkles (when all researchers will tell you that is only a theory that has not yet been proven true for the skin), or Murad Purifying Clay Masque, saying it provides the ideal environment for cellular repair (there is no clay mask that can do this), has sold out completely. Every product has the same hype, the same unsubstantiated claims, the same exaggeration about the beneficial effects of ingredients that are often present only in the tiniest amounts, without even a mention of the standard ingredients and potentially irritating ingredients that are also present. For more information about Murad call (800) 336-8723 or visit the Web site at www.murad.com.

☺ $$$ AHA/BHA Exfoliating Cleanser, Deep Cleansing for All Skin Types ($23 for 6 ounces) is a standard, detergent-based water-soluble cleanser that contains plant oil, synthetic scrub particles, and about 2% AHA and 0.5% salicylic acid (BHA). AHAs and BHA are a problem in cleansers, because you don't want to get them in the eye and because their effectiveness is washed down the drain; however, the pH of this product is too high for it to be effective as an exfoliant. This can be a good, relatively gentle scrub for most skin types except dry.

☹ Clarifying Skin Cleanser ($20 for 6 ounces) is a standard, detergent-based water-soluble cleanser that would have been a decent option for most skin types but it also contains menthol, bitter orange, citronella, lemon, and lime oils, which make it potentially too irritating for all skin types.

☺ **Moisture Rich Skin Cleanser** *($19.50 for 6 ounces)* is a standard, detergent-based water-soluble cleanser with thickening agents and a small quantity of conditioning agents. It isn't what anyone would call rich, though it is a good cleanser for someone with normal to dry skin. There is also a small amount of grapefruit extract in here that can be irritating for some skin types, but the amount is probably too small to be of concern.

☺ **Refreshing Skin Cleanser** *($19.50 for 6 ounces)* is an extremely standard, detergent-based water-soluble cleanser for someone with normal to oily or combination skin.

☺ $$$ **Environmental Shield Facial Cleanser** *($30 for 6 ounces)* is a standard, detergent-based water-soluble cleanser that would have been a decent option for most skin types except that it also contains orange, basil, and grapefruit. That might make it smell like the vitamin C this product is supposed to contain, but the teeny amount of ascorbyl palmitate in here would be washed away before it could have any benefit for skin.

☹ $$$ **Gentle Make-up Remover** *($16.50 for 4.2 ounces)* is an extremely standard, detergent-based wipe-off makeup remover, extremely overpriced for a very ordinary group of ingredients. It does contain a small amount of glycolic acid, but thankfully the pH isn't low enough to make it active on the skin; that would be a huge mistake in something that might get in the eye.

☹ **Clarifying Astringent** *($14.50 for 6 ounces)* contains mostly witch hazel as well as some amount of menthol and lemon; all are completely unnecessary skin irritants.

☹ **Hydrating Toner** *($14.50 for 6 ounces)* contains mostly witch hazel, a completely unnecessary skin irritant. The amount of AHA in here is less than 2% so it is also not effective as an exfoliant.

☹ **Environmental Shield Balancing Toner** *($28 for 6 ounces)* contains mostly witch hazel, along with some amount of menthol, balm mint, and citrus oils. That won't balance anything but it can cause irritation and inflammation. What a shame, because there are some very good water-binding agents in this formula.

☹ **Combination Skin Formula** *($48 for 3.3 ounces)* is a lightweight gel that contains about 7% AHAs and about 1% BHA. It also contain a good deal of alcohol, which makes it a problem for all skin types.

☹ **Oily Prone Skin Formula** *($48 for 3.3 ounces)* is almost identical to the one above and the same review applies.

☹ **Acne Prone Skin Formula for Acne Prone Skin** *($46 for 3.3 ounces)* is a BHA and AHA lotion that also contains a lot of alcohol, which only exacerbates the potential for breakouts from irritation.

☹ **Sensitive Skin Formula** *($48 for 3.3 ounces)* is almost identical to the one above, and that makes calling it a "sensitive skin formula" a bad joke.

☺ $$$ **Sensitive Skin Smoothing Cream** *($48 for 1.7 ounces)* is about a 6% glycolic acid–based moisturizer that also contains a small amount of vitamins, water-binding agents, and anti-irritants. It is overpriced, but very good as an exfoliant for dry skin.

☹ **Skin Smoothing Cream SPF 8** *($48 for 1.7 ounces)* has a low SPF and no UVA-protecting ingredients. It is inconceivable that any line endorsed by a physician would sell an SPF under 15 and not include UVA-protecting ingredients.

☹ **Skin Smoothing Lotion** *($48 for 5 ounces)* is similar to the one above except this one contains orange, cinnamon, and grapefruit oils, all potential and completely unnecessary skin irritants.

☺ **Intensive Formula** *($48 for 3.3 ounces)* is a good 8% AHA in a lightweight moisturizing base for someone with normal to dry skin. It contains its share of anti-irritants and water-binding agents but the price is way out of proportion for what you get. It does contain fragrance.

☹ $$$ **Cellular Eye Gel** *($29 for 0.5 ounce)* is a good lightweight moisturizer for slightly dry skin though the plant extracts are a mix of anti-irritants and irritants (particularly arnica, which should not be used repeatedly on skin).

☺ $$$ **Environmental Shield Essential Night Moisture** *($48 for 1.4 ounces)*. The vitamins in here can be good antioxidants but the amount of them is incredibly small, and the vitamin K in here cannot affect capillaries. Still, this is a good moisturizer for someone with normal to dry skin.

☹ $$$ **Environmental Shield Daily Renewal Complex** *($80 for 1.4 ounces)*. The vitamin C in here is ascorbic acid, considered to be the most irritating and least stable of any of the forms of vitamin C. If you are interested in using a vitamin C product this is not the one to consider. Plus the fragrant citrus oils in here are potentially irritating.

☹ $$$ **Murasome Cellular Serum for All Skin Types** *($42 for 1.4 ounces)* is a good, lightweight moisturizer for normal to slightly dry skin. The plant extracts are a mix of anti-irritants and irritants (particularly arnica, which should not be used repeatedly on skin). It does contain coloring agents.

☹ $$$ **Murasome Eye Complex 10 SPF 8** *($50 for 0.5 ounce)* has a dismal SPF number and cannot be relied on for adequate daily protection. With so many good SPF 15s around, why bother with this one when it comes to protecting your skin from sun damage? And particularly when sunscreen is the most vital part of any skin-care routine, and most likely the only one that really makes a difference in the health of skin?

☹ $$$ **Murasome Night Reform** *($52.50 for 1.4 ounces)* is a good 8% AHA in a lightweight, slightly moisturizing base. The pollen, raspberry, and oat flour in here can be problematic (meaning irritating) for some skin types.

☹ **Perfecting Day Cream SPF 15** *($29 for 2.25 ounces)* doesn't contain the UVA-protecting ingredients avobenzone, zinc oxide, or titanium dioxide, and is not recommended. So much for the concept of "perfecting."

☺ **Perfecting Night Cream** *($31 for 2.25 ounces)* would be a very good moisturizer for someone with dry skin.

☺ **$$$ Perfecting Serum** *($52 for 1 ounce)* is merely a lightweight lotion of water-binding agents, vitamins, and plant oils. It is a very good moisturizer for someone with normal to slightly dry skin.

☺ **Skin Perfecting Lotion** *($27 for 2 ounces)* is a good moisturizer for someone with dry skin. It also contains magnesium ascorbyl palmitate, considered to be a stable form of vitamin C. When used in cream with a 10% concentration, magnesium ascorbyl palmitate was shown to inhibit melanin production. It has also been shown to have protective effect against inflammation caused by UVB sun exposure. However, the amount in here isn't even 1% so its effectiveness for any aspect of skin care is doubtful.

☺ **Skin Soothing Formula** *($9.50 for 0.5 ounce)* is a Vaseline-based moisturizer with lanolin and a tiny amount of BHA. It isn't the right pH for the salicylic acid to be effective, and a BHA product is never considered soothing. However, it is emollient, though Aquaphor (reviewed in this edition) is almost identical (and even better formulated) and far less expensive than this product.

☺ **$$$ Environmental Shield Essential Day Moisture SPF 15** *($40 for 1.4 ounces)* is a very good titanium dioxide–based sunscreen in a good moisturizing base for someone with normal to slightly dry skin. The fragrant citrus oils in here can be skin irritants.

☺ **Daily Defense Oil Free Sunblock SPF 15 (Light Tint)** *($16.50 for 4.2 ounces)* is a titanium dioxide–based sunscreen that would be very good for someone with normal to dry or sensitive skin. The tint is on the peach side, but it disappears into skin and is barely detectable.

☺ **Daily Defense Hydrating Sunscreen SPF 15** *($16.50 for 4.2 ounces)* is an in-part avobenzone-based sunscreen that would be very good for someone with normal to dry or sensitive skin. The pomegranate extract in here is a very good antioxidant but it is not the miracle ingredient described in the brochure.

☺ **$$$ Waterproof Sunblock SPF 30 Face and Body** *($19 for 4.2 ounces)* is a good in-part titanium dioxide–based sunscreen for someone with normal to dry skin.

☺ **$$$ Daily Defense Self Tanner SPF 15 for Face & Body** *($19 for 4.2 ounces)* is a standard, dihydroxyacetone-based self tanner that includes a reliable sunscreen utilizing an in-part avobenzone-base for the active sunscreen agents.

☹ **Acne Management Formula** *($13 for 0.5 ounce)* is a confusing product. While it does contain sulfur as a disinfectant (though that is considered an extremely irritating and potentially problematic way to disinfect blemishes), and AHA and BHA for exfoliation, it also contains a range of thickening ingredients that can clog pores. There are far better ways to exfoliate and disinfect skin than this one.

☹ **Acne Management Masque** (*$32 for 2.5 ounces*) is similar to the Acne Management Formula above, except in the form of a clay mask that also includes camphor, which only adds to the irritation.

☹ **Clarifying Gel** (*$48 for 1.4 ounces*) contains mostly alcohol, which makes it too drying and irritating for all skin types.

☺ **$$$ Purifying Clay Masque** (*$22.50 for 2.25 ounces*) is a standard clay mask with some good water-binding agents. This is as good as any clay mask and can feel good on the skin, but don't expect it to purify anything, it just absorbs oil.

☺ **$$$ Hydrating Gel Masque** (*$22.50 for 2.25 ounces*). This peel-off mask wouldn't be a problem, but several of the plant extracts, including horsetail, pine cone, rosemary, and lemon, can be irritating for most skin types.

☹ **Age Spot and Pigment Lightening Gel** (*$48 for 1.4 ounces*) would be a decent skin-lightening product with its 2% hydroquinone and 8% AHA content, but it also contains a lot of alcohol, and that can cause unnecessary skin dryness and irritation and won't help skin or sun-damage spots (there are no such thing as age spots).

# Nad's Gel Hair Removal

**Nad's Gel Hair Removal** (*$29.95 for one kit*) is a hair remover that uses a method known as sugaring. Sugaring uses sugars with a caramel-like consistency instead of wax to remove hair. It works identically to regular waxing only instead of a wax substance spread over the skin, you're spreading caramel.

I have to say this is one of the first products I've ever run into where the claim of being 100% natural and organic is 100% true. Nad's ingredients are honey, molasses, fructose, vinegar, lemon juice, water, alcohol, and food dye. Now that's what I call natural. But does that make it better than waxing, as the company claims? First, waxing isn't unnatural because wax is a natural substance. And as far as hair removal is concerned, the effect is identical. You spread the Nad's caramel gel over the hair you want removed (there needs to be some hair length or there won't be anything to grab). Then you rip it off and out comes the hair, same as waxing.

The two main positives to sugaring over waxing are, first, sugaring's mess washes away while wax has to be peeled or scratched off (and that isn't easy). Plus caramel doesn't have to be heated while wax does! Easy cleanup and a relatively easier application are the incredible benefits of sugaring.

But before you jump on the bandwagon of Nad's or other sugaring hair-removal systems, there are several concerns about the veracity of the claims that accompany the sugaring method for getting rid of unwanted hair. Nad's states "when you use Nad's, the hair is extracted, including the roots so re-growth is softer, finer and slower." That isn't true. Hormones and genetics determine hair growth and hair thickness, not hair removal. What does happen when you "tweeze" or otherwise pull out hair is that because it has been removed closer to the root the next hair takes longer to get back to the top, unlike shaving, which removes hair only from the surface, so the hair pops back out faster. Also, because each hair follicle has a different rate of growth, the hair can seem softer because there will be less of it as it grows back than what was present when you first waxed or sugared.

There are also claims about sugaring preventing ingrown hairs. Ingrown hairs are unrelated to the way hair is removed. Ingrown hairs occur because after a hair has been removed below the skin's surface, the new hair sometimes has trouble finding its way back to the surface. That applies to hair removal in general, regardless of whether you shave, tweeze, sugar, or wax.

Another claim: "Because of the natural substances in Nad's, there is little chance of irritations. Redness for a short time is normal, depending on how sensitive your skin is." Natural or not, ripping out hair hurts, and for some skin types that can be a problem. What is better about sugaring, however, is that the stuff doesn't have to be heated and so, as a result, it's less irritating—but that isn't about natural.

For more information about Nad's, call (800) 653-9797 or visit the Web site at www.nads.com.

## NARS (Makeup Only)

Francois Nars, a French-born makeup artist/photographer, has continued the trend of makeup artists creating their own lines of products. I'm beginning to wonder if this M.A.C.-clone momentum will ever slow down, as more and more little-known makeup artists are attempting to piggyback off the success of this formidable line. Granted, each one has its own subtleties that set it apart, but these are minor compared to the blatant similarities. So how does NARS measure up? For the most part, you'll be pleased with the foundations, blushes, and the lipstick selection. The brushes are an option, but tend to be pricey and not exceptional enough to warrant the price. There is more shine and outright glitter here than in other lines cut from the same designer cloth, and these don't necessarily offer a smooth application.

One true bonus of most artistry lines of this kind is that often the education provided to the sales staff is superior, with an emphasis on makeup application and artistry, and NARS is such a line. If you ask, you may be offered a makeup lesson with one of the line's on-site artists. As long as you're comfortable with this and the emphasis is on technique as opposed to multiple sales, it can be an invaluable experience. For more information on NARS, call (212) 941-0890 or (888) 903-NARS, or visit the Web site at www.narscosmetics.com.

☺ $$$ <u>FOUNDATION:</u> There are two types of liquid foundation available, each housed in a pump bottle, which can take some getting used to when controlling how much gets used. **Balanced Foundation** *($37)* is an oil-based foundation that has a rich, creamy feel and finish. This is appropriate only for normal to very dry skins that prefer medium coverage. The color range is superior, with only one shade to avoid, Sahara (slightly pink), and some good options for darker skin tones. **Oil Free Foundation** *($30)* claims its finish is semi-matte, but it is actually true matte. This may be an option for normal to oily skins, but the texture is rather heavy, lending itself to medium coverage, and the matte finish is slightly sticky. Again, the color range is impressive—just avoid Sahara, which is too pink for most skin tones. **Gel Fraicheur** *($30)* is really more of a lightweight tinted moisturizer than a foundation. The texture is slightly creamy, blending on very sheer and drying to a soft powder finish. This would be suitable for all but very oily skin, and of the four shades only Antilles is too orange to recommend.

☺ $$$ **Makeup Primer** *($28)* is just a light moisturizer that supposedly "primes" the skin for foundation. There is no reason to layer this number of products on your face (moisturizer, often specialty treatments, then makeup primer, and then foundation). This doesn't help the makeup perform or hold up any better on the skin.

☺ $$$ **CONCEALER:** The lipstick-style **Concealer** *($16)* provides creamy, opaque coverage. NARS claims this is "creamy yet crease-resistant," but it can indeed slip into the lines around the eyes. If you feel you must try this, there are some colors to consider, but avoid Honey, Praline (both too pink), and Toffee (too orange).

☺ $$$ **POWDER:** Both the **Pressed Powder** *($24)* and the **Loose Powder** *($30)* come in several very good shades, with a great smooth texture and a shimmery, very sheer finish. The loose powder is very messy to use, with powder flying all over the place. The shine in both these powders isn't the best for those looking to reduce shine on their face, not adding to it. Of the six shades only Mountain is too ash for most skin tones.

**BLUSH:** There is an impressive, attractive selection of ☺ $$$ **Blush** *($24)* that has a splendid texture and some viable options for a matte or shiny finish. Caution: most of these colors are very strongly pigmented, so use the least amount possible and build from there. Many of these colors would be gorgeous on darker skin tones. **Color Wash** *($24)* is NARS's version of BeneFit's BeneTint liquid blush. There are two shades, and both apply reasonably well and are translucent. This type of blush works best on a normal, smooth-textured skin.

☺ $$$ **The Multiple** *($32)* is a chunky, wind-up stick that has a creamy, somewhat greasy texture and soft, sheer colors that would work for cheeks, eyes, and, in some cases, lips. Although all of the colors have some shine, these are an option for a fun evening look, though the price doesn't hold given everyone from Maybelline to L'Oreal has their own version for a fraction of what this costs!

☹ **EYESHADOW:** Both the **Single Eye Shadow** *($15)* and the **Eye Shadow Duos** *($27)* have an OK, slightly dry texture and are very pigmented, which causes them to blend on unevenly. With colors this strong, you need a smooth, silky texture to artfully apply and blend these. There are a few matte shades to consider, but I wouldn't label any of these a must-have—the majority of shades are too Technicolor-bright (or shiny) for daytime wear.

**EYE AND BROW SHAPER:** The four ☺ $$$ **Eyeliners** *($16)* and four **Eyebrow Pencils** *($16)* are as standard as they come (the Eyeliner pencils are slightly more creamy than the drier-finish Eyebrow Pencils), and absolutely not worth the price tag.

☹ **Glitter Eye Pencil** *($24)* is a fairly creamy, thick pencil infused with flecks of glitter. The glitter tends to chip off onto the face and the price tag on this is just absurd.

☺ $$$ **LIPSTICK AND LIP PENCIL:** For the most part, it's hard to make a bad lipstick and NARS's are just fine; but at most of its counters, none of the **Lipsticks** *($19)* are organized or labeled by their type, and there are three here to consider! The **Satins** are creamy bordering on greasy and are fairly opaque. The **Sheers** are quite glossy and offer very soft color, and the **Semi-Mattes** have an opaque, slightly creamy finish and a good stain. **Lip Gloss** *($19)* features some bold colors in a sticky, thick formula whose price is unwarranted for what you get, which is just a gloss and a rather tacky-feeling one at that. **Lip Lacquer** *($19)* is an improvement over the one above, with a much smoother, non-sticky texture. If you must spend this kind of money for standard lip gloss, choose this one and forgo the Gloss. **Lip Liner Pencil** *($16)* claims it won't bleed or feather, and although this won't hold true for everyone, this one does have a drier finish that should keep those problems in check for a few hours, at least. The color selection is small but good.

☹ **MASCARA:** NARS's **Mascara** *($19)* should, at this price, be the gold standard. Instead, it's merely substandard, taking too much effort to build much length or thickness, and with clumps along the way. **Waterproof Mascara** *($19)* shares similar traits, only this one tends to stick the lashes together and creates a spiky look. It is waterproof, but with the other problems and the high price, why bother?

☺ $$$ **BRUSHES:** NARS is to be commended for designing a practical, user-friendly assortment of **brushes** *($18 to $50)* Almost all of them have a lovely, soft feel and are appropriately shaped for a variety of application techniques. The only ones to steer clear of are the **Brow Brush** *($20)*, which is too scratchy, and the **Retractable Lip Brush** *($18)*, which is really too small for most women's lips.

☺ $$$ **SPECIALTY PRODUCTS:** **Body Glow** *($55)* is just coconut oil with gold shimmer and fragrance. This would be an expensive way to complete your St. Tropez tanned look, which was hopefully from a bottle and not the sun! **Nail Polish** *($15)* truly offers something for everyone, with a color range that goes from classic red to cyberpunk blues and silvers. Finding a nail color to coordinate with your lipstick is almost always chic, and you won't be disappointed here. **Artist's Palette** *($53 to $65)* is NARS's take on Trish McEvoy's makeup planners, only with hers you get to choose the colors. These are overpriced, preselected colors that have limited appeal unless you prefer almost all of your makeup colors to be shiny; however, for the Park Avenue Disco Queen on the run, these may be just the ticket.

## Natura Bisse (Skin Care Only)

If you've heard of or sampled Natura Bisse, I suspect that must mean you've been hanging out at the Neiman Marcus makeup counters where this overpriced, pointless line is sold. It is hyped (and I mean overhyped) as a high-concentration AHA product line, and is supposed to provide the highest concentration of AHAs you can buy. Natura Bisse's Glyco Peeling Plus 50% AHA and Glyco Peeling 25% AHA aren't anywhere near as potent as those percentages imply. Actually, if it was an effective AHA, your skin would start dissolving after a few minutes, and you would be a peeling, oozing, red mass of skin. But you have nothing to worry about from these products, because they are all buffered to a pH of over 4.5 (a fact the company extols on its brochures), which means they can't perform as serious exfoliants and pose little to no risk to your skin, though they do pose a serious risk of wasting your money. This is because AHAs, in order to be effective, need to be in a pH of 3 to 3.5; much over a pH of 4 and they just don't work that well. At a pH over about 3.5, the acid becomes a salt and no longer works to improve cell turnover. I know this sounds like a fine line to cross, but when it comes to pH there is a huge difference between 3.5 and 4.5. Consider that 7 is water but 8 can be an alkaline shampoo or cleanser.

Aside from the AHA claims, there are a host of other gimmicks lurking in this line that range from thymus extract to amniotic fluid, horse protein serum, and a handful of plant extracts. None of those things can benefit skin in any substantial way. There are also products claiming to add oxygen to the skin, but none of them contain enough to give air to one skin cell. For all the hoopla this line makes about advanced skin-care formulations, the SPFs are dismal, and for the most part the sunscreens don't contain UVA-protecting ingredients. So much for up-to-date research on the part of this line! The line may have an elite air about it, but many of the products are poorly formulated. If you're going to overspend on skin care, this is not the place to waste your money. For more information about Natura Bisse, call (800) 7-NATURA or visit www.eve.com.

☹ **China Clay Cleanser Purifying and Cleansing Paste** *($35 for 4.2 ounces)* contains clay and is hard to rinse off. This is a standard, detergent-based water-soluble cleanser with clay, fragrance, and preservatives, and that's it. It's an exceptionally overpriced, ill-advised cleanser.

☺ **$$$ Dry Skin Milk Cleanser** *($24 for 6.5 ounces)* is an OK cleanser for dry skin but it can leave a greasy film on the skin. There is nothing about egg oil that is more beneficial for the skin than any other form of oil.

☻ **Facial Cleansing Gel Foaming Cleanser** *($28 for 7 ounces)* is a standard, detergent-based water-soluble cleanser that also contains a fairly potent film former, styrene, which can be irritating for all skin types.

☺ $$$ **Eye Make-up Remover Hypo-Allergenic Lotion** *($23 for 3.3 ounces)* is just water, a detergent cleansing agent, and plant extracts. It will take off makeup, but there are more effective products available than this overpriced version.

☺ $$$ **Dry Skin Toner Moisturizing Toner** *($24 for 6.5 ounces)* is an OK, ordinary toner. There is a small amount of witch hazel in here that shouldn't be a problem for most skin types but the amniotic fluid in this one, while it may be an OK water-binding agent, offers no special properties for skin over other water-binding agents, and is just an offensive ingredient overall.

☹ **Oily Skin Toner, Astringent** *($24 for 6.5 ounces)* is mostly alcohol and is not recommended for any skin type.

☹ **Glyco-Balance** *($70 for 3.3 ounces)* contains mostly alcohol and is not recommended at any price, and definitely not at this inflated cost, for what amounts to an ineffective AHA product.

☹ **Glyco-Eye** *($62 for 0.8 ounce)* doesn't have a low enough pH to make the AHA in here effective for exfoliation. At this price, and for this tiny amount of product, all the right components should be in place. It doesn't even contain interesting water-binding agents or antioxidants. The minuscule amount of thymus extract in this product has no impact on skin.

☹ **Glyco-Face** *($70 for 2.5 ounces)* is similar to the Glyco-Eye above and the same review applies.

☹ **Glyco-Peeling 25%** *($110 for 12 0.1-ounce ampoules)* contains mostly alcohol, and a pH that is too high for the AHA to be effective as an exfoliant, which is wonderful news, because in an effective pH, this could easily cause burns and damage to skin if not administered by a professional.

☹ **Glyco-Peeling Plus 50%** *($145 for 12 0.1-ounce ampoules)* is similar to the 25% version above, and the same review applies.

☹ **C+C Vitamin Complex Concentrated Serum with Double Vitamin C** *($130 for four 0.2-ounce ampoules)* is an inanely overpriced product that uses ascorbic acid in powder form as the source of vitamin C that you are supposed to mix into a moisturizer. I discuss in Chapter Two of this book whether or not vitamin C is worth the trouble as a skin-care ingredient, but this form is considered to be one of the most irritating and ineffective ways to deliver vitamin C to the skin. The thymus and placenta protein in here are good water-binding agents but no better than lots of other water-binding agents, and mostly these are just offensive ingredients.

⊗ **C+C Vitamin Cream Refirming Cream SPF 10** *($80 for 2.5 ounces)* has a dismal SPF; no UVA-protecting ingredients of avobenzone, titanium dioxide, or zinc oxide; and is not recommended.

⊗ **C+C Vitamin Fluid** *($75 for 1.7 ounces)* contains sunscreen ingredients but no UVA-protecting ingredients and no SPF number, which means it is a waste for sun protection. The orange extract in here may smell like vitamin C but it has no benefit for skin. The vitamin C in here is magnesium ascorbyl phosphate, and that is a preferred form, but there are so many better products that contain it (without the thymus and placenta and wasted SPF).

⊗ **Cytokines Eye Contour Cell Renewal Gel SPF 10** *($68 for 0.8 ounce)* has a dismal SPF and doesn't contain the UVA-protecting ingredients of avobenzone, titanium dioxide, or zinc oxide, and is not recommended. It also contains mostly alcohol, which makes it potentially drying and irritating for all skin types for any part of the face. The thymus and placental extract are good water-binding agents but not better than many other forms of water-binding agents. The topic of cytokines is incredibly complex. In essence, cytokines are released by the lymph system (the immune system) to help regulate metabolism and help fend off all sorts of human problems ranging from cancer to HIV. There is nothing in this product that can positively affect the skin's immune system or growth structure, but it does contain many elements that can hurt the skin's immune response.

⊗ **Cytokines Facial Day Cream Cell Renewal Day Cream SPF 6** *($72 for 1.7 ounces)* has an SPF that isn't even worth mentioning—it is just too embarrassing, and guarantees skin damage—and it doesn't contain the UVA-protecting ingredients of avobenzone, titanium dioxide, or zinc oxide and is not recommended. See the Eye Contour version above for comments about cytokines.

⊗ **Cytokines Top Ten Fluid, Cell Renewal Complex, Skin Growth Factor** *($110 for 1 ounce)* not only can't renew skin, but it contains a good deal of alcohol, which kills skin; I imagine that would put you back at the beginning, as well as create irritation and dryness. See the Eye Contour version above for comments about cytokines.

⊗ **Oxygen Cream for All Skin Types** *($65 for 2.5 ounces)*. You have to sit down for this one. It's a very standard group of thickening agents with some alcohol, and contains hydrogen peroxide (that's right, the stuff you buy at the drugstore for 89 cents for 8 ounces). Hydrogen peroxide can release oxygen to the skin, but once this product is opened, the oxygen is used up (because hydrogen peroxide is a very unstable ingredient). Nor does the oxygen do anything but disinfect. That may be helpful, but it doesn't heal skin or change a wrinkle. The egg oil and lanolin in here are good emollients for dry skin, but what a waste of money for an otherwise boring moisturizer!

☹ **Oxygen Concentrate for All Skin Types** *($110 for 12 ampoules totaling 1.2 ounces)* is similar to the Oxygen Cream above only the second ingredient is alcohol, so this one is irritating, drying, and a waste of money.

☹ **$$$ Oxygen Finishing Mask, for All Skin Types** *($32 for 4.2 ounces)* is a standard clay mask with alcohol as the second ingredient, plus hydrogen peroxide for the oxygen. Irritation and a useless ingredient for a lot of money!

☹ **$$$ Sensitive Cleansing Cream for All Skin Types** *($27 for 7 ounces)* is a standard, detergent-based water-soluble cleanser that would be good for most skin types. It contains a small amount of papaya extract, which can be a skin irritant, but there probably isn't enough to negatively affect the skin.

☺ **$$$ Sensitive Toner for All Skin Types** *($22.50 for 6.5 ounces)* is a good, though exceedingly boring, toner for most skin types. It contains a small amount of papaya extract, which can be a skin irritant, but there probably isn't enough to negatively affect the skin.

☺ **$$$ Sensitive Concentrate Calming Concentrate for All Sensitive Skin Types** *($120 for 6 ampoules totaling 1.2 ounces)* would be a good lightweight moisturizer for someone with normal to slightly dry skin if the price tag doesn't make you dry up first. The plankton and spirulina in here are not miracle ingredients, they are only water-binding agents and possibly anti-irritants, and offer no special properties for skin. The papaya extract in here can be a skin irritant but the amount is probably too small to have any effect.

☹ **$$$ Sensitive Gel Cream Soothing Gel Cream for All Skin Types** *($65 for 2.5 ounces)* is an exceptionally ordinary moisturizer for normal to dry skin with a mere dusting of any interesting ingredients. There are several problematic ingredients for sensitive skin.

☹ **$$$ Sensitive Eye Gel Calming Gel for the Eyes** *($52 for 0.8 ounce)* is similar to the Sensitive Concentrate above and the same basic review applies.

☹ **$$$ Sensitive Night Cream Soothing Night Cream for All Skin Types** *($65 for 2.5 ounces)* is similar to the Gel Cream above, and just as boring, with any potentially interesting ingredients barely present. The same concerns about potentially irritating ingredients for sensitive skin apply to this product as well.

☹ **$$$ Sensitive Mask Soothing Mask for All Skin Types** *($32 for 2.5 ounces)* is basically just thickening agents and film former, with some plant extracts. It does contain a tiny bit of papaya extract, which can be a skin irritant for most skin types, but probably not enough to affect the skin. There are also a small quantity of plant extracts that can be anti-irritants but they are barely present and have no impact on skin. This is just a do-nothing mask.

☹ **Action Complex, Facial Fluid, with Vitamin A+C+E** *($84 for 1 ounce)* lists the second ingredient as alcohol, which makes this potentially irritating and drying for all skin types. The amniotic fluid and thymus extract are water-binding agents, but not the most effective ones around. The minuscule amounts of vitamins in here is barely worth mentioning.

☹ **Double Action Hydroprotective Day Cream for Dry Skin SPF 10** *($58 for 2.5 ounces)* has an SPF 10, and that's bad enough, but this product also doesn't contain the UVA-protecting ingredients of avobenzone, titanium dioxide, or zinc oxide, and is not recommended. It is a decent moisturizing base, but easily replaced with reliable sun protection and a better moisturizing formulation.

☹ **Action Complex Facial Fluid, with Vitamin A+C+E** *($95 for 1 ounce)* contains way too much alcohol amid a bunch of gimmicky ingredients (ranging from amniotic fluid to thymus extract) to be recommended for any skin type.

☺ **$$$ Elastin Refirming Night Cream for Deeply Dry Skin** *($56 for 2.5 ounces)* is a very good, but extremely standard, overpriced moisturizer for very dry skin. The elastin in here is a water-binding agent, and has no effect on the elastin in the skin.

☹ **Essential Shock Concentrate for Mature Skin** *($142 for 12 0.1-ounce ampoules)* is a two-part product, with the ampoules containing amniotic fluid and alcohol, and the bottle containing water-binding agents. If that seems like it's worth $142 for less than 1.2 ounces, nothing I can say will stop you; the only shock will be how nothing about your skin will change unless it may be drier and irritated.

☺ **$$$ Essential Shock Night Cream for Dry Aged Skin** *($74 for 2.5 ounces)* is almost identical to the Elastin Refirming Night Cream above and the same basic comments apply.

☹ **Eye Contour Cream SPF 10** *($52 for 0.8 ounce)* has an inadequate SPF number and it doesn't contain the UVA-protecting ingredients of avobenzone, titanium dioxide, or zinc oxide and is not recommended. It isn't even a very interesting moisturizer on top of the disappointing SPF.

☹ **$$$ Hydroprotective Concentrate for Dry Skin** *($78 for 1.2 ounces)* is just thickeners with lanolin and a tiny amount of collagen and amniotic fluid. This is about as boring and gimmicky as it gets. Amniotic fluid and collagen are good water-binding agents but there are lots of better ones and this formulation leaves the better ones out, along with any antioxidants or soothing agents to boot.

☺ **$$$ Rose Mosqueta Oil for Dry Aged Skin** *($42 for 1 ounce)* is, as the name implies, rose-hip oil with some thickening agents. It can be good for dry skin, but so can any pure oil and for far less money at that.

☹ **Special Lift Immediate Firming Concentrate** *($42 for 0.6 ounce)*. What can I say about a product that contains horse serum proteins, amniotic fluid (from who knows where), and alcohol? Just this: What a complete waste of money!

☹ **Stabilizing Concentrate** *($85 for 12 0.1-ounce ampoules)* won't stabilize anything, and with alcohol as the third ingredient it is primarily drying and irritating for all skin types. It does contain some good water-binding agents but their effectiveness is negated by the alcohol.

☹ **Stabilizing Gel Cream for Oily Skin** *($46 for 2.5 ounces)* contains mostly alcohol, which won't stabilize anyone's skin, though it can be extremely irritating and drying. Aside from that, it is a very mundane, lightweight moisturizer with a small amount of water-binding agents and lots of thickening agents.

☹ **Titian Neck and Chest Firming Serum** *($74 for 1.7 ounces)* is similar to the Stabilizing Concentrate above, and the same review applies.

☹ **Vital Gel Cream for Mature Skin SPF 10** *($80 for 2.5 ounces)* has an SPF 10, which is bad enough, but this product doesn't contain avobenzone, titanium dioxide, or zinc oxide for UVA protection, and is not recommended. It is also an OK moisturizer for dry skin, but absolutely nothing special given the price tag. It does contain an extract from *Opuntia ficus-indica*, the Indian fig or prickly pear cactus. When taken orally, there is some evidence it can alleviate prostate inflammation. But for skin, it can have some emollient properties, and that's it.

☺ **Extreme Sun Protector SPF 30** *($55 for 4.2 ounces)* is an in-part titanium dioxide–based sunscreen. It has an exceptionally mundane moisturizing base that is mostly thickeners, mineral oil, silicone, preservatives, and a teeny amount of vitamins. There are far better sun-protecting options than this one.

☹ **Sun Shield, SPF 20 Refirming Cream for Dry Skin** *($53 for 4.2 ounces)* doesn't contain the UVA-protecting ingredients avobenzone, titanium dioxide, or zinc oxide, and is not recommended.

☹ **Protective Lightening Cream SPF 15** *($80 for 2.5 ounces)* doesn't contain the UVA-protecting ingredients avobenzone, titanium dioxide, or zinc oxide, and is not recommended. It does contain kojic acid in a teeny amount, but it is considered to be unstable and far less effective than hydroquinone. This is a mediocre skin-lightening product, and its lack of UVA protection will only encourage sun damage.

☺ **$$$ Nourishing Lightening Cream** *($80 for 1.7 ounces)* is similar to the Protective Lightening Cream only without the sunscreen. The comments about the melanin-inhibiting properties are the same, though.

☺ **$$$ Intensive Lightening Complex** *($115 for 1 ounce)* is at least a version that does contain 2% hydroquinone, which can definitely inhibit melanin production; however it is in an alcohol base, which makes it too potentially irritating and drying for all skin types. To suggest that there are far better formulations than this for skin lightening is an understatement.

☺ **$$$ Ananas Finishing Mask, for Mature Skin** *($38 for 4.2 ounces)* includes anana, a fancy name for pineapple extract, which can be a skin irritant, though there's not much of that in here so it probably isn't a problem. Other than that, it is just a bunch of thickening agents, which makes it a do-nothing kind of mask.

☺ **$$$ Splendid Finishing Mask for Dry Skin** *($34 for 4.2 ounces)* is similar to the mask above minus the plant extracts, and the same basic review applies.

☹ **$$$ Thermal Mud Finishing Mask for Oily Skin** *($38 for 4.2 ounces)* doesn't contain any mud whatsoever. This is just a bunch of thickening agents with some magnesium aluminum silicate. Almost all of the thickening agents are problematic for oily skin, and while the magnesium aluminum silicate can absorb oil from skin, the thickening agents can be a problem; just using Milk of Magnesia from the drugstore will provide far better results.

## Nature's Cure

Nature's Cure is a two-part acne treatment system, with supposedly homeopathic pills that are supposed to treat acne, and an acne medication cream. There is one group of pills for women and one for men; these are both ☺ **Natural Homeopathic Acne Tablets** and **Acne Medication Cream** *($10.10 for 60 tablets and 1 ounce of cream)*. I can't speak to the tablets other than to say I have yet to see any research supporting the notion that plant extracts and minerals of any kind can somehow change a blemish, or why one formula would work for men versus women. I am even more puzzled that these pills include lactose, when so many people are lactose intolerant and lactose can be a source of allergic reactions. What I can review more specifically is the 5% benzoyl peroxide cream (really a gel). This can be a decent though hardly natural disinfectant for breakouts. It is only part of an acne treatment, however, because you would still need an exfoliant gentle cleanser, and an oil-absorbing mask, but this isn't a bad option.

## Neostrata (Skin Care Only)

Aqua Glycolic, Murad, Alpha Hydrox, M.D. Formulations, Exuviance, Neostrata, and Avon's Anew all sell products with effective AHA concentrations and pH levels. Actually, Neostrata owns Exuviance, with Exuviance being the more upscale line, but only in appearance, not formulation.

What are the differences between all these AHA lines? Although the sales pitches vary, with each one waxing poetic about the quality of its particular company's AHA complex or compound, or its added vitamins or plants, the truth is that the results of all these products are the same. Well-formulated AHAs, meaning the those with an effective concentration and pH, provide good, consistent exfoliation that reduces the thickness of the skin's outer layer, which in turn can solve many skin problems, including dryness, blemishes, sun damage, and skin discolorations. Which product line should you choose? Good question. Alpha Hydrox, Aqua Glycolic, and Neostrata are the most reasonably priced of this group, but other products, such as Avon's

Anew, also contain a good percentage of AHAs. Basically they are all options, and this is where your personal preference plays a major role.

Neostrata products are not all that easy to obtain; they are available mostly through physicians. Call (800) 628-9904 to find a physician in your area who carries the products, or (609) 520-0715 to find out which drugstores in your area carry the products. The Web address is www.neostrata.com.

☹ **Sensitive Skin AHA Facial Cleanser** *($12.95 for 4 ounces)* is a standard, detergent-based water-soluble cleanser that contains 4% AHAs. Although that isn't much, AHAs are wasted in a cleanser and can be a problem if you get the product in your eyes.

☺ **Skin Smoothing Cream** *($12.95 for 1.75 ounces)* contains 8% AHAs. This is a good AHA product in an ordinary but emollient moisturizing base.

☺ **Skin Smoothing Lotion** *($16.95 for 6.8 ounces)* contains 10% AHAs and is quite similar to the cream above, but in lotion form. This is a good AHA product in an ordinary base for slightly dry skin.

☹ **NeoStrata-15 AHA Body and Face Lotion** *($26.95 for 6.8 ounces)* is similar to the one above, only with a higher concentration of AHAs. I do not recommend concentrations of AHAs over 10%. After all, you only have so many skin cells, so the extra irritation that increased AHAs create may be damaging to skin.

☹ **NeoStrata-15 AHA Face Cream** *($25.95 for 1.75 ounces)* is similar to the one above and the same comments apply.

☺ **$$$ Polyhydroxy AHA Eye Cream** *($22.95 for 0.5 ounce)* uses the same mix of AHAs as found in the Exuviance line. This one exfoliates the skin with about an 8% concentration of AHAs in a standard moisturizing base for normal to dry skin.

☺ **Polyhydroxy AHA Ultra Moisturizing Face Cream** *($22.95 for 1.75 ounces)* is similar to the one above, and the same comments apply.

☹ **Daytime Skin Smoothing Cream, SPF 15** *($21.95 for 1.75 ounces)* doesn't contain avobenzone, zinc oxide, or titanium dioxide for UVA protection, and is not recommended.

☹ **Polyhydroxy Daytime Protection Cream Special Care SPF 15** *($22.95 for 1.75 ounces)* doesn't contain avobenzone, zinc oxide, or titanium dioxide, and is not recommended.

☹ **Solution for Oily and Acne Skin** *($16.50 for 4 ounces)* contains 8% AHAs. The alcohol is too irritating and drying for most skin types.

☹ **Gel for Age Spots and Skin Lightening** *($11 for 1.6 ounces)* is a standard 2% hydroquinone skin-lightening product that also contains 10% AHAs. This would be a good product to try on sun-damage (age) spots, except that the second item on the ingredient list is alcohol, which can be drying and irritating to most skin types.

☺ **Sensitive Skin AHA Face Cream** *($17.50 for 1.75 ounces)* is a good emollient moisturizer with about 4% AHAs. It would indeed be good for someone with sensitive skin interested in trying an AHA product.

☺ $$$ **Sensitive Skin AHA Eye Cream** *($16.95 for 0.5 ounce)* is almost identical to the cream above, which means it is completely unnecessary.

☹ **AHA Lip Conditioner** *($3.95 for 0.1 ounce)* doesn't contain avobenzone, zinc oxide, or titanium dioxide for UVA protection, and is not recommended.

## *Neutrogena*

Neutrogena has been around since 1954, when its first clear amber bar of soap was manufactured. How well I remember discovering it when I was a teenager. It didn't leave quite the same soapy film as most bar soaps, and the amber color seemed different enough to establish the notion that it would work to get rid of blemishes. Of course, that wasn't the case. Bar cleansers of any color can be a problem for breakouts; the ingredients that keep bar cleansers in their bar form can clog pores, and the pH is over 8 and that can make breakouts worse.

Since then, Neutrogena has been sold to Johnson & Johnson and it has been busy creating a skin-care line with some products worth considering for all skin types, including some excellent sunscreens, AHA and BHA products, and cleansers. If you are looking for some of the latest gimmicks, like retinol, it has those too and one of them meets the standards you'd think only the more expensive products would deliver. Although the emphasis is still on women who worry about breakouts, ironically that is where the products really are a disappointment. One major point of contention: while several of these products are promoted as being noncomedogenic and being good for acne-prone skin, many of them contain either very irritating ingredients or pore-clogging ingredients. However, that's a caution that applies to many products in the world of skin care that have ingredients that women with blemish-prone skin always need to be wary of.

Neutrogena's makeup line, launched in 1999, is surrounded by its "Beautiful and Beneficial" claims. That means its makeup is supposed to not only make you look better but should be good for your skin too. Throwing in minute amounts of vitamins, plant sugar (melibiose—a moisturizing ingredient), or menthol won't do that for skin. Neutrogena's "makeup as skin care" rhetoric will surely entice consumers, but what is really impressive are some of the makeup's textures, colors, and reliable sun protection. What can be ignored here are the meaningless claims of "noncomedogenic," "hypoallergenic," and "oil-free." There is no justification for those claims, as these products contain lots of ingredients that can generate clogged pores and allergic reactions, and feel oily or greasy on skin!

While Neutrogena's display and packaging are attractive, it would be far more beautiful and beneficial if it would provide testers for its products (as competitor Olay has done with much success), and drop some of the common buzzwords in favor of improving some of its weaker products. Knowing that this line is largely hit-or-miss, if you are still interested in trying it (and there are some beautiful, inexpensive options), pick and choose wisely. For more information about Neutrogena, call (800) 421-6857 or visit the Web site at www.neutrogena.com.

## Neutrogena Skin Care

☹ **Transparent Facial Bar Acne-Prone Skin Formula** *($2.20 for 3.5 ounces)* is a standard, tallow-based bar cleanser. Tallow can clog pores and the detergent cleansing agents in here are fairly drying.

☹ **Transparent Facial Bar Dry Skin Formula (Available in Fragrance or Fragrance-Free)** *($2.20 for 3.5 ounces)* is similar to the bar cleanser above, and the same review applies.

☹ **Transparent Facial Bar Oily Skin Formula (Available in Fragrance or Fragrance-Free)** *($2.20 for 3.5 ounces)* is similar to both bar cleansers above, and the same review applies.

☹ **Transparent Facial Bar Original Formula (Available in Fragrance or Fragrance-Free)** *($2.20 for 3.5 ounces)* is similar to the bar cleansers above, and the same review applies.

☹ **Oil-Free Acne Wash Gentle Yet Effective Cleanser for Acne Treatment** *($6.75 for 6 ounces)* is similar to the Deep Clean cleanser above except with more BHA; this product is not recommended.

☹ **Extra Gentle Cleansing Bar** *($3.99 for 4.5 ounces)* is similar to Dove soap, and even though it is less drying than many bar cleansers, it is still fairly drying, and the ingredients that keep it in a bar form can cause problems for breakouts.

☹ **Antiseptic Cleanser for Acne-Prone Skin Alcohol Free** *($3.78 for 4.5 ounces)* contains a large number of ingredients that are too irritating for all skin types, including camphor, peppermint oil, eucalyptus oil, and benzalkonium chloride. It's nice that it doesn't contain alcohol or fragrance, but these other things are just as irritating to the skin, if not more so.

☹ **Antiseptic Cleanser Alcohol Free Sensitive Skin Formula** *($3.78 for 8 ounces)* contains the same irritating ingredients as the Cleanser above, which makes the name Sensitive Skin Formula meaningless and incredibly misleading.

☺ **Cleansing Wash for Skin Irritated by Drying Medications or Facial Peels** *($6.99 for 6 ounces)* is an ironic product, given how irritating and drying many of Neutrogena's products are for the skin. This is a standard, detergent-based water-soluble cleanser that would work well for most skin types.

☻ **Deep Clean for Normal to Oily Skin** *($5.20 for 6 ounces)* contains sodium C14-16 olefin sulfate as the detergent cleansing agent, which is too irritating for all skin types. This product also contains BHA, and that's a waste in a cleanser both because its effectiveness is washed away and because of the risk of getting it in the eyes.

☻ **Oil-Free Acne Wash Gentle Yet Effective Cleanser for Acne Treatment** *($6.75 for 6 ounces)* is similar to the Deep Clean cleanser below except with more BHA; this product is not recommended.

☻ **Deep Clean Cream Cleanser** *($5.18 for 6 ounces)* contains menthol, a skin irritant, and a small amount of BHA, but the pH isn't low enough for it to be an exfoliant. The creamy base needs to be wiped off and doesn't remove makeup very well. This product has more problems than benefits.

☺ **Extra Gentle Cleanser** *($6.06 for 6.7 ounces)* is indeed gentle, using one of the less irritating detergent cleansing agents. It doesn't remove makeup very well and can leave a slightly greasy film on the skin, but it can be an option for someone with dry skin.

☺ **Non-Drying Cleanser Lotion** *($6 for 5.5 ounces)* is similar to the Extra Gentle Cleanser above and the same comments apply.

☺ **Fresh Foaming Cleanser Soap-Free Cleanser for Combination Skin** *($6 for 5.5 ounces)* is a very good, detergent-based water-soluble cleanser for most skin types. It does contain fragrance.

☺ **Liquid Neutrogena Facial Cleansing Formula (Available in Fragrance or Fragrance-Free)** *($7.50 for 8 ounces)* is a fairly drying water-soluble cleanser that can thoroughly clean the face, but that would be a problem for anyone with sensitive, dry, or combination skin. Even someone with oily skin may find this drying.

☺ **Pore Refining Cleanser** *($7.99 for 6.7 ounces)* adds no new options to the cleansers Neutrogena already has in its lineup. This is a standard, detergent-based water-soluble cleanser that can be slightly drying. It also contains AHA and BHA, which aren't the best in a cleanser because they would just be washed away, but even if that were a problem, the pH of the product is too high for it to be an effective exfoliant.

☺ **Alcohol-Free Toner** *($6 for 8 ounces)* is a very good toner for most skin types.

☻ **Clear Pore Oil-Controlling Astringent Salicylic Acid Acne Medication** *($3.78 for 8 ounces)* would be a decent BHA toner except that it is almost 50% alcohol, and that makes it exceedingly drying and overly irritating for all skin types.

☻ **Pore Refining Toner** *($7.99 for 8.5 ounces)* contains alcohol, witch hazel, eucalyptus, and peppermint—it hurts for me to even write that. This is irritation waiting to happen!

☺ **Combination Skin Moisture Oil-Free** *($9.50 for 4 ounces)*. Supposedly this moisturizer can "put moisture in dry areas [and] take shine out of oily areas." There is no way this product can hold back its moisturizing agents for some areas and absorb oil in oily areas. Everything gets deposited all over. It's a good, standard, light-weight moisturizer for someone with normal to slightly dry skin, and that's about it.

☺ **Healthy Skin Anti-Wrinkle Cream with Retinol** *($12.49 for 1.4 ounces)* climbs aboard the retinol bandwagon and is identical in many ways to Avon's Retinol Recovery Complex or Estee Lauder's Diminish. It can be good as a lightweight but standard moisturizer for someone with normal to dry skin, but that's about it. There is no substantiating research indicating that retinol can behave like Retin-A, but if you're looking for retinol, this is as good a one as any.

☹ **Healthy Skin Anti-Wrinkle Cream SPF 15** *($12.49 for 1.4 ounces)* doesn't contain the UVA-protecting ingredients of titanium dioxide, zinc oxide, or avobenzone, and is not recommended. It does have retinol, but to fight wrinkling, what it really needs is a sunscreen with UVA protection.

☹ **Healthy Skin Face Lotion with SPF 15** *($9.46 for 2.5 ounces)* doesn't contain the UVA-protecting ingredients of titanium dioxide, zinc oxide, or avobenzone, and is not recommended. Neutrogena needs to discontinue this one as it is clearly aware of the UVA issue; many of its other sunscreens excel in that arena.

☺ **Healthy Skin Eye Cream** *($9.46 for 0.5 ounce)*. The little bit of glycolic acid in here and the high pH make this a rather mundane moisturizing cream, not an exfoliant.

☺ **Healthy Skin Face Lotion** *($12.49 for 2.5 ounces)* is a decent 8% AHA moisturizer containing glycolic acid in a standard (but good) moisturizing base for someone with normal to dry skin.

☺ **Healthy Skin Face Lotion Delicate Skin** *($11.49 for 2.5 ounces)* is identical to the original Healthy Skin Face Lotion in almost every way except that the Delicate Skin version contains about a 5% concentration of glycolic acid. It has a good pH, which makes this an option for a more gentle AHA product that still has some effectiveness for exfoliation. It is best for someone with normal to dry skin.

☹ **Intensified Day Moisture SPF 15** *($11.49 for 2.25 ounces)* doesn't contain the UVA-protecting ingredients titanium dioxide, zinc oxide, or avobenzone, and is not recommended.

☺ **Intensified Eye Moisture 12-Hour Hydration** *($7.57 for 0.5 ounce)* is a good moisturizer for normal to dry skin.

☺ **Light Night Cream Won't Clog Pores** *($10.50 for 2.25 ounces)*. Many of the thickeners in this moisturizer could indeed clog pores, and the oils would make the skin feel greasy. This is a very standard, boring moisturizer for someone with normal to dry skin, but I wouldn't call it light.

☺ **Moisture Non-Comedogenic Facial Moisturizer for Sensitive Skin** *($9.50 for 2 ounces)* is almost identical to the Light Night Cream above and the same comments apply.

☹ **Moisture Non-Comedogenic Facial Moisturizer SPF 15 Sheer Tint** *($9.50 for 4 ounces)* doesn't contain the UVA-protecting ingredients titanium dioxide, zinc oxide, or avobenzone, and is not recommended.

☹ **Moisture Non-Comedogenic Facial Moisturizer SPF 15 Untinted** *($9.50 for 4 ounces)* doesn't contain the UVA-protecting ingredients titanium dioxide, zinc oxide, or avobenzone, and is not recommended.

☺ **Pore Refining Cream** *($14.99 for 1 ounce)* is an AHA-type moisturizer, but I wouldn't recommend it to prevent breakouts or clogged pores. The amount of AHA is about 4% to 5%, which is OK for sensitive skin, but the pH isn't appropriate for it to be an effective exfoliant. It does contain retinol, at the same low percentage as all retinol products on the market. Altogether, this is good for dry skin but that's about it.

☺ **Pore Refining Cream SPF 15** *($13.99 for 1 ounce)* is a good in-part avobenzone-based sunscreen in a rather boring, moisturizing base. It does contain AHA but the pH is too high for it to be effective as an exfoliant. It also contains retinol but that has no effect on pores.

☹ **Pore Refining Mattifier** *($11.99 for 0.5 ounce)* is primarily a silicone-based creamy-feeling gel that does make skin look smooth, but it has a fairly silky texture and doesn't create a very convincing matte finish. The tiny amount of BHA in here is not effective for exfoliation due to the high pH of the product. It does contain fragrance. It's worth a try for someone with normal to slightly dry or slightly oily skin, but don't rely on this to hold back an oily feel for very long if at all.

☹ **Oil-Absorbing Acne Mask Natural Clay Mask 5% Benzoyl Peroxide** *($5.70 for 2 ounces)* contains benzoyl peroxide, and that's a great way to disinfect blemish-prone skin, but it would be far better in an irritant-free gel or liquid than in a clay mask used only occasionally.

☹ **Oil Absorbing Drying Gel for Oily Skin Control** *($3.50 for 0.75 ounce).* Alcohol won't control oil, and it is definitely irritating and drying. In fact, all this product can really do is dry and irritate the skin.

☺ **Deep Pore Treatment** *($7 for 2 ounces)* does contain about 1% salicylic acid (BHA) in a nonirritating gel base, though the pH of 4.5 is borderline for being able to exfoliate skin.

☺ **Clear Pore Treatment Nighttime Pore Clarifying Gel Salicylic Acid Acne Treatment** *($6.75 for 2 ounces)* is similar to the one above, only this one contains 2% BHA, and the same review applies.

☹ **Skin Clearing Moisturizer with 2% BHA** *($11.99 for 1 ounce)* is similar to the Clear Pore Treatment above with 2% salicylic acid, only this one is a rather mundane moisturizing base that would be an option for someone with normal to slightly dry skin. The pH of 4.5 makes it minimally passable for reliable exfoliation. It also contains the tiniest amount of retinol imaginable. It does contain fragrance.

☹ **Maximum Strength Oil-Controlling Pads, Salicylic Acid Acne Medication** *($3.80 for 50 pads)* contains almost 50% alcohol, which is too irritating and drying for all skin types.

☺ **Multi-Vitamin Acne Treatment** *($5.12 for 2.5 ounces)* is a lotion with 1.5% salicylic acid along with 4% to 5% glycolic acid. This would be an interesting combination of AHA and BHA to try, given the potential effectiveness of each, though the pH of 4.5 is borderline for being able to exfoliate skin. The vitamins in here have no effect on acne, though they are good moisturizing ingredients.

☺ **On-the-Spot Acne Treatment Tinted Formula 2.5% Benzoyl Peroxide** *($6.75 for 0.75 ounce)* contains benzoyl peroxide, and that's a great way to disinfect blemish-prone skin, but it would be far better in product that didn't have such a strange, peach-colored tint.

☺ **On-the-Spot Acne Treatment Vanishing Formula 2.5% Benzoyl Peroxide** *($6.75 for 0.75 ounce)* is identical to the version above only minus the strange color.

☺ **UVA/UVB Sunblock SPF 45** *($7.99 for 4 ounces)* is an excellent sunscreen with UVA-protecting avobenzone (trade name Parsol 1789); however, the SPF 45 doesn't get you "better" protection, just longer protection. Remember, an SPF 2 blocks about 50% of the UVB rays; an SPF 10 filters out about 85% of the UVB rays; an SPF 15 stops about 95%, and an SPF 30 through SPF 50 stops about 97%, and about the same goes for the UVA part of the protection (but that's determined solely by the active ingredient, not the SPF number).

☺ **Sensitive Skin UVA/UVB Block SPF 17** *(8.99 for 4 ounces)* and **Sensitive Skin UVA/UVB Block SPF 30** *($8.99 for 4 ounces)* are the sunscreens to check out if you have sensitive skin; they have a wonderful smooth feel and would be excellent for normal to dry, sensitive skin. The titanium dioxide (along with zinc oxide) used here has minimal to no chance of causing skin irritation or a sensitizing skin reaction, while other forms of sunscreen ingredients can be a problem for sensitive skin types. It is also important to note that these two Neutrogena versions are fragrance- and color-additive free—wow!

☹ **Dry Oil Spray SPF 15** *($8.39 for 3.5 ounces)* doesn't contain the UVA-protecting ingredients titanium dioxide, zinc oxide, or avobenzone, and is not recommended.

☹ **Kids Sunblock, SPF 30** *($7 for 4 ounces)* doesn't contain the UVA-protecting ingredients titanium dioxide, zinc oxide, or avobenzone, and is not recommended.

☹ **Oil-Free Sunblock, SPF 30** *($9 for 4 ounces)* doesn't contain the UVA-protecting ingredients titanium dioxide, zinc oxide, or avobenzone, and is not recommended.

☹ **Sunblock SPF 30** *($5.50 for 2.25 ounces)* doesn't contain the UVA-protecting ingredients titanium dioxide, zinc oxide, or avobenzone, and is not recommended.

☹ **Sunblock SPF 15** *($7.99 for 4 ounces)* doesn't contain the UVA-protecting ingredients titanium dioxide, zinc oxide, or avobenzone, and is not recommended.

☹ **Sunblock Spray SPF 20** *($7.20 for 4 ounces)* doesn't contain the UVA-protecting ingredients titanium dioxide, zinc oxide, or avobenzone, and is not recommended.

☹ **Sunblock Stick, SPF 25** *($5.30 for 0.42 ounce)* doesn't contain the UVA-protecting ingredients titanium dioxide, zinc oxide, or avobenzone, and is not recommended.

☹ **Transparent Sun Block Gel SPF 30** *($8.39 for 4 ounces)* doesn't contain the UVA-protecting ingredients titanium dioxide, zinc oxide, or avobenzone, and is not recommended.

☹ **Waterproof Sunblock, SPF 15** *($7.30 for 2.25 ounces)* doesn't contain the UVA-protecting ingredients titanium dioxide, zinc oxide, or avobenzone, and is not recommended.

☺ **Sunless Tanning Lotion, SPF 8, Deep Glow, Non-Streaking Formula** *($9 for 4 ounces)* doesn't contain the UVA-protecting ingredients titanium dioxide, zinc oxide, or avobenzone, and is therefore not recommended for outdoor use, but as a self tanner it works as well as any, using dihydroxyacetone as the ingredient to turn skin brown. (By the way, all self tanners can streak, but that has to do with the application, not the formulation.)

☺ **Sunless Tanning Lotion, SPF 8, Light/Medium Natural-Looking Color, Non-Streaking Formula** *($7.19 for 4 ounces)* is similar to the version above and the same comments apply.

☹ **Lip Moisturizer, SPF 15 with PABA-free Sunblock Protection** *($3.29 for 0.15 ounce)* doesn't contain titanium dioxide, avobenzone, or zinc oxide, and is not recommended.

## Neutrogena Makeup

<u>FOUNDATION:</u> ☺ **Healthy Skin Liquid Makeup SPF 20** *($9.99)* is an all titanium dioxide–based SPF that has a slightly dry, matte finish. It blends on sheer and even with 16 shades, and there are lots of options for those with normal to oily skin. The SPF is great, though without testers you are left guessing which color would look best on you until you buy it and take it home. There are several colors to avoid, but that still leaves a good number of shades to choose from. Neutrogena did far better with its lighter shades than it did with the darker ones; most all the colors to avoid are for deeper skin tones. All of these are just too peach or pink for most skin tones: Warm Caramel, Spiced Almond, Rose Cream, Real Pecan, Rich Sable, and Soft Mahogany.

☺ **Skin Clearing Oil Free Compact Foundation** *($11.39)* is a thick, creamy-textured cream-to-powder makeup that uses aluminum starch (can be an irritant though a good absorbent) and some thickening agents that just aren't the best for oily skin—that is, the people to whom this one is being marketed. Although it does have a rather dry matte finish that would please someone with oily skin, the 12 shades are all too peach, pink, or orange to recommend, especially without any testers at the store to see if they can blend unseen into your skin tone. The teeny amount of salicylic acid (BHA) comes with the wrong pH and has virtually no effect on breakouts. If you decide to try this, save your receipt!

☹ **Cream Powder Makeup SPF 20** *($9.99)* doesn't have UVA protection, and I have no idea how they overlooked that one. Most all of the 16 colors are extremely pink, peach, or ash. Plus the texture is very thick and the heavy wax and starch in here just don't feel great on the skin. There are far better cream-to-powder options available.

☹ <u>CONCEALER:</u> **Under Cover Concealer** *($6.29)* comes in a stick, with five shades to choose from, of which two are meant as color correctors (in shades of yellow and green), which do not work to even out the skin tone. The regular shades are fairly peach, which may work for some skin tones, but this concealer easily creases into the lines under the eyes and is just not worth the risk.

☺ <u>POWDER:</u> **Fresh Finish Loose Powder** *($11.75)* and **Fresh Finish Pressed Powder** *($11.75)* have five shades each. Unfortunately, the way these products are packaged, you can't see the shades. They do have a soft, silky finish, and the colors are actually quite attractive, but due to the packaging, the chances of getting the wrong shade are pretty good. By the way, the light-diffusing claim these powders make is completely unrealistic. **SPF 30 Pressed Powder** *($14.29)* is a one-of-a-kind product, a pressed powder with a reliable SPF 30 that uses titanium dioxide as its active ingredient. While Olay debuted a similar product slightly before this one came out, Olay's is an SPF 15, so Neutrogena doubles the ante. Regardless of which one you may test, because both are excellent, I am skeptical that anyone is going to apply a powder sunscreen liberally enough to get the stated SPF protection. However, as a touch-up for makeup as the day goes by to enhance the sun protection you are already wearing (from foundation or moisturizer), this is an excellent idea. (Do keep in mind that an SPF 30, when applied properly, does not equal double *protection,* it only doubles the *length of time* you can stay in the sun and provides only about 3% more protection from UV penetration than SPF 15.) The three available shades are fine, but there are no options for darker skin tones.

☺ **Skin Clearing Oil-Free Pressed Powder** *($11.69)* has a dry, smooth texture and an almost too powdery finish. Plus, the three colors are all too peach for most skin. The inclusion of salicylic acid in a powder is never effective, as the very ingredients that compose a powder have too high a pH to allow the BHA to work as an exfoliant.

☺ <u>BLUSH:</u> **Soft Color Blush** *($9.75)* does have a small amount of shine but also a soft, even finish and an enticing range of nine shades. The hyped vitamins in here are so negligible you can overlook the inane claim that they are somehow good for the skin.

☺ <u>LIPSTICK:</u> **Lip Plush SPF 20** *($7.99)* is a good but fairly greasy-textured lipstick. The SPF lacks any UVA protection, in spite of its impressive number.

☺ <u>MASCARA:</u> **Full Length Defining Mascara** *($6.69)* is a decent mascara but by no means thrilling or a must-have. It builds OK length and doesn't clump or smear, and that's good, but not exciting. **Full Volume Fortifying Mascara** *($6.69)* is a decent mascara that could be much better. It does add some amount of length but little volume and not much thickness, plus it takes awhile to do this. For decent length without clumps or smearing, it performs nicely.

# Neways Skin Care

There are probably many of you who received a slew of spam e-mails in 1999 with headlines emblazoned with the warning that your cosmetics may be killing you. The message then went on to explain why everything from mineral oil to sodium lauryl sulfate, propylene glycol, and even clay (bentonite) were evil and the cosmetics industry was purposely trying to hurt your skin or at the very least help you get cancer. I spent quite a bit of time dispelling the myths propagated in that e-mail (as did many other Web sites, of which my favorite is http://urbanlegends.miningco.com). From every indication (and directly from the company's Web site), the information in that e-mail turned out to be generated by Neways. The brochure for Neways states: "We recognized years ago that there existed a real need for more healthful alternatives to … mass-produced personal care products. … We were astonished to find that potentially unhealthy, toxic, and damaging chemicals are included in many cosmetics, lotions, and treatments applied day after day to the skin and hair. … Believing that most existing companies were not willing to supply safer, more natural products by sacrificing the exorbitant profits made possible by cheap ingredients, we chose to do so ourselves." So almost everyone else is killing you but Neways.

As is usually the case with companies like Neways that make claims about being all natural, they warn you about so-called "dangerous" ingredients by taking information out of context (please see Chapter 1, "Crazy Things You See on the Web" for more information) but then leave out the information about the problematic, completely unnatural ingredients they use. For example, Neways uses sodium C14-16 olefin sulfate in one of its cleansers, which is an extremely irritating ingredient. It also uses the preservatives methylcholorisothiazolinone and methylisothiazolinone, which are so potent they are only allowed in rinse-off products due to the problems they can cause if left on the skin. Even more disingenuous is that Neways uses PVP/hexadecane copolymer and polyacrylamide, forms of plastic that couldn't get much more unnatural if you tried (not to mention suffocating, something Neways really wants you to worry about from other ingredients—which is all bogus). Another Neways ingredient is perfluoropolymethylisopropyl ether—now doesn't that sound like something you can put on a salad? It also uses phenoxyethanol, a formaldehyde-releasing preservative. The spin it puts on other cosmetic companies' contents is clearly not one it uses for itself.

I could go on and on (wait until you read about its product that is supposed to help tanning!) about the absurd claims this company propagates but you'll get the gist in the reviews below. As usual it's not that Neways products are bad but its marketing techniques create a false pretense that lead the consumer down a primrose path that doesn't exist. For more information, call (800) 326-3051 or visit the Web site at www.neways.com.

☹ **1st Impression Cleanser/Clear Up Cleanser** *($10.95 for 4 ounces)* uses sodium C14-16 olefin sulfate as the main detergent cleansing agent, which makes it potentially too drying and irritating for most skin types. Several of the plant extracts in here are also potential skin irritants, including yarrow and papaya, but they would probably be rinsed down the drain before they could have an effect.

☺ **Extra Gentle Cleanser/Veri-Gentle** *($10.95 for 4 ounces)* is a standard detergent-based water-soluble cleanser that can be an option for most skin types. It does contain fragrance.

☺ **TLC/Facial Cleansing Lotion** *($6.95 for 4 ounces)* is a wipe-off cleanser that can leave a greasy film on the skin, though it is an option for someone with dry skin. It is actually a better moisturizer than it is a cleanser. It does contain fragrance.

☺ **$$$ Milky Cleanser** *($16.15 for 4.2 ounces)* is similar to the Facial Cleansing Lotion above and the same basic comments apply.

☺ **Barrier Cream/Protector** *($22.50 for 8 ounces)* is a good, though ordinary moisturizer for normal to dry skin.

☺ **Bio-Mist Activator/Moisture Mist** *($10.50 for 4 ounces)* contains red raspberry leaf and witch hazel, which are potential skin irritants and not recommended.

☺ **$$$ Retention Plus** *($49.45 for 1 ounce)* is a good emollient moisturizer for normal to dry skin. The form of vitamin A in here is not retinol and even if it were, the amount is so microscopic as to be barely present.

☺ **Skin Enhancer Beauty Lotion** *($29.95 for 4 ounces)* is a very good moisturizer for normal to dry skin. The yeast in here is no miracle ingredient and the teeny amount wouldn't raise one grain of flour.

☺ **$$$ Wrinkle Drops** *($80 for 0.5 ounce).* The AHA in here isn't more than 2%, which isn't enough to be an exfoliant. Other than that this is just a good, toner-like moisturizer for someone with normal to slightly dry skin. The elastin in here cannot affect the elastin in your skin.

☺ **$$$ Wrinkle Gard** *($49.95 for 1 ounce)* won't prevent one wrinkle but it is a good emollient moisturizer for normal to dry skin.

☺ **Great Tan SPF 10** *($11.45 for 1.7 ounces).* The SPF number is dismal and it doesn't contain UVA protection, though the dihydroxyacetone in here is the same all self tanners use and there are far less expensive versions to consider.

☺ **Sunbrero SPF 30** *($15.75 for 4.2 ounces)* is a very good, in-part zinc oxide–based sunscreen that would be an option for someone with normal to dry skin.

☺ **Rebound After Sun Lotion** *($41.95 for 4.2 ounces)* is a very good moisturizer for normal to dry skin with some good water-binding agents and a soothing agent, though nothing that will reduce the redness and damage from unprotected sun exposure.

☹ **Lightning Skin Discoloration Drops** *($19.95 for 1 ounce)*. The lemon and sugarcane in here are not AHAs and cannot exfoliate skin. The teeny amount of citrus extract in here has no real impact on skin. This also contains minute amounts of mulberry root extract and magnesium ascorbyl phosphate, which have been shown to inhibit melanin production but not in the amounts this product contains.

☺ **Imperfection Lotion** *($16.55 for 1 ounce)* contains willow bark, which is not the same as salicylic acid (BHA). Please refer to the Cosmetic Ingredient Dictionary in the Appendix for more information. Other than that it is just a good lightweight moisturizer for normal to slightly dry skin.

☻ **Snap Back Stretch Mark and Eye Bag Cream** *($32.55 for 1.7 ounces)*. There is nothing in here that can change sags, bags, or stretch marks any place on your body. It's just an OK moisturizer that contains arnica, a skin irritant that should not be applied repeatedly on skin.

☻ **Tanacity Tanning Accelerator** *($22.45 for 4.2 ounces)*. While this may be a good moisturizer for dry skin, the claims are frightening. "Tanacity may help to prepare your skin for this onslaught of ultra violet rays by enhancing your body's melanin production. This is part of its own protective tanning response. Your skin can be more prepared for exposure of UV rays with Tanacity." This is a dangerous notion because any unprotected sun exposure can lead to sun damage and the best a tan can protect is an SPF 2 or 4.

# Nicole Miller Skin Care

Nicole Miller is a fashion designer who has entered the world of skin care in a way that distantly resembles the efforts of fashion designer Donna Karan. The difference is that Miller seems to have established a following of devotees who believe in the company's mission to bring the wondrous benefits of its products to the world. That's because Nicole Miller Skin Care is a multilayer direct-marketing line along the lines of Amway, Shaklee, and Mary Kay. I am not going to begin to try to review all the details about how you can buy these products at a discount (a big marketing point for this line with a membership fee) or sell them to others as well as encourage others to also sell them, because the nuances of business arrangements like these are far beyond the kind of reviews I do.

The line's primary promise is to offer products to keep women from wrinkling. It seems that almost every plant and vitamin is thrown into these formulations. One of my favorite lines from the company's Web site is this: if "you're already using an eye makeup remover, why not use one that actually repairs and moisturizes your skin? Why not use a moisturizer that has more anti-aging ingredients than most specialty serums?" Makes me wonder what those other specialty serums are that contain these so-called antiaging ingredients Miller is referring to, and do they cost less money?—but I digress.

These products definitely have some of the longest ingredient listings I've ever run into, and that can be a problem for sensitive-skin types, because it just means there are more variables with components that can cause reactions. However, they also include a rather impressive assortment of moisturizers with excellent water-binding agents and good antioxidants.

While it is almost impossible to engage in a critique of every plant used in these formulations (because it is literally a cornucopia), suffice it to say there is no research showing that any of them, from spirulina to red clover and sugarcane extract to cranberry extract, have any antiaging properties that will get rid of one wrinkle on your face. That's not to say, for example, that a pure tincture of red clover may not have a positive effect on eczema, or that aloe doesn't have some anti-inflammatory properties, or that bladderwrack or chamomile can't have some anti-irritant effects on the skin, and on and on. But in the amounts these ingredients are used in cosmetics, watered down and mixed with dozens of other ingredients, preserved, and then packaged in clear glass containers or jars where air floods into the product, there is little evidence that any residual benefit would be left.

In the midst of all these purportedly miraculous ingredients, this line sells only two sunscreens as part of the daily skin-care routine. One is an SPF 6, the other an SPF 8, and neither has UVA-protecting ingredients. I consider that deplorable, as do most medical authorities, ranging from oncologists to the American Academy of Dermatology. Claiming to have a reputable skin-care line with this glaring deficiency in the lineup is nothing less than disturbing. Trusting any of the glorious claims about fighting wrinkles is ill advised, given this glaring omission. It would be like saying you can fight lung cancer and smoke at the same time!

For more information about Nicole Miller Skin Care, visit the Web site at www.nicolemillerskincare.com or call (888) 2-NICOLE.

☺ $$$ **Renew Creamy Cleanser** (*$24 for 4.2 ounces*) is an emollient, cold cream–like product. It needs to be wiped off and can leave a slight greasy film on the skin.

☺ **$$$ Renew Foaming Facial Cleanser** *($24 for 4.2 ounces)* is a standard, detergent-based water-soluble cleanser. It will clean the face and work well for normal to oily skin. This is supposed to contain "hydroxy acid" but the sugarcane and other extracts in here aren't reliable or effective forms of alpha hydroxy acids, nor would they be of much use in a cleanser where they would be rinsed down the drain along with the vitamins and other plant extracts in here.

☺ **$$$ Gentle Care Eye Makeup Remover** *($15 for 4.6 ounces)* is a standard eye-makeup remover. The vitamins and plants in here can't change a wrinkle, but the amount of them is so minimal that even if they could, there wouldn't be enough to have an effect.

☹ **Freshen Balancing Toner** *($20 for 7.4 ounces)*. The tiny bit of lactic acid in here does not make this an effective AHA product. The witch hazel can be a skin irritant.

☹ **Revitalize Hydroxy Creme** *($30 for 1 ounce)* is supposed to be an AHA moisturizer but the pH is too high for it to be effective for that. Other than that, it is a good basic moisturizer for normal to dry skin. There are some great water-binding agents in here.

☹ **Revitalize Gentle Hydroxy Creme** *($30 for 1 ounce)* is almost identical to the version above and the same comments apply.

☻ **Daytime Delivery Moisturizing Creme SPF 8** *($38 for 1.7 ounces)* doesn't contain the UVA-protecting ingredients of avobenzone, zinc oxide, or titanium dioxide, and is not recommended. I won't even get started on the issue of SPF 8.

☻ **Daytime Delivery Moisturizing Lotion SPF 6** *($34 for 1.7 ounces)* doesn't contain the UVA-protecting ingredients of avobenzone, zinc oxide, or titanium dioxide, and is not recommended. If an SPF 8 isn't embarrassing enough for a skin-care line touting miraculous benefits, an SPF 6 makes any other claim utterly inept and pathetic.

☹ **$$$ Night Release Moisturizing Creme** *($40 for 1 ounce)* is supposed to contain AHAs, but the sugarcane, citrus, and apple extracts here are not AHAs, and even if they were, the pH of this product doesn't allow for exfoliation. It would be a good moisturizer for normal to dry skin but that's it.

☺ **$$$ Delicate Repair Eye Gel** *($32 for 0.5 ounce)* is a good silicone-based moisturizer with an interesting and effective array of water-binding agents.

☺ **$$$ Eyewear Refirming Creme** *($24 for 0.5 ounce)* is less elegant than others in the line but it is a good moisturizer for dry skin. It does contain aluminum starch (octenylsuccinate) rather high up in the ingredient listing and that's strange in a moisturizer meant to be used for dry skin around the eyes.

☺ **$$$ Multi-Action Vitamin Complex** *($40 for 1 ounce)* has the same vitamins, if not fewer, than others in the line, so the need for this is at best extraneous, though it would be good for normal to slightly dry skin.

☺ **$$$ Ageless Intensive Recovery Serum** *($44 for 1 ounce)* won't change the aging process for one cell on your face but it is a good moisturizer for normal to slightly dry skin. The amount of BHA in here is less than 1% and the pH is too high for it have any exfoliating benefits.

☺ **$$$ Cellular Delivery Hydrating Mask** *($24 for 4.2 ounces)* would be a good mask for dry skin, but it's really more a moisturizer than anything else.

## Nivea Visage (Skin Care Only)

For more information about Nivea, call (800) 233-2340 or (800) 925-4832 or visit the Web site at www.nivea.com.

☺ **Foaming Facial Cleanser Deep-Cleansing Formula** *($5.49 for 6 ounces)* is a standard, detergent-based water-soluble cleanser that can be an option for normal to dry skin. The tiny amount of lanolin in here has no real impact on skin. It does contain fragrance.

☹ **Gentle Moisturizing Cleanser** *($5.29 for 6.8 ounces)* is a standard, mineral oil–based cleanser that doesn't rinse off very well and doesn't take off all the makeup without the aid of a washcloth. It can be an option, but only for dry skin. It does contain fragrance.

☹ **Eye Make-Up Remover** *($4.99 for 2.5 ounces)* is a standard, but good makeup remover with no coloring agents (don't let the blue-colored tube fool you), and it's also fragrance-free. That's great. The lotion form spreads easily with no greasy or sticky after-feel despite the mineral oil content.

☺ **Alcohol Free Moisturizing Facial Toner** *($5.49 for 6 ounces)* is a soothing, lightly moisturizing, fairly irritant-free toner.

☹ **Anti-Wrinkle and Firming Creme, with Vitamins A and E, SPF 4** *($9.39 for 1.7 ounces)*, with its SPF 4, is just embarrassing. Why would anyone even put that number on their product, and with no UVA-protecting ingredients to boot? The risk of sun damage with this product is certain. As a moisturizer, it is OK but fairly standard, containing mostly thickeners, fragrance, and preservatives. The teeny amount of retinyl palmitate (vitamin A) is almost laughable.

☹ **Q10 Wrinkle Control SPF 4** *($11.29 for 1.7 ounces)* and **Q10 Wrinkle Control Eye SPF 6** *($11.29 for 0.5 ounce)*, both contain coenzyme Q10. Any skin-care company claiming to know something about healthy skin care but still willing to sell such terrible SPF products is either showing its ignorance to the world or turning a blind eye to selling products that truly help skin. What about the coenzyme Q10? It is a dietary supplement with significant research about its positive effects when taken orally. But for the face? It turns out that despite all the research available on coenzyme Q10, there is none establishing its effect on skin other than it being a good antioxidant. Please refer to the section on coenzyme Q10 in Chapter Two of this book for more details. Aside from coenzyme Q10 (which is just one of many good antioxidants used in cosmetics), these aren't bad moisturizers, just very standard, boring ones with no reliable sun protection. The eye cream, however, is more emollient than the face version so the price variation is just bizarre given the similarities between the two products.

☹ **Q10 Wrinkle Control Lotion SPF 15** *($8.99 for 3 ounces)* does not contain the UVA-protecting ingredients titanium dioxide, zinc oxide, or avobenzone, and is not recommended. Even if there was research to support the notion that coenzyme Q10 was good for skin, the sunscreen formulation here would negate any possible benefit by allowing UVA radiation to damage skin.

☺ **Q10 Wrinkle Control Night** *($9.99 for 1.7 ounces)* is a good emollient moisturizer for normal to dry skin. For information about the antioxidant properties of coenzyme Q10, see the Q10 Wrinkle Control SPF 4 review above.

☹ **Daily Nourishing Creme Essential Daily Moisturizer SPF 4** *($5.39 for 1.7 ounces)* also has a very low SPF 4, which is almost a guarantee of sun damage if you're relying on this for daily protection, plus it doesn't contain the UVA-protecting ingredients avobenzone, titanium dioxide, or zinc oxide, and is absolutely not recommended.

☹ **Daily Nourishing Lotion Essential Daily Moisturizer SPF 4** *($6.39 for 3 ounces)* has the same review as the one above.

☹ **Shine Control Mattifying Fluid Oil-Absorbing Moisturizer SPF 4** *($6.39 for 3 ounces)* contains several ingredients that could be problematic for someone with oily skin, and the SPF 4 is too low for anyone to consider wearing during the day. What a shame, because this one does have an in-part titanium dioxide sunscreen base.

☺ **Soothing Eye Gel** *($9.99 for 0.5 ounce)* is a very good lightweight moisturizer for normal to dry skin.

☹ **Tinted Moisturizer SPF 4 (Fair to Light and Medium to Dark)** *($8.99 for 1.7 ounces)* is an exceptionally standard but good moisturizer for normal to dry skin. The fragrance is intense and tends to last on the face longer than you may want it to, and the SPF 4 can be a serious problem for skin if you are relying on this for sun protection, plus it doesn't contain UVA-protecting ingredients. The two shades are slightly on the rosy side, but only slightly, and they disappear to almost nothing when blended on.

☹ **Triple Protection Moisture Lotion, SPF 15** *($9.39 for 3 ounces)* doesn't have much going for it. It may be a decent moisturizer, but it doesn't contain the UVA-protecting ingredients avobenzone, titanium dioxide, or zinc oxide, and is not recommended.

☹ **Cream** *($3.49 for 2 ounces)* is the original Nivea Cream, and it hasn't changed much over the years. It's incredibly basic but it is very good, though heavy, for very dry skin.

☺ **Original Skin Oil** *($4.99 for 8 ounces)* is like mineral oil with a tiny bit of lanolin and Vaseline added. It's incredibly basic, but very good for extremely dry skin.

☺ **Sheer Moisture Spray** *($4.99 for 6.8 ounces),* If the notion of spraying a mist of mineral oil on your face sounds good, then this is the only product I know that does it. This is a very ordinary moisturizer that is an option for dry skin.

## Nivea Vital

This line extension from Nivea is supposed to be special skin care for mature skin. First, not all woman who are "mature" (whatever age that is meant to be) have the same skin type. Second, there isn't anything about these products that is special for older skin. The formulations are good moisturizers but not anything unique or special, and without a sunscreen they aren't even worth your attention as a set. Nivea Vital is only available via mail order, by calling (888) 368-7797.

☺ **Mild Foaming Cleanser, Provitamin B5** *($6.99 for 5 ounces)* is a standard, detergent-based water-soluble cleanser that would work well for most skin types, but would probably be drying for those with dry to very dry skin.

☺ **Daily Moisture Cream, Vitamin Complex** *($10.99 for 1.7 ounces).* If you don't need the sunscreen protection, it would be fine for dry skin for day or night.

☺ **Restorative Night Cream, Vitamin Complex** *($10.99 for 1.7 ounces)* is almost identical to the version above and the same comments apply.

☺ **Firming Vitamin Treatment** *($15.99 for 1 ounce)* is a very good lightweight moisturizer for normal to dry skin.

## Noevir (Skin Care Only)

Noevir's self-declared claim to fame is attributed to Dr. Suzuki (creator of the Noevir product line), who was "one of the few scientists with a Ph.D. in cosmetics research." Actually, the area of cosmetics research is filled with Ph.D.s from all sorts of disciplines: medical, chemical, and cosmetics research. Suzuki hardly stands alone, so that claim is just out of whack. Another quote from the literature: "The medical profession supports Noevir's belief that products with mineral oil and other petroleum-based products are not beneficial to the skin." That could not be further from the truth; there are plenty of studies demonstrating that mineral oil and Vaseline are just fine and quite useful for the skin, and I have never seen any studies or data anywhere indicating the opposite.

What is most disturbing about this line of products that feature all kinds of gimmicky ingredients—from plant extracts (many that are potential skin irritants) to umbilical extract—is that Noevir doesn't have a sunscreen as part of its daily skin-care routine. This philosophy is almost prehistoric. In addition, the brochure announces that Noevir products contain no preservatives or fragrances, even though those substances are listed in black and white on the labels!

Almost every Noevir product has an assortment of collagen, placental protein, vitamin E, spleen extract, thymus extract, umbilical extracts, DNA, plant extracts of every kind, and a host of water-binding agents. While thymus, umbilical, and placenta extract can be a source of water-binding agents or emollients for skin, they cannot generate young skin cells. And DNA, thankfully, cannot affect the DNA in your own skin. The water-binding agents in these products are indeed impressive but they are surrounded by lots of absurd price tags and problematic ingredients, along with clearly untrue marketing claims that are all rather disturbing.

Noevir has several different product groupings and a host of specialty items that are very difficult to tell apart because many of the product names (not to mention the formulas) are strikingly identical. The main distinctions seem to be price and implied quality, because the individual products are not that different from one another. This system of product classification reminds me strongly of Shiseido, another Japanese line; I imagine Noevir began as a way to compete with Shiseido's successful department-store line. For more information about Noevir, call (800) 437-2258 or (800) 872-8888 or visit the Web site at www.noevirusa.com.

☺ $$$ 95 **Herbal Cleansing Massage Cream** *($30 for 3.5 ounces)* is a fairly greasy wipe-off cleanser that is almost identical to several cleansers in this line. Massaging it around the face may feel good, but you can do that with almost any oil-based moisturizer, most of which cost a lot less. This needs to be wiped off, which can be a option for dry skin, although some of the plant extracts can be significant skin irritants, including coltsfoot, balm mint, yarrow, and sage.

☺ $$$ 95 **Herbal Facial Cleanser** *($30 for 3.5 ounces)* is a standard, detergent-based water-soluble cleanser that can be somewhat drying for many skin types. Who thought up these prices for such a basic product? Several of the plant extracts in here can be significant skin irritants, including coltsfoot, balm mint, yarrow, and sage.

☹ 95 **Herbal Cleansing Rinse** *($20 for 5 ounces)* is a standard, alcohol-based toner that also contains some water-binding agents, but they won't counteract the drying and irritating effects of the alcohol.

☹ 95 **Herbal Skin Balancing Lotion** *($30 for 4 ounces)* is a standard, alcohol-based toner that also contains some good water-binding agents, but they won't counteract the drying and irritating effects of the alcohol.

☹ 95 **Herbal Enriched Moisturizer** *($36 for 3.3 ounces)* would be a good moisturizer for normal to dry skin types except that the second ingredient is alcohol, which has no place in a moisturizer. Several of the plant extracts in here can be significant skin irritants, including coltsfoot, balm mint, yarrow, and sage.

☺ $$$ 95 **Herbal Skin Cream** *($40 for 1 ounce)* is a good emollient moisturizer for dry skin. One sales rep explained that using this cream would be like getting baby cells transplanted onto your skin. Nothing could be further from the truth; the placenta protein in here has no special ability to affect skin, it is just a good water-binding agent, and there are many good water-binding agents aside from this offensive choice. Several of the plant extracts in here can be significant skin irritants, including coltsfoot, balm mint, yarrow, and sage.

☺ $$$ 105 **Herbal Cleansing Massage Cream** *($70 for 3.5 ounces)* is virtually identical to many of the other wipe-off cleansers Noevir sells. Wiping off makeup can leave a greasy film on the skin but it can be an option for dry skin. However, given the similarity between the Massage Creams, choose the less-expensive one, because the price for this cleanser is ridiculous. Several of the plant extracts in here can be significant skin irritants, including witch hazel tannin, arnica, yarrow, balm mint, and coltsfoot. For this kind of money, those ingredients should not be in here.

☺ $$$ 105 **Herbal Facial Cleanser** *($56 for 3.5 ounces)* is virtually identical to many of the other detergent-based water-soluble cleansers Noevir sells. It can be drying for most skin types, and it contains tallow, which can cause breakouts. That anyone would charge (or spend) this much money for a cleanser is shocking. Also, several of the plant extracts in here can be significant skin irritants, including witch hazel tannin, ivy, yarrow, balm mint, and coltsfoot.

☹ 105 **Herbal Cleansing Rinse** *($32 for 4 ounces)* is a standard, alcohol-based toner that also contains some water-binding agents, placenta protein, and plant extracts, but they won't counteract the drying and irritating effects of the alcohol.

☹ 105 **Herbal Skin Balancing Lotion** *($62 for 4 ounces)* is virtually identical to all the other alcohol-based toners Noevir sells, with the same list of water-binding agents. Alcohol dries and irritates the skin no matter what else you put in with it.

☹ 105 **Herbal Enriched Moisturizer** *($70 for 2.6 ounces)* is virtually identical to the 95 Herbal Enriched Moisturizer above and the same comments and concerns apply. Why this one is more expensive is anyone's guess.

☺ $$$ 105 **Herbal Skin Cream** *($70 for 0.7 ounce)* is similar to the 95 Herbal Skin Cream above. This is a good emollient moisturizer for dry skin. Several of the plant extracts in here can be significant skin irritants, including coltsfoot, balm mint, yarrow, and sage. This product also contains tallow, which can cause breakouts.

☺ 505 **Revitalizing Balancing Lotion** *($88 for 5 ounces)*. For what is mostly water, glycerin, and alcohol, this is a shocking amount of money. And this product is supposed to be for very dry skin! Several of the plant extracts in here can be significant skin irritants, including coltsfoot, balm mint, yarrow, and sage. The umbilical extract in here cannot make your skin act young, it is just a water-binding agent.

☹ 505 **Hydrating Emulsion** *($132 for 3.3 ounces)* is incredibly overpriced and incredibly similar to the other moisturizers in this line, and alcohol is the fifth ingredient, making it potentially irritating. Other than that, it is just a basic moisturizer with some good water-binding agents and plant oils. That's good, but not for this amount of money.

☺ $$$ **505 Perfecting Cream** *($220 for 1 ounce).* That is the right price—how insulting. This is a good moisturizer for dry skin but there is nothing in here that warrants the price tag. Several of the plant extracts in here can be significant skin irritants, including coltsfoot, yarrow, and sage. The umbilical extract in here cannot make your skin act young, it is just a water-binding agent.

☺ $$$ **Clear Control Clean Wash** *($14 for 2.6 ounces)* is a standard, detergent-based water-soluble cleanser. It would work well for most skin types though it can be drying. It does contain a teeny amount of salicylic acid (BHA), but the pH is too high for it to have any effect as an exfoliant.

☹ **Clear Control Toning Lotion** *($16 for 4 ounces)* is an alcohol-based toner that also contains menthol. That makes it too drying and irritating for all skin types.

☹ **Clear Control Blemish Gel** *($16 for 0.7 ounce)* contains alcohol, which makes this too drying and irritating for all skin types. The BHA in here can exfoliate skin but there are far less irritating, not to mention less expensive, versions to consider.

☺ $$$ **Herbal Skincare Line NHS Deep Cleansing Cream** *($18 for 3.5 ounces)* is a fairly standard wipe-off cleanser that doesn't clean all that deeply. It can leave a film and needs to be wiped off, which can be an option for dry skin. It does contain tallow, which can clog pores, and several of the plant extracts in here can be significant skin irritants, including coltsfoot, balm mint, arnica, yarrow, and sage.

☺ $$$ **Herbal Skincare Line NHS Cleansing Foam** *($18 for 3.8 ounces)* is a standard, detergent-based water-soluble cleanser. It does contain tallow, which can be a problem for breakouts. Several of the plant extracts in here can be significant skin irritants, including coltsfoot, balm mint, arnica, yarrow, and sage.

☹ **Herbal Skincare Line NHS Balancing Lotion Normal to Dry** *($32 for 4 ounces)* is a standard, alcohol-based toner. It does contain some good water-binding agents but they won't counteract the drying and irritating effects of the alcohol. It also contains about 2% AHA, but that's not enough to be effective as an exfoliant.

☹ **Herbal Skincare Line NHS Balancing Lotion Normal to Oily** *($32 for 4 ounces)* is almost identical to the Lotion Normal to Dry above and the same basic comments apply.

☹ **Herbal Skincare Line NHS Enriched Moisture Lotion** *($36 for 3.3 ounces)* lists alcohol as the third ingredient, so this otherwise emollient moisturizer for dry skin can have more problems than benefits. Several of the plant extracts in here can also be significant skin irritants, including coltsfoot, balm mint, yarrow, and sage. It also contains about 2% AHA, which isn't enough to be effective as an exfoliant.

☹ **Herbal Skincare Line NHS Light Moisture Lotion** *($36 for 3.3 ounces)* is similar to the Enriched Moisture Lotion above and the same basic comments apply.

☹ **Whiteness Skincare Toner** *($30 for 4 ounces)* lists alcohol as the second ingredient, and that makes it too irritating and drying for all skin types. However, this does contain magnesium ascorbyl palmitate, a form of vitamin C that when used in a 10% concentration has been shown to inhibit melanin production. Nevertheless, this product has only about a 1% to 2% concentration; in that quantity it's a good antioxidant, but that still won't undo the drying effect of the alcohol. It also contains mulberry bark extract, which does have some value in preventing melanin production, but the research showed that even a pure concentration of it (which this product does not contain) was minimally effective when compared to hydroquinone.

☹ **Whiteness Skincare Emulsion** *($35 for 2.6 ounces)* is similar to the Whiteness Skincare Toner above and the same comments apply.

☹ **Whiteness Skincare Skin Cream** *($45 for 1.7 ounces)* is similar to the Whiteness Skincare Toner above; see that review for information about magnesium ascorbyl phosphate and mulberry bark extract. This is in an emollient base but it contains tallow, which can cause breakouts, and a fair amount of alcohol, which can be a skin irritant.

☺ **Whiteness Skincare Clarifying Masque** *($38 for 2.8 ounces)* is similar to the Whiteness Skincare Toner (see that review for information about magnesium ascorbyl phosphate and mulberry bark extract), only this one contains an even tinier amount of both, making it completely ineffective for skin lightening. By the way, no skin lightener, even the most effective, can have any impact on skin without the consistent use of an effective sunscreen, something Noevir seems to know nothing about.

☹ **Recovery Complex** *($45 for 1 ounce)*. The fruit extracts in here are not the same thing as AHAs, not to mention that the alcohol is a skin irritant and several of the plant extracts in here are also potential skin irritants, including yarrow, sage, balm mint, and thyme.

☺ **$$$ Night Recovery Complex** *($50 for 1 ounce)* is a good lightweight moisturizer for dry skin but there is nothing unique in here that can recover or heal skin.

☺ **$$$ Tirante Face Firming Gel** *($75 for 1.5 ounces)* can't firm anything, it's just a good, though rather basic moisturizer for someone with normal to dry skin.

☺ **$$$ Cleansing Crystals** *($25 for 2.4 ounces)* is a fairly fragrant, standard, detergent-based water-soluble cleanser that uses synthetic scrub particles as the abrasive. The irritating plant extracts of arnica and nettle in here are another concern. The combination can be too drying and irritating for many if not most skin types.

☹ **Advanced Moisture Concentrate** *($65 for 0.83 ounce)*. What a shame they had to stick alcohol in here, because this would be a good, though very overpriced, lightweight moisturizer for normal to dry skin.

☺ $$$ **Extra Moisture Cream** *($40 for 1.2 ounces)* is a very good moisturizer for normal to dry skin. The umbilical extract in here, much like any part of the human or animal body, is a source of proteins, amino acids, and other water-binding agents for skin. It cannot make skin act young just because the source is young. It does contain some potentially irritating and sensitizing plant extracts, including coltsfoot, balm mint, fennel, and sage, though the amounts are probably so small as to have no effect on skin. The glycolic acid and lactic acid in here are in too small an amount to have any exfoliating properties for skin.

☺ $$$ **Eye Treatment Gel** *($65 for 0.52 ounce)* is a good lightweight moisturizer for someone with normal to dry skin. The umbilical and spleen extracts in here serve no special purpose for skin, they are just water-binding agents, period.

☺ $$$ **Intensive Anti-Wrinkle Treatment** *($35 for 0.6 ounce)* is a very good moisturizer for normal to dry skin. The placenta extract in here, much like any part of the human or animal body, is a source of proteins, amino acids, and other water-binding agents for skin. It cannot make skin act young just because the source is young. The amount of glycolic acid (AHA) this contains is too small to have any exfoliating properties for skin. And none of this will get rid of prevent wrinkling.

☹ $$$ **Special Night Cream** *($35 for 0.7 ounce)* is a very standard, heavy moisturizer for someone with dry skin. This is OK but not worth the money.

☻ **Suspension** *($80 for 1 ounce)*. There's too much alcohol in here, and it makes this a problem for all skin types, which is a shame because this would have been a good moisturizer for normal to dry skin.

☹ $$$ **Lip Conditioner** *($9 for 0.12 ounce)* is a good, though standard emollient no-color lipstick.

☻ **Ultimate Peel-Off Masque** *($35 for 2.4 ounces)* places a layer of plastic over your face; after it dries you then peel it off. That can make the skin feel smooth, but this product also contains alcohol and several potentially sensitizing plant extracts, which adds up to dry and irritated skin.

☻ **Clay Masque** *($23 for 3.5 ounces)*. This line puts alcohol in almost everything, and I'm getting tired of warning against it. Except for the alcohol, this could have been a very good clay mask.

## Noxzema (Skin Care Only)

☻ **Original Skin Cream** *($4.31 for 10 ounces)* is one of the most irritating skin-care products around. It contains lye, camphor, menthol, phenol, clove oil, and eucalyptus oil. It hurts my skin just thinking about it.

☻ **Plus Cleansing Cream** *($3.67 for 10 ounces)* is just as seriously irritating as the cream above.

☹ **Plus Cleansing Lotion** *($3.81 for 10.5 ounces)* is just as irritating as the two above, and is not recommended for any skin type.

☺ **Sensitive Cleansing Cream** *($3.67 for 10 ounces)* just isn't a very effective cleanser, but at least they took the irritating ingredients out of this one. It can be an option to clean sensitive, dry skin, if you aren't wearing makeup, though it can leave a film on the skin.

☺ **Sensitive Cleansing Lotion** *($3.25 for 10.5 ounces)* is similar to the Sensitive Cleansing Cream above, and the same review applies.

☹ **Normal Astringent Balanced Deep Cleansing** *($3.19 for 8 ounces)* is mostly alcohol and menthol and is just pure irritation and dryness for skin, nothing more.

☹ **Oily Astringent Salicylic Acid Acne Medication** *($3.19 for 8 ounces)* is mostly alcohol and menthol and is just too irritating for all skin types. The BHA in here is effective for exfoliation but adding that to the irritation from the other ingredients is unwarranted.

☹ **Sensitive Toner** *($3.79 for 8 ounces)* is mostly alcohol, menthol, and fragrance and that would be a problem for all skin types, especially someone with sensitive skin!

☹ **2 in 1 Pads Regular Strength** *($3.67 for 90 pads)* contains a host of irritating ingredients that are damaging to skin, including camphor, menthol, and eucalyptus.

☹ **2 in 1 Pads Maximum Strength** *($3.67 for 90 pads)* is very similar to the Pads above, and the same review applies.

☺ **Skin Fitness Moisture Build Foaming Face Wash** *($4.97 for 6.78 ounces)* is a standard, detergent-based water-soluble cleanser that would work well for someone with normal to oily skin.

☹ **Skin Fitness Pore Purifying Micro-Bead Face Wash** *($4.97 for 6.78 ounces)* contains a few problematic ingredients, including menthol and sodium lauryl sulfate, that can be too irritating for most skin types. Other than that, this is just a standard, detergent-based cleanser with smooth, tiny synthetic beads. There are better ways to scrub the face than this; a washcloth, for example, would be far better.

☹ **Skin Fitness Total Toner Cleansing Discs** *($4.97 for 65 discs)* is a BHA product that contains mostly water and alcohol, and that makes it too drying and irritating for all skin types.

☺ **Skin Fitness Intense Replenishment Oil-Free Moisturizing Cream** *($8.97 for 2 ounces)*. The thickening agents in this product would be a problem for someone with oily skin, and the pH of this product makes the BHA ineffective as an exfoliant.

☺ **Skin Fitness Skin Endurance Oil-Free Moisturizing Lotion** *($8.97 for 4 ounces)* is similar to the one above only in lotion form, and the same comments apply.

# Nu Skin (Skin Care Only)

First I want to say how impressed I was with Nu Skin's straightforward provision of information to the consumer about its ingredient listings. Without hesitation, the company supplied all the information I requested. I wish all companies made their ingredient listings this accessible but, alas, only a handful do. In direct contrast to this consumer-thoughtful assistance, the Nu Skin salespeople were so over-the-top in their presentation that I was left speechless, and for me that is rare. The pressure I experienced to recruit me as a salesperson was intense. Plus, I left with the distinct impression from the salesperson that Nu Skin was busy curing cancer and AIDS and saving the rain forest at the same time rather than making money.

It is far beyond the scope of this book to investigate every claim this company makes for its products, but at least as far as skin care is concerned, I can assure you Nu Skin is not a miracle, a cure, the total answer, or even part of the answer for every woman's skin-care needs. After all, if the products were miraculous for skin care, why did they reformulate and come out with a new line of products making the same claims only with different ingredients? Nevertheless, the people who sell this line want you to believe it can alter your life as well as your skin. Like most of the other lines I've reviewed, this one contains some very good products, some useless ones, and some that are simply overpriced and a waste of money.

What sets Nu Skin apart is its intense direct-marketing strategy and its problems with the law. According to the March 1992 issue of *Drug and Cosmetic Industry* magazine, Nu Skin International has responded to complaints and lawsuits in Ohio, Illinois, Michigan, Florida, and Pennsylvania by voluntarily consenting to change some of its marketing and sales policies. One of the problems was that sales reps, in order to keep their commission percentage up, would overbuy cosmetics and then be stuck with them. After signing agreements with the attorney general's offices in these states, Nu Skin was supposed to refund up to 90 percent of the money its distributors paid for products that went unsold. According to another report in the October 1997 issue of *Cosmetic Dermatology,* Nu Skin International agreed to pay a $1.5 million civil penalty to settle Federal Trade Commission (FTC) charges over claims it made for some of its products. "The FTC alleged that Nu Skin could not produce adequate substantiation for the claims, and that Nu Skin violated a 1994 FTC order requiring the firm to have competent and reliable scientific evidence to support benefit claims for any product they sell." But when you have Christy Brinkley as your new spokesperson, who cares about shoddy business practices?

When it comes to claims, Nu Skin's brochures state that its products have "all of the good and none of the bad," but that depends on how you define "bad." The line has indeed made major improvements in removing the ingredients it used to have in its products, which included peppermint oil, spearmint oil, sulfur, and sulfuric acid. Yet some of the products still contain camphor and many contain fragrance, which are very irritating and known skin sensitizers.

The skin-care presentation I received for the Nu Skin skin-care products was one of the most peculiar I've experienced anywhere. For example, a Clinique toner was set on fire and then compared to the Nu Skin toner that would not light. Of course the reason the Clinique toner was flammable is because it contains alcohol and the Nu Skin one did not ignite because it didn't. But there are lots of skin-care products besides Nu Skin that don't contain alcohol and also therefore aren't flammable. Regardless, flammability doesn't indicate irritation potential anyway. Paper is flammable but it isn't irritating. Camphor doesn't ignite but it is definitely irritating and it shows up in one of Nu Skin's products. I was also shown a pH demonstration indicating that the pH of most bar soaps and cleansers, including expensive ones, was over 8, and most were over 9, but that Nu Skin's bar cleanser was about a pH of 5.5. High pH is definitely a problem for drying and irritating skin, so Nu Skin's bar cleanser is definitely less irritating when it comes to pH. But there are factors besides pH that can cause irritation. The cleansing agent in Nu Skin's bar cleanser is sodium cocoyl isethionate and that can be irritating. Additionally, the ingredients that keep Nu Skin's bar in its solid form can clog pores. I could go on, but this was about as misleading a demonstration as I've seen anywhere in the cosmetics industry.

Another difficulty is that this product line includes almost every gimmick in the book. Some are good for the skin, but most are just for show, to cover all the necessary bases of "natural" skin care: royal bee jelly, human placenta extract, aloe vera, vitamins, wheat germ oil, walnut husks, collagen, jojoba oil, and herbal extracts. As you may have already guessed, the first ingredients—the primary components of the products—are fairly standard ones, such as water, thickeners, water-binding agents, and plant oils.

There are some very good products in the line, but they are not the miracles the company would like you to believe they are. For more information about Nu Skin, call (800) 345-2000 or visit the Web site at www.nuskin.com.

☹ **Cleansing Lotion** *($10.50 for 4.2 ounces)* needs to be wiped off and can leave a greasy feeling on the skin but can be an option for dry skin.

☹ **Facial Cleansing Bar** *($10.30 for 3.5 ounces)* is a standard, detergent-based water-soluble bar cleanser. It can be drying for most skin types.

☺ $$$ **Nu Color Eye Makeup Remover** *($13.15 for 2 ounces)* is a silicone- and plant oil–based wipe-off cleanser that can leave a greasy feel on the skin, but it does work to remove makeup.

☺ $$$ **Exfoliant Scrub Extra Gentle** *($11.95 for 2.5 ounces)* contains mostly water, aloe, glycerin, seashells (as an abrasive), and thickeners. The seashells can be rough on the skin, so calling this product gentle is a stretch, but it is a good exfoliant.

☺ $$$ **Facial Scrub** *($11.45 for 2.5 ounces)* is by far more gentle than the one above, despite the name difference. This one uses walnut-shell powder that does work as a scrub, and it can be good for someone with normal to dry skin.

☹ **MHA Revitalizing Toner** *($10.30 for 4.2 ounces)* could be considered an option for a lightweight AHA and BHA toner except that it contains camphor, which makes it unnecessarily irritating for all skin types.

☹ **pH Balance Facial Toner** *($8.45 for 4.2 ounces)*. The witch hazel and camphor cause irritation, making this toner a problem for all skin types.

☺ **MHA Revitalizing Lotion** *($18 for 1 ounce)* is supposed to be a combination AHA and BHA lotion, but it doesn't have a low-enough pH to make it an effective exfoliant. If this product could exfoliate the skin, and you used it along with the other AHA and BHA combination products in the MHA grouping, you would have a seriously irritated face.

☺ **Interim MHA Diminishing Gel** *($18.40 for 1 ounce)* is an exceptionally standard, lightweight moisturizer for slightly dry skin.

☹ **MHA Revitalizing Lotion with SPF 15** *($19.95 for 1 ounce)* doesn't contain the UVA-protecting ingredients avobenzone, titanium dioxide, and zinc oxide, and is not recommended.

☺ **$$$ Celltrex Skin Hydrating Fluid** *($26.75 for 0.5 ounce)* is a lightweight moisturizer for normal to dry skin. The collagen in this product won't affect the collagen in your skin.

☺ **Enhancer Skin Conditioning Gel** *($29.15 for 2.5 ounces)* is a lightweight gel. The ingredients in this can nicely retain moisture in the skin, but they won't heal anything. The amounts of RNA and royal jelly are too minute to talk about, but in any amount they are strictly gimmicks and offer nothing for the skin.

☺ **$$$ HPX Hydrating Gel** *($49.95 for 1.5 ounces)*. The placenta in this doesn't deserve comment (though it is just a water-binding agent), and the rest just makes this a good moisturizer for normal to slightly dry or combination skin.

☺ **$$$ Intensive Eye Complex Moisturizing Cream** *($40 for 0.75 ounce)* is a very good moisturizer for dry skin. The so-called "barrier repair technology" ingredients are just water-binding agents, which is good for dry skin, but the repair aspect won't change a wrinkle on your face.

☺ **NaPCA Moisture Mist** *($19.80 for 8.4 ounces)* is a lightweight toner of water, slip agent, and water-binding agents. It would be good for most skin types. It does contain about 1% lactic acid, but at that percentage it is a water-binding agent, not an exfoliant. The NaPCA in here refers to a natural component of skin called sodium DL-pyrrolidonecarboxylate; it is a good water-binding agent but no more so than many other natural components of skin used in skin-care products, ranging from glycerin to cholesterol and glycolipids.

☺ **NaPCA Moisturizer** *($19.80 for 2.5 ounces)* is a good lightweight moisturizer for normal to dry skin that does contain sodium PCA (see comments for the Mist above for more explanation).

☺ **Rejuvenating Cream** *($28.45 for 2.5 ounces)* won't rejuvenate the skin, although it can be a good moisturizer for normal to dry skin. You're supposed to believe that the tiny amounts of royal jelly, algae, and RNA in here can rejuvenate your skin; they can't, and there is so little of them in this cream that it's almost silly.

☹ **Tru Face Retinol Skin Perfecting Gel** *($49 for 1 ounce)* does contain retinol; however, the see-through container it comes in guarantees that the retinol will be deteriorated way before you ever use it. Retinol is a highly unstable ingredient and doesn't hold up unless packaged in a relatively airtight container and is completely protected from light.

☺ $$$ **Ideal Eyes Vitamins C & A Eye Refining Creme** *($40 for 0.5 ounce)* is a lightweight cream (it's really more of a serum than a cream) of mostly silicones and slip agents that does contain fractional amounts of vitamin C (as L-ascorbic acid) and vitamin A (retinol). If you're looking for retinol and vitamin C, there are less-expensive versions, but this is as good as any, and is in the right kind of packaging to keep the ingredients stable.

☺ **White Cream** *($28 for 1 ounce)* does contain mulberry extract, which has some value in preventing melanin production, though there is only one study demonstrating this. However, that study showed the pure concentration was minimally effective when compared to hydroquinone, which is considered a far better option for skin lightening. It also contains bearberry extract (containing arbutin), which can also inhibit melanin production, though this has only been shown in vitro. Overall, the amounts of these extracts used in this skin-care product is unlikely to affect skin or melanin.

☺ **White Essence** *($29 for 1 ounce)* is similar to the White Cream version above only in lotion form. The same basic comments apply.

☺ **White Milk Lotion** *($28 for 4.2 ounces)* is similar to the White Cream version above only in lotion form. The same basic comments apply.

☺ **White Skin Lotion** *($26 for 4.2 ounces)* is similar to the White Cream version above only in lotion form. The same basic comments apply.

☹ **White UV Base** *($28 for 1.7 ounces)* doesn't contain the UVA-protecting ingredients avobenzone, titanium dioxide, or zinc oxide, and is not recommended.

☹ **White Masque** *($28 for 3.4 ounces)* is a peel-off type mask that contains even smaller amounts of the mulberry and bearberry extract than in the ones above, making it even that much more ineffective for skin lightening.

☺ $$$ **Skin Brightening Complex** *($17.80 for 0.5 ounce)* uses kojic acid to lighten the skin, but kojic acid is an unstable ingredient and considered not to be as effective as hydroquinone for skin lightening.

☺ **Sunright 28 Ultimate Sunscreen Protection** *($17.45 for 3.4 ounces)* is an effective, in-part titanium dioxide–based sunscreen that can be good for someone with dry skin.

☺ **$$$ Sunright Lip Balm 15** *($5.65 for 0.25 ounce)* is a very emollient lip balm that has a very good, in-part titanium dioxide–based sunscreen.

☹ **Sunright Spray 10** *($20.75 for 4.2 ounces)* has a poor SPF number; doesn't contain the UVA-protecting ingredients avobenzone, titanium dioxide, or zinc oxide; and is not recommended.

☺ **Sunright Prime Pre and Post Sun Moisturizer** *($16.10 for 5 ounces)* is just a good (though very mundane) lightweight moisturizer for dry skin. It has no sunscreen, so you would never apply it before going outside in the sun.

☺ **Sunright Tan Sunless Tanning Lotion** *($17 for 3.4 ounces)* is a standard, dihydroxyacetone-based self tanner that would work as well as any, though there are far cheaper and just-as-effective versions at the drugstore.

☺ **$$$ Clay Pack** *($13.60 for 2.5 ounces)* is a standard clay mask. Again, the vitamins and royal bee jelly are at the end of the ingredient list, meaning you get only a tiny amount. Besides the clay, this product contains no other irritants or drying agents, so it could be a fairly gentle clay mask, or at least as gentle as clay can be on the skin.

☹ **Face Lift with Activator Original Formula** and **Sensitive Skin Formula** *($33.30 for 2.6 ounces of Face Lift Powder and 4.2 ounces of Activator)* is really two separate items you mix together to get the results implied by the name. Basically, the Face Lift Powder is egg white, cornstarch (a possible irritant), and silica (sand). The Activator contains water, benzethonium chloride (a possible skin irritant), aloe vera, soothing agent, and water-binding agent. The Activator swells and irritates the skin, and the egg white and cornstarch in the Face Lift Powder temporarily dry it in place, which supposedly makes it look smoother. It doesn't, at least not for long. Irritation around the eyes can be a problem and might cause more wrinkles.

## Nu Skin 180

☺ **$$$ Nu Skin 180 Anti-Aging Skin Therapy System** *($220 for five-piece kit totaling 10.1 ounces—as this book goes to print only two of the products are sold separately; I was told it is working on selling all the products separately)* is an incredibly overpriced group of products that claim to reprogram your skin by providing the skin with "Barrier Repair Technology." These can't reprogram anything, because if they could that would mean that Nu Skin expected you to only have to buy these products once, use them up, and then your skin would be back to 180 degrees of where it was when you started, meaning younger and less wrinkled. But just as with any other skin-care products like cleansers, moisturizers, or AHA products, you have to continue using the stuff. One of the technology breakthroughs for this line is that its AHA product isn't supposed to be as irritating as others on the market. That lower risk of irritation has more to do with the fact that the pH of the product is over 4, while AHAs work best in a pH of 3. The higher pH, though, would mean a decreased chance of irritation. Although your skin won't have any renewing, these products for the most part would still be quite good, though absurdly overpriced, for someone with normal to dry skin. The studies for these products indicate they make skin look better; what a shock. Are there any studies anywhere in the world showing that a cosmetic made skin look bad?

For all the glorious claims, it turns out the ingredients for these products are actually pretty standard and not as impressive as other Nu Skin formulations from its earlier and current offerings of miracle antiwrinkle products. Though you do have to wonder, if these are now the answer to your wrinkle woes, is Nu Skin going to stop selling its other anti-wrinkle products?

☹ **Triple Action Face Wash** *($35 for 4.2 ounces sold separately)* is part plant oils and part detergent cleansing agent. It can leave a greasy feel on the skin, and the detergent cleansing agent is sodium C14-16 olefin sulfate, which can be irritating for some skin types. It does contain ascorbic acid (vitamin C), but even if that was the reason you thought this cleanser was of some special value, in a wash like this the vitamin C would just be rinsed down the drain or wiped away, and ascorbic acid is not considered the best form of vitamin C to use anyway.

☹ **Skin Energizing Mist** *($29 for 3.4 ounces sold separately)* is a "toner" in spray form that has strontium nitrate as the second ingredient, which is a salt typically used to create a red flash in explosives. It is rather irritating to skin, with no known benefit. Other than that, it contains slip agents, plant extracts, and preservatives.

☺ **UV Block Hydrator SPF 18** *(1 ounce)* is a good in-part zinc oxide–based sunscreen, but for the money you will have to use at least one of these every week or week and a half to apply it liberally enough to get the amount of protection promised.

☺ **Night Repair Complex** *(1 ounce)*. This version does use ascorbyl palmitate as its form of vitamin C, which is more stable than the ones above using L-ascorbic acid or ascorbic acid (and it contains none of the retinol). This would be a good moisturizer for normal to dry skin.

☹ **Cell Renewal Fluid** *(five 0.1-ounce bottles)* is a very overpriced version of AHA with BHA in a pH that is too high to make it all that effective as an exfoliant. It also contains strontium nitrate as the fourth ingredient. See my comments for the Energizing Mist above for my concerns about this ingredient.

# N.V. Perricone, M.D.

In the world of skin care, a growing number of dermatologists and plastic surgeons have crossed the line from physician to cosmetics salesperson. While it is completely reasonable to expect your doctor to be an objective and impartial source for gathering information and options based on the most current, documented, and peer-reviewed published research, it is questionable if that is truly happening when the only option being presented is the doctor's own products. Crossing the line from physician to cosmetics salesperson happens when the physician is both treating and providing personal recommendations to patients, and sidesteps the issue of medical ethics and the use of scientific modalities.

From a scientific perspective this is at best problematic territory, though from a profit viewpoint it's good business and looking better all the time. Highlighting how prevalent and serious an issue this is, an article in the August 1999 issue of the *Tufts University Health & Nutrition Letter* stated that the "American Medical Association has issued guidelines advising physicians not to sell health-related products for profit. When a doctor stands to gain from something a patient buys, it creates a conflict of interest." The American College of Physicians–American Society of Internal Medicine issued ethical guidelines for physicians selling products that were reported on in the *Annals of Internal Medicine*, December 7, 1999. The paper stated that sales of cosmetics and vitamins by physicians are "ethically suspect."

When it comes to skin-care product lines being endorsed and sold by physicians, the most notable of this group are Dr. Sheldon Pinnell of Cellex-C and SkinCeuticals fame, Dr. Murad of Murad skin care (sold for years via infomercial), Dr. George Semel, a plastic surgeon with products available at Nordstrom and Sephora, and now Dr. N. V. Perricone. What all of these doctors have in common is that they sell absurdly expensive skin-care products while making exaggerated claims about what their products can do, based almost exclusively on animal testing, in vitro testing, or no testing at all.

Pinnell is the front-runner in the vitamin C craze, Semel bases his products on DNA as a marvel skin-care ingredient, Murad started with AHA products and now sells every conceivable overly hyped cosmetic ingredient, and Perricone bases his miraculous products on a combination of vitamin C and alpha lipoic acid. All of them want you to believe that their research has found the answer for your wrinkles and that it's available only in their products. Now all you have to do is choose which one to believe and subsequently spend a lot of money.

If Perricone has nothing else, it is indeed an air of authenticity. His résumé is more than impressive. He is certified by the American Board of Dermatology and a member of the Society of Investigative Dermatology, as well as assistant clinical professor of dermatology at the Yale Medical School. What does Perricone want you to believe? His Web site states that his products are the "the only clinical line of skin-care treatments that is researched, created and patented by a Board-Certified Dermatologist and Research Scientist." Pinnell, Murad, and other dermatologists would take issue with that statement. But Perricone's promise to "defy aging and look ten years younger in days without chemical peels, cosmetic surgery or lasers with N.V. Perricone, M.D. all-natural cosmeceutical skin treatments" is where he leaves his medical standing far behind and joins the overhyped world of those selling empty promises and unsubstantiated antiwrinkle products. Where he starts to lie is when his Web site states these "are not cosmetics," because according to the FDA that is exactly what they are.

The two miracle ingredients in this line are ascorbyl palmitate (a form of vitamin C) and alpha lipoic acid. Perricone has even written a book, *The Wrinkle Cure,* explaining why these two ingredients are the be-all and end-all for wrinkles. Getting through all of Perricone's explanations about those two ingredients takes a fairly scholarly or academic background. Even with the chemistry and physiology I've studied, it just isn't easy to understand all that scientific language. After plodding through as much as I could and interviewing other researchers in the field, I have no doubt that the data are impressive. There is a vast quantity of information showing that vitamin C and alpha lipoic acid, when taken *orally* as dietary supplements, have many potential health benefits. Nevertheless, when it comes to getting rid of wrinkles and making a woman look younger, the information is at best theoretical and more realistically inconclusive.

Perricone states in much of what he has written that, when it comes to skin, the studies for vitamin C and alpha lipoic acid were not done on human skin. From his own summary, Perricone states, "In order to prove the physiologic activity of ascorbyl palmitate on collagen production, the molecule was tested on normal human dermal fibroblasts in vitro in two separate cell culture systems." In vitro (test tube) results are always interesting, but that doesn't translate to human skin. In another portion of his Web site he states, "… when looking at the effects of ascorbyl palmitate in the three dimensional system *that mimics human skin,* ascorbyl palmitate showed much greater activity than ascorbic acid. …" (emphasis added). Something that mimics human skin is not the same as living skin.

Where Perricone and I agree is that inflammation and irritation are a problem for skin and a contributing factor to the skin's wrinkling and aging process. He states, "It is important to emphasize that inflammation is an integral part of the aging process. … Any process that causes inflammation in the cell accelerates the aging process, and prevention of inflammation has the opposite effect." He also writes that "all anti-oxidants act as anti-inflammatories." Again he's right. But then how to explain his infatuation with vitamin C and alpha lipoic acid as the only way to protect against irritation and thereby to stop wrinkles? If all antioxidants perform this function, and given there are lots of good ones (many that are considered better than vitamin C and alpha lipoic acid), then according to Perricone's own statement these two are not the only options.

It also deserves notice that while reducing already inflamed and irritated skin is nice, it would be far better for skin *not* to get inflamed or irritated at all. But most of

Perricone's products contain fragrance (a known skin sensitizer), while others contain alcohol or eucalyptus. He also uses sodium lauryl sulfate in his cleansers (it's the second ingredient), which is a known skin irritant. (It is the dermatologic standard for testing comparative irritation levels against other ingredients.)

Further, none of this addresses the issue of sun exposure or UVA damage for skin, something Perricone has completely overlooked. His line doesn't include a facial sunscreen of any kind, and his two body sunscreens don't include UVA-protecting ingredients. It is unbelievable to me that none of Perricone's sunscreens have UVA-protecting ingredients, and that he doesn't have even one for the face. So much for current or even any basic research about skin over the past several years.

One other intriguing aspect of Perricone's work is that he likes glycolic acid and AHAs in general. His research states that "the current trend of daily use of topical glycolic acid thus may provide some photoprotection and resultant decrease of photoaging and perhaps carcinogenesis." What Perricone doesn't say is that for many skin types, AHAs can cause irritation and inflammation, and that the FDA has released research that indicates that repeated use of AHAs can make the skin more sun sensitive! Perricone seems to have a penchant for only presenting one side of a story and not the whole picture.

Several of Perricone's products showcase a group of ingredients identified as "NTP complex." The term is created by Perricone and alludes to some special or rare ingredient compound. However, the ingredient listings for these products show the same cosmetic ingredients available to everyone who wants to use them. NTP is a marketing term and not a unique new ingredient.

So should you run out and buy Perricone's products? I would follow Perricone's own advice, from two of his published papers and presentations on the issue: "The use of topical antioxidants is still very controversial with questions remaining about their efficacy. . . ." In another paper he stated, "The use of antioxidants in the prevention and treatment of . . . aging has just begun. . . . It is simplistic to assume that senescence [aging] is due to one causal factor"—or, from my perspective, is cured by one or even two random ingredients.

Dr. Perricone's products are available at a range of stores including Nordstrom, Bloomingdale's, and Sephora, as well as through several Web sites. For more information, call (888) 823-7837 or visit Perricone's Web site at www.nvperriconemd.com.

⊗ **Alpha Lipoic Acid Nutritive Cleanser** *($27 for 6 ounces)* uses sodium lauryl sulfate as the primary cleansing agent (it is the second ingredient) and is not recommended. Even if this wasn't the case, there is nothing about this basic, detergent-based water-soluble cleanser that is worth the absurd price tag. In a cleanser, the tiny amount of alpha lipoic acid in here, even if you did buy the hype around this ingredient, would be rinsed down the drain.

☹ **Vitamin C Ester Citrus Facial Wash** *($19 for 6 ounces)* is almost identical to the one above, only with ascorbyl palmitate. The same basic comments apply.

☹ **Vitamin C Ester Facial Refresher Splash** *($23 for 6 ounces)* contains eucalyptus and alcohol and is absolutely not recommended.

☺ **$$$ Face Finishing Moisturizer** *($45 for 1.86 ounces)* is a good moisturizer for dry skin, but the only reason to spend this kind of money would be your belief in the claims Perricone has made for the vitamin C and alpha lipoic acid.

☺ **$$$ Alpha Lipoic Acid Evening Facial Emollient with NTP Complex and Retinol** *($80 for 2 ounces)* would cover your bases, though to find Perricone bothering with retinol seems to disprove his own research establishing vitamin C and alpha lipoic acid as the way to rid skin of wrinkles. It's a good moisturizer for dry skin and the buzz-worthy ingredients are in here. But eighty dollars! You could buy eight or ten whole bottles of straight alpha lipoic acid capsules for that.

☺ **$$$ Alpha Lipoic Acid Eye Area Therapy with NTP Complex** *($40 for 0.5 ounce)* is a good lightweight moisturizer for normal to dry skin; to hope for wrinkle-free skin from using this product is to hope for the impossible.

☺ **$$$ Alpha Lipoic Acid Face Firming Activator with NTP Complex** *($85 for 2 ounces)* is about a 5% AHA product with a pH of about 3.5 to 4. It would work well for exfoliating the skin, but to suggest that there are less expensive ways to get that benefit is an understatement.

☺ **$$$ Vitamin C Ester Amine Complex Face Lift with NTP Complex** *($75 for 2 ounces)* is a good moisturizer for normal to dry skin.

☺ **$$$ Vitamin C Ester 15% Concentrated Restorative Cream with NTP Complex** *($75 for 1.86 ounces)* is the one if vitamin C is the goal! Though keep in mind no one knows how much of it the skin needs, if any, or how long it lasts in skin to have an effect. If you do want vitamin C, 15% of an ester sounds good, but from the research, that appears to be meaningless. You would also have to ask yourself, if this has more vitamin C than the other products, why would you need any of the others? It also contains about a 2% concentration of AHA, which isn't enough for an exfoliant. This is a good moisturizer for normal to dry skin.

☺ **$$$ Vitamin C Ester Eye Area Therapy** *($47 for 1 ounce)* contains—are you ready for this?—white blood cell extract. Now I've seen everything. Applying white blood cell extract to the skin can't stimulate any activity of your own white blood cells. This product doesn't deserve a comment but it would be a good lightweight moisturizer for normal to dry skin.

☺ **$$$ Alpha Lipoic Acid Lip Plumper** *($30 for 0.5 ounce)*. It is interesting that Perricone sells two lip-plumper products, one with alpha lipoic acid and the other with ascorbyl palmitate. Which one really works? Both are just lightweight moisturizer with flavoring. The rest is up to you.

☺ **$$$ Vitamin C Ester Lip Plumper** *($30 for 0.5 ounce)* is similar to the Alpha Lipoic Acid Lip Plumper; see the comments above.

☹ **Alpha Lipoic Acid Body Toning Lotion SPF 15 with NTP Complex** *($60 for 6 ounces)* doesn't contain UVA-protecting ingredients and is not recommended.

# Obagi (Skin Care Only)

There's some controversy surrounding Dr. Obagi and his skin-care products that I've written about before. For those of you who aren't familiar with Dr. Zein E. Obagi, he is a dermatologist who created his own skin-care line, to be used in conjunction with his Blue Peel and a prescription for Retin-A. His anti-aging program took off as dermatologists and plastic surgeons alike started to sell his skin-care products and perform his Blue Peel. Yet the Obagi Nu-Derm products are as far from being "dermatologic" as you can imagine. For the most part, there is nothing in these products that cannot be found elsewhere in cosmetics for far less money. And the hype is just absurd for such extraordinarily standard products. The products supposedly contain something called Complex 272, which turns out to be nothing more than saponin. Saponins are constituents of plants known as glycosides and that have a distinctive foaming, soapy characteristic. As a glycoside, saponin can have water-binding properties for skin, and there is some evidence that saponins can have anti-microbial benefits for skin. But there is nothing particularly exciting about any of that, and the teeny amount used in these products is almost laughable.

In contrast, the Blue Peel is completely different and can be used only by dermatologists. Dr. Obagi's Blue Peel is a standard trichloroacetic acid (TCA) peel of a type that has been performed by dermatologists and plastic surgeons for years. TCA is used for peeling the face, neck, hands, and other exposed areas of the body. It causes fewer pigment problems than other doctor-only peels such as phenol, and is considered excellent for "spot" peeling of specific areas. It can be used for medium or light peeling, depending on the concentration and method of application. AHA and BHA peels are considered light peels, and are often done in a series of six. TCA peels are best for fine lines and can be somewhat more effective on deeper wrinkling, but are performed only once every couple of years. Many of the dermatologists I spoke to feel a TCA peel is a viable option for many skin types, despite consumers' fascination with AHA peels. But Obagi doesn't like AHA or BHA peels for some reason, though he doesn't really explain why.

As for the Obagi products, they are sold exclusively through dermatologists' offices and are given the marketing affectation of being "prescribed" by the doctor. However, except for the 4% hydroquinone products in this line, these items are strictly cosmetic and not prescription in the least. There are many reasons why a woman should see a dermatologist. As Obagi states in his brochure, a professionally applied peel, Retin-A or Renova, and an effective skin-lightening product can be the best game plan for reducing the effects of sun damage. The rest of the products, however, are just cosmetics—and are no better or worse than other products being sold today in a wide array of venues. Obagi's customer service number is (800) 636-SKIN, or visit the Web site at www.obagiskinhealth.com.

☺ $$$ **Nu-Derm Foaming Gel Cleanser** *($29 for 6.7 ounces)* isn't all that gentle, but it is a good, detergent-based water-soluble cleanser for someone with normal to oily skin. It does contain fragrance and coloring agents.

☺ $$$ **Nu-Derm Gentle Cleanser** *($29 for 6.7 ounces)* is similar to the Foaming Gel above and the same basic comments apply.

☹ **Nu-Derm Toner** *($29 for 6.7 ounces)*. The potassium alum in this is a potent absorbent and topical disinfectant that can be a skin irritant, and the witch hazel can also be a problem for skin. This product does not return skin to a good pH because the potassium alum has a very high pH, something that is not helpful for skin.

☹ **Nu-Derm Action** *($15 for 2 ounces)* is supposed to "diminish discomfort due to excessive dryness, itching, redness or burning" from the Obagi peel. This is a good moisturizer for dry skin but it is not formulated in any way to reduce irritation any more than any other well-formulated moisturizer. It also contains sodium lauryl sulfate as an emulsifier, but in a product meant to reduce irritation, this extremely irritating ingredient is ill advised.

☺ $$$ **Nu-Derm Tolereen** *($40 for 2 ounces)* is a 0.5% hydrocortisone moisturizer. There are many reasons to use a product that contains hydrocortisone. Minor irritations, skin rashes, allergic reactions, dermatitis, and some inflammations can be calmed quite effectively with an over-the-counter hydrocortisone lotion or cream. Lanacort and Cortaid, which have a 1% hydrocortisone content (both found at drugstores for less than $5 an ounce) work identically if not better to do the same thing, due to their increased concentration. Charging $40 for the same thing at half the strength is unconscionable. Keep in mind that hydrocortisone is for sporadic, infrequent usage only, because with repeated application it can break down the skin's collagen and elastin.

☺ $$$ **Nu-Derm Blender** *($48 for 2 ounces)* is a 4% hydroquinone cream and only available from a physician. It is an absolute option when used in conjunction with a good sunscreen, because it inhibits melanin production and so reduces the appearance of brown discolorations.

☹ $$$ **Nu-Derm Exfoderm** *($48 for 2 ounces)* is just a moisturizer that contains phytic acid as the third ingredient. Phytic acid is a good antioxidant, but not the only one or the best one. Other than that, this is mostly water and thickeners, which makes it a rather mediocre moisturizer for normal to dry skin.

☺ $$$ **Nu-Derm Exfoderm Forte** *($48 for 2 ounces)* is a good 8% AHA product in an extremely standard moisturizer base that is easily replaced by AHA products from lots of other lines that provide the same effect of exfoliation for far less money.

☺ **Nu-Derm Sunblock SPF 25** *($37 for 2 ounces)* is a very good titanium dioxide– and zinc oxide–based sunscreen, in a fairly standard moisturizing base. However, there is nothing about this formulation that can't be replaced by less-expensive versions from Neutrogena at the drugstore.

☹ **Nu-Derm Sunfader** *($50 for 2 ounces)* is a 4% hydroquinone product that also contains a sunscreen with SPF 15. That is an intriguing concept: mixing a skin-lightening agent with sunscreen. However, this sunscreen doesn't contain UVA protecting ingrediets of titanium dioxide, zinc oxide, or avobenzone, and therefore provides inadequate protection.

☺ **$$$ Nu-Derm Eye Cream** *($50 for 1 ounce)* is a standard emollient moisturizer that can be good for dry skin, but it is incredibly overpriced.

# Olay

In the past, when reviewing Oil of Olay products, I often asked, what the heck is an "olay" anyway? It isn't a plant or mineral, so what is it? Of course, there is no such thing as an olay anything. It was just a cute name that must have sounded elegant when this line was first introduced a few decades back. Now it appears that Procter & Gamble, the current owners of the Olay brand, have finally decided that this meaningless name needed to be retired. (It was apparently also a problem that many consumers have a negative association with the word "oil" when used to describe cosmetics.) In their new manifestation, the products are stamped simply "Olay." From my perspective, that is a welcome touch of reality.

Olay's greatest advance by far has been the launch of its makeup line in 1999. Without question, the Olay makeup cosmetics display has one of the best tester units available at the drugstore for most every single product it sells. This in and of itself makes for a refreshingly enjoyable drugstore makeup shopping experience.

What you can expect to find are excellent, lightweight foundations with reliable sun protection, admirable lipstick textures, and, regrettably, a plethora of overly shiny blushes and eyeshadows. The claims surrounding Olay's progression into makeup is right on course with the industry at large, meaning they provide all the language the consumer expects to hear (like non-pore-clogging, all-natural, and hypoallergenic) without any valid research behind it. But in no way does that mean that you should not consider this line; happily, many of the products are attractively priced and perform beautifully—just be prepared to wade through the same pool of marketing claims made by countless other companies. As an aside, it is interesting to note that Cover Girl (also owned by Procter & Gamble) has several similar if not identical product formulations.

For skin care, Olay is still not a very exciting line, lacking any state-of-the-art moisturizing ingredients such as interesting water-binding agents, plant oils, or antioxidants; in fact, many of these formulations are so boring they are hard for me to recommend, but for a basic moisturizer they aren't bad. Olay's Age Defying series all contain salicylic acid (beta hydroxy acid, or BHA). Strangely enough, despite the research accompanying the press release for these products substantiating that a pH of 3 is the effective range for BHA, only two of this line's Age Defying products have a pH of 3, while the other has a pH of 6, which makes it incapable of exfoliation.

ProVital is a line of skin-care products Olay is aiming at the "mature" woman. Grouping women of a certain age into one grand, indefinite bunch euphemistically called mature is insulting. I've said this more times than I can count: age does not determine skin type. There are 50-, 60-, and 70-year-old women with all sorts of skin conditions ranging from breakouts, whiteheads, oily skin, and rosacea to sun damage and blackheads. Dry skin is not the only skin type for older women and they should not all be using the same products. The one area where Olay does excel is in sunscreens with UVA protection, and it was ahead of the pack for this essential part of any skin-care routine.

A new launch for Olay is its Total Effects line of products. One of the only unique aspects of the first moisturizer launched in the summer of 2000 is the price, $17 for 1.7 ounces. That wouldn't be so outlandish in the world of skin care, but, given the formulation, there is nothing here that warrants the price tag. Total Effects is supposed to be the only product that addresses the "seven signs of aging." I'm not sure how Olay accounted for only "seven" signs, because there are dozens and dozens of changes in the skin that reflect "aging." (Actually what appears on the surface of skin is minimally related to aging and primarily related to years and years of sun damage.) Overall, Total Effects offers very little for skin and is easily passed over for far more elegant formulations. For more information about Olay, call (800) 285-5170 or visit the Web site at www.olay.com.

## Olay Skin Care

☺ **Daily Facials Cleansing Cloths, Normal to Oily** *($6.99 for 30 cloths)* is basically a detergent-based water-soluble, wipe-off makeup remover that would be an option if it didn't contain menthol, which adds nothing but irritation to this mode of cleanser, plus the Vaseline in here is not a great option for oily skin types. If the notion of cleansing cloths sounds convenient, Diaparene Baby Wash Cloths, Fragrance-Free ($2.49 for 100 towelettes) or Huggies Baby Wipes Refills, Natural Care, Unscented ($5.29 for 160 towelettes) are far better options than this one and they don't contain fragrance!

☺ **Daily Facials Cleansing Cloths Normal to Dry** *($6.99 for 30 ounces)* is virtually identical to the Normal to Oily version above and the same comments apply.

☹ **Facial Cleansing Lotion** *($3.87 for 6.78 ounces)* is a lightweight cleanser that doesn't quite rinse off without the aid of a washcloth, and it can leave a residue on the skin; it could be OK for someone with dry skin.

☺ **Foaming Face Wash** *($3.87 for 6.78 ounces)* is a standard, detergent-based water-soluble cleanser that cleans the face well and can be good for most skin types.

☺ **Sensitive Skin Foaming Face Wash** *($3.87 for 6.78 ounces)* is similar to the one above only it doesn't remove makeup quite as well.

☹ **Refreshing Toner** *($3.35 for 7.2 ounces)* contains mostly alcohol, which makes it too irritating and drying for all skin types.

☹ **Age Defying Series Daily Renewal Cleanser** *($4.60 for 6.78 ounces)* is a standard, detergent-based water-soluble cleanser that also contains salicylic acid (BHA). The pH of this product is too high for the BHA to be effective as an exfoliant but in this cleanser formulation it is wasted anyway, along with being a potential a problem if it gets in the eyes.

☺ **Age Defying Series Daily Renewal Cream Beta Hydroxy Complex** *($8.91 for 2 ounces)* isn't an exciting formula, but it does have a good pH to make it an effective exfoliant, although the amount of salicylic acid is a mystery. If you are interested in trying a BHA product instead of an AHA, this is a reasonable one to consider, though this is best only for someone with normal to dry skin.

☹ **Age Defying Series Protective Renewal Lotion Beta Hydroxy Complex, SPF 15** *($8.91 for 4 ounces)* does not contain the UVA-protecting ingredients avobenzone, titanium dioxide, or zinc oxide, and is not recommended. It does contain BHA, but the pH of this version is too high for it to be effective as an exfoliant.

☹ **Age Defying Series Revitalizing Eye Gel** *($8.91 for 0.5 ounce)* contains witch hazel as the second ingredient, which can be too irritating for any part of the face, and especially the eye area. Other than that, it is just a very standard gel formula with some water-binding agents (though most are in such minute amounts they don't really count) for normal to slightly dry skin.

☹ **ProVital Perfecting Moisturizer Lightly Tinted Cream** *($8.99 for 1.7 ounces)* is a one-tint product, and that just can't translate to a variety of different skin tones. It is a good, though ordinary, emollient moisturizer for dry skin, but that's about it. The vitamins and water-binding agents are at the very end of the ingredient listing, well after the preservatives, and are barely present to have any effect whatsoever on skin.

☹ **ProVital Night Cream** *($8.99 for 2 ounces)* is similar to the one above only without the tint and slightly less emollient.

☹ **ProVital Protective Moisture Lotion SPF 15** *($8.99 for 4 ounces)* doesn't contain the UVA-protecting ingredients avobenzone, zinc oxide, or titanium dioxide, and is not recommended.

☺ **Moisture Replenishing Cream Daily Care Series** *($5.76 for 2 ounces)* is a good, but very below-standard, moisturizer for someone with dry skin.

☺ **Oil-Free Replenishing Cream, Daily Care Series** *($5.76 for 2 ounces)* won't replenish anything, and the thickening agents can clog pores, which makes this, along with several of the other Olay products, just an exceptionally dated, substandard formulation.

☹ **Sensitive Skin Daily UV Protectant Beauty Fluid SPF 15** *($6.58 for 4 ounces)* doesn't contain the UVA-protecting ingredients avobenzone, zinc oxide, or titanium dioxide, and is not recommended.

☺ **Sensitive Skin Beauty Fluid** *($6.58 for 4 ounces)* is a good though very ordinary moisturizer for normal to dry skin.

☺ **Sensitive Skin Replenishing Cream Daily Care Series** *($5.76 for 2 ounces)* is similar to the one above, only somewhat more emollient, and the same review applies.

☺ **Total Effects Moisturizing Vitamin Complex** *($16.99 for 1.7 ounces)* is supposed to address all of the issues concerning the "signs of aging." However, this product lacks a sunscreen, and without that this product can't address one of the primary ways to prevent most all signs of aging. Aside from that oversight, this product is basically just water, glycerin, silicone, thickeners, film former, more thickeners, vitamins, preservatives, fragrance, and coloring agents. The teeny amounts of vitamin E and panthenol in here show up in thousands of products and are hardly unique. However, what is relatively unique to this otherwise humdrum moisturizer is the inclusion of niacinamide (vitamin B3), in about a 1% to 2% concentration. As I mentioned before, niacinamide in significant concentrations may be helpful for breakouts, though that research is not independent and therefore not all that reliable. So what is niacinamide doing in a moisturizer for wrinkles? That's anyone's guess, but I suspect it has to do with some existing animal studies and in vitro studies on human fibroblasts (cells that produce connective tissue such as collagen), demonstrating that niacinamide may have an effect on skin tumors. However, there is no research for niacinamide in relation to wrinkles or anything else to do with sun-damaged skin. It isn't a bad ingredient, but to suggest that it has special benefit for daily skin care is an overstatement.

☺ **Total Effects Moisturizing Vitamin Complex Fragrance-Free** *($16.99 for 1.7 ounces)* is almost identical to the Total Effects version above only without fragrance or coloring agents. While that is indeed helpful for skin, it doesn't change the mundane formulation.

☺ **Complete UV Protective Moisture Lotion SPF 15** (**Fragrance** and **Fragrance Free**) *($6.59 for 4 ounces)* is a part-zinc-oxide sunscreen, which makes only one of two from Olay with optimal UVA protection. While the sun protection is impressive, the moisturizing base leaves much to be desired. It contains mostly water and wax and no other interesting water-binding agents or antioxidants. That's not bad, it's just not great. Still, the SPF 15 is what really counts for a daytime product anyway.

☺ **Complete UV Protective Moisture Cream SPF 15 (Fragrance** and **Fragrance Free)** *($6.59 for 4 ounces)* is similar to the lotion version above and the same comments apply.

☺ **Night of Olay Night Care Cream** *($5.76 for 2 ounces)* is a good, but extremely ordinary, mundane moisturizer for normal to dry skin.

☺ **Oil-Free Beauty Fluid Daily Care Series** *($7.99 for 6 ounces)* is an ordinary moisturizer that contains more thickeners than anything else. There are far better options for skin care than this antiquated group of ingredients.

☺ **Original Beauty Fluid, Moisture Replenishment Lotion** *($7.99 for 4 ounces)* is a very ordinary moisturizer that contains only water, mineral oil, and thickeners. There is nothing beautiful about this run-of-the-mill, dated formulation.

☹ **Daily UV Protectant Beauty Fluid Daily Care Series Moisture Replenishment Lotion SPF 15** *($7.99 for 6 ounces)* doesn't contain the UVA-protecting ingredients avobenzone, zinc oxide, or titanium dioxide, and is not recommended.

☹ **Daily UV Protectant Cream Daily Care Series SPF 15** *($15.76 for 2 ounces)* doesn't contain the UVA-protecting ingredients avobenzone, zinc oxide, or titanium dioxide, and is not recommended.

# Olay Makeup

☺ <u>**FOUNDATION:**</u> **All Day Moisture Foundation** *($9.99)* is recommended for normal to dry skin and is supposed to moisturize for "11 hours." Why it stops at 11 hours is anyone's guess, but the claim for even a few hours is deceptive. With talc and sodium chloride (salt) as the fourth and fifth ingredients, respectively, this formula is definitely not all that moisturizing. That doesn't make it bad, just a better choice for those with normal to oily skin who prefer a smooth texture and light to medium coverage. There are ten shades available and most of them are great. The ones most skin tones should watch out for are Light Beige (slightly peach) and Medium to Deep Honey (strong yellow). There are a few deeper shades worth checking out!

☺ **Shine Control Foundation** *($9.99)* is nearly identical in application and texture to the one above, with the primary difference being the disappointing colors this one has. Of the ten shades available, these six are too peach or orange for most skin tones: Fair Beige, Light Beige, Light Honey, Deep Beige, Deep Honey, and Medium to Deep Honey.

☺ **All Day Moisture Stick Foundation** *($13.59)* has a cool, wet application that dries to a sheer-to-light-coverage matte finish. The colors tend to be on the peach side but not enough to avoid giving these a try if testers are available (and they usually are). If you have normal to oily skin, this is the best way to use stick foundation, with minimal emollient ingredients being deposited on the skin.

☺ **Complete Radiance Foundation SPF 15** *($13.99)* may be getting a little pricey for a drugstore foundation, yet this one is worth it for its excellent, light-to-medium coverage with a pure titanium dioxide–based sunscreen. There are ten shades available, but no options for very light or very dark skin tones. While that's disappointing, most of the existing neutral shades are very good, with a soft, even texture for someone with normal to dry skin. The only colors to watch out for due to strong overtones of peach, pink, or yellow are Fair Beige, Light Beige, Medium to Deep Honey, and Deep Honey.

☺ **Complete Radiance Compact Foundation SPF 15** *($13.99)* is a pressed-powder foundation with a silky-soft feel. The SPF 15 is part titanium dioxide, which is superb. While this is an option for those who prefer using a powder as their foundation base, I'm concerned that the liberal application necessary to achieve the labeled SPF will not be reached knowing the sheer look most women prefer from powder. Remember, if you can't see it on the skin, or if you wipe it away (blending more off than on), you won't get the protection your skin needs. That said, of the ten colors, the only shades to avoid are Light Beige, Fair Beige, Gold Honey, and Dark Honey.

☺ **Complete Radiance Tinted Moisturizer SPF 15** *($13.59)* is a great in-part zinc oxide–based sunscreen in a boring moisturizer base for someone with normal to dry skin. The three available colors aren't up to par with the other Complete Radiance products, but the coverage is almost imperceptible, so the colors are inconsequential.

☹ **CONCEALER:** Olay's stick **Concealer** *($6.49)* tends to crease in the lines around the eye and the three shades are just awful—these are some of the worst peach shades I've seen in a long time.

**POWDER:** ☺ **Pressed Powder** *($9.99)* is a standard, talc-based powder with a soft, smooth finish that comes in four great, very neutral shades.

☺ **Loose Powder** *($7.99)* makes claims that are really confusing. On the one hand, it claims to have ingredients that can absorb sebum (oil) but on the other it also has emollients to help provide a silky feel. The reality is you simply can't do both (inert ingredients can't figure out what to do or not to do on different parts of the face). Bottom line: this is a good, standard, talc-based powder that comes in two shades, of which one (Medium to Dark) may be too peach for most skin tones.

☹ **BLUSH:** Of the six shades for this fairly powdery **Blush** *($9.99)*, four are extremely shiny and two are matte. These also tend to blend on unevenly, and could certainly benefit from an improved formula.

☹ **EYESHADOW:** The **Eye Shadow** *($3.79)* comes in duo compacts only. All of them are shiny, with poor color combinations and a chalky consistency that will hamper even blending.

☹ <u>EYE AND BROW SHAPER:</u> **Eyeliner** *($5.99)* comes in six shades, two of which are blue, while one is green and another a shiny purple. That makes the color range exceptionally disappointing and limited.

☺ <u>LIPSTICK AND LIP PENCIL:</u> **ColorMoist Lipstick** *($7.99)* is just a very emollient, somewhat greasy lipstick with over 49 colors to choose from. It does glide on easily but you may not be too thrilled if you're prone to having lipstick bleed or feather. **Color Moist Lipstick SPF 15** *($8.89)* is a sheer, moist lipstick that has a glossy finish and offers an in-part titanium dioxide sunscreen! The only drawback is the limited selection of colors. **Lip Shine** *($7.49)* is a very thick, sticky lip gloss that comes in a pot. The texture of this will allow for longer wear and lots of shine, but you have to be willing to put up with the sticky feel. **Lip Pencil** *($6.99)* is a very standard lip pencil that needs sharpening and that features six very nice, usable shades.

<u>MASCARA:</u> ☺ **Beauty Mascara** *($5.99)* creates really impressive long lashes without clumping and it does wash off easily. One downside—it tends to smear a little.

☹ **Aqua Care Mascara** *($5.99)* isn't all that waterproof, not great news for a waterproof mascara, plus it doesn't build much length or thickness.

<u>SPECIALTY PRODUCTS:</u> **Nail Lacquer** *($3.79)* is available in over 24 shades, and the only reason I am mentioning this is because Olay provides a color-matching chart so you can coordinate its nail polish and lipstick colors. Nice touch.

## Ombrelle (Sun Care Only)

The world of sunscreens has changed dramatically over the past two years. Information about UVA protection versus UVB protection has completely changed what we need to consider when buying sunscreens. In the section on sunscreens in Chapter Two, I discuss at length why certain UVA-protecting ingredients are essential when considering which sunscreen to buy. Ombrelle is a small line of sunscreen products that include avobenzone as one of the active ingredients. That makes these products a great option for daily sun protection. For more information about Ombrelle, call (800) 582-8225.

☺ **Ombrelle Spray Mist SPF 15** *($10 for 4 ounces)* is a great sunscreen for both UVA and UVB protection. Unfortunately, it is in an alcohol base, and that can be drying and irritating for the skin when used on a regular basis.

☺ **Ombrelle Sunscreen Lotion SPF 15** *($10 for 4 ounces)* is a great sunscreen for both UVA and UVB protection in a standard, lightweight, moisturizing base. It would be good for someone with normal to slightly dry skin.

☺ **Ombrelle Sunscreen Lotion SPF 30** *($10 for 4 ounces)* is similar to the lotion above only with a higher SPF.

☺ **Kids Spray SPF 28** *($8.69 for 4 ounces).* If a spray form seems like an easier way to get sunscreen on your kids (or on yourself for that matter), spray away—because this is a very good sunscreen with avobenzone! It also contains other sunscreen agents that might be a bit sensitizing for the eye area, but for everywhere else, it should be fine. It is a lightweight formula but it is better for normal to dry skin.

# Origins

Estee Lauder started off the 1990s with a new cosmetics line called Origins, and what a concept it has! Origins uses all of the current fads on the market to create one of the most gimmicky makeup and skin-care collections around. The ad copy is loaded with exotic-sounding botanicals, herbs, and oils. Never mind that there are a host of unnatural ingredients in here that contribute more to the makeup's textures and slip quality than any plant ever could. Perhaps someone thought, why bother with the ordinary when the extraordinary is what gets consumers' attention and money?

Origins (like Aveda and The Body Shop) offers skin-care systems based on every fad in the book and then some, including botanicals, essential oils, recycled packaging (including a recycling service at its counters for the empty bottles and compacts), products that aren't tested on animals, "ancient" skin-care treatments, anti-stress formulas, and aromatherapy. The recycling efforts and animal-free testing are praiseworthy examples. However, the "ancient" and "natural" stuff is the real bait that hooks women. As you might expect, juxtaposed around the "special" oils and herb extracts are exceptionally standard skin-care ingredients, while lots of the plant oils and extracts are potential skin irritants. Further, many of the "natural" ingredients are at the far end of the ingredient lists, meaning they are practically nonexistent.

Origins' basic skin-care theory is that all skin wants to act normal, the way it did when we were young. As we grow up, our skin gets confused or behaves badly, not because it wants to, but because it lacks something. If skin is supplied with the correct plants and oils, according to Origins, "nature's memory" can "retrain" your skin to function the way all skin wants to function—normally. What an enticing concept. Of course, the ingredients that supposedly retrain your skin are derived from the "ancient science of essential oils," which assumes that people who lived long ago had great skin because of this special knowledge. It does sound convincing, but, alas, that's just not how skin works. If it was, then all of the Estee Lauder companies would sell the same formulations, and they don't. But I have to admit that this is one of the most creative skin-care ploys I've ever seen, and that is saying a lot.

Although not much has changed since I last did a full review of Origins' makeup, that is not really a problem. All along, Origins has done a decent job of providing women with neutral liquid foundations, impressive blush shades, and remarkably soft synthetic brushes. Origins also has its fair share of clever products, including practical tinted brow gels, as well as impractical choices (the pre-mascara lash-builder comes to mind). One of the more praiseworthy features is the tester units, which are sensibly organized and inviting to the customer.

Keep in mind that once a plant has been put in a cosmetic and preserved, it has little if any benefit, regardless of whether it had any in the first place. Having said all that, I still think Origins offers some good products; you just have to read between the lines to find out what they are.

For more information about Origins, call 1-800-ORIGINS or visit the Web site at www.origins.com.

# Origins Skin Care

☹ **Cream Bar** *(9.50 for 5.2 ounces)* is a standard bar cleanser with fairly drying detergent cleansing agents, but this one also contains some very irritating and sensitizing plant extracts, including clove, wintergreen, and spruce needle.

☹ **Liquid Clay** *($15 for 5 ounces)* is a standard, detergent-based water-soluble cleanser that also contains a lot of clay, which can be difficult to wash off. But the real drawback to this product is the eucalyptus, sage, and ylang-ylang, which can cause skin irritation.

☹ **Liquid Crystal Extra Gentle Cleanser** *($14 for 6.7 ounces)* contains mostly thickeners and plant oils, which makes it a standard wipe-off cleanser that can leave a greasy film on the face that still needs to be wiped away. That could be an option for dry skin, but the peppermint in here is too irritating for any skin type.

☹ **Mint Wash** *($14 for 6.7 ounces)* includes mint, which is a skin irritant, like the spearmint, orange zest, and lemon peel also in this product. This cleanser can burn the eyes and irritate the skin, and is not recommended.

☹ **Pure Cream Rinseable Cleanser You Can Also Tissue Off** *($14 for 6.7 ounces)* contains peppermint, lime, and tangerine oils, which can burn the eyes and are skin irritants.

☺ **Well-Off Fast and Gentle Eye Makeup Remover** *($11 for 3.4 ounces)* is a standard, detergent-based water-soluble eye-makeup remover. It works, but there is nothing particularly gentle about it.

☹ **Never a Dull Moment Age Erasing Skin Polisher with Fruit Enzymes** *($22.50 for 3.5 ounces)* has a great name, but it's an ordinary product. I've written before about the papain in cosmetics: it just isn't stable enough to exfoliate the skin very well, if at all. Plus there are several ingredients in this product that pose a definite concern about irritation, including eucalyptus, mint, grapefruit, pine, and mango.

☹ **Swept Away Gentle Slougher for All Skins** *($15 for 3.4 ounces)* is a fairly gritty exfoliant that also contains peppermint and grapefruit, both useless as skin-care ingredients because they can irritate and hurt skin. There is absolutely nothing gentle about this product.

☹ **Swept Clean Special Sloughing for Oily-Acting Skin** *($15 for 3.4 ounces)* is almost identical to the Gentle version above except for the addition of menthol, which only makes it more irritating for the skin.

☺ **Comforting Solution If Your Skin Acts Sensitive** *($17 for 5.7 ounces)* is supposed to help sensitive skin defend itself against the environment. It can't protect against the environment; however, it is a soothing toner of sorts. The drawback is that it contains far too many potentially sensitizing plant extracts to ever be considered reliable for sensitive skin.

☹ **Drenching Solution** *($17 for 5 ounces)* contains far too many potentially sensitizing plant extracts, including eucalyptus, sage, spearmint, and jasmine, to be an option for most skin types.

☹ **Managing Solution** *($17 for 5 ounces)* is a toner that is supposed to normalize oil production, but its ingredients—plant water, essential oils, aloe vera, vitamin E, slip agents, and preservatives—won't change oil production. Actually, the fragrant oils and irritating ingredients (including peppermint and lemon) are a problem for all skin types.

☹ **Mending Solution** *($17 for 5 ounces)* is almost identical to the Managing Solution above, only this one is supposed to energize the skin's "look-young systems." No one's skin has "look-young systems." But isn't it amazing that such similar products are supposed to do such disparate things for the skin? Plus, irritating the skin hurts its healing process, which means irritation is a problem if your goal is preventing wrinkles.

☺ **Sprinkler System** *($13.50 for 6.7 ounces)* is a great name for a rather standard toner. It's OK for someone with normal to slightly dry skin, but the plants in here, including coriander and cinnamon, can be problematic for many skin types.

☹ **Tuning Solution** *($17 for 5 ounces)* is supposed to rebalance the oily and dry areas of your face. It doesn't contain anything capable of doing that, but it does contain lemon and eucalyptus, among other extracts that can be irritating for the skin.

☺ **Clearance Time** *($22.50 for 1 ounce)* includes sugarcane extract, but that's not the same as AHAs, and it can't exfoliate skin. However, this product does contain salicylic acid (BHA, about 1% concentration), and that can exfoliate skin, though the pH is just passable for this purpose. Other than that, this is a very good moisturizing base. It does contain fragrant plant extracts.

☹ **Starting Over** *($22.50 for 1 ounce)* is supposed to improve cell renewal, and while the sugarcane extract is supposed to make you think you are getting an AHA product, you aren't. Even if you were, there isn't enough of the extract at the right pH for this moisturizer to work as an exfoliant.

☺ **Constant Comforter** *($22 for 1.7 ounces)* is a good emollient moisturizer for normal to dry skin, but it won't calm anything; in fact, many of the plant oils and extracts are potential skin sensitizers, including lavender, lemon, lime, and rosemary.

☹ **$$$ Eye Doctor** *($25 for 0.5 ounce)* is similar to the Constant Comforter above and the same basic comments and concerns apply.

☹ **Fine Tuner If Your Skin Acts Confused** *($22 for 1.7 ounces)* is supposed to even out combination skin. None of its ingredients can change oily skin, although some of them can make oily skin feel oilier, including plant oils and shea butter, both of which can be a problem for someone with any amount of oily skin. This is a good moisturizer for normal to dry skin, but it's a confused product. Many of the plant extracts in here can be skin irritants.

☺ **$$$ Line Chaser Stop Sign for Lines** *($25 for 0.5 ounce)* can't stop wrinkles, but it is a very good lightweight moisturizer for normal to slightly dry skin. Finally, an Origins products that leaves out the irritating plant extracts!

☺ **Night-A-Mins** *($27.50 for 1.7 ounces)* is named and packaged to look like oral vitamins. Night-A-Mins definitely contain a group of vitamins, but as you now know, they are more gimmicky than effective and not the least bit nutritious for the skin, though they are good antioxidants. This would be a good moisturizer for someone with normal to dry skin, but that's about it. It does contain fragrant plant extracts.

☹ **Oil Manager If Your Skin Acts Oily** *($22 for 1.7 ounces)* contains nothing that can stop oil or close pores. It does contain some plant oils, as well as thickening agents that can clog pores, which would be a problem for someone with oily skin. What was Origins thinking?

☺ **Steady Drencher If Your Skin Acts Dry** *($22 for 1.7 ounces)* is a good emollient moisturizer for someone with dry skin. The anti-irritants in here are wasted because several of the plant extracts can also be irritants.

☺ **Time Mender** *($22 for 1.7 ounces)* is a very good moisturizer for dry skin. The company claims that this product can firm the skin, but all the plant oils and water-binding agents in the world can't do that. The anti-irritants in here are wasted because several of the plant extracts can also be irritants.

☺ **Urgent Moisture** *($25 for 1.7 ounces)* is a rather ordinary moisturizer for normal to dry skin. It does contain a minuscule amount of water-binding agents and soothing agents that have little to no impact on skin, and it does contain fragrance.

☺ **Have a Nice Day Cream SPF 15** *($28.50 for 1.7 ounces)* is a very good in-part titanium dioxide based sunscreen. The fairly mundane moisturizing base could make this appropriate for someone with normal to dry skin but the peppermint, lemon, grapefruit, and spearmint extracts in here make it a strong potential for irritation, and with so many well-formulated sunscreens around these days, why settle for any potential risk to your skin?

☺ **Have a Nice Day Lotion SPF 15** *($28.50 for 1.7 ounces)* is similar to the Have a Nice Day above except in lotion form, though the same concerns apply to this one. There are better ways to have a nice day than with this product.

☺ **Let the Sunshine SPF 14** *($13.50 for 5 ounces)* is a very good, titanium dioxide–based sunscreen, but Neutrogena has better options for less money that don't contain fragrance.

☺ **$$$ Silent Treatment Instant UV Face Protector SPF 15** *($15 for 1.7 ounces)* is a titanium dioxide–based sunscreen suspended in a silicone base. It is a great idea, but it can leave a slightly white cast on the skin. I was very concerned to see that this product contains lavender oil, which can cause photosensitivity (if you go out in the sun wearing lavender oil, you can get an allergic reaction).

☺ **Summer Vacation: The Natural-Looking Self Tanner** *($17.50 for 5 ounces)*, like all self tanners, uses dihydroxyacetone to turn the skin brown. This works as well as any of them.

☺ **$$$ Clear Improvement Active Charcoal Mask to Clear Pores** *($16.50 for 3.4 ounces)* is a standard clay mask. Charcoal has unique absorption and disinfecting properties but there is so little of it in here that it doesn't have much impact on skin.

☺ **$$$ Drink Up 10 Minute Moisture Mask** *($17.50 for 3.4 ounces)* definitely contains oils and should feel nice as a mask if you have dry skin, but no more so than applying a regular moisturizer over the skin and letting it stay in place for ten minutes. This does contain fragrant plant extracts.

☹ **$$$ No Puffery** *($20 for 0.64 ounce)* claims it can release trapped fluids and toxins from the skin, but that is not possible. Meanwhile it does contain plant extracts, including almond meal, ivy, yarrow, and horsetail, that can cause irritation and make eyes look more puffy.

☹ **Out of Trouble** *($17.50 for 3.4 ounces)* is meant to be a way to solve blemishes and blackheads. I wish it could, but this formulation is what's in trouble. Zinc oxide and titanium dioxide can clog pores and cause breakouts, camphor and sulfur can cause irritation and redness, and there isn't enough BHA at the right pH to have an impact on exfoliating the skin.

☹ **Spot Remover to Clear Up Acne Blemishes** *($10 for 0.3 ounce)* is a standard salicylic acid (BHA) and alcohol solution. Without the alcohol, this product may have been an option, but there are far better BHA options for less money in far less irritating bases to consider than this one.

☹ **Zero Oil Instant Matte Finish for Shiny Places** *($10 for 0.64 ounce)* cannot stop oil production, but sodium magnesium silicate can absorb oil much as talc does. However this product also contains camphor, which can be skin irritant. This is pretty much a modified version of Phillips' Milk of Magnesia, which can do the same sort of thing, only better. There is no reason to use camphor on skin.

☹ **Cover Your Mouth SPF 8** *($6.50)* is not something you should put anywhere on your skin, much less near your mouth. Not only is the SPF 8 inadequate, but this one contains peppermint, which can irritate lips.

☹ **Lip Remedy** *($10 for 0.17 ounce)* isn't much of a remedy. This lip product contains a long list of thickeners, plant oil, more thickeners, and preservatives, which wouldn't be bad except that it also contains menthol and camphor, which are irritants and not helpful for lips or skin. There are better emollient lip balms available that can help smooth dry lips.

☺ **Mind Your Mouth** *($6.50 for 0.15 ounce)* is a very emollient, standard lip gloss. It doesn't contain sunscreen, but it is very good for dry lips any time of year, as long as it isn't daytime.

# Origins Makeup

**FOUNDATION:** Original Skin is the clever name for Origins' foundations, although it is hardly accurate. This stuff doesn't look like original skin, it looks like foundation—a nice foundation, but foundation nevertheless. The salesperson told me Original Skin would make my skin look like a baby's bottom and let it breathe the way it does without foundation. Although I thought Original Skin was pretty good, it did not make my skin look like a baby's bottom, nor was the product more breathable than other foundations. It also did not hide tiny lines (foundation almost always makes lines look more prominent). Don't expect anything unique in terms of ingredients, either; besides some plant extracts and a small amount of plant oils, this is just a good, standard foundation. Please note that the names of the foundations reviewed below are perfectly accurate descriptions. Also, all of the foundations below are best for normal to oily skin (the salespeople will tell you that all skin types can use them, but they are not very emollient or moisturizing).

☺ **Some Coverage** *($14.50)* is almost watery, like a liquid, but it goes on sheer and blends more evenly than you would expect. The shades to consider avoiding are Porcelain, Blushing, Beige, Rosy, Golden, and Sable, which are all to pink or peach for most skin tones.

☺ **More Coverage** *($14.50)* provides just that: more coverage than the Some Coverage foundation above but it is still only light coverage. These shades can be too pink, orange, peach, rose, or ash for most skin types: Porcelain, Rosy, and Golden.

☺ **Most Coverage** *($14.50)* ups the coverage another notch than the More Coverage but it still is light-to-medium coverage. These shades can be too pink, orange, peach, rose, or ash for most skin types: Porcelain, Rosy, and Golden.

☺ **Sunny Disposition Liquid Bronzer** *($15)* is a very sheer, pink/bronze tint that would work well on warm or sallow skin tones that want a tanned appearance.

☹ **As Good As It Gets** *($20)* sounds like the ultimate makeup convenience: foundation, concealer, and powder in one. It comes up short on all counts and remains a loose powder that goes on rather thick, with eight slightly shiny, slightly peachy shades. If you blend it on well, it can have a sheer to light coverage with a silky finish, but in order to get all of the extra features, you're supposed to mix it with a moisturizer, which can get messy and streaky. Used alone, it performs much like any standard loose powder with shine, and to me, that's as good as this foundation gets!

☺ **$$$ Original Skin Pressed Makeup** *($22.50)* is a pressed-powder foundation with a smooth, slightly dry texture and sheer colors that apply easily and blend well. Upon first glance, the available colors all seemed quite peach and pink; however, this is sheer enough for that not to be much of a concern—just be sure to check these out in natural light before buying.

☺ <u>CONCEALER:</u> **Original Skin Concealer** *($10)* has a smooth, light texture, and some OK colors, but all of the shades are slightly shiny, which isn't best for under the eye when it comes to smoothing out lines or helping the area to look even with the foundation (unless your foundation is shiny).

☺ **$$$ <u>POWDER:</u> Original Skin Loose Powder** *($17)* has a wonderfully smooth texture and a soft, dry finish, in seven exceptional colors, including options for darker skin tones. **Original Skin Pressed Powder** *($17.50)* shares the same characteristics as the Loose Powder, but is slightly drier; there is one shade to avoid, Cedar, which can be too peach for most skin tones. **Sunny Disposition Powder Bronzer** *($17.50)* is a fine option for bronzing powder; the color is appropriate for most skin tones and the shiny speckles are barely present.

☺ <u>BLUSH:</u> **Brush-On Color** *($14)* has a slightly dry texture that still blends on soft and sheer. There are some attractive matte colors to choose from, and some minimally shiny shades to consider as well. **Pinch Your Cheeks** *($10)* conjures up images of small children running from that too-affectionate aunt who visits once a year! In reality, this is a liquid stain for the cheeks that blends nicely (once you get the hang of it, so be careful), and offers a transparent, plummy-pink blush. This works best on normal, even-textured skin.

☺ <u>EYESHADOW:</u> Origins has divided its shadows into two groups: the **Eyeshadows** *($11)* have a matte finish and slightly dry texture that is not the best for classic blending but the colors are beautifully soft and muted. **Eye Accents** *($11)* are a much larger group of shades meant to "harmonize or highlight" and they do that with—guess what? right—varying degrees of shine. The less intense versions are easily discernible and would be an option for nighttime accenting. **Shadow Stick** *($12.50)* is described as "a powdery pencil for eyes." It does have a soft powder finish but tends to ball up enough to make creating a seamlessly smooth line a challenge you may not want to accept.

☺ <u>EYE AND BROW SHAPER:</u> **Kohl Mine** *($6.50)* consists of short bullets of color in a slide-up tube that create an intense, creamy line that applies and blends smoothly. This consistency is prone to smearing, but for a "smoky" look they could work well. The very standard **Eye Pencil** *($11)* comes in a limited though attractive group of colors. Ditto for the **Brow Pencil** *($11)*. **Just Browsing** *($12)* is a lightweight, softly tinted brow gel with an OK brush that works to add natural color and definition to the eyebrow. All of the shades are great, and while the finish is minimally sticky, overall it works well. **Brow Fix** *($12)* is basically clear mascara for the brows and, though overpriced, will work to keep them groomed and in place.

☺ <u>LIPSTICK AND LIP PENCIL:</u> I wish Origins would tweak its **Lip Color** *($11)* formula just a bit. The texture and greasy finish of these just can't compete with the myriad lipsticks in most other lines, from Chanel to Almay. The color selection is top-notch, but not worth the effort (due to fading) or if you're trying to prevent lip colors from bleeding. **Matte, Sheer,** and **Shimmer Sticks** *($12)* are the original "chubby sticks" that many lines sport these days. Why these ever caught on is anyone's guess. They need constant sharpening, most are too soft to get a controlled lip line, and that brings us back to what they really are: a standard, creamy lipstick in pencil form. The **Matte Stick** is not matte in the least, and is actually rather greasy. The **Sheer Stick** is even greasier than the Matte version and with less pigment. The **Shimmer Stick** is just creamy and iridescent. **Bite Your Lips** *($12.50 for full size or set of three minis; $6 for individual minis)* are nothing more that sheer, glossy lip tints that tend to slip on and then slide off. **Lip Gloss** *($11)* is just as good as any gloss at the drugstore selling for half the price. **Lip Pencil** *($11)* is a standard pencil with a dry texture and very little stain, which means it should fade at the same rate your lipstick does.

<u>MASCARA:</u> ☺ **Fringe Benefits Mascara** *($12)* is a good mascara that builds long lashes evenly without smearing. I wouldn't choose this over less-expensive options, but that name is so darn cute!

☹ **Underwear for Lashes** *($12)* has very little purpose other than to coat fragile lashes with an extra layer of clear mascara. For some, this may make a slight difference in their lashes' thickness, but there are scores of mascaras out there that can do that all by themselves.

☺ $$$ <u>BRUSHES:</u> Origins' **brushes** *($15 to $50)* are synthetic—which for many animal-rights activists is a strong selling point. What helps even more is that, for synthetics, they are exquisitely soft, and dense enough to pick up and apply product professionally. What's a detriment is the fact that many of these brushes are too big and full to use with precision and ease when applying eyeshadows, blushes, and powders. They're worth a look if you want good synthetic hair, and the ones to consider include: **Powder Eyeliner** *($15)*, which can work for a wider line; **Eyeshadow**

Placement *($17.50)* and **Eyeshadow Contour** *($15)*; the retractable **Lip Brush** *($15)*; and, as an extra option, the **Brush On-the-Go** *($25)*.

# *Orlane*

Women who buy Orlane products aren't wondering whether they can afford the $500 to $1,000 or more it costs to take care of their skin the Orlane way; they just want to be assured that what they're getting is the best of the best, regardless of cost. Orlane's slick, sapphire blue packaging with silver letters is stunning. Its opulent, elegant appearance communicates prestige. But there has to be more to skin care than brilliant packaging, right? How does Orlane seduce a woman into believing its cosmetics chemists know something no one else does?

Orlane's pitch is that a Nobel laureate created "anagesium," one of the ingredients in its Anagenese line of products. Now, *that* is a great angle. Of course, I haven't received any information on who the person is or was, or what the research revealed. But it definitely sounds good.

Orlane says that anagesium is a combination of proteins that is supposed to provide some outstanding benefit to the skin. However, the ingredient lists reveal the truth: there are no unique proteins, or unique anything, in any of the Orlane products. Every product contains standard ingredients just like those used by the rest of the industry. Most of Orlane's products contain proteins and amino acids, which can help keep water in the skin, but they are not the only ingredients that can do that, and Orlane is not the only cosmetics company using them.

Maybe I shouldn't say that all of Orlane's ingredients are standard. Two hard-to-miss components are brain and spleen extract. What the consumer is supposed to swallow (no pun intended) is that a hunk of dead cow brain or spleen can have some rejuvenating effect on the skin. La Prairie makes the same body-parts ingredient claims, but there is no evidence or research to support this contention.

All of Orlane's brochures feature gushing phrases such as "optimum functioning of the epidermis," "natural molecules called Oxytoners," and "creates the proper environment for the skin." It all sounds so impressive—until you take a closer look and notice that the claims just don't jibe with the accurate information on the ingredient list. No facts, no actual research, no proof is given in anything I've read from the company. It is all hyperbole. Charts for Orlane's Anagenese Total Time Fighting Care proclaim that it has produced a 52 percent reduction in wrinkles. But nowhere are there details of how that study was done, how many women were in it, what age group was tested, whether the study was double-blind, and who measured the before-and-after results. A 52 percent reduction might appeal to your emotions and hopes, but without more data it's a meaningless number.

It is hard for me to imagine that a woman could sincerely believe that spending this kind of money on skin-care products will prevent wrinkles or aging skin or make her skin more beautiful. Women who can afford the so-called "best" products still have to get face-lifts and eye tucks. But believe these claims they do—Orlane's sales are not hurting.

To be fair, and I always try to be, the line does have several creams and lotions that have a wonderfully silky texture. Orlane has one of the largest selection of skin-care products of any line I've ever reviewed. As I mentioned, most Orlane products contain fancy water-binding ingredients in the form of proteins and amino acids, and although they aren't unusual, they are indeed interesting. Proteins work primarily by staying on top of the skin and preventing dehydration, while amino acids are better able to penetrate the skin and protect against moisture loss a little more deeply. That's about it, though. Do I think that translates into some extraordinary benefit for the skin? No. But they do feel nice and can keep the skin moist.

Orlane's makeup products try to continue the overblown hype started by its skin care (which is really this line's focus), but in spite of the technical names and too-good-to-be-true claims, there is little here to extol, and the good products are marred by disproportionate price tags. For more information on Orlane, call (800) 775-2541, or visit www.eve.com.

# Orlane Skin Care

☺ $$$ **Wash-Off Cleansing Cream for All Skin Types** (*$29 for 6.8 ounces*) is a standard, detergent-based water-soluble cleanser that would be an option for someone with normal to dry skin. The lanolin and isopropyl palmitate in here do not make this appropriate for all skin types. It does contain fragrance.

☹ **Gentle Exfoliating Cream for All Skins** (*$28 for 2.5 ounces*) is a wipe-off cleanser with thickeners and plant oils and a small amount of detergent-cleansing agent, and uses synthetic particles (polyvinyl chloride) as the abrasive. It's an OK, standard scrub that would be an option for normal to dry skin.

☺ $$$ **Soothing Lotion Alcohol-Free for Dry or Sensitive Skin** (*$29 for 6.8 ounces*) isn't the best for sensitive skin, but it is a good irritant-free toner for all skin types.

☹ $$$ **B21 Bio-Energic Cleansing Preparation Care for Face** (*$40 for 6.8 ounces*) is a standard mineral oil–based wipe-off cleanser that also includes plant oils and fragrance. This can leave a greasy film on the skin, so it can be an option for dry skin, but this is a very mundane formula that is easily replaced by similar versions ranging from Olay to Pond's.

☺ $$$ **B21 Oligo Vit-A-Min, Vitalizing Cleanser for Dry or Sensitive Skin Types** (*$32.50 for 8.4 ounces*) is similar to the one above only slightly less greasy. It does have a host of water-binding agents and vitamins, but they come well after the preservative and hardly amount to anything. This does contain fragrance.

☺ $$$ **Gentle Cleansing Milk for Dry Sensitive Skins** *($32 for 6.8 ounces)* is similar to the Vitalizing Cleanser above and the same basic review applies. There is nothing about this cleanser that makes it better for sensitive skin types. It does contain fragrance.

☺ $$$ **B21 Oligo Vit-A-Min Vitalizing Scrub for Dry or Sensitive Skin Types** *($30 for 1.7 ounces)* is a wipe-off cleanser with thickeners and plant oils and a small amount of detergent cleansing agent. It does contain menthol and fragrance, which makes it inappropriate for sensitive or dry skin types. The long list of vitamins and water-binding agents comes well after the preservatives, which means that these will have at best an insignificant effect on skin.

☺ $$$ **B21 Bio-Energic Vivifying Lotion for All Skins** *($40 for 6.8 ounces)* would be a good, nonirritating toner for most skin types. The serum protein in this is just a fancy name for a good but fairly standard water-binding agent. The urea in here is about a 1% to 2% concentration, which makes it a mild exfoliating agent for skin.

☺ $$$ **B21 Oligo Vit-A-Min Vitalizing Lotion for Dry and Sensitive Skin Types** *($35 for 8.4 ounces)*. The very minute amount of urea in here has no effect for exfoliation. Other than that, this is a very commonplace but good toner for normal to dry skin.

☺ $$$ **B21 Bio-Energic Absolute Skin Recovery Care** *($130 for 1.7 ounces)*. The leech extract and aorta and spleen extract have no unique benefit for skin. This can be a good, though fairly ordinary moisturizer for someone with dry skin; its smattering of bells and whistles makes it sound far more exotic than it really is.

☺ $$$ **B21 Absolute Skin Recovery Care Eye Contour** *($75 for 0.5 ounce)* is a mineral oil–based moisturizer. This can be a good, though fairly ordinary moisturizer for someone with dry skin; the bells-and-whistles ingredients make it sound far more exotic than it really is.

☺ $$$ **B21 Bio-Energic Absolute Youth Concentrate Age Defense-Protective Oxytoning Care** *($300 for 1.7 ounces)* is a good moisturizer for normal to dry skin but the minute amount of yeast in here has no "oxytoning" properties for skin. Even if this could provide oxygen, given that oxygen generates free-radical damage, that would just cause skin damage. There is nothing to encourage youthful skin in this product. Just the price is enough to add a wrinkle or two to your face and there's nothing in here to change that.

☺ $$$ **B21 Bio-Energic Protective Oxytoning System for All Skin Types** *($300 for 0.7 ounce)*. The yeast won't provide oxygen to the skin (see comments above for the Youth Cream). Hematin is a bluish-black substance containing iron that is obtained from blood and provides the red color to blood; it has no known effect on skin. There are lots of ingredients in here that would be problematic for someone with oily skin but it can be an option for normal to dry skin.

☺ $$$ **B21 Bio-Energic Extreme Line-Reducing Care** *($150 for 1.7 ounces)* is a good moisturizer for normal to dry skin, but there is nothing in here that will reduce one line on your face; it is just a good moisturizer.

☺ $$$ **B21 Bio-Energic Intensive Firming Care** *($120 for 1.7 ounces)* is a good moisturizer for normal to slightly dry skin. This does contain a tiny bit of arnica, which hopefully isn't enough to be a problem for most skin types.

☺ $$$ **B21 Bio-Energic Intensive Nurturing Care, Nightly Concentrate for Dry and Very Dry Skin** *($120 for 1.7 ounces)* is a good (though not worth the money) moisturizer for normal to dry skin. The teeny amount of royal bee jelly here has no effect on skin.

☺ $$$ **B21 Bio-Energic Morning Recovery Concentrate** *($60 for 1 ounce)* is a lightweight lotion. It's a good, albeit strange, moisturizer for normal to minimally dry skin, though I suspect you're supposed to believe miraculous things about this combination of ingredients.

☺ $$$ **B21 Bio-Energic Points Vulnerable Creme for All Skins** *($70 for 1 ounce)* is a good, fairly basic moisturizer for dry skin. The spleen extract in here has no special beneficial properties for skin. If you're going to splurge on a moisturizer, there are better-formulated versions than this one in the Orlane lineup.

☺ $$$ **B21 Bio-Energic Ultra-Light Cream for the Day** *($75 for 1.7 ounces)* is a good, though extremely average moisturizer for someone with normal to dry skin.

☹ **B21 Oligo Eye Balm for Sensitive, Fragile and Allergic Skin Types** *($40 for 0.68 ounce)*. There is a trace of water-binding agents here, but the amount is so minuscule as to be completely inconsequential for skin. The talc in here, rather high up on the ingredient listing, and a host of other problematic ingredients including fragrance and plant extracts, make this inappropriate for allergic skin types.

☺ $$$ **B21 Oligo Gentle Soothing Cream for Sensitive Fragile & Allergic Skin Types** *($63 for 1.7 ounces)* is a very good moisturizer for dry skin.

☺ $$$ **B21 Oligo Light Smoothing Cream** *($63 for 1.7 ounces)* is a good, though standard moisturizer for dry skin. The interesting ingredients are so far down the ingredient list as to be almost undetectable.

☺ $$$ **B21 Bio-Energic Protective and Moisturizing Base** *($75 for 1.7 ounces)* is a mineral oil–based moisturizer. It's a good though very ordinary basic moisturizer for dry skin. Most of the really interesting ingredients come at the end of the ingredient listing and are barely present.

☺ $$$ **B21 Bio-Energic Super Moisturizing Concentrate Day and Night** *($95 for 1.7 ounces)* is a good though exceptionally ordinary moisturizer for dry skin.

☹ **B21 Sol-Energic Serum Soleil Visage Energizing System Before and After**

Sun *($120 for 1 ounce)* is supposed to encourage protection from the sun while you tan, which is not humanly possible, and completely disingenuous.

☹ **B21 Sol-Energic Serum Soleil Visage Energizing System Before and After Sun** *($120 for 1 ounce)* does not contain enough sun protection, nor does it have any UVA protection, though it does contain PABA, considered to be one of the more irritating sunscreen agents and one rarely used by most companies.

☺ **$$$ B21 Oligo Vit-A-Min Vitalizing Masque** *($32.50 for 1.7 ounces)* is a standard clay mask with several thickeners, preservatives, and fragrance. It doesn't get much more basic than this, although it's an option for normal to slightly oily skin.

☺ **$$$ B21 Bio-Energic Line Reducing Lip Care** *($50 for 0.33 ounce)* is just water, mineral oil, thickeners, silicone, some water-binding agents, preservatives, and fragrance. That's good for dry skin but it won't change one line on your lips.

☺ **$$$ Normalane Foam Cleansing Gel for Mixed and Oily Skins** *($25 for 4.2 ounces)* is a very standard, detergent-based water-soluble cleanser that can be good for someone with normal to oily skin. It does contain fragrance.

☹ **$$$ Normalane Astringent Soothing Lotion for Mixed and Oily Skins** *($25 for 6.8 ounces)*. The balm mint this contains can be a skin irritant, and that's a problem for all skin types. The teeny amount of tea tree oil in here is not even vaguely enough to have any effect for skin. The pH of this product isn't low enough for the BHA to work as an exfoliant. This toner has more problems than it has benefits.

☹ **Normalane Correcting Gel, Mixed and Oily Skins** *($22.50 for 0.5 ounce)*. The tiny bit of tea tree oil has no effect on the skin. It can be quite irritating to leave detergent cleansing agent on the skin, as recommended here.

☹ **$$$ Normalane Night Balancing Gel** *($30 for 1 ounce)* contains balm mint, which can be a skin irritant. The teeny bits of tea tree oil and yeast in here have no effect on the skin.

☹ **Normalane Daytime Mat-Finish Base** *($30 for 1 ounce)* includes talc and magnesium aluminum silicate, which can help absorb oil, but several of the other ingredients (including coconut oil high up on the ingredient list) can cause oil shine to show up faster than you want. The balm mint in here can be a skin irritant, and the teeny amount of tea tree oil has no impact on skin.

☹ **Normalane Balancing Mask for Mixed and Oily Skins** *($35 for 1.7 ounces)* is a standard clay mask with some thickeners and water-binding agents. Some of these thickeners can be problematic for someone with oily skin, and the balm mint can be a skin irritant.

☹ **Extrait Vitale Multi-Active Revitalizer with Apple Alpha-Acids** *($70 for 1.7 ounces)* contains apple extract, which is unrelated to AHA, at least in terms of having any exfoliating properties. It also contains cornstarch, which can be a skin irritant. It does contain lactic acid, but less than 1%, so that has no effect as an exfoliant either. Aside from that, this is an exceptionally standard moisturizer that contains mostly water, thickeners, and mineral oil.

☺ $$$ **Extrait Vital Biological Cream for Dry and Very Dry Skins** *($60 for 1.7 ounces)* is a good emollient moisturizer for someone with dry skin.

☺ $$$ **Extrait Vital Biological Fluid** *($65 for 2.5 ounces)* is a very good moisturizer for normal to dry skin.

☺ $$$ **Extrait Vital Eye Contour Serum** *($42 for 0.33 ounce)* is a very good emollient moisturizer for someone with dry skin. I don't have to discuss the spleen or calfskin extract, right?

☺ $$$ **Anagenese Eye Contour Cream Total Time Fighting Care for All Skins** *($40 for 0.5 ounce)* contains something called hirudinea extract, which translates to leech extract, and if this has an impact on skin, a search of the dermatologic and other skin-care databases shows no such benefit. The tiny amount of vitamins and water-binding agents in here are hardly worth noting, while the cornstarch makes this somewhat problematic for the eye area.

☺ $$$ **Anagenese Total Time Fighting Serum** *($52.50 for 1.7 ounces)* is a standard, lightweight moisturizer that is good for someone with normal to slightly dry skin. All of the interesting ingredients come well after the preservatives and fragrance, making them inconsequential for skin.

☺ $$$ **Hydro-Climat Moisture Shell Multiprotective Fluid** *($60 for 1.7 ounces)* is a very standard moisturizer. This is good for dry skin, but mostly a waste of your money. The dusting of vitamins and water-binding agents in here have no effect on skin.

☹ **Claircilane Whitening Formula Hydro Whitening Creme for All Types** *($75 for 1.7 ounces)* contains magnesium ascorbyl phosphate, which is a stable derivative of ascorbic acid. When used in a cream with a 10% concentration, it can inhibit melanin production. However, this product contains less than 2%, and thus has minimal to no effect on the color of skin.

☹ **Claircilane Hydro Whitening Masque for All Skins** *($55 for 1.7 ounces)* is similar to the one above and the same comments apply.

☹ **Claircilane Hydro Whitening Serum for All Skins** *($100 for 1 ounce)* is similar to the one above and the same comments apply.

☺ $$$ **After Sun Creme for Face** *($30 for 1.7 ounce)* is just a good moisturizer for dry skin.

☺ $$$ **Creme Solaire Total Block Sun Cream For the Face 30+ UVA 11** *($30 for 1.7 ounces)* is a very good, in-part titanium dioxide– and zinc oxide–based sunscreen for someone with dry skin.

☹ **Progressive Tanning Cream SPF 6 for Fair Skin** *($20 for 4.2 ounces).* When a cosmetics line sells a product that encourages tanning, the one thing known for certain to cause wrinkles and skin damage, and then gouges consumers by selling absurdly expensive skin-care products, that's as unethical as it gets in the cosmetics industry.

☹ **Safe Tanning Cream SPF 10 Maximum Protection for Sensitive Skin** *($20 for 4.2 ounces)* has an SPF 10, which is hardly maximum protection, and while this one does contain zinc oxide as part of the sunscreen protection, with so many good SPF 15s on the market, why bother with it?

☺ **Safe Tanning Cream SPF 18 Ultra Sun Protection for Delicate Skin** *($20 for 4.2 ounces)* is a good, in-part zinc oxide–based sunscreen with a great SPF number. However, the notion that this one is for delicate skin doesn't prove true; it is just a good moisturizing base for normal to dry skin.

☹ **Self-Tanning Moisture Balm SPF 4** *($25 for 4.2 ounces)* not only has a terrible SPF, but also this product doesn't contain avobenzone, zinc oxide, or titanium dioxide for UVA protection, and is absolutely not recommended. It does contain dihydroxyacetone, the ingredient in all self tanners that can turn skin brown, but there are far better options than this one in all price categories, and those have the appropriate SPF, too.

☹ **Stick Solaire, Total Sunscreen 30, Ultra Protection for Fragile and Delicate Areas** *($16.50 for 0.28 ounce)* lists the first ingredient as castor oil (it appears as the plant name *Ricinus communis*), which can have a slightly sticky feel, as well as some heavy waxes that aren't the best for delicate skin. Though this is a part titanium dioxide–based sunscreen, it also contains PABA, which is a very sensitizing sunscreen agent rarely used by cosmetics companies.

# Orlane Makeup

<u>FOUNDATION:</u> ☹ **B21 Treatment Foundation** *($50)* is a creamy, sheer makeup that dries to a soft matte finish. All of the six shades have a slight to heavy peach undertone that most skin tones would do well to avoid. **Satilane** *($35)* is semi-creamy and leaves a minimal matte finish with sheer to light coverage. The six colors are mostly forgettable, with four of them—Porcelaine, Miel Fonce, Topaz, and Biscuit—being too pink, peach, or rose for most skin tones.

☺ **$$$ Compact Cake Foundation, Dual Effect** *($42.50)* is a very good though standard powder foundation that has a super-soft and luxurious texture. The finish of this leaves a bit of a sheen, making it appropriate for normal to slightly dry skin, and the six colors are almost all wonderful. Only Ambre 05, which is too orange, should be avoided.

☹ <u>CONCEALER:</u> **Conceal Creme** *($18)* is an OK concealer that comes in two colors. Clair is good for light to medium skin tones, but Tres Clair is too pink for just about everyone. As this book went to press, Orlane was launching a new concealer due out in December 2000. I will review it in my newsletter in 2001.

<u>POWDER:</u> ☺ **$$$ Translucent Powder** *($35)* is a talc-based powder with a

small amount of plant oil. The texture is silky and the three available shades are excellent. There are also two bronzer shades for this powder but both are too shiny to recommend, and look artificial.

☹ **Velvet Pressed Powder** *($32)* has a silky, weightless texture but all six shades are shiny—truly a waste in a product that is meant to eliminate shine! **Normalane Shine Powder** *($35)* is a talc-based "specialty" powder that is meant for oilier skins. There are two shades available, and they're OK, but the claim that this powder can pH-balance the skin is not possible, as the pH of this is too high to do that.

☺ $$$ <u>BLUSH:</u> **Velvet Blusher** *($35)* has a relatively standard dry, smooth texture, but beware, because all of the colors are exceedingly shiny.

☹ <u>EYESHADOW:</u> **Velvet Eyeshadow** *($30 for duos)* is quite shiny and most of the duo color combinations have not been seen since *Dynasty* was topping the Nielsen ratings. **Fluid Eyeshadow** *($25)* is just a creamy, overpriced, ultra-shiny eyeshadow with a slight powder finish.

<u>EYE AND BROW SHAPER:</u> ☺ $$$ **Crayon Extraordinaire** *($20)* is a very standard pencil with a creamy texture and a sponge tip. The price is the only thing that's extraordinary about this one.

☹ **Crayon Multi-Beaute** *($20)* is nothing more than another multipurpose chubby pencil, only this one's texture is slightly sticky and all of the colors speak shine, loud and clear. **Eyebrow Pencil** *($18)* has a dry, hard texture that applies sheer and easily smudges.

☺ $$$ **Extra Liner** *($28)* is a good liquid liner, but not worth this outlandish price tag. **Eyebrow Fixing Shine** *($22.50)* is a sheer golden brow gel that gives a slightly glossy look to the brows. It works, but so do countless others for one-fifth the price.

☺ $$$ <u>LIPSTICK AND LIP PENCIL:</u> **Extraordinary Lipstick** *($20)* supposedly features mattes and creams, but closer inspection reveals nothing more than standard creamy lipsticks that have a glossy, iridescent finish and minimal stain. **Fluid Lip Color** *($22.50)* is a "liquid" lipstick that applies wet and dries to a natural, slightly greasy finish. The colors are mostly shiny and have enough pigment to last a little longer than usual. One caution: if you have any lines around your lips, this will travel to them easily. **Lip Lining Pencil** *($16.50)* is a boringly standard pencil that has very little going for it other than great packaging. **Lip Gloss** *($16.50)* comes in a pot or with a wand applicator and has a pleasant texture and the requisite shiny finish, but so do other glosses in all price ranges.

<u>MASCARA:</u> ☺ $$$ **Lengthening Treatment Mascara** *($25)* will lengthen your lashes with some effort. It tends to make lashes look somewhat spiky, which isn't the best. **Treatment Mascara Velvety Finish** *($22.50)* plays up the fact that it contains plant marrow (bamboo extract) to grant lush lashes, which sounds beguiling, but the reality is that with or without the bamboo, this is a do-nothing mascara that never

gets as far as the claims for it. It does lengthen and slightly thickens, and while that's good, at this price it should be great.

# *Osmotics*

If you haven't heard about Osmotics' Blue Copper Firming Elasticity Repair, you will. It is receiving a great deal of buzz on the Internet and in fashion magazines. It is right up there with vitamin A (retinol), vitamin C, and alpha lipoic acid, among other starlets in the world of skin-care ingredients, all boasting about cell repair and getting rid of wrinkles. Osmotics' entire Blue Copper claim is based on the research of ProCyte Corporation, a company located in Redmond, Washington. According to an article in *The Seattle Times*, ProCyte originally set its sights on products designed to help in wound care. ProCyte had some setbacks with the FDA regarding the results of some pertinent clinical studies for a wound-care pharmaceutical product it was hoping to market. Approval in the world of pharmaceuticals is no easy matter, but no such guidelines apply in the world of cosmetics. According to ProCyte, it was looking for niche opportunities and cosmetics was one such arena.

It would be far too cumbersome for me to delve into the endless list of promises made for Blue Copper Firming Elasticity Repair and about the research ProCyte has done on the effectiveness of this ingredient; the one study published doesn't support the claims anyway (I'll explain that in a moment). What I find most amazing is that a ProCyte-related company, Skin Biology, is competing with Osmotics by selling a product called Protect & Restore Skin Renewal Cream *($17.95 for 2 ounces)* that is identical to Osmotics' Blue Copper Firming Elasticity Repair that's priced at $95 for 2 ounces. Regardless of the lack of substantiation for either of these products, why choose the expensive version and not go with the less inexpensive, yet identical version?

According to the information on ProCyte's Web site, "Skin renewal creams that increase collagen, elastin, and proteoglycans [in the skin] and increase the amount of subcutaneous fat (the very thin layer under the skin) both firm the skin and increase its thickness. Creams such as Blue Copper Firming Elasticity Repair and Protect & Restore produce these effects. The effectiveness of both types of creams on skin renewal has been proven in independent, published clinical studies." Why then is the Osmotics version $77 more? That's anyone's guess. But if you were going to accept the research ProCyte has done and are interested, there would be no reason to even consider the Osmotics version, given that both are literally from the same source. While Osmotics wants you to believe it "sets itself apart from other cosmetics companies by using patented delivery technologies combined with essential antioxidant vitamins and minerals," clearly that is not the case, or Protect & Restore would not be available.

As an aside, before I go on with Osmotics, if you want more information about

Protect & Restore Skin Renewal Cream, call Skin Biology at (800) 405-1912. By the way, Skin Biology also sells a decent AHA product called Glycolic-8 Skin Exfoliating Lotion *($10.95 for 1 ounce)*. It isn't a bargain but it is a well-formulated AHA product for dry skin.

Actually, allow me to belabor the issue a bit more by mentioning that the study proving the effectiveness of the Osmotics and the Skin Biology products is at best limited. The study only looked at a control group (meaning nothing was applied to the skin), a placebo group (these used the base formula without the Blue Copper stuff), and a group using the same base formula with the Blue Copper ingredient. While the study seems to be on the up-and-up, the only information you can garner from it is that, as an ingredient, copper works to help skin heal. However, the study did not compare other ingredients, such as vitamin C, vitamin A, superoxide dismutase (copper stimulates the production of superoxide dismutase), a range of other antioxidants, or even a silicone-based product, to the copper formula. Do those other ingredients in the base formula do the same thing? That wasn't part of the study, so there is no way to know. All the study showed is that the base formula didn't work as well without the copper. In the long run, damaged skin can use some help healing, and I suspect there are lots of ingredients that can help that process; copper is possibly one such ingredient.

While Blue Copper Firming Elasticity Repair is getting attention for Osmotics, the company isn't willing to put all its eggs in one antiaging basket. Kinetin is its new "revolutionary discovery from science and technology in the battle against aging." Wow. And Blue Copper hasn't even been around for more than a couple of years. Nevertheless, Kinetin's claims make Blue Copper look like a waste of time and money. The Osmotics brochure declares that "Kinetin delays and partially reverses clinical signs of photodamaged and age-related changes of human cells, while restoring skin's normal barrier function." Isn't that what Blue Copper was supposed to do? But I digress. Even more fantastic is the claim that "Kinetin is the first cosmetic skin-care product to have clinically validated claims [and] is the only product which has undergone the identical study protocols applied to Renova. ... Exhaustive tests proved both the safety and effectiveness of Kinetin, whose performance was equivalent to, and in many categories was superior to, that of Renova." As it turns out, the studies researching Renova's effectiveness against wrinkles were hardly stunning. In fact, they were at best of the milquetoast variety. According to the press release concerning the clinical trials for Renova, "only a small percentage of [Renova] users, about 16% in one study and less than that in another, were pleased with their results. More than two-thirds thought the results were either mediocre or nonexistent." That makes Kinetin's comparison hardly exciting. One thing Renova definitely has over Osmotics, though, is the recognition of the importance of sunscreen that showed up in the press release accompanying the FDA approval of the product, which said, "[Renova is] useless when it comes to preventing wrinkles without a sunscreen." Osmotics doesn't seem to know that. For more information about Kinetin, please read the review for Kinerase in this chapter.

I'm almost done, but I would like to cover just a few more points. Sadly, while at face value all this research makes blue copper sound like every woman's answer to wrinkle fighting, there is a good deal of research Osmotics has ignored. None of the Osmotics daily sun-care products contain UVA protection, which makes all other battle plans against wrinkles ineffective. Another piece of information in the Osmotics brochure says, "An oily skin can be a blessing because it is more resistant to aging due to an abundant supply of the skin's own protective oil secretions. This lipid layer is the skin's first defense against free radicals." That is about as far from the truth as suggesting that there is any such thing as a safe tan. Sun damage is the primary cause of wrinkles and all the oil in the world won't stop one iota of damage. The notion that oily skin ages less than dry skin is sheer nonsense and is no longer believed by anyone researching issues of skin aging.

I do, however, agree with the notion that "a common mistake in treating oily skin is the use of harsh, stripping cleansers, scrubs, and alcohol-based products [because] this over-treatment can dry out the surface of the skin." Yet, Osmotics didn't seem to notice that some of its "gentle" products contain irritating ingredients, including mint.

Wait, I almost forgot to mention the Antioxidant Skin Care Derms, which is supposedly one more "radical leap in skin-care technology." It uses L-ascorbic acid, the same stuff in Cellex-C, and makes the same intense claims about rebuilding collagen. But why would you need this product if you use the other products? Most cosmetics companies can't resist jumping on the vitamin C bandwagon, and Osmotics is no exception. As Osmotics tells it, this "is the one step that every woman or man over the age of 25 should add to their current skin-care regime." Vitamin C may be an interesting cosmetic ingredient, but there are lots of products that contain it and there is no evidence it has any effect in getting rid of wrinkles. (As far as the cosmetics industry is concerned, everything that sounds natural and vitaminlike gets rid of wrinkles.) For more information on Osmotics, call (800) 440-1411 or visit the Web site at www.osmotics.com.

☺ $$$ **Balancing Cleanser for Normal to Oily Skin** ($27 for 6 ounces) is a standard, detergent-based water-soluble cleanser that contains mint, which can be irritating for all skin types. This product also contains a scrub element that for many skin types can be too harsh to use twice a day; for occasional use it is an option.

☺ $$$ **Calming Cleansing Milk for Sensitive Skin** ($27 for 6 ounces) definitely contains several anti-irritant–type ingredients, but aside from that it is just a standard, detergent-based water-soluble cleanser that would be fine for normal to dry skin. However, the price can't be calming to anyone, given the extremely standard, boring ingredients this product contains.

☺ $$$ **Hydrating Cleanser for Normal to Dry Skin** *($27 for 6 ounces)* isn't hydrating in the least. It is a standard, detergent-based water-soluble cleanser similar to many other cleansers available for far less money. It does contain a small amount of water-binding agents, which is nice, but for dry skin they really can't compete with the drying effect of the cleansing ingredients on the skin. This product would be a fine cleanser for someone with normal to oily skin who isn't allergic to the plant extracts in it.

☹ $$$ **Balancing Tonic Facial Mist** *($35 for 6.8 ounces)* would actually be quite good as a toner for most skin types if it weren't for the mint in it. Unfortunately mint is an irritating ingredient and serves no purpose for the skin.

☺ $$$ **Firming Tonic Facial Mist** *($35 for 6.8 ounces)* is similar to the Balancing Tonic above, minus the mint. That makes this toner fine for most skin types that aren't allergic to the plant extracts.

☺ $$$ **Facial Renewal** *($75 for 1.7 ounces)* definitely contains AHA (glycolic and lactic acid) in about an 8% to 10% concentration. It is in a standard moisturizing base and would be fine for someone with dry skin. However, be aware that there are effective AHA products out there for far less money!

☹ **Antioxidant Eye Therapy** *($55 for 0.5 ounce)* would be a lightweight moisturizer to consider, but why anyone would put mint and lemongrass, both potential skin irritants, in a product meant to be used around the eye is anyone's guess. The risk of irritation to the eye area is a problem.

☺ $$$ **Blue Copper Firming Elasticity Repair** *($95 for 2 ounces)*. The claims around this product are enough to make me want to become a rainmaker. This overpriced miracle product reads like the answer to every man or woman's antiwrinkle skin-care need, but so do most of Osmotics' products. Why would you need any of these other products if you could use this? Copper has been shown to be effective in healing serious wounds, but that is unrelated to daily skin care or to preventing wrinkles.

☺ $$$ **Kinetin Cellular Renewal Serum** *($78 for 1.7 ounces)* is a good moisturizer for dry skin that contains lots of ingredients that show up in other skin-care products, such as plant oils, antioxidants, and soothing agents. Please refer to the review for Kinerase in this chapter for more information about Kinetin.

☺ $$$ **Kinetin Intensive Eye Repair** *($75 for 0.5 ounce)* is similar to the one above and the same basic comments apply.

☺ $$$ **Intensive Moisture Therapy** *($65 for 2 ounces)*. The plant extracts can be a problem for some skin types, but for the most part this is a very good moisturizer for dry skin; it's the price that is obnoxious.

☹ **Balancing Complex SPF 15** *($55 for 4.25 ounces)* doesn't contain the UVA-protecting ingredients avobenzone, zinc oxide, or titanium dioxide, and is not recommended.

☹ **Daily Eye Protection SPF 15** *($55 for 0.5 ounce)* doesn't contain the UVA-protecting ingredients avobenzone, zinc oxide, or titanium dioxide, and is not recommended.

☹ **Hydrating Complex SPF 15** *($50 for 4.25 ounces)* doesn't contain the UVA-protecting ingredients avobenzone, zinc oxide, or titanium dioxide, and is not recommended.

☺ **Protection Extreme Total Body SPF 15** *($30 for 4.25 ounces)* does contain UVA protection and that would make it a consideration. Be aware that the price discourages correct usage, because it takes at least one ounce of a sunscreen to adequately cover the body and provide the labeled SPF protection. At a little over 4 ounces, this product would last about four days.

☺ **Protection Extreme Total Body SPF 25** *($32 for 4.25 ounces)* is similar to the one above and the same comments apply.

☺ $$$ **Extremely Natural Self Bronzer** *($28 for 3.7 ounces)* is not natural in the least. Rather, it is a standard dihydroxyacetone-based self tanner that would work as well as any. For the money and formulation, there would be no reason not to use Neutrogena's or Coppertone's self tanners instead.

☹ $$$ **Facial Refining Masque** *($30 for 2 ounces)*. This standard group of ingredients can make skin feel smooth and make this mask an option for dry skin. However, it won't refine anything and a few of the plant extracts in this product can be a problem for some skin types.

☹ $$$ **Antioxidant Skin Care Derms** *($48 for six treatments)* does have a form of vitamin C that you can patch onto your skin; however, it uses ascorbic acid, which is considered the least stable and most irritating form.

# Oxy Balance (Skin Care Only)

In the lineup of acne products at the drugstore, Oxy Balance actually has some of the better choices, at least when it comes to good topical disinfectants that include benzoyl peroxide. But be careful; you still have to pick and choose in order to avoid some irritating and drying mistakes. Still, there are some good topical disinfectants in this line to consider. To find where Oxy Balance is distributed, call (800) 245-1040.

☹ **Oxy 10 Maximum Medicated Face Wash** *($4.99 for 8 ounces)* is a standard, detergent-based water-soluble cleanser with 10% benzoyl peroxide. While benzoyl peroxide is a great topical disinfectant, in a cleanser the effective ingredients would be washed down the drain before they could go to work. To compensate for that problem, the directions on this cleanser state to "massage gently onto face for 1 to 2 minutes." Even if you had the time to do that, you would be massaging the cleansing agents onto the skin for that length of time too, which can cause fairly serious irritation and dryness and that is not helpful for breakouts.

☹ **Deep Pore Cleansing Pads, Acne Medication with Salicylic Acid** *($4.77 for 90 pads)* would be a good BHA product except that it contains a lot of menthol and alcohol, which are way too irritating for any skin type.

☹ **Gentle Deep Pore Cleansing Pads Acne Medication with Salicylic Acid** *($4.77 for 90 pads)* is similar to the one above and the same warning applies. Calling this "gentle" is just bizarre.

☹ **Maximum Deep Pore Cleansing Pads, Acne Medication with Salicylic Acid** *($4.77 for 90 pads)* is similar to the one above, and the same warning applies.

☺ **All Night Deep Pore Treatment** *($4.84 for 2 ounces)* is a good salicylic acid (BHA) product in a very lightweight base that shouldn't be a problem for most skin types. The pH is just slightly high for this to be a truly effective exfoliant, but only slightly, and it is still definitely an option to consider.

☺ **Oxy 10 Acne Medication Sensitive Skin Formula** *($4.52 for 1 ounce)* is a very good 5% benzoyl-peroxide disinfectant with no other irritants added. But you would always want to start with the lower concentration of benzoyl peroxide, and then you would try this one if you found the milder one not to be as effective as you were wanting.

☺ **Oxy 10 Acne Medication Invisible Formula** *($4.52 for 1 ounce)* is similar to the one above except in a 10% strength. This is an option if the lower strengths of benzoyl peroxide (2.5% and 5%) have not proven to be effective. The next step beyond this formula would be a topical antibiotic prescription you would get from a dermatologist.

☹ **Oxy 10 Acne Medication Cover Up Formula** *($4.66 for 1 ounce)* is similar to the one above, except this one is tinted; unfortunately the color leaves much to be desired.

# Pan Oxyl (Skin Care Only)

These two acne products are found at drugstores but are best left on the shelf. For more information, call (800) 327-3858.

☹ **Pan Oxyl Bar Benzoyl Peroxide 5% Regular Strength** *($5.11 for 4 ounces)* is a detergent-based water-soluble bar cleanser that adds 5% benzoyl peroxide to the mix. The ingredients that keep bar cleansers in their bar form can clog pores, and benzoyl peroxide is wasted in a cleanser because it would just be washed down the drain.

☹ **Pan Oxyl Bar Benzoyl Peroxide 10%, Maximum Strength** *($5.53 for 4 ounces)* is similar to the one above, only this one has 10% benzoyl peroxide.

# *Parthena (Skin Care Only)*

Parthena is clearly aimed at the burgeoning needs of baby boomers—"the forgotten woman," as its brochure states, though "forgotten" is hardly the case for women over 40. Given the thousands of antiaging products being sold, the over-40 woman is not only remembered, she is relentlessly pursued and reminded that she is aging and that there are miracles to help her get over that plight!

Another incongruous statement in the Parthena brochure is that the creators of this line "began to notice a trend in department stores: clients no longer wanted expensive, complicated, and time-consuming regimes, that in our opinion, just did not deliver the results they promised." Uncomplicated?! There are over 12 antiwrinkle products in this line, plus the routine includes separate products for day versus night, a kit for the face and another for the eyes, while there's not a sunscreen anywhere to be found.

Part of Parthena's pitch is that some of its products contain plant hormones, in this case, wild yam extract. Unfortunately (or perhaps fortunately), wild yam cannot act like progesterone when applied on skin. According to *The PDR Family Guide to Natural Medicines & Healing Therapies* and the *American Journal of Obstetrics and Gynecology*, volume 18, 1999, as well as the definitive book on the subject from Dr. John Lee, *What Your Doctor May Not Tell You About Menopause: The Breakthrough Book on Natural Progesterone* (Warner Books, 1996), wild yam is used in the production of artificial [synthetic] progesterone, but it will not yield the hormone in the absence of a chemical conversion process that the body can't supply, though it can be created in a laboratory. That means the use of wild yam on skin is a waste of your time and energy, and makes other creams that do contain USP progesterone a far more interesting consideration.

For more information, call (800) 660-0666 or visit the Web site at www.parthena cosmetics.com or www.hsn.com.

☹ **Echinacea and Camphor Antibacterial Wash** *($19.50 for 8 ounces)* contains camphor, a substance that irritates skin and is a particular problem for the eye area.

☺ **Sense & Sensibility Milk Orchid Cleanser** *($19.50 for 8 ounces)* is basically cold cream with AHAs. You have to wipe off your makeup with a tissue or washcloth to get this off and it can leave a greasy film on the skin, though that can be an option for dry skin. The pH of this cleanser isn't low enough for it to work as an exfoliant.

☺ **$$$ Soothing Eye Makeup Remover** *($16 for 4 ounces)* is a standard, detergent-based makeup remover that would work as well as any.

☺ **Cool Off Moisture Magnet Mist** *($7.50 for 2 ounces)* is basically just a toner, and the witch hazel could be an irritant, but the amount of any of the ingredients other than the water is at best negligible. The wild yam extract in here does not contain progesterone or anything else that would act like progesterone. According to *The PDR Family Guide to Natural Medicines & Healing Therapies* and the *American Journal of Obstetrics and Gynecology*, volume 18, 1999, wild yam is used in the production of artificial [synthetic] progesterone but it will not yield the hormone in the absence of a chemical conversion process that the body can't supply, though it can be created in a laboratory.

☺ **Rapid Skin Exfoliation System for Skin, Eyes, and Lips** *($49.95 for three 2-ounce bottles plus a skin lightener)* is a three-part system that starts you off with a 5% AHA concentration for two to three weeks, then a 10% concentration for two to three weeks, and finally a 15% concentration for another two to three weeks. You then rotate back to the 5% concentration and start all over again. Building up to gradually higher concentrations of AHAs is an interesting concept. The logic for this approach is to slowly increase exfoliation so your skin has a chance to get used to the potential irritation. However, I completely disagree that the goal with AHAs is increased superexfoliation. If anything, increased exfoliation with high concentrations of AHAs is risky for skin due to the fact it is irritating, and besides, how much exfoliation does the skin need? For these products, though, this whole discussion is moot, because the first two bottles have a pH of 5 and so they can't exfoliate the skin; the other one has a pH of 4, which makes it just passable as a good exfoliant.

☺ **Skin Lightening Cream** *($24.50 for 1 ounce)* does contain a good amount of hydroquinone, as well as kojic acid and anti-irritants. There is sunscreen in here but it is minimal and provides no UVA protection. Hydroquinone is considered to be the most effective melanin-inhibiting ingredient, while kojic acid is considered to be unstable and rather irritating in comparison.

☹ **All in One Improvement Cream** *($37.50 for 6 ounces)* is an interesting mixture of AHA and sunscreen for a distressing price. Again, who needs this many AHA products? But the pH is too high for this to be an effective exfoliant and the sunscreen doesn't use avobenzone, titanium dioxide, or zinc oxide, so it is ineffective for UVA protection, too.

☺ **Anhydrous Extreme** *($24.95 for 4 ounces)* is a very good moisturizer for dry skin. The minuscule amount of wild yam in here has no hormonal impact on skin.

☺ **Longevity Daily Line Smoothing Fluid** *($24.50 for 1 ounce)* would be a good moisturizer for someone with normal to dry skin. The wild yam extract in here does not contain progesterone or anything else that would act like progesterone.

☺ **Longevity Resource Cream** *($37.50 for 4 ounces)* is similar to the one above, only in cream form.

☹ **Stress Line Reducing Cream** *($16 for 0.5 ounce)* is another AHA product. It's supposed to contain sunscreen, but it neither states the SPF nor contains UVA protection, and the pH is too high for the AHA to be effective as an exfoliant.

☺ **Eye Power Lift** *($19.95 for 2 ounces)* is just a lightweight moisturizer for normal to dry skin; it won't lift skin anywhere.

☹ **Hydro-Enzymatic Line Digesting Mask** *($24.99 for 4 ounces)* is a great name for a product that is nothing more than a standard plasticizing mask that digests little more than your money! It contains mostly witch hazel, alcohol, and some enzymes. You already know about witch hazel and alcohol being irritants, and while enzymes have some ability to exfoliate skin, the problems posed by the other ingredients are harmful for skin.

☺ **$$$ Metamorphosis** *($37.50 for four ampoules, total of 1 ounce)* is more wild yam with a host of other gimmicks like bioengineered placenta extract (meaning fake placenta), collagen, shark cartilage powder, and a host of vitamins. None of this will change anything, but this is a good lightweight moisturizer for normal to slightly dry skin. It is supposed to be worn under the All in One Cream, which clearly isn't so complete or you wouldn't need this stuff underneath. It also contains wild yam extract, which has no hormonal effect on skin.

☹ **Sulfur and Mint Vacuum Mask** *($16 for 4 ounces)* has a name that speaks for itself. Mint (menthol) is a skin irritant that, combined with sulfur, can cause more problems than it can help.

## Paula Dorf Cosmetics (Makeup Only)

Paula Dorf is well known among some cosmetics companies as a makeup artist par excellence for ads and commercials. With that reputation in place, Dorf has now entered the fray where other makeup artists turned entrepreneurs, such as Bobbi Brown, Laura Mercier, and Jeanine Lobell (of Stila) have set up shop. Dorf has stamped her signature of approval on a handsome line of products. Are these cosmetics inherently better because a makeup artist approves and stands behind them? Well, yes and no. On the one hand, a makeup artist's line usually consists of excellent, neutral-toned foundations, matte blush and eyeshadow colors, a vast palette of lipstick choices, and—the crowning jewel—a stunning collection of well-made makeup brushes, and Dorf's line does excel in those areas.

On the other hand, there is a lot to be said for technique and skill, because the best makeup artists can make complicated, redundant makeup application steps look like a breeze. Regrettably, Dorf excels here as well. You will notice a preponderance of unnecessary application tools and products that seem like a good idea but will only become part of every woman's graveyard of impulse cosmetics buys. My suggestion is to ignore these "unique" items unless you can reasonably see yourself using them on a regular basis. Beyond that, this is a line that has good potential, especially if some of the gimmicky products are weeded out. There is more than enough here to make this line worth stopping for if you happen to come across a display. Although Paula Dorf may not yet be a household name, the line is expanding to more stores and is already a presence on the Internet, so you will undoubtedly be seeing more of it, nestled among the "me too" clamor of her peers. For more information on Paula Dorf Cosmetics, call 888-472-8523 or visit the Web site at www.pauladorf.com.

☺ $$$ <u>FOUNDATION:</u> **Moisture Foundation Oil-Free** *($34)*. The somewhat confusing combination of "oil-free" and "moisturizing" in the name may leave you wondering exactly who is supposed to use this foundation. It turns out to be a very good, lightweight, matte-finish foundation that is appropriate for someone with normal to oily skin seeking sheer to light coverage. The 12-shade color selection is quite nice. The only colors to consider avoiding are Cream, Sand, and Cocoa; they may be too peach for most skin tones.

☺ $$$ **Face Tint SPF 15** *($34)* is a very sheer, tinted moisturizer that contains no UVA protectants, so it is not recommended for sun protection. However, for a slight hint of color, it can work well, even though most of the six shades are slightly peach or pink.

☺ **Perfect Primer** *($24)* is not a foundation; it is a lightweight moisturizer with a film-forming agent that can leave a somewhat matte finish on the skin. It is meant to provide an even canvas for makeup application. If you are already using a light moisturizer over dry areas, this is an extra step, and the oil-control and lifting claims are not substantiated either by the standard ingredients on the list or their performance.

<u>CONCEALER:</u> ☹ **Total Camouflage** *($22)* has two shades of concealer in a single pot. The texture is rather thick and greasy and the color combinations are strange. Each duo has one neutral color and a corresponding shade of peach or pink. Although this claims to "last all day" and be "lightweight," the emollience of this one assures fading and creasing as the day wears on. Besides, with so many reliable neutral concealer options out there, who wants to waste time blending two separate colors, especially ones that have no relation to skin tone? **Magic Stick** *($15)* is a very greasy, opaque concealer in a lipstick-style tube. There is only one color, a peach tone, and this, coupled with the heaviness of the product, makes it difficult to recommend. Dorf's claim that "one color fits all skin tones" is embarrassing.

<u>POWDER:</u> ☺ $$$ **Pressed Powder** *($25)* has a beautiful, smooth texture that blends on evenly over the skin. All of the colors are workable, including some excellent matte bronze shades for women of color.

☺ $$$ **All-Over Glimmer Dust** *($20)* is simply very shiny loose powder with either gold or silver pigment. This could work for an evening look but it is messy and easy to overdo.

☺ $$$ <u>BLUSH:</u> **Cheek Color Powder** *($17)* has a wonderful texture and a soft, dry finish. The colors are a nice range of matte neutrals and they blend on sheer, allowing you to build on the intensity. **Cheek Color Creme** *($17)* is a small but superior group of cream-to-powder blushes. This dries to a sheer, almost translucent powdery finish, and the colors are great.

EYESHADOW: ☺ $$$ Eyecolor ($16) is billed by Paula Dorf as the "creamiest powder shadow," and although that sounds divine, its drier, matte texture contradicts that claim. These are still nice eyeshadows, with a good selection of matte shades that go on evenly and should wear well. The shiny shades are all here too, and easily identified. ☹ Eye Primer ($20) is a very thick, waxy eyeshadow base that is completely unnecessary. This will only create a whitish ring around the eye area and, owing to its creaminess, creasing is guaranteed. Eye Color Glimmers ($17) are a small collection of creamy, shiny eyeshadows. The shine is glaring and the texture of these can make blending difficult.

EYE AND BROW SHAPER: Topping the list of unnecessary makeup products is this one, called ☹ Transformer ($14); this mostly watery substance is supposed to transform eyeshadow to a liquid liner. Funny—tap water does the same thing and it's virtually free.

☺ Eye Pencil ($14) is a standard pencil with a slightly creamy, smooth application. The pigment base is strong, so even though these are creamier they should last longer (they may also be harder to remove). $$$ Brow Duet ($20) is a dry-textured matte brow powder that is packaged with two shades. There are three duos suited to most brow colors from blonde to black, and they apply softly and easily. Each set's colors are similar, so you may find you can use both or, as I suspect will happen for most women, you will prefer one shade over the other. Perfect Brow ($12) is a clear mascara for the lashes or the brows and it does work to keep the brow in place. There are much less expensive options for this kind of look, the least pricey of which is grooming the brows with some hairspray on an old toothbrush.

LIPSTICK AND LIP PENCIL: The ☺ $$$ Lipstick ($16) makes the most universal of all lipstick claims: that it wears "all day long." Well, it might if you reapply at regular intervals, but otherwise this is a standard, greasy lipstick that has a lot of slip and a glossy finish. Lip Pencil ($14) comes in a nice range of colors. Due to a higher pigment level, these do tend to stain the lips more than usual so they tend to stay longer than most. Lip Gloss ($15) is nothing but a standard, fairly sticky gloss in one of the smallest packages I've seen. There is no reason to spend this much on such a very basic product. Moisture Stick with Vitamin E ($14) is a standard waxy lip balm that works as well as any to soothe dry, cracked lips. The vitamin E in here is only a dusting so it serves little purpose.

☹ Perfect Illusion ($18) is supposed to plump your lips and stop lipstick from feathering. It falls flat on both counts. When tested, it took less than an hour for even a soft matte lipstick to break through into lines, and there was no difference in the size of your lips whatsoever.

<u>MASCARA:</u> ☺ **Mascara** *($14)* builds nice, long, and clump-free lashes but it does take some effort to get there. Don't expect much thickness, in spite of this being labeled a "thickening formula."

☹ **Cake Mascara** *($20)* says on the box it's from "Hollywood's Golden Age," and while that may be true in terms of mascara's history, by no means does that make this anything you should consider today. Why Dorf thought this was a good idea is a mystery. It is awkward and messy to use, builds no length or thickness, and, given the way you have to hold the fan-shaped brush, is very to easy to get it in the eye. Trying to apply this became quite amusing, but the laughter was only because I knew I would be returning this waste-of-time mascara the next time I went to the cosmetics counters.

☺ $$$ <u>BRUSHES:</u> There is a great array of **brushes** *($6 to $60, and $95 to $150 for partial sets)* to consider. Most of these are quite good, particularly the eyeshadow and eyelining options. There is an unusually wide range of synthetic brushes that are softer and smoother than the norm, and these may be an option for foundation or concealer and even shadow application.

However, there are several gimmicky brushes you can easily ignore, such as the ☺ $$$ **Foundation Brush** *($35)*, because if there are makeup artists who use this technique of applying foundation I haven't met any, and the ☺ $$$ **Cream Cheek Brush** *($35)*, when a sponge or your fingers work just as well. The ☹ **Mascara Fan Brush** *($16)* and the ☹ **Brow Brush** *($17)* are too stiff and scratchy, while the **Lip Brush** *($17)* is too small for most women's lips, and takes forever to completely apply color. The ☺ $$$ **Blush** *($40)* and the **Powder** *($60)* brushes are very soft but too loosely packed for the money; denser brushes are far better for applying color evenly.

## Paula's Choice/Paula's Select

By now many of you are aware that I created my own skin-care line called Paula's Choice, and a makeup line called Paula's Select. Some of you may find that shocking, while others, about 70,000 of you as this book went to press, thought I had formulated a great, inexpensive line of skin-care and makeup products. It's not that I haven't had returns—not everyone's skin can tolerate everything—but for the most part it has been a great venture, and the feedback and the relationship with the people who buy my products has been incredibly satisfying.

For those of you not familiar with my work, you may be wondering just why I decided to create a line of skin-care products at all. Isn't that like Ralph Nader designing and selling cars? Good question (except, personally, I wish Ralph would come out with a reliable group of automobiles!).

Believe me when I say I did not undertake this endeavor without a great deal of thought. Actually it is where I started more than 20 years ago, when I owned my own cosmetics stores that included my own skin-care line. If anything, I feel I have come full circle, except now I know far more than I did back then! Basically, after 20 years of analyzing and reviewing hundreds of cosmetics lines and thousands upon thousands of skin-care and makeup products, it seemed like a natural extension of my work. As you already know, I have been continually frustrated by the endless array of products making claims that are either untrue or misleading. And even when I find products that meet my criteria for performance they often fall short in other ways. For example, many products I otherwise like contain fragrance (a major cause of skin irritation), coloring agents, problematic preservatives, irritating or sensitizing plant extracts; are tested on animals; have (for AHAs and BHA) the wrong pH or concentration to be effective; or, more often than not, are just absurdly overpriced.

Paula's Choice is a line of skin-care products that I have formulated to meet my criteria. None of my products contain coloring agents, fragrance (not even masking fragrances), or any of the irritating ingredients I've been warning about for years, and they aren't tested on animals. I make no exaggerated claims and, better yet, these products are inexpensive—every product is under $14, and they come in generous-sized containers. Paula's Select is a range of cosmetics that I feel can create a classic makeup look that can go from day to night and work beautifully for women trying to create a sophisticated, professional image.

A few women have voiced concerns that I would be abandoning my cosmetics and hair-care research, as well as my objectivity, for cosmetics sales. This is not my intent. I truly believe that offering women inexpensive, high-quality skin-care products that live up to my expectations is a service that should not get in the way of my judgment. However, all of you will be the best judges of whether I indeed remain objective. I believe the reviews in this book speak louder than anything I could say directly to you. Clearly there are plenty of products I recommend that aren't mine because there are many good options that can have a positive effect on skin, and that's what women need.

I am committed to maintaining my standards. There will always be great products for me to recommend, and terrible, overpriced products for me to caution you about. My products are one option from what my research indicates are reliable and effective products: nothing more, nothing less.

I debated at length about how to review my products. After all, this is an area where it is the hardest for me to be impartial. I attempted as best I could to review them as if they weren't my own, and decided to just give it a go, trying to be as objective as I could possibly be. Basically, this section is just a way to give you a better understanding of my products. I did decide to leave them unrated (without faces), because I couldn't possibly be *that* impartial! Paula's Choice and Paula's Select products are available by calling (800) 831-4088 or (206) 444-1622. You can also order through my Web site at www.cosmeticscop.com.

# *Paula's Choice*

**One Step Face Cleanser for Normal to Oily/Combination Skin** *($10.95 for 8 ounces)* is a standard detergent cleanser that takes off all makeup, including eye makeup, without irritating or drying the skin.

**One Step Face Cleanser for Normal to Dry Skin** *($10.95 for 8 ounces)* is a standard detergent cleanser that takes off all makeup, including eye makeup, without irritating or drying the skin. It contains some glycerin to soften and soothe skin.

**Final Touch Toner for Normal to Oily/Combination Skin** *($9.95 for 8 ounces)* is a nonirritating toner. It should leave a clean, soothing feeling on the skin.

**Final Touch Toner for Normal to Dry Skin** *($9.95 for 8 ounces)* is a nonirritating, moisturizing toner. It should leave a clean, soothing feeling on the skin.

**Essential Moisturizing Sunscreen SPF 15** *($11.95 for 6 ounces)* is a partly titanium dioxide–based sunscreen that contains thickeners, plant oil, vitamins (antioxidants), and preservatives. This is a good emollient moisturizer for someone with dry skin.

**Essential Non-Greasy Sunscreen SPF 15** *($11.95 for 6 ounces)* is an avobenzone-based sunscreen in a lightweight lotion form. It is irritant-free and leaves a matte finish on the skin.

**Essential Pure Block Sunscreen SPF 15** *($12.95 for 6 ounces)* uses only titanium dioxide and zinc oxide as the active sunscreen agents. That makes it a very good option for someone with sensitive skin, though it can be effective for any skin type except blemish-prone skin.

**Completely Non-Greasy Moisturizing Lotion** *($12.95 for 4 ounces)* is a good lightweight moisturizer for someone with normal to oily skin. It can also be used around the eye area if that area needs moisturizer.

**Completely Emollient Moisturizer** *($12.95 for 4 ounces)* is a good emollient moisturizer for someone with normal to dry skin. It can also be used around the eye area if that area needs moisturizer.

**Extra Emollient Moisturizer for Extra Dry Skin** *($12.95 for 4 ounces)* is formulated so it can also be used around the eyes. It is best for someone with dry to very dry skin. It is very emollient and has great water-binding agents and anti-irritants.

**Remarkable Skin Lightening Lotion for All Skin Types** *($12.95 for 4 ounces)* takes account of all the research I've seen that indicates that hydroquinone is most effective in inhibiting melanin production when it is used in a conjunction with an effective sunscreen. Strengths of 1% to 2% concentrations are available over the counter while 4% to 12% concentrations are available from physicians. My product contains 2% hydroquinone with 7.4% glycolic acid (AHA) in a lightweight moisturizing base with a pH of 3.5. This product can be used on the face, hands, arms, legs, or neck, and is best for someone with normal to dry skin.

**Blemish Fighting Solution for All Skin Types** *($12.95 for 4 ounces)* is a 2.5% benzoyl peroxide solution in a lightweight base. It also contains anti-irritants. For years, I have been recommending 3% hydrogen peroxide to disinfect blemishes, and that is a good option for some, but for others, 2.5% benzoyl peroxide lotion or gel is the next step in trying to win the battle against breakouts. This **cannot** be used with Retin-A, Renova, or Differin.

**Extra Strength Blemish Fighting Solution** *($12.95 for 4 ounces)* combats blemishes by stopping problem-causing bacteria with 5% benzoyl peroxide. It also contains anti-irritants that can reduce redness and irritation. This formulation leaves no residue on the skin. This **cannot** be used with Retin-A, Renova, or Differin.

**8% Alpha Hydroxy Acid Solution** *($12.95 for 4 ounces)* is an 8% gel/serum-type AHA with a pH of 3.2. It also contains an anti-irritant, water-binding agents, and preservatives. It can be mixed with other moisturizers or used under sunscreens. It is an effective exfoliating product for the face or body.

**1% Beta Hydroxy Acid Solution** *($12.95 for 4 ounces)* gently exfoliates the skin and unclogs pores without leaving the skin feeling greasy or dry. There are no waxy ingredients to clog pores or make skin feel layered with too many products, and it includes anti-irritants to help soothe the skin. This is best for someone with blemishes and blackheads with normal to dry skin. It can be especially helpful for someone with rosacea. There is anecdotal information that BHA, due to its relationship to aspirin (both are salicylates), can reduce redness and inflammation while gently exfoliating. This **can** be used with Retin-A, Renova, or Differin. It has a pH of 3.2.

**2% Beta Hydroxy Acid Solution** *($12.95 for 4 ounces)* is similar to the 1% Beta Hydroxy Acid Solution in terms of performance but this one is double the strength and in a liquid base. It is better for more stubborn blemish problems. It has a pH of 3.2.

**All Day Cover Moisturizing Sunscreen SPF 30+ with Antioxidants Waterproof** *($11.95 for 6 ounces)* is similar to my Essential Moisturizing Sunscreen SPF 15. I put slightly more antioxidants in this one and more SPF protection (it's still part titanium dioxide), and made it waterproof.

**All Day Cover Non-Greasy Sunscreen SPF 30+ with Antioxidants Waterproof** *($11.95 for 6 ounces)* is similar to my Essential Nongreasy Sunscreen SPF 15. I put slightly more antioxidants in this one and more SPF protection (it's still part avobenzone), and made it waterproof.

**Almost the Real Thing Self-Tanning Gel** *($12.95 for 6 ounces)* provides a fast, natural-looking tan. This is a gel formula that works well for all skin types. It is tinted with a caramel coloring so it is easy to see where it has been applied, helping you achieve a more even application.

**Total Protection Lip Care SPF 15** *($6.95 for 0.5 ounce)* is a very good emollient lip balm, but that isn't so unusual. What is special about this product is that it has an in-part titanium dioxide base. That helps with sun protection and prevents dry lips.

**Exfoliating Lip Treatment** *($7.95 for 0.5 ounce)* is a unique way to get dry skin off your lips without irritation. You use a tiny amount and rub it into your lips, then keep rubbing until the excess skin starts to flake off. Simply brush off what remains, and then apply the Total Protection Lip Care SPF 15 above or another emollient lip balm.

**Oil-Absorbing Facial Mask Oily/Combination Skin** *($9.95 for 6 ounces)* absorbs excess oil from the surface of the skin and from within the pore without irritation or dryness. There are no clays to dehydrate skin or waxy ingredients to clog pores. This mask is best for someone with oily or blemish-prone skin.

## *Paula's Select*

FOUNDATION: Available Spring 2001.

CONCEALER: **No Slip Concealer** *($6.95)* is a creaseless concealer with a soft matte finish in four neutral shades.

POWDER: **Soft Pressed Powder** *($9.95)* can be used as a finishing powder over foundation or alone as a powder-based foundation for all skin types. It can also be used wet or dry. It has a silky-soft texture and, I think, eight great neutral shades with a light matte finish.

BLUSH: **Soft Matte Blush** *($7.95)*. I've chosen ten shades of blush that have a good velvety, matte, light texture that does not fade or dissipate throughout the day. They go on smooth and even, and I think you'll find the colors are quite workable and can blend on soft or dramatic, depending on what you need.

LIPSTICK AND LIP PENCIL: **Soft Matte Lipstick** *($6.95)*. I decided to start my lipstick line with my favorite texture of lipstick, an opaque matte-finish lipstick (there are 14 shades). **Soft Cream Lipstick** *($6.95)* has an emollient, smooth feel with a silky texture and opaque coverage and it is available in ten shades. **Long-Lasting Anti-Feather Lipliner** *($5.95)* is a standard, twist-up lip liner that I chose to match my soft matte lipsticks. These have a smooth texture but aren't greasy, and they can help prevent feathering (which most pencils that have this kind of texture can do). I've also included a clear Long-Lasting Lipliner that is similar to a discontinued version from The Body Shop called No Wander. This can help keep most lipsticks from bleeding (though it won't stop exceptionally greasy, glossy lipsticks from feathering). **Soft Shine Moisturizing Lip Gloss** *($5.95)* is a good basic gloss that doesn't feel too sticky or thick on the lips.

MASCARA: **Lush Mascara** *($6.95)* will create long, thick lashes without clumping, flaking, or smearing, and it will last all day. It's water soluble for easy removal.

Epic Lengths Mascara *($6.95)* has great lengthening ability without the intense thickening action of the Lush version.

<u>BRUSHES:</u> My brushes are very soft and dense, and hold their shape, as well as place color evenly with minimal to no flaking of powder. The **Powder Brush** *($14.95)*, **Blush Brush** *($11.95)*, two **Eyeshadow Brushes**, **Small** and **Large** *($8.95 each)*, a **Brow Brush** *($6.95)*, an **Eyeliner** *($6.95)*, and a **Lip Brush** *($5.95)* are all great options. There is also a convenient **Brush Carrying Case** *($12.95)* that can hold up to eight brushes. I also have Paula's Select **Makeup Application Sponges** for applying foundation *($2.95 for ten round latex sponges)*.

# Peter Thomas Roth

Peter Thomas Roth has created a skin-care empire, or at least an empire in the making. What makes it so illustrious is the large number of products: it is unusual for a new spa or specialty line to start out with such a vast array. Actually, to call this line of skin-care products large is an understatement—it is huge. Over 80 skin-care products are listed in the catalog, and that doesn't include new ones I'm sure they will be launched! In terms of product formulation, the company has done a good job of staying current with the industry, something a lot of far more expensive, fancier lines haven't done.

What is most fascinating to me is that, in some ways, this is a rather straightforward line with uncomplicated formulations. Many of them are quite good and state-of-the-art. Most all of the acne, AHA, BHA, sunscreen, and moisturizing products contain what they should to be effective and helpful for skin. Not surprisingly, many are also redundant, with only minor changes in formulation, but that doesn't make them bad, it just makes this line overcrowded and confusing for the consumer or aesthetician.

Another novel aspect of this line is that there are few (if any) nonsense ingredients. These products conspicuously lack the exotic, potentially irritating, sensitizing, and often unnecessary plant extracts, plant oils, and fragrances that show up in most expensive skin-care lines, especially spa lines. Many of the products do not contain coloring agents, fragrance, or a long list of ingredients. The simplicity is as impressive as it is refreshing.

What you will notice immediately is that the prices are ridiculous. Almost every product in the Peter Thomas Roth line is easily replaced by far less expensive versions. However, this is a line worth looking at, because if you're the type of consumer who is going to overspend on skin care, you may as well get products that can do something for the skin. For more information on Peter Thomas Roth, call (800) PTR SKIN.

☺ $$$ **Chamomile Cleansing Lotion** *($30 for 8 ounces)* is a very standard, detergent-based water-soluble cleanser that uses a few cleansing agents I wouldn't exactly call gentle. Still, this would be very good for someone with normal to oily skin.

☺ $$$ **Gentle Cleansing Lotion** (*$30 for 8 ounces*) is similar to the one above minus the stronger detergent cleansing agents and with a little bit of safflower oil added. It would be a very good cleanser for someone with normal to dry skin.

☺ $$$ **Foaming Face Wash** (*$30 for 8 ounces*) is similar to the one above only with lemon oil, an unnecessary skin irritant, which does not make this better for oily skin. However, the amount is small enough so it probably doesn't pose much of a problem for skin.

☺ $$$ **Extra Strength Cleansing Gel Oil-Free for Oily, Combination or Problem Skin** (*$30 for 8 ounces*) is a very standard, detergent-based water-soluble cleanser that would be very good for someone with normal to oily skin.

☺ $$$ **Sensitive Skin Cleansing Gel** (*$30 for 8 ounces*) is similar to the ones above, only with a reduced amount of detergent cleansing agents. It would be good for someone with normal to somewhat dry or oily skin.

☺ $$$ **Combination Skin Cleansing Gel** (*$30 for 8 ounces*) is similar to the Sensitive Skin version above and the same review applies.

☹ $$$ **Silky Cleansing Cream** (*$30 for 8 ounces*) is a standard emollient, cold cream–like, wipe-off cleanser. For very dry skin it would be an option, but no better than lots of other similar cleansers at the drugstore.

☺ $$$ **Glycolic Acid 3% Face Wash** (*$30 for 8 ounces*) is similar to the Foaming Face Wash only without the lemon oil. The minimal amount of AHA in here and the high pH make this ineffective as an exfoliant (which isn't the best in a cleanser anyway) so it is just fine to consider. This would be a good cleanser for someone with normal to oily skin.

☺ $$$ **Beta Hydroxy Acid 2% Acne Wash** (*$32 for 8 ounces*) is an exceptionally standard, detergent-based water-soluble cleanser that would be an option for normal to oily skin. The BHA in here is not effective as an exfoliant due to the high pH of the product.

☹ $$$ **Medicated BPO 5% Acne Wash** (*$28 for 8 ounces*) is an exceptionally standard, detergent-based water-soluble cleanser that would be an option for normal to oily skin. The benzoyl peroxide is a good topical disinfectant but it would just be washed down the drain before it had a chance to have an effect. And if you left the cleanser on the face for a period of time, that cleansing agent would overly irritate and hurt the skin.

☹ **AHA/BHA Face & Body Polish** (*$30 for 8 ounces*) contains sodium C14-16 olefin sulfate as its second ingredient, which is too drying and potentially irritating for all skin types. The amount of AHA in here is not enough to be an exfoliant and the pH is too high for it to have any exfoliating properties even if there were enough.

☹ **Botanical Buffing Beads** *($30 for 8 ounces)* has a gentle synthetic abrasive but the detergent cleansing agent is too drying and irritating for all skin types.

☹ **Pumice Medicated Acne Scrub with 2.5% Benzoyl Peroxide** *($30 for 8 ounces)* uses pumice as the scrub, which can be too abrasive for all skin types. The benzoyl peroxide in here would be washed off before it had a chance to have an effect.

☹ **Silica Face & Body Polish** *($30 for 8 ounces)* uses sodium C14-16 olefin sulfate as the cleansing agent, which is too drying and irritating for all skin types.

☹ **Silica Strawberry Scrub** *($30 for 8 ounces)* uses pumice and ground-up plastic as the abrasive, but the pumice can be too irritating for most skin types.

☺ **$$$ Aloe Tonic Mist** *($30 for 8 ounces)* is a rather simple, though nonirritating toner. It would work well as a toner for most skin types.

☺ **$$$ Conditioning Tonic** *($30 for 8 ounces)* is an incredibly simple formulation of water, slip agent, preservative, and about 0.5% BHA, period! The pH is too high for this to be effective as an exfoliant. Clinique has a version that is better for half the price.

☹ **Glycolic Acid Clarifying Tonic** *($30 for 8 ounces)* contains alcohol and is not recommended.

☺ **$$$ Oxygen Mist** *($35 for 8 ounces)*. The claim that this product can provide any more oxygen to the skin than what is already available in the air is sort of funny, except, of course, to the people who have wasted their money on it. Even if this was a great way to deliver oxygen, it doesn't explain the potential problems generated from oxidative damage, which is what the world of antioxidant ingredients is all about.

☺ **$$$ Power C Firming Spritz** *($35 for 8 ounces)*. If you're looking for a vitamin C product, this one would work well as a toner, though I am skeptical that this form of vitamin C is stable in this formula.

☺ **$$$ Glycolic Acid 5% Moisturizer** *($40 for 2 ounces)* is a good AHA product for someone with sensitive, dry skin, but Pond's Age Defying Cream (with the red cap) has an almost identical formula.

☺ **$$$ Glycolic Acid 10% Moisturizer** *($40 for 2 ounces)* is similar to the one above, and would be a very good AHA moisturizer for someone with normal to dry skin. This is a very plain, ordinary ingredient listing, but it is a good exfoliant.

☺ **$$$ Glycolic Acid 10% Hydrating Gel** *($45 for 2 ounces)* is quite similar to Alpha Hydrox's oil-free version, which costs about $10 for 1.7 ounces. This one is definitely a good AHA formula for someone with normal to oily skin and it does have very good water-binding agents.

☹ **Glycolic Acid 10% Clarifying Gel** *($45 for 2 ounces)* contains both BHA and AHA, but it also contains alcohol and is not recommended. Also, the amount of BHA in here is not enough for it to be effective as an exfoliant.

☺ **$$$ AHA 12% Hydrating Ceramide Repair Gel** *($45 for 2 ounces)* is similar to the Hydrating Gel above only it adds a tiny amount of water-binding agents and a variety of AHAs. The additional AHA ingredients are unnecessary and don't work as well as the glycolic or lactic acid, but this would still be a good AHA product for someone with normal to oily skin.

☺ $$$ Glycolic Acid 3% Eye Complex ($48 for 0.75 ounce) is a good emollient moisturizer for dry skin, but the 3% AHA isn't enough to exfoliate skin and nor is the pH low enough to create that effect anyway.

☹ $$$ AHA/Kojic Acid Under Eye Brightener ($48 for 0.75 ounce) is a good emollient moisturizer for dry skin (similar to the one above), only this one adds kojic acid. Kojic acid can have some effect on reducing melanin content, but it is not a stable ingredient and is considered not as effective as hydroquinone.

☺ $$$ Ceramide Moisture Renewal ($45 for 2 ounces) is a very good emollient moisturizer for dry skin. Ceramide is a good water-binding agent, but it is no more a must-have ingredient for skin than dozens of other good water-binding agents.

☺ $$$ Ceramide Night Renewal ($50 for 2 ounces) is similar to the one above and the same comments apply.

☺ $$$ Ceramide Ultra-Rich Night Renewal ($55 for 2 ounces) is similar to the two versions above only with more plant oils and emollients, which makes it better for someone with dry to very dry skin.

☺ $$$ Ceramide Eye Complex ($48 for 0.75 ounce) is a very good emollient moisturizer for dry skin.

☻ Co-Oxygen Q-10 Wrinkle Repair ($110 for 2.3 ounces) is an incredibly confused product. For one thing, it is a very standard, basic, Vaseline-based moisturizer with thickeners and glycerin (which is just fine for dry skin, but Lubriderm would be just as good if not better for that). It also contains hydrogen peroxide, which minimally releases oxygen, but you could accomplish that far better by buying an 89-cent bottle at the drugstore. The other issue is that while the coenzyme Q10 this product contains is a good antioxidant, the hydrogen peroxide releases oxygen, so they would at best cancel each other out. There is also a minuscule amount of BHA in here, but the pH is too high for it to be effective as an exfoliant. If you're looking for a coenzyme Q10 product, Nivea's version is far less confused and far better formulated than this one.

☺ Environmental Repair Hydrating Gel ($35 for 2 ounces) won't repair anything, but it is a good, lightweight moisturizer for normal to slightly dry or oily skin.

☹ $$$ Oil-Free Moisturizer ($40 for 2 ounces). The interesting ingredients are barely present, which makes this a very basic, mundane moisturizer for someone with normal to slightly dry skin.

☺ $$$ Power C 10 Serum Liquid ($75 for 1 ounce) contains 10% L-ascorbic acid, along with slip agents, water-binding agent, and preservatives, so if you want a vitamin C product this is an option for most skin types, though why anyone needs this is more a result of the power of marketing and publicity than skin-care health.

☺ $$$ **Power C 10 Anti-Oxidant Serum Gel** *($80 for 1 ounce)* is similar to the one above, only this one has additional antioxidants and some plant extracts. It would also be an option for a vitamin C product in a gel formula for most skin types.

☺ $$$ **Power C 20 Anti-Oxidant Serum Gel** *($80 for 1 ounce)* is similar to the Serum Gel above only with more of the vitamin C.

☺ $$$ **Power C Eye Complex** *($48 for 0.75 ounce)* is a good moisturizer for dry skin. It contains magnesium ascorbyl palmitate, which has some effectiveness at inhibiting melanin in skin, but not in this small amount.

☺ $$$ **Power C Souffle** *($85 for 1.5 ounces)* is similar to the Eye Complex above and the same comments apply.

☹ $$$ **Power C Instant Glow** *($110 for 0.8 ounce)* contains 10% ascorbyl palmitate in a standard group of thickening agents and preservatives. Ascorbyl palmitate is a good antioxidant, and 10% is a nice amount, but the price tag is bizarre and the benefit to skin just theoretical. This won't change a wrinkle and it isn't even a very good moisturizer.

☹ $$$ **Power C Ultra Lite Skin Luminizer** *($110 for 1 ounce)* is similar to the Instant Glow above only with about a 5% concentration of ascorbyl palmitate in a slightly more emollient base.

☺ $$$ **Power K Eye Rescue** *($100 for 0.5 ounce)*. The primary claim for vitamin K's use in cosmetics is to reduce the appearance of dark circles and reduce the appearance of surface capillaries. Yet there is no independent research showing vitamin K to be effective for any aspect of skin care. The study quoted as proof for this was done by the patent holder and the company selling vitamin K products. This is a good moisturizer with good water-binding agents and antioxidants, which is great for dry skin, but it's not worth this price tag. It does contain magnesium ascorbyl phosphate, which can inhibit melanin production in a concentration of 10%, but this doesn't even have a 1% concentration.

☺ $$$ **Power K Skin Brightener** *($110 for 1 ounce)* is similar to the Power K version above and the same comments apply.

☹ $$$ **Retinolique Forte (5%)** *($85 for 1 ounce)* definitely contains a form of vitamin A, but it is not the one all the current research is talking about, namely retinol. This one contains retinyl propionate, and whether or not it can make a difference in skin at any concentration is unknown but very unlikely, given its distant relationship to retinol.

☺ $$$ **Potent Botanical Skin Brightening Gel Complex** *($45 for 2 ounces)* is a lightweight gel that contains kojic acid. Kojic acid can have some effect on reducing melanin content, but it is not a stable ingredient and is considered not as effective as hydroquinone. This also contains ascorbic acid, which is not considered to be stable or effective for skin lightening. However, this does contain azelaic acid, which by itself is considered a weak skin-lightening agent, though it can compare to hydroquinone when combined with high concentrations of glycolic acid and this product has that. This is a mixed bag but a definite option for skin lightening.

☺ $$$ **Potent Botanical Skin Brightening Lotion Complex** (*$45 for 2 ounces*) is similar to the Gel Complex version above only with 10% AHA, and this one is in lotion form.

☺ $$$ **Potent Skin Lightening Gel Complex** (*$50 for 2 ounces*) is similar to the Brightening Lotion above only with the addition of hydroquinone. This is a definite option to consider for skin lightening.

☺ $$$ **Potent Skin Lightening Lotion Complex** (*$50 for 2 ounces*) is almost identical to the Gel Complex above except it is in a lightweight lotion form and has some water-binding agents and vitamins.

☺ $$$ **Ultra Gentle Skin Lightening Gel Complex** (*$50 for 2 ounces*) is similar to the Gel Complex above only the pH is too high for the AHA to have an exfoliating effect on skin. Due to the hydroquinone and azelaic acid in here, it is still an effective option for skin lightening.

☹ **AHA/BHA Acne Clearing Gel** (*$45 for 2 ounces*) contains alcohol, which is too drying and irritating for all skin types. There are effective AHA and BHA products available for far less money that don't add this or other irritating ingredients to their formulations.

☺ **BPO Gel 2.5%** (*$20 for 3 ounces*) is a very good benzoyl peroxide product in a lightweight gel base for disinfecting areas of skin that tend to break out.

☺ **BPO Gel 5%** (*$22 for 3 ounces*) is similar to the one above only with a stronger concentration, and the same comments apply.

☺ $$$ **BPO Gel 10%** (*$24 for 3 ounces*) is similar to the one above only with a stronger concentration, and the same comments apply.

☹ **BPO Gel 10% and Sulfur** (*$30 for 3 ounces.*) Adding sulfur to this product only makes it harder on skin, causing redness, irritation, and flaky skin.

☹ **Therapeutic Sulfur Masque** (*$40 for 5 ounces*) contains sulfur, along with clay, thickening agents, and preservatives. I do not recommend sulfur for breakouts, as this ingredient can be quite irritating and drying for most skin types, and the high pH it creates can actually increase bacteria growth in skin.

☹ **Sulfur Cooling Masque** (*$40 for 5 ounces*) has the same problems as the one above, plus this one also contains eucalyptus. Ouch!

☺ **Daily Defense Moisture Cream SPF 20** (*$25 for 4 ounces*) is a good, part titanium dioxide–based sunscreen; it also contains some thickening agents and a tiny amount of vitamins and preservatives. To say the least, there are similar if not better versions than this for far less money.

☺ **Oil-Free Sunblock SPF 20** *($25 for 4 ounces)* is almost identical to the Cream version above and the same review applies. The wax thickeners in this product aren't oil, but they may not make someone with oily skin happy.

☺ **Oil-Free Sunblock SPF 30** *($25 for 4 ounces)* is almost identical to the SPF 20 version above and the same comments apply.

☺ **Water Resistant Sunblock SPF 20** *($25 for 4 ounces)* is similar to the ones above only with a water-resistant formula.

☺ **Water Resistant Sunblock SPF 30** *($25 for 4 ounces)* is similar to the SPF 20 version above and the same comments apply.

☹ **Oil-Free Hydrating Sunscreen Gel SPF 20** *($25 for 4 ounces)* does not contain UVA-protecting ingredients, but it does contain alcohol, and is not recommended.

☹ **Max Daily Defense Moisture Cream SPF 30** *($25 for 4 ounces)* is similar to the SPF 20 version above and the same comments apply.

☺ **Max Sheer All-Day Moisture Defense Lotion SPF 30** *($37 for 1.7 ounces)*. I can't make this point strongly enough: this sunscreen in many ways is no different from products from Ombrelle or Neutrogena for a fraction of the price. This is a good, in-part avobenzone-based sunscreen in a good moisturizing base that includes water-binding agents and vitamins.

☺ **Tinted Protective Day Cream SPF 30** *($40 for 2.3 ounces)* has a color that isn't for everyone, but it disappears well into the skin so it doesn't have much effect. Other than that, it is a very good sunscreen with titanium dioxide and zinc oxide as the active sunscreen agents.

☺ **Titanium Dioxide Sunblock SPF 15** *($25 for 4 ounces)* is a very good, but very ordinary, pure titanium dioxide–based sunscreen.

☺ **Titanium Dioxide Sunblock SPF 30** *($6.26 for 1 ounce)* is similar to the SPF 15 version above, and the same comments apply.

☺ **Ultra Lite Oil-Free Sunblock SPF 30 with Parsol 1789** *($25 for 4 ounces)* is a good sunscreen with in-part avobenzone and titanium dioxide. The name for this product implies it would be good for oily skin and it is not. It is rather emollient and creamy and far better for someone with normal to dry skin.

☹ **Cucumber Gel Masque** *($40 for 4.5 ounces)* contains several irritating ingredients, including pineapple, orange, and lemon, and is not recommended.

☺ **$$$ Hydrating Nutrient Masque** *($40 for 5 ounces)* is a standard clay mask with several thickeners and a small amount of plant oil. It isn't all that hydrating, but it is a good, albeit ordinary, clay mask.

☺ **$$$ Aloe-Cort Cream** *($25 for 2 ounces)* is a very standard 1% hydrocortisone cream, which makes it virtually identical to Lanacort or Cortaid found at the drugstore for half the price.

☺ $$$ **Post-Peel Healing Balm** *($25 for 0.8 ounce)* is almost identical to the Aloe-Cort above and the same comments apply.

☺ $$$ **Soothing Repair Ointment** *($45 for 2 ounces)* contains 2% lidocaine. Lidocaine is synthesized from cocaine and is a popular and very effective anesthetic. It can also be a skin irritant or sensitizer, not to mention that there are far cheaper versions at the drugstore.

## *Pevonia Botanica Skin Care*

Pevonia has become quite a popular spa/salon line of exclusive (read: expensive) skin-care products. Its vast range of products uses just about every hyped marketing angle the cosmetics industry has to offer. From plants and DNA to oxygen and vitamins, there is a little bit of everything here, along with products to reduce thighs, plump up breasts, and, of course, get rid of wrinkles, de-puff eyes, cure acne, and leave you spiritually elevated.

"Experience a realm of skin care far beyond the norm. Each and every pore is drenched with nature's most selective, unadulterated plant extracts; every sensitizer and photosensitizer has been meticulously eliminated." That's quite a claim, but then, one might wonder, how does Pevonia rationalize the use of diazolidinyl urea (a formaldehyde-releasing preservative), triethanolamine, camphor, lemon oil, pine extract, and sodium C14-16 olefin sulfate in its products? Perhaps that's why Pevonia made it so difficult for me to review its ingredient listings.

Pevonia makes a range of other claims that aren't true in the least. For example, Pevonia states that its products are "non-comedogenic" even though they contain several ingredients that can clog pores or trigger breakouts, such as capric triglyceride and irritants like lemon oil. Pevonia boasts that its products "contain no artificial fragrance." That may indeed be true, but because all fragrance is potentially irritating and sensitizing for skin, it has no benefit for skin, whether the source of the fragrance is synthetic, artificial, or natural. "No chemical fillers" is another promise many women think sounds wonderful. Yet Pevonia's products are full of chemical fillers, from triglycerides to stearic acid, polysorbate, carbomer, and polyethylene glycol (PEG).

As is true for most companies with a natural bent, Pevonia brags that its products "contain no mineral oil [and] no lanolin." With so many companies picking up on the absurd, unsubstantiated myth that these two ingredients are somehow bad for skin, it's possible it will be just a matter of time before the entire industry starts leaving these ingredients out of their formulations. Lanolin, an animal derivative, might pose a problem of principle for vegans, but other than that it is an excellent moisturizer for very dehydrated, parched skin. It can be an allergen for some sensitive skin types, but it is not a "bad" or "evil" ingredient. Likewise, mineral oil is an exceptional ingredient for dry skin and its demise in skin-care products would be sad to see.

What gets lost in all the marketing mumbo jumbo and foolishness is the one definite and rather poignant strength of this line: Pevonia's rather simple but elegant formulations. Forget the far-fetched, distorted claims, and you'll see that there are some interesting ingredient combinations to be found here. If you are going to spend money on expensive skin care, it is far better to consider a line that has state-of-the-art combinations of water-binding agents, antioxidants, emollients, and sunscreens with effective UVA protection. Pevonia is definitely more interesting than some of the other overpriced spa and prestige lines I've reviewed, such as Decleor Paris, Guinot, Givenchy, Yon Ka Paris, Phytomer, and Osmotics, among others, which don't have anywhere near the impressive formulations that Pevonia has. For a nice change, some of these products are indeed well-formulated and not a complete waste of money.

For more information about Pevonia, call (800) PEVONIA or visit its Web site at www.pevonia.com.

## Dry Skin Line—Ligne Sevactive

☺ **Sevactive Cleanser** *($19.75 for 6.8 ounces)* is just a cold cream. This can leave a greasy film on the skin and needs to be wiped off though it can be an option for dry skin.

☺ **Sevactive Lotion** *($19.75 for 6.8 ounces)* is a very simple toner that is more like applying fragrance to the skin than anything else. It also contains a minuscule amount of lettuce extract, which can be an anti-irritant, but has no real impact on skin in this amount.

☺ **Sevactive Care Cream** *($28.25 for 1.7 ounces)*. Other than the plant extracts of pine needle, rosemary, and orange, which can be skin irritants, this is a good, though extremely ordinary moisturizer for dry skin.

☹ $$$ **Sevactive Mask** *($29.25 for 1.7 ounces)* would be an option for dry skin but the plant extracts of arnica and horsetail are skin irritants and definitely not an option for sensitive skin.

☹ **Sevactive Face Oil "Jouvence"** *($27.75 for 1 ounce)* is just hazelnut oil with fragrance and a teeny amount of vitamin. Skip the fragrance, which can be a skin sensitizer, and just use some pure hazelnut oil that you buy at the grocery store for far less money.

## Sensitive Skin Line—Ligne Lavandou

☺ **Lavandou Cleanser** *($19.75 for 6.8 ounces)* is almost identical to the Sevactive Cleanser above and the same basic review applies.

☺ **Lavandou Lotion** *($19.75 for 6.8 ounces)* is a very simple toner and is more like applying fragrance to the skin than anything else. It also contains a minuscule amount of lettuce extract, which can be an anti-irritant but has no real impact on skin in this amount.

☺ $$$ **Lavandou Care Cream** *($38.25 for 1.7 ounces)* is a good though ordinary moisturizer for very dry skin. It contains grapefruit extract, which is not the best for sensitive skin.

☺ $$$ **Lavandou Mask** *($30.75 for 1.7 ounces)* is a standard clay mask. The amount of fragrance in here can be a problem for some skin types, while the amount of vitamins is barely detectable, but it can be a good, albeit ordinary clay mask for normal to slightly dry skin.

☹ $$$ **Propolis Concentrate** *($44 for 1 ounce)* does contain propolis, with some water, thickeners, fragrance, and preservative. Propolis is a brownish resinous material collected by bees that is then used in the formation of the hive. It has antibacterial and anti-inflammatory properties for skin. The belief that this is a miracle skin-care ingredient is myth and not based on any research or data.

☹ **Lavandou Face Oil "Douceur"** *($25.25 for 1 ounce)* is just hazelnut oil with fragrance and a teeny amount of vitamin. Skip the fragrance, which can be a skin sensitizer, and just use some pure hazelnut oil that you buy at the grocery store for far less money.

### Normal to Combination Skin Line—Ligne Fondamentale

☹ **Fundamental Cleanser** *($19.75 for 6.8 ounces)* is a greasy cleanser that is inappropriate for combination skin, plus the grapefruit oil and pine and lemon extracts can cause irritation.

☹ **Fundamental Lotion** *($19.75 for 6.8 ounces)*. This standard toner contains witch hazel, which can be a skin irritant. It does contain lactic acid, but the amount is so tiny it is not effective as an exfoliant. This is a very ordinary toner with problems for most all skin types.

☹ **Fundamental Care Cream** *($35 for 1.7 ounces)*. This moisturizer is too emollient for combination skin and the arnica extract and lemongrass oil here make it potentially irritating for all skin types.

☺ $$$ **Fundamental Mask** *($29.75 for 1.7 ounces)* is a standard clay mask. It doesn't get more basic than this, though the pine and rosemary oil can be irritants.

### Oily Skin Line—Ligne Purilys

☹ **Phyto-Gel Cleanser, Ligne Purilys** *($24 for 6.8 ounces)* uses sodium C14-16 olefin sulfate as the main cleansing agent, which makes it too drying for most skin types. It also contains lemon and pine extract, which only add to the irritation.

☺ $$$ **Oily Skin Toning Lotion, Ligne Purilys** *($22 for 6.8 ounces)*. There is no reason to put geranium oil on oily skin, and the amount of lactic acid (AHA) in here isn't enough for it to be effective as an exfoliant. Other than that, it would be an OK toner, but this is really just rose water (water, fragrance, and glycerin), only with geranium oil instead of rose oil. This is more of a "why bother?" product than anything else.

☹ **Purilys Care Cream** *($26.25 for 1.7 ounces)*. The formulation for this one is a bit shocking, especially given that it is supposed to be for oily skin. First, why does someone with oily skin need a moisturizer (though if you use some of these products on oily skin, you are likely to have dry, irritated skin)? Second, what possible use could irritating ingredients such as grapefruit oil and pine and lemon extracts have for skin? And finally, why use thickening agents such as triglycerides that are best suited for dry skin?

☹ **Purilys Mask** *($24.25 for 1.7 ounces)* would just be a very standard but OK clay mask for oily skin if it weren't for the mandarin oil and pine and lemon extracts high up on the ingredient listing. These irritants make it problematic for all skin types.

## RS2 Line—Ligne Rose (Rosacea and Sensitive Skin)

☺ $$$ **RS2 Gentle Cleanser** *($26 for 6.8 ounces)* is just a very good, standard detergent-based water-soluble cleanser that would work well for most skin types. However, the notion that this or any of the products in the Ligne Rose is appropriate for sensitive skin of any kind, particularly rosacea, is nonsense. The basic need of anyone with sensitive skin is not to use products that contain fragrance, and this product and all the Ligne Rose products contain lots of fragrance, including frankincense and rose. This product does contain good anti-irritants but they would be combating the effect of the fragrance in here, not helping your skin.

☹ $$$ **RS2 Gentle Lotion** *($22 for 6.8 ounces)*. The irritating fragrance in here and the guarana extract—a plant that contains two and a half times more caffeine than coffee, that can have constricting properties on skin, and can therefore be a potent skin irritant make this problematic for anyone with sensitive skin or rosacea.

☺ $$$ **RS2 Concentrate** *($48 for 1.7 ounces)* still contains fragrance, but if that isn't a problem for you, this is a rather boring but good lightweight lotion for normal to slightly dry skin. The anti-irritants in here end up being useless, as they would only be fighting the irritation caused from the fragrance.

☺ $$$ **RS2 Care Cream** *($48 for 1.7 ounces)* is a very emollient, though basic moisturizer for someone with normal to dry skin. This is easily replaced with Lubriderm or Cetaphil moisturizers at the drugstore and then you wouldn't have to worry about the fragrance or price.

## Eye Line—Ligne Yeux

☹ **Eye Make-up Remover Lotion, Ligne Yeux** *($22 for 6.8 ounces)* doesn't remove makeup very well. This product also contains arnica, which is just bizarre to put in a product meant to be used around the eye, as arnica is not supposed to come into contact with mucous membranes.

☺ **$$$ Eye Gel** *($29.75 for 0.7 ounce)* is a good, lightweight, moisturizer for slightly dry skin. The orange extract in here (rather high up on the ingredient listing) can be an irritant for sensitive skin, particularly around the eyes.

☺ **$$$ Collastin Eye Fluid** *($48.25 for 1 ounce)*. The bottom line: this is a very good moisturizer for dry skin but the claims for this product are overblown. First, the plant extracts in here aren't AHAs and don't work for exfoliation, and then, even if they did, their concentration and the product's pH aren't correct for that function. This moisturizer does contain collagen and elastin, but aren't we long past believing that those two ingredients in a cosmetic can affect those elements in our skin?

☺ **$$$ Eye Cream, Ligne Yeux** *($34 for 0.7 ounce)* is a very good, albeit pricey moisturizer for dry skin.

## Oxygenating Line—Soin Optimale

☺ **$$$ C Complexe, Soin O2ptimal** *($67 for 1 ounce)* contains no oxygen, unless you consider water a source of oxygen. The form of vitamin C in this product is ascorbyl glucosamine, and it is a good antioxidant, which is strange when you consider this product was supposed to put oxygen into the skin, not eliminate it. Of course no skin-care product can provide oxygen for skin.

☹ **$$$ Combination Skin Care Cream, Soin O2ptimal** *($49 for 1.7 ounces)* doesn't have any oxygen, unless you buy the notion that water is a source of oxygen. This overpriced moisturizer would be a good moisturizer for dry skin, but the lemon oil in here makes it problematic for irritation.

☹ **$$$ Dry Skin Care Cream, Soin O2ptimal** *($55 for 1.7 ounces)* doesn't contain oxygen, so in that regard the same comment applies here as for the one above but it is very good for dry skin. It also contains algae, propolis, and royal bee jelly, but on skin they only work as anti-irritants; they don't have any rare, miraculous skin benefits. One more point: this does contain vitamin C, but in the form of ascorbic acid, a particularly irritating, unstable form.

☺ **$$$ Sensitive Skin Care Cream, Soin O2ptimal** *($55 for 1.7 ounces)* is a very good moisturizer for dry skin, but you already know it doesn't contain any oxygen, right? It does contain celandine, a plant extract that has anti-viral properties, though it has no known benefit for skin.

## Lightening Line—Ligne Radiance

☺ **$$$ Radiance Lightening Gel** *($33.75 for 1 ounce)* is a very good, skin-lightening gel that contains mostly water, AHA, kojic acid, hydroquinone, glycerin, thickener, and preservatives. Kojic acid and hydroquinone can both have a positive effect on inhibiting melanin production. However, without the use of a sunscreen, skin-lightening products are ineffective (unprotected sun exposure always stimulates melanin production, causing skin discolorations).

☹ **Radiance Lightening Fluid** *($33.75 for 1 ounce)* is an AHA and BHA solution, though the pH is too high for them to be effective as exfoliants. It does not contain any skin-lightening (melanin inhibiting) ingredients.

☺ **$$$ Radiance Lightening Mask** *($29.75 for 1.7 ounces)* is a clay mask that contains AHA and BHA. The pH of this mask isn't low enough for the AHA or BHA to have any effect as exfoliants. Also, it is far better for skin if you use an AHA or BHA on a regular basis, not occasionally as you would with a mask (that is, if this mask had a good pH). It does not contain any skin-lightening (melanin inhibiting) ingredients.

☺ **$$$ Radiance Glycocides Cream** *($42.25 for 1.7 ounces)* is a good 10% to 12% AHA cream that would be good for dry skin, but that doesn't help inhibit melanin discolorations. AHAs exfoliate skin, and that's helpful and definitely can improve the appearance of skin, but it takes hydroquinone to reduce melanin production.

## Acne/Problematic Skin Line—Ligne Clarifyl

☹ **Clarigel Exfoliating Cleanser** *($25.25 for 6.8 ounces)* uses sodium C14-16 olefin sulfate, which is an extremely irritating and drying detergent cleansing agent. This does contain triclosan, which can have some effect as a disinfectant against bacteria, but it would be washed off before it had much of a chance to have any effect.

☹ **Clarifyl Toning Lotion** *($19.25 for 6.8 ounces)* contains witch hazel and camphor, which are completely unnecessary skin irritants, and it is therefore not recommended.

☺ **Clarifyl Care Cream** *($33.75 for 2.5 ounces)*. The pH for this lightweight moisturizer is too high for the glycolic acid to be effective as an exfoliant. Keep in mind that for breakouts, this would be far better if it contained BHA (provided it also had the right pH, that is).

☹ **Clarifyl Purifying Mask** *($33.75 for 2.5 ounces)* is a clay mask that contains sulfur and camphor, which are unnecessary irritants for all skin types. Sulfur can have disinfecting properties, but there are far less irritating ways to disinfect against breakouts.

☹ **Clarifyl Spot Treatment** *($32.25 for 1 ounce)* contains camphor and alcohol and is not recommended.

## Special Line—Ligne Speciale

☹ Exfoliant Moussant Gentle Exfoliating Cleanser, Ligne Speciale *($22 for 5 ounces)* uses pumice powder as the exfoliant, which makes this a fairly scratchy scrub. The thickening agents in here, including titanium dioxide, clay, and rice powder, are hard to rinse off.

☺ $$$ Reactive Skin Care Cream, Ligne Speciale *($55 for 1.7 ounces)*. This simple, ordinary moisturizing formula for dry skin would be good for sensitive skin due to its basic ingredients. But the price? That's just a burn.

☺ $$$ Intensive Care Neck Cream *($40.25 for 1.7 ounces)*. I can't stress strongly enough that there is absolutely nothing in here that is intensive or makes it better for the neck. This is just an ordinary moisturizer for normal to slightly dry skin, and that's it.

☺ Exclusive Formula *($27.75 for 1.7 ounces)*. There is nothing in here that makes it exclusive, it is just a good, rather basic emollient moisturizer for dry skin. Several of the plant extracts in here can be skin irritants.

## Sun Line—Chemical-Free Sunscreens—Ligne Soleil

☺ Sunblock Dry to Sensitive Skin, SPF 15 *($28.25 for 2.5 ounces)* is a good, titanium dioxide–based sunscreen that would indeed work well for dry skin. The tea tree oil in here is confusing, as it is a topical disinfectant and not the best for sensitive skin.

☺ Sunblock Combination to Oily Skin, SPF 15 *($28.25 for 2.5 ounces)* is a good sunscreen that contains zinc oxide in part, but this is inappropriate for oily skin of any type. The emollients and thickeners in here are suitable for dry skin.

☺ $$$ Sunblock Eye & Lip, SPF 15 *($17.25 for 0.5 ounce)* is similar to the Sunblock Dry to Sensitive Skin above and the same comments apply.

☺ Sunblock Body Milk, SPF 15 *($29.25 for 5 ounces)* is similar to those above, and the same basic comments apply.

☺ Phyto-Aromatic Mist *($22.25 for 8.5 ounces)* is just a toner in a spray container. This would be a good, irritant-free toner, but it serves no purpose in a sun-care lineup. It contains nothing that would help reduce or change sun damage.

## Biologica Line—Ligne Classique

☺ $$$ Collagen Cream *($46.25 for 1.7 ounces)* is a good emollient moisturizer for dry skin, but the collagen in here can't affect the collagen in skin; it is just a moisturizing ingredient.

☺ $$$ Elastin Cream *($47.25 for 1.7 ounces)* is almost identical to the Collagen version above, only with this one you're supposed to believe the elastin in here will affect the elastin in your skin.

☺ **$$$ Dioxyribonucleic Acid Cream, Ligne Classique** *($50 for 1.7 ounces)* contains DNA. That makes it sound like this product can affect the genetic material in your own skin cells, but it can't. Even if it could, that would be dangerous for the health of your skin. Other than that, this is a very good moisturizer.

## Concentrates—Les Essentiels

☹ **$$$ Liposomes Gel Concentrate** *($58.25 for 1 ounce)* is a strange formulation to analyze because it includes liposomes on the ingredient listing, yet there is no ingredient called "liposome." Liposomes are actually a delivery system that combines water-soluble and oil-soluble groups of ingredients. Despite this glitch, this does seem to be a good, though extremely basic, lightweight moisturizer for slightly dry skin.

☹ **$$$ Firm-Active Concentrate, Les Essentials** *($50 for 1 ounce)* contains something called amnioserine, an ingredient derived from the amniotic fluid of animals, and a couple of thickening agents, fragrance, and preservatives. Amniotic fluid can be a good water-binding agent but its association to a fetus does not mean it will make your skin act young.

☹ **$$$ Collagen Concentrate** *($44.25 for 1 ounce)*. Collagen in a product can't affect the collagen in your skin, but it can be effective as a water-binding agent. That's good, but not worth this price.

☹ **$$$ Elastin Concentrate** *($44.25 for 1 ounce)* is similar to the Collagen Concentrate above, only you're supposed to believe this one will fix the elastin in your skin. It can't.

☹ **$$$ Deoxyribonucleic Acid Cream, Les Essentials** *($47 for 1 ounce)* contains DNA. That makes it sound like this product can affect the genetic material in your own skin cells, but it can't. Other than that, this a lightweight, ordinary moisturizer for slightly dry skin.

# *philosophy*

philosophy has an upscale, department-store élan, with a touch of Zen, family values, and a heavy dose of twenty-something attitude thrown into the mix. It's hard to tell if you are shopping a cosmetics line or looking for a new religious experience. philosophy's philosophy is clearly to capture the attention of women in all age ranges, but chiefly those between 18 and 30, as evidenced by the large number of acne products as opposed to wrinkle creams. Younger women who are not yet fighting off the unwanted advance of time seem to want more from life than just beauty. They also want meaning and fun. philosophy meets that need with a brochure that looks like a volume of poetry, not a sales catalog. The only graphics are a series of photographs, circa 1950 and up, of children, parents, and grandparents, on outings or enjoying life. No glamour shots to be found anywhere. Unbelievable.

Skin care is philosophy's real raison d'être, and its line is more entertaining than anything else. The company preaches about cause and effect, offers the product it says you need to create the effect, and gives it a fetching name. It's hard to not be curious about something named "hope and a prayer" (philosophy likes to use lowercase letters for product names). philosophy has statements that appear on each and every product. Its sunscreen with SPF 15 is called "the naked truth," and the label reads "philosophy: if withholding the truth is an act of love, then is telling the truth only an act of courage?" Wow. Heavy. What that has to do with sunscreen is anyone's guess, but it's a great marketing gimmick. The eyeshadows are romantically called "windows of the soul." The rest of the label reads, "philosophy: to know the true story of the soul, look deeply into the eyes," presumably past the eyeshadow. I've never seen products with such riveting copy.

Most of the basic information in the philosophy brochure is actually quite good, such as advice about weight loss, sun care, exercise, and relaxation, and basic facts about skin aging. But there's also a fair share of nonsense about vitamins and botanicals being the beneficial ingredients in these products. On a less whimsical note, some extremely misleading information is tossed around, and that is not a philosophy I care for. The brochure recommends that you determine how sensitive your skin is by whether or not you tan. If your skin always burns, it claims, you know you have sensitive skin; if you usually tan, you can use most products. That isn't the least bit accurate. What about women of color? Don't they have sensitive skin sometimes? Sensitive skin has little to do with a woman's ability to tolerate sun exposure.

philosophy's makeup, which started as a smaller palette of neutral shades with some of the smoothest textures around, has blossomed into something larger. While I wish I could say that all of the new additions are well worth the wait, what's new is not really much of an improvement. The original, matte colors are still nicely represented, but now there are almost as many shiny, vivid shades. These shades are eye-catching, so much so that when you wear them they are likely to be the only thing people notice about your makeup—not a philosophy I encourage anyone to adopt! There have also been some disappointing additions with philosophy's mascara, concealer, and more of those mini-makeup sets. This is quickly becoming a line that stresses the perceived value of makeup "kits," and many women will be convinced. But try to step back and ask yourself how many of these colors/products you will (realistically) use. For more information about philosophy, call (888) 2-NEWAGE (doesn't that phone number just figure?) or visit the Web site at www.philosophy.com.

## *philosophy skin care*

⊗ **on a clear day cleanser** *($14 for 4 ounces)* is a very strong, detergent-based water-soluble cleanser that uses sodium lauryl sulfate as the cleansing agent. Sodium lauryl sulfate is a potent skin irritant, and makes this not recommended.

☺ **real purity cleanser** *($15 for 6 ounces)* is a standard, detergent-based water-soluble cleanser that would work well for most skin types. It does contain several fragrant plant oils that can be potential skin irritants, as well as black pepper oil, something that has no purpose in skin care and definitely not in a cleanser that can get in the eyes.

☺ **the health bar** *($9 for 3.2 ounces)* is a standard bar soap with oatmeal, which can have anti-irritant properties and exfoliate skin as a gentle abrasive; however, the cleansing agents in this soap can be fairly drying.

☹ **change me, make-up remover** *($12 for 4 ounces)* is a standard, detergent-based makeup remover that would work as well as any. The sage extract in here can be a skin irritant.

☹ **$$$ deeply superficial enzyme scrub** *($18 for 2 ounces)* is a scrub that uses cornmeal as the exfoliating ingredient. The tiny amount of papaya in here does contain the enzyme papain, but it is unstable and present in too minuscule an amount to have any exfoliating properties.

☹ **$$$ under your skin, face and body scrub** *($18 for 4 ounces)* is a gel-based scrub that uses synthetic particles as the abrasive. It does work without being too abrasive, but this is extremely standard and doesn't work any better than baking soda mixed with Cetaphil Gentle Skin Cleanser.

☹ **the great awakening** *($25 for 1 ounce of gel and 2 ounces of foam)* might better be called a rude awakening. It's supposed to be a two-part facial: the gel is a cleanser to prepare the skin, and the foam is meant to bring oxygen to the skin. How does it do that? Easy: with hydrogen peroxide. Yes, the good old 3% hydrogen peroxide you buy at the drugstore in a brown bottle for 89 cents. But even if this were a good way to deliver oxygen to the skin (and it isn't), hydrogen peroxide deteriorates almost immediately on exposure to air and sunlight, which means the extra oxygen would be gone after you first opened it. That's why I call charging $25 for hydrogen peroxide and a teensy bit of basic cleanser a rude awakening. Ironically, this product also contains catalase, an enzyme that decomposes hydrogen peroxide into water and oxygen to prevent it from causing oxidative damage in the body. So why use the hydrogen peroxide in the first place only to make it ineffective?

☹ **$$$ dark shadows eye brightener** *($25 for 0.5 ounce)* contains vitamin K. The only research establishing vitamin K as being able to reduce dark circles is from another company that makes vitamin K products and is the patent holder for the ingredient. It has never been substantiated in independent research. This is a good (though basic) lightweight moisturizer for someone with slightly dry skin, but that's it.

☺ **$$$ eye believe** *($25 for 0.5 ounce)* is a good moisturizer for dry skin, with several very good water-binding agents.

☺ **hope in a bottle oil-free moisturizer normal to oily skin** *($30 for 2 ounces)* is a good 1% to 2% BHA product in a lightweight moisturizing base. It is an option for exfoliation for most skin types.

☹ **hope in a jar moisturizer for normal to dry skin** *($30 for 2 ounces)* is about a 6% AHA in a minimally moisturizing base, except that the pH isn't low enough for it to exfoliate the skin.

☺ **$$$ hope and a prayer topical vitamin C** *($45 for 1 ounce)* is philosophy's attempt to keep abreast of the vitamin C craze. The gimmick here is that you mix this product up every time you use it; the kit comes with a bottle of vitamin C powder and a bottle of silicone-based liquid. Of course you're supposed to believe this concoction keeps the vitamin C fresh, but that doesn't answer the question about why that's necessary (there are plenty of stable and effective forms of vitamin C that don't require this process). It is important to note that the only effective aspect of this form of vitamin C—ascorbyl palmitate—is as an antioxidant, yet it's hardly the only one (there are lots and lots of antioxidants), much less the best form of vitamin C available in cosmetics.

☺ **the present oil-free moisturizer sensitive skin** *($20 for 2 ounces)* is just thickeners and silicone, and that's nice for normal to slightly dry skin, but it is really basic and ordinary. The lavender oil in here doesn't make this the best for sensitive skin types.

☺ **thin skin, rich moisturizer** *($24 for 2 ounces)* is a good emollient moisturizer for someone with dry skin, but there is nothing special about this moisturizer regardless of how thick or thin your skin is.

☺ **$$$ between the lines topical vitamin A** *($20 for 0.5 ounce)* is a good lightweight moisturizer that is supposed to go under a more emollient moisturizer. The vitamin A in here is several steps removed from retinol, which is the hyped ingredient that has a modicum of research hinting that it is helpful for skin.

☺ **$$$ help me** *($45 for 1.05 ounces)*. philosophy has joined the retinol mania with this version that is quite similar to L'Oreal's Line Eraser, which is available for a quarter of the price.

☹ **the damage is done glycolic acid cream** *($24 for 2 ounces)* is about a 6% AHA product, but it doesn't have a low enough pH to work as an exfoliant.

☺ **the healthy tan self tanning gel** *($16 for 4 ounces)* is a standard self tanner that uses the same ingredient every other self tanner does to turn the skin brown. This one would work as well as any.

☹ **in the buff** *($20 for 6 ounces)* doesn't contain the UVA-protecting ingredients of avobenzone, zinc oxide, or titanium dioxide, and is not recommended.

☹ **shelter for the face SPF 15** *($16 for 2 ounces)* doesn't contain the UVA-protecting ingredients avobenzone, zinc oxide, or titanium dioxide, and is not recommended.

☹ **shelter for the body SPF 15** *($16 for 4 ounces)* doesn't contain the UVA-protecting ingredients avobenzone, zinc oxide, or titanium dioxide, and is not recommended.

☹ **a pigment of your imagination** *($20 for 1 ounce)* contains two reliable skin-lightening agents, but the alcohol can be irritating and not just what you should be imagining is taking care of your skin.

☺ **when lightening strikes** *($45 for 4 ounces)* is a good, hydroquinone-based skin-lightening product.

☹ **exit strategy facial cream for skin that burns** *($12 for 1 ounce)*. Several of the thickeners in this product can cause breakouts, and that's not great. The sulfur in here can be a disinfectant, but a very irritating one, and camphor is just plain irritating.

☺ $$$ **never let them see you shine oil absorbing serum** *($12 for 1 ounce)* is nothing more than milk of magnesia. This product contains mostly water, slip agent, magnesium, absorbent, preservatives, and fragrance.

☹ **out of control blemish gel for skin that tans** *($18 for 1 ounce)* is mostly alcohol with some AHA and BHA. The alcohol is unnecessarily drying and irritating for all skin types.

☹ **rescue mission deep cleansing mask** *($16 for 1 ounce)* is a clay mask that contains eucalyptus and orange oil, which are too irritating for all skin types.

☺ $$$ **stuck in the mud** *($18 for 2 ounces)* is a good basic clay mask that also contains a tiny bit of charcoal, which does help in oil absorption.

☺ $$$ **kiss me lip balm** *($8 for 0.5 ounce)* is little more than Vaseline and lanolin in a pot. It's fine for dry lips.

☺ $$$ **kiss me red lip balm** *($8 for 0.5 ounce)* is the same as the lip balm above only in an intense red shade.

## *philosophy makeup*

☺ $$$ <u>FOUNDATION:</u> There is still only one foundation available, and it is a far cry from the former liquid foundation, which has been discontinued. The sole option now is a thick, loose powder foundation named **complete me SPF 15** *($30)*. It is quite similar to Origins' As Good As It Gets, only the 12 shades here are much more neutral. The sunscreen is zinc oxide, but even with that plus, this is not an easy or convenient way to apply foundation, and the high mineral content in here may be irritating to some skin types. Being a powder, this has a dry texture, yet you are left with more of a sheen than a matte finish. If this still sounds appealing to you and you have normal to slightly oily skin, you may want to check this one out.

☺ <u>CONCEALER:</u> **trust me SPF 15** *($15)* has a great, titanium dioxide–based sunscreen but the consistency is heavy and creamy and will crease by the time you are done applying your makeup! What a shame, because the colors are excellent, but if you aren't worried about creasing and you have dry skin, it is a consideration.

☺ $$$ <u>BLUSH:</u> Once known as "he makes me blush" and now renamed as the politically correct **you make me blush** *($16),* this is still quite nice, with an attractive color selection and a soft, sheer application. The price is steep given the wide availability of far more affordable blushes, but these are an option. **The supernaturals cheek, lip tint and lip lacquer** *($15)* is a liquid stain that can go from sheer to an intense reddish-pink. Like any liquid blush, this will achieve the best results for those with smooth, flawless. As a lip stain, it holds up reasonably well.

☺ **EYESHADOW: windows of the soul** *($15)* is the most ingenious and poetic name for a cosmetic I've ever seen! Nevertheless, it doesn't take long to discover that, clever name notwithstanding, these are just standard, talc-based shadows with a wonderful smooth texture that blend on easily. There are more shiny shades than in the past, but the mattes are still the strong point to look for.

☺ **EYE AND BROW SHAPER: the coloring crayon for eyes** *($12.50)* is a standard, creamy pencil that is not preferred to philosophy's excellent dark, matte eyeshadow options.

☺ **LIPSTICK AND LIP PENCIL: word of mouth lipstick** *($15)* is available in a matte or cream formula. The mattes are smooth and softly matte, which is great, while the creamy formula tends to be quite glossy and doesn't hold up well. **The coloring crayon for lips** *($12.50)* are a small collection of standard lip pencils.

☹ **word of mouth lipstick spf 15** *($15)* is very greasy and the sunscreen offers no reliable UVA protection.

☺ **MASCARA: the supernaturals lash darkener** *($15)* is sort of a mascara hybrid; it does almost no lengthening or thickening to speak of but does darken the lashes. If you love the lashes you were born with but want a little extra depth, it's worth a try.

☺ **BRUSHES:** philosophy has a small band of **brushes** *($10 to $25 each; $80 for complete set)* that are satin-soft and nicely tapered. However, most of them are inferior in shape and density when compared to those from neighboring lines like Trish McEvoy, Bobbi Brown, Stila, M.A.C., and others. The only ones to strongly consider are the **blush** *($25)* and **shadow** *($20)*—both are acceptable and correctly sized.

☺ $$$ **SPECIALTY PRODUCTS:** philosophy established its color line with an all-in-one kit known as **the coloring book** *($160).* It is comprised of ten eyeshadows, four blushes, five lip colors, and two eye/lip pencils along with a set of brushes, and I imagine it seemed utterly practical at first glance but may now be collecting dust next to that unread copy of *War and Peace.* For those of you who embraced the idea and concept of these "books," or complete sets of makeup, there are now two new volumes, largely made up of philosophy's newer, trend-driven shades. They look sharp but the same caveats apply—think long and hard before you spend this much for a supposed convenience. **the pocketbook** *($47.50)* is a small, tri-fold wallet of products including one blush, one eyeshadow, one lipstick, and a small, almost unusable, tiny brush set. There are better and more reasonable ways to put together a usable makeup bag. **finger paints** *($40)* are a small palette of shiny, creamy colors meant to serve as lip, cheek, or eye tints. The three sets come with a lacquer that you can use to go from merely shiny to beaming with glossiness. It's adorably packaged but the price is unwarranted for such small amounts of product.

# pHisoDerm (Skin Care Only)

For more information about pHisoDerm, call (800) 745-2429.

☹ **4 Way Daily Acne Cleanser** *($3.79 for 6 ounces)* uses sodium C14-16 olefin sulfate as the detergent cleansing agent, which is too drying and irritating for all skin types.

☺ **Daily Cleanser and Conditioner, for Normal to Oily Skin** *($7.93 for 14 ounces)* is a standard, detergent-based water-soluble cleanser with a small amount of mineral oil. The mineral oil isn't the best for oily skin, but this cleanser does work well for someone with normal to dry skin. It does contain fragrance.

☺ **Daily Skin Cleanser and Conditioner, for Normal to Dry** *($7.93 for 14 ounces)* is similar to the Normal to Oily version above only with more mineral oil, and the same basic comments apply.

☺ **Daily Skin Cleanser and Conditioner, Sensitive Skin Formula, for Sensitive Skin** *($7.93 for 14 ounces)* is similar to the Normal to Oily version above only this one doesn't include fragrance, and that makes it better for sensitive skin, though it is really fine for all skin types.

☺ **Gentle Skin Cleanser for Baby** *($5.41 for 8 ounces)* is similar to the Normal to Dry version above and the same basic comments apply. There is nothing in this product that makes it more appropriate for a baby's skin. If anything, the Sensitive Skin version above would be far better because it doesn't include fragrance.

☹ **Sensitive Skin Cleansing Bar** *($1.99 for 3.3 ounces)* is a standard, tallow-based bar cleanser that includes Vaseline and lanolin. Tallow and lanolin are both known skin sensitizers, and make the name of this product completely inappropriate.

☺ **Blemish Patch** *($6.95 for 24 patches)* is pHisoderm's attempt at duplicating the Biore Strips. These are just as effective (or ineffective). Not everyone finds these products all that effective for blackheads, and they do come with cautions for potential for irritation. The salicylic acid in here is ineffective for exfoliation.

☹ **Phisopuff** *($3.18)* is a round puff of scrubbing material that can be too irritating and abrasive for all skin types.

# Physicians Formula

There aren't really any doctors at Physicians Formula (the founder of the company was an allergist, Dr. Frank Crandell, but that was back in 1937), and no physicians currently sell or endorse it either. The line brags that there are a lot of potentially irritating ingredients it doesn't use that other lines do. As great as that sounds, some of the products in this line do contain ingredients that can pose serious irritation and skin sensitivity problems, including alcohol, sodium lauryl sulfate, camphor, and menthol, among others. Despite the nonsensical name and bogus identity, Physicians Formula does have some products in all categories that I can recommend but also some problematic ones, particularly its makeup products. Almost every product category is lacking in some respect: there are foundations that have great sun protection but awful colors, or silky-feeling powders in a mosaic of colors that are unrelated to skin color. It is unlikely that you'll come across a line that is more in love with the concept of correcting skin color with a wash of products than this one, and that alone may prod you to skip this line's makeup altogether. The lipsticks have been eliminated save for two compacts, the mascaras are borderline pathetic, and most of the new products have an incredibly shiny or metallic finish. That may be right in step with current trends, but it's assuredly not what the doctor ordered!

For more information on Physicians Formula, call (800) 227-0333 or visit the Web site at www.physiciansformula.com.

# Physicians Formula Skin Care

☺ **Oil-Control Deep Pore Cleansing Gel for Normal to Oily Skin** (*$6.95 for 8 ounces*) is a standard, detergent-based water-soluble cleanser that can work well for most skin types.

☹ **Oil-Control Facial Bar for Normal to Oily Skin** (*$3.50 for 3.5 ounces*) contains several ingredients that can clog pores and irritate skin.

☹ **Oil Free Eye Makeup Remover Pads for Normal to Oily Skin** (*$4.75 for 60 pads*) combines a detergent-based water-soluble makeup remover with ready-to-go pads, but this also contains witch hazel and rose water high up on the ingredient list, which are a problem for repeated use on the eyes.

☺ **Vital Lash Oil Free Eye Makeup Remover for Normal to Oily Skin** (*$4.50 for 2 ounces*) is a standard, detergent-based water-soluble makeup remover. It works as well as any.

☹ **Oil-Control Conditioning Skin Toner for Normal to Oily Skin** (*$6.95 for 8 ounces*) is an alcohol-based toner that also contains camphor and menthol. This is extremely drying and irritating for all skin types.

☺ **Oil-Control Oil-Free Moisturizer for Normal to Oily Skin** (*$8.50 for 4 ounces*). I can't imagine why the company thinks thickening agents with clay and a little bit of magnesium are oil-controlling. The thickening agents in here can clog pores and make the skin feel oily, though for a very boring, matte-finish moisturizer it is an option, just not a very good one.

☺ **Oil-Control Shine Away for Normal to Oily Skin** *($6.95 for 1 ounce)* contains a film former as the main ingredient. Film formers place a thin, plastic-like layer over the skin that can feel smooth and have some ability to absorb oil. For the money, this is one you can test drive but it is minimally effective at holding back oil.

☺ **Oil Free Nourishing Eye Gel for Normal to Oily Skin** *($5.95 for 0.5 ounce).* Caffeine's high tannin content can make it irritating on skin with repeated use, and the ivy extract in here can be a skin irritant.

☺ **Shine Away Acne Control Primer for Normal to Oily Skin** *($6.95 for 1 ounce)* is similar to the product above, only with the addition of salicylic acid. The BHA would be a good addition, but this product has too high a pH for it to be an effective exfoliant.

☹ **Deep Cleaning Face Mask for Normal to Oily Skin** *($5.95 for 2.75 ounces)* is a standard clay mask. The clay is drying, and the alcohol and witch hazel will only make things worse. This mask won't deep-clean, but it can deeply irritate the skin.

☺ **Gentle Cleansing Lotion for Normal to Dry Skin** *($7.25 for 8 ounces)* is a standard mineral oil– and Vaseline-based wipe-off cleanser that can leave a greasy film on the skin. It is only an option for very dry skin.

☹ **Gentle Cleansing Facial Bar for Normal to Dry Skin** *($3.75 for 3.5 ounces)* is a detergent-based water-soluble cleansing bar that can be drying for most skin types. It does contain tiny quantities of plant oil and water-binding agents, but that won't take care of the dryness caused by the other ingredients.

☹ **Pore Refining Skin Freshener, for Normal to Dry Skin** *($6.95 for 8 ounces)* is mostly just alcohol and fragrance. This is an irritation and inflammation waiting to happen.

☺ **Extra Rich Rehydrating Moisturizer for Normal to Dry Skin** *($8.50 for 4 ounces)* isn't rich or interesting, just a very below-par moisturizer for normal to dry skin.

☺ **Elastin Collagen Moisture Lotion for Normal to Dry Skin** *($8.50 for 4 ounces).* This very emollient moisturizer would be good for dry skin. It contains elastin and collagen, but they are just water-binding agents, nothing more.

☺ **Enriched Cleansing Concentrate for Dry to Very Dry Skin** *($5.95 for 4 ounces)* is a standard, mineral oil–based, wipe-off cleanser that contains plant oil and Vaseline. It is really just cold cream and can leave a greasy film on the skin, which can be an option for dry skin.

☺ **Gentle Cleansing Cream for Dry to Very Dry Skin** *($5.95 for 4 ounces)* is similar to the Enriched Cleansing Concentrate above, only with more Vaseline, which makes it even greasier. The same basic comments apply.

☺ **Eye Makeup Remover Lotion for Normal to Dry Skin** *($4.50 for 2 ounces)* is just mostly mineral oil, some thickeners, and Vaseline. There is little reason to use this if you are already using a wipe-off, greasy makeup remover for the rest of your face. There is nothing in this product that makes it better for the eye area.

☺ Gentle Refreshing Toner for Dry to Very Dry Skin *($6.95 for 8 ounces)* is a good toner. This product does contain ginseng, which can be a skin irritant.

☹ Collagen Cream Concentrate for Dry to Very Dry Skin *($8.95 for 2 ounces)* is a good emollient moisturizer for dry skin, but the water-binding agents and vitamins are barely present and have no real impact on skin.

☹ Intensive Therapy Moisture Cream for Dry to Very Dry Skin *($8 for 2 ounces)* would be good for dry skin, but it is exceptionally ordinary.

☹ Nourishing Night Cream for Dry to Very Dry Skin *($5.95 for 1 ounce)* is an extremely emollient, dull moisturizer for someone with dry skin.

☹ Emollient Oil for Dry to Very Dry Skin *($5.25 for 2 ounces)* is primarily safflower oil, which you can easily use from your kitchen cabinet for less money and ip the fragrance that is in here.

☺ Beauty Buffers Exfoliating Scrub All Skin Types *($5.95 for 2 ounces)* is a standard, detergent-based water-soluble scrub that uses synthetic particles as the scrub agent. This can exfoliate the skin, but the number of thickening agents here makes it problematic for oily skin, though it can be good for someone with normal to slightly dry skin.

☹ Eye Makeup Remover Pads for All Skin Types *($4.75 for 60 pads)* is just a mineral oil–based eye-makeup remover that can leave a greasy film on the skin, which won't make someone with oily skin very happy.

☹ Luxury Eye Cream All Skin Types *($5.95 for 0.5 ounce)* is a very good, though ordinary emollient moisturizer for someone with dry skin, not for all skin types as the name implies.

☹ Self Defense Protective Moisturizing Lotion with SPF 15 for Normal to Dry Skin *($6.95 for 2 ounces)* doesn't contain the UVA-protecting ingredients avobenzone, titanium dioxide, or zinc oxide, and is not recommended.

☹ Self Defense Protective Moisturizing Lotion with Sunscreen with SPF 15 for Normal to Oily Skin *($6.95 for 2 ounces)* doesn't contain the UVA-protecting ingredients avobenzone, titanium dioxide, or zinc oxide, and is not recommended.

☹ Self Defense Color Corrective Moisturizing Lotion with Sunscreen SPF 15 for All Skin Types *($6.95 for 2 ounces)* doesn't contain the UVA-protecting ingredients avobenzone, titanium dioxide, or zinc oxide, and is not recommended. I won't even get into the strange color shades this product comes in.

☹ Sun Shield Oil Free Formula SPF 20 for Normal to Oily Skin *($7.25 for 4 ounces)* doesn't contain the UVA-protecting ingredients avobenzone, titanium dioxide, or zinc oxide, and is not recommended.

☹ Sun Shield Moisture Formula SPF 20 for Normal to Dry Skin *($7.25 for 4* *ounces)* doesn't contain the UVA-protecting ingredients avobenzone, titanium diox-ide, or zinc oxide, and is not recommended.

☺ **Sun Shield for Faces Formula SPF 20 for All Skin Types** *($7.25 for 2 ounces)* doesn't contain the UVA-protecting ingredients avobenzone, titanium dioxide, or zinc oxide, and is not recommended.

☹ **Sun Shield Sport Non-Stick Formula Dry Lotion Sunscreen, SPF 15** *($7.50 for 5 ounces)* doesn't contain the UVA-protecting ingredients avobenzone, titanium dioxide, or zinc oxide, and is not recommended.

☺ **Sun Shield Sensitive Skin Formula Chemical Free Sunscreen SPF 25** *($8.50 for 4 ounces)* is indeed a pure titanium dioxide–based sunscreen in a moisturizing base. Finally a great sunscreen in this lineup! It can leave a slightly white film on the skin, but it provides excellent protection!

☺ **Sun Shield for Faces Sensitive Skin Formula SPF 15 for All Skin Types** *($8 for 2 ounces)* is similar to the one above, only in a much less moisturizing formula. This would be better for someone with normal to slightly dry skin.

☹ **Sun Shield Sunless Tanning Lotion, SPF 20, for All Skin Types** *($7.50 for 4 ounces)* contains dihydroxyacetone, which is the ingredient in all self tanners that turns skin brown, but it doesn't contain the UVA-protecting ingredients avobenzone, titanium dioxide, or zinc oxide, and for an effective SPF that's essential.

☹ **Sun Shield Lip Care SPF 15** *($1.95 for 0.15 ounce)* doesn't contain the UVA-protecting ingredients avobenzone, titanium dioxide, or zinc oxide, and is not recommended.

☺ **Vital Defense Sun Stick For Faces SPF 30 for All Skin Types** *($6.95 for 0.55 ounce)* is an in-part titanium dioxide–based sunscreen in a fairly standard, almost matte base. Considering the amount of this product you get and how much you have to use to get the indicated protection, this is a very overpriced sunscreen.

☹ **Vital Defense Moisture Concentrate with SPF 15 for Dry to Very Dry Skin** *($8.50 for 2 ounces)* doesn't contain avobenzone, titanium dioxide, or zinc oxide, and is not recommended.

☹ **Vital Defense Moisture Cream SPF 15** *($8.25 for 2 ounces)* doesn't contain avobenzone, titanium dioxide, or zinc oxide, and is not recommended.

☺ **Vital Defense Oil Free Lotion with SPF 15 for Normal to Oily Skin** *($8 for 6 ounces)* is similar to the Self Defense Lotion for Normal to Oily Skin above, and the same review applies.

☹ **Vital Defense Tinted Moisturizer SPF 15 in Light, Medium, and Dark** *($8.25 for 2 ounces)* doesn't contain the UVA-protecting ingredients avobenzone, titanium dioxide, or zinc oxide, and is not recommended.

☹ **Vital Defense Lip Treatment SPF 15** *($3.50 for 0.15 ounce)* doesn't contain the UVA-protecting ingredients avobenzone, titanium dioxide, or zinc oxide, and is not recommended.

# *Physicians Formula Makeup*

**FOUNDATION:** Physicians Formula's foundations leave me frustrated. On the one hand, many of them have reliable SPF 15 protection, which is great. Yet, at the same time, these are some of the poorest colors and lackluster textures around.

☹ **Le Velvet Film Makeup SPF 15** *($5.14 refill; $3.09 for compact)* is a cream-to-powder foundation that goes on surprisingly moist and creamy and can be blended out fairly sheer. The SPF is part titanium dioxide, which is great, but the finish is somewhat chalky. Even if testers were available, most of the shades are just too pink, peach, or orange to recommend.

☹ **Le Velvet Powder Finish Makeup SPF 15** *($5.14 refill; $3.09 for compact)* is similar to the one above, only this has a lighter, smoother texture (it's silicone based) that looks more natural on the skin. The colors are all a problem though, with strong rose or peach tones prevailing, which is a shame because the SPF does contain part titanium dioxide.

☺ **Refill Sponges** *($2.50)* are for both the Le Velvet makeups but can work well with any foundation, and are superior to the wedge-shaped sponges normally sold at the drugstore.

☹ **Sun Shield Liquid Makeup SPF 15** *($5.19)* is a standard liquid foundation whose SPF does not offer UVA-protecting ingredients. On top of that, the six colors are noticeably pink, peach, or rose.

☹ **Oil Control Matte Makeup** *($5.19)* is indeed oil free, but with equally disappointing colors, and a texture that can feel heavy and thick on the skin, and that does not make for a pretty picture.

☹ **Sheer Moisture Light Diffusing Makeup** *($5.19)* has a smooth, moist finish but the phrase "light diffusing" only refers to the sparkles in the makeup. Shine does reflect light but if you were hoping that will reduce the appearance of wrinkles, it won't; it actually makes them look worse.

☺ **Beauty Spiral Skin Brightening Liquid Foundation** *($9.89)* is a sheer, light-textured foundation that has an uneven, slightly pasty finish due to the high amount of titanium dioxide it contains. The four shades are passable, but this one should go back to the drawing board one more time. **Beauty Spiral Brightening Foundation** *($9.89)* is a cream-to-powder foundation that has an incredibly sheer application and an almost imperceptible finish, which makes it almost a "why bother?", though if you are looking for an ultra-sheer finish this could be an option. The "spiral" aspect of these two products is just the way the colors are swirled in the foundations (both liquid and powder). It's eye-catching, but it serves no function for improving application, and there's nothing brightening about either of these.

☹ **Capsulation Fresh Foundation Capsules** *($11.89 for approximately 24 cap-*

*sules)* is a silicone- and talc-based foundation packaged in small plastic bubbles, similar to Elizabeth Arden's Ceramide Capsule packaging. This mess of a foundation is supposed to be more sanitary and clean, but ends up being a waste on all fronts. The capsules contain a set amount of product and, once opened, the instructions say to discard them (they cannot be "closed"), which wastes an absurd amount of foundation for those who want to use it sparingly. The ad copy makes this sound like a brilliant idea but the reality is a headache waiting to happen.

☹ **2-in-1 Perfecting Foundation and Concealer SPF 15***($9.89)* comes in a compact and features a cream-to-powder foundation with a small amount of concealer. The colors are strongly peach to orange and have an unpleasant, thick texture. Kudos for the great, titanium dioxide–based SPF, but that's hardly consolation for the negative points.

☹ **Makeup Artist Palette SPF 15** *($8.89)* comes in a compact and has a peach-toned, creamy foundation as its centerpiece, surrounded by mauve, yellow, and green creamy color correctors. If there are makeup artists out there who regularly use this method, I have yet to meet them, and if they do exist, you don't want to meet them and have them use something like this on your face. Mauve, yellow, and green leave a strange shade on the skin and can't affect the overall color tone of your face.

☹ <u>CONCEALER:</u> Few, if any, companies have such a broad variety of color-correcting concealers. All these really do is place a strange and far from natural color on the skin, and the texture of all of these ensures a less than subtle finish. **Gentle Cover Concealer Stick** *($4.69)* is a lipstick-style concealer that is very creamy, feels heavy, and is hard to blend on the skin. The flesh-toned shades are too peachy-pink, and the color correctors should be avoided. **Concealer Twins SPF 15** *($5.89)* are dual-sided, lipstick-style concealers whose color combinations and textures are undesirable. The SPF is great, but not enough to warrant trying this product. **Gentle Cover Cream Concealer SPF 10** *($4.69)* comes in a compact and will easily crease into any lines around the eye. The colors are the same as the Gentle Cover Stick Concealer, and the same comments apply. **Powder Finish Concealer Stick SPF 15** *($4.69)* is another creamy stick concealer with titanium dioxide as one of the actives for sun protection, which is nice, but the only flesh-toned shade is too pink to look natural, and the powder finish here is minimal—this tends to stay creamy and can easily crease. **Beauty Spiral Perfecting Concealer** *($6.89)* comes in the typically bad assortment of colors like the rest of the Physicians Formula concealers do, meaning one substandard flesh tone and two color-correcting shades (yellow and green). This one has an unusually dry, powdery finish yet still manages to slip into lines, and looks chalky on the skin. **Beauty Spiral Perfecting Cream Concealer** *($6.89)* comes in a bottle with a wand applicator and has a much lighter texture and softer application than all of the other concealers in this line. However, right in step with the other concealers, this also comes in terrible colors that do not resemble skin in the least.

**POWDER:** ☹ **Translucent Loose Powder** *($9.95)* is a talc-based powder with a dry, powdery finish and an unnecessarily messy container. Add to this a slight shine and a color that is far from translucent (it's peach) and this becomes one to avoid. **Powder Palette Multi-Colored Pressed Powder/Corrector** *($11.89)* is a kaleidoscopic arrangement of different colors that all come off as the same color on the skin, as it should be. The colors are a strange lot—you'll find neutral bronze tones along with greens, whites, and, believe it or not, grays! The only one worth recommending is the Translucent version, which would be a good, talc-based powder for lighter skin tones that are normal to dry. **Pearls of Perfection Multi-Colored Face Powder** *($11.89)* are large pots of colored powder beads, available in bronze, flesh, and shiny high-lighting shades. They're fun in concept, but the execution is messy and not worth the effort. **Geometric Colors 3-in-1 Face Powder** *($11.89)* features a pressed powder, blush, and eyeshadow, geometrically arranged in one compact. There are no dividers, so the colors will run into each other, making application with the appropriate brush difficult to impossible, plus they all have a slight to heavy shine.

☺ **Dust of Gold, Bronze, or Crystal** *($9.95)* are very shiny loose powders that have a smooth texture and a relatively subtle, glittery finish. These adhere well to the skin and are best used for special evening makeup. The same three colors are also available in lotion form *($9.95)* and the same comments apply.

**BLUSH:** ☺ **Blush Palette Multi-Colored Blusher** *($9.89)* comes in either mauve or brown tones, each with five shades arranged (without dividers) in one compact. These just end up as one color when applied on the skin, and the center color is quite shiny, which makes these fun to admire but impractical to wear (the shine doesn't get applied evenly over the cheek). Still, if you're curious, better to try these before investing in identical products from Guerlain or Givenchy!

☺ **Matte Blush** *($5.75)* is a great find, if you can find it. Many of the stores I visited did not seem to carry it, but according to the company it is still available. These aren't too silky, but do apply smoothly and are matte. The colors (three in all) are muted but work well.

**EYESHADOW:** ☺ **Quad Eyeshadow** *($5.49)* has some of the best, neutral color combinations around, with a texture that applies and blends beautifully.

☺ **Eyebrightener Multi-Colored Eyelighter** *($7.39 single; $7.99 for duos)* is definitely eye-catching. Unfortunately, this variegated display of colors ends up placing a sweep of intense, metallic shine on the eyelid.

☺ **EYE AND BROW SHAPER:** **Eyeliner Palette Multi-Colored Cake Liner** *($9.89)* is a great concept. This is a traditional cake liner that you use wet with a brush to create a line. The only negative is that it tends to flake all over the place, and chips and flakes off as you wear it. **Eye Definer Automatic Eye Pencil** *($4.89)* is a twist-up eye pencil that is greasier than most, which means it can smear and smudge easily. **Eyebrightener Brightening Liquid Eyeliner** *($5.29)* is a standard liquid liner with a good, firm brush and a sheer application that dries to a metallic finish. The consistency is not the best, and this is not the most attractive look I can think of, but for an interesting evening look it's an option. **Eyebrightener Pencil Duo** *($5.29)* is a standard dual-ended pencil with two colors, shiny black and shiny white. For shine, they'll work as well as any other pencil. **Gentlewear Eye Pencil** *($4.75)* is a thick pencil that is hard to sharpen and use for a controlled line. Also, the four colors are mostly shiny and creamy enough to smear easily. The matte versions are an option but unfortunately the packaging does not indicate what type of finish each color has. **FineLine Brow Pencil** *($3.89)* comes in four decent shades and has a standard, dry texture. **Brow Corrector** *($5.99)* is a standard, sticky brow gel with a very sheer tint. This is an OK option for grooming and minimally—and I mean minimally—coloring the brows, and the price is acceptable.

LIPSTICK AND LIP PENCIL: ☺ **Lip Spectrum 100 Lipsticks in One** *($9.89)* comes in a compact and features one creamy lip color coupled with two tints—sheer black and iridescent white. The idea is to use the black tint to deepen the color and the shiny white to lighten it. How anyone could get even five lipstick colors out of this much less a hundred is anyone's guess. The concept isn't a bad one, but it's so much easier to just buy the right lip color in the first place.

☹ **LipLash Splash** *($6.69)* is a dual-ended product with an iridescent, peppermint flavored gloss on one end and a shiny, clear mascara on the other. Gloss and mascara together? Why?

MASCARA: ☺ **Eyebrightener Mascara** *($4.84)* is a very good mascara for lengthening and a slight amount of thickening. It has a slight tendency to clump, but for the most part it does a nice job of defining lashes.

☹ **To Any Lengths Lash Extending Mascara** *($4.84)* and **Full Lash Mascara** *($4.84)* both take you to great lengths just to achieve any significant length or thickness, plus they tend to smear! **Plentifull Length-Plus Lengthening Mascara** *($4.84)* and **Plentifull Full Lash Thickening Mascara** *($4.84)* neither lengthen nor thicken. The one thing these give you plenty of is smudging way before the day is done. **Month 2-Month Mascara** *($5.84)* is two mascaras packaged together rather than just one, and is intended to provide a freshness system. You note the date when you start one of the tubes and after a month you dispose of it and start the next one. The two ophthalmologists I spoke to both said they had never heard of mascara going bad in a month, and instead recommended (as I do) discarding mascara after three to four months. One month just seems wasteful, although this is such a dull, do-nothing mascara you may want to chuck it immediately! **AquaWear Mascara** *($4.84)* will build some length but no thickness, and what is especially disappointing is that it's not waterproof in the least.

# *Phytomer*

Phytomer is perhaps the most wanton in terms of its claims versus extremely unimpressive ingredient formulations. What I find even more startling is the way a cosmetics line can carry on about its superior formulations, remarkable ingredients, and unequaled ability to erase wrinkles, and yet not include a sunscreen product as part of a daily skin-care routine. In fact, of the sunscreens Phytomer does carry, not one has UVA protection. What's even more outrageous is that this line has the audacity to sell sunscreens meant for beachwear with SPFs of 2, 4, and 8! Unbelievable. Isn't that like an oncologist who specializes in lung cancer selling cigarettes? Either way, regardless of how you feel about the information I present, I remain completely skeptical of a company's "quality" if it can't at least get the sunscreen issue straight.

Phytomer's claim to fame is the ocean, or to be more precise, algae and salt water from the sea. In fact, algae shows up in almost every one of the Phytomer products. Algae is unquestionably a stylish ingredient these days. If Estee Lauder's Creme de La Mer can get away with selling algae, mineral oil, and thickening agents at over $1,000 for 16 ounces, why shouldn't Phytomer have an opportunity? And Phytomer's prices are actually less daunting. Does the sea offer any special advantage for skin? Do salt water and sea plants repair skin? I guess you would have to go on faith with this one, because while there is indeed research indicating algae derivatives can have anti-inflammatory and anti-irritant benefit for skin, as well as water-binding properties, they aren't the only ingredients that can do that. Plus, even if algae was a miracle ingredient for skin, algae as a cosmetic ingredient is cheap, and I mean really cheap, so the price is even more ludicrous! Seawater leaves me speechless. It is great to swim in the ocean or sea, but that water is not automatically helpful to skin and, if anything, needs to be rinsed off after you're done swimming to prevent dry skin and dry hair.

Aside from the algae and seawater, Phytomer also uses the same standard plant extracts, plant oils, thickening agents, water-binding agents, and other standard ingredients found throughout the cosmetics industry, and many of the nonalgae plant extracts used are skin irritants (which would seem to negate the benefit of the algae). What is always surprising to me is to find that a company bragging about its natural attitude would include incredibly unnatural coloring agents, thickening ingredients, and slip agents. That is just one of those little "natural ingredient" issues I get a chuckle out of.

On the exotic side, Phytomer's spa products include thalassotherapy and balneotherapy. These terms, and the related spa services they represent, exaggerate the benefits of seawater and marine by-products for therapeutic use. For example, balneotherapy is just a fancy way to refer to soaking in a bath, and thalassotherapy refers to the use of sea products for skin care.

As far as skin healing–type spa services go, if you aren't allergic to the ingredients used, it can be a relaxing experience, and relaxation goes a long way to making everyone feel better. But even though relaxation is guaranteed, the promise of pain-free, healed skin is a stretch. Spa services often promise the world—enhanced immune-system functioning, improved lymph and blood circulation stimulation, increased cell turnover, muscle relaxation, and who knows what else. Soaking in a bath, almost regardless of what the water contains, can do a world of good. However, allergic or irritating reactions should not be ignored, and oversoaking, especially in winter, can make skin dry. One more point: hot baths can cause capillaries to surface or look more prominent. The rest of the claims are about belief, not fact. For more information about Phytomer, call (800) 227-8051 or visit the Web site at www.phytomer.tm.fr.

☺ **$$$ Gentle Cleansing Cream** *($27 for 5 ounces)* is a standard, detergent-based water-soluble cleanser clearly similar to Cetaphil Gentle Skin Cleanser. In fact it is almost identical except that this one contains menthol, a completely unnecessary skin irritant. That makes Cetaphil not only far more reasonably priced, but far more gentle on the skin.

☺ **$$$ Gentle Cleansing Milk** *($25 for 6.8 ounces)* is more of a wipe-off cleanser than anything else. There is no reason to chose this cleanser over Neutrogena's Extra Gentle Cleanser for less than half the price and that doesn't contain fragrance.

☺ **$$$ Neutralizing Cleanser** *($34 for 6.8 ounces)* is almost identical to the Gentle Cleansing Milk except for a tiny amount of yeast and algae extract. This product can't neutralize anything; it is merely a wipe-off cleanser, nothing more, nothing less.

☺ **$$$ Purifying Cleansing Gel** *($26 for 5 ounces)* is a standard, detergent-based water-soluble cleanser with some algae. Again, the faith in algae is up to you because that would be the only reason to consider spending this kind of money on such an exceptionally standard cleanser that is easily replaced at the drugstore for one-third the price.

☺ **$$$ Phormidiane Cleanser-Toner** *($26 for 6.8 ounces)* is a standard, rather boring toner. It's up to you if you think algae has some magical benefit for the skin.

☹ **Seaweed Soap** *($11.50 for 5.3 ounces)* is, as the name implies, soap, tallow, and a strong detergent cleansing agent, with a tiny amount of seaweed. This can be too drying for most skin types and the tallow can clog pores.

☺ **$$$ Purifying Gommage Exfoliant** *($28 for 1.7 ounces)*. The bits of clay can feel slightly abrasive, but this is pretty waxy stuff and several of the plant extracts in here can be skin irritants, including yarrow, coltsfoot, and birch.

☺ **$$$ Vegetal Exfoliant with Natural Enzymes** *($28 for 1.7 ounces)*. Papain is a very unstable enzyme, which means its ability to exfoliate is limited. For enzymatic exfoliation, bromelain is far more stable, although I'm not convinced that enzymes are generally the best way to exfoliate; even so the amount of papain in here is negligible.

☹ **$$$ Refreshing Seawater Spray** *($31 for 4.25 ounces).* At least the name is clear—this is regular water and seawater. Charging this much money for water out of the ocean is amazing, but if you are looking for salt water (though I can't imagine why), here it is.

☹ **$$$ Rosee Visage Face Dew** *($25 for 8.5 ounces)* is basically water, rose water (glycerin and fragrance), slip agents, preservatives, fragrance, and salt water. This has none of the water-binding agents or soothing agents that would make this product interesting for skin care.

☻ **Intensive Exfoliant Clarifying with AHA** *($12.75 for 1.7 ounces)* lists the second ingredient as alcohol, which makes this too irritating and drying for all skin types.

☹ **$$$ Decongestant Micro Emulsion** *($37 for 0.5 ounce)* is a good, though exceptionally mundane and overpriced, moisturizing formula.

☹ **Eau Marine Lotion** *($38 for 8.5 ounces)* includes the tiniest amount of seawater, which isn't great because salt can be a skin irritant. It also contains arnica, witch hazel, and ivy, all potential skin irritants.

☹ **$$$ Extreme Climate Skin Cream** *($62 for 1.7 ounces)* is a very good but very standard moisturizer for dry skin.

☺ **Hydrating Moisture Base Skin Cream** *($31 for 1.7 ounces)* is a good moisturizer for normal to dry skin, but it is incredibly mundane and unimpressive, though for the money this is a better formulation for less money than the Extreme Climate version above.

☹ **$$$ Hydration Reinforcement Moisture Supplement Cream** *($58 for 1.7 ounces)* is a good moisturizer, but for the money the lack of any interesting water-binding agents or antioxidants make this a real "why bother."

☹ **$$$ Intensive Hydrating Formula Cream Anti-Pollution** *($55 for 1.7 ounces)* is simply a moisturizer for dry skin and a rather ordinary one at that. Why someone would think a bunch of standard thickening agents, glycerin, silicone, plant oil, algae, preservatives, fragrance, and coloring agents can stop pollution from impacting the face is anyone's guess.

☹ **$$$ Lift Contour Replenishing Formula** *($45 for 0.5 ounce)* is a product that's very hard to deal with. This gel is simply water, glycerin, thickeners, mulberry extract, a tiny amount of soothing agent, preservatives, and coloring agents. Wow! I'm sure Phytomer is relieved most people don't know how to read an ingredient label. The tiny amount of mulberry extract in this one cannot inhibit melanin production. The listing of liposomes on the ingredient label is either a mistake or just foolish, because liposomes are not an ingredient but a delivery system.

☻ **Moisturizing Micro Emulsion** *($37 for 0.5 ounce)* contains lemon, orange, and grapefruit oil, all of which are too irritating for skin and the rest of the formula is just wax and silicone. Gee, it doesn't get much more poorly formulated than this.

☺ **$$$ Neutralizing Cream** (*$49 for 1.7 ounces*) is almost identical to many of Phytomer's moisturizers. The tiny amount of yeast in this product can have some minimal antioxidant benefits. But if you were interested in yeast, there are other products you could choose using that ingredient that at least also include other interesting ingredients too, because this product has none.

☺ **$$$ Nourishing Micro Emulsion** (*$37 for 0.5 ounce*) is basically just wax, silicone, and fragrant oils. There is nothing nourishing or particularly helpful about this product for any skin type.

☺ **$$$ Nutri-Complex Skin Care Fluid** (*$50 for 0.5 ounce*). Are you ready for this? This product merely contains algae, protein, castor oil, gum, and fragrance. Unbelievable. It would end up being a good moisturizer for dry skin, but it just isn't worth it. How much algae does one person need anyway? The protein is just a good water-binding agent, it doesn't have any effect on the protein in skin.

☺ **Purifying Emulsion Shine Free for Oily Skin** (*$30 for 1.7 ounces*) contains several ingredients that could be problematic for oily skin, including plant oils, arnica, and orris root, which are skin irritants. Other than that, this is a good moisturizer for dry skin. There isn't enough tea tree oil in this product to work as a disinfectant for breakouts, however.

☺ **$$$ Purifying Micro Emulsion** (*$37 for 0.5 ounce*). There are no words for how below-average a formulation this is, and the lemon oil in here should be for furniture, not for skin.

☺ **$$$ Reconditioning Skin Cream Replenishing Formula** (*$55 for 1.7 ounces*) is the line's most interesting formulation, but that isn't saying much; it would be good for dry skin.

☺ **$$$ Replenishing Complex to Smooth Fine Lines** (*$90 for 1.05 ounces*) is similar to the product above and the same review applies.

☺ **$$$ Replenishing Micro Emulsion** (*$37 for 0.5 ounce*) is a very boring and easily avoidable moisturizer for any skin type.

☺ **$$$ Soothing Skin Cream for Sensitive and Blotchy Skin** (*$63 for 1.7 ounces*). The plant extracts in here can be anti-irritants, which may help reduce redness.

☺ **$$$ Gentle Mask for Sensitive Skin** (*$31 for 1.7 ounces*) is a standard clay mask. Fragrance in products for sensitive skin is always problematic, but this could be a good mask for someone with normal to slightly dry skin.

☺ **$$$ Hydrating Seaweed Facial Mask** (*$26 for 1.7 ounces*) is similar to the one above, minus the emollients. It would be OK for someone with normal to slightly oily skin.

☺ **$$$ Intensive Nourishing Mask** (*$30 for 1.7 ounces*) is similar to the Gentle Mask for Sensitive Skin above, and the same basic review applies.

☹ **Purifying Facial Mask** (*$25 for 1.7 ounces*) is a standard clay mask that also contains several ingredients that are problematic for oily skin, including plant oils, plus skin irritants like arnica and peppermint. It does contain tea tree oil, but in this amount it would be ineffective as a topical disinfectant.

☹ **Replenishing Foaming Mask** *($48 for 1.7 ounces)* contains alcohol and lemon high up on the ingredient list and is not recommended.

☹ **Whitening Cleansing Milk** *($26 for 6.8 ounces)*. If you are a reader of ingredient listings, it would only take a quick once-over to notice that the ingredients for this cleanser are almost identical to the Gentle Cleansing Milk above. Only the name has changed—and, of course, the price. Notably what this cleanser does not contain is any skin-lightening ingredients whatsoever, though even if it did, they would be wiped or washed off before they had a chance to have an effect!

☺ $$$ **Whitening Day Cream** *($45 for 1.7 ounces)* does contain some of the more popular "natural" ingredients for inhibiting melanin production, including kojic acid, licorice extract, and mulberry extract. These are an option, though in the amount used in this formula, it is doubtful they would have any effect on skin. Regardless, no whitening product can produce positive results without an effective sunscreen, and Phytomer doesn't have anything to offer in that regard.

☺ $$$ **Whitening Night Cream** *($52 for 1.7 ounces)* is similar to the Whitening Day Cream and the same review applies.

☺ $$$ **Whitening Mask** *($57 for seven treatments)*. There are no melanin-inhibiting ingredients in this mask, which makes it useless for the purpose of lightening skin. Other than that, it is merely citric acid with baking soda, titanium dioxide, and algae. Titanium dioxide can make the skin *look* white, but it can't do anything to the color of skin itself.

☺ $$$ **5-Day Urban Treatment** *($55 for 1.7 ounces)* has a standard group of ingredients, including water, lots of thickeners, silicone, algae, fragrance, and preservatives, so I'm not clear why this would be a treatment of any kind or warrant a special price or package.

☺ $$$ **Protective Aromatic** *($37 for 0.5 ounce)* is just thickeners, fragrance, algae, and preservatives, none of which will protect anything.

☹ **Moisturizing Sun Lotion SPF 8** *($33 for 4.25 ounces)*. No one really thinks an SPF 8 is appropriate anymore, right? SPF 15 is the standard for any kind of sun product.

☹ **Tanning Gel for Use with Tanning Beds SPF 2** *($28 for 4.25 ounces)*. They've got to be kidding! A product that encourages using tanning beds? This is one of the more unconscionable skin-care products I've seen.

☹ **Intensive Tanning Oil SPF 4** *($33 for 4.25 ounces)*. What is this company thinking? A product that encourages tanning is as bad as the one above for people using tanning beds.

# Pond's (Skin Care Only)

Pond's spent over $36 million to advertise its line of AHA products, called Age Defying Complex, so it has likely caught your attention by now. Six-page ads in major fashion magazines and several sultry television commercials are the company's way of letting you know it has seriously joined the AHA competition. The ads carry on about tests showing that Pond's AHA products improved the skin of women who used them over a six-month period. Of course, the ads don't mention whether any other AHA products were tested or what other products the women were using beforehand. They probably figured that most women wouldn't want to be bothered with such details. So the ads don't really give you any information you can use to make a decision. Having said all that, and even though I consider the ads to be totally bogus, I do happen to think that Pond's has created two very good AHA moisturizers. Sadly, the other Pond's products are far less interesting and desirable. For more information about Pond's, call (800) 743-8640 or visit the Web site at www.unilever.com.

☺ **Cleansing and Make-Up Remover Towelettes** *($3.97 for 30 towelettes).* Though I am not a fan of wiping off makeup, these towelettes from Pond's are a fine option. This does contain some benzyl alcohol, but in such a small amount it is only there as a preservative. If you think these are a clever way to remove makeup, an even cheaper version is fragrance-free baby wipes. They come in far larger packs for about the same money and contain almost identical ingredients! The ginseng extract in the Pond's version can be a skin irritant.

☺ **Clear Cold Cream** *($4.50 for 4 ounces)* is a clear, thick version of regular opaque, white cold cream. Neither rinses off; they need to be wiped off and can leave a greasy residue on the skin. This one does contain a tiny amount of glycolic acid but not enough to do anything for the skin. It can be an option for dry skin.

☹ **Cold Cream Deep Cleanser** *($5.49 for 6.1 ounces)* is a classic cold cream: greasy and thick, and very occlusive and heavy on skin.

☹ **Clear Solutions Deep Pore Foaming Cleanser** *($5.69 for 6 ounces)* is a standard, detergent-based water-soluble cleanser that uses sodium C14-16 olefin sulfate as one of the cleansing agents, which is far too drying and irritating for the skin.

☹ **Fresh Start Daily Wash** *($5.99 for 5 ounces)* contains menthol, and the red beads in here can feel irritating on skin.

☹ **Self-Foaming Facial Cleanser** *($6.99 for 4 ounces)* uses sodium C14-16 olefin sulfate as the detergent cleansing agent, which makes it too drying and irritating for all skin types.

☺ **Cleansing Lotion** *($4.39 for 4 ounces)* is a water-soluble cleanser that doesn't remove makeup all that well without the help of a washcloth, though it can be good when you aren't wearing makeup, or for someone with dry skin.

☹ **Clear Solutions Deep Pore Scrub** *($5.69 for 3 ounces)* is a standard, detergent-based water-soluble cleanser that uses ground-up plastic as the scrub material. It is an option for topical exfoliation, though the cleansing agent can be too drying for some skin types.

☹ **Clarifying Astringent** *($4.39 for 7 ounces)* is a standard, alcohol-based toner that also contains witch hazel, menthol, and eucalyptus, all of which can seriously irritate the skin.

☹ **Clear Solutions Pore Clarifying Astringent** *($4.39 for 7 ounces)* is a problem waiting to happen. It contains mostly water, alcohol, witch hazel, menthol, and eucalyptus oil. Ouch!

☺ **Age Defying Complex SPF 4** *($10.99 for 2 ounces)* and **Age Defying Complex for Delicate Skin SPF 4** *($11.59 for 2 ounces)* are both very good AHA products. Although the two creams are labeled differently (one for delicate skin and the other presumably for all skin types), they are practically identical except for the amount of AHAs: the Delicate Skin formula contains 4% AHAs; the other, 8%. However, the SPF is just embarrassing and is not even vaguely capable of protecting skin from sun damage.

☺ **Age Defying Lotion SPF 4** *($10.99 for 3 ounces)* and **Age Defying Lotion for Delicate Skin SPF 4** *($12.49 for 3 ounces)* are similar to the products above, only in lotion form, and the same review applies. They contain 8% and 4% AHAs, respectively.

☹ **Age Defying Eye Cream SPF 8** *($10.99 for 0.5 ounce)* contains about 2% to 3% glycolic acid in a very lightweight, standard moisturizing base, with vitamins and silicone. At this concentration, it isn't much of an exfoliant, and everything else about it is pretty unimpressive for skin, including the very poor SPF and lack of UVA-protecting ingredients.

☹ **Prevent and Correct Cream Age Defying System SPF 8** *($16.99 for two products, totaling 2.5 ounces)* is simply a repackaging of the Age Defying Complex AHA cream and a sunscreen. The sunscreen part is called Prevent, and its SPF is 8, which isn't great, especially as it doesn't contain avobenzone, zinc oxide, or titanium dioxide for UVA protection, and is not recommended. You can buy a good SPF 15 sunscreen for a lot less and buy the Age Defying Complex individually for less, and get more of both.

☹ **Prevent and Correct Lotion Age Defying System with Alpha Nutrium SPF 8** *($14.99 for 4.25 ounces)* is identical to the one above, only in lotion form.

☺ **Clear Solutions Combination Skin Moisturizer** *($5.69 for 4 ounces)*. As a combination AHA (about 4% to 5% lactic acid) and BHA (about 0.5%) product, this is a good option. It should, however, be used alone, not with any of the other products in the Clear Solutions lineup, which are fairly drying and irritating products.

☺ **Dry Skin Cream, Extra Rich Skin Cream** *($4.39 for 3.9 ounces)* is a standard mineral oil– and Vaseline-based moisturizer with thickeners and preservatives. It would be good for dry skin, but its ingredients are very ordinary and boring.

☺ **Nourishing Moisturizer Cream** *($5.99 for 2 ounces)* can't nourish the skin and it definitely isn't oil-free, but it is a good moisturizer for normal to dry skin. The teeny amounts of vitamins and water-binding agents in here are barely worth mentioning.

☺ **Nourishing Moisturizer Lotion** *($5.99 for 4 ounces)* is similar to the Cream version above only in lotion form.

☺ **Nourishing Moisture Lotion with SPF 15** *($5.99 for 2.5 ounces)* won't nourish anyone's skin, but it does contain a good in-part titanium dioxide–based SPF 15 in a lightweight moisturizing base for someone with normal to dry skin.

☺ **Overnight Nourishing Complex Cream** *($6.29 for 2 ounces)* is similar to the Nourishing Moisturizer Cream above, and the same comments apply.

☺ **$$$ Revitalizing Eye Capsules** *($10.99 for 20 capsules totaling 0.26 ounce)* are capsules that contain silicones, slip agents, vitamins, and water-binding agents. If you want a lightweight silky moisturizer for slightly dry skin, this one is great, though overpriced.

☺ **$$$ Skin Smoothing Capsules** *($10.99 for 26 capsules)*. The results won't be dramatic, but this is certainly a good product for someone with slightly dry skin.

☹ **Revitalizing Eye Gel with Vitamin E** *($5.99 for 0.5 ounce)*. Witch hazel is a possible skin irritant and a problem in a product meant to be used near the delicate skin around the eyes.

☹ **Soothing Cucumber Eye Treatments** *($7.56 for 24 pads)* is a very lightweight gel with a tiny amount of cucumber extract. The orange peel in here may smell like vitamin C but it's a skin irritant.

☹ **Clear Solutions Overnight Blemish Reducers** *($5.99 for 24 dots)* are patches coated with film former, a hairspray-like ingredient, along with 0.5% BHA and about the same quantity of AHA, as well as some plant extracts, tea tree oil, and slip agents. The AHA and BHA are useless as exfoliants because the pH is too high (not to mention that 0.5% is really at the low end for any effectiveness). Also, AHA and BHA need some time to work to prevent breakouts; their effectiveness isn't the overnight kind. Tea tree oil can be an alternative to benzoyl peroxide as a disinfectant but probably not at this tiny concentration. There are far better ways to treat acne, but I imagine teenagers will find this product way too tempting to pass up.

# *Prescriptives*

Estee Lauder owns Clinique, Prescriptives, and Origins, among many other lines, ranging from Bobbi Brown, M.A.C., Stila, Donna Karan, and Aveda to Jane at the drugstore. But just to stay with the original three Estee Lauder line extensions for a minute, notice that first Estee Lauder introduced Day Wear SPF 15, next Clinique introduces Weather Everything SPF 15, and then Prescriptives launches Any Wear SPF 15. See a pattern? Here's another example: Estee Lauder brings out Diminish Retinol Treatment and then Prescriptives launches its retinol product, LSW. Estee Lauder creates Nutritious and shortly afterward Origins has its look-alike version called Night-a-Mins. This happens with almost every imaginable product among the original Estee Lauder family of line extensions. But Estee Lauder's intention isn't to be direct with the consumer about this, just to cover all the bases in terms of appealing to every consumer group.

So where does Prescriptives appear on the map of cosmetics niche marketing? While Estee Lauder certainly appeals to the upscale baby boomers and older, and Clinique the young adult struggling with the pressures of adulthood, Prescriptives aims for the thirty-something urban sophisticate who needs a bit more scientific convincing and a slick image. Think of what comes to mind when you hear the name "Prescriptives." A physician's prescription, maybe? Even some of the packaging has a medical or clinical appearance. What a great gimmick.

Prescriptives specializes and excels in offering a huge selection of excellent foundations, eyeshadows, blush, and lipsticks. The color displays are well organized into what Prescriptives has termed "color families." It also offers a now-familiar procedure called color-printing, which supposedly allows the salesperson to determine the foundation shade that exactly matches your skin. While that is ultimately the goal, color printing does not replace the need to check the foundation color in daylight! One glaring shortcoming of Prescriptives' foundations is that there are a preponderance of inappropriate colors that are noticeably pink or peach. You can spot these a mile away—they are the full tester bottles while the more normal skin-tone choices are half gone.

In terms of skin care, you'll find a mixed bag of options here, with the strong points being the same ones as for most of the Estee Lauder companies: great moisturizers, OK toners, good sunscreens, and a mixed review for cleansers. For more information about Prescriptives, call (212) 572-4400. In late winter 2001, Prescriptives' Web site will be www.gloss.com.

## Prescriptives Skin Care

☺ **All Clean Fresh Foaming Cleanser** *($19.50 for 6.7 ounces)* is a standard, detergent-based cleanser that can be somewhat drying, but can also work well for someone with normal to oily skin. The plant extracts in here are fragrance.

☺ **All Clean Rich Cream Cleanser** *($19.50 for 6.7 ounces)* is a standard, wipe-off cleanser that can leave a greasy film on the skin, though it is an option for someone with dry skin.

☹ **All Clean Sparkling Gel** *($18.50 for 6.7 ounces)* is a standard, detergent-based water-soluble cleanser that uses tea-lauryl sulfate as the main cleansing agent, which makes it potentially too drying and irritating for all skin types. It also contains small amounts of grapefruit, lemon oil, and spearmint oil, which can irritate or burn the eye area.

☺ $$$ **Quick Remover for Face Makeup** *($18.50 for 4.2 ounces)* is just a wipe-off makeup remover that can leave a slight film on the skin.

☺ **Eye Makeup Remover** *($15 for 4 ounces)* is a standard eye-makeup remover. It will work as well as any.

☺ $$$ **Px Purifying Scrub** *($18.50 for 3.6 ounces)* is really more of a standard clay mask (which is one of the uses recommended) than a scrub. It also contains menthol, which can be a skin irritant.

☹ **Immediate Matte Skin Conditioning Tonic** *($18.50 for 6.7 ounces)* contains alcohol and peppermint, which are drying and irritating for all skin types. The only thing immediate about this product is not to use it.

☹ **Immediate Glow Skin Conditioning Tonic** *($18.50 for 6.7 ounces)*. Menthol can give the skin a glow, but it's also an irritant; other than that, it's just an ordinary toner.

☺ **All You Need Action Moisturizer for Normal to Dry Skin** *($32.50 for 1.7 ounces)* doesn't have an SPF rating, so it isn't all you need for daytime. It would be fine as a nighttime moisturizer for someone with normal to somewhat dry skin, but it's nothing exceptional. This is Prescriptives' attempt at an AHA product, but it contains fruit extract, which isn't the same thing as a true AHA. Even if it were, there isn't enough in the product for it to work as an exfoliant, nor does the product have a low enough pH for any exfoliant to work.

☺ $$$ **All You Need Action Moisturizer for Dry Skin** *($32.50 for 1.2 ounces)* is similar to the Normal to Dry Skin version above only more emollient, but the same basic review applies.

☺ $$$ **All You Need Action Moisturizer Oil-Free** *($32.50 for 1.2 ounces)* is similar to the moisturizer above, only this one includes a more effective form of AHA, just not enough of it to be an exfoliant. There are also several potentially irritating plant extracts in here, including sage, sandalwood, and coriander.

☺ **Px Comfort Lotion** *($30 for 1.7 ounces)* would be a very good moisturizer for someone with dry skin.

☺ $$$ **Px Comfort Cream 24 Hour Care for Sensitive Skin** *($37.50 for 1.7 ounces)* is a good moisturizer for someone with dry skin. Fragrant plant extracts always pose a particular irritation potential for someone with sensitive skin, but aside from that this is a good moisturizer for dry skin.

☺ $$$ **Px Concentrate** *($60 for 1 ounce)* is a very good, lotion-type moisturizer for normal to dry skin.

☺ $$$ Px **Eye Specialist Visible Action Gel** *($32.50 for 0.5 ounce)* would be a good, lightweight moisturizer for normal to slightly dry skin, though the caffeine's high tannin content can cause skin irritation with repeated use.

☺ Px **Flight Cream** *($28 for 1.7 ounces)* is supposed to help skin when it's subjected to the rigors of flying conditions. It is a good standard moisturizer for dry skin, but nothing more. It also contains balm mint, which can be a skin irritant.

☺ $$$ Px **Retinol LSW** *($50 for 1 ounce)* makes claims about retinol being a "poor man's" Retin-A or Renova—LSW stands for lines, spots, and wrinkles—though at $50 for 1 ounce, this isn't about being an inexpensive substitute; after all, real Retin-A costs about $51 for 1.58 ounces (funny, that's almost twice as much to boot, and that's for the strongest-strength product). Even if retinol were an acceptable but second-rate alternative to Retin-A, why would you want to spend all this money on a product that performs only second or third best? Still, you can easily give retinol (the technical name for vitamin A) a try with Neutrogena Healthy Skin Anti-Wrinkle Cream with Retinol ($10.89 for 1.4 ounces) or L'Oreal Line Eraser ($12 for 1 ounce) for a small fraction of the price.

☺ $$$ Px **Uplift Active Firming Cream** *($45 for 1 ounce)* is a lightweight cream with the proclaimed virtue of actively firming the skin, instantly and for the long term. Wow! That's a lot to accomplish for some pretty standard cosmetic ingredients. Despite the claims about firming and long-term moisturization, you are supposed to wear it in conjunction with Prescriptives Super Line Preventor or All You Need Action Moisturizer, and that still leaves you without sun protection. Uplift isn't all that uplifting, but it is a good lightweight moisturizer for someone with normal to slightly dry skin.

☺ $$$ Px **Uplift Firming Eye Cream** *($35 for 0.5 ounce)* is similar to the one above, only it adds caffeine to the mix. Due to caffeine's high tannin content it can be a skin irritant with repeated use.

☹ Px **Blemish Specialist Fast Acting Lotion, Spot Treatment for Acne** *($17 for 1 ounce)* is just another alcohol-based blemish product. It contains some glycerin and a soothing agent, but that won't counteract the irritation from the alcohol.

☺ $$$ Px **Insulation Anti-Oxidant Vitamin Cream with SPF 15** *($40 for 1.7 ounces)* is one overpriced sunscreen, but it does contain titanium dioxide as one of the active sunscreen ingredients, and in a rather good moisturizing base.

☺ **Any Wear SPF 15** *($19.50 for 1 ounce)* is a very good sunscreen for someone with dry skin, mainly because it is part titanium dioxide in a good moisturizing base.

☺ $$$ **Super Line Preventor** *($45 for 1 ounce* is a good moisturizer for normal to slightly dry skin but that's about it.

☺ $$$ **Vibrant Instant Eye Brightener** *($37.50 for 0.5 ounce)* is just a standard, lightweight moisturizer for normal to dry skin. The added caffeine can be a skin irritant with repeated use and the fish cartilage in here does not have any rare properties for skin. The Px Uplift Firming Eye Cream above is a far better formulation.

☺ $$$ **Vibrant Vitamin Infuser for Dull, Stressed Skin** *($45 for 1.7 ounces)* is a good standard moisturizer for dry skin, available in cream or lotion. It doesn't infuse the skin with anything that you won't find in lots and lots of products. This product does contain a tiny amount of mulberry root extract, which is backed by some research demonstrating it can inhibit melanin production, but not in the amount used in this product.

☺ **Magic Illuminating Liquid Potion** *($30)* comes in a small, vial-like bottle with a sponge tip applicator. When applied to the skin it dries to a soft, sheer shine (OK, not sparkly, but definitely shiny). It is supposed to be a "holographic" liquid (I swear that's what the information sheet from Prescriptives calls it). By any name it is just soft, sheer shine.

☺ **Magic Illuminating Cream Potion** *($35)* is a cream-to-powder compact in a soft pink shade that has a shiny effect (OK, OK, luminescent, not glitter), with a sheer finish.

☺ **Magic Cooling Wand** *($28)* comes in a tube that looks like a large concealer stick, and gives a slight white, sheer color. It has the most minimal of effects on the skin, but it does go on cool and dries to a no-appearance finish. I'm sure it's good for something, but though the cooling sensation is nice, the promise of taking away puffiness doesn't come true.

☹ **Magic Cooling Globe** *($30)* is the most magical product in the group, because it took a great deal of magic for the salesperson to explain this to me and keep a straight face. Are you sitting down? This is a glass bulb filled with water and antifreeze. That's it. You're supposed to put it in the refrigerator and then rub it over your face to reduce puffiness. Like you can't just use a cool compress? Talk about magical thinking!

☺ $$$ **Magic Invisible Line Smoother** *($35 for 0.5 ounce)* is a thick cream that is virtually identical to Lancome's Touche Optim' Age ($22.50 for 0.52 ounce) and M.A.C.'s Matte Creme Matifiance ($16.50 for 0.75 ounce), with the same matte-cream texture that is reminiscent of a sheer, soft spackle. It definitely can give the appearance of smoother skin, but it is temporary, lasting only a few hours depending on what you wear over it and how much you move your face.

# Prescriptives Makeup

**FOUNDATION:** ☺ $$$ **Virtual Skin Oil Free SPF 10** *($30)* claims to have an undetectable finish and is supposed to fit like a "second skin." While this sounds great, this is just foundation—albeit a very good one with sheer to light coverage and a natural finish. The color range is impressive and this does blend out beautifully. The only colors to avoid are: Real Cream, Real Ivory (both slightly pink), Real Cameo (very pink), Real Bisque, Tan and Fawn (both slightly orange), and Real Camellia (slightly pink). The SPF of 10 is without UVA-protecting ingredients and should not be relied on.

☺ $$$ **Photochrome Compact Makeup SPF 15** *($35)* is a cream-to-powder foundation with a good, titanium-dioxide–based sunscreen. The claims about this one having "self-adjusting, photochromatic pigments" don't hold up in any light, but this is still a good option for someone with normal to slightly dry skin wanting medium coverage and a powdery finish. This formula blends very well, but dries quickly, calling for a deft hand when it comes to application. Avoid Warm Ivory (slightly pink) and Warm Ginger (slightly orange, but may work if blended on sheer).

☻ $$$ **Luxe Soft Glow Moisture Makeup SPF 15** *($30)* is quite similar to M.A.C.'s recently launched Hyper Real Foundation ($24) in that both are light-weight, natural finish foundations that leave behind a subtle layer of iridescence. The same "light-reflecting" and "makes-skin-glow-from-within" claims are attached to Luxe but no matter how you slice it, shine is shine and even though this is soft, it can look glaring in daylight. The SPF is without UVA protection (for shame!) and the 24 colors have the same shade names as most of the other Prescriptives foundations, save for the prefix 'Rich'. As usual, the Yellow/Orange shades are the ones to consider while the Red/Orange, Red, and Blue/Red shades, though sheer, are mostly too pink, peach, orange, or rose to recommend. Consider avoiding Rich Peach, Rich Fawn, Rich Honey, Rich Petal, Rich Cameo, Rich Suede, and Rich Rose. There are few options for very dark skin. Although this is recommended for normal to dry skin, the high talc content (it's the fifth ingredient) makes it a better option for normal to slightly dry or slightly oily skin—but think twice about adding this much shine to your routine.

☺ $$$ **100% Oil Free Makeup SPF 15***($30)* is a great true-matte foundation that offers medium to full coverage and a beautiful assortment of colors, by far the best neutral selection in Prescriptives' lineup. The SPF of 15 is minus any UVA protection, so a good sunscreen would still be necessary under this, which means more layers, not the best for someone with normal to oily skin. The only colors to watch out for are Fresh Ivory (slightly peach), Fresh Tan (slightly orange), Fresh Cameo and Rose (slightly pink), and Fresh Blush (very pink).

☺ $$$ **Custom Blend Foundation Oil Free** *($55)* is similar to the Makeup + reviewed above only with a slightly lighter texture. This is best for a normal to dry skin; despite the name, the texture of this would not make someone with oily skin happy.

☺ $$$ **Custom Blend Foundation Moisturizing Formula** *($55)* would be great for a normal to dry skin needing light to medium coverage and it does have an emollient feel on the skin. Both Custom Blend formulations are great alternatives if you are having trouble finding the right color out there in the world of foundations.

But be patient and don't rush the process, and be sure you find a salesperson who has been doing this technique for a while. While this may just be the best match in a foundation you've ever found, you still have to check the color in the daylight and it may take several tries until you get the shade you want.

☺ $$$ **Matchstick Foundation SPF 15** *($35)* is Prescriptives' contribution to the stick foundation trend. In some ways it has come out ahead, as this has a reliable SPF 15, but it is still only best for someone with slightly dry to slightly oily skin, as the very ingredients that keep this in solid form may clog pores. The coverage can go from sheer to full, but keep in mind if this is used as a sheer foundation then sun protection may be compromised. This dries quickly to a soft powdery finish, but tends to let a lot of shine show through on oilier areas. All of the colors are fairly neutral; just watch out for Cool Shell (slightly pink), Warm Vellum and Ivory (both slightly peach), and Cool Desert (peach).

☺ $$$ **Invisible Finish Foundation SPF 15** *($29)* is a sheer, tinted foundation that has a great, soft texture that feels wonderful on the skin, especially if you have normal to slightly dry or slightly oily skin. Of the 14 shades only a few are a problem: Sheer Cameo, Sheer Camellia, Sheer Antelope, Sheer Fawn, and Sheer Rose are all too pink, peach, or ash for most skin types. But alas, the SPF 15 doesn't include UVA protection, and it is not recommended for sun protection, but if you don't mind wearing a sunscreen with UVA protection underneath it, then the ultralight coverage is worth trying.

<u>CONCEALER:</u> ☺ **Camouflage Cream** *($15)* has a creamy, smooth application and only a slight chance of creasing. Of the 14 shades only Red Light, Blue Red Medium, Red Medium, and Red Orange Dark should be avoided.

☹ $$$ **Concealing Wand Corrector/Concealer** *($25)* is a standard pencil that is dual-ended. One half is a creamy (bordering on greasy) concealer whose colors are all slightly pink or peach; the other end is a color corrector that has the same texture as the concealer, except these are slightly shiny, and both ends leave a creamy finish that could easily crease. The intended effect is to blend the two together over imperfections to "optically airbrush the face," but you are better off with a reliable, neutral concealer with a natural finish that doesn't draw attention to what is being hidden.

☺ **Concealing Wand Highlighter** *($14)* is virtually identical to the one above, only this features one color and is smaller in size. There is only one shade, a pearlescent white, and for those who prefer using a creamy pencil to softly accent the brow bone and the like, this would be an option.

<u>POWDER:</u> ☹ $$$ **All-Skins Loose Powder** *($25)* is a standard talc-free powder with a small amount of shine. It has a smooth feel with a dry finish. The shimmer in here won't help you reduce the shine on your skin if that's the reason you are looking for a loose powder.

☺ **$$$ Virtual Skin Pressed Powder** *($23)* is an overpriced but good pressed powder with a slightly heavier application than most and a great range of colors. **Powder Play Loose Color** *($18)* consists of salt-shaker vials of loose powder, all with a smooth texture and a very shiny finish. They're a fun possibility, but the shine is way too intense for anything other than an evening look. **Magic Liquid Powder** *($30)* is, as the name implies, a powder with a wet finish that dries to a sheer powder feel. It works well, and the cool feel is nice. This is an intriguing product to test, but don't count on anything even vaguely magical (wait until you hear the claims the salesperson will bestow at the counter).

☺ <u>BLUSH:</u> **Powder Cheekcolor** *($14.50)* comes in beautiful shades and most have no visible shine, although some of the colors tend to go on quite sheer. **All Skins Face Colors Refillable** *(blush tins $14.50 each, compact $5)* is a two-in-one blush container. What a great concept. You can pick a contour and a blush color, two different blush colors, or a blush and a pressed powder of your choice. One caution: most of the colors have a slight amount of shine, although not enough to be a problem. **$$$ Mystick Swivel Stick Cream Blush** *($25)* is an aptly named product with a small color selection that features both sheer and vivid tones. The texture is somewhat dry, making this harder to blend than a more creamy-finish version, but for close-to-flawless skin types, this is an option. (If you want a less expensive version, L'Oreal's QuickStick is virtually identical.)

☺ <u>EYESHADOW:</u> **Pick 2 Eyeshadow** *($11 each; $5 for the compact)* is a great concept that allows you to choose two colors out of a sea of choices. This almost always ensures you will end up using both shades, and there are some wonderful matte colors available. As is the current trend, many shiny shades have crept back into the fray, but that choice is up to you. All of the colors have a soft texture and blend on evenly, although the pigmentation is on the lighter side, so some fading may be apparent at day's end.

☹ **$$$ Eye Paint** *($22.50)* is strictly for those who enjoy using vivid, rainbow-bright colors. This is Prescriptives' revision of its Eyeshadow Trios, which used to offer three coordinating matte shades. Now you are supposed to decide between royal blue with yellow and turquoise or orange and cranberry hues. How disappointing! In spite of the colors, the same basic comments apply here as for the eyeshadows above. **Eyelights** *($15)* are cream-to-powder eye colors in a tube. These go on quite smoothly and tend to not crease, but every color is extremely shiny.

☹ <u>EYE AND BROW SHAPER:</u> **Eyelining Pencil** *($13)* is a standard pencil with a decent color selection. The application is on the greasy side, and there are dozens of better pencils available for a fraction of the cost. **Softlining Pencil** *($14.50)* is a powdery eyeliner in pencil form with an effortless application (sans sharpening!). This is almost too creamy, and could easily smudge or fade, so test this one out at the store first and wear it for awhile before making a decision. **Automatic Eye Pencil** *($13)* is exactly that: a pencil that doesn't need sharpening. This is great but very standard and hardly unique, as lines from Almay to Revlon have their identical version for far less. **Skinny Dip Liquid Eyeliner** *($12)* has the cutest "fountain pen" packaging and is a decent liquid eyeliner, but the brush is hard to control, giving you a thick line no matter what you do. **Brow Shaping Pencil** *($13.50)* comes in some workable colors but has a rather dry, hard texture and is not the best for an even application. **$$$ Diffusion Liner** *($18)* is a standard pencil that comes in three flesh-toned colors and has an iridescent finish. Prescriptives recommends these for optically altering the shape of eyebrows and lips, or for filling in wrinkles, but that would be a mistake. Shine draws attention to problems, it doesn't alter them. The claims that get attributed to iridescence are incredible, but they seem to be convincing a lot of women that sparkles actually do something other than add shine to the face.

☺ LIPSTICK AND LIP PENCIL: **$$$ Lavish Lipstick SPF 15** *($16)* has a great name and a veritable kaleidoscope of colors. The application is smooth and light, with a greasy finish. The claim of long wear may have something to do with the fact that these are quite pigmented, but the "anti-feathering" claim is contradicted by the standard greasy application. This does get points for having a reliable SPF 15. The **$$$ Soft Suede Lipstick** *($16)* offers great colors and an unusually smooth, semi-matte finish. This one will stick around longer than the one above. **Sheer Lipstick** *($15)* is pretty standard and nothing exceptional. **$$$ Potent Lipstick** *($16)* is Prescriptives ultra-matte lipstick, but it is not as matte as many others, though it does nicely stain the lips and tends to not roll or chip off. This is worth a look if you've had challenges in the past with a matte lipstick. **Lip Gloss** *($12.50)* is a standard wand-applicator gloss with a nice selection of colors. **Lip Lacquer** *($15)* offers a creamier, more opaque formula with a non-sticky, "wet" finish. **Lip Polish** *($12.50)* is virtually identical to the Lip Gloss above only this one has glitter particles in it. **Lip Coloring Pencil** *($13)* is nothing to get excited about—it's a standard, twist-up pencil with OK colors. This one tends to drag at the lips and go on unevenly.

☺ MASCARA: **Intensified Mascara** *($15)* and **Dramatic Mascara** *($15)*, while not terrible, are completely lackluster and ordinary, and despite the different names they perform the same. Don't expect any dramatic or noticeable lengthening or thickening from either. They don't smear or clump, which is nice, so if you don't want thicker or longer lashes, these may be an option.

☺ **$$$ BRUSHES:** The makeup **brushes** *($15 to $50)* for the most part have a satiny soft feel, and most of the shapes are quite workable, while others are not for everyone. The eyeshadow and eyeliner brushes are particularly great, with good density and shapes.

The only ones to consider avoiding are the ☹ $$$ **Powder Brush** *($32.50)*, which is too floppy and big for most faces; the **Buff Brush** *($42.50)*, both unnecessary and cumbersome, and the **Lip Brush** *($15)*, which is very pointed and would take forever to apply lip color evenly.

## Prestige Cosmetics (Makeup Only)

Prestige, a lower-priced drugstore line, is more than capable of holding its own against some of the big names at the department store. In many drugstores, Prestige has its own sleek display unit, and the product's packaging (and often its performance) is quite similar to M.A.C. as well as other makeup artist/designer lines. It used to be that the variety of Prestige products varied remarkably from store to store, but this has seemingly changed; some of the unfavorable products have now been done away with, and there is more consistency than ever before. For more information, call (800) 722-7488.

☺ <u>CONCEALER:</u> **Extreme Cover Concealer Creme** *($5.99)* comes in a generously sized pot and features four good colors. It is supposed to provide heavier coverage, but it doesn't have enough staying power to do that, at least not any more than any other concealer. It can also slip into the lines under the eye unless you really set it with powder—and that can make the undereye area look heavy, caked, and lined. **Correctives Everyday Cover Concealer** *($3.99)* is a standard, lipstick-style concealer with coverage that is almost identical to the one above. Unfortunately, it also has the same problems. However, if your eye area is unlined, the colors make this worthy of a try—but stay away from the yellow, mauve, and mint green color-correcting shades. In any format, these never work the way you would like them too.

☺ <u>BLUSH:</u> Now known simply as **Blush** *($3.19)*, you'll be surprised how well these lovely matte colors compare to far more expensive versions. These have a smooth, even texture, and many of the shades are richly pigmented, which is great for darker skin tones. The only shiny shade to watch out for among all the mattes is Silk.

☺ <u>EYESHADOW:</u> Prestige's **Eyeshadows** *($3.19)* can be a little trickier to navigate than the Blush above, but there are some impressive matte shades here, and since these are sold as singles, you can pick and choose the ones *you* want and will use. The shiny-to-matte shade ratio is about 50/50, and the matte colors are decidedly more silky than the shinier ones.

☺ <u>EYE AND BROW SHAPER:</u> **Eye Liner** *($2.69)* is a standard pencil that has a good, soft but dry texture and comes in many colors—if you like variety with your pencils, these will satisfy and not break the bank. **Waterproof Eye Pencils** *($3.99)* go on fairly creamy but do stay on well. They aren't any more waterproof than most pencils are. **Waterproof Mechanical Eye Pencils** *($3.99)* are just "no sharpening necessary" versions of the one above that needs sharpening. **Liquid Eyeliner** *($4.49)* comes in an inkwell package and has a great, firm, but not-too-stiff brush that lays down a thin or thick line. It's dramatic, and there are some colors to eschew (blue, purple) but for the most part this is an excellent liquid liner that dries quickly and doesn't chip. **Brow Liner** *($2.69)* is nothing more than your basic brow pencil with a dry finish and soft application. What's great for brow-pencil lovers is the incredibly reasonable price! There is a mini brow brush on the cap, which is a nice little extra.

☺ <u>**LIPSTICK AND LIP PENCIL:**</u> The **Lipsticks** *($3.59)* are available in standard creams or sheers. Both have mediocre staying power (with the Creams outlasting the Sheers, as expected) and are good, basic lipsticks. The packaging has improved and it is now much easier to see the actual color of the lipstick as opposed to just a poor swatch of color. **Creamy Matte Lipstick Crayon** *($4.49)* is reminiscent of Elizabeth Arden's discontinued Lip Talkers. This thick but sleek lip crayon is almost identical in texture, application, and glossy finish. It is not matte, but it isn't greasy—just suitably creamy with enough of a stain to help the color hold up longer than normal. This can still bleed into lines around the mouth, so those who have problems with that may wish to skip this one. **Lip Pencils** *($2.69)*, like the Eye Pencils, come in a good assortment of colors and are overall standard and very affordable for those who don't mind sharpening. **Waterproof Lipstick Pencils** *($3.99)* are identical to the Eye Pencil version. They go on creamy, stay well, and aren't any more waterproof than your average pencil. **Waterproof Mechanical Lip Pencils** *($3.99)* are just non-sharpening versions of the one above. As twist-up pencils, these perform nicely. **Aromatherapy Lip Gloss** *($2.69)* is a pot of standard lip gloss with a fairly intense fragrance that not everyone will find all that therapeutic but it is still a good basic gloss.

☺ <u>**BRUSHES:**</u> Prestige has a small but good collection of **Makeup Brushes** *($1.99 to $8.39)*. They are soft and relatively firm, with good flexibility. If you're in need of brushes and on a budget, these are certainly worth considering.

## *Principal Secret*

Is there something about acting talent or being beautiful that is equal to knowledge? I guess there must be, because having celebrities endorse products is big business the world over. It is simply amazing to me that Victoria Principal can convince women that they can have great skin like she does by using her skin-care routine. In fact, Victoria Principal's infomercial is one of the most successful ever. But I should stick with the facts and not get bogged down by the phenomena of marketing and advertising spectacles and the public's unwavering acceptance of it all.

Victoria Principal's skin-care products were formulated and manufactured by Aida Thibiant, a Beverly Hills aesthetician who has run a successful skin-care boutique and cosmetics manufacturing business there for years. Because the Guthy Renker Corporation that markets and distributes the line felt they no longer needed Thibiant to establish Principal's credentials, they severed ties with her in 1995. That isn't good or bad, it just means it isn't Principal's own skin-care genius behind these products.

This is a line with deals, or at least that's what they appear to be on the surface; look a little deeper and these are just expensive products. You can get the Gentle Deep Cleanser, Eye Relief, and Time Release Moisture for $59.85. Or a seven-piece kit called Total Skin Care that includes Gentle Deep Cleanser, Eye Relief, Time Release Moisture, Gentle Exfoliating Scrub, Invisible Toning Mask, Intensive Serum with AHAs, and AHA Booster Complex for $109.95. Then there is a grouping of makeup products also arranged in varying kits. The makeup and skin care just end up being incredibly overpriced for what you get.

I should mention that several of these products aren't bad, and a few are actually quite nice, specifically for someone with normal to dry skin. (Someone with oily, sensitive, or blemished skin could have problems finding options.) But no one needs six to ten different products to take care of her face and body. Did I forget to mention that the claims are exaggerated?

In the following reviews, all prices listed are retail. If you decide to use these products, joining the club is a good idea, because you will need to reorder frequently; most of the products come only in 0.25- to 6-ounce sizes. Six ounces of any cleanser won't last more than two months. For more information about Principal Secret products, call (800) 545-5595.

## *Principal Secret Skin Care*

☺ $$$ **Advanced Gentle 4-in-1 Cleanser** *($24 for 6 ounces).* There is nothing advanced about this standard, detergent-based water-soluble cleanser. The teeny amount of vitamins in here would just be washed away before they could have an effect on skin. This does contain fragrant oil. It would work fine for most skin types, but could easily be replaced by lots of far less expensive cleansers at the drugstore and cosmetics counters.

☺ $$$ **Gentle Deep Cleanser** *($22 for 6 ounces)* is a standard, detergent-based water-soluble cleanser that is similar to the one above only without the vitamins.

☺ $$$ **Gentle Exfoliating Scrub** *($20 for 4 ounces)* is a standard, detergent-based water-soluble cleanser that uses ground-up plastic as the scrub agent. It would work well for most skin types.

☹ $$$ **Gentle Deep Revitalizing Scrub** *($22 for 4 ounces)* is a standard, detergent-based water-soluble cleanser that uses pumice as the scrub agent; it works, but this can be too rough on skin.

☺ $$$ **AHA Booster Complex** *($45 for 1 ounce).* Because the handful of exotic-sounding ingredients are at the very end of the ingredient list, it means they're almost nonexistent. However, this is a good (though absurdly overpriced) 4% AHA product. It would be good for someone with sensitive skin, but it is almost indistinguishable from Pond's Age Defying Cream for Sensitive Skin, which costs one-fourth as much.

☺ $$$ **Intensive Serum with AHAs** *($45 for 0.5 ounce)*. There is nothing intense about this product except the price. The plant extracts in here are not AHA ingredients and they cannot exfoliate the skin. This product also contains urea, which can be an exfoliant, but not in this teeny amount.

☺ $$$ **Advanced Continuous Lift** *($45 for 0.5 ounce)*. The plant extracts are a strange mix of irritants and anti-irritants, which is just a waste. Other than that, it is a good moisturizer for normal to dry skin. The vitamin K in here has no special effect on skin.

☹ **Advanced Continuous Moisture with SPF 8** *($37 for 2 ounces)* has a dismal SPF and no UVA-protecting ingredients of titanium dioxide, zinc oxide, or avobenzone, and is not recommended.

☺ $$$ **Advanced Eyesaver Gel** *($32 for 0.5 ounce)* is a good, lightweight moisturizer for normal to dry skin. The vitamin K in here has no special effect on skin, but at least this version only uses plant extracts known for their anti-irritant properties.

☹ **Advanced Gentle Enzyme Treatment** *($49 for 1 ounce)* shows the second ingredient as aluminum starch (octenylsuccinate), which isn't gentle—it's an absorbent that can be a skin irritant. The teeny amount of papain in here is not effective as an exfoliant.

☺ $$$ **Advanced Lipline Anti-Feathering Lip Treatment** *($22 for 0.5 ounce)* does have a matte finish but it is minimally effective at preventing lipstick from feathering.

☺ **Extra Nurturing Cream** *($40 for 2 ounces)* is a good moisturizer for dry skin.

☺ $$$ **Eye Relief** *($30 for 0.5 ounce)* is a light gel with a light feel. It isn't very emollient, but it does include good water-binding ingredients. It would be good for someone with normal to slightly dry skin. The label claims that it can prevent the formation of wrinkles, but there is absolutely nothing in here that is capable of that.

☹ **Oil-Control Hydrator with SPF 8** *($38 for 2 ounces)* has an SPF of 8, and with so many good SPF 15s around, why even think about this one, which also doesn't contain any UVA-protecting ingredients of avobenzone, zinc oxide, or titanium dioxide, and is not recommended.

☹ **Time Release Moisture with SPF 8** *($35 for 2 ounces)* has the same review as the one above.

☹ **Time Release Tinted Moisture** *($35 for 2 ounces)* has the same review as the one above.

☺ $$$ **Sun Block SPF 20** *($17 for 4 ounces)* is a part titanium dioxide–based sunscreen in a lightweight moisturizing base. It would be good for someone with normal to slightly dry skin.

☻ **Blemish Buster Mask** *($25 for 2 ounces)* contains cornstarch, which can cause breakouts, as the third ingredient, as well as several other ingredients that can clog pores. It also contains menthol and eucalyptus, which are unnecessary skin irritants. The sulfur in here can disinfect but it is extremely drying and irritating, too. There are more gentle ways to disinfect the skin.

☻ **Blemish Buster Solution** *($20 for 0.5 ounce)* is just alcohol, sulfur, and zinc. It can irritate the skin and, like many other much less expensive acne products with the same ingredients, it won't get rid of acne. Sulfur can be a disinfectant, but there are far gentler ones to try besides this, and the price is ludicrous.

☺ **$$$ Invisible Toning Masque** *($23 for 2 ounces)* is a moisturizing mask that won't tone anything. It closely resembles the Extra Nurturing Cream. It seems unnecessary, since so many of the other products contain the exact same ingredients.

☻ **Liptensive Lip Balm with SPF 15** *($10 for 0.16 ounce)* doesn't contain avobenzone, zinc oxide, or titanium dioxide for UVA protection, and is not recommended.

# Color Principal Makeup

**FOUNDATION:** ☻ **Cream Foundation SPF 15** *($29)* does not have UVA-protecting ingredients, though this cream-to-powder foundation does go on creamy and dries to a soft powder finish. There are four compacts of two shades each, with the idea being to mix the two shades (if need be) to exactly match your skin. Yet all of the four duos have a slight to strong peachy tint that is unflattering to most skin tones. Plus, having to mix the right portions of foundation every morning is not the most convenient method of applying makeup.

☺ **$$$ Time Release Tinted Moisture Plus SPF 15** *($27)* at least has a good UVA-protecting ingredient, but is otherwise a fairly emollient, tinted moisturizer whose colors leave much to be desired. Of the four shades, only Sheer Beige looks like skin. The others are incredibly peachy or rose, and although this is sheer, it's noticeable enough to matter.

☺ **CONCEALER:** **Perfect Concealer SPF 8** *($15)* has no UVA-protecting ingredients and the SPF 8 is inadequate for daylong protection, but for a creamy, smooth concealer with good coverage, with just minimal chance of creasing into lines, this one is an optoin.

☻ **POWDER:** **Pressed Powder SPF 8** *($20)* does not have UVA-protecting ingredients, and even if it did, getting SPF protection from a powder takes opaque coverage; a light dusting won't do it. This is a talc-free formula that has a silky, though fairly powdery application and a slight amount of shine with each of the four colors. If powdering to increase shine appeals to you, this will do nicely, but it's a real "why bother?" and doesn't begin to compare to Neutrogena's SPF 30 and Olay's SPF 15 pressed powders, available at almost half this price with UVA protection, a better color selection, and lots of other benefits this one leave outs. **Marbleized Bronzing Powder** *($17.95)* was described to me as being matte, yet lo and behold, when I opened the compacts it was all about shine. What a disappointment—the colors themselves are great for light to medium skin tones, but tan-looking skin isn't about shine.

☺ $$$ <u>BLUSH:</u> **Blush Duo** *($22)* comes in an attractive black case with two shades of blush, one matte and the other shiny. They have a silky-soft feel and go on even and smooth, but so do lots of other blushes for far less money and without the shine.

☺ $$$ <u>EYESHADOW:</u> **Eye Shadow Quad** *($29)* is a set of four eyeshadow shades that are coordinated nicely, are surprisingly matte, and have a soft, even application—but $29 for such tiny amounts! These aren't *that* nice.

☺ <u>EYE AND BROW SHAPER:</u> **Defining Eye Liner** *($10)* is just a standard, two-ended eye pencil with a smooth, slightly creamy finish. **Golden Shimmer Eyeliner** *($7.95)* is a creamy, twist-up pencil that colors your eye area a pale, shiny golden color that will accentuate any wrinkles or lines you may have.

☺ <u>LIPSTICK AND LIP PENCIL:</u> **Lipstick** *($15)* has a creamy, slightly glossy finish. These work as well as any. **Liptensive Lip Tint** *($15)* is similar to the lipstick above, only with less color. Its texture is creamy without being too glossy or greasy. **Defining Lip Liner** *($10)* is a standard, two-ended lip liner. The colors are fine and the application creamy but not greasy.

☺ $$$ <u>MASCARA:</u> **Double Duty Mascara** *($19)* is a very overpriced mascara. It does build a good deal of thickness and length, but it tends to clump, and the mascara tube gets incredibly gunky and gooey. The mascaras come in a two-ended format, with a black shade on one end and brown on the other. The other has black mascara at both ends! The two sides and different wand shapes don't improve the application.

## *ProActiv (Skin Care Only)*

ProActiv is a small group of products aimed at those with breakouts. It was created and endorsed by two dermatologists, Dr. Katie Rodan and Dr. Kathy Fields, who market these products via infomercial. Their promise of results is so overexaggerated that someone should take these doctors to task for their unmedical and unethical perspective. While I don't doubt these doctors' dermatologic expertise, the notion that these products are the be-all and end-all for acne is at best misleading and, coming from doctors, probably unethical. A percentage of people will get benefit from this routine, but it's definitely not for everyone, and any dermatologist knows this (just check out the American Academy of Dermatology Web site at www.aad.com, for example, on their recommendations for battling blemishes). It also goes without saying that less expensive versions of all the ProActiv products are available.

Some of the ProActiv products are very good but some of the formulations are lacking some essentials. Plus, many of the products contain fragrance, which is particularly problematic from a so-called dermatologic line. Finally, the prices are steep for what you get, unless of course you join their club. In order to get your first order at the discount price for $39.95 plus shipping, you need to agree to automatic shipments of the same four products for $39.95 plus shipping every two months. If you want to pick and choose which products work best for you, the price goes up considerably. My constant reminder to all of you trying to take good care of your skin is to pick and choose carefully. For more information, call (800) 950-4695 or visit the Web site at www.proactiv.com.

☺ $$$ **Renewing Cleanser** *($16 for 4 ounces)* contains 2.5% benzoyl peroxide. Though benzoyl peroxide is an effective disinfectant for breakouts, putting it in a cleanser doesn't make much sense. You risk getting the disinfectant in the eyes and the effectiveness is rinsed down the drain before it can work. To counter that issue, the directions suggest leaving the cleanser on for five minutes. Even assuming you have the time to do this, leaving the cleansing agent base on your skin for five minutes can be irritating to skin.

☺ $$$ **Revitalizing Toner** *($16 for 4 ounces)* is a potentially good AHA liquid. However, when it comes to most kinds of breakouts, current research indicates that BHA (salicylic acid) is the best way to exfoliate for breakout prevention, because it can work on the surface of skin as well as within the pore, while AHAs exfoliate primarily on the surface of skin. The witch hazel in here is in such a small amount it probably has no irritating effect on skin.

☺ $$$ **Oil Free Moisture with SPF 15** *($25 for 1.7 ounces)* is a good, in-part titanium dioxide–based sunscreen. This is pricey for such an exceptionally basic sunscreen. It does have a fairly matte finish, but the titanium dioxide can be a problem for someone with breakouts.

☺ **Repairing Lotion** *($22.95 for 2 ounces)* contains 2.5% benzoyl peroxide. This is a fine benzoyl peroxide product, but it doesn't repair anything in the skin; it only disinfects. There's nothing special or unique about this benzoyl peroxide lotion; you can find several products just like it in the acne section of your local drugstore.

☹ **Daily Oil Control** *($18 for 1.7 ounces)* contains mostly alcohol and a form of aluminum starch found in deodorants. There are better ways to deal with oil than this irritating combination.

☹ **Refining Mask** *($20 for 2.5 ounces)* is a standard clay mask that also contains at least 6% pure sulfur. Sulfur can be a good, mild antibacterial agent, but it is also a pretty good skin irritant. There are far better ways to disinfect skin than this.

☺ **Skin Lightening Lotion** *($22 for 1 ounce)* is a very good, 2% hydroquinone skin-lightening lotion. It also contains about 4% AHA and kojic acid, which can both have a beneficial impact on skin discolorations.

## *Profaces (Makeup Only)*

Profaces is primarily a small Web site makeup store. Unlike many companies, it is very willing to send samples of its products. And in terms of quality, its products are definitely up there with the best of them. The eyeshadows and blushes are silky-soft, with smooth, even coverage, and the shades are beautifully neutral and matte. You can customize the kits with the colors of your choice, but you have to choose from the representations on the screen. That isn't the most reliable way to duplicate color, but that is always the risk with mail-order products.

An overlapping of shades in the kits is a bit confusing. The "light to medium" kits have several colors that show up in the "medium to dark" kits, which is a strange overlap, but you can still pick and choose, so it isn't a big issue. The brushes are great but there are some you will want to avoid, especially in the brush kit. I didn't think the prices were as much of a bargain as Profaces says they are, but these are reliable color products worth looking at. For more information, call (888) 881-2001 or visit the Web site at www.profaces.com.

☺ $$$ **4 Color Compact Kit** *($39.95)* is a small compact makeup kit that contains three eyeshadows and one blush.

☺ $$$ **10 Color Light to Medium, Medium to Dark Kits** *($89.95 each)*. These two separate kits each contain ten colors supposedly suitable for light to medium or medium to dark skin types; the colors can be used interchangeably for eyes, brows, eyeliner, or blush.

☺ $$$ **12 Color Brush Kit** *($149.95)* contains 12 colors plus nine brushes. This kit cannot be customized.

☺ $$$ **12 Color Brush Kit plus 4 Color Compact Kit** *($169.95)* contains 12 colors plus nine brushes and the 4 Color Compact Kit described above. These kits cannot be customized.

☺ $$$ **5 Color Kit** *($119.95)* contains a combination of 15 colors that can be used for the eyes, brows, eyeliner, and blush.

☺ $$$ **Makeup Brushes in Leather Pouch** *($110)* contains eight brushes, of which six are quite usable. The blush brush, three eyeshadow brushes, lipstick brush, and eyeliner brush are excellent. However, the sponge brush is not practical, as it would easily break down with subsequent washings and is not as useful in comparison to a disposable makeup applicator sponge. The brow brush is a stiff, scratchy version that would hurt the skin. The leather brush pouch by itself is $25, so you could buy the case and then only the brushes you need.

Brushes are also sold individually and range in price between $6.50 and $20. Some are worth checking into, particularly the blush, contour, powder, and eyeshadow brushes, most of which are priced between $18 and $20. However the **Mini Brow Brush** *($7)* is stiff and scratchy, the **Smoothie Blender Brush** *($6)* and **Flocked Sponge Shadow Brush** *($4)* are just expensive sponge applicators, the **Metal Lash Comb** *($9.50)* and **Brow/Lash Groomer** *($6)* don't work as well as a toothbrush, and the **Deluxe Spooly Mascara Brush** *($6.50)* can be free if you simply wash out an old mascara wand from used-up mascara that you haven't thrown away yet.

## PropapH (Skin Care Only)

I remember this line of acne products from when I was a kid, and it hasn't changed since way back then. They are just as irritating and problematic for skin today as they were in the '70s! The company's phone number is (800) 645-4664 or you can visit the Web site at www.propaph.com.

☹ **Foaming Face Wash Acne Medication and Moisturizer** *($2.99 for 8 ounces)* is a detergent-based water-soluble cleanser, but this one contains menthol, which is too irritating, and salicylic acid, which is wasted in a cleanser. The fruit acids in here are not the same thing as alpha hydroxy acids and have no exfoliating benefits for skin.

☹ **Astringent and Cleanser Acne Medication and Moisturizer Maximum Strength** *($3.79 for 10 ounces)* contains salicylic acid, which would have made this a nice product if it didn't also contain menthol, peppermint, and alcohol. This is a burn for the skin, causing more problems than it could ever hope to help.

☹ **Astringent Cleanser Acne Medication and Moisturizer Maximum Strength** *($3.79 for 10 ounces)* is similar to the one above, and the same review applies.

☹ **Astringent Cleanser Acne Medication and Moisturizer Normal to Sensitive Skin** *($4.21 for 12 ounces)* is similar to the one above, and the same review applies.

☹ **Overnight Pore Clarifier Acne Treatment and Moisturizer** *($3.79 for 2 ounces)* doesn't contain unnecessary irritants, but the pH of this part–salicylic acid, part–AHA based product (and it's not a great mix of these, I should mention), isn't low enough for it to be an effective exfoliant.

☹ **Peel-Off Acne Mask Acne Treatment and Moisturizer** *($4.21 for 2.66 ounces)* is similar to the one above only in mask form, and it contains alcohol.

## Purpose (Skin Care Only)

The Purpose line of skin-care products is owned by Johnson & Johnson, a company that, prior to 1987, was better known for baby care and Band-Aids than for skin care products. That has changed. These days Johnson & Johnson has become well known for its controversial foray into the world of serious wrinkle treatment with Retin-A and Renova. Leaving no stone unturned, Johnson & Johnson made great strides convincing physicians that a prescription for Retin-A and Renova should be accompanied by the Purpose line of products. That marketing campaign was heeded, and now J&J has added the Neutrogena, RoC, and Clean & Clear lines. Your face could easily live without most of the Purpose products, although the Dual Purpose Sunscreen is a consideration for daily sun protection. For more information about Purpose products, call (800) 526-3967 or visit the Web site at www.jnj.com.

☹ **Gentle Cleansing Bar** *($3.17 for 6 ounces)* is just a standard bar cleanser that contains tallow and a strong detergent cleansing agent with a little glycerin added, but that won't counteract the drying effect of the soap. Also, the tallow can cause breakouts.

☺ **Gentle Cleansing Wash** *($4.95 for 6 ounces)* is a standard but good detergent-based water-soluble cleanser. It is an option for someone with oily skin.

☹ **Alpha Hydroxy Moisture Lotion with SPF 15** *($10.05 for 4 ounces)* and **Alpha Hydroxy Moisture Cream with SPF 15** *($9.84 for 2 ounces)* contain about 8% glycolic acid in a pH of about 3 to 4. That makes them decent AHA products for someone with normal to dry skin. Now if only the SPF contained avobenzone, titanium dioxide, or zinc oxide for UVA protection, you would have a decent two-in-one AHA with a reliable SPF. Alas, it doesn't, so although this one comes close, it's still miles away from the real thing.

☺ **Dry Skin Cream** *($5.61 for 3 ounces)* is a very standard but good moisturizer for someone with dry skin.

☺ **Dual Treatment Moisturizer with SPF 15 Protection** *($7.89 for 4 ounces)* is a good in-part titanium dioxide–based sunscreen in a rather mediocre moisturizing base that would be an option for someone with normal to slightly dry skin.

# R Pro (Makeup Only)

R Pro began as a small line of makeup products distributed by Revlon to beauty-supply stores that are open to the public. The line is currently undergoing some changes that may make it a chore to track down the products you're interested in or the stores that carry them. I was told by Revlon's consumer relations department that R Pro had been sold to a company called Colomer USA. Apparently, Colomer USA is in the process of reconfiguring the product lineup and distribution of R Pro makeup, but trying to learn out anything more specific than that was impossible. Sadly, what were once the line's strong points (blushes and eyeshadow singles) are very hard to find. Revlon claims nothing has been discontinued, but it sure feels that way when you're out searching for it. There are still some products worth checking out and the prices are attractive, but they are not worth going on a wild goose chase for when you can easily locate comparable products at your neighborhood drugstore. For more

The Reviews R

information about R Pro, call Colomer USA at (800) 933-4303. (The products reviewed below were consistent with R Pro's current brochure.)

☺ <u>POWDER:</u> **Pressed Powder** *($7.99)* and **Loose Powder** *($8.99)* are both talc-based and come in an attractive range of colors that have a smooth, soft finish. The way these are packaged makes it hard to see the color, and most stores do not offer testers, so it becomes a guessing game to find your best color.

☻ <u>EYESHADOW:</u> **Eyeshadow Trio** *($5.99)* is a well coordinated group of mostly neutral colors, but almost all of them are shiny (look closely), and the application isn't nearly as smooth and even as the not-discontinued-but-nonexistent Eyeshadow Singles. By the way, the R Pro brochure says to always apply eyeshadows *after* mascara, and that must be a misprint because it is a bad idea. Applying shadow after mascara poses a problem when excess shadow falls onto the (mascaraed) lashes, not to mention the risk of smudging or flaking off mascara while applying the eye design.

☺ <u>EYE AND BROW SHAPER:</u> **Eye Pencil** *($4.99)* and **Brow Pencil** *($3.99)* are very standard but good pencils available in good colors. It would be better if these were twist-ups, but they're fine as far as pencils go. **Liquid Eyeliner** *($4.99)* is about as standard as they come. This has a pen-tip applicator that works well to create a solid, dramatic line.

☺ <u>LIPSTICK AND LIP PENCIL:</u> R Pro's lipsticks are available in three types, but the Mattes are next to impossible to track down. What you'll find in most stores are the **Frosts** *($4.99)* and **Cremes** *($4.99)*. The Frosts are just that: iridescent lipsticks that go on sheer. The Cremes have a good, creamy-opaque texture and smooth application. **Lip Pencil** *($4.99)* is very standard but has an agreeable price and a pleasing range of colors. If they were twist-ups, I'd suggest stocking up!

☻ <u>MASCARA:</u> R Pro's **Mascara** *($5.99)* isn't terrible, just unimpressive—plus it tends to clump and takes forever to build any length or definition. Wait, maybe it *is* terrible.

☺ <u>BRUSHES:</u> Brushes are a strong point for this modestly appointed line. There are some great, affordable options here, from the **Blush Brush** *($8.99)* to a clever **Retractable Blush Brush** *($8.99)* and **Eyeshadow Brushes** *($4.99 to $5.99)*. The only ones to be cautious of are the **Face Brush** *($8.99)*, which is just huge and hard to adjust and control for different areas of the face, and the **Lipstick Brush** *($6.99)*, which has a cumbersome, too-long handle, though there are scarcely any of these to be found, as far locating one goes.

# Rachel Perry (Skin Care Only)

Health food stores have been selling Rachel Perry products for years. This is one of the original "natural" cosmetics lines, and it is now also available at some large drugstore chains. Rachel Perry products contain many, if not more, of the same natural-sounding ingredients included in more highbrow natural-product lines such as Aveda, Clarins, and Origins. For the consumer on a budget who is interested in the ballyhoo surrounding botanical skin-care products, this line could satisfy that curiosity without hurting the pocketbook. But watch out for your skin, because there are skin irritants and allergens lurking everywhere in these products, plus with ingredients like myristyl myristate, TEA cocoyl glutamate, and butylene glycol, there are lots and lots of unnatural ingredients in these products; actually they are mostly synthetically derived. For more information about Rachel Perry products, call (800) 966-8888 or visit the Web site at www.rachelperry.net.

☹ **Citrus-Aloe Cleanser and Face Wash, for Normal to Dry Skin** *($10.50 for 4 ounces).* The oils make this more of a wipe-off product than a face wash. It can leave a greasy residue on the skin. The reason for the rating is that several of the plant extracts in here, including arnica, sage, and clary, are potent skin irritants.

☹ **Tangerine Dream Foaming Facial Cleanser with Alpha-Hydroxy Acids for All Skin Types** *($10.50 for 6 ounces)* is a standard, detergent-based water-soluble cleanser that contains about 3% AHAs. At only 3%, they wouldn't be effective as an exfoliant anyway, but even if they were, AHAs are wasted in a cleanser, because their effectiveness is rinsed down the drain. Plus, several of the plant extracts and the menthol in here can be skin irritants.

☹ **Peach & Papaya Gentle Facial Scrub** *($10.50 for 2 ounces)* contains menthol, lemon peel, balm mint, and several other potentially irritating ingredients. Even papaya does nothing for the skin except cause irritation. Ouch!

☺ **$$$ Sea Kelp-Herbal Facial Scrub** *($10.50 for 2.5 ounces)* is a pretty thick mess to use as a scrub. It would be cheaper and better for the skin to use plain cornmeal, sea salt, or almond meal, without any of the fragrance or irritating plant extracts this product contains.

☹ **Lemon Mint Astringent, for Normal to Oily Skin** *($9.50 for 8 ounces)* has more than its share of irritating ingredients, including mint, lemongrass, peppermint, and witch hazel.

☹ **Perfectly Clear Herbal Antiseptic, for Oily or Acne Prone Skin** *($10.50 for 8 ounces)* is mostly alcohol, but contains a host of even more irritating ingredients, including camphor, eucalyptus oil, menthol, peppermint oil, and clove oil. This product is a skin rash waiting to happen.

☺ **Violet Rose Skin Toner** *($9.50 for 8 ounces).* Several of the plant extracts in here, including arnica, yarrow, and juniper, are skin irritants.

☺ **Visible Transition 10% Alpha-Hydroxy Serum** *($27.50 for 1.1 ounces)* has a good concentration of AHAs, but the pH is too high for it to be effective as an exfoliant.

☺ **Bee Pollen-Jojoba Maximum Moisture Cream** (*$12.50 for 2 ounces*). This rather basic moisturizer contains several potentially irritating plant extracts, including arnica and juniper.

☺ **Calendula-Cucumber Oil Free Moisturizer** (*$13.50 for 4 ounces*) might be oil-free, but this basic moisturizing formula is still better for normal to slightly dry skin than for someone with oily skin. The product does list information about sun protection but it doesn't indicate an SPF or the active ingredients and can't be relied on for that claim.

☺ **Elastin and Collagen Firming Treatment** (*$14.50 for 2 ounces*). The collagen and elastin won't firm anything, but the witch hazel can cause irritation, as can several of the other plant extracts including ivy, yarrow, ginseng, and horsetail.

☺ **Ginseng and Collagen Wrinkle Treatment** (*$14.50 for 2 ounces*). The vitamins are way down on the list, but they can provide some antioxidant benefit. This would be a good moisturizer for dry skin, but several of the plant extracts in here can be skin irritants, including arnica and ginseng.

☺ **Hi Potency "E" Special Treatment Line Control** (*$14.50 for 2 ounces*). Vitamins are good antioxidants, and this one has a lot of them, though no one knows how much of them it takes one way or the other. This stuff also won't control lines, but it is a very good moisturizer for dry skin. Be aware that vitamin E can be an allergen for many people.

☺ **$$$ Immediately Visible Eye Renewal Gel-Cream with Liposomes** (*$22.50 for 0.5 ounce*). Bee pollen can be a good antioxidant but it can also be an allergen, while algae is a good antioxidant and anti-irritant but won't change a wrinkle on your face.

☹ **Lecithin-Aloe Moisture Retention Cream for Normal-Combination Skin** (*$12.50 for 2 ounces*) includes enough oil so that it isn't good for combination skin, and the amount of sunscreen is minimal and doesn't provide UVA protection. It also contains arnica and balm mint, which are both skin irritants.

☺ **$$$ Clay and Ginseng Texturizing Mask** (*$10.50 for 2 ounces*) is a standard clay mask, and several of the plant extracts may be too irritating, particularly combined with the drying effect of the clay. The RNA won't affect your skin cells, but it sounds impressive.

☺ **Lip Lover** (*$2.53 for 0.2 ounce*) is a good, emollient, and even tasty group of lip balms in a host of flavors.

## Ré Vive (Skin Care Only)

There is no doubt that the founder of Ré Vive, Dr. Greg Brown, has some impressive credentials. According to his curriculum vitae, he is a board-certified general and plastic surgeon who trained at Vanderbilt, Harvard, and Emory Universities, and received his medical degree from the University of Louisville. Given this estimable medical background and the products he is marketing, he can join the ranks of Dr. Howard Murad (of Murad infomercial fame), Dr. Sheldon Pinnell (of Cellex-C and SkinCeuticals), and Dr. N. V. Perricone (with products bearing his name) as a physician-turned-skin-care-salesperson. Now there is one more doctor telling you his research is the way to go for the fountain of youth, and it will cost you a pretty penny (lots of pretty pennies) if you decide this one's got the answer.

Brown says that the answer to "rejuvenated, young-looking skin is bioengineered products." The Web site for Ré Vive products states that in Brown's "experiments using human Epidermal Growing [sic] Factor (EGF) to stimulate wounds to heal faster …'I saw evidence of absolute [healing] acceleration the first day and I became impassioned.' " Wow, sounds great. These products must be flying out of Neiman Marcus, where they're being sold, but that's only because these are cosmetics, and cosmetics companies don't have to tell you the rest of the story.

Dr. Bruce A. Mast, M.D., Division of Plastic and Reconstructive Surgery, Department of Surgery, at the University of Florida, Gainesville, in his class on wound healing, has stated that "Brown's research, done at the University of Louisville back in 1989 (published in the *New England Journal of Medicine* at that time), did show Epidermal Growth Factor (EGF) to have a positive effect on wound healing, however, a study from the University of West Virginia by Dr. I. Kellman Cohen, et al., showed no positive effect on wound healing with EGF." Mast went on to say, "As a result of the contradictory information the research on EGF for wound healing has gone by the wayside and the primary research for wound healing is looking at TGF-A, TGF-B, and PDGF."

Note: EGF promotes proliferation of epithelial (skin) cells; TGF-A (Transforming Growth Factor–Alpha) may be important for normal wound healing, TGF-B (Transforming Growth Factor–Beta) promotes the growth of fibroblasts (collagen), and PDGF (Platelet Derived Growth Factor) promotes the growth of blood clotting factor. The more well-known HGFs for skin are EGF, TGF-A, and TGF-B (there are at least 100 different family members for TGF-B growth factor).

It is important to make clear that the topic of HGF is exceedingly complicated. The physiological intricacies of HGFs defy a layperson's comprehension. Nonetheless, because the use of HGF seems to be a direction some skin-care companies are taking (including Ré Vive, Jan Marini, Osmotics, and Kinerase—Kinerase uses plant growth factors), and because there is a large body of research showing its efficacy for wound healing (but not for wrinkles), it does deserve more comment. Grasping the full depth of this issue, however, is not within the scope of my work.

So what is Epidermal Growth Factor (EGF) anyway ? It's a cytokine. I know, what's a cytokine? A cytokine is any substance released by a cell or cells that causes some action to take place on another cell or cells. EGF is part of a much larger group of cytokines known as Human Growth Factors (HGFs). HGFs are proteins (proteins are the primary components of all living cells and include many substances, such as enzymes, hormones, and antibodies, that are necessary for all life functions). These HGF proteins bind to receptor sites on the cell surface (receptor sites are the way cells communicate with any substance to know what or what not to do). HGFs need to communicate with cells to instruct them to activate the production of new cells or to tell a cell to create new cells that have different functions. Many HGFs are quite versatile, with the ability to stimulate cellular division in numerous different cell types, while other HGFs are specific to a particular cell type, say blood cells or bone cells.

The main problem for HGFs when they are taken internally, as in certain cancer treatments (Interleukin and Interferon are cytokines), is that they can be highly mitogenic (causing cell division) and at certain concentrations and lengths of application can cause cells to overproliferate and cause problems, one result of which is cancer.

But what about the effect on skin? What happens when you put EGFs on skin? According to Dr. Mast, "the biggest reason not to use these [EGFs] is that they could accelerate the growth of skin cancer by stimulating the overproduction of skin cells." And the reason not to use TGF-B, the ingredient used in the products in Jan Marini's line, Mast says, is because "TGF-B primarily stimulates fibroblasts [collagen], which can encourage scarring. Scars are excessive collagen; if you make too much collagen you get a scar or a knot on the skin."

All of the research on the issue of HGFs for skin has primarily looked at the issue of wound healing. But Ré Vive and other product lines purporting to use these substances aren't just talking about wound healing and short-term use, they're talking about wrinkles and ongoing use. Ré Vive wants you to believe that EGF "stimulates skin cells to revert to their adolescent renewal pattern." Now if that isn't the fountain of youth I don't know what is. Despite this outlandish statement, there are no studies showing this to be even remotely possible. According to Mast (and many other physicians I've interviewed), "Wound healing is unrelated to wrinkles, and the growth hormones have no effect on making skin act young."

There is one other body of research concerning the HGFs that are being touted as being the answer for wrinkles. Here is what the research shows. Based on established scientific protocol, you can create "living" skin cells in a petri dish. It is known that normal human skin cells divide a predictable number of times and then die. Skin cells grow and divide rapidly early on, then the division rate slows as we age. Finally the cells cease replicating. In vitro (a glass dish), you can re-create the skin cell's life process and accelerate the effect, so you can watch the growth process of cells in a short period of time (weeks, as opposed to a normal person's life span). If you leave these skin cells alone they go through a normal life span and eventually stop replicating. However, when you add some forms of growth factors (GFs), the skin cells live far longer than they would on their own. While that sounds like your skin would stay young forever, the other part of the picture is that if you add too much GF the skin cells die off sooner than they would if you hadn't added any. This part of the information is often left out of the impressive data companies like to publicize in regard to their products.

The research into HGFs and GFs is without question intriguing, but the risk to skin is just too great if these products really do work. However, what I suspect to be true is that these products can't even remotely do what they claim, despite the inclusion of the EGF or TGF-B on the ingredient labels. These are almost without question not active forms of these "drugs," because if they did work the risk to skin would be scary.

Incidentally, aside from all the purported, astonishing benefit realized from Dr. Brown's research so many years ago, it is clear that he ignored other research about sun damage and sun protection. His only SPF product doesn't include UVA-protecting ingredients.

For more information about Ré Vive, call (800) 937-9146 or visit the Web site at www.revivecosmetics.com.

☺ $$$ **Eye Renewal Cream** *($85 for 0.5 ounce)* is a decent, but ordinary moisturizer, aside from the EGF, of course.

☺ $$$ **Lip and Perioral Renewal Cream** *($105 for 0.5 ounce)*. Other than being a nice, silky-soft moisturizer (due to the high content of silicone), the decision about EGF is up to you.

☺ $$$ **Renewal Cream** *($120 for 2 ounces)* contains about 4% to 5% AHA (glycolic acid) and the pH is around 4. That makes it a good AHA exfoliant in a very good moisturizing base. If you're spending this kind of money on a rather average AHA product, it's because of marketing, not skin knowledge.

☹ **Fermitif Neck Renewal Cream SPF 15** *($105 for 2.5)* does not contain UVA-protecting ingredients and is not recommended.

☹ **Sensitif Cellular Repair Cream SPF 15** *($165 for 2 ounces)* does not contain UVA-protecting ingredients and is not recommended.

# reflect.com

Procter & Gamble's reflect.com Web site has a mind-boggling goal, or at least on the surface it's mind-boggling. After you fill out a questionnaire, with questions like "My personality is best represented by…"; "If I were a house I would be…"; "I am most likely to dream about…"; "I like to wear…"; and "My life can best be described as…," you then end up getting a Web page aimed at your preferences. Depending on how you answer, you may get a vivacious, funky home; a bubbly teen-oriented site; or a subdued forty-something site filled with flowers.

From there, you answer more questions about your skin type and then end up creating your own specially formulated products allegedly created specifically for your skin's individual needs. According to Procter & Gamble, the reflect.com line offers over 50,000 possible formula and packaging combinations. To say I was skeptical would be an understatement. First, you can't legally formulate a "special sunscreen," for example; each time a woman decides to add or leave something out, and ship it out in a week (the company's claim regarding their quick delivery time). According to the FDA, if you change even a fragrance or a level of one ingredient you must go through all the stability testing required by the FDA for sunscreens, and the same would be true for any product containing an active ingredient.

It turns out that you really aren't creating your own products, despite the fact that you have to answer dozens (and I mean dozens) of questions before you can even see what kind of products this site has to offer. In reality the options for skin care didn't change one iota regardless of what I punched in about my skin and lifestyle (though the colors and graphics on the Web pages changed—nice but not helpful in the least for my skin!—and there were products still yet to be launched, particularly products for breakouts). What you are really creating is your choice of packaging wrapper (not the style of bottle), that is, just the color of the package. Plus, you can also identify the fragrance you want. And what you absolutely *can't* do is opt for no fragrance. So much for creating your own products. Out of 50,000 options and all the song and dance about formulated specially for me, and I can't choose a fragrance-free version?

The makeup part of the site is even more frustrating than the skin care. It's not that the product formulations are bad—there are some good options for lipstick, blush, and eyeshadows, though the loose powder's fragrance can knock you over—but the endless questions and processing of information is exhausting. Just show me what you've got and let me buy a product! Here's the strangest aspect: after providing the required information I was given a final choice of only two colors for the foundation, pressed powder, and concealer—one shade being light and the other rather dark. That's an option? The lipstick selection was even more frustrating, because I couldn't tell what decision the site had made for me. Was I getting a frosted or matte shade? Was it creamy, glossy, or sheer? The lipstick options for each of the lipstick types were so vague as to almost seem, well, sneaky. Why couldn't they just be direct about everything, like let me see the products, tell me how they perform, and leave it at that? But no, not reflect.com. And every time I wanted to view a different product or see alternative selections I had to answer another series of questions. What is so complicated about lip liner that you need to answer five questions? Even more exasperating was that no matter how I answered the questions, I still got the same lip liner. Was reflect.com really thinking no one would notice that there is absolutely nothing being created just for you in any way, shape, or form?

So what do you get at the end of this experience? Not surprisingly, these products seemed virtually identical to many of those by Olay, another company owned by Procter & Gamble. The sunscreens, cleansers, and moisturizers are all available for less money at the drugstore, so the only benefit of getting them on the Web site is the fun of filling out forms, if you call that fun. The makeup has some strong points, but the shopping experience is not worth the effort. For more information, call (800) 243-2288 or visit the Web site at www.reflect.com.

(Note: As this book goes to press I had received samples of the eyeshadows—great matte shades with a soft, sheer application—and blush—silky smooth with a sheen that is less obvious than most when applied—but these were not yet available on the site.)

## reflect.com Skin Care

☺ **Facial Cleanser, Creamy Lotion Cleanser** *($17 for 6.7 ounces)* is a standard wipe-off cleanser that can work well for dry skin. It is quite similar to Neutrogena's Extra Gentle Skin Cleanser that's available at half the price.

☺ **Facial Cleanser, Foaming Cleanser** *($17 for 6.7 ounces)* is a standard, detergent-based water-soluble cleanser that would work well for most skin types.

☺ **Facial Cleansing Cloths** *($18.50 for 30 cloths)* are gentle cloths covered with detergent cleansing agents, and they work well to wipe off makeup. While this is not the way I would encourage women to remove makeup, it is an option, but for the money and what you get with these, you could be using fragrance-free baby wipes that are even more gentle for skin.

☹ **Facial Cleanser with 2% Salicylic Acid** *($17 for 6.7 ounces)* contains 2% salicylic acid, which can be a problem if it gets in the eyes, though the pH of this cleanser is too high to make it effective for exfoliation. The cleansing agent for this one is sodium lauryl sulfate, and it also contains menthol, which makes it potentially too irritating for all skin types.

☺ **Facial Scrub** *($16.50 for 5 ounces)* is a standard, detergent-based water-soluble cleanser with synthetic scrub particles that would work well for most skin types, but mostly normal to oily.

☺ **Facial Moisturizer UV Facial Cream SPF 15** *($25 for 1.7 ounces)* is a good, part zinc oxide–based moisturizer for normal to dry skin. The moisturizing ingredients are fairly ordinary. Olay has a virtually identical version at the drugstore for half the price.

☺ **Facial Moisturizer UV Facial Lotion SPF 15** *($19.50 for 6.7 ounces)* is almost identical to the Cream version above, only you get more of this and for less money. Go figure.

☹ **Facial Moisturizer Lotion** *($19.50 for 6.7 ounces)* is a very ordinary moisturizer that would be minimally OK for normal to slightly dry skin. There are far more state-of-the-art and elegant formulations available for far less at the drugstore.

☹ **Facial Moisturizer Facial Cream** *($25 for 1.7 ounces)*. The pH of this product is too low for it to be effective as an exfoliant, and the moisturizing part is so ordinary as to be almost embarrassing. There is very little reason to see this as an option for any skin type, as there are far better choices from Neutrogena, Lubriderm, or Eucerin to consider in place of this do-nothing, overpriced concoction.

☺ **Facial Moisturizer for Combination or Blemish Prone Skin** *($29.50 for 1 ounce)*. Niacinamide is vitamin B3. There are a handful of studies demonstrating that when a 4% concentration of niacinamide is applied topically in gel form, it can have similar effects as a topical antibiotic; however, this research is primarily from the company that makes this product (Papulex, 4% Niacinamide), and it can still cause dryness and inflammation. This is an option as an experiment to see how it affects your skin.

☹ **$$$ Facial Treatment Eye Gel** *($28 for 0.5 ounce)*. Witch hazel contains alcohol, and that can be drying, while cucumber extract is not the best for eyes any more than applying cucumber slices would be. If you have any lines or dry skin around your eyes, this would not improve things.

☺ **$$$ Facial Mask for Combination Skin** *($24 for 5 ounces)* is a standard clay mask that contains mostly clay and fragrance. It would work as well as any.

# *reflect.com Makeup*

**FOUNDATION:** ☹ **$$$ Liquid Refine Foundation** *($29.50)* has a very smooth, sheer-to-light coverage application, with a soft matte finish. The color selection is tricky, because you are only given two rather disparate options (your suggested shade and then another shade that appears to be very dark), but reflect.com is great about sending out samples if you ask. For some people, getting a foundation with your name on it may be worth the money and the trouble of navigating this site, though for the cost there are far better foundations for less at the cosmetics counters ranging from Clinique to Club Monaco, not to mention the great options at the drugstore, especially from Olay's line of makeup products. **Cream-to-Powder Foundation** *($16.50)* is labeled as being a liquid-to-powder finish, but this is a creamy application with a powder finish. It works well and has a smooth, even application, but the color choices I have seen are fairly peachy pink. The limitation of color selection is the same for all the products—you don't get to see a range of colors, you just see the computer's recommendation for you.

**CONCEALER:** ☹ **Concealer Stick** *($14)* is a traditional, lipstick-style concealer that creases into the lines around the eyes and can look rather cakey. Of the three shades I've seen, all were too peach or pink for most skin tones. **Concealer Cream** *($14)* comes in a squeeze container but has the same texture and problems as the stick version.

☺ $$$ **POWDER: Pressed Powder** *($16.50)* is a standard, talc-based pressed powder with a smooth application and soft texture. There appear to be only a handful of colors, but navigating the site is confusing and it's hard to tell how many colors there really are. But steer away from the notion that pink is ever a category to click or you will end up with a very unnatural-looking product. **Loose Powder** *($16.50)* is highly fragranced (it can be overwhelming), but the feel of this standard talc powder is silky-smooth. The color choice is hard to determine because the site doesn't show a range of colors. However, watch out for the pink shades: they are exceptionally peachy pink and do not look like real skin.

☺ **LIPSTICK AND LIP LINER: Lipstick** *($12)* has a wonderful creamy, slightly glossy finish and a seemingly endless parade of colors. **Long Lasting Lipstick** *($12)* goes on almost wet and dries to a solid matte finish. This ultra-matte formula is a good option for non-transfer-resistant lipstick, because it doesn't budge once it has dried in place and it doesn't chip or flake either. A definite plus! **Lip Liner** *($12)* is a standard lip liner that needs sharpening. It has a nice, slightly creamy feel.

## Rejuveness (Skin Care Only)

You may have noticed ads in fashion magazines for a product called Rejuveness, claiming that it can magically heal scars. ☺ **Rejuveness** *($39.50 to $295, depending on the size ordered)*, and other products like it, are nothing more than pliable sheets of silicone, quite similar to the silicone used in so many skin- and hair-care products because of its texture and water-binding properties. It is not clear how these sheets of silicone work. They may increase the amount of water in the scar, and continuous rehydration of scars may soften the tissue, making it more elastic and pliable, thus encouraging natural skin-cell production and the flattening process. But work they do, and rather successfully (although I use the word "successfully" with caution).

Silicone sheets appear to be most effective for hypertrophic or keloidal scarring. As wonderful as this sounds, and as close to wonderful as it is, there are disadvantages. Users purchase one relatively inexpensive sheet of silicone that is worn over and over again. You have to wear these sheets of silicone over the scar for prolonged periods of time, which means that you might not want to wear one on your face or other exposed parts of your body, at least not during the day. You need to keep the sheet clean, too, which requires some amount of care and maintenance time. Also, the silicone sheet can stick to the skin (wearing camisoles or T-shirts can help), and skin reactions such as rashes or irritation can occur.

What's even more difficult and uncomfortable is that you have to wear the covering for long periods—for hours at a time, over a span of at least two to nine months—in order to see a difference. But patience pays off: the longer you wear it, the more likely it is that the scar will dissipate to some extent. Of course, these sheets work best over new scars, but they also can make a difference with old ones. Even acne scarring—thick, raised scars, not pits—can be reduced if the scars have been around for less than 16 years. As wonderful and hopeful as this all sounds, be aware that the word "reduce" can be a suspect term. Do not give these a try if you are hoping for extraordinary results, of the kind the advertising implies. Dr. Loren Engrav, associate director and chief of plastic surgery for the University of Washington burn unit at Harborview Medical Center, Seattle, explains that the "silicone strips are standard treatment for helping dissipate scars, and though the results may be good, they are absolutely not a miracle."

Some women buy the sheets to use over stretch marks, but there is no clinical evidence that this product will have any effect on them whatsoever, and the Rejuveness company will not guarantee its product for this use. These sheets use a flattening process, not a raising process, which would be required for stretch marks. For raised scars this isn't for everyone, but if you are willing to be persistent, it is absolutely worth a try. For more information, call (800) 588-7455 or visit the Web site at www.rejuveness.com.

## *Rejuvenique*

Some of you have told me that on occasion my reviews can sound unnecessarily crass or insolent. Believe it or not, I actually tone down my more brutal comments in the reviews you finally read, but you should hear me in my office! That's when I let loose with my real feelings of utter frustration and abject disillusionment. I aspire to be less jarred by the idiotic claims and poor skin-care and makeup products being sold to women, but I'm not very successful at it. The cosmetics industry can be so offensive to me that there are times I literally scream! This is definitely one of those times.

The Rejuvenique products deserve no less than a trouncing. Linda Evans is the spokesperson for Rejuvenique and she should be ashamed to represent such nonsense. Her surgically altered visage beaming on the box and brochures for these products, in nicely retouched pictures, is there as part of a tried-and-true campaign to convince a naive, trusting consumer that this beautiful face is a result of the products being sold. It isn't.

What is Rejuvenique? It is a set of skin-care products packaged with a face machine costing $200 that's sold at Target and via infomercial. The skin-care products are ordinary enough, although they carry the same amazing claims as every other skin-care product being sold. What makes this nonsense more bizarre is the Rejuvenique Mask. This Halloween-looking blue mask is worn as you would wear any mask, only this one has electric pulsations being sent through 261 metal contact points that press against the skin. And, you guessed it, these electrical pulses are meant to achieve "a smooth, toned, radiant look without undergoing time consuming procedures, harsh chemicals or other expensive invasive measures." Is there any research anywhere showing that this kind of electrical stimulation changes one wrinkle? I couldn't find a trace of it, and it turns out that even the company doesn't believe this works, but I'll get to that in a second. Does Linda Evans look as wrinkle-free as she does because of this machine? No way! It isn't remotely possible. But what I found most shocking about all this is that there is no warning about the risk of electrical impulses stimulating circulation and increasing the risk of triggering surfaced broken capillaries!

The only reason skin may look smoother from this mask is because of the irritation the electrical shocks cause, producing temporary swelling, which is why the recommendation is to use the machine three to four days a week, twice a day for 15 minutes. Once the swelling goes down the face won't look different. There is an interesting disclaimer in the booklet that comes with the Rejuvenique products and mask. It says, "It is not intended [for] any permanent physical changes." Well, at least that's honest—but that information wasn't easy to find, and every other claim made here sounds different from that one small hidden statement. For more information on Rejuvenique, the numbers are (800) 543-5427 or (800) 934-7455, or visit the Web site at www.facetone.com. However, I don't recommend that you call or even think about surfing in that direction.

☺ **Facial Toning System** (*$199; includes Rejuvenique Mask, Purifying Cleanser (4 ounces), Vitamin C Serum (1 ounce), Eye Toner (1 ounce), and Facial Moisturizer (2 ounces).*

☺ **$$$ Purifying Cleanser** (*$18.50 for 4 ounces*) is a very standard, very overpriced detergent-based water-soluble cleanser that would work well enough.

☺ **Vitamin C Serum** (*$50 for 1 ounce*) contains water and ascorbic acid. If you are interested in trying a vitamin C product, for the money, this is one of the worst! Ascorbic acid is considered irritating and unstable, though if that is what you are looking for, try Avon's version for less than half the price.

☺ **Eye Toner** (*$22 for 1 ounce*) is an OK moisturizer for normal to slightly dry skin, and this amount of film former can make things look "tighter," but it won't work well under makeup.

☺ **Facial Moisturizer** (*$24 for 2 ounces*) is a good basic moisturizer for normal to dry skin.

☺ **Enriched Toning Gel** *($5 for 4 ounces)* is a "a conductive gel" meant to help the electrical shock of the mask be transmitted to your skin. The gel is just the same "gel-like" thickening agent used in all clear products of this nature, sort of like what they use to administer an EKG.

# *Remede*

Remede is a skin-care line I've received a lot of questions about. I suspect many have learned about it through small feature editorials in fashion magazines. It is also available through Bliss Spa, the New York–based mecca for skin care and overall head-to-toe pampering. Remede is sold as a line with "patented technology delivering more of what your skin needs—vitamins, botanicals, hydration and oxygen—for daily reparative rejuvenation." If there is something patented in these formulations, it is beyond me what it could be. These are some of the most ordinary, standard formulations I've ever seen (not to mention there are no sunscreens). And the prices?! If you're wondering whether or not any of these products are worth the flagrantly out-of-line price tag the answer, in one word, is NO. There are a number of things about most of these products that are too irritating, distorted, and preposterous for words, so I'll just jump to the reviews and let that be explanation enough. For more information, call (888) 873-6333 or visit the Web site at www.blissout.com.

☹ $$$ **Milky Wash** *($28 for 6.8 ounces)* is a very standard detergent cleanser that contains mostly thickeners, sodium lauryl sulfate (yes, that's the irritating one), honey, milk, and preservatives. The honey and milk are useless for skin, and I suspect there isn't that much SLS in here to be a problem for skin. What is all too clear is that this is a poor but pricey imitation of Cetaphil.

☺ $$$ **Rinseable Cold Cream Deep Cleanser for All Skin Types** *($32 for 6.8 ounces)* at least has an accurate description—this cleanser is just an incredibly overpriced cold cream that contains water, mineral oil, Vaseline, and a host of thickeners, and there is nothing rinseable about it. Why anyone would use this over Pond's Cold Cream is a puzzle; maybe they simply didn't notice the price tag and believed the absurd hype on the label about how this product can dissolve blackheads. The thickeners and grease in here would make anyone with oily skin cringe.

☹ $$$ **Dissolve** *($22 for 3.4 ounces)* may be a pretty color, but it is just slippery cold cream. Using pure mineral oil or safflower oil would not only be cheaper, it would give you almost exactly the same thing, minus only the fragrance and coloring agents.

☺ $$$ **Sweep** *($36 for 2.7 ounces)*. Marble may be great on counters and floors, but ground up in a skin-care product, it is not in the least an improvement over baking soda and Cetaphil Gentle Skin Cleanser.

☹ $$$ **Spot Detox Clarifying Treatment for Problem Skin** *($49 for 1 ounce)* is supposed to "eliminate blemishes and the dreaded dark spots they leave behind." This product can't do either. The pH of this product is not low enough for the AHA or BHA to be effective for exfoliation, plus the cornstarch in here can clog pores. Tea tree oil can be a disinfectant but it is not as effective as benzoyl peroxide, and is definitely not effective in the teeny amount found in this product. Kojic acid can inhibit melanin production, but that is unrelated to the scarring or discoloration left behind from a blemish.

☺ $$$ **Complexion Polish** *($48 for 2.7 ounces)*. The pH for this exceptionally ordinary product just makes it over the line as an AHA option for someone with normal to dry skin; however, in terms of every other aspect it has nothing over Neutrogena's Healthy Skin, Alpha Hydrox products, or Pond's Age Defying Cream, which are all available at the drugstore!

☺ $$$ **Alchemy** *($72 for 1.7 ounces)*. The only thing about this product related to alchemy is the price—it would take mumbo jumbo to get someone to spend this much money on a standard moisturizing formula for dry skin.

☺ $$$ **Energy for All Skin Types** *($65 for 2.7 ounces)*. You have to sit down for this one—the energy in here is hydrogen peroxide, which is supposed to provide oxygen to the skin. Hydrogen peroxide is the stuff you buy at the drugstore for 89 cents. The amount of vitamins and water-binding agents is negligible, making this a very standard moisturizer for normal to dry skin. I feel bad for the women who think their $65 bought something special. One more point: given that oxygen generates free-radical damage, how do they explain that adding it is not helpful for skin?

☺ $$$ **Energy for Oily Skin** *($65 for 2.7 ounces)* is almost identical to the one above, including the second ingredient isopropyl palmitate, a wax known to cause breakouts. The same basic review applies.

☺ $$$ **Resistance Anti-Oxidant Firming Complex** *($65 for 1 ounce)*. This light-weight moisturizer would be very good for someone with normal to slightly dry or slightly oily skin, though it makes me wonder if you need to use it to combat the damage caused from the hydrogen peroxide in the two Energy products above? The witch hazel in here is in such a small amount it probably isn't a problem for skin.

☺ $$$ **Eyebright** *($52 for 1 ounce)* has a list of ingredients so long and in such small print it hurt my eyes. This would be a very good moisturizer for dry skin, but keep in mind that most all of the unique water-binding ingredients and vitamins come well after the preservative content, making them less than a fraction of the product. The vitamin K in here can't change dark circles under the eye.

☺ $$$ **Eye Repair Balm for All Skin Types** *($38 for 0.68 ounce)* could have been a good emollient moisturizer for dry skin, except for some reason this product contains sulfur and arnica, which are incredibly irritating especially for the eye area.

☹ **Rescue** *($47 for 1 ounce)*. While the basic moisturizing ingredients are quite good, there are several plant oils and plant extracts in here that are strong sensitizers, including lemon oil, grapefruit oil, orange oil, lime oil, citronella oil, lavender oil, lemon extract, and pine extract. This product is not recommended.

☹ **Serum Intensif Rescue for All Skin Types** *($47 for 1 ounce)* contains several plant extracts that can be irritating for most skin types, including horsetail, pine, and lemon, as well as lemon oil, grapefruit oil, orange oil, lime oil, mandarin oil, and citronella oil. This product is not recommended.

☺ **$$$ Hydralock Lip with SR-38** *($22 for 0.5 ounce)* is a fairly emollient, though standard lip gloss that contains water, coconut oil, Vaseline, cocoa butter, thickeners, and preservatives. Twenty-two dollars for lip gloss? Wow!!!

## Renew Skin Care Formula

Renew Skin Care Formula products are nothing more than a poor assortment of AHA products with a cleanser and a poor version of a vitamin C liquid. These "amazing new face-lift-in-a-jar" products clearly are not so amazing. Amazing products should perform amazingly, don't you think? I wonder how many women have been duped by this ad, with a smiling Terri Welles telling you to expect unbelievable results. I've seen it in almost every local newspaper all over the United States and Canada. What a sad, expensive mistake for many women. Not only are these products a waste of money, but they are unnecessarily expensive and poorly formulated (at least when it comes to the AHA and vitamin C products), and the line does not include a sunscreen, so women are left with no way to really stop wrinkling and take good care of their skin. All this from some "famous" plastic surgeon. I would hate to be this doctor's patient. What dermatologist or plastic surgeon would encourage all this nonsense without discussing Retin-A, Renova, well-formulated AHA products, or sunscreen?

I haven't been able to locate a phone number for this company.

Note: This line comes in a kit that cost $65 for the six products below.

☹ **Glycolic Facial Shampoo** *(2 ounces)* is a standard, detergent-based water-soluble cleanser, except the cleansing agent is extremely drying for most skin types. Plus, it contains citrus oils, which can irritate the skin and eyes. It also contains a small amount of glycolic acid, but its effectiveness is washed down the drain before it can work.

☹ **Fruity Skin Tonic** *(2 ounces)* is a glycolic acid–based toner, but this product has the wrong pH to be an effective exfoliant, and the citrus ingredients in here provide no benefit but can definitely irritate the skin.

☺ **Oil-Free Moisture Gel** *(2 ounces)* could be a good lightweight AHA product in a light moisturizing base, but the pH isn't adequate for exfoliating the skin.

☺ **Topical Vitamin C** *(0.25 ounce)* is just what the name says, but it isn't that different from Avon's product Anew Formula C Treatment Capsules. Vitamin C won't save skin or change it.

☺ **Wrinkle Cream with Topical C and AHAs** *(0.25 ounce)*. The amount of AHA in this product isn't even 2%, which makes it a moisturizing ingredient, not an exfoliant. The vitamin C, though in a different form from that used in the product above, is also unstable and has no proven effect on the skin; and I have no comment about the egg white.

☺ **Vitamin Enriched Natural Moisture Factor** *(0.5 ounce)* would be a good moisturizer for someone with normal to dry skin, but that's about it.

# Revlon

As one of the leading mass-market cosmetics lines in the world, Revlon has done an excellent job lately with product innovation and keeping up with current research on formulating products with the appropriate sunscreen agents. In fact, the majority of Revlon's foundations can boast reliable sun protection along with mostly neutral colors and some of the best textures around. As a result, it has become much more pleasurable to shop Revlon at the drugstore. The mainstay of Revlon's success over the past several years has been its two major color lines, Age Defying (for the 35 and over crowd) and ColorStay (for the under-35, oily-skin crowd). Both age groups are served well, as these lines offer excellent options. Age Defying is best for normal to very dry skin, while ColorStay, whose namesake lip color spawned a new generation of lipstick consistency that is both ultra-matte and dry, is great for normal to oily skins. Revlon is still strongly in the running against such trendy lines as Hard Candy and Urban Decay, with its small collection of StreetWear Makeup. Although not for more conservative tastes, if lime green lip gloss is what you're after, the prices here are much more friendly than at the department store, and product quality is just as good, if not better.

Revlon's weaker spots can be seen (or felt) among its ColorStay Blush, Wet/Dry Eyeshadows (which are all shiny), and some poor concealers and mascaras that are merely average, especially when compared to competitors such as L'Oreal and Maybelline. Still, Revlon has earned its reputation for its superior products, and, for now, those help to offset the deficiencies. There's more than enough here to consider when you want to (and I quote Revlon's tag line) "feel like a woman" (though personally, I think we already understand that feeling like a woman means more than just wearing makeup).

When it comes to skin care, however, it seems Revlon's proverbial head has been in the sand, as it's ignored some advances and new information about skin care. Revlon's standard lines—Eterna '27', Natural Collagen Complex, and Moon Drops are still around with nary a change in over 15 years. Today's world of skin care has much that's new to offer, leaving these products back somewhere with beehive hairdos and go-go boots. For more information, call (800) 4-REVLON or visit the Web site at www.revlon.com.

# Revlon Skin Care

☺ **Moon Drops Extra Gentle Cleansing Cream Water-Rinseable for Sensitive/ Delicate** *($5.99 for 4 ounces)* is a standard, mineral oil–based wipe-off cleanser that can leave a greasy film on the skin. This isn't water rinseable in the least, though it can be an option for someone with dry skin

☹ **Moon Drops Replenishing Cleansing Lotion Water Rinseable for Normal to Dry** *($5.99 for 8 ounces)* is similar to the one above and the same basic review applies.

☹ **ColorStay Makeup Remover Pads** *($5.47 for 80 pads)* is a standard, detergent-based water-soluble makeup remover that definitely will help you (and you will need help) to get the ColorStay products off. However, I usually advise against wipe-off products, as they can encourage skin to sag.

☹ **Age Defying Performance Skin Care Face Cream, SPF 15** *($12.61 for 1.75 ounces)* and **Age Defying Performance Skin Care Oil-Free Face Lotion, SPF 15** *($12.61 for 1.7 ounces)* are both average moisturizers but poor sunscreens; neither contains the UVA-protecting ingredients of avobenzone, titanium dioxide, or zinc oxide, and therefore neither is recommended.

☺ **Eterna '27' All Day Moisture Lotion** *($11.99 for 2 ounces)* is a very emollient, good moisturizer for dry skin.

☺ **Eterna '27' All Day Moisture Cream** *($11.99 for 1 ounce)* is very similar to the lotion above but with still more thickeners and mineral oil. It would be good for dry skin.

☹ **Eterna '27' with Exclusive Progenitin** *($15.69 for 2 ounces)* contains pregnenolone acetate, often derived from animal urine. Pregnenolone acetate is a precursor to other hormones and can affect levels of progesterone and estrogen in the body when taken orally. When applied to skin it may work as a water-binding agent. There is no information on whether absorption through skin is possible.

☹ **Moon Drops Nourishing Moisture Lotion SPF 6 Normal to Dry** *($6.93 for 4 ounces)*, with its SPF 6, is bad enough, but this product also doesn't contain the UVA-protecting ingredients of avobenzone, zinc oxide, or titanium dioxide, and is not recommended.

☹ **Moon Drops Soothing Moisture Cream SPF 6 Extra Moist for Sensitive/ Delicate Skin** *($5.99 for 4 ounces)* is similar to the one above, and the same review applies.

# Revlon Makeup

**FOUNDATION:** Revlon seldom has testers for its foundations, but many stores do sell sample packs with three shades so you can experience the colors for a minimal investment.

☺ **Age Defying Makeup with SPF 10** *($11.98)* is best for someone with normal to dry skin (the formula contains oil), and provides light to almost medium coverage. The SPF is titanium dioxide–based, but the number is marginally low. However, if you're willing to wear an SPF 15 underneath, the makeup's texture and 12 shades are quite good.

☺ **Age Defying Makeup and Concealer SPF 20** *($13.89)* is an excellent option for foundation and sunscreen in one. The sunscreen base is titanium dioxide with zinc oxide, and the SPF number is impressive for a foundation. The foundation part is a cream-to-powder makeup that has a smooth, even finish and some great colors, though nothing for very light or very dark skin tones. The concealer part has the same SPF but is fairly greasy and can easily crease into lines under the eyes. Medium skin tones may find some of the concealer colors are too dark to cover circles under the eye, yet these shortcomings are minor compared to the strong positives, and this would work well for normal to dry skin, with eight shades to choose from.

☺ **Age Defying All Day Lifting Foundation SPF 20** *($13.89).* It probably won't surprise any of you when I say that this foundation won't lift your skin anywhere. However, it is an excellent emollient foundation for normal to dry skin that can provide medium to opaque coverage. It also has a brilliant SPF, using titanium dioxide as the only active sunscreen ingredient. There are ten shades to consider, but none for very light or very dark skin tones, which is very disappointing. Avoid Honey Beige, Cool Beige, and Sand Beige, which may all be too pink or peach for most skin tones.

☺ **ColorStay Makeup SPF 6** *($12.28)* is beyond matte, beyond no shine, and far beyond the claim of "it won't come off on him." It won't come off even when you want it to, as this is one of the most stubborn makeups I have ever tested. Get it on right the first time, because once it dries, it won't budge. If you get even the slightest wrong color it can look like a chalky mask, and removing it at night takes some effort, including several attempts with your cleanser and washcloth. Therefore, it is only appropriate for someone with truly oily skin and a deft hand at blending who is looking for medium to heavy coverage. Revlon has expanded the number of shades to 16, but all of the deeper shades, from Tawny through Mocha, are way too copper, orange, or red for darker skins. Also, the deeper colors are without sun protection, but the SPF 6 (titanium dioxide–based) is really too low to count anyway. The remaining shades for light to medium skin tones fare better, but watch out for Ivory and Natural Beige—both are slightly pink. Medium skin tones have the best selection of neutral colors with this one.

☺ **ColorStay Lite Makeup SPF 15** *($12.59)* is Revlon's answer to the negative comments it received on its original ColorStay makeup above. This Lite version is an excellent matte foundation, and is a must-try if you have oily skin! Even better, all of the 12 colors are excellent—not a bad one in the bunch, though Ivory can be too peach for some skin types—but that's really nitpicking! The SPF is pure titanium dioxide, and some women may find that exacerbates breakouts, but therein is the agony of using sun protection when you have oily skin. One complaint: the container for this foundation is a poor design. It stands on its head, which isn't helpful for this very liquidy makeup as it tends to easily spill out when opened.

☺ **ColorStay Compact Makeup SPF 25 Nonchemical** *($13.89)* is, far as I'm aware, the highest SPF-rated foundation available. The "nonchemical" in the name means that the excellent SPF uses pure titanium dioxide as the only active ingredient. What is unique about this makeup is that the consistency is more like a liquidy powder delivered through a screen that you press on with a sponge to bring up the foundation. It spreads over the skin like a thick liquid foundation but quickly dissolves into a sheer-to-medium coverage, ultra-matte foundation with a slightly powdery finish. In the true spirit of ColorStay, it doesn't budge once it is in place. While it smoothes over the skin easily, if you have any dry skin patches it can tend to make things look more flaky. There are now 12 shades, and testers are scarce, so you're left alone to wonder which color is best. If you're curious, try this: purchase a few possible shades from a store with a liberal return policy (Rite Aid comes to mind).

☺ **ColorStay Stick Makeup SPF 15** *($13.89)* glides on smooth and slightly creamy, and then dries to a soft, translucent finish. It can have light to medium coverage, comes in ten great colors, and has a really great SPF that is part titanium dioxide and part zinc oxide. The noncomedogenic claim is bogus, but this is absolutely worth a try if you want a soft, matte, slightly powdery finish that is far less drying than the compact version. However, please be aware that while this version can be great for someone with normal to slightly dry or slightly oily skin, it doesn't have the staying power of the other ColorStay foundations. It can slip and let oil show through like most stick foundations do.

☺ **New Complexion Makeup SPF 4** *($11.58)* has an embarrassingly low titanium dioxide–based SPF but does have a very light texture that blends evenly and dries to a natural, light-coverage finish. There are some neutral colors for medium skin tones to consider, but the lightest shades are too pink and the deeper shades are glaringly orange or copper.

☺ **New Complexion One Step Makeup SPF 15** *($12.59)* is a cream-to-powder foundation with titanium dioxide as the only sunscreen agent, which is great. This one is surprisingly similar, if not identical to Clinique's City Base Compact Foundation SPF 15 *($20)*. I simply could not tell the difference in a side-by-side face test of the two products. They applied, felt, looked, and wore the same. Revlon has 12 shades to choose from (Clinique has ten), and the shades are, for the most part, fairly neutral, although the range of tones is strange. The selection of lighter shades is extremely limited for Revlon, and the darker colors are all a bit coppery. If you have a more medium skin tone, you're in luck, and if you have normal to slightly dry skin you'll do well with this product. Avoid Natural Beige, Cool Beige, Warm Beige, and Sun Beige.

☺ **New Complexion Even Out Makeup Oil-Free SPF 20** *($11.58)* is a mixed bag that tries to be a little bit of everything and comes up far too short in most departments and way ahead in others. The sunscreen is excellent and one of the better combinations for dry skin on the market, using both zinc oxide and titanium dioxide. Yet the color selection, with half of the nine shades being too peach, pink, or ash, is disappointing. The consistency is rather light and moist, which is great for a sheer finish if you have dry skin. However, this also contains salicylic acid (BHA), which is a waste in a foundation in which the pH is too high for it to even be effective. All in all, there are more problems than positives with this one and I wouldn't choose it over Revlon's New Complexion One Step reviewed above. If you want to brave the odds, the only colors that look like skin are Sand Beige, Caramel, Nude Beige, and Natural Tan.

<u>CONCEALER:</u> ☹ **New Complexion Oil Free Concealer SPF 12** *($9.49)* has a great titanium dioxide–based SPF and is a good matte concealer with a smooth, dry finish that isn't prone to creasing. However, most of the seven shades are too peach, pink, or yellow for most skin tones, so if you decide to try this, double-check the color in daylight. **New Complexion Correct and Conceal Blemish Stick** *($9.79)* contains 1% BHA, which isn't the best in a makeup product, but again, not to worry—the pH of this product is over 5 and that means it has no exfoliation properties. While that isn't problematic for the skin, it isn't helpful either. What is potentially irritating to the skin is the menthol in this concealer and, to top it all off, the colors for these are best described as strange.

☺ **ColorStay Concealer SPF 6** *($9.49)* is awesome and ranks up there with the best of them. It absolutely doesn't crease, stays on very well, isn't as heavy or thick as the ColorStay original foundation, and comes in six very good neutral colors. It does provide opaque coverage and can be a problem if you want to hide instead of accentuate lines under the eyes, but it takes good care of dark circles all day long.

<u>POWDER:</u> ☹ **Love Pat Pressed Powder** *($9.99)* has colors that are too pink or peach for most skin tones and is not worth considering. **ColorStay Powder** *($12.59)* is virtually identical in every way imaginable to Almay's Amazing Lasting Powder

reviewed at the beginning of this book. My review for the Revlon version is exactly the same too: don't bother.

☺ **New Complexion Powder Normal to Oily Skin** *($11.49)* is a standard, talc-based powder with a decent color selection, but nothing about this powder will control oil—it's just a good, standard, dry-finish powder. It blends on smooth and soft and comes in a decent assortment of shades. **Age Defying Smoothing Powder** *($12.59)* has a very silky texture and a dry finish that can look a bit too chalky, especially over normal to dry skin. It works best if applied with a brush only, and the color range has options for very light (almost white) skin tones. The nine shades fall short by not offering any options for dark skin tones. **Age Defying Pressed Loose Powder** *($11.98)* is a puzzle. Pressed loose powder is a contradiction in terms, isn't it? This product is a lightweight pressed powder that applies rather sheer but also slightly chalky. It feels silky and the colors are just OK but some are worth a consideration. **New Complexion Bronzing Powder** *($11.59)* is a talc-based, pressed-powder bronzer that comes in a very natural-looking tan shade with minimal shine. It would work best on light to medium skin tones. **Street Wear All Over Face Glitter** *($4.99)* is just a face highlighter with lots of sparkling glitter that's as good as anything else for all-over shine.

    BLUSH: ☺ **Age Defying Cheek Color** *($11.98)* is a cream blush with a slightly powdery finish. Cream blushes tend to be hard to blend and usually dissipate during the day, and this one is no exception. Unless you have flawless skin, this will tend to accentuate every dent or imperfection. If you have perfect, even skin, you may like this blush—it does have a nice, smooth texture and a great color selection. **Naturally Glamorous Blush-On** *($11.98)* is a powder blush with a great color selection and smooth application. These colors are too shiny: Sandalwood Beige and Pure Radiance. **New Complexion Blushing Cheek Powder** *($11.48)* has a dry, floury texture that isn't the softest around but nevertheless can be counted on for a very sheer, even application. The six shades are all worthwhile and matte.

    ☹ **ColorStay Cheekcolor Oil Free** *($12.59)* is a cream-to-powder blush that takes a lot of patience to apply and remove. It blends well but dries to an immovable, sticky finish. It's not for everyone, and would assuredly undo a carefully blended foundation—it is almost impossible to blend over powder.

    ☺ **Smooth-On Blush** *($8.89)* is a powder blush with a luscious, silky texture and a soft, sheer finish. It isn't much for depth or brightness, and unfortunately many of the colors are deceptively shiny—check them in the daylight and you'll see what I mean.

    ☹ EYESHADOW: **Wet/Dry Eyeshadows** *($3.99 singles; $4.19 duos; $6.49 quads)* are quite similar in texture and performance to Estee Lauder's Wet/Dry Eyeshadows, but Revlon's are all shiny, and that just doesn't wear well, wet or dry. The notion of applying eyeshadows wet for a more intense, opaque effect is interesting, but opaque shine will only magnify any wrinkles, and tends to flake off much easier than matte shades would. As an option, there is one matte quad set, called In the Buff, whose colors are nicely coordinated, but the rest just have too much shine. **ColorStay Eyecolor** *($7.99)* comes in a tube, which is not my favorite way of applying eyeshadow, since blendability is essential and that isn't easy with such a dry, unmovable eye color. These colors are all about as stubborn as they come. They "grab" to the skin before you can blend them. And forget about adding more than one color or applying it again, because once this formula sets, any efforts to blend result in clumps and eyeshadow fingerprints! The only positive is that they will definitely last throughout the day without fading.

EYE AND BROW SHAPER: ☺ **Timer Liner Eye Pencils** *($6.69)* are very good, standard pencils that apply and blend easily. **ColorStay Eyeliner** *($6.79)* is also a standard pencil that comes in a twist-up container. It eventually sets and stays put but may still smear and goes on somewhat choppy. **Softstroke Powderliner** *($6.79)* has a great powdery texture and a matte finish that has great staying powder. The only drawback is the sharpening this one needs. **Wet/Dry Eyeliner** *($6.49)* is a standard pencil that is slightly creamy and that can smudge if used dry. Wet application dries to a more solid finish but also gives a more dramatic look. **ColorStay Brow Color** *($8.19)* is a two-ended product: one end is a mascara-like wand with color to stroke on the brow, and the other end is a pencil. In some ways this is the best of both worlds, particularly if you already use a brow pencil and a brow groomer to thicken and tint the brow. This one's brow gel goes on easily and stays well, while the pencil is just a pencil, nothing special, and it doesn't stay any better than other pencils.

☹ **ColorStay Liquid Liner** *($7.19)* has a strange, hard applicator that scratches at the eyelid as you put it on. Why Revlon would make this brush is beyond me. It does stay well, but getting it on is less than ideal.

LIPSTICK AND LIP PENCIL: ☺ Most of the **Moon Drops Moisture Creme and Frosts** *($8.39)* and **Super Lustrous Creme and Frosts** *($8.39)* have great colors (including some one-of-a-kind vivids) and an emollient, creamy texture. **ColorStay Lip Shine** *($7.99)* is a dual-ended product with one end being a liquid lipstick and the other a silicone-based gloss. You're supposed to apply the lipcolor, wait three minutes for it to "set," and then apply the wet-looking gloss. Well, you could wait an hour for this creamy lipstick to set and miss work, and it still feels creamy. It lasts well by itself and isn't anywhere near as greasy as true lip gloss, but once you apply the glossy component, the color tends to slip and bleed and you're right back with the same old problem. **ColorStay Lip Tint SPF 15** *($7.39)* isn't anywhere near as drying as the original ColorStay Lipstick, but the sunscreen is lacking any effective UVA-blocking ingredients. Other than that, this is more of a glossy lipstick, with only slightly better staying power than other glosses. **MoistureStay Lipcolor** *($9.49)* is moist and relatively matte, a nice combination for someone who wanted to like ColorStay Lipstick but found it to be too lip-crackingly dry. **MoistureStay Protective LipTint SPF 25** *($9.49)* is just standard lip-gloss with a sheer, wet finish and no significant UVA protection. **StreetWear Lip Gloss** and **StreetWear Lipstick** *(both $2.99)* are nothing new in regard to formula or performance—it's the wild colors that are the stars here, and anyone who appreciates nontraditional shades would do well to start here before checking out similarly themed items from the department store. **New Complexion Condition and Color Lip Stick** *($7.89)* is a dual-ended, thick pencil that has two similar lip colors. One end is thicker and quite greasy, the other end is thinner at the tip and is nicely creamy. If you don't mind sharpening, these they can be a convenient way to mix and match colors. **Time Liner Lip Pencil** *($7.29)* is an automatic pencil with a good texture and suitable colors, and **ColorStay Lip Liner** *($7.39)* is packaged the same but is undeniably tenacious and far less greasy than most.

☺ **ColorStay Lipstick** *($7.39)* is slightly less ultra-matte than the original version, which does reduce the chipping/peeling problem many women had (the lipstick tended to ball up or come off in chunks, which made wearing it not nearly as pretty as Cindy Crawford made it seem in commercials). It still peels off from the inside out, and that's still not a pretty picture. There have been numerous knockoffs of this ultra-matte finish, but without adding extra oils or emollients (the very things which make lipstick fleeting) to prevent the peeling issue, no one has been able to perfect the formula for a comfortable ultra-matte lipstick that wears evenly. **ColorStay Liquid Lip** *($9.19)* is supposed to be a transfer-resistant lipgloss that comes in a tube with a wand applicator. It applies fairly greasy, as does any gloss, and then, after what seems like several minutes, it slightly "sets." But the finish stays moist, is not transfer-resistant in the least, and can tend to roll off. Do not expect this to be the sheer, moist stain the ads proclaim. **Line and Shine** *($9.49)* and **Line and Matte** *($9.49)* are both two-in-one products that have a standard lip pencil on one end and a liquid lip color on the other. The Shine version is just semi-opaque lip gloss, and the Matte version is not really matte but is creamy with a slightly powdery finish. With both, you get a little convenience in exchange for a tiny amount of each respective product. **MoistureStay Lip Liner** *($7.89)* is an automatic pencil but it has an awkward, flat-wide tip that is seldom seen—and for good reason, as it is difficult to apply with precision.

**MASCARA:** ☺ **Lashfull Mascara** *($6.79)* goes on well and makes it through the entire day without incident. **ColorStay Lash Color** *($6.99)* goes on quickly and definitely lengthens but, even with the newly designed brush, tends to clump. **Everylash Mascara** *($6.69)* is virtually identical in look and performance to Almay's Stay Smooth Mascara. You'll get some noticeable length rather quickly but there is little clumping, so the comb, though nice, isn't really necessary, and not as helpful as an old, clean mascara wand. **ColorStay Waterproof Mascara** *($6.99)* turns out to be the best of Revlon's waterproof options, building substantial length and decent thickness with no clumps. It is mostly waterproof, but does break down slightly with enough water exposure. **ColorStay Extra Thick Lashes Mascara** *($6.99)* takes awhile to build any length, but with patience you do get relatively long, thick lashes without clumping or smearing. The brush isn't an advantage and has a tendency to feel scratchy if you get it to close to the rim of the eye.

☺ **Everylash Waterproof Mascara** *($6.69)* meets basic expectations in terms of length, but it takes some effort for this to just be a standard, nicely waterproof mascara. **Lashfull Waterproof Mascara** *($6.79)* builds OK length but absolutely no "power thickness" to speak of. It doesn't clump or smear and the waterproof claim turns out to be true.

## *Rimmel (Makeup Only)*

Rimmel is a London-based company under the ownership of Coty, which may explain why the Coty line of makeup has all but disappeared and is now being replaced with this import. According to the press release surrounding the U.S. launch of Rimmel, it is the top-selling makeup line in England. Given the very low price point and several good products to choose from (though nothing groundbreaking), that may indeed be true. What are worth paying attention to if you happen to come across this line are the blushes, eyeshadows, and powders. The foundations are worth a look as well, but without testers it is always a guessing game as to which color would be best for you. However, at these prices, why not buy two or three shades and experiment? The pencils and lipsticks are basic but worth a look, and there are dozens of nail polishes to consider. My only significant complaint about Rimmel is the packaging. The lipstick caps do not fit very securely and can come off relatively easily, and the tops to the blush and eyeshadows are awkward and tricky to remove. However, these are small technicalities that are easy enough to live with, especially at these prices! For more information about Rimmel, call Coty at (212) 850-2300 or visit the Web site at www.coty.com.

**FOUNDATION:** ☺ **Stay Matte Foundation** *($2.97)* is recommended for normal to oily skin but the moist texture and slightly creamy finish would be more suitable for normal to dry skin. This provides light-to-medium coverage and comes in a tube, which makes it a bit hard to control the amount that comes out. There are eight shades, and half are too pink or peach for most skin tones. Avoid Sand, Soft Beige, Warm Honey, and Amber. Porcelain is slightly pink, but may work for some lighter skin tones, and Bronze is a good, neutral shade for darker complexions.

☺ **Light Finish Foundation** *($2.97)* has a similar texture and finish to the one above, only this is slightly less creamy. The coverage is sheer to light, but unfortunately six of the eight shades are too pink, peach, or orange for most skin tones. The only shades to consider are Nude (for light skin) and Natural Beige (for medium skin).

☺ <u>POWDER:</u> **Stay Matte Pressed Powder** *($2.97)* is talc-based and has a light, silky texture that goes on smooth even though it isn't quite as dry a finish as the name implies. Oilier skin types may see shine before too long, but normal to dry skin should enjoy the feel of this one. There are four shades, with no options for darker skins, and Toast is too orange for most skin tones. **Light Finish Compact Powder** *($3.97)* is talc-based and has a slightly drier texture and finish than the one above. However, the three shades are packaged in such a way that it is almost impossible to see the color, making this an iffy proposition for selecting the right color, which is a shame because the available colors are impressive.

☺ <u>BLUSH:</u> Rimmel's powder-based **Blush** *($1.97)* comes in a small compact and features predominantly warm-toned shades, all with a shiny finish. If only these were matte, they would be a steal, as the texture and blendability are wonderful.

<u>EYESHADOW:</u> ☺ **Special Eyes Mono Eyeshadow** *($1.97)* has a silky, slightly powdery (it can be a bit messy to apply), but easy-to-blend texture, and some worthwhile matte options among many pastel blue or shiny colors. The matte shades to consider are Planet, Matte White, and Blonde.

☹ **Special Eyes Duos** *($1.97)* and **Trios** *($2.97)* feature the same texture as the Special Eyes Mono Eyeshadow, but most of the colors are shiny. The trios are easy to pass up, with lots of iridescence and hard-to-combine colors. These duos are matte and worth a look: Orchid and Spice.

<u>EYE AND BROW SHAPER:</u> ☺ **Eye Liner Pencil** *($1.97)*, **Soft Kohl Kajal Pencil** *($1.97)*, and **Professional Eyebrow Pencil** *($1.97)* are standard in every sense of the word. They need to be sharpened and have a dry finish, which can mean less smudging.

☹ **Liquid Eye Liner** *($1.97)* is standard liquid liner that comes with a long, skinny brush that can be hard to control over the lashline. Plus, the formula tends to easily smear and fade.

<u>LIPSTICK AND LIP PENCIL:</u> ☺ **Lasting Finish Lipstick** *($3.97)* has a soft, creamy texture and slightly glossy finish. **Rich Moisture Lipstick** *($3.97)* is a very good, creamy lipstick that goes on smoothly and is less slippery than the Lasting Finish. **Sheer Finish Lipstick** *($3.97)* is just that, a sheer tint for lips with a glossy finish. **1000 Kisses Stay On Lip Liner Pencil** *($1.97)* is a standard pencil that needs to be sharpened. It has a smooth and comfortably creamy texture and stays on as well as any other pencil.

☹ **1000 Kisses Lipstick** *($3.97)* is Rimmel's take on an ultra-matte lipstick and it is slightly matte with a texture that tends to ball up and chip off over time, like most other ultra-matte lipsticks. **Lip Liner Pencil** *($1.97)* has a dry texture and stiff feel, making application somewhat uncomfortable.

<u>MASCARA:</u> ☺ **Extra Super Lash Mascara** *($1.97)* goes on well and builds impressive length but no thickness to speak of. It doesn't clump or smear either. **Exaggerate Mascara** *($3.97)* is the one to choose for a quick, clean application with lots of length and decent thickness without clumps or smears.

☹ **Endless Lash Mascara** *($2.97)* takes a seemingly endless amount of time to build what amounts to unimpressive length, no thickness, and some smearing.

☺ <u>BRUSHES:</u> In addition to some standard sponges and powder puffs, Rimmel offers two brushes. The **Powder Brush** *($2.97)* is reasonably dense and full, but could be softer and more tapered to fit the contours of the face. The **Blush Brush** *($3.97)* is floppy, sparse, and too small for the cheek area. Why it costs more than the Powder Brush is a mystery.

## RoC (Skin Care Only)

Johnson & Johnson, owner of Purpose, Neutrogena, Clean & Clear, Retin-A, and Renova, has launched RoC in the United States (it was previously available in other countries such as Canada and Australia). Several products are available in Canada only and those products follow the section for the products available in both the United States and Canada.

RoC prides itself on gentle, sensitive skin care. This line does contain far fewer irritating ingredients than most cosmetics lines (such as no fragrance or coloring agents!). There are a handful of exceptions, but for the most part, these simple formulations are distinctive for their concern in preventing skin irritation or skin sensitivity. The product line as a whole is definitely a consideration for sensitive or dry-skin types, though if you have oily or blemish-prone skin there really aren't any options or solutions among these products. For more information about ROC in Canada, call (519) 836-6500; in the US, call (800) 526-3967 or visit the Web site at www.roc.com.

☺ **Cleanser + Toner in One** *($7.99 for 6.76 ounces)* isn't much of a toner or cleanser. It is more of a wipe-off cleanser and it doesn't tone a thing. It could be good for someone with dry skin, but it doesn't take off makeup very well without a lot of wiping. [In Canada this product is called **Cleanser and Refresher for Face and Eyes 2 in 1** *($16 for 200 ml)*.]

☺ **Gentle Skin Toner** *($7.99 for 6.76 ounces)* is a fairly standard toner for cleansing, but it is not great for soothing or adding water-binding agents to skin. [In Canada this is called **Skin Toner, Dry Skins** *($14.50 for 200 ml)*.]

☺ **ChronoBlock Active Preventive Daily Moisturizing Cream SPF 15** *($16.99* *for 1.35 ounces)* is a very good, in-part avobenzone-based sunscreen in a good but rather mundane moisturizing base for someone with normal to dry skin. The teeny amount of retinol in here is unlikely to have an effect on skin. [In Canada this is called **Chrono Block Daily Moisturizing Care SPF 15** *($32 for 40 ml).*]

☺ **Hydra + Effet Reservoir for Normal Skin** *($15.69 for 1.35 ounces)* is a good, though fairly standard moisturizer for normal to slightly dry skin. Why anyone would put talc in a moisturizer is difficult to comprehend. [In Canada this is called **Hydra + Effet Rèservoir Light Texture** *($23.50 for 40 ml).*]

☺ **Hydra + Effet Reservoir for Dry Skin** *($15.69 for 1.35 ounces)* is almost identical to the one above, though this one uses ammonium starch (octenylsuccinate), which functions much the way talc does but isn't great for dry skin and can be a skin irritant. [In Canada this is called **Hydra + Effet Rèservoir Enriched Texture** *($23.50 for 40 ml).*]

☺ **Hydra + Light Mat Cream** *($12.17 for 1.35 ounces)* is almost identical to the Hydra + Effet above only with more film former, which can have a more matte feel on the skin. [In Canada this is called **Hydra+ Mat, for Combination Skins** *($23.50 for 40 ml).*]

☺ **Melibiose Active Firming Treatment for Normal Skin** *($13.99 for 1.35 ounces)* does contain melibiose, an interesting chemical (a sugar much like lactose, which this product also contains) that has some interesting research (all done in vitro—in a test tube) showing that it protects other skin substances from breaking down. That's great, but just because something works in a test tube doesn't mean it will work for real skin on real people. Other than that, melibiose is a saccharide and its main function for skin is as a water-binding agents. This is a good moisturizer for dry skin (not normal skin). [In Canada this is called **Melibiose Anti-Aging Action Light Texture** *($30 for 40 ml).*]

☺ **Melibiose Active Firming Treatment, for Dry Skin** *($13.99 for 1.35 ounces)* is almost identical to the Normal Skin version above and the same comments apply. [In Canada this is called **Melibiose Anti-Ageing Action-Enriched Texture** *($30 for 40 ml).*]

☺ **Melibiose Eye Contour Cream** *($13.99 for 0.51 ounce)* is almost identical to the Normal Skin version above and the same comments apply. [In Canada this is called **Melibiose Anti-Ageing Action Eye Contour** *($24 for 15 ml).*]

☹ **Retinol Actif Pur Anti-Wrinkle Treatment, Day-SPF 10** *($15.99 for 1.01 ounces)* has an SPF of 10 and no UVA-protecting ingredients, and that makes this is a waste of money. There's retinol in here, but it is a waste if you're looking for retinol and sun protection. [In Canada this is called **Rètinol Actif Pur Jour - Moisturizing Anti-Wrinkle Day Care** *($32.75 for 30 ml).*]

☺ **Retinol Actif Pur Anti-Wrinkle Treatment, for Night** *($15.99 for 1.01 ounces)* does contain retinol (about 0.1%), with only water and thickening agents. This is the same amount as in Neutrogena's Healthy Skin with Retinol, which has a more elegant, moisturizing base. If you're going to try a retinol product, go for Neutrogena's instead, and you get more product for less money.

☺ **Retinol Actif Pur-Eye Contour Cream** *($15.99 for 0.51 ounce)* is virtually identical to the one above, only this has a whole 0.5 ounce less of product for some reason. Maybe they thought you wouldn't read the ingredient label and notice. [In Canada this is called **Rètinol Actif Pur Eye and Lip Contour** *($28.75 for 15 ml).*]

☹ **Retinol Actif Pur-Anti-Age Hand Treatment, SPF 10** *($7.99 for 1.69 ounces)* is a waste of your money since it is only an SPF 10 and does not contain UVA-protecting ingredients.

## RoC (Canada Only)

These products are only available in Canada. All prices listed are in Canadian dollars.

☺ **Cleansing Milk Pure and Balancing, Normal to Combination Skin** *($14.50 for 200 ml)* contains problematic ingredients that are known for blocking pores. This product is not recommended for combination skin, though as a wipe-off cleanser for normal to dry skin it is an option.

☺ **Cleansing Milk Pure and Soothing, Dry Skin** *($14.50 for 200 ml)* contains lanolin oil, which can leave a greasy film on the skin and is a potential allergen for some people. This is a wipe-off cleanser that can leave a greasy film on the skin.

☺ **Rinse-off Facial Cleanser** *($14.50 for 125 ml)* is a good, standard, detergent-based water-soluble cleanser that isn't the best at removing makeup but can be good for normal to dry skin.

☺ **Eye Makeup Remover Lotion** *($14.50 for 125 ml)* is a standard detergent-based water-soluble wipe-off cleanser; it would work as well as any.

☺ **Gentle Exfoliating Cream** *($14 for 50 ml)* is a mineral oil–based scrub that uses synthetic scrub particles. This one can leave a greasy film on the skin.

☹ **Skin Toner Refreshing and Balancing, Normal to Combination Skin** *($14.50 for 200 ml)* contains alcohol as the second ingredient; it is a skin irritant and not recommended for any skin type.

☹ **Hydra + Teint Tinted Moisturizing Cream: Clair, Hale, Dore** *($23.50 for 40 ml)* comes in colors that are too peach for most all skin tones.

☺ **Revitalizing Night Cream** *($30 for 40 ml)* is a good moisturizer for someone with dry skin.

☺ **Hydra + Masque Moisturizing Mask** *($20 for 40 ml).* The clay can be drying and the witch hazel irritating, but as a mask that's on your skin only briefly, it can be OK for someone with normal to slightly oily skin.

☺ **$$$ Retinol Actif Pur Night Treatment Cream** *($35.75 for 30 ml)* is a good emollient moisturizer for dry skin, and it does contain retinol if that's the ingredient du jour you are looking for.

☻ **Retinol Actif Pur Radiance Anti-Wrinkle Mask** *($25 for 40 ml)* contains only a negligible amount of retinol, so even if that could make a difference in the skin, it can't in here. This is just glycerin and thickeners, boring but OK and hardly worth the trouble.

☺ **Nutri + Protect - Amino Moisturizing Cream, Dry Skin** *($22.00 for 50 ml* is a very emollient, though ordinary moisturizer for dry skin.

☺ **Nutri + Lips - Lip Protector** *($7.25 for 3 grams)* is a good but basic emollient for dry skin. The teeny amount of vitamin E in here has no impact on skin.

# *Sage Skin Care*

The hope of eliminating acne is an enticing one, and this line's promise of "zerozits," which is also the name of the company's Web site, is nothing less than brilliant marketing. This is a Web-site company with what appeared on the surface to be a great deal of information. However it ended up being a very tricky process to review these products. First and foremost, the products I ordered did not come with ingredient lists! The slapped-on labels (several askew on the packaging) were in total disregard of any acceptable FDA cosmetics-labeling regulations. When I requested ingredient listings, I did receive some sort of ingredient listings, but they didn't meet the FDA's labeling regulations and I didn't feel the ingredients matched the fragrance or consistency of the products. For example, most of the products had a noticeable fragrance, yet no fragrances were listed; preservatives were listed on some products as merely "preservatives" (they need to be spelled out); and the AHA ingredient was listed simply as "alpha" and the beta hydroxy acid was listed as "beta." None of that is acceptable or accurate. After my review of this line first appeared in my newsletter, the flood of comments on Internet beauty message boards seemed to have gotten the attention of the owner, and now ingredient listings are in accordance with FDA regulations—but what took so long?

Aside from the packaging flaws, there are parts of the "zerozits" Web page that are curious. Sage Skin Care is owned by Barbara Strickland, "a para-medical esthetician with 17 years experience," but there is no licensing or special training associated with that identification, at least not according to the FDA. Sage claims to use "the finest natural ingredients and combine them with technological advances to give you the safest, freshest, non-acne causing products available." Yet these products contain a host of unnatural ingredients, ranging from benzoyl peroxide to polyethylene (that's plastic), sunscreen ingredients, and carbomer, and none of these are plant-oriented in the least. What is of greater concern is the information presented and whether or not it is valid for addressing the issues around breakouts. That is more of a mixed bag, with some real hokey "sage" advice, some more practical realistic ideas and products, among a wide range of other misleading, unsubstantiated, and even risky recommendations and concepts.

On the positive side, the basic layout of Sage's acne game plan is extremely valid. Gentle cleansing, exfoliating, disinfecting, absorbing oil, and sun protection comprise a great approach, and most of those elements are offered in effective formulations. The prices here are out of line for what you get, but the method is fundamental to treating acne. Moreover, like any acne treatment, it can't work for everyone and it can't produce "zerozits." Breakouts are typically a function of hormones and how your skin type, pores, and the bacteria in the skin react, and not everyone will respond perfectly to the same formulations.

My biggest concern is that some of the advice on this site is a problem for skin. For example, Strickland advises applying her "Gelloid Moisturizer after [the] SPF 25," or applying any of her other products over sunscreen. This advice is great if you want a sunburn or wrinkles. But if you want to prevent those things, sunscreen should be the last thing you put on. You must never dilute or put something over sunscreen that would weaken its integrity, because that would degrade its effectiveness. (If you're wondering whether foundation dilutes sunscreen, it depends on how you put it on. If you are blending foundation over the skin without over-wiping, there isn't a problem. However, overblending a foundation or heavily wiping it over the skin can cut the efficacy of the sunscreen underneath.)

Another suggestion from Sage: "Retin-A, Renova, or Avita [a tretinoin cream like Renova] should be kept in the refrigerator—these products work faster when cold." I have seen no research showing whether or not this is true. However, any pharmaceutical or cosmetic in a cream form (which all of these are) can deteriorate and break down in temperatures over 90 degrees Fahrenheit or under 40 degrees Fahrenheit. Certain liquid prescription items are best kept in a refrigerator, but those come with specific instructions.

And another: "Use an ice cube to ice your face for one minute. Icing reduces swelling and inflammation and allows your products to penetrate more quickly. . . ." The directions explain to take the ice and apply it directly to the face. Ice should never be applied directly on skin anywhere—it can cause a burn response and damage skin. Ice for athletic injuries is always applied indirectly, wrapped in a protective barrier to prevent damage or over-freezing the skin. Further, because the ice constricts skin, and thereby the pores, pulling circulation away from the surface, it doesn't help penetration in the least!

And still another: "Remember a zit takes 90 days to form." Anyone who has a menstrual cycle knows this isn't true, it takes about 21 to 28 days to create a blemish. An important exception to that is the likelihood, according to Dr. Zoe Draelos in the February 1999 issue of *Cosmetic Dermatology,* of an irritated response triggering immediate breakouts. "The acne eruption observed in patients following the use of certain [cosmetics] is probably not acne, but rather a[n] irritant contact dermatitis. . . . This is why the reaction occurs almost immediately . . . [while] acne is a disease process that takes time to develop."

The Sage Web site has a page with a lengthy list of cosmetic ingredients rated for their irritation and comedogenicity (whether or not they may cause breakouts) potential. Where this information came from is not cited. However, what I surmise is that this is a very old listing excerpted from research originally conducted by a Dr. Robert Fulton. Fulton's book, *Dr. Fulton's Step by Step Guide to Acne,* was published in 1983. At the time, Fulton's research regarding the causes for breakouts was unprecedented. Fulton applied cosmetic ingredients to rabbit ears and waited to see what happened. As promising as this research was, it has since never been repeated and is rarely cited, for several reasons (which I explain in Chapter Two in the section "Will It Make Me Break Out?").

Sage is fairly pricey stuff, but there are options here to consider. For more information about Sage, call (888) 434-6660 or visit the Web site at www.zerozits.com.

☹ $$$ **Corrective Grains Regular, Corrective Grains Extra Gentle,** and **Corrective Grains Extra Strength** *($30 for 8 ounces each)* are three detergent-based water-soluble cleansers that all use ground-up plastic as the abrasive, and they all work as well as any. They do contain fragrance and coloring agents. These also contain benzoyl peroxide, but that is wasted in a cleanser because the disinfecting properties would just be rinsed down the drain.

☺ $$$ **Facial Shampoo, Facial Shampoo Extra Gentle,** and **Facial Shampoo Extra Strength** *($30 for 8 ounces each)* are each exceptionally standard, detergent-based water-soluble cleansers that work well for cleaning the skin.

☺ **SPF 25 Sunblock** *($21 for 4 ounces)* has a good SPF with part titanium dioxide as one of the active sunscreen agents. It is in a lightweight lotion formula that is a good option for someone with normal to oily skin. Please keep in mind that the recommendation to apply this before the other products in this line is dangerous advice. Sunscreen is the absolutely final thing you apply to your skin.

☺ $$$ **Gelloid Moisturizer and Masque** *($40 for 4 ounces)* is a fairly emollient moisturizer that would only be appropriate for dry skin types. The lanolin in here can cause breakouts.

☹ $$$ **Biological Redefining Masque** *($40 for 4 ounces)* is a standard clay mask with aloe and thickeners. It also contains menthol and tangerine oil, which can be skin irritants. It's an OK mask for oily skin, but this is a lot of money for clay and some problematic ingredients.

☹ **Glycolic Acid 12% Smoothing Cream** *($60 for 2 ounces)* has a pH of 5, so it doesn't work well if at all as an exfoliant. It also contains salicylic acid, but that also requires a pH of around 3 to 4 to be effective as an exfoliant.

☹ **Glycolic Acid Smoothing Cream 20%** *($60 for 2 ounces)* also has a pH of 5, which is great because at this strength the risk of irritation would be significant.

☹ **Glycolic Acid Smoothing Gel** *($60 for 2 ounces)* is similar to the two above only in a gel formulation instead of a cream, and the same comments apply.

☺ **Miracle Zit 2.5%** *($20 for 4 ounces)* is not a miracle, it's just a standard, 2.5% benzoyl peroxide gel that is great for disinfecting blemishes.

☺ **Miracle Zit 5%** *($20 for 4 ounces)* is similar to the one above only with a 5% benzoyl peroxide concentration.

☺ **Miracle Zit 10%** *($20 for 4 ounces)* is similar to the one above only with a 10% benzoyl peroxide concentration.

☹ **XX Miracle Zit 10% with Sulfur** *($20 for 4 ounces)* is similar to the one above only with a 10% benzoyl peroxide concentration and sulfur. Sulfur is a mild disinfectant but a potent skin irritant. Plus, it is highly alkaline, which raises the pH on skin, and can encourage the growth of bacteria.

☺ **Fix Zit 2.5%** *($20 for 4 ounces)* is similar to the XX Miracle Zit 2.5% version above only in a light, moisturizing lotion base. It is a good option for someone with dry skin struggling with breakouts.

☺ **Fix Zit 5%** *($20 for 4 ounces)* is similar to the Miracle Zit 5% version above only in a light, moisturizing lotion base. It is a good option for someone with dry skin struggling with breakouts.

☹ **Fix Zit XX Strength 10%** *($23 for 4 ounces)* is similar to the XX Miracle Zit above and the same comments apply.

☹ **Bleaching Lotion with Kojic Acid** *($45 for 2 ounces)*. Kojic acid is a more irritating, less stable ingredient for skin lightening than other options. However, it is still considered an option. The rating is due to the alcohol content in this product that can be irritating for all skin types.

☺ **Emulsion/Moisturizer** *($50 for 4 ounces)* is a very good moisturizer for normal to dry skin.

☹ **Old Lady Cream** *($40 for 2 ounces)* is just water, mineral oil, Vaseline, thickeners, and preservatives. This is a lot of money for what amounts to little more than Nivea Hand Cream or Aquaphor (reviewed in this book).

# Sea Breeze (Skin Care Only)

Like so many lines aimed at those struggling with breakouts, Sea Breeze adds the most absurd combination of irritating, skin-damaging ingredients to its products. I suspect all these companies think consumers who have acne-prone skin want a cool, tingling feel from their acne products. While that may or may not be true, the truth is that cool and tingling means irritating and skin damaging, and that these ingredients are bad for all skin types, especially someone with acne. After all, what color is acne? Red. And what color do these irritating ingredients make the skin? Redder. That's not smart, that's painful. Irritation also reduces the skin's ability to fight infection, and that too would cause more breakouts. The phone number for Sea Breeze is (800) 831-2684, or visit the Web site at www.seabreezezone.com.

☹ **Facial Cleansing Bar, for Normal to Oily Skin** *($2.99 for 3.25 ounces)* is a standard, tallow-based bar cleanser. The tallow can clog pores, which just doesn't make sense in a product for oily skin, and the cleansing agents can be fairly drying. It does contain fragrance.

☹ **Whipped Facial Cleanser** *($4.99 for 6 ounces)* contains camphor, a skin irritant, in an otherwise fairly ineffective skin cleanser.

☺ **Foaming Face Wash for Normal to Oily Skin** *($3.78 for 6 ounces)* is a detergent-based water-soluble cleanser that would be an option for someone with oily skin.

☺ **Foaming Face Wash for Sensitive Skin** *($3.78 for 6 ounces)* is a detergent-based water-soluble cleanser that would be an option for someone with oily skin.

☹ **Exfoliating Facial Scrub** *($3.78 for 3.5 ounces)* would have been an OK synthetic scrub, but they just had to add camphor to it so it would irritate the skin.

☹ **Astringent for Oily Skin** *($3.78 for 10 ounces)* is the product for you if you want red, irritated skin; it contains an amazing list of toxic ingredients, including alcohol, camphor, clove, eucalyptus, and peppermint.

☹ **Astringent for Sensitive Skin** *($3.78 for 10 ounces)* is similar to the one above, which makes this product's label for sensitive skin inexcusable.

☹ **Astringent Original Formula** *($4.99 for 16 ounces)* is similar to the one above, and the same review applies.

☹ **Breezers Astringent Facial Towelettes** *($4.19 for 24 towelettes)* are towelettes with astringent that is similar to the one above, and the same review applies.

☺ **Alcohol-Free Toner** *($3.99 for 10 ounces)* is actually a very good irritant-free toner. The fragrance is a bit much, but no more so than lots of other lines.

## Sears Studio Makeup

**FOUNDATION:** ☹ **Moisturizing Foundation** *($7.50)* would be a decent consideration for a light-to-medium-coverage foundation for normal to dry skin if it weren't for the fact that most of the 12 colors are way too peach or ash for most skin tones.

☹ **Oil-Free Foundation** *($7.50)* does have a more matte finish than the Moisturizing Foundation, but not by much. It would be acceptable for someone with normal to slightly oily skin but the colors are only slightly better than the Moisturizing one, which leaves little reason to give this one a try.

☹ **Wet Dry Foundation** *($7.50)* has an extremely powdery, dry finish (which doesn't work well as a foundation), plus a slight amount of shine. While shiny foundation may be a preference for some women, the shades of these powders are too peach or ash for most all skin tones. Only #2, #3, #4, and #5 are an option.

☹ **Color Corrector** *($7.50)*, like all color correctors, is a group of yellow, mint, and apricot concealers. Adding yellow, mint, or apricot to the skin doesn't change its color, but merely adds a strange color to the skin.

☹ **PRESSED POWDER: Pressed Powder** *($7.50)* has strange colors, which is one problem; the other is that all the shades are shiny, which makes them useless for setting makeup and reducing shine. **Loose Powder** *($7.50)* comes in four shades and all four are shiny. The trend for everything being shiny in the cosmetics world is just odd, but clearly the consumer must be falling for this one since more and more products are sparkling and iridescent. **Bronzing Powder** *($7.50)* has a great, silky texture and the colors are nice, but the shades of tan you would be getting are all shiny. Has anybody ever noticed that tan skin doesn't sparkle?

☹ **BLUSH: Blush** *($7.50)* has a nice range of colors with a rather dry, hard finish, which wouldn't be great for dry skin types. Regardless of the texture, all the colors are iridescent.

☹ **EYESHADOW: Eyeshadow** *($7.50)*, much like the Blush, is individually packaged eyeshadows that have an attractive range of colors. Unfortunately, the texture is too choppy for smooth application, plus all the colors are iridescent. **4-1 Eyecolor Kit** *($12.50)* has the same problems as the single eyeshadows.

☺ **EYE AND BROW SHAPER: Eye Liner** *($7.50)* is a definite consideration. There is a nice array of color options and the finish is on the dry side, which can prevent smearing. **Eye Brow Pencil** *($7.50)* is a pencil, and the same positive comments about the Eye Liner apply here.

☺ **LIPSTICK AND LIP PENCIL: Lipstick** *($7.50)*. If you are interested in a large selection of lipsticks, this line excels. The Creme Lipsticks have a great smooth, creamy finish; the Matte Lipsticks have a soft, slightly matte finish; the Sheer Lipsticks are far more glossy than anything else; and the Frost Lipsticks have a sheer finish with a good deal of iridescence. **Lip Liner** *($7.50)* has a large selection of shades to choose from, all with a smooth, dry finish. **Lip Gloss** *($7.50)*. The glosses are fairly standard and just as worth checking out as any other gloss.

☺ **MASCARA: Mascara** *($7.50)* is just OK. It doesn't build much length, definition, or thickness, but it doesn't smear or clump. If you don't need the volume, this wouldn't be a bad mascara to consider.

# Sears T.I.M.E.

Sears must like being in the makeup business because it has added another group of products to its existing in-house lines, Circle of Beauty and Studio Makeup. Now you have T.I.M.E., which stands for ☹ The Instant Makeup Expert ($20). The concept is a good one. A small blue makeup bag folds out flat with three sections and comes filled with preset groupings of colors—Tawny, Brown, Wine, Plum, and Pink. Each kit comes with a blush, a two-sided eyeshadow, lipstick, lip liner, eyeliner, mascara, and nail polish, all for the low price of $20. I wish I could say that these are a great bargain as well a time saver by having all the colors prearranged into makeup outfits for you, but they aren't. A handful of the sets do have some good color-coordinated colors but most have a strange mixture of shades. One of the Tawny sets has a shiny gold and forest green eyeshadow and a peach blush. One of the Wine sets has a shiny gray eyeshadow matched with vivid, rose-colored eyeshadow. Most of the eyeshadows are intensely shiny and go on somewhat choppy. The blushes do have a soft, smooth texture and the mascara is decent, building OK length and thickness with no smearing or flaking, but you're better off buying the blush separately, and there are more exciting mascaras around. The eye and lip pencils are fairly standard, though slightly on the creamy side, which isn't bad for the lip pencil; eye pencils are better slightly on the drier side. To purchase the T.I.M.E. kit products separately the prices are: ☺ Mascara ($6); ☺ Lip Liner ($6); ☺ Blush ($7.50); ☹ Eyeshadow ($6); Nail Polish ($3.50); and ☺ Lip Stick ($7.50). Also available as an option outside what's available in the kits are ☺ High Beam Eye Powders ($7.50), which are just what the name implies—shiny, brightly colored powders. These iridescent shades are in a tube applicator that isn't the most helpful to use, but these will shine well if that's what you are looking for.

# Selleca Solution (Skin Care Only)

It seems celebrities are believed no matter what they are endorsing. All it takes is celebrity status to convince consumers that something is worth buying, which is clearly the situation with Selleca Solution products. The first major problem with this small line is the glaring lack of a sunscreen. The second issue is the very limited range of products, with no differentiation between skin types. There is really only one specific skin type represented here, namely normal to somewhat dry skin. The last problem is that these products are especially standard, boring formulas in very small quantities for way too much money.

What you are supposed to believe about these products, besides that they make Connie look great, is that sea algae extract works wonders. Even if algae could have some benefit for skin (it can't, but let's just say it can), there isn't enough in here to even notice. Don't get me wrong: these aren't bad products, just a waste of time and energy for the consumer—but lots of consumers won't know that.

Please note that the first price is retail and the second is the club members' price. It is lower, but this isn't a club worth joining, because either way the products are truly overpriced. For more information about Selleca Solution, call (800) 365-1974 or check out the Web site at www.choicemall.com.

☺ $$$ **Soothing Cleanser with Chamomile** *($28, $19.50 for 6 ounces)* is a standard, detergent-based cleanser that would be almost identical to Cetaphil Gentle Skin Cleanser except that this one contains fragrant oils, including rose, clove, and sandalwood, that can cause allergic reactions and skin sensitivities. By the way, Cetaphil retails at about $10 for 16 ounces and you don't have to join a club.

☺ $$$ **Gentle Eye Makeup Remover** *($25, $17.50 for 4 ounces)* is a good, standard eye-makeup remover, effective, but overpriced.

☹ $$$ **Daily Difference Moisturizer** *($42, $29.50 for 2 ounces)* lacks sunscreen. Without sunscreen, when it comes to use for day wear, the only difference this moisturizer can make is to cause more wrinkles by leaving the skin unprotected from the sun. At night it would be a good moisturizer for normal to dry skin. There is a tiny amount of algae in here, but don't count on seaweed being a cure for wrinkles.

☺ $$$ **Firming Eye Gel** *($35, $24.50 for 0.5 ounce)* is a very lightweight, almost do-nothing gel moisturizer. It can be OK for very slightly dry skin, but for the most part you're buying some gel thickening agents and a teeny bit of algae.

☺ $$$ **Hydrating Eye Cream** *($38, $26.50 for 0.5 ounce)* is a good emollient moisturizer for dry skin.

☺ $$$ **Nighttime Miracle Cream** *($47, $32.50 for 1.7 ounces)*. Calling this a miracle is a piece of fiction that makes *Star Trek* look like fact. This cream for normal to dry skin contains mostly water, thickeners, water-binding agents, Vaseline, algae extract, fragrance (several that can be skin irritants), silicone, and preservatives. That's good, but it's also almost identical to the Daily Difference Moisturizer above. So how come that one isn't a miracle too?

☹ $$$ **Quick Lift Facial Firming Gel** *($55, $38.50 for 0.5 ounce)* is virtually identical to the Firming Eye Gel. The redundancy and change in price is bizarre. Did they think no one would notice?

☺ **Essential Moisture Body Lotion** *($35, $19.50 for 6 ounces)* doesn't even come close to improving on moisturizers like Lubriderm, and the price difference is substantial enough not to ignore.

# *Sephora*

Sephora takes shopping for cosmetics to a whole new level. It is a mixture of glamour, fun and exotic high-cost and low-cost cosmetics shopping all rolled together in one. If there is a beauty product you're looking for, the chances are it's here, along with some you didn't even know existed. From tweezers to hair accessories, professional scissors, and manicure tools, there are lots of body-tending choices to peruse. Under one roof you can shop Clinique, NARS, Stila, Decleor Paris, Peter Thomas Roth, Shu Uemura, Vincent Longo, and many, many others, including Sephora's own line of makeup and an array of perfumes.

While all this may sound relatively standard, what isn't standard is the fact that the salespeople are not paid on commission, so there is no pressure to buy from anyone, not even the manager, who spent a good deal of time helping me without ever pushing or hustling a sale. In comparison, department store salespeople are not only paid on commission, they must meet their counter's sales quotas (thousands of dollars a month) or their jobs can be on the line—not a fun prospect for the salesperson, but it does explain why lots of women shopping for cosmetics feel put upon by sales associates. The other positive here, and this is a big positive, is that the testers for the products are easily accessible, with no one standing over you while you play.

Sephora's line of color cosmetics is one of the largest I've ever seen. Talk about every color under the sun! This is a veritable rainbow of options. Aside from that, it only has brushes, lipsticks, lip pencils, nail polishes, and an all-purpose lip and eye pencil, but the colors are just astounding. Were you wanting to find a specific shadow of navy blue, or yellow lipstick with matching lipliner and polish? Then look no further. If you can locate a Sephora store near you (there are almost 50 and more opening every month), it is worth a visit. But try to be restrained; the shopping here is tempting and it's too easy to splurge or indulge unnecessarily. For more information about Sephora, call (415) 392-1545, or for store locations check out the Web site at www.sephora.com.

☺ **Lipstick** *($9)* has a texture that is pretty standard—creamy with a rather glossy finish. But with this line's over 200 shades of lipstick (sheers and opaques), you can have quite a time matching outfits to your heart's content.

☺ **Lip and Eye Pencil** *($3.50)* are tiny, standard pencils, but the color variations are too tempting to ignore. If you're going to try one of the lipsticks, don't leave without a matching pencil.

☺ **Pencils for Eyes, Cheeks, and Lips** *($4.50)*. I wouldn't use these as blush, but the chubby pencil (which is tricky to sharpen) is a fun accessory for lips. As an eyeshadow it can be pretty greasy and crease, and as a blush it's hard to apply it smoothly. But if the fun colors are more important, why not?

☺ **Nail Polish** *($3.50)* are the teeniest bottles of polish I've seen, so don't be too impressed by the price. But the color selection is just amazing.

☺ **Brushes** *(from $5 to $42)* come in a range that is just amazing, and some of them are exceptional. In particular, check out the eyeshadow brushes here. The brushes that come up short, and overpriced, are the blush and powder brushes, which just aren't as silky and soft as you would want for the face, especially considering the steep price tag.

## Serious Skin Care

Serious Skin Care has changed a lot since it first launched as a line featuring a small group of acne products. Its successful infomercial has created lots of additional products, and its simple three- or four-step routine has become complicated and the claims more overblown. It's not that there aren't some good products in this line, because there are, it's just that several of these are fairly serious when it comes to irritation, while others can clog pores. There are products to consider, so just be sure to choose carefully. For more information about Serious Skin Care, call (800) 540-8662 or visit the Web site at www.hsn.com.

☹ **Acne Wash** *($16.50 for 4.2 ounces)* contains peppermint, and that serves no purpose other than to irritate and inflame skin, especially if splashing this off causes some to get in the eyes.

☹ **Glycolic Cleanser** *($18 for 4 ounces)* is a standard, detergent-based cleanser that contains about 5% to 6% glycolic acid (AHA). In a moisturizer or gel that would be fine, but in a cleanser the effective ingredients would just be rinsed down the drain (and the chances of getting it in the eyes are pretty good and a problem). To get around the problem of the AHA being washed down the drain, the instructions suggest leaving this product on the face for two to five minutes. Of course, that also means leaving the detergent cleansing agents on the skin for two to five minutes too, and running a strong risk of irritation or skin sensitivity.

☹ **Mother of Pearl Soap** *($16.50 for four bars)* is a standard, tallow-based bar cleanser (tallow can clog pores) that also contains emollients, which can be a problem for lots of skin types. There is mother of pearl in here, but it is rinsed down the drain, so even if it had some purpose other than shine, it would be eliminated when you were done washing.

☹ **Sulfur Soap** *($16.95 for four bars)* is almost identical to the soap above except that it contains sulfur. If you are considering trying sulfur for disinfecting it would be better not to have it in a cleanser where its effectiveness would be rinsed down the drain.

☹ **Tea Tree Oil Soap Bar** *($16.95 for four bars)* is a fairly standard, detergent-based bar cleanser. It contains the tiniest amount of tea tree oil, which isn't going to help acne (it takes far more tea tree oil than this for it to work as a disinfectant), and the cleansing agents can be drying, while the ingredients that keep the bar in its bar form can clog pores.

☺ **$$$ Eye Sweep** *($15 for 2 ounces)* is a standard, detergent-based gel makeup remover. It also contains sodium lauryl sulfate, a very irritating detergent cleansing agent, and though it doesn't contain much of this, it can be a problem over the eye area.

☹ **Serious Buff Polish** *($19.95 for 4 ounces)* is a standard, detergent-based cleanser with walnut shells, ground-up plastic (polyethylene) and a tiny quantity of AHAs. It will work as a scrub, but not nearly as well as Cetaphil Gentle Skin Cleanser and baking soda mixed together. This product also contains several potentially irritating ingredients that can hurt skin, including lemon oil, citrus oil, and balm mint oil.

☹ **Toner** *($14.95 for 4 ounces)* is an irritating mix of alcohol and eucalyptus. The AHA in this one is good, but the other ingredients can hurt skin.

☺ **Glycolic Renewal Gel** *($20 for 4 ounces)* is a good gel/liquid 8% AHA product with about 0.5% BHA (salicylic acid). This is a good option for someone with normal to oily/combination skin for exfoliation. The plant extracts in here can be good anti-irritants.

☺ **1 Million I.U. Vitamin A Cream** *($26.50 for 2 ounces)* contains 1 million international units (I.U.) of vitamin A. While 1 million is an impressive number, there is no evidence that the form of vitamin A in this product (retinyl palmitate) is anything other than a good moisturizer and antioxidant for skin. Hanging your hopes on vitamins sounds healthy, but there is no evidence that they can make a difference, especially not when it comes to breakouts. Other than that, this is a fairly ordinary Vaseline-based moisturizer with some thickeners, silicone, fragrance, and preservatives.

☺ **A Force Vitamin A Serum** *($25 for 1 ounce)* is a serum version of the above and the same basic comments for the vitamin A apply here as well. This formula is an option as a lightweight moisturizer for normal to slightly dry skin.

☺ **Mega Mins** *($28 for 1 ounce)* is almost identical to the Vitamin A Serum above and the same comments apply.

☺ **Emu & Aloe Soothing Cream** *($24.50 for 2 ounces)* is a good, though exceptionally standard moisturizer for dry skin. If you want emu oil this product has it, but that's about all it has. The notion that emu oil is the best oil for skin isn't true, it is just a good emollient similar to other oils—though for many reasons, plant-derived oils are better for skin. There are far better moisturizing formulations than this one.

☺ **$$$ Eye Help** *($19.95 for 0.05 ounce)* is a very ordinary moisturizer for normal to dry skin. The plant extracts are good anti-irritants.

☺ **$$$ Refirm Firming Eye Gel** *($16.50 for 0.5 ounce)* is a good moisturizer for someone with normal to dry skin, though the film-forming agent in here can feel slightly sticky. The collagen in here can have no effect on the collagen in your skin.

☺ **Reverse Lift 2000** *($26.50 for 2 ounces)*. The hyped ingredients in this product include wild yam extract. According to the *American Journal of Obstetrics and Gynecology*, volume 18, 1999, "Wild yam is used in the production of artificial [synthetic] progesterone but it will not yield the hormone in the absence of a chemical conversion process that the body can't supply, though it can be created in a laboratory." It also contains pregnenolone acetate, a precursor to other hormones that can affect levels of progesterone and estrogen in the body when taken orally. When applied to skin it may work as a water-binding agent. There is no information about whether absorption through skin is possible. This also contains royal jelly, which may have an antibacterial benefit, but in this amount it has no real impact on skin at all. And the menthol in here just adds irritation and a misleading sensation that something is happening to skin.

☺ **Super Hydrate** *($19.95 for 4 ounces)* is a good, lightweight gel/serum moisturizer for normal to slightly dry skin though it is more of a toner than a moisturizer.

☺ **Aqua Plus Hydrating** *($24.50 for 2 ounces)* is a good moisturizer for someone with normal to dry skin.

☹ **Serious Shade Sun Block, SPF 15** *($16.50 for 4 ounces)* doesn't contain the UVA-protecting ingredients avobenzone, zinc oxide, or titanium dioxide, and is not recommended.

☺ **A-Copper Serum** *($24.50 for 2 ounces)* does contain copper, which has been shown to have some effect in wound healing and hair regrowth, but that does not translate to general skin care. And aside from that, this is just a good lightweight moisturizer for normal to slightly dry skin.

☹ **Acne Treatment Pads** *($19.95 for 45 pads)* contain a lot of alcohol, which can hurt skin and negate the effectiveness of the BHA in this product.

☺ **Clarifying Treatment with 2% Salicylic Acid** *($19.95 for 4 ounces)* is just that: 2% salicylic acid in a liquid base of water, glycerin, and slip agent. If you want to try a salicylic acid exfoliant for acne, this is one to check out.

☺ **Clearz-It with 5% Benzoyl Peroxide** *($19.95 for 4 ounces)* is, as the name implies, 5% benzoyl peroxide in a liquid base of water, glycerin, and slip agent. It is a great option, although 5% benzoyl peroxide is a little strong to start with, particularly when used with all these other irritating products. I would suggest starting off with a more gentle 2.5% benzoyl peroxide product and seeing if that works, and then moving on to a 5% and then a 10% version to see how those work for you.

☹ **Dry-Lo** *($24.95 for 1 ounce)* contains several irritating ingredients that can hurt the skin's healing process, including alcohol and camphor.

☺ **Fading Fluid** *($22.50 for 2 ounces)* is an OK hydroquinone-based skin-lightening product, but it also contains sodium sulfite and sodium bisulfite, which are both potential skin irritants. There are gentler hydroquinone products to consider than this one.

☺ **Lighten Up Skin Lightener** *($15 for 2 ounces)* contains 1% hydroquinone in a lightweight lotion, and that makes it a far better option than the one above.

☹ **Lipo-Fix** *($19.95 for 0.23 ounce)* contains witch hazel, grapefruit oil, lavender oil, and orange oil, which won't fix anything but can cause irritation and dryness.

☺ **$$$ Phase Out** *($19.95 for 0.5 ounce)* is supposed to be "specifically for the problem of dark circles underneath the eyes," yet there is nothing in here unique or special for dark circles. There is vitamin K in here, but that has no effect on dark circles. It also contains arnica, which is an irritant that should not be used repeatedly on skin.

☺ **Pure E** *($24 for 4 ounces)* includes such a teeny amount of vitamin E that is hardly worth mentioning. This is a very standard moisturizer for dry skin.

☺ **Triple Acting Glycolic Mask** *($12 for 2.5 ounces)* is just a standard clay mask with amounts of AHA and BHA that are too small to be effective as exfoliants.

☺ **Unplugged** *($22 for 2 ounces)* contains isolutrol, which is supposed to be effective in unclogging pores. A paper published in the *Australasian Journal of Dermatology* in February 1995 explained that in one study a comparison of isolutrol (extracted from the gallbladder or liver of sharks) with 5% benzoyl peroxide "showed that both isolutrol and benzoyl peroxide significantly improved patients' acne by reducing the number of inflamed lesions. [However,] Isolutrol did not significantly reduce the numbers of non-inflamed lesions whereas benzoyl peroxide did. Fewer side-effects were experienced by patients treated with isolutrol when compared with benzoyl peroxide." In essence, benzoyl peroxide is still the better option, though for some skin types that are sensitive to benzoyl peroxide this may be an option.

☺ **$$$ Zero Shine** *($14.95 for 0.05 ounce)* is merely powder with silicone. That wouldn't be bad, but it is hardly special; the problem is that it contains eucalyptus oil, which can be a skin irritant.

☺ **$$$ Mini Facial Peel Program** *($28 for six towelettes)* is a good 10% AHA product that would work well for exfoliation, especially for someone with oily skin, but how much exfoliation can one face take? The price is overkill, and the number of exfoliating products in this line is overkill too.

## Shade Guard (see Coppertone)

## Shaklee (Skin Care Only)

Shaklee has a line of skin-care products called Enfuselle. Its claims about these products portray them as nothing less than outstanding. Statements about patented formulations and the substantial research that was supposed to be published from two independent labs are the basis of its primary marketing push. The Shaklee brochure states, "In collaboration with physicians from the Dermatology Division of the Scripps Clinic and Research Foundation, Enfuselle products have been clinically tested at the independent laboratories of the California Skin Research Institute for safety and performance." The studies were never published—well, at least not other than in the Shaklee brochure—and without documentation of the actual study (though independent substantiating research is truly the standard), research cited by a company that did its own study is just not reliable. It is no more accurate than a child relating the results of his or her report card and, as any parent knows, you need to see it yourself to get the real story. Patented formulations may sound impressive but patents never ever indicate efficacy. Patents are about the way an ingredient or ingredients are put together, regardless of the effectiveness on skin.

About the results, Shaklee's brochure states its products showed a "154% increase in skin elasticity and firmness in 4 weeks, 88% reduction in the appearance of fine lines in 2 weeks, 104% reduction in the appearance of facial wrinkles in 8 weeks." Yet those kinds of numbers are meaningless. As a Ph.D. in statistics pointed out to me, if that were true, and if the elasticity in your skin increased 154%, your skin would be so elastic it would bounce. A 104% reduction in wrinkles? Not only would your wrinkles disappear in eight weeks, but your skin would be lifted up an additional 4%. So wouldn't that mean some of your skin would be gathered around your forehead? Or if you continue the products for another eight weeks, would the percentage improvement continue, creating raised, swollen skin instead of wrinkles?

Aside from the strange numbers, the way the tests were performed renders the information useless. The Shaklee brochure states as much: "The results of the Enfuselle clinical tests dramatically reflect the difference between one side of the face being untreated and exposed to changing climatic conditions, and the other side of the face being treated with Enfuselle under the same climatic conditions." That's all true. If the skin is dry, and you leave one side of the face without any moisturizer, it's going to look wrinkly and dehydrated. So much for scientific research.

While the claims for these products are as exaggerated and overblown as any in the cosmetics industry, there are definitely a lot of Shaklee salespeople who believe this is the gospel (of course they also felt that way about the products the Enfuselle line replaced). However, I never said the products were bad, at least not all of them, because many are impressive, at least as far as moisturizers go. However, given that all of the ingredients found in the Shaklee products show up in lots and lots of other skin-care products, these simply can't live up to the claims about getting rid of wrinkles or stopping the skin from aging, and definitely not any better than a host of other products with similar to identical formulations.

Shaklee is very proud of the antioxidants used in its products, and that seems to be the reality behind the brouhaha about them, because they all do contain antioxidants. Antioxidants are theoretically good for skin, and most skin-care products contain them; however, there is no research anywhere proving that they can affect or stop aging or change one wrinkle on your face, or even that one particular form or combination of them is the best.

As it turns out, nothing in these products makes them unique in any way, and a few have serious problems that you need to be aware of. Several of the products contain potentially irritating ingredients that are just bad for skin and completely unnecessary. Further, for all the patented ingredients and "serious scientific" research that is supposed to be supporting the claims, whoever these scientists are, they don't have any information about UVA sun protection, because none of the sun products contain avobenzone, zinc oxide, or titanium dioxide. (A Shaklee representative told me the sun products were tested and approved by the FDA for UVA protection, yet according to the FDA—www.fda.gov—no such standard exists.) Plus there are no disinfectants or exfoliants for breakouts. Shaklee needs to go back to the drawing board with this line. For more information about Shaklee, call (800) 742-5533 or visit the Web site at www.enfuselle.com.

☹ **Gentle Action Cleansing Bar** (*$15.25 for 4.5 ounces*) is a standard bar cleanser that can be drying to the skin, and the ingredients that keep the bar in its form can clog pores.

☺ **Hydrating Cleansing Lotion** (*$16.50 for 6 ounces*) is a standard, wipe-off, creamy cleanser that can leave a slight film behind on the skin; it could be an option for dry skin.

☺ **Purifying Cleansing Gel** (*$16.50 for 6 ounces*) is a good, detergent-based water-soluble cleanser for most skin types. There are a handful of antioxidants in this formula, just as in most of the Enfuselle products, but even if these could somehow be effective in fighting wrinkles, in this one they would simply be rinsed down the drain.

☺ $$$ **Eye Makeup Remover** (*$9.15 for 2 ounces*) is an extremely standard, detergent-based eye-makeup remover. It can work, but why bother wiping off makeup if the cleansers above could do the job?

☹ **Refining Polisher** (*$16.50 for 2.5 ounces*) contains menthol and alcohol, which are too irritating for all skin types. It does contain something called bilberry fruit extract, but that is not an AHA and has no exfoliating properties.

☹ **Hydrating Toner** (*$12.75 for 6 ounces*) contains both witch hazel and menthol, which makes it too irritating for all skin types.

☹ **Purifying Toner** (*$12.75 for 6 ounces*) is almost identical to the one above, and the same comments apply.

☺ **Balancing Moisturizer** (*$19.95 for 2 ounces*) does contain good antioxidants, but so do lots of other skin-care products. This is a good moisturizer for normal to dry skin but it won't change a wrinkle.

☺ $$$ **Eye Treatment** (*$19.95 for 0.5 ounce*) is similar to the Balancing Moisturizer above, and the same comments apply.

☺ **Hydrating Moisturizer** (*$19.95 for 1.7 ounces*) is similar to the Balancing Moisturizer above, and the same comments apply.

☹ **Time Repair A.M. SPF 15** *($45 for 2 ounces)* doesn't contain the UVA-protecting ingredients avobenzone, titanium dioxide, or zinc oxide, and is not recommended.

☹ **Body, SPF 15** *($16.50 for 4 ounces)* doesn't contain avobenzone, titanium dioxide, or zinc oxide for UVA protection, and is not recommended.

☹ **Body SPF 30** *($16.50 for 4 ounces)* doesn't contain avobenzone, titanium dioxide, or zinc oxide for UVA protection, and is not recommended.

☺ **$$$ Calming Complex** *($45 for 2 ounces)*. If it weren't for the alcohol, this would be a good lightweight moisturizer for normal to slightly dry skin.

☺ **$$$ C+E Repair P.M.** *($45 for 1 ounce)* contains mostly silicone and vitamins. Silicones leave a nice silky feel on the skin, but that's about it. If you're looking for a vitamin C product, this one isn't it. The vitamin C in here is ascorbic acid, and that is considered to be one of the more unstable and irritating versions of the vitamin.

☺ **$$$ Infusing Mineral Masque** *($16.50 for 2.5 ounces)* is a standard clay mask with a tiny amount of BHA (salicylic acid); however, the pH is too high for it to work as an exfoliant. It also contains menthol, which is a completely unnecessary skin irritant.

# *Shiseido*

Shiseido is the largest and one of the oldest cosmetics companies in Japan. Because of its size and marketing adroitness, Shiseido has been able to successfully penetrate other markets, particularly the United States, where it is found in most major, upscale department stores. The claims made about the company's products run the gamut from the benefits of natural ingredients to almost every anti-aging trick in the book, and the prices reflect the high-end appeal Shiseido strives for.

In 2000, Shiseido launched its line called The Skin Care, which added another group of products to its already existing lines of Benefiance, Vital Perfection, Pureness, and Bio-Performance, available at Shiseido counters in department stores, as well as its 5S boutique line opening around the country. There is only one way to sum all this up … what in the world are all these products for? It is difficult to understand why there should be so much blatant redundancy along with endless repetitive claims about getting rid of wrinkles. It's almost impossible to sum up all the premises behind Shiseido assertions for this array of unnecessary products, but just to give you an idea the following is a good example of what you can expect from Shiseido's claims.

The products from The Skin Care are based on Shiseido's "Basement membrane and Epidermal communication Skincare Treatment Theory [B.E.S.T] … skincare for the 21st century and beyond … " Shiseido claims to have an ingredient in these products called "phyto-vitalizing factor" that is supposed to promote restoration of the skin's "basement membrane." Phyto-vitalizing factor sounds very impressive, but the only unique ingredient in a few of these products is thiotaurine, an antioxidant. Taurine is an amino acid that has great antioxidant properties. There is a lot of research that shows that taurine is an excellent dietary supplement for many human body functions (and also particularly for cats), ranging from the heart (superior in some studies to coenzyme Q10) to the bile ducts. Animal protein is the only natural source of taurine (it is not found in vegetable protein), so attributing the term "phyto," which means "plant," to thiotaurine is a misnomer. If you take taurine orally, that's great—but how that translates to skin is unknown. There is no research demonstrating that thiotaurine is better or preferred over lots of other antioxidants used in cosmetics these days. And even if this was the be-all and end-all of antioxidants, the notion that thiotaurine in the minuscule amounts used in these products could change cell production is a stretch of reality. It is also questionable to find Shiseido making claims about repairing skin when several SPF products for this line (considering that sun is one of the major reasons skin gets damaged in the first place) are a dismal SPF 10.

Shiseido's eclectic array of makeup products has its strong and weak points. Its strengths lie in the texture and variety of foundations and lipsticks, while its weaknesses are seen in almost every other area, from poor concealers and mascaras (except the waterproof version) to the striking lack of matte eyeshadows. The tester unit for the makeup is large and imposing but not user-friendly, so be prepared to ask for assistance. Artistic leanings aside, Shiseido only needs to look to any of its neighbors in the cosmetics department to see what it is missing.

Even though this is a line you could easily pass up, there are some items to consider—but ignore the scientific-sounding claims. For more information on Shiseido, call (800) 354-2160, or (212) 805-2300 or visit the Web site at www. shiseido.com.

## Shiseido Skin Care

☺ $$$ **Benefiance Creamy Cleansing Emulsion** *($27 for 6.7 ounces)* is a very standard, mineral oil– and Vaseline-based wipe-off cleanser that can leave a greasy residue on the skin, though it may be an option for someone with dry skin. It does contain fragrance.

☺ $$$ **Benefiance Creamy Cleansing Foam** *($27 for 4.4 ounces)* is a very standard, detergent-based water-soluble cleanser that can be drying for most skin types due to the high alkaline content. It does contain fragrance.

☺ $$$ **Benefiance Balancing Softener** *($34 for 5 ounces)* is a good (though extremely mundane) irritant-free toner. There are some water-binding agents at the very end of the ingredient list, which makes them completely irrelevant for skin.

☻ **Benefiance Enriched Balancing Softener** (*$34 for 5 ounces*) is similar to the product above, except that it contains alcohol, which can irritate and dry the skin.

☻ **Benefiance Daytime Protective Emulsion SPF 8** (*$35 for 2.5 ounces*), besides having a lowly SPF 8, doesn't contain the UVA-protecting ingredients avobenzone, zinc oxide, or titanium dioxide, and is absolutely not recommended.

☻ **Benefiance Daytime Protective Cream SPF 8** (*$35 for 1.4 ounces*) is similar to the Emulsion SPF 8 above and the same comments apply.

☺ **$$$ Benefiance Revitalizing Eye Cream** (*$40 for 0.51 ounce*) is a good emollient moisturizer for dry skin.

☺ **Benefiance Revitalizing Emulsion** (*$40 for 2.5 ounces*) is an exceptionally ordinary moisturizer for someone with normal to dry skin.

☺ **$$$ Benefiance Revitalizing Cream** (*$40 for 1.3 ounces*) is almost identical to the Revitalizing Emulsion above and the same basic comments apply.

☺ **$$$ Benefiance Enriched Revitalizing Cream** (*$125 for 1.4 ounces*) is a good moisturizer for normal to dry skin, but not worth the money. The tiny amount of placenta extract in here has no special benefit for skin.

☻ **Benefiance Energizing Essence** (*$47 for 1 ounce*) is an alcohol-based serum, and that makes it potentially irritating to skin; it is not recommended.

☻ **Benefiance Neck Firming Cream** (*$40 for 1.8 ounces*) is specially for the neck, but what makes it special for this is a mystery. However, what isn't a mystery is that this cream contains alcohol, menthol, witch hazel, ginseng, and caffeine, which are all irritating and drying for every part of the body.

☺ **$$$ Benefiance Firming Massage Mask** (*$37 for 1.9 ounces*) is a peel-off mask that uses a form of plastic to create a layer over the skin. This doesn't firm anything, but skin always feels smoother when one of these kinds of masks are peeled off the face. It does contain fragrance.

☺ **$$$ Pureness Cleansing Foam Oil-Control** (*$15 for 3.7 ounces*) is almost identical to the Benefiance Creamy Cleansing Foam above and the same basic comments apply. It does contain fragrance.

☻ **Pureness Cleansing Gel** (*$15 for 5.4 ounces*) is a standard, detergent-based water-soluble cleanser that uses sodium lauryl sulfate, which is extremely drying and irritating for most skin types, as the cleansing agent.

☺ **Pureness Cleansing Water** (*$15 for 5 ounces*) is an irritant-free toner. It's OK for most skin types, but just very ordinary and more of a do-nothing kind of product.

☻ **Pureness Balancing Lotion** (*$18 for 6.7 ounces*) is an alcohol-based toner that won't balance anything, though it will irritate the skin. It also contains a small amount of sodium phenolsulfate, which can be a skin irritant and cause breakouts.

☻ **Pureness Balancing Lotion Oil-Control** (*$18 for 6.7 ounces*) is an alcohol-based toner that also contains clays, sulfur, and salicylic acid. It won't control oil, but it can be drying and irritating for most skin types.

☺ **Pureness Exfoliating Treatment Gel** *($18 for 3.6 ounces)* uses synthetic scrub particles (ground-up plastic) as the exfoliant in a water-soluble base. It can be a good scrub with minimal cleansing ability for normal to dry skin. It does contain fragrance.

☹ **Pureness Moisturizing Cream** *($20 for 1.3 ounces)* is part of the Pureness line of products, and is supposed to be ideal for getting rid of breakouts, yet this product contains several ingredients that are notorious for clogging pores, including tallow and stearic acid. Plus the second ingredient is plant oil; that's good for dry skin, but not oily skin!

☹ **Pureness Moisturizing Emulsion** *($20 for 1.6 ounces)* is similar to the Cream above, only this one contains Vaseline, which is even more problematic for oily skin.

☹ **Pureness Moisturizing Gel Oil-Free** *($20 for 1.6 ounces)* contains mostly alcohol as well as sodium phenolsulfonate, which makes it too irritating and drying for all skin types.

☺ **Pureness Blemish Control Cream** *($15 for 0.53 ounce)*. Sulfur is a disinfectant, but also a skin irritant. This is not the best way to control breakouts, and the alcohol in here can also add to the irritation.

☹ **Pureness Hydro Purifying Masque, Peel-Off** *($18 for 2.7 ounces)* is basically plastic and alcohol. It dries on the face like a film and then you peel it off. It can make the face feel smooth after you remove the layer of plastic, but the alcohol can be drying and irritating for all skin types.

☺ $$$ **Pureness Oil-Blotting Paper** *($10 for 100 sheets)* is just what the name implies. You press these small sheets over your face to help absorb oil during the day. The sheets are coated with a light layer of clay that can absorb oil. It's an option, but plain old powder and permanent-wave end papers do essentially the same thing.

☺ $$$ **Vital Perfection Cleansing Cream** *($22 for 3.9 ounces)* is a standard, mineral oil– and Vaseline-based cold cream that must be wiped off the face, and can leave a greasy film on the skin. It can be an option for dry skin but it doesn't get much more ordinary than this. It does contain fragrance.

☺ $$$ **Vital Perfection Cleansing Foam** *($22 for 4.5 ounces)* is almost identical to the Benefiance Creamy Cleansing Foam above, and the same review applies.

☺ $$$ **Vital Perfection Advanced Makeup Cleansing Gel** *($23 for 4.2 ounces)* is a mineral oil–based eye-makeup remover with detergent cleansing agents. It works, but plain mineral oil for far less would do the same thing, and that would also help you avoid the fragrance this product contains.

☺ $$$ **Vital Perfection Balancing Softener** *($30 for 5 ounces)* is a good, irritant-free toner. It would be good for someone with normal to dry skin.

☹ **Vital Perfection T-Zone Balancing Toner** *($25 for 2.5 ounces)* is almost identical to the Pureness Balancing Lotion above and the same review applies.

☹ **Vital Perfection Daytime Protection Moisturizer SPF 8** *($30 for 1.4 ounces)* has a disappointing SPF, though it does contain in part titanium dioxide, and with so many great SPF 15s available, why bother with this?

☺ **Vital Perfection Moisture Active Cream** *($32 for 1.3 ounces)* is a good emollient moisturizer for dry skin. Vital Perfection is a line of products meant for someone with oily skin that has a dry surface; I suspect that if the cleansing products in this group weren't so drying, you wouldn't have a dry surface! Even more to the point, why would someone with any amount of oil want to put the Vaseline and the form of tallow this contains on her skin? There are other ways to treat a dry skin surface than adding oil and fat to it. It does contain fragrance.

☺ **Vital Perfection Moisture Active Emulsion** *($32 for 2.3 ounces)* is similar to the Moisture Active Cream above minus the tallow but with added plant oils; this is good for dry skin but not at all for oily or combination skin. It does contain fragrance.

☺ **Vital Perfection Moisture Active Lotion** *($32 for 2.3 ounces)* is a more lightweight version of the Moisture Active Emulsion above, owing to the alcohol in here. That lessens the emolliency, but the alcohol just adds irritation and dryness to the mix.

☺ **$$$ Vital Perfection Daily Eye Primer** *($30 for 0.5 ounce)* is a good, basic moisturizer for normal to dry skin, but it's incredibly ordinary and there are far better options available for the money.

☹ **Vital Protection Soothing Lotion** *($27 for 5 ounces)* isn't in the least soothing; it contains menthol and zinc sulfate, which can be skin irritants.

☺ **$$$ Vital Perfection Hydro-Intensive Mask** *($28 for 1.4 ounces)*. This very ordinary mask can be drying for some skin types, plus the oils in here can be problematic for oily skin types.

☹ **Vital Perfection Rinse-Off Clarifying Mask** *($25 for 3 ounces)* is basically just clay and alcohol. It can be drying and irritating for most skin types.

☺ **$$$ Vital Perfection Protective Lip Conditioner SPF 4** *($20 for 0.14 ounce)* doesn't have much of a sunscreen, so there isn't much else to say about this otherwise very emollient lip balm that doesn't contain any UVA protection.

☺ **$$$ Bio-Performance Advanced Super Revitalizer Cream** *($60 for 1.7 ounces)* is a very standard moisturizer for someone with dry skin. However, silicone and Vaseline for $60 is a burn, and the teeny amount of water-binding agents in here makes them barely detectable.

☹ **Bio-Performance Advanced Super Revitalizer Whitening Formula** *($60 for 1.7 ounces)* contains none of the ingredients known to lighten skin, such as hydroquinone, magnesium ascorbyl palmitate, azelaic acid, or kojic acid, which makes this product a complete waste of time and money.

☺ **$$$ Bio-Performance Intensive Clarifying Essence** *($65 for 1.3 ounces)*. The good stuff comes well after the preservatives, and so adds up to only a negligible amount. If you're going to splurge on a moisturizer for normal to dry skin, this is not the one to consider.

☹ $$$ **B.H.-24-Day/Night Essence** *($65 for two 0.5-ounce containers)* consists of two very small bottles, each containing a liquid that is supposed to be worn under your regular moisturizer. The large amount of alcohol in both liquids is an irritant. Basically, this is an overpriced toner; if the moisturizer you are using is a good one, you shouldn't need a second undercoat. And if you have dry skin, you shouldn't be using a moisturizer with alcohol. The collagen in these products cannot affect the collagen in your skin.

☺ **Gentle Sun Block Cream SPF 22** *($20 for 3.8 ounces)* is a very good, pure titanium dioxide–based sunscreen in a slightly matte base that includes talc. It is an option for normal to slightly oily skin.

☺ **Sun Block Face Cream SPF 35** *($22 for 1.7 ounces)* is a very good, in-part titanium dioxide–based sunscreen for someone with dry skin, but the rather ordinary moisturizing base isn't the most exciting.

☹ **Sun Block Lip Treatment, SPF 15** *($15 for 1 ounce)* doesn't contain the UVA-protecting ingredients avobenzone, titanium dioxide, or zinc oxide, and is not recommended.

☺ $$$ **Sun Block Stick SPF 35** *($18 for 0.31 ounce)* is a very good, in-part titanium dioxide–based sunscreen with a small amount of tint for someone with dry skin. Unfortunately, the amount you get in this product wouldn't last you more than a day if you were to use it properly.

☺ $$$ **Translucent Sun Block Stick SPF 30** *($20 for 0.31 ounce)* is similar to the SPF 35 above and the same comments apply.

☹ **Sun Protection Emulsion SPF 8 Waterproof** *($16 for 5 ounces)* has a paltry, low SPF 8; doesn't contain the UVA-protecting ingredients of avobenzone, zinc oxide, or titanium dioxide; and is not recommended.

☺ **Ultra Light Sun Block Lotion SPF 30** *($25 for 3.3 ounces)* is a very good, in-part titanium dioxide–based sunscreen in a slightly moisturizing base. It would be best for someone with normal to oily skin.

☹ **Self-Tanning Moisturizing Gel** *($18 for 5 ounces)* contains too much alcohol and that can be drying to the skin; nevertheless it does contain dihydroxyacetone, the same ingredient in all self tanners that turns the skin brown.

## Shiseido *The* Skin Care

☹ $$$ **Gentle Cleansing Cream** *($23.50 for 4.3 ounces)* lists alcohol as the third ingredient, and that doesn't make it gentle—it makes it problematic for causing dry or irritated skin.

☺ **$$$ Gentle Cleansing Foam** *($23.50 for 4.8 ounces)* is a standard, detergent-based cleanser that can be drying for most skin types, though it may be an option for someone with oily skin. It does contain fragrance.

☹ **Gentle Cleansing Foam** *($23.50 for 5 ounces)* has alcohol as the third ingredient, so the name Gentle doesn't apply and this product isn't recommended.

☹ **Hydro Refining Softener** *($30 for 5 ounces)* has alcohol as the second ingredient, which makes this too irritating and drying for all skin types.

☺ **$$$ Soothing Spray** *($20 for 2.5 ounces)*. This few cents' worth of ingredients is OK for most skin types, but it is also just a very ordinary and do-nothing kind of product.

☹ **Day Essential Moisturizer SPF 10** *($34 for 2.5 ounces)* is a sunscreen that does contain avobenzone for UVA protection, but at SPF 10 it's just a waste. With all the many great SPF 15 products available (and that's the standard recommended by the American Academy of Dermatology), an SPF 10 is inadequate for basic healthy skin care. If it's going to be essential, it should at least meet the basic criterion for sun-damage protection.

☹ **Day Essential Moisturizer, Enriched SPF 10** *($34 for 2.5 ounces)* is similar to the one above and the same comments apply.

☹ **Day Essential Moisturizer, Light SPF 10** *($34 for 2.5 ounces)* is similar to the one above and the same comments apply.

☺ **Day Protective Moisturizer SPF 15** *($30 for 1.4 ounces)* is a very good, titanium dioxide–based sunscreen, although the price is completely unwarranted (Neutrogena has similar products for far less). It would work well for someone with normal to slightly dry or slightly oily skin. It does contain fragrance.

☺ **Night Essential Moisturizer** *($36 for 2.5 ounces)* is about as boring a moisturizer as you can find, with a mere dusting of interesting water-binding agents. Why bother? It does contain thiotaurine, a good antioxidant, but the amount is so negligible as to make it barely present, and there are lots of great antioxidants—this is not the only one.

☺ **Night Essential Moisturizer, Enriched** *($36 for 2.5 ounces)* is similar to the one above, only this version contains Vaseline (yes, Vaseline). This does make it better for dry skin but there isn't much reason to spend this kind of money on such an ordinary moisturizer.

☺ **Night Essential Moisturizer, Light** *($36 for 2.5 ounces)* is a good, standard (though overpriced) moisturizer for dry skin.

☺ **$$$ Eye Revitalizer** *($35 for 0.53 ounce)* is a good basic moisturizer for normal to dry skin, but there is nothing in here special for the eye area; it is simply a standard moisturizer with the same formulation used for the face moisturizers in this group of products.

☺ **$$$ Moisture Relaxing Mask** *($30 for 1.7 ounces)* is a standard, plasticizing-type mask. Other than the plastic-type ingredients in it, this mask is virtually identical in formulation to the various moisturizers in this line.

☹ **T-Zone Balancing Gel** *($25 for 1 ounce)* gives the second ingredient as alcohol, and it also contains menthol. That won't balance anything, but it will cause irritated, red, flaky skin. The third ingredient is cornstarch, which can be a problem for clogging pores.

# Shiseido Makeup

FOUNDATION: ☺ **$$$ Stick Foundation** *($30)* has a very creamy, smooth texture and can go from sheer to full coverage. It is best for dry to very dry skin because it is too emollient for other skin types. All of the following colors can be too pink or orange for most skin tones: Natural Fair Ivory, Natural Light Ivory, Natural Deep Ivory, Natural Light Beige, Natural Deep Beige, Natural Light Pink, and Natural Fair Pink. There is also a shade called Controlling Green that is not recommended for any skin tone, as this color never looks natural, either by itself or with foundation.

☺ **$$$ Fluid Foundation** *($30)* has an agreeable, light texture with sheer to light coverage and a natural finish. This formula is best suited to normal to dry skin and does have some great colors to consider. Avoid these shades, all of which can be too peach or pink for most skin tones: 14, B2, B4, B6, P2, P4, and P6.

☺ **$$$ Benefiance Enriched Revitalizing Foundation SPF 15** *($40)* is a good sheer foundation that blends evenly, leaving a soft matte finish. It also uses in-part titanium dioxide as one of the active sunscreen ingredients. There are 13 great shades, with only three to avoid: B2, B4, and P2 are either too pink or too peach. In many ways this product is quite similar to Neutrogena's with an SPF 20. It is basically a liquid foundation with talc. One word of warning: the salespeople recommend this for dry or combination skin, but it is not appropriate for dry skin.

☺ **$$$ Creme Powder Compact Foundation** *($35)* looks like a cream but has a silky, light finish. That's nice, but all the shades have some amount of shine, plus the color range leans toward the pink and peach side and won't work for everyone.

☺ **$$$ Dual Compact Powdery Foundation** *($30)* is a standard, talc-based pressed powder that can be used wet or dry (though wet can go on streaky and smeary). It comes in an excellent assortment of sheer colors, and you can wear it as a foundation although it is more a pressed powder than anything else.

☹ **Liquid Compact Foundation SPF 15** *($35)* isn't liquid at all but, rather, a very dry finish, cream-to-powder foundation. The SPF 15 with titanium dioxide is excellent. All that would make this a foundation to consider if the colors weren't so blatantly peachy pink. The only shades that look like real skin color are 02 and 04!

☹ **Shiseido PreMakeup Cream SPF 8** *($24.50 for 1.4 ounces)* is really just a good moisturizer for someone with normal to dry skin, despite the claims that it will hold makeup and fill in lines. The demonstration on the back of my hand was not the least bit convincing. Even the salesperson commented that it didn't look like it was working the way she was taught by the line representative who trained her. Although this SPF 8 cream does contain titanium dioxide, the SPF number leaves much to be desired.

☺ $$$ **Vital Perfection Tinted Moisturizer SPF 10** *($26)* has good, titanium dioxide–based UVA protection, but SPF 15 would be a lot better. True to the nature of tinted moisturizers, this blends on very sheer and is best for minimal coverage. Although this has oil, there is talc in here too, which leaves a slight powdery finish on the skin. Of the four shades, only #40 is too orange to consider.

☺ **Sun Block Compact SPF 32** *($25)* offers a smooth, medium-coverage pressed-powder finish with very good UVA protection. However, knowing the way powder is applied, it is doubtful you would be getting the designated SPF. A smart way to use this would be to partner it with a good sunscreen in lotion form to ensure even protection AND a matte finish. There are only two shades here, but they are both acceptable.

☹ <u>CONCEALER:</u> **Concealer for Circles** *($18)* comes in only two shades; 01 is too peach for most skin tones, and 02 is too gold for most skin tones. I wish the colors were better, because the texture of this product is smooth and it blends well. **Concealer for Lines** *($18)* is a standard pencil that comes in two light shades; one is rather peach and the other pink. They don't hide lines in the least, they just look like a very different color from the foundation, and they can easily crease.

☺ $$$ <u>POWDER:</u> **Natural Pressed Powder** *($23.50)* is a standard, talc-based powder that goes on very sheer and soft, and the colors are great. It can be a little too emollient for those with oily skin. **Rich Matte Film** *($29)* is a loose powder with a suede-like texture and a soft, even finish. There is only one shade, called Translucent, and it is very light and opaque enough to only make it suitable for very fair skin tones.

☺ $$$ <u>BLUSH:</u> **Singles** *($24.50)* offer a decent selection of silky matte shades that blend on quite sheer. There are a few shiny shades to watch out for. **Modulative Blush** *($29)* is a compact with three shades of blush in the same tone. These are matte and apply well, blending into one sheer color on the face.

☹ <u>EYESHADOW:</u> Shiseido has made the decision to discontinue its single eyeshadows in favor of the **Duos** *($22.50)*. That is a shame, because many of the single shadows were sheer and matte, whereas the existing duos are all shiny and have a powdery texture that tends to flake off. **Shadow Play** *($23)* consists of one set of three shiny, white shadows that are no doubt in line with the shinefest being seen in most cosmetics lines today. Give these a try only if you want your eyeshadow to speak louder than you do.

**EYE AND BROW SHAPER:** ☺ The **Eye Liner Pencil** *($13.50)* has a smooth application that stays creamy and tends to smudge. **Eye Brow Pencil** *($12)* has a drier, powdery application that should stay in place after it is blended. **$$$ Eyebrow Shapeliner** *($20)* is an extremely overpriced, lightly tinted brow gel that has a sticky texture and a poor brush applicator. **$$$ Eyebrow Shadow Liner** *($23)* feature two shades of brown to black matte powder in a compact. These can be used for filling in the brows or lining the eyes. The brush included is too loose to apply eye or brow color with any precision, and much less expensive options are plentiful. **$$$ Shadow Liner** *($26)* is virtually identical to the one above, only this has three shades of almost the same color, which tend to flake, making this difficult to use. **Liquid Liner** *($18.50)* does allow for drawing a thin line, but the brush is hard to control. This is intense color that dries slowly but should stay put.

☹ **Fine Liner** *($24; refills $9)* is a liquid eyeliner with a brush that is only capable of applying a thick line. The color is seeped into the brush much like a fountain pen, making it hard to control how much comes out at once. Strangely enough, the only available color, olive green, is labeled as being black!

**LIPSTICK AND LIP PENCIL:** ☺ Shiseido offers an imposing selection of lip colors, with some good formulas and wonderful textures. **$$$ Advanced Performance Lipstick** *($17)* is a standard but good creamy lipstick with a glossy finish. **Matte Variations Lipstick** *($15)* is really just a good creamy, full-coverage lipstick that feels great and has enough stain to last reasonably well. **$$$ Staying Power Lipstick** *($18.50)* is a richly pigmented lipstick that can't outperform similar ultra-matte versions from Revlon's ColorStay to Maybelline's Great Wear. Shiseido's version goes on smoothly, but leaves a greasy finish that assures only minimal staying power, although the colors do tend to stain the lips. There is an unnecessary **Staying Power Lipstick Remover** *($13.50)* that is supposed to be a special remover for the Staying Powder Lipstick, but the lipstick comes off all by itself or after wiping with a tissue, just like any other lipstick. **$$$ Advanced Performance Lip Gloss** *($16)* is not so much a gloss as it is just a greasy, sheer lipstick. The colors are bright and soft, but don't expect them to stick around too long. **Lip Liner Pencil** *($13.50)* is a standard, dry pencil that applies well and has a noticeable stain, so fading won't be as obvious.

**MASCARA:** ☺ **$$$ Advanced Performance Mascara** *($18)* is OK, but nothing special or worthy of this price tag. **Optimal Volume Mascara** *($17)* tends to clump and make lashes look spiky and uneven instead of full. That's disappointing, because it does build decent length and thickness.

☺ **$$$ Waterproof Mascara** *($18)* does stay on under water and builds nicely thick and long lashes with minimal effort and clumping.

☹ **BRUSHES:** Shiseido offers a small **Brush Set** *($49)* that features six makeup tools that most anyone would have difficulty with. All of the brushes are either too small, too floppy, or too poorly constructed to do much good. These are overpriced, to say the least.

## Shu Uemura

Shu Uemura is a makeup artist who started his skin-care line back in 1968. His Tokyo-based line has been available in the United States for the past ten years. It isn't widely known, but it gets attention in fashion magazines and is sold at Barneys in New York and Los Angeles, at Nordstrom in San Francisco, and at the Shu Uemura boutique in Los Angeles and New York. The line has an exclusive yet simple flair. The products are plainly packaged and the descriptions are straightforward and re-freshingly uncomplicated. Unfortunately, I can't say the same for the prices.

Shu Uemura's literature claims that "recent environmental conditions for our skin have taken a turn for the worse, due to the aggravating air pollution, the increase of social stresses, and the recent trends in foods and lifestyle. . . . [The products are] composed effectively to promote the skin's natural metabolism without giving it more nourishing materials than it needs."

None of these products can provide nourishment for the skin, nor can they counteract the effects of pollution or stress, because we don't know what those effects are. More to the point, none of these products contains anything new or different, just the same old standard stuff, *and* without a sunscreen. (So much for preventing environmental damage.) Several of the products do contain DNA. We all know put-ting DNA on the skin, or even taking DNA pills, can't affect our own DNA, right? If it could, you would be risking cancer and all kinds of possible mutations. It is just a gimmick—nothing more, nothing less.

Where Uemura does excel is in eyeshadows, blushes, and brushes. Many of the colors aren't much to look at, but the textures are some of the most exquisite around. It is worth the trouble to check out the application of these shades just to see how creamy, smooth, and evenly they cover. And don't forget to check out this vast collec-tion of brushes. Some of the prices are just absurd, but it is one of the most extensive collections of brush sizes being sold anywhere. For more information about Shu Uemura, call (800) 743-8205 or visit the Web site at www.shu-uemura.co.jp.

## Shu Uemura Skin Care

☺ $$$ **Cleansing Beauty Oil Balancer** (*$40 for 8.4 ounces*) is a lot of money for mineral oil and corn oil. It will cut through makeup as you wipe it off, but you could just use pure mineral oil and save lots of money and get the same results. It is sup-posed to be washed off, but why do two steps when a gentle water-soluble cleanser can do it all in one step?

☹ **Cleansing Beauty Oil Fresher** *($40 for 8.4 ounces)* is almost identical to the product above, and the same review applies.

☹ **Cleansing Oil Foam** *($15 for 1.9 ounces)* is almost identical to the ones above and the same review applies.

☺ **Cleansing Water** *($25 for 8.4 ounces)* is a detergent-based gel cleanser that would be good for most skin types, though it can be on the drying side.

☺ $$$ **Gommage Extra Gentle Facial Peeling Cream** *($38 for 2.3 ounces)* will exfoliate the skin, but it can also leave a greasy film. The talc and clay can cause dryness and irritation, so I would be skeptical of the term "gentle."

☺ $$$ **Moisture Lotion** *($35 for 8.4 ounces)* is a good toner for normal to dry skin.

☺ $$$ **Refreshing Lotion** *($35 for 8.4 ounces)* isn't all that refreshing, but it is a good lightweight toner for slightly dry skin, similar to the Moisture Lotion above.

☺ $$$ **Absolute Cream** *($40 for 1.05 ounces)* is a good moisturizer for dry skin.

☺ $$$ **Moisture Fluid** *($40 for 1.6 ounces)* is similar to the Absolute Cream above only in lotion form and the same basic review applies.

☺ $$$ **Principe 21 Bio-Energizing Concentrate** *($60 for 1 ounce)* is supposed to contain revolutionary ingredients to increase cell production (the cosmetics industry has more revolutionary ingredients than the world of medicine). It is actually far less impressive than the other moisturizers in this group of products. There is a teeny amount of aminobutyric acid in here, which is an amino acid that can be a good water-binding agent and may have anti-inflammatory properties.

☺ $$$ **Utowa Beaute Douce Eye Pads** *($33 for 12 packets)* is one of the Utowa products that are supposed to "act in harmony with the biorhythms of your skin" as well as replace lost elasticity and deliver a range of other wishes for skin. The ingredients don't live up to those claims in the least. While there are lots of water-binding agents in this product, it contains more alcohol than any of those, and that makes it potentially irritating for skin.

☹ **Utowa Beaute Douce Moisture Mask** *($66 for eight packets)* contains too much alcohol to be recommended for any skin type.

☹ **Utowa Day/Night Double Concentrate** *($125 for 1 ounce each of Day Concentrate and Night Concentrate)* includes no sunscreen, and without that there is little reason to bother with the Day part, plus the Day part contains alcohol as the third ingredient, which makes it too drying for all skin types. The Night Concentrate has the same problem.

☹ **Cicica Water** *($9.50 for 1.7 ounces)* is, despite the claims, just nitrogen and slip agents. Nitrogen is a gas, and not bad when present in plant food or water, but it's a do-nothing ingredient for your skin, because it would just be released into the atmosphere.

☺ $$$ **Balancing Mask** *($33 for 2.2 ounces)* is supposed to be ideal for oily skin, but the thickening agents and plant oils in here would be a problem, leaving the face more oily and running the risk of clogging pores. It could be good for someone with dry skin.

# Shu Uemura Makeup

<u>FOUNDATION:</u> There are seven foundation types in this line, and all but three have an exceptionally narrow range of colors. Trying to find your shade among four or five selections is a frustrating experience. Consolidation would be a good idea for this line, or increasing the color options. There are many choices for very light to medium skins, but virtually nothing for darker skin tones.

☺ $$$ **Foundation Fluide S SPF 8** *($26)* is a titanium dioxide–based sunscreen, but the SPF would be far better if it were an SPF 15 because as is you can't rely on it for daily sun-damage protection. This one does go on sheer and smooth and of the eight colors, half are quite good. Avoid #130, #165, #355, and #575.

☺ $$$ **Foundation Fluid N SPF 8** *($26)* is a liquid foundation with an even, soft finish. The SPF is titanium dioxide–based, but the number is disappointing and means this can't be relied on for daily protection. The color range is large (30 shades!) and quite good, and the texture is one of the better options in this line for normal to dry skin. The colors to avoid are: #185, #325, #375, #584, #754, and #775.

☺ $$$ **UV Powder Foundation SPF 26** *($30)* This smooth, sheer, talc-free powder has four great colors, and now officially lists titanium dioxide as the active sunscreen agent. Although there are more and more powders with sun protection available, keep in mind that it takes a liberal application to get the SPF protection indicated on the label. A light dusting of powder will not provide adequate sun protection. By the way, Neutrogena's SPF 30 Pressed Powder *($14.29)* is available for about half this price, and has even better all-day protection.

☺ $$$ **UV Cream Foundation SPF 31** *($30)* is an in-part titanium dioxide–based compact foundation. It has a smooth, fairly greasy cream-to-powder finish and a small range of five colors that are all excellent. It would be best for someone with normal to dry skin.

☺ $$$ **UV Liquid Foundation SPF 21** *($30)* has a great in-part titanium diox-ide–based sunscreen and a light, fluid texture that dries to a matte finish This is appropriate for those with normal to oily skin who prefer medium coverage and have the knack for blending this systematically—the formula spreads well and dries quickly. Of the five colors, these two should be avoided: Pink 118 and Beige 250.

☻ **Make-Up Cake** *($22)* is a very thick, heavy, mineral oil–based foundation that isn't the best unless you want opaque, noticeable coverage that won't hold up past the lunch hour.

☺ **Nobara Waterproof Cream Foundation** *($19.50)* is a cream-to-powder foundation with a matte powder finish. Unfortunately the powder finish doesn't hold up; the waxes and oil in here show through fairly quickly, so it's only appropriate for normal to dry skin. The 13 shades are mostly neutral, but there are some obvious pink and peach ones to watch out for. It isn't anymore waterproof than any other cream-to-powder base makeup.

☹ **CONCEALER: Cover Crayon** *($18)* is a two-ended pencil concealer. Both pencils and all four shades are too peach or pink for most all skin tones. **Mark Concealer** *($19)* comes in a tube and has a smooth but very opaque texture and dry finish. This is potent stuff and very easy to overdo, and then it just looks heavy. There are three shades, and the only one to avoid is Pink 5. **Base Control** *($26)* is a group of color correctors using a mineral-oil base that go on extremely sheer but add a strange color to the skin and don't help correct color problems. Isn't that what foundation is for? This just adds another layer to the skin, and if you have any other skin type than dry, this is going to feel greasy.

**POWDER:** ☺ **$$$ Face Powder** *($25)* is a standard, talc-based loose powder with a soft, dry finish. Most of the colors are excellent, but avoid peach, purple, pink 100, pink 200,  pink 300, and pink 5.

☹ **Compact Powder** *($30)* has a smooth finish but strange colors. The one called "One Colorless" works, but the rest simply don't look like skin color.

☺ **$$$ Face Powder C with Puff** *($50)* is a talc-based loose powder that comes in a generous 3.5-ounce tub, though I doubt anyone really needs this much powder. Even a 1-ounce container of loose powder can last for months and months. There are three colors; one is shiny and the other two are for pale skin only.

**BLUSH:** ☺ **$$$ Glow On** *($18)* has an ultra-sheer, soft finish. There are a huge range of colors to choose from, and some excellent matte shades. The shiny ones are clearly identified.

☺ **$$$ Luminizer** *($20)* is a sheer and creamy twist-up highlighter stick that can be used anywhere. It leaves a shiny finish on the skin that will eventually appear greasy and doesn't have great staying potential.

**EYESHADOW:** ☺ **Pressed Eyeshadows** *($15)* have one of the most silky-smooth textures, and they go on beautifully, without streaking or flaking. Most powders this smooth have a difficult time clinging evenly, but not these. The color selection features close to 80 shades, with half of those being matte! The remaining shiny shades are labeled as being Iridescent, Perle, or Metallic.

☹ **Cream Eyeshadow** *($12)* are creamy to the point of being greasy, and although they are sheer, they are also messy to use, easily crease and smear, and are definitely not for anyone who wants their eye makeup to last.

☺ **Etincell Iridescent Eyeshadow** *($15)* is finely milled shiny powder for eyes that comes in small pots. For intense shine, they'll work, but the mess these can create is a nuisance.

☺ <u>EYE AND BROW SHAPER:</u> The price for these ordinary pencils is just beyond belief; I had to check the numbers twice just to be sure I wasn't seeing things. The pencils are decent, but the prices are completely indecent. $$$ **Retractable Eyeliner** *($28; $15 for refills)* and **Retractable Eyebrow Pencil** *($37)* are standard, twist-up pencils with a smooth application. **Eyebrow Pencil** *($15)* is a very standard pencil that goes on almost the same as the retractable. **Kajal Eye Liner** *($13)* comes in two shades and is a fairly greasy pencil, which means it can easily smear and smudge. $$$ **Hard Formula Eyebrow Pencil** *($20)* is just that, hard to get on. It does have a more dry appearance on the brow but it can also be more difficult to apply.

☺ <u>LIPSTICK AND LIP PENCIL:</u> **Lip Rouge** *($15)* has three types of finishes: Sheer, which isn't all that sheer but does have a good creamy, slightly glossy finish; Matte, which is fairly creamy and not really all that matte; and Neutral, which is a standard, cream-finish lip color. Be careful, lots of these colors are shiny. $$$ **Powder Lipstick Rouge** *($27)* is Shu Uemura's version of Revlon's ColorStay Lipstick and it has lots in common with it. This one has a dry finish and, like the new version of ColorStay, doesn't feel powdery; it also tends not to flake or chip like some ultra-matte lipsticks can. But there's is no reason to spend $27 on this one instead of $7.39 for the ColorStay version. $$$ **Lip Gloss** *($20)* is a group of standard, incredibly overpriced pot glosses that have a slightly sticky texture. **Pencil Lipliner** *($15)* and $$$ **Retractable Lipliner** *($28; $15 for refills)* are almost identical. Both are very standard lip pencils with smooth applications, but the one you don't have to sharpen is by far easier to use.

<u>MASCARA:</u> ☺ $$$ **Mascara Basic** *($27)* is wildly overpriced but does go on evenly and quickly. It builds lots of length but very little thickness, but it stays on well throughout the day.

☹ $$$ **Mascara** *($20)* comes in circus-clown colors that have little appeal, unless having green eyelashes excites you. The brown shade is misleading—it's actually a coppery red!

☺ $$$ <u>BRUSHES:</u> *($5 to $260).* There is an amazing selection of **Brushes** in the Shu Uemura lineup, with dozens to choose from. Their prices are beyond belief. There is no reason to spend over $15 to $20 on any makeup brush. Despite the claims about exotic hair sources, a brush doesn't have to be sable or badger to work. Fortunately, the line has many reasonably priced brushes too.

# Signature Club A (see Adrien Arpel)

# Sisley

I often wonder what it would be like to be a fly on the wall at a meeting of Sisley marketing executives when they sit down to establish the prices for their products. I imagine it must go something like this: "Let's see, this product is really similar to a drugstore moisturizer that costs $9 for 6 ounces, but if we package it in an elegant box, put it in a matching jar with a shiny black cap, play up the European know-how angle with French words and accents on the label, and stick in some exotic-sounding plant extracts and oils, we can probably charge $145 for 2 ounces. Women just love that kind of foolishness." Even if that isn't what they are really saying behind closed doors, it comes through loud and clear on the product label and in the brochures. What is perhaps most distressing is that the Sisley formulations are some of the most embarrassingly ordinary yet outrageously and insultingly overpriced I've seen. I can emphatically state that there is nothing in these products you can't find at the drugstore from lines such as Nivea, Pond's, Neutrogena, Eucerin, and L'Oreal; and actually, those lines have far better and more interesting products than this one does.

When it comes to skin-care information, Sisley's is best described as spurious. For example, it states that "oily skin, which is thicker [there is no research anywhere showing this to be true]... is very well protected and ages less quickly than other skin types." That myth was put to rest years ago with the research about sun damage. Oily skin prevents dry skin, but dry skin is unrelated to skin's wrinkling or to the processes involved in aging.

Sisley's makeup is a bit more straightforward than its skin care, at least in terms of exaggerated claims, but the shockingly high prices are still intact and made all the more insulting by makeup that barely makes it across the finish line in terms of texture and performance. Let me assure you that there is absolutely nothing within Sisley's makeup line that is worth the imposing price tags. It is more or less an adjunct to an expertly packaged, slickly marketed skin-care line that, if you dig beneath the surface and expose the roots, is just good old-fashioned smoke and mirrors. For more information about Sisley, call (214) 528-8006 or visit the Web site at www.sisley.tm.fr.

# Sisley Skin Care

☺ $$$ **Botanical Cleansing Milk with Hawthorn for Dry/Sensitive Skin** (*$65 for 8.4 ounces*) is an exceptionally mundane, mineral oil–based cold cream. It can leave a greasy film on the skin, and if you are of the mind to waste this kind of money on a product that has more in common with Pond's Cold Cream than anything else, go right ahead if you have dry skin. The hawthorn extract in here can dilate capillaries, which may be a problem for some skin types. It does contain fragrance.

☹ **Botanical Cleansing Milk with Sage for Combination/Oily Skin** *($65 for 8.4 ounces)* is similar to the product above, only with sage, a skin irritant. Everything about this product is unacceptable for someone with oily skin.

☹ **Botanical Soapless Cleanser for All Skin Types** *($55 for 4 ounces)* is indeed soapless, but it does contain several very drying and potentially irritating standard detergent cleansing agents, including sodium lauryl sulfate as the first ingredient!

☹ **Buff and Wash Botanical Facial Gel for Daily Use** *($74 for 3.5 ounces)* contains standard synthetic scrub particles (ground-up plastic) in a base of thickening agents, castor oil, mineral oil, and a tiny amount of plant oils. It also contains a good amount of lemon, and that can be a skin irritant. For this price, the sheer mediocrity of this standard scrub for dry skin is just shocking.

☺ **$$$ Botanical Gentle Facial Buffing Cream, for All Skin Types** *($60 for 1.3 ounces)* is just wax, clay, and synthetic scrub particles (ground-up plastic). The clay makes it fairly drying and not appropriate for most skin types. It can be an option for normal to slightly oily skin, although the waxes in here are problematic for clogging pores.

☺ **$$$ Botanical Eye and Lip Special Cleansing Lotion** *($65 for 4.2 ounces)* is a standar, detergent-based makeup remover, and when I say standard I mean very standard! It does contain fragrance.

☹ **Botanical Floral Spray Mist** *($61 for 4.2 ounces)* is just water, witch hazel, and preservatives for the most absurd amount of money I've ever seen. Witch hazel is a skin irritant, as is the orange water in here.

☹ **Botanical Floral Toning Lotion for Dry/Sensitive Skin** *($60 for 8.4 ounces)* is similar to the Mist above, and the same review applies.

☹ **Botanical Grapefruit Toning Lotion, for Combination/Oily Skin** *($61 for 8.4 ounces)* contains alcohol and grapefruit, which are useless for oily skin. These two ingredients can leave skin feeling irritated, dry, and red.

☹ **Botanical Lotion with Tropical Resins for Combination/Oily Skin** *($56 for 4.2 ounces)* contains too much alcohol to be recommended for any skin type. The tropical resins are just standard plant extracts and some are irritants while others are anti-irritants.

☺ **$$$ Hydra-Flash with B-Hydroxyacid and Natural Plant Extracts for All Skin Types** *($160 for 2.1 ounces)* contains no beta hydroxy acid of any kind. This is just an extremely overpriced, standard moisturizer for dry skin. If you're going to overspend on skin care, this is not the product to even vaguely consider.

☹ **Botanical Day Cream with Lily for Normal to Oily Skin** *($115 for 1.6 ounces)* has isopropyl myristate as its second ingredient, and the fifth is mineral oil. Why anyone with oily skin would want to spend this kind of money on ingredients known to make oily skin worse is anyone's guess. It contains horse serum but your guess about that ingredient is as good as mine.

☹ **Botanical Fluid Compound with Tropical Resins, for Combination/Oily Skin** *($127 for 1.7 ounces)* contains even more oil than the one above and the same basic comments apply.

☺ $$$ **Botanical Intensive Day Cream** *($220 for 1.7 ounces)* isn't even remotely intensive, and as a day cream it is actually a problem, because it has no sunscreen. Some plant extracts appear at the very end of the ingredient list, which makes them nonexistent at best. If you can get over the price—wait, there is no reason to get over this price. The plant extracts in here are primarily skin irritants including juniper, *Centella asiatica,* and marjoram.

☺ $$$ **Botanical Intensive Night Cream for All Skin Types** *($248 for 1.6 ounces).* I don't have any good words for how out-of-date and beyond dull this moisturizer is. The price would be laughable if there weren't women out there wasting their hard-earned money on this do-nothing product.

☺ $$$ **Botanical Night Cream for Dry/Sensitive Skin** *($137 for 1.5 ounces)* is a Vaseline-based moisturizer with thickeners, plant oil, and minimal water-binding agents. It also contains arnica, a plant extract that can be irritating for most skin types, but especially for sensitive skin.

☺ $$$ **Botanical Moisturizer with Cucumber** *($115 for 1.5 ounces)* is a standard, mineral oil–based moisturizer with absolutely nothing else of any consequence.

☺ $$$ **Botanical Night Cream with Collagen and Woodmallow** *($137 for 1.6 ounces)* is a mineral oil– and lanolin-based moisturizer. It would be good for dry skin, but the price is what's painful for this 50-cent formula. The teeny amount of collagen in here has no impact on skin, and the mallow can be an anti-inflammatory but in this minuscule amount it can have no effect on skin at all.

☺ $$$ **Botanical Protective Day Cream for Dry/Sensitive Skin** *($115 for 1.6 ounces)* is similar to the one above, and the same review applies, only without sunscreen this product is completely inappropriate for daytime.

☺ $$$ **Botanical Restorative Facial Cream with Shea Butter for Day and Night** *($137 for 1.6 ounces)* is similar to the Botanical Night Cream above with the addition of shea butter; that is a good emollient, but it's hardly unique to this product.

☺ $$$ **Botanical Tensor Immediate Lift** *($143 for 1.05 ounces).* These plants won't lift your skin anywhere, though krameria can be a skin irritant, tormentil is a red dye, and the Chinese herb rehemannia has no known benefit for skin, while there's a slight potential for irritation from the witch hazel in here. This is a standard moisturizer for dry skin that is priced as if it contained something special, but it doesn't.

☺ $$$ **Botanical Night Complex for All Skin Types** *($237 for 1 ounce)* isn't all that botanical—most of the plant stuff is at the end of the ingredient list—but even if it were, that wouldn't make it better for the skin. This is a really average moisturizer that would be OK for someone with normal to dry skin.

☺ $$$ **Botanical Throat Cream** (*$127 for 1.5 ounces*) is a mineral oil–based moisturizer with thickeners, plant oil, fragrance, and preservatives. The handful of plant extracts in here can be skin irritants, including lady's mantle and krameria.

☺ $$$ **Ecological Compound Day and Night for All Skin Types** (*$176 for 4.2 ounces*) is a mineral oil–based moisturizer with just thickening agents, fragrance, preservatives, and plant extracts (of which most are skin irritants). Someone at Sisley has to be laughing at the women willing to spend this kind of money on wax and mineral oil.

☺ $$$ **Botanical Tinted Moisturizer for All Skin Types** (*$78 for 1.4 ounces*) has a tint that isn't for everyone and is just water, mineral oil, plant oil, preservatives, and fragrance. Gee, I didn't think it could get more boring, but it just did.

☺ $$$ **Sisleya** (*$300 for 1.7 ounces*). It's up to the consumer to decide if minuscule amounts of algae, shiitake mushroom extract, *Gingko biloba* extract, butcher's broom extract, and vitamins are worth this kind of money (but most all of these show up in other skin-care products for a fraction of this price). All of those can have an anti-inflammatory effect on skin, though the horsetail in here can be a skin irritant. The vitamins in this one are a mere dusting and barely present to have any effect whatsoever for skin.

☹ **Botanical Facial Sun Cream SPF 8** (*$154 for 2 ounces*) is sun damage waiting to happen. Not only is the SPF inadequate for daily wear, it does not contain the UVA-protecting ingredients of titanium dioxide, zinc oxide, or avobenzone, and is not recommended.

☺ $$$ **Botanical Sun Block SPF 20** (*$100 for 1.5 ounces*) is a good, though incredibly overpriced, in-part titanium dioxide–based sunscreen. To suggest that there are equally good (if not better) sunscreens at the drugstore for a fraction of the price is an understatement.

☹ **Botanical Sun Oil SPF 5** (*$100 for 1.5 ounces*) comes with a brochure that states this product "encourages an even, long-lasting tan while screening out harmful sun rays." This dangerous notion is like suggesting you can smoke cigarettes while filtering out the harmful tars that cause lung cancer. This type of product is injurious to skin, and it is completely unethical for a skin-care company to promote.

☺ $$$ **Botanical Self Tanning Lotion Medium** (*$93 for 3.5 ounces*), like all self tanners, uses dihydroxyacetone to turn the skin brown. Unlike other self tanners, this one is the most expensive one I've reviewed and the most ordinary for the money.

☹ **Botanical Facial Mask, with Tropical Resins for Combination/Oily Skins** (*$71 for 1.5 ounces*) is a standard clay mask that contains several ingredients, including isopropyl myristate, that are problematic for someone with oily skin. It also contains fragrance. The plant extracts in here are a mix of irritants (frankincense and myrrh) and anti-irritants, like burdock.

☺ $$$ **Radiant Glow Mask** *($71 for 2.15 ounces)* is just water, wax, and clay. It is a very standard, very boring clay mask that would be an option for normal to dry skin, but I just can't imagine why anyone would want to spend this kind of money on such futility.

☺ $$$ **Botanical Eye and Lip Contour Complex** *($137 for 0.5 ounce)*. What a waste of money for an ordinary lightweight moisturizer.

☺ $$$ **Botanical Eye and Lip Contour Balm** *($93 for 1 ounce)*. You really do have to sit down for this one. This contains water, witch hazel, tomato extract, thickeners, and preservatives. Honest! How this line has the effrontery to charge this kind of money for this kind of nonsense is just astounding.

# Sisley Makeup

**FOUNDATION:** ☺ $$$ **Transmat** *($68)* is a lightweight but creamy foundation with a natural, sheer finish. The six shades leave many skin tones without a choice, but given the ludicrous price for this very basic makeup, that's not so bad. Avoid #1 and #5, both of which are too peach for most skin tones.

☹ **Botanical Tinted Moisturizer** *($78)* also has a creamy texture and leaves a moist finish. The four shades are quite pink or peachy and at this price it is not recommended.

☹ **CONCEALER:** **Phytocernes Concealer** *($61)* has a price that is insulting. Are there really women buying this stuff? It has a greasy, easy-to-crease texture and just barely OK colors.

☹ **POWDER:** **Pressed Powder Compact** *($71)* is nothing more than standard pressed powder. It feels silky and nice, but why tempt yourself with this when those features are so easily obtained from most every powder in my Best Products lists at a small fraction of the price? Not to mention that all the shades are too rosy or ash for most skin tones. **Translucent Loose Face Powder** *($56)* also feels great, but of the three colors only #1 is an option, and only then if you have money to burn. **Sun Glow Pressed Powder** *($71)* is the same shiny, orange-toned bronzing powder seen in dozens of other lines that wouldn't have the audacity to charge this much money for such a poor product.

**BLUSH AND EYESHADOW:** ☺ $$$ **Double Blush** *($56)* is a bargain by Sisley's standards—you get two blush tones (although one is more for highlighting) in one compact. These have a dry, soft texture and a few are noticeably shiny but they work.

☺ $$$ **Eye Shadow Singles** *($20)* have a very nice texture and apply darker than they look, but almost every one of them is shiny. What a perfect way to play up any lines around the eyes you had hoped to alleviate with one of Sisley's $100+ eye creams. For a similar line-emphasizing effect, Sisley has **Golden Touch** *($25)*, a cream-to-powder highlighter for eyes, cheeks, or wherever you want to artificially shine.

☹ <u>EYE AND BROW SHAPER:</u> **Eye Pencil** *($34)* and the **Brow Pencil** *($34)* are hopelessly ordinary and greasy enough to smear or smudge shortly after you apply them.

<u>LIPSTICK AND LIP PENCIL:</u> The regular ☺ $$$ **Lipstick** *($34)* and **Long Lasting Lipstick** *($34)* are practically indistinguishable. Both have a very greasy texture and glossy finish that would test even the most lenient definition of "long lasting."

☺ $$$ **Phyto Brilliant Lip Gloss** *($25)* is a standard lip gloss in a tube. It offers minimal stickiness and a maximum price. **Lip Liner** *($34)* is a standard pencil that leans to the greasy side of creamy but does have a good stain. Contrary to the claim, these won't do much to help stop feathering.

☹ <u>MASCARA:</u> **Phyto-Protein Mascara** *($47)* is, without a doubt, one of the most expensive mascaras I've ever purchased. It absolutely created long, thick lashes without clumping, but after just a couple of hours it smeared and started crumbling. What a shame and what a waste of money!

☺ $$$ <u>BRUSHES:</u> Sisley's **Brushes** *($30 to $44)* are a small group of good brushes that are nicely shaped and properly sized. There is nothing too exceptional here, but if you simply must have Sisley brushes, you won't be disappointed.

# *SkinCeuticals*

SkinCeuticals is the line Dr. Sheldon Pinnell started after his falling out with Cellex-C. The history here is that Cellex-C is in a legal battle with Dr. Sheldon Pinnell. Cellex-C is a line of skin-care products that centers around a $70-an-ounce product containing a form of vitamin C called L-ascorbic acid that was researched by Pinnell, although Duke University holds the patent. However, Cellex-C does not feel that Pinnell is the only one who knew about L-ascorbic acid and denies the patent is valid, since Cellex-C was already using the L-ascorbic acid technology. According to Cellex-C, they were "already using L-ascorbic acid in 1991, almost one year before the Duke University patent was issued. Those formulations included 10% L-ascorbic acid at a pH of 2.5 plus tyrosine and zinc, just as they do today. The Duke patent was not even issued until August 1992!"

Before these conflicts arose, Pinnell was in a joint business venture with Cellex-C, endorsing the product and sharing in its success. And successful it was. But by October 1997, the joint venture between Pinnell and Cellex-C had fallen apart. Pinnell then opened his own company, SkinCeuticals, claiming it was the only company using truly stabilized vitamin C, the L-ascorbic acid he claims he invented.

According to Pinnell, Cellex-C is using some dreadful form that is completely unacceptable. How that changed from when he first got involved is unclear.

Cellex-C sued Pinnell and his new company for $100 million in damages caused by the false information SkinCeuticals allegedly released about Cellex-C. Not surprisingly, Cellex-C has also issued a cyber-libel suit for $70 million (Canadian) against SkinCeuticals (and Pinnell) for broadcasting libelous material over the Internet. Lawsuit or not, Pinnell feels his research demonstrates his L-ascorbic acid is a unique skin rejuvenator, the only one the skin can use, and the only ingredient to build collagen and prevent skin degradation. Cellex-C disagrees.

All of this hullabaloo revolves around Pinnell's research on L-ascorbic acid that showed it reduced the effect of sunburn on hairless pigs. Now doesn't that make you want to run out and spend $70 an ounce for a product? Considering the original issue of the stability of the vitamin, and given that Pinnell was willing to endorse products he knew were unstable and therefore ineffective in the first place, why should we now accept that his new line is going to be more reputable or supposedly miraculous?

What is absolutely clear is that there are no published studies showing that vitamin C in any form is paramount or of any vital importance on human skin, much less in the fight against wrinkles. The propaganda about this ingredient, or any "must have" cosmetic ingredient, is established for the sake of selling skin-care products, not for offering women truly viable options about the health of their skin. There are lots of good antioxidants, and vitamin C in any or all of its forms is not the only one. According to Jeffrey Blumberg, Ph.D., associate director and professor, Antioxidants Research Laboratory at Tufts University, in all the years he's been researching in this field to find the "best," there isn't one.

A brochure for the SkinCeuticals line, which features more than 20 products, states, "Each product contains a unique blend of botanical extracts which help restore a youthful, radiant experience." Any time scientists start bandying about cosmetics-babble like "botanicals" and restoring a "youthful radiant experience" (whatever that means), medical and ethical lines have been crossed. And where is the research substantiating any long-term effects of Pinnell's rather expensive products, or even his now-stable L-ascorbic acid? Vitamin C may help skin, but lots of other ingredients do too.

The entire arena of antioxidants is so new, and there are as yet no definitive findings to warrant the cost or tumult. Antioxidants won't get rid of wrinkles or replace sunscreen. They can offer increased sun protection, which is important, but that's it. Of course, that doesn't stop companies from making claims about reversing aging, building collagen, feeding the skin, and healing sun damage, despite the fact that, as Pinnell states in his own paper, published in *Les Nouvelles Esthetiques,* February 1996, "conclusive studies of the effect of this solution [topical vitamin C to reduce sun damage] have not yet been conducted."

In some ways SkinCeuticals is indeed a better line than Cellex-C, not because of the vitamin C issue, which is now so overblown and exaggerated it's become more of a joke than a skin-care treatment, but because SkinCeuticals is less complicated, with far fewer products and relatively fewer wild claims. The sunscreen formulations do all contain part zinc oxide, and while that is great, the price is unreasonable. If you are interested in sunscreens that contain zinc oxide, Olay and Basis both have very good options for a fraction of the price.

A strong point of SkinCeuticals, as is often true for so-called "physician lines," is that most of the products contain no coloring agents. That is indeed better for skin. The downside is that this line gives the impression that it is fragrance-free, although many of the plant extracts and plant oils in these products are there for their fragrance and nothing else. For more information about this line, call (800) 811-1660 or (972) 279-4552 or visit the Web site at www.skinceuticals.com.

☺ **Delicate Cleanser** *($24 for 8 ounces)* isn't all that delicate—it is just an over-priced cold cream–type cleanser for dry skin that can leave a slightly greasy film on the skin. It contains something called mixed fruit acids, but this term is meaningless and doesn't tell you what you would really be putting on your face. Regardless, the pH of this product makes the fruit acids ineffective as exfoliants even if they were the right forms of glycolic or lactic acid. The plant extracts in here, including yarrow and ginseng, can be skin irritants.

☺ **Simply Clean** *($24 for 8 ounces)* is a standard detergent-based cleanser that would work for normal to oily skin, but the price is uncalled-for given this very basic formulation. It also contains fruit acids and the same comments for the Delicate Cleanser above apply for those here as well.

☺ **Equalizing Toner** *($22 for 8 ounces)*. If there were information as to what the mixed fruit acids were, this might be a decent liquid AHA. But without that information you have no idea what you are putting on your skin, and the pH is too high for this to be an effective exfoliant.

☹**Revitalizing Toner** *($22 for 8 ounces)* has witch hazel as the second ingredient, and that makes it too potentially drying or irritating for all skin types. Several of the plant extracts in here can be skin irritants, including thyme, lavender, and horsetail.

☺ **$$$ Renew Overnight, Oily** *($45 for 2 ounces)* lists the second ingredient as mixed fruit acid, and so the same problem exists for this one as with the "mixed fruit acids" in the others above. Besides, how many AHA products does one face need? Even if the fruit acids were known AHA or BHA ingredients, the pH isn't high enough for them to make this an effective exfoliant. Other than that, while this is a good moisturizer for normal to dry skin, several ingredients make it problematic for oily skin.

☺ **$$$ Renew Overnight, Dry** *($45 for 2 ounces)* is almost identical to the Renew Overnight, Oily above and the same comments apply.

The Reviews S

☺ $$$ **Eye Cream** *($53 for 0.67 ounce)* is a good moisturizer for dry skin, and if you are a believer in the vitamin C craze, this product will give you what you are looking for and damage your pocketbook at the same time.

☺ **Eye Renewal Gel** *($27 for 1 ounce)* is a good, lightweight moisturizer for slightly dry skin, but the vague "mixed fruit acid" is useless for skin, especially as the pH of this product isn't low enough for it to be effective as an exfoliant.

☺ $$$ **Eye Gel** *($42 for 0.5 ounce)*. This lightweight eye gel is good for slightly dry skin, and if you want vitamin C, this product contains it.

☺ $$$ **Hydrating B5 Gel** *($55 for 1 ounce)*. This one is up to you; it is a good lightweight moisturizer, but B5 offers nothing that's any more special for skin than lots of other vitamins that show up in skin-care products that cost far less. The claim is that this product is essential for use with the vitamin C products in this line. Now that's confusing! Does that mean that L-ascorbic acid (vitamin C) isn't the big deal, but that you need to layer products to get the miracle results? One more thing: this product is supposed to restore hyaluronic acid, "your skin's natural moisturizer." The skin has dozens and dozens of substances that act as "natural" moisturizers, ranging from glycerin to cholesterol, amino acids, saccharides, and on and on. There is nothing about hyaluronic acid that makes it superior to lots of other water-binding agents.

☺ $$$ **Intense Line Defense** *($50 for 1 ounce)*. This simple group of ingredients is similar to the Hydrating B5 Gel above and the same basic comments apply. You have to decide if the water-binding agent in here, a form of hyaluronic acid, is the answer for your wrinkles versus the vitamin B5 or L-ascorbic acid in the other antiwrinkle products in the SkinCeutical ensemble.

☺ $$$ **Phyto Corrective Gel** *($45 for 1 ounce)* is similar to the Intense Line Defense above only minus the useless mixed fruit extract.

☹ $$$ **Intensive Moisture Replenisher** *($45 for 1.67 ounces)* is a good basic moisturizer for dry skin, with one of the most absurd price tags, given this basic group of ingredients. It does have a small amount of sunscreen, but it doesn't even come close to an SPF 15, so even mentioning that it has this tiny amount of protection is deceptive for a line of supposedly "doctor-endorsed" products.

☹ $$$ **Vita-E** *($45 for 1.67 ounces)* does contain sunscreen ingredients, but is not rated with an SPF. But wait a second, now vitamin E is the great ingredient. This doctor needs to makeup his mind; which is it—vitamin B? vitamin C? vitamin E? AHAs? Maybe they should just put them all together in one product and leave it at that.

☺ $$$ **Skin Firming Cream** *($85 for 1.67 ounces)* has more L-ascorbic acid, but other than that, it's just an overpriced, standard moisturizer for dry skin. The zinc sulfate in here can be a skin irritant.

☹ $$$ **SkinC Serum 10** *($60 for 1 ounce)*. I'm concerned about the zinc sulfate in this product, because it can be a minor skin irritant, but perhaps that swells the skin slightly and makes wrinkles look diminished. It is probably in here as a preservative and if so there's not enough of it to be a problem for skin. Again, if you are looking for vitamin C, this one has plenty, even though how much of it the skin needs and what the outcome is of using it have never been determined.

☺ $$$ **SkinC Serum 15** *($75 for 1 ounce)* is almost identical to the one above only with more ascorbic acid. Given that no specific amount of vitamin C has been established as being effective for skin, this one is as good a guess as the one above.

☺ **Daily Sun Defense SPF 20** *($28 for 3 ounces)* is a good in-part zinc-oxide sunscreen. It would work well for normal to dry skin. Aside from that, this standard ingredient listing does not warrant its price tag. In fact, Olay Complete UV Protection Moisture Lotion SPF 15 ($9.99 for 6 ounces) contains 3% zinc oxide and works equally well for dry skin. Moreover, because you are more likely to use the correct amount of sunscreen with a less-expensive product, the Olay is ultimately the better choice.

☺ **Ultimate UV Defense SPF 30** *($34 for 3 ounces)* is a good, in-part zinc-oxide sunscreen. It would work well for normal to slightly dry skin. It contains several ingredients that could be problematic for oily skin (such as carnauba wax and beeswax) and for dry skin (such as aluminum starch-octenylsuccinate). Other than that, this standard ingredient listing does not warrant the price tag, and Eucerin with SPF 25 will provide you with close to the same protection and the same zinc oxide active ingredient for UVA protection.

☺ **Ultimate UV Defense SPF 45** *($34 for 3 ounces)* is similar to the SPF 30 above and the same basic comments apply.

☺ $$$ **Clarifying Clay Masque** *($33 for 2 ounces)* is an exceptionally standard clay mask. It does contain fruit acids, but they are useless for anything other than looking interesting and sounding natural on an ingredient label.

☹ **Vitamin C Tightening Mask** *($75 for 8 ounces)* contains egg white, cornstarch, tapioca, disinfectant, and preservatives. Is anyone else as offended by this ingredient listing, the tightening claim, and the price tag as I am? And a doctor is endorsing this line!

# *Primacy by SkinCeuticals*

Primacy is a group of four exceedingly overpriced products that primarily claim to be the best at preventing free-radical damage. While the zinc sulfate, vitamin C, and vitamin E may indeed be great antioxidants (though this has not been established for application on human skin; it is all strictly theoretical), there is no research establishing whether or not these can change or prevent one wrinkle.

☺ $$$ C + AHA *($115 for 1 ounce)*. The pH of 3 makes the glycolic and lactic acid effective exfoliants, but the belief in the zinc and vitamin C in here as being the be-all and end-all for skin care is up to you and your pocketbook.

☹ C + E *($115 for 1 ounce)* lists the third ingredient as alcohol, which makes this product too irritating and drying for all skin types. One of the concepts that is fairly well established in skin aging is the matter of inflammation and irritation being damaging to skin, so why it would ever be an option to use unnecessary irritating ingredients is beyond me.

☺ $$$ Serum 20 *($95 for 1 ounce)*. If you are looking for these antioxidants then here they are, but the selection of these over many others ignores a great deal of research.

☺ $$$ Phyto + *($65 for 1 ounce)* is supposed to be effective for inhibiting melanin production to reduce the appearance of brown discolorations on skin. Kojic acid can inhibit melanin production but it is a highly unstable ingredient, and considered more irritating than hydroquinone. Arbutin is a naturally occurring form of hydroquinone, and can suppress melanin production; however, unlike the huge body of research for hydroquinone, arbutin's effectiveness has only been shown in vitro. It also contains bearberry, a plant that contains arbutin.

# SmashBox

The name SmashBox refers to an antique accordion-style camera, which is the icon for the SmashBox studio, a Hollywood-based photography studio. How SmashBox's makeup got launched is a question worth asking, because there is very little that is even remotely exciting about the products and they are ridiculously overpriced. The company's creators, Dean and Davis Factor, have their heritage in makeup: their great-grandfather was legendary makeup artist Max Factor. However, I suspect that if Max Factor knew what his great-grandsons had created, he might be crestfallen. The pencils are incredibly standard, the blushes are almost too soft to show depth on darker skin, the eyeshadows are almost all shiny, and many of the newer products are miles behind what the rest of the industry is moving forward with. Even its latest foundation with SPF was formulated without any UVA-protecting ingredients.

It turns out SmashBox isn't so smashing after all, and pales in comparison to other makeup-artist/designer lines like M.A.C., Bobbi Brown, Stila, Trish McEvoy, and Laura Mercier. So what gives? The line is clearly aimed at the twenty- to thirty-something crowd, offering all the requisite hooks, such as celebrities who claim to use their products (and everyone else's too, of course), hip color names, and enough shine and shimmer to merit a star on the Hollywood Walk of Fame. Of course, the most significant element of all this is whether you want to spend your money on clever marketing with Generation X appeal or on really great products. SmashBox seems to be relying on the former. The plus side, for those in the mood to play with some good foundations and a parade of iridescent colors from blush to lipstick, is that the tester unit is nicely set up for experimentation. For more information about SmashBox, call (888) 558-1490 or visit the Web site at www.smashbox.com.

The three skin-care products here seem to have been a complete afterthought, and the line would be better off without them. ☺ $$$ **Cleanser** *($26 for 3.5 ounces)* is a standard detergent-based face wash that cleans well, but can be somewhat drying for some skin types. It is best for someone with normal to oily skin. ☺ **Smashing Eye Makeup Remover** *($14 for 4 ounces)* is an extremely standard detergent-based wipe-off eye-makeup remover that would work as well as any. ☺ $$$ **Moisturizer** *($28 for 3.5 ounces)* is about as ordinary as a moisturizer can get. It isn't even worth mentioning, but I couldn't exactly pretend it doesn't exist. You should.

<u>FOUNDATION:</u> SmashBox's main strengths are its foundations. The colors and textures are worth a look, although there are few options for very light and darker skin tones.

☺ $$$ **Anti-Shine Foundation** *($26)* is an intriguing product. It is mostly water and magnesium with a hint of color. Magnesium (that's what you find in Milk of Magnesia) absorbs oil very well and does not feel as heavy on the skin as clays do. This formula goes on extremely matte and dry and has great staying power. The colors (or lack thereof) can be a problem, but they go on sheer, and clearly this product is more about shine control than coverage. I wouldn't bet on this for a true foundation, but for those who need an oil-controlling product with some longevity, this is a definite option. It now comes packaged in a tube as opposed to the original cumbersome glass jar.

☺ $$$ **Liquid Foundation** *($28)* is a water-based foundation containing a small amount of oil, making it best for someone with normal to dry skin. It blends on evenly, allowing for light to medium coverage, and with a silky-soft finish. Of the nine shades, the only one to avoid is Sand.

☺ $$$ **Foundation Stick** *($28)* has a creamy, slick texture that can blend out sheer and soft—but it takes some patience to get it to do that. It is similar to most cream-to-powder makeups, making it ideal for normal skin, but any dry patches will look more noticeable when this type of product is applied and the ingredients that keep this in a stick form are not great for oily or blemish-prone skin types. There are eight shades, and the ones to avoid are: Ivory (can be slightly pink), Sand, and Warm Beige (slightly peach).

☺ $$$ **Wet/Dry Foundation** *($32)* is a talc-based, pressed-powder foundation that is much better used dry than wet. It has a smooth, slightly dry texture and five mostly neutral shade; only Sand is too peach for most skin tones.

☺ **$$$ Studio Matte Oil-Free Foundation SPF 15** *($28)* would have been a slam dunk for normal to oily skin craving a matte-finish, lightweight foundation, but alas, this one is without any UVA-protecting ingredients. The texture and finish are reminiscent of Revlon's ColorStay Lite Makeup, which is nicely equipped with a full-spectrum SPF 15 and sells for roughly half this price. However, those who insist on SmashBox will find eight neutral colors to choose from, but no options for darker skin tones.

☹ <u>**CONCEALER:**</u> **Retouch** *($12)* is a thick pencil concealer that goes on creamy and heavy, and will definitely crease into any lines around the eyes. Of the three shades, only #1 is neutral and would work for lighter skin tones.

☺ **$$$** <u>**POWDER:**</u> **Loose Powder** *($28)* is talc-based and has a soft, powdered-sugar texture that goes on soft and light. There are only two colors to choose from, which is almost no choice at all, and both of these are only appropriate for lighter skin tones. **Pressed Powder** *($24)* is also talc-based, and offers more shades than the Loose, with a sheer, silky texture and a soft finish.

☺ **$$$** <u>**BLUSH:**</u> **Blush Compact** *($24)* has some beautiful colors and a very sheer application that will not show up well on darker skin tones. Cost aside, this is an option for lighter skins, though unless you want shiny cheeks, stay away from Viola, Amethyst, and Opal (a shiny white). **Soft Lights** *($26)* is a small collection of large-pan blushes (similar to M.A.C.'s) that offer more color intensity than the one above, but still not enough for dark skins. All of the colors are slightly shiny. For the money, I would just visit the M.A.C. counter.

☺ <u>**EYESHADOWS:**</u> **Single Eye Shadow** *($14)* was what SmashBox sorely needed the last time this line was reviewed, and sad to say, most of the more than 40 colors now available are shiny and go on sheer but choppy. **$$$ Eye Shadow Duos** *($24)* share the same comments, except that many of the pairings are strange (shiny pink and purple) and hard to work with. For fantasy makeup, these are contenders, but you'll still have to put up with sheer colors that don't cover or cling well. There is one matte duo, and it is a good pairing: Fleetwood/Chocolate. **$$$ Cream Eye Shadow** *($18)* is for women who want a cream eyeshadow. Why anyone would want one is another story altogether. As is true for most cream eyeshadows, this one tends to crease and is hard to blend evenly across the eye. The number of shades has expanded and iridescence reigns supreme here. The same is true for **$$$ Highlighters** *($24),* which are five shades of cream-to-powder color that can be worn anywhere to add iridescence to the face, eyes, or lips.

☺ <u>**EYE AND BROW SHAPER:**</u> **Eye Pencil** *($12)* is a standard pencil that comes in a handful of good colors. The texture and application are drier than most, which means these aren't the easiest to apply, but it does decrease the chance of smearing. **$$$ Cream Eye Liner** *($22)* is an interesting notion that sounds better than it ends up working. On the one hand, the creamy, slick texture goes on very smooth and intense. However, these then tend to fade, smear, and run, which makes them not worth the effort, especially at this price. **$$$ Key Lights *($18)*** are standard, thick pencils that are supposed to put the wearer in her "key light," which is photographer's jargon for finding a subject's perfect lighting. What a clever way to describe what amounts to a shiny pencil. **$$$ Brow Tech *($22)*** is made to sound as if it is a revolutionary product for brows. It's merely a split-pan compact with a matte brow powder that you mix with the other half, which is a clear wax. The effect is billed as "supermodel brows," but this look can be achieved with any good brow pencil (where the waxes and pigments are premixed) or a matte eyeshadow set with brow gel or, for a glossy look, a dab of Vaseline. It can also end up looking like a greasy mess if you aren't careful, so experiment with this one first if you want to see how the look works for you.

<u>**LIPSTICK AND LIP PENCIL:**</u> ☺ **Lipstick** *($14)* is available in four finishes: frost, gloss, matte, and sheer. All of them, including the mattes, lean toward the greasy side of creamy, and almost half of the colors are frosted, though the color range is enormous. **Lip Gloss** *($14)* is standard gloss in a tube that has a non-sticky feel and all iridescent colors. For gloss, it's as good as any. **Lip Pencil** *($12)* are standard pencils with a creamy texture and dry finish. They'll work as well as most other pencils in all price ranges.

☺ **Anti-Shine Lipstick** *($14)* turns out to be a mockery of its name: it is obviously shiny and this one needs to be either retooled or renamed.

☺ <u>**MASCARA:**</u> SmashBox's **Mascara** *($14)* has greatly improved since the last edition of this book. Although it took some effort, this builds impressive length and stays on well and is now deserving of a smiling face.

☹ **$$$** <u>**BRUSHES:**</u> The small assortment of **brushes** *($18 to $42)* have come down a bit in price and there are some options to consider, but most of these are either too soft or too large, or their use is too limited to warrant spending this amount of money. The ones to consider are the **$$$ #3 Large Eyeshadow** *($30)*, **#12 Brow Brush** *($19)*, and **#9 Eyeliner Brush** *($18)*, with the eyeliner one being one of the better types of this brush around. It is thin enough to use for both upper and lower lash lines, and you can make the line as thin or thick as you like using almost any eyeshadow.

# *Sonia Kashuk (Makeup Only)*

Target is an interesting place for international makeup artist Sonia Kashuk to launch her line of makeup products. Kashuk has been doing fashion magazine and runway makeup for years and has been a consultant to cosmetics companies too. She also co-wrote *Basic Face,* Cindy Crawford's book on makeup application. While *Ba-*

The Reviews S

*sic Face* was little more than a Crawford photofest, the fundamental makeup information was quite good. (Kashuk probably more than just co-wrote that book, but that's another story.)

Perhaps the only drawbacks with this line, which has many more strong points than weak ones, are that its display allows for no testers, and that the packaging, though attractive (a shiny, slick, silver-plastic casing that has a great mirrorlike surface) doesn't let you see the colors. What a shame, because all the neighboring product lines have far more enticing "see me, feel me" displays. I hope that doesn't hurt this line because there are some good products to consider. For more information, visit www.soniakashuk.com.

☺ <u>FOUNDATION:</u> **Perfecting Liquid Foundation** *($9.99)* is a very sheer-to-light coverage liquid foundation for someone with normal to dry skin; thanks to the amount of silicone and mineral oil it contains, it has a great soft texture. However, the price is not as reasonable as it may appear. There is only 0.6 ounce of foundation here, while most every other foundation sold at drugstores and department stores contains at least a full ounce or more, and that makes Kashuk's one of the most pricey drugstore foundations being sold. Six shades are available, but the packaging is such that it is almost impossible to see the real color. That makes getting the right shade even trickier.

☺ <u>CONCEALER:</u> **Confidential Concealer** *($4.99)* has a soft, creamy texture that you may find has a bit too much slip, which means sheer to light coverage. It does eventually blend well and has a satiny finish, but it can crease, and keep creasing—so if you have lines, be warned. There are only two colors, which seems strange from a makeup artist's line, and while Light is great, Medium is too peach for most skin tones.

☺ <u>POWDER:</u> **Dual Coverage Powder Foundation** *($9.99)* is an extremely standard (but good) talc-based pressed powder that has a soft, silky finish. There are six shades, but because you can't see the color getting the right shade is a guessing game. **Bare Minimum Pressed Powder** *($7.99)* is almost indistinguishable from the Dual Coverage Powder Foundation above and the same comments apply. There are three shades to choose from. **Barely There Loose Powder** *($7.99)* is a standard, talc-based loose powder that comes in one shade called Naked that is an extremely light, almost translucent shade. It has a wonderful silky feel and would work well for very light skin tones.

☺ <u>BLUSH:</u> **Beautifying Blush Powder** *($7.99)* has a great silky feel and goes on quite smooth but almost too sheer. The colors are not visible through the packaging so the five shades require a guessing game as to which one is best. There are also two shades of **Beautifying Blush Cream** *($7.99)* available; these are slightly greasy and shiny, though for a cream blush this works well enough and the shine is relatively subtle.

**EYESHADOW:** ☺ **Enhance Eye Color** *($4.99)* shares the same packaging problem as the rest of the line, making it hard to view the colors for these eyeshadows. That's a disappointment, because several are matte and go on quite softly (similar to the sheer application of Clinique's eyeshadows), and there are good brown tones available. There are about 12 shades to choose from if you don't mind guessing which tone is right for you.

☹ **Enlighten Eye Cream** *($5.99)* consists of small tubes of exceedingly iridescent eyeshadow. These have a cream-to-powder texture that lays down opaque shine that tends to easily crease into the fold of the eye.

☺ **EYE AND BROW SHAPER: Eye Definer** *($4.99)* is a standard, fairly greasy pencil that requires sharpening. There are only two shades (though I'm told other Target stores might have more) that can easily smear if you are lining under the eye. **Eye Smudge** *($4.99)* is a standard pencil that is almost indistinguishable from the Eye Definer except for a slightly thicker application. Both types of pencils can easily be smudged, so the name difference appears to be one of marketing, not application.

**LIPSTICK AND LIP PENCIL:** ☺ **Luxury Lip Color** *($5.99)* is a good cross between a gloss and an opaque lipstick. It gives good coverage but has a very slippery, greasy finish. Again, the 16 shades available are hidden, but if you don't mind guessing, there are some great choices. **Lip Definer** *($4.99)* is identical to the Eye Definer, though the somewhat greasy application is not a problem for the lips, unless you have a problem with lipstick feathering. The four shades are attractive and the color representation on the tip is rather accurate.

☹ **Lip Glossing** *($5.99)* is a standard lip gloss that has a slippery texture and a small assortment of sheer colors. For gloss, it's fine, but it does have a rather surprisingly unpleasant taste.

☺ **MASCARA: Lashify Mascara** *($5.99)* is a very good mascara that builds reasonable length and some thickness without clumping or smearing. With a little effort it can make lashes really long and thick.

**BRUSHES:** There are a handful of brushes available. Their feel isn't as soft and velvety as some of the more expensive brushes you may find, but for the money, they are a consideration. The options are as follows: ☹ **Powder Brush** *($8.99)*, ☹ **Blush Brush** *($8.99)*, ☺ **Lip Brush** *($6.99)*, ☺ **Eye Liner Brush** *($4.99)*, and ☺ **Eyeshadow Brush** *($4.99)*.

# Sothys Paris (Skin Care Only)

It would take an entire book unto itself to deal with all of the exaggerated claims attributed to Sothys Paris's exceedingly ordinary, overly hyped products. Sothys Paris has the same élan and prestige that are associated with other high-end French lines, and, from my perspective, this line relies on prestige and has very little to offer in product content. As is typical with many cosmetics lines that don't yet know about the insidious risk of sun damage, Sothys Paris's daily skin-care routine recommendations do not include the use of a reliable sunscreen. Dozens of moisturizers later and not one UVA-protecting SPF 15 product in its daily skin-care regimens means your face is just asking for wrinkles. There are many other areas where Sothys Paris falls short. The blemish products either contain useless irritants or pore-clogging ingredients, but no disinfectant or effective exfoliant; the cleansers use cleansing agents known for their irritation or are little more than expensive cold creams; and the AHA products are poorly formulated and completely ineffective for exfoliation. There are great moisturizers, and lots of them, but for the money they are fairly basic.

Sothys Paris does an outstanding job of making its products sound remarkable and scientifically sound. For example, the Desquacreme Deep Pore Cleanser is supposed "to increase the complexion's receptiveness by unclogging and desincrustating [sic] the follicular ostium as well as eliminating dead cells." As impressive as that sounds, and although I have no idea how skin becomes "receptive," this simply says it exfoliates skin in the pore and on the surface of skin. Then the copy carries on to say "due to its high content of poamino acid salts, Desquacreme improves and regulates sebaceous secretions." While there are amino acids in this cleanser, they can't regulate oil production in any way, shape, or form; these are water-binding agents, and that's it. What the copy doesn't mention is that Desquacreme contains sodium lauryl sulfate as the main cleansing agent, which is a serious skin sensitizer and potential irritant and not recommended for any skin type. I guess they decided to leave that part out. I wish I had space to explain to you why the claims for the rest of these products are so bogus, but there just isn't room.

Suffice it to say there are far better and less-expensive products to choose from. If you're looking for pricey skin-care products to splurge on, this is not the line to shop. For more information about Sothys Paris, call (800) 325-0503 or visit the Web site at www.sothys.com.

The groupings below follow Sothys Paris's arrangement.

### Normal or Combination Skin

⊗ **Normalizing Beauty Milk Skin Cleanser for Normal or Combination Skin** (*$26 for 6.7 ounces*) includes grapefruit, a skin irritant that serves no purpose for any skin type, plus several ingredients that would be problematic for someone with combination skin, including coconut oil, acetylated lanolin, and sorbitan palmitate.

⊗ **Normalizing Lotion for Normal or Combination Skin** (*$24 for 6.7 ounces*) contains mostly witch hazel, and that won't normalize anything though it will cause irritation.

☺ **Day Cream for Normal or Combination Skins** *($35 for 1.7 ounces)* has as its second ingredient isopropyl palmitate, which, along with the acetylated lanolin in this cream, is known for clogging pores. This product is not recommended for combination skin, though it is an OK moisturizer for someone with normal to dry skin.

☺ **$$$ Night Cream for Normal or Combination Skins** *($39 for 1.7 ounces)* contains several ingredients that can be a problem for combination skin types, including plant oil and acetylated lanolin, but for dry skin it's an OK moisturizer. The collagen in here is a water-binding agent only, it can't affect the collagen in your skin.

☹ **Vitality Serum for Normal or Combination Skins** *($50 for 1 ounce)* is just slip agent, witch hazel, a teeny amount of water-binding agents, fragrance, and preservatives. This is an absurd amount of money for ingredients that don't add up to a few pennies; it's more of a poorly formulated toner than anything else!

☺ **$$$ Beauty Mask for Normal to Combination Skin** *($31 for 1.7 ounces)* contains plant oil, which isn't the best for combination skin; other than that, it is just a good, standard clay mask for normal to dry skin.

## Dry Skin

☺ **$$$ Softening Skin Cleanser for Dry Skin** *($26 for 6.7 ounces)* contains the tiniest amount of aloe imaginable. Other than that, this is extremely standard, but an option for someone with dry skin.

☺ **$$$ Nutrithys Day Cream for Dry Skin** *($35 for 1.7 ounces)* is only suitable for use at night as an ordinary moisturizer, since it is without a reliable SPF or UVA protection.

☺ **$$$ Nutrithys Nourishing Serum for Dry Skins** *($50 for 1 ounce)* is a good, but exceptionally standard, emollient moisturizer. It isn't nourishing in the least, and the interesting ingredients come well after the preservative on the ingredient label, meaning they are barely present.

## Oily Skin

☹ **Desquacreme Deep Pore Cleanser** *($29 for 6.7 ounces)* contains sodium lauryl sulfate as one of the main cleansing agents, which is a skin sensitizer, a potential irritant, and not recommended for any skin type.

☹ **Purifying Lotion for Oily Skin with Blemish Problems** *($26 for 6.7 ounces)* contains camphor and witch hazel, which are skin irritants and don't help skin in the least.

☹ **Matt Cream, for Oily Skin with Blemish Problems** *($35 for 1.7 ounces)* contains lanolin wax and mineral oil, absolutely a terrible problem for oily, blemish-prone skin.

☹ **Active Cream for Oily Skin with Blemish Problems** *($39 for 1.7 ounces)* is mostly waxy thickening agents (including a form of lanolin) and plant extracts, none of which are helpful for oily or blemish-prone skin. If anything, this product can clog pores.

☹ **Clarifying Mask, Mask for Oily/Acne Skins** *($29 for 1.7 ounces)* is a very basic clay mask with some thickening agents that can be a problem for blemish-prone, oily-skin types, including zinc oxide, caprylic/capric triglyceride, and mineral oil.

## Sensitive Skin

☺ **$$$ Comfort Soothing Skin Cleanser, Avocado Extract, for Sensitive Skins** *($26 for 6.7 ounces)* is just a wipe-off cleanser that can leave a greasy film on the skin, though it can be an option for dry skin, but not at this absurd price.

☺ **$$$ Soothing Skin Lotion, with Allantoin Extract, for Sensitive Skin** *($26 for 6.7 ounces)* contains the tiniest amount of allantoin (0.3%), although it is indeed a standard anti-irritant. It is an option for most skin types.

☺ **Immuniscience Cream for Sensitive Skin** *($36 for 1.7 ounces)* is a very good moisturizer for dry skin. It's nice that this doesn't contain fragrance, and that the plant extracts in here are not irritants (though the tiny amount of bee pollen can be a problem for some skin types). So overall, this is a very good moisturizer for normal to dry skin and is one of the better-formulated products in the entire Sothys Paris line up.

☺ **Immuniscience Fluid for Ultra-Sensitive Skin** *($36 for 1.7 ounces)* is similar to the one above and the same basic comments apply.

☹ **Immuniscience Mask for Sensitive Skin** *($30 for 1.7 ounces)* is a standard clay mask with plant oil, but it also contains arnica, a skin irritant, fairly high up on the ingredient listing, which can cause redness and irritation.

## Cleansers General

☹ **Morning Cleanser** *($28 for 4.2 ounces)* is a standard detergent-based cleanser that uses some of the more irritating cleansing agents. This product does contain emollient and plant oil, which is confusing. While the cleansing agents dry out the skin, the emollients grease it back up?

☹ **Eye Make-Up Removing Gel** *($20 for 2.5 ounces)* contains mostly thickeners and slip agents. It is a standard wipe-off makeup remover that isn't as effective as most for removing makeup.

☺ **$$$ Eye Make-Up Removing Lotion for All Skin Types** *($25 for 6.7 ounces)* contains mostly thickeners and plant oil. It is as standard a wipe-off makeup remover as you can get.

## Time-Interceptor Line/Intensive Care

☹ **Alpha Serum 3% AHAs** *($32 for 1.7 ounces)* is honest about the amount of AHA it contains, but in this quantity it isn't effective as an exfoliant.

☺ **Time Interceptor Alpha-Serum Intensive Care with AHA** *($67 for 1 ounce)* contains less than 3% AHA, which makes it ineffective as an exfoliant; other than that it is just a good moisturizer for dry skin.

☺ **Time Interceptor Mask with AHA, 3% AHAs** *($32 for 1.7 ounces)* is nothing more than a good, ordinary moisturizer for dry skin. It's nice Sothys Paris told us how much AHA this product contains, but I guess they didn't know that it takes at least a 5% concentration for products like these to be effective for exfoliation.

☹ **Noctuelle with AHA, Universal Night Creme 8% AHAs** *($60 for 1.7 ounces)*. While this does include 8% AHA, the right amount for exfoliation, the pH of this product is too high for it to work as an exfoliant. At this price you should be getting an AHA product that works to exfoliate!

☺ **$$$ Two Phase Firming Complex** *($77 for 0.5 ounce each of Gel and Moisturizer)* are two standard moisturizers for normal to slightly dry skin. The Energizing Gel-Serum won't energize anything but it is a good moisturizer. The Firming Gel-Serum won't firm one millimeter of skin but it is a good moisturizer and similar to the Energizing version. The Firming version does contain arnica, which can be a problem when applied repeatedly to skin.

☹ **Repairing Serum, Regulating Intensive Care** *($50 for 1 ounce)* contains alcohol as the second ingredient, and that inhibits the skin's repair process; it doesn't help skin of any skin type.

☺ **$$$ Hydrogel Moisturizing Intensive Care Liposomes** *($62 for 1.7 ounces)* is a good, though extremely standard, moisturizer for dry skin.

☺ **$$$ Retinol-15 Night Cream, Time Interceptor Line** *($48 for 1 ounce)* does contain retinol, in a rather standard group of thickening agents, silicone, and preservatives. While the evidence about retinol being an alternative to Retin-A or Renova is at best highly speculative, this one has the appropriate packaging for a retinol product, because retinol is a very unstable ingredient. However, there is nothing about this product that makes it one iota better than L'Oreal's Line Erase with Retinol that sells for $12 for 1 ounce.

☺ **$$$ Retinol-30** *($48 for 1 ounce)* is similar to the product above and the same review applies.

## Fragile Capillaries

☹ **Clearness Serum, Fragile Capillaries Line** *($50 for 1 ounce)*. I can't think of why you would need this for skin, and arnica can only make skin red and worsen the presence of capillaries.

☺ **Rougeur Diffuses Special Creme for Dry Skin** *($34 for 1.7 ounces)* is as ordinary a moisturizer for dry skin as it gets.

☺ **Rougeur Diffuses Day Creme** *($32 for 1.7 ounces)* is similar to the Special Creme above only with problematic ingredients that include sodium lauryl sulfate, which can be a skin irritant. It also contains leech extract. Taken orally, leech extract has been shown to prevent clotting, but there is no research indicating it's of any benefit topically on skin.

☹ **Beauty Mask, Diffused Redness Line for Delicate and Fragile Skins** *($31 for 1.7 ounces)* is a standard clay mask with plant oil, but it also contains arnica fairly high up on the ingredient listing, a skin irritant that can cause redness and irritation.

## Moisturizing

☺ **$$$ Hydroptimale Cream for Dehydrated Skin** *($49 for 1.7 ounces)*. The interesting ingredients are at the end of the list, but there are a lot of them, which makes this one of the better options for dry skin if you're dead set on shopping this line; just watch out for the fragrance.

☺ **$$$ Hydroptimale Gel for Normal Skin** *($45 for 1.7 ounces)* is almost identical to the Creme version above, and the same basic comments apply.

## Refirming

☹ **$$$ Capital Fermete Comfort for Dry Skin** *($47 for 4.2 ounces)*. This very standard moisturizer would be an option for dry skin but the interesting ingredients are so far at the end of the ingredient list they have no real benefit for skin.

☹ **$$$ Capital Fermete Light Texture for Dry Skin** *($47 for 4.2 ounces)* is similar to the Comfort version above and the same comments apply.

## Radiant Complexion Oxygenating Line

☺ **$$$ Oxyliance Creme for Normal/Dry Skin** *($52 for 1.7 ounces)* is somehow supposed to provide oxygen to the skin. It can't, as it doesn't contain any, which is fine because if it did it would have no impact on skin (the skin can't absorb oxygen this way), and definitely not any more than the oxygen already present in the air. This is a good, emollient moisturizer for dry skin, but that's about it.

☹ **$$$ Oxyliance Fluid for Combination Skin** *($52 for 1.7 ounces)* is similar to the Normal to Dry version above, which makes this one very problematic for combination skin. It's still an option for someone with normal to dry skin.

☹ **Source de Radiance Oxygenating Serum** *($55 for 1 ounce)* contains several problematic plant extracts high up on the ingredient list, including rosemary, horsetail, pine cone, and lemon, and the ingredient after that is fragrance! What a waste, and there is no oxygen in this product to boot, just irritation. The minuscule amount of vitamin C in here has no impact on skin.

## Sun Products

☺ **SPF 25 Sunblock** *($23 for 2.5 ounces)* is a very good in-part titanium dioxide–based sunscreen in a standard emollient base for normal to dry skin.

☹ **Active Sun Spray, SPF 4** *($25 for 5.1 ounces)* has a pathetically low SPF number that would encourage someone to seriously hurt their skin.

☹ **Hydrating Tanning Lotion, SPF 8** *($25 for 5.1 ounces)* has a low SPF number and would allow tanning, just as the Sothys Paris brochure states, even though any minimal amount of tanning is a serious risk to skin.

### All Skin Types

☺ **$$$ Active PhytoContour Anti-Wrinkles, Anti-Circles Eye Serum** *($47 for 0.5 ounce)* is an exceedingly ordinary, emollient moisturizer for dry skin. The interesting ingredients are so far at the end of the ingredient listing they are not even worth mentioning.

☹ **Bio-Relaxing Eye Contour Gel** *($31 for 0.5 ounce)*. This ordinary, lightweight moisturizer can irritate the skin due to several problematic plant extracts including ivy, lady's mantle, witch hazel, and sage.

☺ **Hydrobase Light Moisture Base** *($33 for 1.7 ounces)* is a very standard moisturizer. There is about 1% lactic acid in this product, but that's not enough for it to be effective as anything but a water-binding agent.

☺ **Placentyl Cell Renewal Cream, with Vegetable Protein** *($37 for 1.7 ounces)* is a very ordinary moisturizer of water and thickeners, and it doesn't contain any protein or placentyl anything. The name is far more interesting than the product.

## St. Ives (Skin Care Only)

For more information about St. Ives products, call (800) 333-0005 or visit the Web site at www.stives.com.

☺ **Age-Defying Hydroxy Cleanser** *($3.34 for 12 ounces)* is a standard, mineral oil–based, wipe-off cleanser that can leave a greasy film on the skin. That can be an option for someone with dry skin. This does contain about a 2% concentration of AHAs and about 0.5% of BHA, but in these amounts, and in the high pH of this product, they are inadequate as exfoliants. This does contain fragrance.

☺ **Makeup Remover & Facial Cleanser** *($2.32 for 7.5 ounces)* is a standard mineral oil– and lanolin oil–based wipe-off cleanser that can leave a greasy film on the skin. That can be an option for someone with dry skin. It does contain fragrant plant extracts and coloring agents.

☺ **Swiss Formula Peaches and Cream Renewal Wash** *($3.34 for 12 ounces)* is a standard, detergent-based water-soluble cleanser that would be an option for someone with normal to oily skin. It does contain about 1% BHA, which is a problem in a cleanser because it can get in the eyes, even though the pH of this product is too high for the BHA to be effective as an exfoliant. BHA works better when the effective ingredient isn't just washed down the drain. This does contain fragrance and coloring agents.

The Reviews S

☹ **Purifying Clear Pore Cleanser** *($3.99 for 12 ounces)* is similar to the Cream Renewal Wash above and the same basic comments apply, although this version adds eucalyptus, lemon, thyme, and bergamot to the mix, making this too irritating for all skin types.

☹ **Medicated Apricot Scrub With Soothing Elder Flower** *($2.32 for 6 ounces)* includes sodium lauryl sulfate among the cleansing agents, which makes it too potentially irritating for all skin types. It also contains lanolin oil, making it a problem for oily or blemish-prone skin types. The medicated part of this product is supposed to be the salicylic acid (BHA) it contains. However, BHA is an exfoliant and there is nothing medicated about that. Even so, the pH of this product is too high for the BHA to be effective as an exfoliant.

☹ **Invigorating Apricot Scrub with Soothing Elder Flower** *($2.32 for 6 ounces)* is almost identical to the Medicated Apricot Scrub, just minus the salicylic acid. The same basic comments apply.

☹ **Shine Control Refreshing Toner** *($3.99 for 12 ounces)* lists its second ingredient as alcohol, which doesn't make this refreshing in the least, though it does make it drying and irritating for all skin types. It also contain eucalyptus, lemon, thyme, and tangerine, which just adds fuel to the fire.

☺ **Age-Defying Hydroxy Moisture Lotion** *($2.32 for 6 ounces)* contains about 5% AHA and 1% BHA in a moisturizing base. While this would have been a good AHA and BHA product, the pH is too high for it to be effective as an exfoliant, though it is an option for just a good moisturizer if you have dry skin.

☺ **Collagen-Elastin Essential Moisturizer** *($3.19 for 18 ounces)* is a very good moisturizer for dry skin. The vitamins in here are in such a teeny concentration as to be completely inconsequential for skin. Collagen and elastin in a skin-care product cannot affect the collagen or elastin in your skin.

☺ **Hypo-Allergenic Oil-Free Moisturizer** *($2.99 for 4 ounces)* contains way too many problematic ingredients to even begin to rate as halfway close to being hypoallergenic, which is a meaningless term anyway. This is a very good moisturizer for normal to dry skin.

☹ **Protective Nourishing Moisturizer with Vitamins and SPF 15** *($2.79 for 4 ounces)* doesn't contain the UVA-protecting ingredients titanium dioxide, zinc oxide, or avobenzone, and is not recommended.

☹ **Alpha Hydroxy Exfoliating Peel-Off Masque** *($2.32 for 6 ounces)* lists the second ingredient as alcohol, which makes this too irritating and drying for all skin types.

☺ **Cucumber & Elastin Eye & Face Stress Gel** *($2.79 for 4 ounces)* includes fragrant plant extracts that are problematic for the eye area. If you don't have a problem with plant sensitivities, this is a good lightweight moisturizer for normal to slightly dry skin.

☺ **Vitamin K Dark Circle Diminisher Under Eye Treatment** *($8.99 for 0.5 ounce)* might be an intriguing product to consider, especially if you are aware that a recent study published in the December 1999 issue of *Cosmetic Dermatology* seemed to demonstrate that vitamin K could reduce dark circles under the eye. However, what you may not know is that the study's results are, at best, questionable, having been conducted by the company that manufactures the ingredient, and by the doctor, Melvin Elson, who holds the patent for it. The study merely looked at 28 women who applied this vitamin K cream and then a few weeks later reported on how they liked it. That isn't a scientific study by any standard; it isn't double-blind, nor were the results measured by any known protocols. It's nice when a woman says her skin looks better, but lots of women feel their skin looks better after using new products. As it stands, there is no independent research showing vitamin K to be effective for any aspect of skin care. Previously, Elson's research (also questionable and not substantiated by any independent source) pointed to vitamin K for improving the appearance of surfaced capillaries. It didn't work for that problem, and this version, other than being a good moisturizer, won't fare any better at reducing dark circles.

☺ **Vitamin A Anti-Wrinkle Serum** *($6.99 for 14 0.16-ounce capsules)* has no advantage over any of the other retinol products being sold from Neutrogena, Avon, RoC, Alpha Hydrox, or L'Oreal, not to mention little price advantage over similar versions being sold at the department store. The capsule is nice for issues of stability, but other product lines take care of this issue by using a patented version of stable retinol and appropriate packaging (an aluminum squeeze container prevents problems as well). The serum would work as well as any of the retinol products available, and that number is growing by the hour.

☺ **Multi Vitamin Retinol Anti-Wrinkle Cream** *($10.99 for 0.5 ounce)* is a good moisturizer, and just in case you thought retinol wasn't as impressive as a whole bevy of vitamins, this version does have all the latest buzzword vitamins, and takes care of that concern. This would be an option for normal to dry skin.

☹ **Coenzyme Q10 Eye Cream** *($8.99 for 0.5 ounce)* is a rather standard, ordinary moisturizer for normal to dry skin that contains a teeny amount of coenzyme Q10. Coenzyme Q10 can be a good antioxidant for skin, but it is not the best antioxidant for skin care or a miracle ingredient for wrinkles.

☹ **Coenzyme Q10 Wrinkle Corrector with SPF 15** *($8.99 for 2 ounces)* does not contain the UVA-protecting ingredients titanium dioxide, zinc oxide, or avobenzone, and is not recommended.

# Stila

Stila, which means "to pen" in Italian, was the brainchild of Los Angeles–based makeup artist Jeanine Lobell. According to Lobell, she wanted to launch a cosmetics line that would allow all women to be able to use makeup quickly and effortlessly, thus allowing more time for the hundreds of other things that must be accomplished each day. So what were the other lines trying to do, make life more difficult? Nonetheless, with a little ingenuity and marketing smarts, Stila has captured a large piece of the cosmetics pie—enough to be sought after and purchased by one the biggest fishes in the cosmetics pond, the Estee Lauder Company. So what was it that caught the eye of the Estee Lauder execs (aside from the fact that they have been on a buying frenzy over the past few years that includes Aveda, Bobbi Brown, and M.A.C.)? Probably a cute, youthful, twenty-something trademark, the "Stila Girl," and the fact that several of the products were appealingly innovative and clever, attracting a younger, makeup-aware audience. After all, that's something not every line can boast.

Stila has some very good (albeit overpriced) products, and a few that even rise above the horizon far enough to be deemed truly one-of-a-kind or as close to that label as you can get in this copycat industry. Lobell's products excel in the same way other artistry lines do: by offering a very workable palette of neutral foundations and concealers; matte, neutral eyeshadows; and other staples found in any makeup artist's kit. This is a line not to pass by, so go ahead and take a peek . . . but do check out other options before making a final purchasing decision for some of the more ordinary options offered here. For more information about Stila, call 1-888-999-9039 or visit the Web site at www.stilacosmetics.com.

☺ **H₂ Off Cleansing Cloths** *($25 for 40 cloths)* is basically a standard and I mean a really, really standard detergent-based makeup remover, except you get these cloths instead of using your own cotton. Now isn't that special! If the notion of cleansing cloths sounds convenient, these hold no advantage whatsoever over Diaparene Baby Wash Cloths, Fragrance-Free ($2.49 for 100 towelettes) or Huggies Baby Wipes Refills, Natural Care, Unscented ($5.29 for 160 towelettes).

☺ **FOUNDATION:** There are now three types of foundation available, although there are still no viable color options for darker skin tones. **$$$ Complete Coverage** *($40)* is housed in an aluminum tube. This is an exceptionally creamy makeup that blends very well and has a lovely, smooth finish. The name implies fuller coverage than what you actually end up with, which is really just medium cover. This is best for normal to dry skin. Almost all of the shades are gorgeous and truly neutral. The only ones to avoid are shade H and shade I, which are too orange for most skin tones. **$$$ Oil-Free Liquid Makeup** *($30)* is preferred to the one above if you want a sheer-to-light-coverage foundation that is slightly creamy and dries to a natural, sheer finish. The colors are superior—there's not a bad one in the bunch—making this excellent for normal to slightly dry or slightly oily skin types. **Illuminating Powder Foundation** *($22 for powder; $20 for compact)* bills itself as "the first powder to bring radiance to the skin." While this is a satiny, smooth powder with a slight sheen to it (the radiance, perhaps?), it is nothing more than a standard pressed-powder foundation that offers light coverage and works best on normal to slightly oily skin types. All of the available colors are just fine. **Caution:** although this is labeled as SPF 12, there are no active sunscreen ingredients listed. Stila confirmed the SPF 12 is accurate, but without an active ingredient, it is unreliable for daily sun protection.

☺ $$$ <u>CONCEALER:</u> **Eye Concealer** *($16)* comes in a round pot and is a rather thick, creamy concealer that provides great coverage and a slightly powdery finish. Unfortunately, this is still creamy enough to crease, and unless you're very careful with the application it can look heavy. **Cover-Up Stick** *($17)* is a roll-up stick concealer that has replaced the former Face Concealer. Alas, this also has a creamy, slightly greasy texture that will easily lend itself to creasing. This is fine to use if you need heavier coverage over birthmarks or broken capillaries, as the colors are almost all excellent, although this is not a matte-finish concealer, as stated. Avoid shade F, which is too orange.

☺ $$$ <u>POWDER:</u> **Loose Powder** *($27)* has a velvety-soft texture and a smooth, dry finish, which is exactly what a good powder should have. The color selection is limited, and the container (saltshaker style) is not my favorite, but if that doesn't bother you, give it a try. Avoid Warm, which is too orange for most skin tones. **Pressed Powder** *($32)* is not as impressive as the Loose Powder. It has a slightly dry texture and a soft finish. The color selection is extremely limited, with nothing for medium to dark skin tones. **Stila Sun** *($36)* is an overpriced bronzing powder with a lovely texture and two decent colors—but beware: these are shiny.

☹ <u>BLUSH:</u> Stila features a good selection of **Blush** *($15)* colors that have a slightly dry texture, which can make blending difficult. There are some choice matte shades and a very shiny color, but all are sheer, and the lack of smoothness is disappointing. $$$ **Convertible Color** *($28)* is basically a sheer, creamy formula that feels more like a lipstick. It comes packaged in a compact meant to be used on both lips and cheeks for a simple, easy, "finger-painted" look. The texture is creamy bordering on greasy, and the colors are sheer but still bright. This is not for everyone, but if greasy cheeks appeal to you and price isn't an issue, why not?

<u>EYESHADOW:</u> ☺ Stila's **Eyeshadows** *($15)*, in contrast to the blush, have a gorgeous, smooth texture that blends very well. Sadly, there are only a handful of matte shades, but those are great. The shiny shades are quite iridescent and really only for a special evening look.

☹ **Eye Rouge** *($13)* offers two pale, pastel colors that leave a shiny finish. The names are almost too cute to pass up, but the shine is intense! $$$ **Eye Gloss** *($18)* makes you guess that if Stila can have success with greasy blush, why not showcase greasy eyeshadow too? This is strictly Vaseline with pigment and glitter, and just not worth the money for the mess.

☺ <u>EYE AND BROW SHAPER:</u> **Brow Set** *($15)* offers two slightly shiny brown shades in one pan for lining the eyes and shaping the brows, but the two colors will not work for everyone. It is an option, but the price is steep for what you get, and there are better color options for brows in Stila's regular matte eyeshadows that have the identical texture as this.

<u>LIPSTICK AND LIP PENCIL:</u> ☺ The small selection of lipstick colors is available in $$$ **Creams** *($16)*, which are more glossy than creamy, and $$$ **Mattes** *($16)*, which are more creamy than matte. Both have a good amount of stain that helps keep the color on the lips. $$$ **Lip Shine** *($17)* comes in a squeeze tube with a slightly sticky feel and a wide range of colors to choose from. **Pencil** *($14)* for the eyes and lips is standard only in application; unlike other pencils, the pencil part is made of recycled paper. $$$ **Lip Polish** *($24)* is a lip gloss in a self-dispensing brush applicator, for more money than this clever packaging is really worth. A few clicks at the base release a flow of gloss onto the lip-brush applicator. It's nifty and convenient, but it is just a gloss. $$$ **Lip Rouge** *($26)* claims to be a magic marker for the lips. I wouldn't call it indelible, but it has some excellent staying power, just not what you would expect for the money. (This is similar to Lip Ink, reviewed in this edition.) Inside a fountain pen–style package, a very pigmented liquid is fed into a brush tip, which is applied to the lips; it then sets into a long-lasting, feel-like-nothing stain. One word of warning: it dries up easily and the hard brush tip makes application almost painful.

☹ $$$ **Pocket Palette** *($36)* is more lip gloss (four shades to be exact) in a compact. These are just small amounts of lip gloss in a compact, and that makes it overpriced for what you get!

☹ <u>MASCARA:</u> The **Mascara** *($16)* goes on terribly, and never really accomplishes any length or thickness without creating a clumpy mess. Even after wiping down the wand, this was still problematic.

☺ $$$ <u>BRUSHES:</u> There are several great **brushes** *($17 to $53)* to be found here, most with a soft but firm feel and excellent shapes. Stop by and check these out if you are shopping for brushes, but try to avoid the **Precision Liner** *($15)*, which is too thick and soft to create a fine line; the **Precision Crease** *($17)*, which is too floppy for detailed crease work; and the **Eyebrow Brush** *($17)*, which is too stiff. The **Blush Brush** *($25)* is not as soft as it could be, but is still an option.

☹ $$$ <u>SPECIALTY PRODUCTS:</u> **All Over Shimmer** *($28)* is a slick cream that feels somewhat powdery but never quite dries and doesn't stay in place. It is easy to rub off or smear even after you think it has absorbed in. The colors are loaded with shine, and they will do nicely to add shine to the skin, but this can also flake while you're wearing it.

☺ $$$ **Nail Shimmer** *($12)* is only being mentioned because there are so many colors, and any of these would be an option to coordinate with the lipsticks. **Flaunt** *($45)* is a large container of shimmery, fragranced body powder. For those times when you feel like shining up from head to toe and want a whiff of scent too, throw common sense out the window and flaunt! **4-Pan Compact** *($12)* is a sturdy cardboard compact that you can fill with the eyeshadow and blush tins of your choice. These are a great option if you're stuck on Stila.

## Stridex (Skin Care Only)

Although I can't think of a reason why, but just in case, for more information on Stridex products, call (800) 761-1078.

☹ **Facewipes to Go** *($5.49 for 32 cloths)* contain citric acid, menthol, and alcohol high up on the ingredient listing, making this a problem for all skin types. There is nothing beneficial about irritating skin; if anything, it can hurt the skin's immune response, making blemishes harder to heal.

☹ **Antibacterial Cleansing Bar with Triclosan Maximum Strength** *($1.99 for 3.5 ounces)* is a confusing product, because one of the main ingredients is acetylated lanolin alcohol, which can clog pores. Plus, the detergent cleansing agents in this product are fairly strong and drying.

☹ **Clear Antibacterial Foam Face Wash** *($4.93 for 6 ounces)* contains alcohol and menthol along with a solvent that makes this too irritating and drying for all skin types.

☹ **Dual Textured Super Size Pads Maximum Strength** *($3.44 for 32 pads)* has alcohol and menthol added; for this BHA product, that becomes too irritating to even think of using.

☹ **Maximum Strength Pads** *($3.44 for 55 pads)* is similar to the one above, and the same review applies.

☹ **Invisible Clear Gel Maximum Strength** *($4.93 for 1 ounce)* doesn't contain much alcohol, so it may be an option for someone wanting an effective BHA product, but be careful.

☹ **Pads for Sensitive Skin with Aloe Acne Medication with Salicylic Acid** *($3.44 for 55 pads)* is a puzzle: how a company can rationalize calling a product with menthol and a 28% alcohol content good for sensitive skin is beyond me.

☹ **Regular Strength Pads** *($2.99 for 55 pads)* contains menthol and alcohol, and is way too irritating for all skin types.

☹ **Super Scrub Pads, Oil Fighting Formula** *($3.44 for 55 pads)* is similar to the one above, only it contains even more alcohol.

## Suave (Skin Care Only)

More often than not, I'm a big fan of inexpensive skin-care and makeup products. If the same thing exists for less money, unless you can't live without the image and packaging, there is no reason to spend extra cash. I was hoping that concept would hold up for the Suave line of skin-care products, but, alas, it doesn't. What a shame, because the prices for these products are great. Two of the cleansers are an option for some durable skin types, but you have to get past the bad taste they leave in your mouth and the slight irritation over the eyes; the moisturizers are dated, pointless formulations; and there is no sunscreen. For more information about Suave, call (312) 661-0222 or (800) 782-8301 or visit the Web site at www.suave.com.

☺ **Balancing Facial Cleansing Gel** *($2.75 for 8 ounces)* is supposed to gently clean and maintain the skin's moisture balance. It does clean, but it doesn't maintain any moisture balance, though this standard, detergent-based cleanser can be an option for someone with normal to oily skin. It does contain fragrance.

☺ **Foaming Face Wash** *($2.75 for 8 ounces)* is similar to the Cleansing Gel, and the same basic comments apply. It does contain fragrance.

☹ **Greaseless Medicated Cleansing Cream** *($1.99 for 10 ounces)* includes enough irritating ingredients to cause problems for almost anyone's face. It contains, in part, clove oil, camphor, phenol (I didn't think anyone was using phenol anymore), eucalyptus oil, and menthol. This product is absolutely not recommended. Suave must think "medicated" and "irritating" are synonymous.

☺ **Water Rinseable Cold Cream** *($1.99 for 4 ounces)* is a standard wipe-off cold cream made with mineral oil and wax that is not rinseable, as it can leave a greasy film on the skin. However, this can be an option for someone with dry skin.

☹ **Exfoliating Peach Facial Scrub** *($1.99 for 12 ounces)* is a strange mixture of talc, thickeners, walnut shells, detergent cleanser, and plant oils. Several of the plant oils, especially lemon oil, can be irritating, and the talc feels tacky on the skin. Despite the low, low price, there are much better ways to exfoliate the skin than this.

☹ **Clarifying Facial Astringent** *($1.93 for 10 ounces)* is mainly water and alcohol, plus a touch of menthol. Ouch!

☹ **Oil Controlling Facial Astringent** *($1.93 for 10 ounces)* is similar to the Clarifying version above, only this one adds fuel to the fire with peppermint, clove, and camphor.

☹ **Age Defense Renewing Cream, 8% Alpha Hydroxy Complex** *($3.47 for 4 ounces)* contains glycolic acid but it doesn't have a low enough pH to be an effective exfoliant.

☹ **Age Defense Renewing Lotion** *($3.47 for 4 ounces)* is similar to the Cream version above and the same comments apply.

☺ **Replenishing Moisture Cream** *($3.47 for 2 ounces)* isn't a bad moisturizer, just an incredibly boring, ordinary one.

☺ **Replenishing Moisture Lotion** *($3.47 for 4 ounces)* is similar to the Moisture Cream, but with fewer thickening agents.

☺ **Replenishing Moisture Lotion for Sensitive Skin** *($3.47 for 4 ounces)* is an OK but fairly ordinary moisturizer for someone with normal to slightly dry skin.

# T. Le Clerc (Makeup Only)

Theophile Le Clerc, a French pharmacist, was fond of creating makeup at his Paris drugstore and his best-known "invention" turned out to be loose powder. While that doesn't sound too exciting, the resurgence of this very standard, very overpriced talc-based powder has unleashed the floodgates for this small company to expand in the United States. As such, there is now a complete makeup line to complement the original powders, which, inexplicably, turn up in beauty magazines month after month. The hype surrounding this line makes it seem very tempting, but let me assure you there is nothing here that is at all deserving of such steep price tags. The powders are mostly talc and rice starch, and the Loose version is highly fragranced. Rice starch doesn't add anything special to the formula, and can actually cause problems for those with sensitive skin or a tendency toward breakouts. There are dozens and dozens of powders that perform the same as these, at prices from $5 to $30. What's true about T. Le Clerc's powders (and the accompanying makeup) is that there is no extra value or quality for the cost. In fact, if you weigh price against performance for this line, you may leave as disappointed as a Parisian without a paramour. For additional information about T. Le Clerc, call (800) 788-4731.

**FOUNDATION:** ☺ **$$$ Matte Fluid Foundation** *($37)* has a good, even texture and a natural matte finish. It can go on thick, and provides medium coverage that may feel heavy. There are only six colors, with nothing for very light or dark skin, and most are a problem due to overtones of peach, pink, or strong yellow. The shades to consider are Banane and Ocre.

☺ **$$$ Powder Compact Foundation** *($45)* is a standard pressed powder–type foundation that has a very soft texture and a satin finish with a small amount of shine. The formula is talc-free and all six colors are worthwhile. The only drawback is the steep price.

☹ **CONCEALER:** T. Le Clerc's **Concealer** *($19)* is problematic on several counts. Its creamy-bordering-on-greasy texture will crease into any lines under the eye, and it's almost too sheer to provide any coverage and yet somehow still manages to look caked. Even more dismal are the colors, which are either too peach or too pink.

☺ **$$$ POWDER:** **Loose Powder** *($45)* is a talc-based powder that also contains a small amount of rice starch. It has a very fine, dry texture and will work as well as any powder, price notwithstanding. The 20 shades may seem like a real bonus, but most of them are unusually impractical, being all manner of pink, rose, peach, green, lavender, and so on. If you're intent on trying this one, the colors to consider are Translucide, Ivoire, Nacre, Camelia, and Peche. **Pressed Powder** *($45)* has the same talc-based texture and matte finish as the Powder Compact Foundation above but comes in 15 colors, and the same warnings apply with shade selection. Havane and Ebene could be considered for contour or bronzing colors, but the only neutral shades to consider are Translucide, Ivoire, and Peche.

☺ $$$ <u>BLUSH:</u> **Powder Blush** *($25)* has a wonderfully silky texture and the colors are densely pigmented, which is great for darker skin tones. Deplorably, almost all of the colors have a slight to intense shine that is too obvious for daytime wear.

☹ $$$ <u>EYESHADOW:</u> **Powder Eyeshadow** *($23)* are sold as tonally similar duos, with no divider between the colors, which makes selecting one of the colors to wear almost impossible as the brush will pick up both shades. The texture is dry and powdery, but blends better than you might expect. All the duos are intensely shiny, and while they may work for an evening look, they're ill suited for the light of day.

<u>EYE AND BROW SHAPER:</u> ☺ **Eye Pencil** *($15)* is a standard pencil that has a creamy, easy-glide texture, and a dry finish. There are several colors to choose from.

☹ **Eyebrow Pencil** *($17)* has an impossibly hard, dry texture that is painful to apply and not worth the bother or expense.

<u>LIPSTICK AND LIP PENCIL:</u> ☺ **Satin Lipsticks** *($20)* are creamy lipsticks with a very glossy finish and a slight stain. The color range is stunning, with some great reds. $$$ **Matte Lipstick** *($23)* is definitely not matte but, rather, creamy and slick, with a slightly greasy finish. They are richly pigmented, so the color will linger once the emolliency has worn off. $$$ **Lip Gloss** *($19)* features a small selection of sheer colors with a light, non-sticky texture. The price is way out of line for gloss, in spite of the positives. **Lip Pencil** *($15)* is utterly standard and any other pencil from Prestige Cosmetics or Wet 'n' Wild would work just as well.

☹ **All Over Glitter Pencil** *($22.50)* is a thick pencil infused with large flecks of glitter. It's messy to use and the glitter tends to stick exactly where you don't want it.

☺ $$$ <u>MASCARA:</u> **Mascara** *($19)* goes on well, building great length and some thickness with only minimal clumping, and it lasts all day without smudging or flaking. There are even blue and purple shades for those so inclined!

☹ <u>BRUSHES:</u> The makeup **brushes** *($35)* are either too large or too poorly constructed to recommend for practical, everyday use. If brushes in this price range are acceptable to you, check out the countless options at Trish McEvoy or Stila, which are often sold alongside this line at Barneys New York stores.

# Tend Skin

Specifically aimed at reducing or preventing the red bumps caused by shaving is this toner-like product called **Tend Skin** *($50 for 16 ounces)*. It contains isopropyl alcohol (70%), propylene glycol, acetylsalicylate, and glycerin. This is a very interesting formulation that is ridiculously overpriced, while the alcohol part makes it self-defeating. Alcohol causes irritation and redness, the very problems this product is supposed to address. How absurd! As it turns out, Tend Skin is nothing more than aspirin (that's what acetylsalicylate is) suspended in alcohol with a slip agent (glycerin). Aspirin is an anti-inflammatory, and a very effective one at that. The notion that you can put it on your skin to reduce irritation is intriguing and completely worth trying. However, the $50 is best kept in your pocket, because there is no reason why you can't put this concoction together yourself with a small bottle, one or two aspirins, a quarter cup of tap or distilled water, and perhaps a touch of glycerin (which can be purchased at a drugstore; just ask your pharmacist). The drawback to creating this yourself is guessing at the proportions, but with a little experimenting you should be able to produce an interesting toner for ingrown hairs and for areas that get inflamed after shaving, including the face (for men), bikini line, legs, and underarms. You can apply your moisturizer after the aspirin solution is absorbed into the skin.

If you find the bumps do not respond well to the aspirin, try an over-the-counter cortisone cream to reduce the redness and irritation. However, if the bumps get infected you will need to disinfect them with an over-the-counter antibiotic like Neosporin, Polysporin, or Bacitracin. All three are excellent for quick relief from the discomfort of small topical infections. For more information about Tend Skin, call (800) 232-8189 or visit the Web site at www.tendskin-distributor.com.

## TheraCel (Skin Care Only)

On many occasions I've heard from readers who provide product reviews that echo mine exactly or almost exactly. Even when they disagree, readers provide insights that I always appreciate. In the case of TheraCel, I heard from two readers who had completely different experiences. Here are their comments. For more information about TheraCel, call (800)943-5844.

*Dear Paula,*

I am 32 years old and have very fair skin. I do everything I can possibly do to keep my skin in good shape. I have read many informative books (including yours) on such maintenance. Through your books, I have grown somewhat savvy about being taken by the beauty industry and I use your books as a personal guide before trying new products. On occasion, however, I must admit that I have let myself be lured into the seductive promises of the infomercial. Those darn before-and-after pictures get me every time. Such is the case with the TheraCel infomercial.

I'm sure you have seen (and cringed when you saw) Shelley Hack in Paris with this "breakthrough product." I watched her and TheraCel's creator, Ardiss Boyd, and they both seemed so down-to-earth and honest that I was sold.

When I got the products in the mail, an instructional video came along. I watched it and did exactly what it said to do. The kit contained a bar of soap, a night moisturizer, a day moisturizer, and these vials of "serum." You are supposed to wash your face with this soap until it is "squeaky clean." This right away made me a little nervous, but I trusted it was a good product so I did as it instructed. As you may suspect, my skin felt very tight and dried out. The next step was to apply one third of the serum vial onto my face in even, light strokes, and keep my face still for ten minutes. This should have tipped me off that something was faulty with a product that is supposed to moisturize your skin and does not allow you to move it. Reluctantly, I applied this watery fluid in the instructed fashion and waited. As it dried during those ten minutes, it felt as though there was a light solution of water and egg whites tightening my face. When it was completely dry, I curiously touched my face and it felt like there was a piece of cellophane over it.

Now that my skin was thoroughly dried out, and artificially tightened, the next step was the day moisturizer. I hoped, at this point, that this product would somehow make this whole experience reach some kind of balance and undo all the bad effects that it had already done to my skin, so I applied this watery "moisturizer." My skin continued to feel tight, but I had spent all of this money and I really wanted it to work so I gave it a week, hoping for a positive change.

During this time, I did not see any positive results with my skin, let alone the "instant results" that the infomercial had so generously promised. In fact, my skin got very dry and flaky, the lines I was hoping to get rid of around my eyes looked more defined, and a rash developed under my chin and around my eyes. Needless to say, the product got shipped back and the company credited my account. A few days after that, a company representative called my house to see how I was "enjoying" the product. I politely told her about my experiences and was not surprised when she confided in me that many people she had talked to had some similar statements. I didn't feel quite so naive upon realizing that there were quite a few trusting souls who saw that same infomercial and bought it; however, my heart goes out to them, knowing they had comparable unpleasant experiences with this line, and I hope they sent the products back as well.

I don't know if you were going to review this product for your newsletter, but I thought you might be interested in my experiences with it. I feel that if you do review this line, you will find similar discoveries and will be able to warn your readers about this, in my opinion, bogus product line. This is the last time I ever try a new product until you have reviewed it first. Keep up the good work, Paula!

Theracelled Out, via e-mail

And now for another reader's comments:

*Dear Paula,*

Thank you for considering evaluating the skin-care line TheraCel. I do not work for TheraCel. I just recently bought the product (from their infomercial) and am interested in your opinion.

I have found the product really does reduce lines after only ten minutes! The Advanced Procellular Formula is the key to it. I am 38 years old and the results were quite dramatic. The delicate skin under my eyes was turned into perfect baby skin!

There are three products you get in the initial starter kit: night serum, moisturizer, and the stuff that gives the miraculous (no joking) results, the Advanced Procellular Formula (vials).

The only problems are:

1. The product is drying to my slightly oily skin type.

2. The products are too expensive for the average person. Ninety-nine dollars for a 30-day supply of the Advanced Procellular Formula vials alone is a bit much!

3. Deep lines on the throat are not affected (even though the product directs the user to apply only to the face).

4. The night serum and moisturizer do little to moisturize.

I also wonder where they get the placental protein and embryo extract from. (Could it be from aborted humans, or is it just chicken eggs?) What on earth is emu oil? Maybe you could develop a similar product and work out the kinks in this version.

Renee, Boise, Idaho

To Theracelled Out, Renee, and all my readers:

My review of the TheraCel products reflects both Renee's and Theracelled Out's experiences, at least in terms of the products' overall performance. However, I find the notion of "miracle" skin-care products or *any* antiaging skin-care routine that doesn't include an effective sunscreen to be unethical and harmful! I also found TheraCel's ingredient list to be most likely incomplete. There is no way these products can perform and feel the way they do—that is, the plastic layer on the skin and the watery mess of the serums—and contain what the label says, not to mention the lack of any preservatives. The only product that seems to have an accurate ingredient list is the bar soap.

In regard to the improvement Renee had with the Advanced Procellular Formula, there will always be women who experience success with this kind of product. The improvement may be a result of the extremely lightweight nature of the products as well as the film-forming ingredients. Hairspray-like ingredients can make skin look smoother, but they also leave the face feeling sticky and dry, as both women experienced. About the placental and embryo stuff, the company says it is from animals, but they weren't sure which ones. For more information, visit www.wellquest intl.com

☹ **Emu Cleansing Bar** *($49.95 for six 2-ounce bars)* is a standard, tallow-based bar with detergent cleansing agents and a tiny amount of emu oil (an emu is a bird native to New Zealand). Emu oil has no miraculous properties to help skin.

☺ **$$$ Advanced Procellular Moisturizer** *($49.95 for 2 ounces)* is accompanied by an ingredient list that is probably incomplete. Aloe can be considered a soothing agent, and beta-glucan is a decent antioxidant, but they can't keep water in the skin or provide any emolliency. This product also won't generate cell production, as the name seems to promise. As a toner this could be a viable option, but not to keep moisture in the skin.

☺ **Emu Promoist** *($39.95 for 2 ounces)* is identical to the moisturizer above except this one has emu oil. Again, I doubt the ingredient list is complete, but in any case this is a lot of money for some bird oil, vitamin A, and aloe. This would be a good toner for someone with normal to dry skin, but not a good moisturizer by itself.

☹ **$$$ Advanced Procellular Formula** *($99.95 for ten 0.07-ounce vials)* has an ingredient list that is personally offensive to me. It reads as follows: serum protein, placental protein, embryo extract, hydrolyzed collagen. While protein and collagen can be good water-binding agents, animal placentas and embryos seem inappropriate and unnecessary given the excellent plant sources available for these ingredients. This product also leaves a tacky, stiff feeling on the skin, like that caused by a film-forming ingredient, which leads me to believe the ingredient list isn't accurate.

☹ **$$$ Advanced Procellular Night Serum** *($49.95 for 2 ounces)* is just aloe, beta-glucan, and a marine source of elastin. Again, I doubt this list is complete; if it is, spoilage would be a major issue. This $50 product would last for only a week or two, even in your refrigerator. If you have normal to slightly dry skin, this could be a good toner, but that's about it.

☹ **$$$ Emu Oil** *($120 for 4 ounces; $200 for 8 ounces)* is pure emu oil. Women believed for a while that mink oil was the answer for wrinkles, so why not emu oil? Though if you were interested for some reason, this kind of product is available at some health food stores for far less.

## *Three Custom Color*

What is unique about this company is that it lives up to its claim that it can match a lipstick color and texture from any line you send it. And it doesn't even have to be the entire lipstick. Just a small color swatch is all they need, along with the name of the lipstick brand and color. I sent them a random M.A.C. lipstick and they duplicated the color and texture to a T. It was almost impossible to tell the two products apart! For those of you who have been disappointed that a favorite lipstick is no longer available, this shopping experience is worth a consideration. However, the matching does come at a price: two tubes of a custom-blended color cost $50.

If you would rather play with Three Custom Color's own ready-to-wear makeup products, they have over 22 shades of **lipstick** *($15)* available in a rather creamy, opaque finish; 22 shades of a standard **lip gloss** *($15);* ten shades of a very standard, somewhat dry finish lip pencil that needs sharpening *($12.50);* and 10 shades of a cream-to-powder **blush** with a soft, smooth finish *($15).* All the shades are nicely divided into warm and cool color groupings.

Because the demand for color palettes has become quite popular, Three Custom Color provides an interesting, though pricey kit option (each kit is $45) for those who consider themselves lipstick devotees. There are six kits: two lipstick and two lip-gloss groupings, each with ten shades organized by warm and cool shades; there is also a red lipstick grouping with shades of just the color red. Then there is the Special Effects Palette with nine more unusual shades so you can blend away to your heart's content and create any potential makeup look you can think of. The colors in this group include white, black, silver, shimmery white frost, opalescent, copper, and gold. You get very little of each color, the lipsticks tend to be more glossy than creamy, and the glosses are just standard glosses, but the kit concept definitely works for some women.

For more information, call Three Custom Color at (888) 262-7714 or visit the Web site at www.threecustom.com.

# *Tommy Hilfiger*

I may be one of the few people in the world who doesn't own a single item of clothing or paraphernalia with the Hilfiger logo on it—until now, that is, since I've purchased this new skin-care and makeup line of products. With the abundance of new makeup lines available, I was curious to see what made this line interesting. Nothing much, as it turns out. There are definitely some good products here and the prices are fairly reasonable. The look is young and upbeat. This is a line that definitely expects to be selling to women under the age of 30—there isn't a wrinkle cream or antiaging product to be found, at least not yet. I also imagine Hilfiger expects to sell to men as well; the skin-care packaging is decidedly unisex or even masculine in appearance, with nothing feminine or elegant about it. If there can be a crossover in the world of cosmetics, this line may be able to carry it off.

For more information about Tommy Hilfiger makeup and skin care, call (800) 798-8858 or visit the Web site at www.tommy.com.

## Tommy Hilfiger Skin Care

☹ **Clean Break Daily Cleanser** (*$12 for 5 ounces*) is a wipe-off cleanser that can leave a slight greasy feel on the skin.

☺ **Clean Scheme Gel Cleanser** (*$12 for 5 ounces*) is just a very standard, detergent-based cleanser that would be fine for normal to oily skin.

☹ **Get Lost Eye and Makeup Erase** (*$10 for 3.4 ounces*) works as a wipe-off makeup remover.

☹ **Polished Clean Face Scrub** (*$14 for 3.4 ounces*) is a fairly drying and rather abrasive scrub that can be a problem for most skin types.

☺ **Dew Point Face Lotion** (*$20 for 3.4 ounces*) is an exceptionally standard moisturizer for dry skin.

☹ **Portable Tan Self Tanner and Bronzer** (*$14 for 1.7 ounces*) uses the same self-tanning ingredient as all self tanners, but the bronzer part has a strange ashy, almost greenish-brown color that isn't tan-looking at all.

☹ **Spot Clearing Acne Treatment Gel** (*$10 for 0.85 ounce*) contains alcohol, which is problematic for blemishes, and the pH isn't low enough for it to be very effective for exfoliation.

☹ **Stop Light Face Protector SPF 30** (*$8 for 0.21 ounce*) doesn't have UVA protection, but what's even more of a concern is that the pricing makes this one of the more expensive sunscreens available. For one ounce of this stuff it would cost $40! Can you imagine?

## Tommy Hilfiger Makeup

☺ **FOUNDATION: Set It Up Oil-Free Foundation SPF 15** (*$15*) is a very good, soft matte–finish foundation that blends on evenly and smooth with light to medium coverage; the problem is that the SPF doesn't include any UVA-protecting ingredients. What a shame the SPF is lacking, because this is a great option for normal to oily skin types, and without complete sun protection, it still requires another sunscreen underneath and that can be a problem for oily skin. The 18 shades are mostly impressive, but there are no options for very light skin tones, though there are several for dark to very dark skin tones. Still, for those of you who use Prescriptives' Virtual Skin foundation, this is nearly identical in formulation and texture, and for half the price! The only colors to be cautious with are: Light Porcelain (slightly pink), Light Buff (slight peach), and Medium Sand (too peach for most skin tones).

☺ <u>CONCEALER:</u> **Fixer Upper Concealer** *($10)* is a very good, creamy, smooth liquid concealer that dries to an opaque, fairly natural finish with minimal risk of creasing. The six shades are all fine. Be aware that the squeeze tube means you can waste product by squeezing out more than you need, though once you get the knack of it, it shouldn't be a problem for long.

☺ <u>POWDER:</u> **Powder Up Pressed Powder** *($15)* is a standard but good pressed powder with eight suitable neutral shades and a silky, slightly dry texture. It applies easily and the finish is sheer. Darker skin tones will find some good options, but avoid Cider, which is too orange for most skin tones.

☺ <u>BLUSH:</u> **Glow for It Cheek Color** *($15)* has a smooth, matte, somewhat dry finish and a great range of colors; the one shade of purple is curious, but I'm sure someone will be interested. Much like the eyeshadows, the blush colors go on much softer than you would think, but that does help to create a softer look.

☺ <u>EYESHADOW:</u> **Double Feature Wet/Dry Eye Color** *($10)* comes in a large range of colors ranging from shiny white to a nice grouping of neutral brown tones. The colors have a silky feel (some with intense shine but several with minimal shine) and go on very soft. It can take some effort to build any depth of color, but if you use them wet that helps boost the intensity.

☺ <u>EYE AND BROW SHAPER:</u> **Retroliner Liquid Eyeliner** *($10)* is just a good liquid liner that has a relatively solid finish. It works well and goes on easily. **Borderline Eye Pencil** *($10)* has a great name, though it's an exceptionally standard pencil with a slightly creamy texture. There are ten shades with only a few that fall in the outrageous category. **Fast Talk Lip Shine** *($10)* is just iridescent gloss in a tube. **Small Talk Lip Pencil** *($10)* is a clever name for an exceptionally standard pencil with a slightly dry texture and ten great shades.

<u>LIPSTICK AND LIP LINER:</u> ☺ **Fresh Talk Conditioning Lipcolor** *($10)* has a very standard, sheer, glossy finish but a very good and large range of colors. **Sweet Stix Flavored Lip Color** *($10)* are standard, slightly greasy lipsticks that taste like fruits or desserts. If these appeal to you, check out Jane's MegaBites Flavorful Lip Color *($2.99)*—they're basically the same thing for one-third the price.

☺ **All Talk Lip Crayon** *($10)* is a chubby pencil that can be used as lipstick or lip liner. It's hard to sharpen and offers little advantage over a regular lipstick with the same creamy finish.

<u>MASCARA:</u> ☺ **Big Deal Volumizing Lash Color** *($10)* comes in two standard colors and also the rather unique options of green, blue, and purple. Regardless of color, I just can't comment on the need for vivid pastel eyelashes. This is a good basic mascara that builds decent length and some thickness with no clumping or smearing. However, it is not a big deal or particularly volumizing.

<u>BRUSHES:</u> ☺ **Powder Brush** *($20)* is really too large and not all that soft.

☺ **Blush Brush** *($15)* is OK, but just OK; it works, but the size is almost too small, though the texture is good. ☺ **Eyeshadow Brush** *($10)* is a great, versatile brush with a good texture. ☹ **Eyeliner Brush** *($10)* is too thick to be an eyeliner and too floppy to be an eyeshadow brush. ☺ **Eye Definer Brush** *($10)* is a good standard wedge brush for brows or lining.

# Tony & Tina

Tony & Tina is a line of cosmetics that, much like Hard Candy and Urban Decay, had its beginning with nail polish. Graduating to a full-blown cosmetics line is not an easy task, and a smaller company assuredly needs a good angle to attract attention. Tony & Tina definitely has found a distinctive approach that sets it apart from the rest: this line is "dedicated to promoting our conscious evolution through Vibrational Remedies." The company's earnest belief is that all living things give off energy, which in turn can be influenced or controlled by certain colors and aromas. Whether or not it is plausible to apply a certain shade of lipstick or blush to obtain "conscious evolution" or "positively manipulate energy," or "discover … endless potential" is a matter for discussion, but it is important to keep in mind that we're talking about makeup here, not a religious epiphany. However, for those who subscribe to the notion of cosmic energy and color therapy, that can certainly be enjoyed with or without Tony & Tina. Once you get past the embellishments, there is really not much here to meditate on, unless your preference is for all manner of shine and sparkle (does conscious evolution require glitter?).

The packaging is artful and the counter displays are nicely accessible; you are free to play and achieve all the bliss you can handle. The nail polishes, as expected, are the standout products in this line, and they do dazzle, but Tony & Tina's notion that this is "the first step towards realizing our powers as healers" needs to get a grip. In the meantime, you'll find colors both subdued and shocking for every product grouping. For more information about Tony & Tina, call (212) 226-3992 or visit the Web site at www.tonytina.com.

☹ **Herbal Aromatherapy Cleanser Normal/Dry Skin** *($24 for 8 ounces)* definitely contains lots of oils and emollients, which makes it little more than a cold cream, albeit an overpriced one. However, it also contains eucalyptus, witch hazel, and other plant extracts that make it potentially irritating for all skin types, and especially for the eye area.

☺ **Herbal Aromatherapy Make Up Remover** *($18 for 8 ounces)*. Aromatherapy is nice for your nose but a problem for your skin. This makeup remover is a decent toner with good water-binding agents but the fragrance is not helpful for skin.

☺ **$$$ CONCEALER: Therapeutic Eye Base** *($22)* comes in only one shade and is sold as a multipurpose product to prevent fine lines, soothe puffy eyes, and function as a concealer. What this turns out to be is a slightly wet, cream-to-powder concealer with semi-opaque coverage and a slightly shiny finish, which as a base isn't the best idea. This may be an option, but only if your skin matches this particular color. The antiaging claim is linked to apple seed enzyme, and even if this were a miracle ingredient (it's not—enzymes are OK exfoliants on skin but that's about it), there isn't enough of that in here to diminish anything.

**BLUSH AND EYESHADOW:** ☺ **Multi-Purpose Face Color** *($9 each; $10 for compact)* are *very* small discs of creamy color that fit into a compact holding up to six shades. These are meant for use on eyes, cheeks, or lips. The texture is light and these go on sheer, but—like any cream—will tend to crease around the eye area. $$$ **Cosmetic** *($24)* is a small pot of highly iridescent loose powder. Tony & Tina claims it is "all you need, all day," which is OK if glitter is part of your skin's major needs. $$$ **Color Frequency Eye Shadow** *($18)* is a group of shadows that have a far better gimmick than performance. Actually the marketing copy for Frequency far surpasses any simple definition of the word "gimmick." The incredible concept for this product is that it contains chamomile and vitamins "for the physical," and color "for the metaphysical … [to] awaken your intuition with Color Frequency Eye Shadow. Clinically proven to aid in personal revelation." Eyeshadow can aid in personal revelation? Enlightenment via makeup—can spirituality get any more superficial than this? The amount of chamomile and vitamins is at best negligible and these exceptionally standard, overpriced eyeshadows (I guess personal revelation doesn't come cheap) are in a single-disc compact with two shades, available in either high shimmer, standard (which is slightly shimmery), flat (meaning matte), or wet/dry formulations. The texture is powdery and sheer for the shiny shades and dry to chalky on the wet/dry (and matte) colors. To suggest that there are far superior options in other lines from Jane to M.A.C. for far less and without the New Age pretense is an understatement.

☹ **Cosmic Lights** *($12)* uses "pure Crystalina" to create these eight shades of sparkly powder, similar to the Cosmetic above. The only difference is that these have a rough, grainy texture and do not adhere well to skin. That's not surprising, given that crystalina is made of an iridescent translucent Mylar flake (yes, like Mylar bags or balloons), and it explains why it isn't so skin friendly, but it undeniably does shine.

☺ $$$ **EYE AND BROW: I&I Herbal Eye Pencil** *($16 without sparkles/$18 with sparkles)* is a standard, and I mean really standard, pencil that has a creamy texture and glides on easily. These have a powdery finish, and are best used for a smoky look, as they smudge easily. These also promise to firm skin with cucumber, but like the other claims here that's just bogus.

**LIPSTICK AND LIP PENCIL:** ☺ **Mood Balance Lipstick** *($15)* comes in a package that goes on and on about the lavender, rosemary and St. John's wort the lipstick contains, but it is merely window dressing for a rather standard, boring group of lipsticks. There are three finishes—creamy, semi-matte, and gloss—and all are barely distinguishable from each other. They all have a creamy texture and slightly glossy finish, although some are more opaque. **Herbal Aromatherapy Lip Gloss** *($14)* is just standard, non-sticky lip gloss with some OK, high-shine colors to choose from.

☺ $$$ **Herbal Lip Pencil** *($16)*. Once you get around all the hype about this pencil being "therapeutic," what you find is the same old lip liner that every other line has been selling for years. $$$ **Lip Sparkle** *($18)* consists of chunky pencils infused with glitter, which lends this standard, creamy pencil an uninviting, grainy texture—but the shine is here for those who crave it.

☺ $$$ <u>MASCARA:</u> **Herbal Eye Mascara** *($18)* was my favorite product in this line. Although overpriced, it went on beautifully and built long, separated, lightly thickened lashes with minimal effort. It also held up well and did not smear throughout the day.

☺ $$$ <u>BRUSHES:</u> Tony & Tina sought the assistance Shu Uemura for its collection of **brushes** *($36 to $98)*, and the benefit is apparent. These are wonderfully full, soft brushes with workable shapes. What a shame they are so exorbitantly priced! If you survive the sticker shock, you will find some definite options here, but you can absolutely ignore the **Brow Brush** *($32)*, which is insanely overpriced for what you get, and the **Lip Brush** *($48)*, also way too pricey for a standard, very small brush.

☺ <u>SPECIALTY PRODUCTS:</u> **Nail Paint** *($10)* is basic nail polish with some of the most imaginative colors and textures I've ever seen. For those of you wishing for shiny, polyester-infused blues, and fuchsias with tiny heart-shaped sparkles, welcome home! **Hair Wand** *($15)* is Tony & Tina's take on the hair-mascara trend, and there are suitable colors here, though all are very shiny. Perhaps they didn't notice that most people don't have iridescent hair or roots.

# Tova (Skin Care Only)

This is the line that made 1950s Oscar-winner Ernest Borgnine look like a new man—at least that's what the ads originally claimed when this line was first launched years ago by his wife, Tova Borgnine. Tova is now a line of products featured on QVC. The essence of these skin-care products is presumably an ingredient called "cactine 1." This ingredient is extracted from cactus plants supposedly once developed by the Aztecs. Because of its cactus origin, cactine is supposed to help skin do what these desert plants can do: namely, protect itself against water loss. Interesting concept, but there is no supportive evidence for this, and botany experts say cacti can go without water for many different reasons, not just because of one ingredient. A closer look at Tova reveals ingredients that are more standard than anything else.

What is decidedly not standard are the prices ($19 to $40), which lean toward the higher end of the cosmetics spectrum.

I get the feeling the popularity of this line has mostly to do with the moisturizing products designed for women with dry skin (along with some amount of celebrity élan). These are very emollient products with good absorption, not fancy or state of the art, but good and reliable. If you have dry skin or if you buy the theory on cactine, some of these may be worth checking out. Avoid buying sets of these products (one of the skin-care groupings sells for $166), because you are more than likely to end up with products that are a total waste of money and not great for your skin. For more information about Tova's products, call (800) 852-9999 or visit the Web site at www.beautybytova.com.

☹ **Cactine Beauty Bar** *($24 for 3.8 ounces)* is an overpriced, standard bar cleanser. The ingredients that keep the bar in its solid form can clog pores, and the cleansing agents can be drying.

☹ **Cactine Skin Renual Cleanser** *($22 for 6.7 ounces)* is a detergent-based cleanser with some plant oil, preservatives, and fragrance. It can leave a greasy film on the skin, but of more concern is the cleansing agent used here, sodium lauryl sulfate, which is a fairly potent skin sensitizer. It does contains some AHAs, but in too small a quantity to be effective as an exfoliant. And in a cleanser they would be useless anyway because their effectiveness would be washed away.

☺ $$$ **Cactine Eye Makeup Remover** *($29 for 6.7 ounces)* is a standard, detergent-based, incredibly ordinary eye-makeup remover. It will take off eye makeup but no better than hundreds of other products priced far more reasonably. It does contain fragrance.

☹ **Cactine Cream Scrub** *($24.50 for 3.2 ounces)* is almost identical to the Renual Cleanser above except for the addition of synthetic plastic scrub particles. The same problems apply for this product.

☹ **Cactine Skin Refresher** *($20 for 6.7 ounces)*. The witch hazel in here is too irritating for all skin types, and the fragrant oils can be sensitizing.

☹ **Cactine Skin Toner** *($18 for 6.73 ounces)* is almost identical to the Skin Refresher above, except this one contains alcohol, which is even worse for the skin.

☺ $$$ **Cactine CelRenual** *($41 for 1 ounce)* is very good moisturizer for someone with normal to slightly dry skin. The elastin and collagen in here can have no effect on the collagen and elastin in your skin.

☺ $$$ **Cactine EyeRenual Treatment** *($31 for 0.5 ounce)* is similar to the one above and the same review applies.

☺ $$$ **Cactine Eye Lift** *($28 for 0.5 ounce)* won't lift anything, but it is a good moisturizer for normal to dry skin. The pH of this product isn't low enough for the salicylic acid to work well as an exfoliant, and I would question using a BHA in an eye product anyway.

☺ $$$ **Cactine Firming Eye Cream** *($34.50 for 0.5 ounce)* has a huge ingredient list that includes everything but the kitchen sink. This is a very good moisturizer for normal to dry skin, but there is nothing in here that will firm skin.

☺ **Cactine Firming Throat Cream** *($34.50 for 4 ounces)* is similar to the CelRenual treatment above and the same comments apply.

☻ **Cactine Emollient** *($23.50 for 1 ounce)* is a Vaseline-based moisturizer that also contains plant oil, lanolin, and waxes. This is a very greasy, very thick moisturizer that would be good, though standard, for someone with dry skin.

☻ **Cactine Moisture Milk** *($19.50 for 3.38 ounces)* is a good though very standard moisturizer for normal to slightly dry skin.

☻ **Cactine Moisture Rich Cream** *($26.50 for 1 ounce)* is a good, though ordinary moisturizer for someone with dry skin.

☻ **Cactine Skin Renual Cream** *($31 for 1.7 ounces)* is supposed to be an AHA product, but it contains neither enough AHA or the right pH for it to be an effective exfoliant.

☹ **Cactine Masque** *($29.50 for 4 ounces)* contains primarily witch hazel, which can be a skin irritant; it also has rice starch, which can be sensitizing. The teeny amount of cactine in here, and I mean minuscule, makes this a real waste of time.

☺ $$$ **Cactine Moisture Masque** *($29.50 for 4 ounces)*. While this might be good for dry skin, it is no different from other moisturizers in this line.

☹ **Fragrance Free Block, SPF 30** *($18.50 for 4 ounces)* doesn't contain avobenzone, titanium dioxide, or zinc oxide for UVA protection, and is not recommended.

☻ $$$ **Cactine Lip Renual Masque and Lip Renual Serum** *($21.50 for both 1 ounce of the Masque and 0.25 ounce of the Serum)* is mostly wax that can rub off dry skin, but the witch hazel and rice starch can be irritating. The serum is mostly film former and water-binding agents. That can make the lips feel tight and slightly smoother, and hold lipstick in place, but it can also eventually cause dryness because there are no emollients in the product.

# Trish McEvoy

Trish McEvoy's line of skin-care and makeup products is competing nicely with her neighbors at the department store, such as M.A.C., Bobbi Brown, and Stila. But unlike those other companies, she is the stand-alone who hasn't sold out to Estee Lauder. That may or may not be a good thing, but the line definitely retains McEvoy's full attention and style. New counter displays that are not only user friendly but are also clearly labeled and some nice line additions are standouts, and make Trish McEvoy worth checking out more than ever. The prices may still lead you back over to M.A.C., though.

The large brush selection is impressive, with some of the best selection and range available, and the great lipsticks, large matte eyeshadow selection, and beautiful blushes (both cream and powder), as well as some good foundation choices, are all notable. One very unique aspect of the Trish McEvoy line is her Face Planner. These day planners have plastic boards inserted on binder rings that you can fill with whatever product you choose. With three sizes to choose from, these pricey makeup books warrant a visit to the Trish McEvoy counter just to check them out and see if they would work for you.

One drawback is Trish McEvoy's skin-care line. It is still a disappointment. Most of the skin-care products go beyond ordinary to downright boring. On one hand, I was thrilled to see a department-store line that didn't include an obnoxious list of plants or sea extracts, but on the other I was disappointed to find such standard formulations with such unreasonable price tags. For more information, call (800) 431-4306.

## *Trish McEvoy Skin Care*

☺ **$$$ Essential Cleanser** *($38 for 8 ounces)* is a standard, detergent-based water-soluble cleanser that is an option for someone with normal to oily skin. The price for this cleanser is completely unwarranted. There are dozens of other cleansers that are equal to if not far better than this one.

☹ **Essential Wash** *($38 for 8 ounces)* uses sodium C14-16 olefin sulfate as the main detergent cleansing ingredient, and that makes this cleanser potentially irritating and drying for all skin types. There are far more gentle ways to effectively clean the skin for far less money.

☹ **Gentle Cleansing Lotion** *($38 for 8 ounces)* is almost identical to the Essential Wash above and the same comments apply.

☹ **Glycolic Wash** *($38 for 8 ounces)* has a pH of 5, and so that means the glycolic acid in here can't work as an exfoliant, which is good news, because you don't want to get an effective AHA product splashed into the eye. Plus the main cleansing agent is sodium C14-16 olefin sulfate, which makes it potentially too drying and irritating for all skin types.

☹ **Moisture Retaining Bar** *($22.50 for 3.7 ounces)* is a standard, tallow-based bar cleanser that can be drying and potentially cause breakouts due to the ingredients that keep the bar in a solid form. The Vaseline in here won't help undo the drying effects of the cleansing agents. Plus, if you want this type of cleanser, Dove Cleansing Bar is actually a better option.

☹ **Astringent Cleansing Bar** *($22.50 for 3.5 ounces)* is a standard, tallow-based bar cleanser that can be drying and potentially cause breakouts due to the ingredients that keep the bar in a solid form.

☺ $$$ **Eye Makeup Remover** *($18.50 for 2 ounces)* is a fairly standard, detergent-based eye-makeup remover that would work as well as any.

☺ **Oil-Controlling Gel** *($28 for 2 ounces)* is similar in many ways to plain milk of magnesia. It contains merely water, a form of magnesium, slip agent, preservative, and coloring agents. It will work to absorb oil, but so will just plain milk of magnesia for far less.

☺ $$$ **Dry Skin Normalizer** *($55 for 2 ounces)*. The interesting ingredients are here in such teeny amounts that they are barely worth mentioning. The plant extracts are a mix of irritants (like ivy) and anti-irritants (chamomile).

☺ **Enriched Moisturizer** *($38 for 2 ounces)* is almost identical to the Dry Skin Normalizer above and the same comments apply.

☺ **Light Moisturizer** *($38 for 2 ounces)* is an exceptionally ordinary moisturizer for normal to slightly dry skin. It's OK, though there are far better options than this overpriced version.

☺ $$$ **Moisture Gel (Oil-Free)** *($19 for 1 ounce)* is a silicone-based, lightweight moisturizer that is more boring than it is helpful. The silicone can feel good on skin, but it would be better if this product contained some water-binding agents or soothing ingredients that were more interesting than what is in here. The plant extracts in here are a mix of irritants (ivy) and anti-irritants (chamomile) and, therefore, are just a waste.

☺ $$$ **Glycolic Face Cream** *($38 for 1 ounce)* is about a 4% AHA concentration, which would be fine for someone with sensitive skin, however, the pH of 5 makes it ineffective as an exfoliant.

☺ **Glycolic Lotion** *($38 for 2 ounces)* would be a very good (but overpriced) 8% AHA for someone with oily skin, and this one has a pH that makes it reliable for exfoliation.

☺ $$$ **Line Refiner** *($25 for 0.18 ounce)* won't change a line on your face, but it is a very good moisturizer for someone with dry skin.

☺ **Protective Shield Moisturizer SPF 15** *($38 for 2 ounces)* is a very good, in-part titanium dioxide–based sunscreen for normal to slightly dry skin. The moisturizing base is exceedingly mundane and there is nothing about this formulation that warrants the price; it's easily replaced by many others for a fraction of the price.

☺ **Sport Cream SPF 30** *($19 for 4 ounces)* is a very good, in-part zinc oxide–based sunscreen that will provide UVA protection for someone with normal to slightly dry skin.

☹ **Sunscreen Spray SPF 15** *($18 for 4.5 ounces)* doesn't contain the UVA-protecting ingredients of avobenzone, zinc oxide, or titanium dioxide, and is not recommended.

# Trish McEvoy Makeup

**FOUNDATION:** ☺ **$$$ Natural Tint Foundation Oil-Free** *($35)* goes on evenly and smoothly, and is quite sheer. Most of the colors are good, with only a handful to really stay away from. For the money, this is just an ordinary foundation with nothing really to highlight. Avoid these colors: C1, C2, C4, N6, and W6.

☺ **$$$ Cream Powder Makeup** *($40)* is just what it says—a creamy-feeling makeup that spreads smoothly and sheer and then leaves a soft, powdery finish. It can be OK for dry skin types, but could be a problem for someone who tends to break out. It contains plenty of wax (including carnauba), and the second ingredient is isopropyl myristate, which can clog pores. Most of the colors are very good but these colors should be avoided: C2, C3, C6, W4, W5, W6, and N4.

☺ **$$$ Cream Powder Makeup Oil-Free SPF 8** *($40)* may not contain oil but it contains plenty of waxes that can be a problem for someone with oily or blemish-prone skin. Also, the low SPF does not have UVA protection. This does have a soft, powdery, smooth finish and can work well for someone with normal to slightly oily or slightly dry skin. Most of the colors are very good but these colors should be avoided: C2, C3, C6, W5, W6, and N4.

☺ **$$$ Dual Powder** *($28)* is meant to provide all-over face color as an alternative to traditional foundation. This product has a dry, powdery finish even though it does have a silky feel. This can be great for a regular pressed powder.

☺ **$$$ Foundation Sticks** *($38)* are one of the new products to consider, and are another good option for a stick foundation. This one has a creamy, soft application that has sheer to medium coverage. Most all of the 16 shades available are superior, with an excellent selection for very light to very dark skin tones. The only ones to be cautious of are Beige, Warm Beige, and Warm Bronze; these can be too peach for some skin tones. This one would be an option for someone with normal to dry skin.

☺ **$$$ Face Shine** *($28)* is a cream-to-powder that has a more greasy finish and adds the requisite trendy shine women seem to want.

☺ **$$$ CONCEALER: Protective Shield Cover-up** *($23)* gives great coverage and blends out nicely to a subtle finish, but it does tend to crease and some of the colors are poor. Avoid Light, 1C, 2E, and 2C.

**POWDER:** ☺ **$$$ Loose Powder** *($20)* is talc-based, with a very silky, soft texture, but the four color choices are appropriate only for light to medium skin tones. Did someone forget that this line has foundation colors for dark to very dark skin tones? What are those women supposed to use?

☺ **$$$ All Over Face Powder** *($28)* is a group of rather ordinary talc-based powders.

**BLUSH:** ☺ **$$$ Sheer Blush** *($20)* is a group of soft matte shades that really do go on quite sheer. The regular colors are nice but fairly ordinary, and there are a few strange or shiny colors to watch out for.

☺ $$$ **Lip & Cheek Pencils** *($18.50)* are very fat pencils that are soft enough to be used as lipsticks or blushes. They feel like very glossy lipsticks or very creamy blushes. The pencils are convenient if you can somehow figure out how to keep them sharpened all the time.

☺ $$$ **Cream Blush Sticks** *($32)* deliver a very creamy, almost greasy, stick-applicator blush. It blends out to just a hint of color and works great for a soft wash of color.

**EYESHADOW:** ☺ $$$ Four types of eyeshadows might sound like overkill, but in this case you can ignore the categories and just look for the colors you like, because they are all fairly similar. The **Glazes** have some amount of shine; the **Shapers** are supposed to be softer colors; the **Definers** are intense, deep colors for liner; and the **Enhancers** are medium shades for the crease *($18 each)*. All of the colors are interchangeable and the matte ones are, of course, the best. Most of the eyeshadows, particularly the darker shades, are a bit on the "wet" side and tend to crease.

☺ $$$ **Face Essentials Kit** *($35)* is a compact quad group of colors with strips for blush, eyeliner, and two eyeshadows. The way the colors are organized makes it hard to prevent the blush brush from getting into the eyeshadows, and the colors tend to flake into one another. Additionally, anytime you buy sets, you rarely end up using all the colors, which makes this kind of product a waste of money. On the other hand, some of the color groupings are beautifully matte, and the color that is meant to be used as the blush can be used around the eyes, so if you find a selection that meets all your needs, this can be an essential kit for you.

☺ $$$ **EYE AND BROW SHAPER:** The **Eye Pencils** *($15)* are incredibly standard, in a very typical assortment of colors.

**LIPSTICK AND LIP PENCIL:** ☺ $$$ **Sheers** *($16)* are like a gloss, with the same staying power. **Sheers with SPF 15** *($16)* are identical to the Sheers except they contain sunscreen but no UVA protection. **Lip Colors** *($16)* are creamy lipsticks with good staying power, a wonderful texture, smooth application, and a very impressive color selection. **Semi-Matte** *($16)* has a good opaque, creamy finish. **Highlights Lip Gloss** *($16)* comes in a tube applicator and offers an interesting array of colors, including red, a shiny lavender, and a shiny gold, as well as soft, pale shades of pink, mauve, and peach. These glosses go on very thick and rich, looking more wet than glossy. **Lip Essential** *($20)* is a compact of four lip colors and texture types. One is glossy, the others creamy, semi-matte, and sheer. It works, but I prefer a traditional lipstick tube. **Lip Pencils** *($16)* come in a nice assortment of colors, and one side of the pencil is a lip brush. It's a nice touch, but Max Factor sells almost the exact same pencil for a quarter of the price.

☹ **Matte Over** *($16)* is supposed to be used as a lipstick base to help keep lipstick on longer or as a top coat to make any cream lipstick look matte. Either way, it is a problem. Used as a base it tends to peel, and used over lipstick it is just messy.

☺ $$$ <u>MASCARA:</u> The Mascara *($16)* stays on wonderfully and doesn't smear or clump; it also builds decent length and some amount of thickness.

☺ $$$ <u>BRUSHES:</u> It takes good professional brushes to apply makeup well and there are definitely some options in this group. The prices range from $18 to $38, but most are overpriced and have far less pricey counterparts elsewhere. Stay away from the blush and powder brushes—the texture is stiff and coarse. (I was told they were getting new ones due to this problem but as this book went to press the old ones were still there.)

☺ $$$ <u>SPECIALTY:</u> **Face Planner** *($35 to $45 for the case, $12 to $14 for the pages)* is a very clever way to assemble a makeup bag that resembles a day planner. A two-ring binder inside a pouch holds "pages" that can be filled with the color of your choice. It's pricey, but this is an intriguing assortment and exceedingly convenient, especially if you're loyal to Trish McEvoy's color line of eyeshadows and blushes.

# *Trucco (Makeup Only)*

Trucco is a small line of makeup products developed by the hair-care company Sebastian International. The brochures for Trucco have the "no-rules Generation X" edginess seen in lines such as Urban Decay or Hard Candy, yet the products are decidedly more tame and, dare I say, mainstream. The tag line for Trucco is "Addicted to Color," and although there are a few products here worth checking out if you come across a salon or boutique that carries this line, nothing here merits even a mild case of addiction. What you may want to investigate are the foundations and powders, which offer some good neutral colors, and the decent selection of matte eyeshadows and blushes. The rest of the lineup is a mixture of standard fare, ranging from problematic mascaras to a bevy of shine-inducing products. Product cost for Trucco varies from location to location, as salons that sell it set their own retail price. Therefore, consider the prices listed here to be an average and decide from there whether or not Sebastian's Trucco makeup is as appealing to you as its enormous selection of hair-care products. For more information about Trucco, call (800) 829-7322 or visit the Web site at www.sebastian-intl.com.

<u>FOUNDATION:</u> ☺ **Pro Coverage Opaque Foundation SPF 8** *($20.75)* is a slightly thick but smooth-textured foundation that does provide a UVA-protecting ingredient (titanium dioxide) along with its disappointingly low SPF (SPF 15 is the standard). The foundation blends on well and provides light to medium coverage and a satiny-soft finish. It would be suitable for normal to dry skin, and of the eight shades (with nothing for very light or very dark skins), only Bisque, Tan, and Sand are too peach for most skin tones. Olive, Beige, and Ivory are lovely neutral colors.

☺ **Prepair Duo Powder Foundation** *($21.50)* is a standard, talc-based powder foundation with a smooth, soft texture and medium coverage that blends very nicely. There are six colors, with no options for darker skin, and Mood is the only one to steer clear of; it is too orange for most skins.

☺ **Studio Creme Foundation SPF 12** *($21.50)* is a creamy makeup that comes in a compact and almost dries to a powder finish. The SPF is not indicated on the ingredient list, which makes this misleading and definitely unreliable for sun protection. There are only three shades, which is shortsighted, and Compromise is too peach for most skin tones.

☺ **Tinted Moisturizer SPF 8** *($14.25)* does not offer any UVA-protecting ingredients and is just a basic, very sheer but emollient tint for the face. The two available shades are fine.

☹ **CONCEALER: Micro-Encapsulated Concealer** *($10.95)* comes in a pot and has a creamy, almost greasy texture that is only capable of light coverage and can easily crease into any lines around the eyes. The colors are right-on, but the negatives offset that. **All Purpose Color Corrector** *($14.75)* is similar to the Concealer, but the intent is to use this very peach-toned cream to neutralize unwanted skin tones, and the end result is exactly what you might expect: peach-tinted-looking skin.

**POWDER:** ☺ $$$ **Touch Up Pressed Powder** *($15.50)* is talc-based, with a dry, soft texture and sheer application. Of the three colors, two are very light and one is best used as a matte bronzing powder instead of an all-over face powder. **Final Touch Loose Powder** *($13.75)* is talc-based and has a smooth, even texture and three very good colors suited to lighter skin tones.

☹ $$$ **Rock Candy** *($15.95)* is very shiny loose powder that is messy to use but does indeed add sparkle.

☺ **BLUSH: Powdered Blush** *($10.50 singles; $18.35 trios)* has a soft and sheer, slightly dry texture that blends decently but not as easily as many other powder blushes. The singles have a small but good group of matte shades, and the trios present blush, contour, and highlighter colors in one compact. Those can be a convenient option, but there are no dividers between the colors, so once you've used them they tend to spill over onto each other. The colors are well coordinated, but watch out for the very shiny Flirt. **Face Cremes** *($9.95)* are creamy, glittery colors for eyes, lips, and cheeks. Due to the glitter particles, the texture is somewhat rough. If you're interested in this type of product, a better place to start would be M.A.C.'s Creme Colors *($14)*.

☺ **EYESHADOW: Eye Colour** *($9.25)* are single eyeshadows with a smooth texture that is a bit stubborn when it comes to blending evenly. The shiny colors are labeled as Reflectives while the Mattes are called just that; they're not entirely matte but the shine is very soft.

**EYE AND BROW SHAPER:** ☺ **Pro Eye Contour Pencil** *($8.75)* is a very standard pencil that glides on well and has a soft, dry finish. **Graphic Liquid Eyeliner** *($11.65)* has a great, quick-drying formula that goes on solid and heavy. Be careful when applying it, as the brush is too stiff and scratchy. If you can handle the discomfort of the applicator, which does make getting an even line tricky, it does wear well!

☺ **$$$ Hi-Brow Trio** *($28)* is virtually identical to Hard Candy's Training Brow Compact *($28)*. Trucco's offers three matte colors (light, medium, and dark) that have a dry finish and apply well, but most women would do just fine with one matte color for the brows, and these are too dry to double as eyeshadow. This may be worth it to makeup artists without any budget constraints but others will get limited use from two of the three shades. **Brow Shaper** *($11)* is your basic, everyday clear brow gel that works as well as any.

☺ **LIPSTICK AND LIP PENCIL: Identity Lipsticks** *($10.95)* are marketed with a transcendent flair but in reality are just ordinary lipsticks. The **Cremes** are very creamy and rich with a glossy finish and mostly iridescent colors. The **Mattes** are not matte in the least but are nicely creamy and opaque. The texture is somewhat sticky, and feels that way on the lips. The **Sheers** have an SPF 12 sans UVA-protecting ingredients, but can be relied on for an emollient, very glossy lip tint with lots of colors to choose from. **Divinyls Lip Gloss** *($7.50)* is for serious gloss fans. This is a rich, thick, slightly sticky gloss that comes in a tube and leaves an extremely wet-looking finish. The colors go from bold to subtle, and many have iridescence. **Lip Contour Pencil** *($8.75)* is as standard as it gets. This pencil needs sharpening and has a creamy and relatively solid finish.

☹ **MASCARA: In Focus Mascara** *($15.50)* goes on a little too wet and can make lashes look heavy and limp. It builds some length, but the side effects are not fun to live with. **In Focus Waterproof Mascara** *($15.50)* is just fine for average length and no thickness. Don't get caught in the rain with this one; it breaks down readily with water.

## Ultima II

Ultima II's makeup is in need of some serious renovation and restructuring. The tester units have been compacted to include products from several different categories, and what used to be a wonderful group of foundation colors has been whittled down to what amounts to an insignificant handful of options. A few categories, such as Vital Radiance, have been eliminated altogether, while others, such as The Nakeds, are hanging on by a thread. What's most disappointing, but nevertheless seems to be giving women what they crave, are the Glowtion products. What began as one innocuous, sheer, and shiny face tint has multiplied into an ever-expanding range of shiny companion products. For women who loved the luminescent shine they got from the original Glowtion, this is good news—they can now get more of that from companion products including compact foundations, powders, lip glosses, and lipsticks. That much shine can serve as a beacon for passing ships! I imagine before too long there will even be Glowtion mascara available so the lashes won't feel all alone and boringly matte.

What's most disappointing is that Revlon, which owns Ultima II, seems to have taken an indifferent attitude toward the line and its products. Several calls to Revlon's customer service number made me feel as if I were running in circles, as I was consistently told to phone J.C. Penney's (the department store that carries the line), and then when I did, the salespeople at J.C. Penney's told me to call Revlon. What's even more confusing is that Ultima II is haphazardly distributed through several drugstores, which usually receive just the newer products while the original ones are left to gather dust at J.C. Penney's nationwide. There are still some good stragglers left here to consider, but come prepared, as this is not an easy line to navigate and you'll more than likely need some assistance, if you can find anyone who knows something about the line, because Revlon is not offering any help to their counter people. For more information about Ultima II, you can attempt to contact Revlon at (800) 4-REVLON or (212) 572-5000 or visit the Web site at www.ultimaII.com. Be aware that while Ultima's Web site does exist, it's nothing more than a title page with no other product or company information.

Note: The "CHR" acronym stands for Collagen Hydrating Response. The CHR products all do contain tiny amounts of collagen. But collagen is merely a good water-binding agent for skin; it cannot affect the collagen in your skin or what causes wrinkles, or alter them in any way, shape, or form.

# Ultima II Skin Care

☹ $$$ **CHR Cream Cleanser** *($18.50 for 4 ounces)* is a standard, mineral oil–based cleanser that must be wiped off and that can leave a greasy film on the skin, though it may be an option for someone with dry skin.

☺ $$$ **CHR Double Action Gentle Cleanser for Dry Skin** *($17.50 for 4.8 ounces)* is a standard, detergent-based water-soluble cleanser that can work well for most skin types. The minuscule amounts of plant oil and water-binding agents in this product do not help dry skin very much. It does contain fragrance.

☺ **Vital Radiance Foaming Face Wash for Normal to Dry Skin** *($17.50 for 5 ounces)* is almost identical to the CHR Double Action Gentle Cleanser above and the same comments apply.

☺ **Vital Radiance Foaming Face Wash for Normal to Oily Skin** *($17.50 for 5 ounces)* is a standard, detergent-based cleanser that can work well for normal to oily skin. It does contain sodium lauryl sulfate, but less than 2%, so it probably won't be a problem for causing irritation or dryness.

☺ **Eye Makeup Remover for Sensitive Eyes** *($12.50 for 3.6 ounces)* is a standard, detergent-based eye-makeup remover. There are too many detergent cleansing agents in here to make it good for sensitive eyes.

☺ **Going Going Gone Makeup Remover** *($13.50 for 4 ounces)* is just a mineral oil–based cold cream that can leave a greasy film on the skin, though it can be an option for dry skin.

☹ **Vital Radiance Skin Renewing Exfoliator for All Skin Types** *($17.50 for 4.7 ounces)* lists the third ingredient as sodium lauryl sulfate, which makes this too potentially irritating and drying for all skin types.

☹ **CHR Double Action Gentle Toner for Dry Skin** *($17.50 for 8 ounces)* contains menthol, which makes it anything but gentle for any skin type, much less dry skin.

☺ **Vital Radiance Skin Renewing Toner Normal to Dry Skin** *($17.50 for 8 ounces)* is a very good toner with about 2% salicylic acid (BHA). The pH of this product is about 4, which makes it just borderline effective as an exfoliant. Other than that it contains very good water-binding agents and vitamins. It does contain fragrance and coloring agents.

☹ **Vital Radiance Skin Renewing Toner Normal to Oily Skin** *($17.50 for 8 ounces)* is similar to the Normal to Dry Skin version above only this one contains witch hazel as the second ingredient, which makes it potentially too irritating and drying for all skin types.

☹ **CHR Double Action, Day Lotion with Ceramides SPF 15** *($45 for 1.7 ounces)* doesn't contain the UVA-protecting ingredients avobenzone, zinc oxide, or titanium dioxide, and is not recommended.

☺ **CHR Lotion Concentrate** *($32.50 for 3 ounces)* is about as ordinary as moisturizers get. The teeny amount of collagen in here is inconsequential for skin.

☺ **CHR Cream Concentrate** *($32.50 for 2 ounces)* is a very standard, boring moisturizer for someone with dry skin. The teeny amount of collagen in here has no impact on skin.

☺ **$$$ CHR Double Action Night Cream** *($42.50 for 2 ounces)* is similar to the Cream Concentrate above, and the same review applies.

☺ **$$$ CHR Double Action Eye Cream** *($22.50 for 0.5 ounce)* is similar to the Cream Concentrate above, and the same review applies.

☺ **Glowtion Skin Brightening Moisture Cream SPF 15** *($21.50 for 2 ounces)* is a very good, in-part avobenzone-based sunscreen in a very good emollient moisturizing base for someone with normal to dry skin. The shine this product imparts on the skin is not for everyone and it definitely doesn't hide flaws.

☺ **Glowtion Skin Brightening Moisturizer SPF 25** *($21.50 for 2 ounces)* is similar to the Glowtion Cream SPF 15 above, only this one is in lotion form with a higher SPF; the same basic comments still apply.

The Reviews U

☹ **ProCollagen Eyes with Sunscreen** *($27.50 for 0.8 ounce)* doesn't contain the UVA-protecting ingredients avobenzone, zinc oxide, or titanium dioxide, and for some strange reason no SPF is indicated. Without any way to know the amount of protection you're getting, you'd do well to avoid this product, especially as it has no UVA protection; it is not recommended.

☹ **ProCollagen Face and Throat with Sunscreen** *($40 for 2 ounces)* is similar to the ProCollagen Eyes above, and the same comments apply.

☺ **Under-It-All Makeup Perfector SPF 25** *($13.50 for 1.25 ounces)* is a very good, titanium dioxide– and zinc oxide–based sunscreen in a very good moisturizing base with interesting water-binding agents and vitamins for someone with normal to dry skin.

☹ **Under Makeup Moisture Cream** *($22 for 2 ounces)* is a very ordinary emollient moisturizer for dry skin.

☹ **Under Makeup Moisture Lotion** *($27.50 for 4 ounces)* is identical to the Under Makeup Cream above except that it is slightly less emollient, but the same basic comments apply.

☹ **Vital Radiance Skin Perfecting Lotion SPF 15** *($22.50 for 1.5 ounces)* and **Vital Radiance Skin Perfecting Cream SPF 15** *($22.50 for 1.5 ounces)* are supposed to be beta hydroxy acid (BHA—salicylic acid) formulations with SPF. Even if they had a low pH to make the BHA effective (they don't), the sunscreen agents don't include the UVA-protecting ingredients of titanium dioxide, zinc oxide, or avobenzone to assure protection against UVA sun damage. Without those ingredients, these two aren't vital; at best they're trivial and unimportant.

☹ **Vital Radiance Skin Renewing Eye Reviver SPF 8** *($22.50 for 0.4 ounce)* has a dismal SPF number and doesn't contain the UVA-protecting ingredients titanium dioxide, zinc oxide, or avobenzone; it is not recommended.

☺ **Vital Radiance Skin Renewing Night Serum** *($25 for 0.95 ounce)* is a very good, lightweight moisturizing lotion. The seaweed in here can be good soothing agents, but they don't repair skin.

☹ **$$$ Brighten Up, Tighten Up Eye Cream** *($20 for 0.5 ounce)* is a very good moisturizer/concealer for dry skin. The ingredient list is immense; if you want to try almost every water-binding agent in the book, this is the product to buy. Of course, it won't do anything a hundred other moisturizers can't do, and unfortunately the colors are unrelated to skin tone.

## Ultima II Makeup

**FOUNDATION:** ☹ **Ultimate Coverage** *($18.50)* comes in a jar and is a thick, full-coverage foundation that blends on quite well for such a heavy-duty product.

This has been pared down to four shades, all with a rosy cast, which makes this almost impossible to recommend, though it may be worth a look if you really need this much coverage.

☺ **Beautiful Nutrient Nourishing Makeup SPF 15** *($21.50)* has a great, in-part titanium dioxide–based sunscreen. This foundation has sheer coverage and a soft, lightweight texture that can feel a bit slippery while you're blending it. There are now 11 shades, with no options for darker skins. These shades are too peach, rose, or orange for most skin tones: Alabaster, Dawn, Almond, and Aurora Beige.

☺ **Beautiful Nutrient Nourishing Compact Makeup SPF 12** *($23.50)* is a cream-to-powder foundation that is more cream than powder. It applies very well and the SPF is titanium dioxide, but while the SPF 12 is close to the standard, an SPF 15 is preferred. There are nine shades here that appear to be less neutral than they really end up being when applied on skin. These shades may be too peach or rose for most skin tones: Alabaster, Natural, Honey, and Ginger.

☺ **WonderWear Foundation SPF 6** *($21.50)* goes on matte and must be blended quickly to avoid streaks—and then it wears and wears and wears! This is Ultima II's version of Revlon's ColorStay Makeup, and they share the same problems: they dry into place almost immediately, they're hard to remove, and if you get this on your nails it will wreck your manicure. It does last all day for someone with oily skin, but there are definite drawbacks along with the benefits. The SPF is far too low to rely on for protection. Of the 16 shades, most are neutral; these colors are too peach or rose for most skin tones: Alabaster, Sand, Honey, Fawn, Almond, and Mocha (which is very orange). Forget this one and consider Revlon's ColorStay Lite SPF 15 instead (it costs less and does supply the appropriate SPF requirements).

☺ **WonderWear Cream Makeup SPF 6** *($21.50)* has titanium dioxide as its sunscreen, but the SPF number is too low to offer adequate protection. This is a creamy foundation that provides full, opaque coverage; it's not for foundation beginners—and even foundation pros may shy away from such a thick, hard-to-blend texture. Still, the six colors are decent, except for Ginger, which is too ash for most skin tones.

☹ **The Nakeds Line Smoothing Makeup SPF 10** *($20)* won't smooth lines, and in spite of the claim to the contrary, can settle into fine lines, like most any creamy foundation can. The SPF is titanium dioxide, but the seven colors are too peach or ash to recommend.

☹ **Glowtion SPF 25** *($20 lotion or cream)* is a tinted moisturizer with an in-part titanium dioxide sunscreen and a great SPF number. What's problematic are the five shades, for both cream and lotion are all iridescent and peach- to orange-toned. The shine is on the subtle side, but still obvious.

☹ **Glowtion to Go Compact Tinted Moisturizer SPF 15** *($21.50)* has a very good, part zinc-oxide and part titanium-dioxide sunscreen, but this is otherwise an awful pink-coppery iridescent cream-to-powder makeup that lays on shine that would be noticeable across a crowded room.

☺ **Glowtion Skin Brightening Makeup** *($17.50)* has ten absolutely wonderful colors and a smooth texture that are waylaid by this foundation's iridescent finish! Perhaps I can concede to a touch of shine for a special occasion.

☺ **CONCEALER: WonderWear Concealer SPF 6** *($14.50)* has a smooth, even application that is neither too dry nor greasy, and that makes it an excellent choice. There is only a small chance this will slip into the lines around the eyes. Of the three shades, Ivory may be too pink for some skin tones. The sunscreen, though the SPF is too low, is titanium dioxide.

☹ **POWDER: The Nakeds Loose Powder** *($21.50)* comes in a huge tub but has shine, which fundamentally defeats the purpose of powder. **The Nakeds Pressed Powder** *($16.50)* is talc-based and feels feather-soft, but the three available colors are too peach or pink to recommend. **WonderWear Pressed Powder** *($16.50)* takes the negatives from the two above powders (shine and poor colors) and rolls them together into a third unimpressive powder.

☺ $$$ **BLUSH: Nourishing Blush Stick** *($17)* is a twist-up, cream-to-powder blush that has a soft, beautiful texture and a sheer, even application. Although I generally do not recommend cream blush over powder, this is one to consider, and the colors are plentiful. Only Coral Sun and Warm Shimmer are shiny. **WonderWear Cheek Color** *($16.50)* has a smooth, even, but dry texture and some excellent colors. Most of them leave a soft sheen on the skin that isn't as obvious as most shiny powders deliver. **The Nakeds Cheek Color** *($16.50)* has an exceptional, soft-matte application but has been edited down to only three shades, all warm tones.

**EYESHADOW:** ☺ **Fade Not, Crease Not Eyeshadow Base** *($13.50)* is a silicone-based, pink-toned primer for the eyes. It does have a silky texture that dries to a soft powder finish, but with mineral oil as the second ingredient, the fading and creasing you were hoping to eliminate will only increase.

☺ $$$ **WonderWear Eye Color** *($15.50 duos; $20 quads)* has some workable duos to choose from, and these go on soft and matte. The quads have some worthwhile color combinations, but often include one or more shiny colors. The shade selection for Ultima II's eyeshadows is nowhere near as good as it used to be; even some of the endearingly odd shades have vanished.

☹ **Fade Not, Crease Not Shadow Liner** *($13.50)* is a dual-ended product that features an ultra-shiny, cream-to-powder eyeshadow on one end and a creamy eye pencil on the other. The cream eyeshadow will crease within minutes of applying it, plus the pencil is very small and just a pencil that needs to be sharpened.

**EYE AND BROW SHAPER:** ☺ **WonderWear EyeSexxxy Longwearing Eyeliner** *($12)* is an extremely standard pencil that does not need sharpening and is about as long wearing as most other pencils.

☻ **BrowSexxxy** *($12)* is a twist-up brow pencil with a too-creamy finish that wouldn't be the best choice for creating a natural-looking eyebrow.

**LIPSTICK AND LIP PENCIL:** ☹ **Glowtion Luminous Lipcolor SPF 15** *($11.50)* does not have UVA-protecting ingredients and is quite greasy and sheer, with loads of iridescence.

☺ **The Nakeds Lipstick** *($13.50)* is a good creamy, slightly glossy lipstick that now offers only a handful of colors, all warm tones. **Full Moisture Lipcolor SPF 25** *($13.50)* also is without UVA-protecting ingredients, which is a shame, because the SPF rating is great. This is just a slick, slightly greasy lipstick that has a glossy finish and some amount of stain. **Glowtion Lip Brightener SPF 15** *($11.50)* has inadequate UVA protection but is a nice sheer, lightly tinted iridescent lip gloss. **Lipsexxxy Lipliner** *($12)* is a standard, twist-up lip pencil that comes in a decent array of colors and applies smoothly.

☻ **Full Moisture Lipliner** *($12)* makes the "anti-feathering" claim that just begs to be put to the test, but when I did it was obvious this very moist and creamy lip pencil would easily pave the way for lip color to bleed. Plus, the opening and tip of this pencil are flat and wide, a shape that's difficult to work with when precisely outlining the lips is the goal.

**MASCARA:** ☺ **WonderWear Mascara** *($13)* builds long lashes with no clumping or smearing but it doesn't have any more staying power than other mascaras. While the claim of keeping mascara on for 18 hours sounds impressive, lots of mascaras can do that.

☺ **LashFinder Mascara** *($11)* is quite adept at building lots of length, but it does take time to get anywhere. Thickness is hard to come by, but if that's not what you're after, this lengthens and defines without clumps and lasts well.

☹ **Beautiful Nutrient Mascara** *($13.50)* is just an OK mascara; it doesn't build much length or thickness and tends to clump and smear a bit.

## *Ultimate Hairaway*

☻ **Ultimate Hairaway** *($39.95 per 2-ounce bottle)* is another hair-growth-inhibiting product that claims to be all-natural, even though the ingredient list is as far from natural as you can get. It contains water, extractable fruit derivatives (whatever that's supposed to mean), polypropylene glycol, glycerol, disaccharides, urea, dithiothreitol, EDTA, methylparaben, and propylparaben. What could be inhibiting hair growth in this product? It isn't the natural-sounding fruit derivatives. It's probably the dithiothreitol. Dithiothreitol is related to thioglycolic compounds, which are standard, highly alkaline ingredients that can dissolve hair and potentially irritate skin.

Depending on your sense of humor, you may find Ultimate Hairaway's suggestion that you "first remove hair from the roots, as with waxing, sugaring, tweezing, or electrolysis" before you apply this product terribly funny. They claim Ultimate Hairaway isn't a depilatory, which is why the hair has to come off first. Rather, it is supposed to inhibit hair growth, eventually phasing out the need for hair-removal procedures. Given the variable cycle of hair growth and the fact that you are supposed to use another method to remove the hair, it would be long before you had any idea it wasn't working. Tweezing and waxing already make hair growth seem slower, because the hair has to grow longer to get back to the surface when it's been removed from the root. Moreover, electrolysis is already the only hair-removal system approved by the FDA as being able to stop hair growth, but Ultimate Hairaway fails to mention that.

Another claim Ultimate Hairaway makes is that it works like "male pattern baldness, inhibit[ing] hair growth." While that comment simplifies the issue, the description in the brochure is much more complicated and hard to follow. According to the booklet, "the top of a healthy papilla [*papilla* is a term that refers to the bump or bulge where a hair grows] is naturally cornified . . . [*cornified* refers to the conversion of skin cells into a keratinized material, such as hair or nails]. When the hair is removed, the sides of the papilla are exposed and susceptible to the treatment. [That may be true, though I doubt it, but regardless, the papilla isn't where the hair grows from.] . . . Male pattern baldness is caused by renegade type apocrine glands that develop and connect to the duct of the sebaceous gland and introduce naturally occurring secretions into the hair follicle. The opening of hair follicles at the skin's surface is often blocked by shampoo, conditioner, gels, hairspray, sweat, oils, sebum, etc. This blockage disallows these natural secretions to escape. These acidic secretions, having no place to go, seep their way to the base of the hair follicle and slowly cornify the sides of the papilla, preventing penetration of hair cells. Ultimate Hairaway can duplicate the cause of baldness on the desired area." Wow!

Let me try to interpret this mumbo jumbo. First, male pattern baldness is caused by the hormone dihydroxytestosterone (DHT), which binds to the base of hair follicles and causes them to shrink and deteriorate. *Apocrine glands* refers to any glandular secretion, anywhere in the body. I have no idea what that has to do with the hair shaft, because it isn't how the hair follicle functions (unless they are referring to DHT, but they don't say that). Then they start talking about how some hair-care products can clog a hair follicle and, I suppose, cut off its blood supply and reduce growth. Now, that is true, but hardly something you would want to encourage, because you would also be clogging the pores at the same time. The rest of the stuff I can't decipher. I've never heard of this acidic secretion issue that cornifies the hair follicle itself. It sounds like their product blocks the pilosebaceous unit (the hair follicle and oil gland combined are the pilosebaceous unit) to stop unwanted hair growth. Are they suggesting that you can artificially create acidic secretions in the hair follicle (secretions I haven't seen any evidence of) to stop hair growth? Does that mean AHAs (which are highly acidic) can stop hair growth? None of this is substantiated by one ounce of published research, and none of the dermatologists I spoke to confirmed or even understood what any of this means.

Perhaps the final joke is the last statement in the Ultimate Hairaway brochure: "If you prefer to shave to control unwanted body hair, simply apply [Ultimate Hairaway] twice a day for one week and then once a day thereafter until the desired results are acquired. Shave as necessary." See, they were talking about mechanically removing hair by shaving (or any other method) all along; it just took them a very long time to say that.

# University Medical Skin Care

What was true for this line in the last edition of this book is still true. University Medical Skin Care just about wins the prize for the most ignominious claims and assertions about its products. First, there is no university associated with University Medical Skin Care(in the first edition this line even quoted a physician in its ads, and when I interviewed this doctor he said he never heard of these products—and this misinformation has since been deleted from the marketing materials I've seen for University Medical Skin Care). However, even if there were a host of doctors backing up the name University Medical Skin Care, they would all have to have their licenses revoked for endorsing such a distorted, worthless group of products. Many forms of cosmetics advertising are offensive to me, but the kind with false medical pretensions always takes the cake. If you find the claims enticing and the prices seemingly benign, just keep in mind that in almost all of these products there is nothing that can live up to even a small percentage of the claims being made for them. After all, how many products in the same line can promise to erase wrinkles before we catch on that none of them are telling the truth, because if even a single one could erase wrinkles, why would you need more than that? Here is my review of this line for your information, although there is really no reason to consider any of these products. For more information about University Medical Skin Care, call (800) 535-0000 or visit the Web site at www.universitymedical.com.

☺ $$$ **Face Lift Prima Hydroxy Daily Cleanser** *($19.99 for 4.1 ounces)* is just a detergent-based cleanser with some plant extracts. There are no AHA ingredients in here to affect the skin (sugarcane and sugar maple are not alpha hydroxy acids). It does contain some orange and lemon extract, which can be irritating to the skin and eyes.

☺ **Face Lift Cell Regeneration Cream** *($24.99 for 1.5 ounces)* is supposed to renew elastin and collagen, and give the skin oxygen to heal and plump cells. If this product worked, you wouldn't need any of the other ones in this line. The oxygen in here is just taken up by the atmosphere, and so can't add anything to the skin, nor can it penetrate skin. Plus, given that the other products in this line boast antioxidants (ingredients that ward off oxygen), how do they rationalize trying to give the skin more oxygen? Moreover, given the vast number of products in the world of cosmetics claiming to build collagen and elastin, it is amazing how many wrinkles still exist. This is a good, lightweight moisturizer with very good water-binding agents, but that's about it.

☺ $$$ Face Lift Under Eye Therapy *($24.99 for 0.5 ounce)* is a good moisturizer for the eye area if you have somewhat dry skin. The "lifting" ingredient is yeast, but that won't lift a thing. If yeast could lift the skin anywhere, we would all just be rubbing plain old yeast extract on our faces.

☺ Overnight Moisturizer with Lavender Aromatherapy *($14.99 for 2.5 ounces)* does smell nice, but it is better to wear lavender as fragrance than have it in a product you put on your face. Lavender, like all fragrant plants and oils, can be a skin irritant. Plus, this product also contains several other irritating plant oils including lemon, bergamot, and orange oil. Other than that, this is a good, though standard moisturizer for dry skin. It also contains colostrum, which is the "pre-milk" that female mammals secrete prior to producing milk. Colostrum contains immunoglobulins (disease resistance factors) that are helpful to newborns. While there is a small body of evidence indicating that adult consumption of colostrum may have disease-fighting potential, this is hardly substantiated, and there is no known benefit when it is applied topically to skin.

☺ Advanced Retinol-A *($13.97 for 1 ounce)* actually doesn't contain retinol at all; rather, it contains another form of vitamin A, retinyl palmitate, which is several generations removed from retinol (itself already several generations removed from the active ingredient in Renova and Retin-A). This is a good moisturizer for dry skin, but the name is just blatantly misleading marketing information.

☻ Face Lift Anti-Oxidant Moisturizer SPF 15 *($19.99 for 3.4 ounces)* does not contain the required UVA-protecting ingredients avobenzone, zinc oxide, or titanium dioxide, and is not recommended.

☺ Face Lift Deep Wrinkle Mask *($19.99 for 3.4 ounces)* is merely water, glycerin, thickening agents, and some plant extracts. The claims, though, are far more exotic, with promises of plumping up depleted cells in deep wrinkles, immediate tightening and firming, drawing moisture into the skin, and delivering essential minerals and antioxidants. There aren't any essential minerals in here and the algae is just a good soothing agent. The plumping up is true, but any product with water and glycerin will do that.

☺ Face Lift Ultra Skin Lightener *($19.99 for 2 ounces)* does contain hydroquinone, the classic ingredient for lightening skin, which would make it a decent skin-lightening product. But I would be far more enthusiastic about this product if it stated how much hydroquinone, though I suspect from the ingredient listing it is about 1% or 2%, which is just fine.

☹ **Brown Spot Lightener Patch** *($10.97 for six patches)* does contain hydroquinone, which is effective for inhibiting melanin production in skin, but there is no benefit in getting it delivered in a patch. Moreover, the minimal amount of hydroquinone in this one, and the need to use it daily to maintain the lightening effect, make it one of the most expensive and probably least effective hydroquinone products on the market.

☺ **Face Lift Vitamin C Anti-Wrinkle Patch** *($19.99 for eight patches)* does contain vitamin C, but the notion that it is clinically proven to do something about wrinkles is not true. There is no clinical evidence proving vitamin C does much of anything for the skin except reduce irritation and offer a tiny amount of UVB protection. These glycerin-coated patches with vitamins C and E (a teeny, tiny amount at best) are moisturizing, but that's about it.

☺ **Face Lift Youth Serum C** *($24.99 for 1 ounce)*. Don't you wonder why you would need this product to "diminish appearance of fine lines and wrinkles" and "help strengthen elastin and collagen" if the other products in this overextended, overhyped line worked? This is supposed to be an AHA product, only it doesn't contain any. It does contain some sugarcane extract, but that isn't the same thing as glycolic acid or lactic acid. This product does not contain vitamin C, though it does contain irritating lemon and orange extracts, as well as other skin irritants.

☹ **Ease** *($24.99 for 2 ounces)* is one of those products aimed at baby boomers who are worried about the effects of menopause on their skin, and is one of a growing number of products being sold with plant extracts that supposedly contain estrogen or progesterone. It does contain yam extract, but there is no research showing this provides any benefit for skin, or has any bioavailable plant hormones that can be delivered to the skin (please see Chapter Two of this book for the section on "Battling Hormones" for more detailed information).

☺ **Face Lift Ultimate Lip Experience** *($8.25 for 0.35 ounce)* contains Vaseline and mineral oil, which are emollient—but the claims of lifting the lips with this stuff are bizarre. Plus, there is no SPF rating despite the claim on the package stating UVA and UVB sun protection. This is just lip gloss, period.

☹ **The Original Thigh Cream** *($19.99 for 4.1 ounces)* does contain aminophylline, which was the original ingredient in the first thigh-cream product to be sold. But if you recall any of the information I've written in the past about "thigh creams" you will have already laughed at seeing the name of this product. Sadly, it didn't work back then (that was over eight years ago) and it still doesn't work today. If it did, who would have cellulite? And wouldn't there would be a lot more products containing this nonexclusive ingredient?

☹ **The Original Tummy Cream** *($19.99 for 4.1 ounces)* takes its place with thigh creams to take away cellulite and tummy creams to tighten up the skin there. Well, why not? If you believe a cream can magically eliminate fat on your thighs, there should be something you can buy to magically take care of your stomach.

# Urban Decay (Makeup Only)

Urban Decay prides itself on having "… created entirely new looks and options in beauty to appeal to fashion-forward women and men with a yen for experimentation and self-expression." While I have no qualms with anyone expressing themselves, I strongly feel it is wise to think twice about what wearing bizarre colors (black metallic nail polish, glittery peacock-blue eyeliner, or gold lamé body paint) is really saying to the world about you. Depending on your age, hair style, and clothing choices, you will either be thought of as oddly cool, flamboyant, or eccentrically out of place.

Nevertheless, self-expression is a highly personal thing, and if Urban Decay's philosophy of "no rules, no formulas, just a lot of pretty pots, tubes, and vials of shimmery, shiny stuff" really speaks to your beauty ideals, by all means dive right in and snatch those temporary body tattoo decals they sell. In the end, you have the power to control how others perceive you and this line does present a whole new set of options.

Urban Decay's formulations have actually improved in some respects. Along with the revised packaging, you'll find some changes—some for the better, others not so good, and still others for the worse. What definitely has not changed is the lineup of unusual nail-polish shades and the prevailing attitude to "express that extraordinary beauty of yours any way you damn well please." Talk about in-your-face makeup! This line has its image down pat, and it is up to you whether or not to comply with that image, a decision that only you can make. For more information on Urban Decay, call (800) 784-8722 or visit the Web site at www.urbandecay.com.

Please note: as this book went to press, Urban Decay was in the midst of a revamp, and the reviews below reflect the combination of old and new products that are still for sale.

☺ <u>FOUNDATION:</u> **Surreal Skin Makeup 4 in 1 Powder** *($25).* It must be the name that's surreal, because it can't be the quality of this fairly standard, talc-based powder that has a slightly thicker consistency so it can cover more like a foundation. It does have subtle shine, so those with oily skin need to consider the downside of adding more shine. If you have dry skin, a pressed-powder foundation can make skin look and feel drier. That only leaves normal skin types for this version. The six shades are just fine, but there is nothing special about this product—there are lots of other powders that work just as well and even better for far less.

☹ <u>CONCEALER:</u> **Camouflage Concealer** *($14)* is a very emollient, slightly waxy concealer that features a split pan of flesh-toned color and a mint green color. The mint shade is useless, and while the flesh tones are just fine, this will assuredly crease and is absolutely not a good idea for blemishes, contrary to what the instructions recommend.

<u>EYESHADOW:</u> ☺ You will notice, at least as this book goes to press, two different types of packaging for the **Eye Shadow** *($14)*. The colors in the plain cardboard package have an excellent texture, and blend smoothly. They are color-rich, so if you opt for these ultra-shiny shades, apply them sparingly. The glittery shades have a drier texture and tend to flake. The newer silver boxes have the same colors but a different, less pleasing formula that is not as silky. **PotHoles** *($14)* is the name for a small grouping of dark, shiny shadows meant for lining the eyes. They are richly pigmented, but the shine is glaring.

☹ **F/X Powder** *($18)* is a test-tube vial of loose powder that is supposed to have a holographic effect on the skin; all it does is add shine. The texture is grainy and does not adhere that well, so you're left with shine everywhere but where you wanted it to go.

<u>EYE AND BROW SHAPER:</u> ☺ **Eye Pencil** *($12)* is quite standard and has a creamy finish that smears easily. **Liquid Eye Liner** *($14)* has a good, firm brush that applies the color evenly. The plain cardboard packaging has a formula that tends to chip off, while the newer silver-packaged liners have a formula that is much better and stays on very well. Even though the product itself is nice, the colors are truly bizarre and are either metallic or shiny.

☹ **Sparkle Sticks** *($17)* are thick pencils that need sharpening and have a very creamy texture that is infused with large flecks of glitter. Shine aside, this can become an unsightly mess in no time, smearing all over and shedding glitter where you may not want it.

<u>LIPSTICK AND LIP PENCIL:</u> ☺ Urban Decay's **Lipstick** *($12)* features a wide range of unimpressive colors, although there are some decent options mixed in, particularly amid the reds. As this book goes to press, the old packaging (plain cardboard) is a creamy, opaque formula with a good, creamy, iridescent finish. The newer formula (silver box) is less opaque and more greasy than creamy, which is a shame. **Skitz-O-Styx** *($14)* are overpriced, two-toned lipsticks that are very shiny and greasy. **Lip Gunk** *($12)* is a clever name for a standard gloss with a uniquely odd range of colors. The old packaging's formula has a thick, sticky texture and the new packaging's formula is smoother and less sticky.

☺ **Lip Pencils** *($12)*. These are extremely standard pencils that need sharpening, though the small color selection is more intensely pigmented than most.

☺ <u>MASCARA:</u> *($12)* is an OK mascara that builds minimal length and thickness and tends not to smear. This isn't exciting as a mascara, but the colors are. If you want magenta lashes, this would be one of the few places to find that option.

☺ $$$ <u>BRUSHES:</u> Urban Decay has a small range of synthetic **brushes** *($15 to $35)*. They are mostly excellent, and made with firm, soft Taklon (a synthetic, hair-like fiber), with enough density to apply color efficiently. The only ones to be wary of are the **Liner/Shadow Brush** *($15)*, whose shape is not the best for liner but would work well for spot-applying concealer, and the **Concealer Brush** *($15)* itself, which has a strange square tip and is too flimsy for much accuracy or even blending.

☺ <u>SPECIALTY PRODUCTS:</u> **Nail Enamel** *($9.50)* features all the funky, crazy colors you could possibly ever want, in a completely ordinary formula. If the colors strike your fancy, that's what you're really paying for. **Nail Graffiti** *($6.50)* are simply stencils for nails that take the edgy colors to the next level of shocking. **Body Jewelry** *($6.50)*, **Body Paint** *($28)*, **Body Paint to Go** *($12)*, and **Disco Inferno Black Light Pen** *($12)* are all further options for bringing out your rebellious, savvy, street-club, iconoclast look. **Body Haze** *($18)* has been improved. The old version (in plain cardboard) was dry, thick, and hard to blend. The new formula is smooth and slightly creamy and applies evenly. All of the colors are shiny, glittery, and best for an impetuous evening look. **UD40** *($18)* are vivid, highly pigmented, goopy cream colors for the hair (or body). For an extreme look with no commitment, they can be a fun change, but the colors work best in a punk band or on one of those nights where emulating Courtney Love seems like a good idea. **Liquid FX SPF 15** *($16)* is nothing more than an iridescent tint for the face and body. The effect is glow with glitter and the SPF is without UVA protection.

# Uvavita (Skin Care Only)

It is always makes me incredulous to see what warrants attention or headlines in the cosmetics world. In this case, it was grape seed oil that did it. With this, what would otherwise be a completely unimpressive, innocuous, do-nothing group of products somehow becomes a miracle treatment for skin because of that single ingredient. Grape seed oil is now the answer for wrinkles because it is supposed to be the final answer for fighting free-radical damage. Or anyway that's Uvavita's hook. Its products do contain grape seed oil. It probably won't shock you to learn that grape seed oil won't change or prevent a wrinkle on anyone's face, but even if it could, the minimal amount of it used in these products means that it isn't even all that helpful as an antioxidant. And despite the "uva" in the company name, you don't want me to get started on the fact that this small group of products doesn't include a sunscreen. [For your information, "uva" is the spanish word for grape.]

A lot of the buzz on anything involving grape extracts is from a story in *Con-*

*sumer Reports* for November 1999 that ranked grape juice just above green tea and blueberries as having strong antioxidant properties. However the benefits reported in both *Consumer Reports* and a lead story in *USA Today* for February 2, 2000, had to do with drinking the stuff, not putting it on the skin. There are no published studies indicating that grapes in any form, applied topically, can affect the wrinkling process (and vineyard workers are hardly wrinkle-free). But when it comes to skin care, there are lots of unpublished studies that "prove" all kinds of things. Uvavita loves pointing to a Dr. Stephen Herber of the St. Helena Institute for Plastic Surgery [not surprisingly, St. Helena is in the heart of California's wine country], who conducted a study on the benefits of grape seed. This "study," and I use the word loosely, had 16 volunteers use pure milled grape seed extract as a topical application to their facial skin twice each day for six weeks. The results? What a surprise! Herber found that 88% of the volunteers reported improved texture to their facial skin. Other reported effects include evening-out of complexion pigmentation and excessive oil, a decrease in breakouts, and a decrease in dryness. It only takes a cursory look to notice that this study wasn't done double-blind, that a placebo wasn't used (so we don't know if the results would be the same with a similar or dissimilar type of extract), and that we have no idea of the status of the participants' skin before they started, or what their relation to the product line or researcher was. Even if you buy the results of this study, the study itself used a pure concentration of the substance on the skin, and Uvavita products use minuscule amounts of grape extract or grape oil. There is no information on whether this watered-down version has any benefit whatsoever.

As I've stated before, antioxidants are a big issue, and I do feel strongly that the new millennium will see incredible strides in this area. Right now, it's too early to suggest that we know which antioxidant is the best, how much of it is needed, or whether or not they work on the surface of skin to affect wrinkling, and products that say they know best are a waste of money and don't help your skin. For more information, call (707) 967-8482 or visit the Web site at www.uvavita.com.

Please note: Most all of the Uvavita products contain a tiny amount of phenol, an extremely irritating preservative that is rarely used in cosmetics anymore. As a matter of fact, this is one of the only product lines in this entire book that utilizes it.

☺ $$$ **Day Antioxidant Moisturizer** *($53 for 2 ounces)* is an exceptionally ordinary moisturizer for normal to dry skin. The minuscule amounts of water-binding agents and vitamins in this product make them inconsequential for skin. What the tiny amount of grape seed oil can do is up to you.

☺ $$$ **Night Antioxidant Nourishing Cream** *($56 for 2 ounces)* is similar to the Day Antioxidant above and the same basic comments apply. The teeny amount of collagen in this product has no impact on skin.

☺ $$$ **Exfoliating Body Scrub** *($34 for 6 ounces)* is a fairly gentle, extremely standard, detergent-based, overpriced body scrub that uses crushed grape seeds as the abrasive. This one is a leap of faith that the crushed grape seeds have any special properties for skin, though even if they did, they would be rinsed down the drain before they could have any benefit.

☹ $$$ **Exfoliating Dead Sea Mask** (*$40 for 8 ounces*) is a standard a clay mask with the most minuscule amount of grape seed oil imaginable. Aside from the grape seed oil, this product contains Dead Sea mud. While Dead Sea mud may have some benefit for certain skin diseases and it can absorb oil (just like any other source of earth minerals can), there is no research anywhere indicating it has any other unique benefit for skin.

☺ **Hydrating Body Lotion** (*$30 for 6 ounces*) is just a decent moisturizer with a minuscule amount of grape seed extract.

# Vaseline Intensive Care and Dermasil (Skin Care Only)

For more information about Vaseline or Dermasil products, call (800) 743-8640.

☺ **Advanced Healing Lotion** (*$2.89 for 11 ounces*) is an exceptionally standard, Vaseline-based moisturizer for dry skin.

☹ **Aloe & Naturals Lotion** (*$2.29 for 3.3 ounces*) contains eucalyptus, orange oil, and sage, which makes it potentially irritating for all skin types.

☺ **Dermasil Dry Skin Treatment Cream** (*$7.79 for 4 ounces*) is an exceptionally standard, though good, Vaseline-based moisturizer for dry skin.

☺ **Dermatology Formula** (*$2.29 for 11 ounces*) is a very emollient, though very standard, mundane moisturizer for someone with dry skin.

☺ **Dry Skin Lotion** (*$2.29 for 3.3 ounces*) does have an SPF 5, which is just appalling, especially as it doesn't contain UVA-protecting ingredients. This is a decent moisturizer for dry skin but the sunscreen is just a waste.

☹ **Petroleum Jelly Cream Enriched with Vitamin E** (*$2.99 for 4.5 ounces*) has, as its second ingredient, aluminum starch, which can be a skin irritant and shouldn't be in a product aimed at dry skin.

☺ **Solutions Skin Repair** (*$2.99 for 3.5 ounces*) is a good, though standard moisturizer for dry skin but it can't repair skin.

# Vichy (Skin Care Only/Canada Only)

Vichy is a line of skin-care products owned by L'Oreal. Much like L'Oreal, Vichy retails at drugstores, the prices are relatively inexpensive, and there are some impressive product selections. The areas where Vichy excels are its moisturizers and sunscreens, though it falls short in its acne and cleansing products. Vichy has chosen to set itself apart from other lines on the basis of the special water they use that comes from a mineral spring in the town of Vichy, France (of course if the water is so special and great for skin it can make you wonder why all the L'Oreal product lines don't use it). Is there actually something to the use of Vichy spring water for skin care? According to articles in the *International Journal of Cosmetic Science,* 1996 (18, 269–277), and *Nouvelles Dermatologiques,* 1998 (volume 17), it seems Vichy water has been used for local application in the treatment of certain dermatitis. Rather than having some mysterious quality, the most likely reason for Vichy water being of help is due to the high fluoride content of the water. Two journal articles, one published in the *American Journal of Kidney Disorders,* August 1987 (10:2, 136–139), the other in *Pathologie et Biologie* (Paris), January 1986 (34[1]:33–39), indicate that Vichy water is "a highly mineralized water containing 8.5 mg/L of fluoride." Fluoride is a potent antimicrobial agent. Dermatitis conditions such as rosacea and psoriasis can be helped by topical antimicrobial agents, so it isn't surprising that the fluoride in the Vichy water may transfer some of that benefit to skin. However, whether or not any of that benefit is retained once the Vichy water is mixed into a skin-care product is unknown.

What is clearly misleading here are the claims about these products being hypoallergenic (the fragrance in most all of these products negates any notion of these products having a reduced potential for allergic reactions). The company also claims they are dermatologist tested, but if a dermatologist tested them, he or she didn't know much about skin care in regard to irritation, how an effective AHA or BHA product is formulated, or what ingredients can be a problem for combination skin.

The far more logical reason to shop Vichy is for some of its well-formulated products; the spring water used in the products is a gimmick that makes for a great story but very little in the way of skin care. For more information, call (514) 335-8000 or (888) 45-VICHY or visit the Web site at www.vichy.com.

☺ **Purete Thermale Demaquillant Integral One-Step Cleanser for Face and Eyes 3-in-1** *($15.50 for 200 ml)* is mostly a wipe-off cleanser with a teeny amount of detergent-cleansing agent. It is an option for normal to dry skin with minimal risk of leaving a greasy film on the skin. It does contain fragrance.

☹ **Dermatological Cleansing Bar** *($7.95 for 100 g)* is a standard, detergent-based bar cleanser that can be drying, and the ingredients that keep the bar in its bar form can clog pores.

☺ **Normaderm Express Cleansing Gel, for Acne Prone Skin** *($9.99 for 150 ml)* is a standard, detergent-based cleanser with a teeny amount of AHA and an even teenier amout of disinfectant. The amount of AHA isn't enough to exfoliate the skin, and the disinfectant would be rinsed down the drain before it had much of an effect on the skin. It's still a decent cleanser for normal to oily skin. It does contain fragrance.

☹ **Normaderm Express 2-in-One Lotion, for Acne Prone Skin** *($11.99 for 150 ml)* is mostly alcohol, and that hurts all skin types.

☺ **Purete Thermale Dermo-Protective Cleansing Milk Dry Skin** *($14.95 for 200 ml)* is a standard, wipe-off cleanser that can leave a greasy film behind on the skin, though this can be an option for someone with dry skin. It does contain fragrance.

☺ **Purete Thermale Dermo-Protective Cleansing Milk Normal & Combination Skin** *($14.95 for 200 ml)* is almost identical to the Dry Skin version above, which makes it a problem for someone with combination skin. It does contain fragrance.

☺ **Purete Thermale Hydra-Purifying Cleansing Gel** *($14.95 for 125 ml)* is a standard, detergent-based water-soluble cleanser that would work well for most skin types but is probably best for someone with normal to oily skin.

☺ **Demaquillant Yeux Sensibles Eye Makeup Remover for Sensitive Eyes** *($13.50 for 150 ml)* is a standard, detergent-based cleanser that contains way too many cleansing agents as well as fragrance, which does not make it better for sensitive eyes, though as a standard makeup remover it works as well as any.

☺ **Purete Thermale Gentle Exfoliating Gel** *($13.50 for 50 ml)* is a standard, detergent-based scrub that uses synthetic scrub particles (ground-up plastic) as the abrasive. It isn't all that gentle, but it can exfoliate. This also contains salicylic acid, but the pH of this one is too high for it to be effective as an exfoliant. This does contain fragrance and coloring agents.

☹ **Purete Thermale Dermo Protective Toning Lotion, for Dry Skin** *($14.95 for 200 ml)* contains witch hazel, which can be a skin irritant.

☹ **Purete Thermale Dermo Protective Toning Lotion, for Normal to Combination Skin** *($13.50 for 200 ml)* contains even more witch hazel than the one above, and is not recommended.

☺ **Thermal Spa Water** *($4.88 for 50 ml)*. The fluoride content of the water may have some antimicrobial benefit if you have dermatitis, but for healthy skin it is not of help.

☺ **Adaptive Skin Balancing System, for Combination Skin** *($21.50 for 40 ml)*. The interesting ingredients for this product are so far at the end of the ingredient list that they are completely inconsequential for skin. Plus, there is absolutely nothing in this product that can balance oily or dry skin. It is just an OK, rather ho-hum moisturizer for normal to dry skin.

☹ **Lift-Activ** *($28 for 50 ml)*. The cornstarch in here may make the skin feel tighter but it is also drying and irritating for the skin. What a waste, because every other aspect of this product makes for a good moisturizer.

☹ **Lift-Activ Eyes** *($26 for 15 ml)* is similar to the one above, and the same review applies.

☹ **Lift-Activ Lotion** *($18.95 for 40 ml)* is almost identical to the one above; the same review applies.

☹ **Lift-Activ Night Intensive Detoxifying Firming Care** *($35 for 50 ml)* is similar to the other Lift products above, and the same comments apply.

☹ **Lift-Activ Dry Skin** *($32 for 50 ml)* is similar to the other Lift products above and the same comments apply.

☺ **Lumiactive Rejuvenating Daily Filter-Care** *($26 for 50 ml)* is a very good, UVA-protecting sunscreen that contains both avobenzone and Mexoryl SX™. It also contains a small amount of AHA, but not enough to be effective as an exfoliant, especially not with the high pH this one has.

☺ **Lumineuse Sheer Radiance Tinted Moisturizer, Dry Skin** *($22 for 30 ml)* has a tint color that isn't the best, but this is a good emollient moisturizer for dry skin. It also contains some plant extracts that you're supposed to believe act like AHAs, but they don't.

☺ **Lumineuse Sheer Radiance Tinted Moisturizer, Normal to Combination Skin** *($22 for 30 ml)* is similar to the one above, only this product contains ingredients that can be a problem for combination skin, including several plant oils.

☺ **Nutritive 1 Balanced Nutrient Cream for Dry Skin** *($26 for 40 ml)* is a good, basic moisturizer for dry skin. The minuscule amounts of vitamins and water-binding agents in here make them inconsequential for skin.

☺ **Nutritive 2 Reinforced Nutrient Cream for Very Dry Skin** *($26 for 40 ml)*. This is a very heavy, very ordinary moisturizer for dry skin that is easily replaced with just plain Vaseline, and then you wouldn't have the fragrance and heavy wax ingredients.

☺ **Optalia Restructuring Eye Gel** *($28.50 for 15 ml)* is a good lightweight moisturizer for normal to slightly dry skin. However, the really interesting ingredients come well after the preservative, making them barely helpful for skin.

☺ **Regenium Night Renewal Cream** *($31 for 40 ml)* is an emollient moisturizer for normal to dry skin.

☺ **Thermal S1: Long Lasting Hydration** *($24 for 50 ml)* is a very good moisturizer for dry skin.

☺ **Thermal S2: Long Lasting Hydration for Very Dehydrated Skin** *($24 for 50 ml)* is similar to the one above, and the same basic review applies.

☺ **Thermal S2 Lotion: Long Lasting Hydration** *($24 for 50 ml)* is similar to the one above, and the same review applies.

☺ **Therma S Oil Free Lotion** *($24 for 100 ml)* is a good lightweight moisturizer for normal to slightly dry skin, but it contains cornstarch, which can be a problem for clogging pores.

☹ **Thermal S Mat** *($24 for 50 ml)* contains alcohol high up on the ingredient listing, which makes this too irritating and drying for all skin types.

☺ **Capital Soleil Protective Gel-Cream SPF 15** *($15.50 for 120 ml)* is a very good sunscreen for normal to dry skin; it contains three of the four known UVA-protecting ingredients: titanium dioxide, avobenzone, and Mexoryl SX™.

☺ **Capital Soleil Protective Lotion SPF 15** *($15.50 for 120 ml)* is a very good UVA-protecting sunscreen for normal to dry skin; it contains titanium dioxide, avobenzone, and Mexoryl SX™.

☺ **Capital Soleil Sunblock Cream for the Face SPF 25** *($15.50 for 50 ml)* is a very good sunscreen for normal to dry skin; it contains titanium dioxide, avobenzone, and Mexoryl SX™.

☺ **Capital Soleil Sunblock Lotion SPF 25** *($15.50 for 120 ml)* is a very good sunscreen for normal to dry skin; it contains titanium dioxide, avobenzone, and Mexoryl SX™.

☺ **Capital Soleil Total Sunblock Lotion SPF 30** *($15.50 for 120 ml)* is a very good sunscreen for normal to dry skin; it contains titanium dioxide, avobenzone, and Mexoryl SX™.

☺ **Capital Soleil Total Sunblock Cream SPF 45** *($15.50 for 50 ml)* is a very good sunscreen for normal to dry skin; it contains titanium dioxide, avobenzone, and Mexoryl SX™.

☺ **Capital Soleil Total Sunblock Cream SPF 60** *($19.50 for 50 ml)* is a very good sunscreen for all the same reasons the other Vichy sunscreens are so great, but the SPF 60 just doesn't make sense. The SPF 60 tells the average fair-skinned individual that they can stay in the sun for 20 hours, but there are very few places in the world that have that amount of daylight. SPF 60 doesn't offer "better" or more intensive protection, just unnecessarily longer protection.

☺ **Capital Soleil Sunblock Lotion for Children SPF 25** *($15.50 for 120 ml)* is a very good sunscreen for normal to dry skin that contains titanium dioxide, avobenzone, and Mexoryl SX™; however, there is nothing about this product that makes it more appropriate for children.

☺ **Capital Soleil Sunblock Lotion for Children SPF 35** *($19.50 for 120 ml)* is similar to the Children SPF 25 above, and the same comments apply.

☺ **$$$ Capital Soleil Sunblock Stick SPF 25** *($9 for 3 ml tube)* does contain titanium dioxide; however, given that all the other sunscreens from Vichy also contain avobenzone and Mexoryl SX™ (which really add to the UVA protection you get), this one is not the pick over the ones above.

☹ **Capital Soleil Self-Tan Cream-Gel for Face SPF 7** *($18 for 50 ml)* does contain very good UVA protection, but the SPF number is not enough for daily protection. The self-tanning ingredient used here is the same as in the one below, and it works, but do not rely on this for sun protection.

☺ **Capital Soleil Self-Tan Milk for the Body** *($18 for 100 ml)* is a standard, dihydroxyacetone-based self tanner, the same ingredient used in all self tanners. This one will work as well as any.

☺ **Capital Soleil After Sun Calming Reparative Gel for Sunburn** (*$18 for 100 ml*) is a very good moisturizer for normal to dry skin, but the claim that it "encourages repair of DNA caused by the sun" is absolutely not possible. There is not one ingredient in here that can repair one skin cell from the damage caused by sunlight.

☹ **Heliocalm Soothing and Hydrating After-Sun Milk** (*$15.50 for 150 ml*) would have been a great moisturizer, but this one contains menthol, a skin irritant that can hurt the skin's healing process.

☺ **Heliocalm Calming Reparative Gel for Face and Body** (*$15.50 for 100 ml*) is a very good lightweight gel. This won't repair anything, but it is a good moisturizer for someone with normal to slightly dry skin.

☺ **Normaderm Express Tinted Treatment Cream, for Acne Prone Skin** (*$11.99 for 30 ml*) has a tint that isn't the best color, and although this product is meant to be an AHA exfoliant, which might be helpful, it doesn't contain enough AHA to do that.

☺ **$$$ RETI-C Intensive Care, Retinol, Anti-Wrinkle Vitamin C, Radiance** (*$33 for 30 ml*) is here for all those women who will think that they now have the best of both worlds, a product with both retinol and vitamin C in one place. While this product definitely contains retinol, the vitamin C in here is ascorbic acid, which is considered to be one of the more irritating and unstable forms. Also, this one contains aluminum starch (octenylsuccinate), cornstarch, and magnesium sulfate, which are all absorbent and drying and not the best in a product meant to help with making skin look less wrinkled.

☹ **Normaderm Express (Tinted and Non-Tinted) Treatment Cream, for Acne Prone Skin** (*$12.50 for 30 ml*) includes a teeny amount of glycolic acid that is not enough to exfoliate skin, and the titanium dioxide and cornstarch in here can clog pores. Neither of these formulations are of much use to someone with blemish-prone skin.

☹ **Normaderm Patch Express, for Acne Prone Skin** (*$10.99 for 24 patches*) contains a tiny amount of disinfectant and some BHA. The disinfectant is OK but not the best for breakouts, and the pH isn't low enough for the BHA to be effective as an exfoliant.

☹ **Normaderm Stick Express Treatment Stick for Imperfections, for Acne Prone Skin** (*$9.99 for 0.28 g*) contains lots of ingredients that would be a problem for blemish-prone skin, including castor oil, titanium dioxide, thick waxes, and aluminum chlorohydrate (that's deodorant!).

☺ **$$$ Purifying Thermal Mask** (*$19.95 for 50 ml*) is a very standard clay mask that can be good for normal to oily skin.

☺ $$$ **Rehydrating Thermal Mask** *($19.95 for 50 ml)* is a fairly emollient moisturizer that is being used as a mask, which is just fine.

# *Victoria Jackson Cosmetics*

Victoria Jackson Cosmetics was one of the first cosmetics lines to be sold via infomercial, and as a result remains one of the most successful ones to hit the airwaves. Armed with everything from celebrity endorsements to impressive before-and-after pictures of several women, Jackson's presentation is impressive, and it's hard to not fall under Jackson's concept of what it takes to look beautiful. Almost everything you need for a complete makeup application is included with the **Introductory Kit** *($119.85; $234.35)*, (the pricing depends on whether you're a member of the Jackson buying club but I'll get to that later). From a brush set to mascara, and everything in between, it's all here. There's even a how-to video and reorder forms inserted "because we're so sure you'll be happy with Victoria Jackson cosmetics."

The hook with all of Jackson's kits is that the prices for individual products ordered separately are far steeper than what you end up paying (item for item) when you order the kits. For example, the foundation is sold by itself for $24.95, although you receive the same item for $12.95 if you order one of the kits that includes this product. Actually, all of Victoria Jackson's products have two prices. If you are so inclined to order a certain number of products, you can get the cheaper price every time.

But what about the products? The majority of the makeup items are fine, although nothing special or worthy of "must-have" status; a few don't work well at all. Overall, although some additional kits with new colors are available, along with a few other minor additions, the makeup has not changed much since it was last reviewed. Still, I liked some of these products very much and the prices (if you buy more than $20 at a time) are quite reasonable.

Once you've placed your order, you will begin receiving the product catalog. Among several regular and seasonal "money saving specials" are a group of eyeshadows, eye pencils, blushes, and lipsticks divided into **Morning, Noon, and Night Color Kits** *($41.95; $82.75)*. There are three different intensities of makeup (a total of 12 products) designed to correspond with the different light levels throughout the day. Along these same lines, the Morning colors are softest, Noon a bit more intense, and Night includes "dramatic" colors. This is more makeup than anyone needs, and it assumes that you need different makeup colors for morning than you would for the afternoon, and then different again at night. There are easier ways to turn morning makeup into night without purchasing an entirely new set of products. Besides, within these kits and almost every other color kit Jackson "personally selects" for you, there are shiny eyeshadows and greasy lipsticks. The blushes and pencils are nice, but these end up costing more if purchased outside of the kits.

Jackson's **Vanity Kit** *($52.95)* is dubbed the Ultimate Space-Saving Makeup Kit. It does look great in the picture and it does end up occupying only a small amount of room on your vanity. Yet for all the convenience and orderliness this kit provides, the containers are not refillable, so once products start running out, replacing them becomes an expensive proposition because you have to start all over again.

The makeup demonstration videotape that came with the Introductory Kit was good and understandable, although I didn't always agree with Victoria Jackson's application techniques. For example, she recommends applying eyeliner and brow color before eyeshadows, but that means the shadows will more than likely undo or mess those up. A more annoying feature of the tape is that over half of it feels like you are sitting through another ad, listening to Ms. Jackson and a guest celebrity talk about how great the products are. If you've got the tape, you already have the products; now you want to learn how to use them. Sigh. I suppose sometimes it's hard to stop selling.

The first price listed for the products below is the "whoelsale price," the second price listed is for the "retail price," which is the price you pay if you spend more than $20. It's an interesting concept but given the ease of ordering $20 worth, there really is no reason for the two-price level, though I suspect some women will think they are getting a great deal. For more information on Victoria Jackson Cosmetics' products, call (800) V-MAKEUP or visit the Web site at www.vmakeup.com.

# *Victoria Jackson Skin Care*

☺ **Facial Cleanser and Eye Makeup Remover** *($9.25, $13.50 for 4 ounces)* is a standard, detergent-based wipe-off cleanser. You are supposed to wipe off your makeup using this watery cleanser applied to a cotton ball, and then rinse off any residue. Wiping off makeup pulls at the skin and over time can cause it to sag.

☹ **$$$ Sensitive Facial Scrub** *($12.95, $19.95 for 4.7 ounces)* claims that this product is oil-free, but there are several ingredients in here that would not make someone with oily or combination skin happy. This is a group of thickeners with cornmeal as the scrub agent. You would be far better off with baking soda and some Cetaphil Gentle Skin Cleanser than with this waxy scrub.

☺ **Toning Mist** *($9.75, $14.50 for 4 ounces)* is a very good nonirritating toner.

☺ **$$$ Eye Repair Gel** *($12.50, $19.50 for 0.5 ounce)* would be a good lightweight moisturizer for the skin around the eyes.

☹ **Moisture Enhancer with Sunscreen SPF 8** *($12.75, $19.50 for 1.9 ounces)*. SPF 8 already doesn't count, but then this product doesn't contain avobenzone, zinc oxide, or titanium dioxide for UVA protection, and is not recommended.

☺ **Moisturizer** *($13.75, 20.50 for 2 ounces)* would be a very good moisturizer for someone with dry skin.

☺ **Nourishing Skin Revitalizer** *($12.95, 19.95 for 1 ounce)* isn't all that revitalizing, but it is a good moisturizer for someone with dry skin.

☺ **Skin Renewal System** *($30.95, $39.95 for 0.14 ounce of Extra-Intensive Eye Cream and 1.25 ounces of Extra-Intensive Night Cream)* is somewhat unusual. The Night Cream is in the bottom half of the jar, and the Eye Cream is in the top half. Very cute. However, the ingredients in each are not all that different, so the division seems unnecessary. Both creams are very good moisturizers for dry skin.

☹ **Firming Gel Masque** *($11.95, $17.50 for 4 ounces)* won't firm anything, and the second ingredient is a strong skin irritant. If your skin looks tighter after you take this mask off, it's due to the irritation.

☹ **Moisturizing Lip Conditioner SPF 15** *($9.95, $15.95)* doesn't contain avobenzone, zinc oxide, or titanium dioxide, and is not recommended for sun protection.

# Victoria Jackson Makeup

☺ <u>**FOUNDATION:**</u> There is only one type of **$$$ Foundation** *($14.95; $25.95)*; it comes in a single compact that holds two shades for each of four categories of skin tones: Light, Medium, Tan, and Dark. The colors are marginally good, with the medium shades being a tad ashy green and the Light shades being a bit pink. There are two options for darker skin tones, and Mahogany is quite dark but slightly shiny. To create the right color for your skin, you are supposed to mix the two shades together, which is fine if you know how to mix them in the right proportions. If you don't, you're likely to have trouble. The foundation's texture is quite thick, and the application is not what I would call sheer, as the commercial claims. It's Vaseline-based with several waxes and is fairly greasy. Oily and combination skins, or anyone who tends toward breakouts, would not do well with this one.

☹ <u>**CONCEALER:**</u> There is no individually packed concealer in the Victoria Jackson line. Instead, she suggests using the lighter of the two foundation shades for the under-eye area. That would be fine if the foundation wasn't as greasy as it is. This easily slips into lines around the eyes, and any liner you use afterward will probably smear.

☺ <u>**POWDER:**</u> **$$$ Pressed Powder** *($11.95; $17.95)* comes in three shades and is talc-based. The colors are all fine and the texture is sheer and light.

☺ <u>**BLUSH:**</u> Each color-family kit (Peach, Pink, Red, and all of the "theme" kits) comes with a **$$$ Blush Compact** *($11.95; $20.95)* that contains two colors. One shade is either a pale pastel or vivid shade and the other is either a vivid or earthy-brown tone. The textures and colors are very good, although some of the color combinations do not work well with the rest of the kit's shades, and that can make blending one color into the next a challenge.

☺ <u>**EYESHADOW:**</u> The **$$$ Eyeshadow Compact** *($11.95; $20.95)* is a single compact with four different colors. Most of the color combinations are excellent, but there are a few odd mixes that would look a little off if applied for the same eye design. However, almost all of the colors are slightly to heavily shiny.

☺ <u>EYE AND BROW SHAPER:</u> All of the **Eye Pencils** *($7; $10.95)* and the **Taupe Brow Pencil** *($7; $10.95)* are standard but workable, with a fairly dry texture. In most of the kits, you'll receive two twist-up eye pencils in black and brown. The Taupe Brow Pencil (which is not going to work for everyone) is available in the Introductory Kit. The **Beauty Survival Kit** *($42.95)* and the **Vanity Kit** *($52.95)* each contain the Eye Pencils but not Taupe Brow Pencil (which is hardly a problem).

<u>LIPSTICK AND LIP PENCIL:</u> ☺ Each Victoria Jackson Cosmetics color kit includes a $$$ **Lip Compact** *($11.95; $18.95)* that contains four different colors. In the original Peach, Pink, and Red kits, you get three fairly greasy lip colors and a lipcolor powder. The lip powder is a problem because it tends to cake on the lips and dry them out when used alone or for an extended period of time. The rest of Jackson's color kits contain the Lip Compacts in varying color combinations, and all four colors are the standard, greasy lipstick formula, and no lipcolor powder. Each kit includes a matching **Lip Pencil** *($7; $10.95)* that is just a standard, creamy, twist-up pencil. $$$ **Tube Lipsticks** *($9.95; $15.95 singles; $24.95; $47.85 for a set of three)* are simply a traditional tube version of Jackson's lip compact colors. The shades are lettered and numbered to correspond with the order of colors (from left to right) in the compact. For example, in the Peach Kit, the first color on the left has a tube counterpart named Autumn Sand P1. It's a clever way to tell the oftentimes similar colors apart, but these remain fairly standard, opaque, and greasy lipsticks that are not for those prone to lip colors bleeding. By the way, although these single colors are divided into four finishes (matte, gloss, satin, and frost) they are largely indistinguishable and the mattes are just as greasy as the others.

☺ $$$ **At Long Last** *($9.95; $15.95)* is a very creamy, full-coverage tube lipstick whose colors are not about subtlety. The 12 shades stay on reasonably well (definitely longer than Jackson's other lipsticks) and offer an assortment of reds, browns, and deep plums that would be especially flattering on darker skin tones. This is still creamy enough to bleed into lines around the mouth, but nevertheless it's a good lipstick.

☺ <u>MASCARA:</u> The Introductory Kit comes with **Dual Black Mascara** *($8.50; $13.95)* with one end a clear lash conditioner and the other end black mascara. The mascara is good but the conditioner part is just glycerin and film former. It won't do much for the lashes, and you won't notice any difference when you use it. Victoria Jackson Cosmetics' traditional black **Mascara** *($14.95)* is great all by itself.

☹ **Waterproof Mascara** *($9.50; $14.95)* goes on slightly heavy and sticky, clumping lashes together, and feels rather heavy, and then it isn't all that waterproof.

☹ <u>BRUSHES:</u> Victoria Jackson Cosmetics includes a set of brushes in the Introductory Kit that are adequate but not great. A **Retractable Brush Set** *($40)* that includes a retractable blush and a lip brush is very overpriced for what you get, and the blush brush can feel rough on the skin. The **Professional Brush Set** *($18.95)* includes a lip brush, an eyebrow brush/comb, a two-sided eyeshadow brush, and a blush brush. The bristles on all of these are sparse and not firm enough to hold color well. There are better brushes on the market.

## Victoria's Secret Cosmetics (Makeup Only)

Victoria's Secret Cosmetics (makeup products only) clearly tries to have the same sleek, coy sexuality the rest of the Victoria's Secret merchandise is known for. And in what better environment to offer makeup! Victoria's Secret is all about a woman feeling sexy and beautiful, head to toe. Donning a silky teddy or lacy corset almost begs for full, glossed, pouty lips and softly blushed cheeks. Plus, what woman can pass a cosmetics counter and not start to play, which is exactly what was taking place on several of my visits to a few Victoria's Secret stores—women were shopping for makeup and the lingerie part of the store was empty. It will be hard not to stop and try these products: the large, imposing display is easily accessible, and the sales staff eager and almost too enthusiastic. Plus, the polished silvery containers and boxes are indeed beautiful and the names sweet and winsome. Draw Me a Line Lip Pencil and Keep Your Secret Cream Concealer are irresistibly cute. But cute doesn't always mean quality, and beyond the packaging, there needs to be good product quality that works. It would be easy to get waylaid by the impulse buying this line (or any line for that matter) can attract, but let me encourage you to pick and choose wisely. What won't be a secret after you read my review are which products work and which ones don't. For more information about Victoria's Secret Cosmetics, call (800) 888-8200 or visit the Web site at www.victoriassecret.com.

**FOUNDATION:** ☺ **Seamless Cover Oil-Free Cream-to-Powder Makeup SPF 10** *($19.50)* has a creamy-slick texture that quickly dries to a nice matte finish, and the SPF 10 is a decent titanium dioxide base. The 12 colors for this haven't gotten much better than they were when I first reviewed this line, but their excessive shininess has thankfully been eliminated. These shades are too peach, pink, or rose: 02, 05, 06, 07, 08, 09, 10, and 12.

☹ **Seamless Cover Moisture Rich Cream-to-Powder Makeup SPF 10** *($19.50)* has ten poor colors, but, even more disappointing, it lacks any UVA-protecting ingredients. The texture is rather thick and creamy, which isn't bad, just heavy and hard to blend.

☹ **Liquid Lingerie Moisture Rich Makeup SPF 10** *($17.50)* has a very soft, sheer finish, but the color selection is poor; of the ten shades, half are too pink, peach, or ash to recommend, plus the SPF (which should be an SPF 15) doesn't include UVA-protecting ingredients.

☺ **Liquid Lingerie Oil-Free Makeup SPF 10** *($17.50)* has all the benefits the Moisture Rich version above lacks, including far better colors—there are 15 of them, including shades for very light and dark skins—and a titanium dioxide–based sunscreen (though a higher SPF would be better). The application isn't as sheer as the name implies, but you do get light to medium coverage with a dry, smooth finish! This one is worth checking out if you have normal to oily skin, but watch out for shades 06, 08, 12, and 13.

<u>CONCEALER:</u> ☺ **Keep Your Secret Cream Concealer** *($10)* comes in a tube with four excellent shades! It does have a smooth, even finish, but it can crease, so test this one before you consider buying.

☹ **All an Illusion Skin Tone Primer** *($17.50)* is your standard group of green-peach- and lavender-toned color-correctors. They don't change skin tone, they only add a strange cast to the skin and interact even more strangely with your foundation. Even if you're sold on this kind of product, this one contains isopropyl myristate (the second ingredient), which is known to cause breakouts. **Trick Stick Corrector Crayon** *($10)* has the same concept as the Primer, only in pencil form, and for some reason comes in only two shades, yellow and green. **Thick Stick Concealer Crayon** *($10)* is a chubby pencil with three shades, of which two are way too peach for most all skin tones. The Light shade is just fine, but the texture is heavy and hard to blend, and it tends to easily crease into lines.

☺ <u>POWDER:</u> **Powdered Silk Finishing Powder** *($15)* is a standard, talc-based pressed powder with a wonderful, smooth, silky texture. Of the eight shades #2, #5, #6, and #8 can be too rose, peach, or pink. The other four shades are excellent skin tones.

<u>BLUSH:</u> $$$ ☺ **Sudden Blush Sheer Blushing Powder** *($15)* has a gorgeous silky texture, with a beautiful range of mostly matte shades—only Honey and Wine are noticeably shiny.

☹ **Dream Dust Face & Body Shimmer Powder** *($17.50)* is actually not all that shiny or iridescent and the texture is not as soft and even as that of the other powders in this line. While I'm not a fan of shiny, this product wouldn't past muster even if I did like shine.

☺ <u>EYESHADOW:</u> **Silky Wear Eye Colour** *($11)* is a good-looking group of very workable eyeshadow colors. Unfortunately, most of the shades are iridescent, even though the salesperson tried to convince me otherwise. The only matte shades were In the Buff, Hazelnut Cream, Java, Shell, Love at First Sight (this one is pink), and Bisque. **Party of 4 Eye Colour Quad** *($15)* is a set of four shiny shades of white, off-white, cream, and tan. For shiny this is fine, but how much shine can any one face handle?

☺ <u>EYE AND BROW SHAPER:</u> **Pencil Me in Brow Pencil** *($10)* has an exceptionally dry finish, which can make brows look less "penciled," but this one is hard to get on in the first place. All in all this is just a very standard brow pencil with a comb on one end to soften the application. **Draw Me a Line Eye Pencil** *($10)* is a standard, rather creamy-finish pencil. It will definitely tend to smear along the lower lashes, though it will be easier to apply over eyeshadow. **Unruffled** *($12.50)* is a brow mascara that comes in a clear gel (like a gel hairspray) and two colors—blonde and dark brown. The color choice is limited, but this one works well enough. **Stroke of Brilliance Shimmery Liquid Eyeliner** *($12)* will work as well as any if you want shiny gold or shiny black eyeliner.

<u>LIPSTICK AND LIP PENCIL:</u> ☺ **Smooth Talk Creamy Lip Colour** *($12.50)* is a huge array of lipsticks with a great color selection. The application is definitely creamy, so if you have any lines around your lips this one will bleed in an instant, but if not, these are a great option.

☺ **Pure Reflection Ultra Shine Lipstick** *($13)* has a slippery, greasy texture that will slide off with even the softest kiss. The colors are almost all iridescent and are an option if that's the look you are going for, but it isn't the best for wear or texture. **Liquid Gleam Shiny Lipstick** *($11)* is a high-gloss lip gloss with sparkles that comes in a tube. **Mirror Mirror Shiny Lipgloss** *($10)* is similar to Liquid Gleam, only this one comes in a pot. **Draw Me a Line Lip Pencil** *($10)* is a large range of standard lip pencils that have a creamier application than most. **Quick Draw Lip Crayon** *($11)* is a chubby pencil that works as a lipstick, but has a very smeary, glossy application. **Mouth to Mouth Long Wear Lip Colour** *($12.50)* isn't all that long-wearing. The colors for this one are also limited, and the shades are too dark for lighter skin tones.

☹ **Pleasingly Plump** *($12)* is supposed to be a type of "spackle" that fills in the lips, making them smooth and perfect. It doesn't work. It's just a matte-finish concealer that sits on the surface of the lips for several minutes until it settles into the lines. It doesn't fill in anything or change the appearance of lips. **Party of 4 Lipgloss Quad** *($15)* is a group of four lip glosses ranging from black to white. It's supposed to change the color of any lipstick you own. It will indeed do that, but it also gives the lipstick a bizarre color quality.

<u>MASCARA:</u> ☺ **Stroke of Brilliance Mascara** *($12)* is a group of glittery mascaras. They don't make lashes very long or thick, but they do add a bit of silvery or purply iridescent color. I imagine there is a reason for this (everything these days is about shine), but I wouldn't recommend it.

☹ **Brush with Greatness Thickening Mascara** *($12)* and **Exaggeration Lengthening Mascara** *($12)* both leave much to be desired. The Lengthening Mascara doesn't lengthen in the least, and the Thickening Mascara doesn't thicken, though it does work somewhat better than the Lengthening, but only somewhat. Neither of these is worth the money. **Push Up Plumping Lash Primer** *($12)* has a name that conjures up countless double entendres, but is merely a useless, sticky lash primer that would be easy to overlook if Victoria's Secret Cosmetics could find some way to ask, say, Lancome for its "secret" to superior mascaras!

☺ <u>BRUSHES:</u> If there is one solid area of interest for this line, it is the handful of handsome, silver-handled brushes. The feel is soft and the density great for application. The **Face Powder Brush** *($17.50)*, **Blush Brush** *($14.50)*, and **Retractable Blush Brush** *($14.50)* are very good, as are the **Eye Colour** *($10.50)* and the **Retractable Lip Brush** *($8.50)*. The only one I question is the **Eye/Lip Definer Brush** *($8.50)*; it is really too small for the mouth and too big to use for the eyes, but if you are in need of this specific size brush (say, to smudge eyeliner), it is an option.

# Vincent Longo (Makeup Only)

Vincent Longo is a fashion makeup artist with a long list of celebrity and supermodel clients. To give a little background, Australian-born Vincent Longo has been in the business for quite a while. He studied makeup artistry in Italy and eventually migrated to New York, where he was the featured makeup artist for one of Cindy Crawford's first professional photo shoots, circa 1981. He now joins the ranks of Bobbi Brown, Stila, Lorac, Trish McEvoy, and NARS with his own line of makeup products. Plus, checking out Longo gives you a reason to visit a Sephora store near you, the primary place where you can find Longo's creations.

From a comparative point of view, Longo's line has strength in its foundation textures and colors, but the rest of the line is fairly standard and in some cases (as in blush shades) woefully lacking. The eyeshadows have potential and feel great but, in contrast to the ones available from his competitors, almost all of Longo's shadows have shine. The brushes aren't of the quality you might expect from an artistry line, and the mascara is lackluster. For now, get excited about Vincent Longo, the makeup artist, but don't feel any dire need to go out of your way to investigate the products that bear his name.

Longo doesn't have a Web site, but he has quite a visible presence on www.eve.com, a beauty Web site retailing cosmetics from dozens and dozens of different lines. For more information on Vincent Longo, call (800) 773-9332 or visit www.eve.com.

<u>FOUNDATION:</u> ☺ **$$$ Water Canvas** *($40)* is Longo's trademark product, and though it has an interesting texture it is not exclusive to Longo's line. Olay's All Day Moisture Stick Foundation ($10.99) and Dior's Teint Glace ($35); do come in stick form, but have the exact same feel, texture, and application. What all of these have in common is a foundation that feels like liquid powder; it has a watery texture, not a creamy feel, and then dries to a satiny-smooth, matte, slightly powdery finish,

great for someone with normal to oily/combination skin or slightly dry skin looking for light to medium coverage. These all have beautiful textures and aren't the least bit greasy. Be aware that Longo's version can roll and chip out of the container. When you're spending this much money on foundation you don't want to waste any. Nevertheless, for color choice Longo wins hands down, with 16 shades, of which most are excellent. The only ones to avoid are Cafe Soleil, Golden Beige, and Honey Pecan; these can be too peach or ash for most skin tones.

☺ $$$ **Dew Finish Liquid Canvas** *($30)* is a fairly standard liquid foundation with no outstanding features, at least not in comparison to the Water Canvas above. It has a soft, smooth texture and a semi-matte finish, with sheer to light coverage. This would work well for normal to slightly dry or oily skin and the color range, nine shades in all, is mostly terrific; Porcelain (slightly pink), Medium Beige, and Golden are the only shades to be cautious with.

☹ <u>CONCEALER:</u> **Cream Concealer** *($16)* is disappointing, especially when compared to Longo's foundations. It's very thick and creamy, and the colors, though mostly adequate, are nothing to get excited about. This will crease and crease and crease if you have even a hint of lines around your eyes.

<u>POWDER:</u> ☺ $$$ **Loose Powder** *($30)* is supposed to contain "triple milled silk fibers," and as luscious as that sounds, this is a standard, talc-based powder with a fairly standard feel and finish. There is nothing special about it. Of the five shades, only Golden Oriental should be avoided.

☹ $$$ **Pressed Powder** *($26)* is a talc-free pressed powder that has an undeniably silky texture and a smooth, seamless application. What a shame three of the six colors are just not realistic skin tones! These may be worth a look if you can find a match, but steer clear of Translucent (almost pure white), Topaz (too peach), and Golden Banana (too yellow for most skin tones). **Bronzer** *($16)* has a great texture and two believable colors, but is too shiny to recommend.

<u>BLUSH:</u> The ☺ $$$ **Powder Blush** *($16)* has a beautiful, smooth texture and a very small selection of sheer colors, which is a shame. The **Creme Blush** *($16)* has a small but good collection of intensely pigmented shades that blend on surprisingly sheer, though slightly greasy, leaving a slight cream-to-powder texture. If you're adept at cream blush, give this one a try.

☹ $$$ **Duo Powder Blush** *($18)* is a two-sided blush, with a matte cheek color and a shiny highlighter. It is difficult to separate the two with a brush, so you will end up with shine even if you're careful, which leaves me unimpressed.

<u>EYESHADOW:</u> ☹ $$$ The **Powder Eyeshadow** *($16)* consists of matte, glimmer, or frost finishes, with a preference toward the ultra-shiny. That's a shame, because these all have a smooth, easy-to-blend texture and are dense enough to show up well on darker skin tones. The mattes in this collection are beautiful, and most are deeper

colors, suitable for contour or lining. **Cremed Powder Eyeshadow** *($16)* has a slightly heavy texture that is more powdery than creamy. The color selection is extremely limiting, but if you like the look, they are an option. However, if you have any problem with eyeshadow creasing, this will do it faster than most.

☹ **Eyeshadow Trio** *($20)* all have a silky, slightly creamy texture and apply beautifully. It's too bad the color combinations are set up to run in opposition to each other and that the three shades (all in one tin) tend to spill into each other, making application difficult. **Creme Eyeshadow** *($16)* offers almost no color choices and has a slick texture and soft powdery finish with lots of shine and glitter.

☺ **EYE AND BROW SHAPER: Eye Pencil** *($14)* is a standard pencil with a creamy texture and slightly shiny finish that tends to drag along the skin. $$$ **Brush-On Brow** *($16)* offers only three rather dry-finish shades of powder, and although the colors are all matte and apply well, the selection is limiting. If you find a good match here, test these out, but any non-shiny matte shade of eyeshadow in the right color will produce the same results.

**LIPSTICK AND LIP PENCIL:** ☺ $$$ Vincent Longo's lipstick selection is large and not organized in any recognizable way. There are eight purported finishes, and they are strewn throughout the collection with no rhyme or reason, a frustration to say the least if you're trying to make a selection. The **Lipstick** *($18)* formulas (Gloss, Stain, Sheer, Crème, Crème Frost, Frost, Satin Matte, and Matte) for the most part are fine, though very standard and assuredly overpriced for rather standard formulations. **Gloss** is simply a sheer lip color with a very glossy finish; **Stain** is more akin to the Gloss, and leaves no stain at all; **Sheer** is more opaque than sheer and has a slightly greasy finish; **Creme** is nicely creamy and opaque with a slightly glossy finish; **Creme Frost** is identical to the Creme, only these have iridescence; **Frost** is similar to the Creme Frosts, only these are even shinier; **Satin Matte** is accurately named (these have a slick texture, are opaque, and have a nice stain); and **Matte** is more creamy than matte, and offers full, smooth coverage and a slight stain.

☺ **Lip Liner** *($14)*. This is a lot of money for an extremely standard pencil that needs sharpening. It tends to be on the creamy side, making it more likely to bleed into the lines around the mouth. The finish has a subtle shine.

**MASCARA:** Longo's ☺ $$$ **Mascara** *($16)* is only an option if you want minimal length and no thickness, otherwise it is no competition for many of the superior lengthening and thickening mascaras found at the drugstore.

☺ $$$ **Waterproof Mascara** *($16)* builds decent length and holds up well under water. It goes on relatively easily and removes nicely with minimal pulling.

☺ $$$ **BRUSHES:** I was a bit surprised at the mostly unexceptional **brushes** *($10 to $35)* available from this line. While some may find these shapes and textures workable, I have found far better options from M.A.C. to Laura Mercier than what is offered here. One plus is that most of the brushes are available in short- and long-handled versions. The short-handled brushes can work well for travel, and the prices aren't atrocious, but for far silkier, more lush-feeling brushes this isn't the line to choose.

☺ $$$ <u>SPECIALTY PRODUCTS:</u> **Divine Shimmer Creme & Diva Dust** *($38 per set)*. Everyone else has shimmer in their collection, so why not Vincent Longo? These can be a (costly) consideration for an evening look. One is a shiny cream that disappears as a cream-to-powder texture that does work well for covering the body (using a powder can be messy for head to toe application). Diva Dust is a shiny, translucent loose powder, very standard, very shiny, and very overpriced. **Faerie Cream** *($20)* is a moisturizing lotion that has a sheer but shimmery application.

# Wet 'n' Wild (Makeup Only)

Wet 'n' Wild is one of the few cosmetics companies around that prides itself on being extraordinarily cheap. But don't let its hokey name and its "cheap"-looking packaging deter you, because there are some great options to be found here. Clearly Wet 'n' Wild isn't the most exciting drugstore line, but for pressed powder and definitely for lipsticks there are some items worthy of your attention, and you'll assuredly leave with money to spare. For more information about Wet 'n' Wild, call (800) 325-6133.

<u>FOUNDATION:</u> ☹ **Twisted Cream Foundation Stick** *($2.99)* is a standard, cream-to-powder foundation with a poor, choppy texture and an extremely limited color selection. The coverage is very sheer with a dry finish, and it tends to disappear into the skin, as if you hadn't applied it at all.

☺ **Keep It Real Oil Free Foundation** *($2.99)* has a smooth, satiny texture and goes on sheer and light. This tends to stay moist once it has dried, making it appropriate for normal to dry skin only. Of the five colors, only Bare is neutral; the rest are too peach, rose, or orange to recommend.

☹ **Moisturizing Liquid Makeup** *($1.99)* has an OK texture and finish, but all of the colors are too glaringly pink or rose to even consider.

<u>CONCEALER:</u> ☹ **Coverall Stick** *($1.49)* is very greasy easily creases under the eye, and the shades look nothing like real skin. How's that for "three strikes, you're out"?

☹ **Blemish Block** *($1.49)* is meant to be a medicated concealer for blemishes, and in reality is a transparent, shiny tint that uses willow bark extract as the blemish-fighter. Willow bark is distantly related to salicylic acid, but there isn't enough of it in here to exfoliate skin, nor is the pH of this product low enough to make it effective if there were enough.

☺ <u>POWDER:</u> **Pressed Powder** *($2.49)* is a standard, talc-based powder, but that is not a bad thing, considering the smooth, silky feel and even application it has.

The shades are slightly shiny, making these best for those not worried about applying shine to the skin, and in that case this one is a contender. **Bronzer** *($2.79)* comes in two shades—one is matte (#701, a very believable tan color) and the other is orange and shiny (#702). The matte shade has an exceptional texture and would work beautifully as a bronzer or blush/contour color for most skin tones.

☺ **BLUSH: Twist-Up Blush Stick** *($1.99)* is a great option for those who prefer cream-to-powder blush. These apply and blend well (much better than the Twisted Foundation Stick), and the colors are sheer and bright. Comparatively, you could pick up four of these for the price of one department store blush stick, and you won't see much difference. These do leave a slight sheen on the skin, and Flirt is an opalescent shimmer that would be best used for evening makeup, if at all. **Silk Finish Blush** *($1.86)* offers some excellent soft colors, a few of which are matte. If you find a suitable shade, these work about as well as any other powder blush you may have tried.

☺ **EYESHADOW: Silk Finish Creative Eye Shadow** *($2.99)* is indeed silky and very smooth. The creative part comes into play when trying to figure out how to coordinate the four disparate colors that come in each compact! These are also slightly shiny, but not enough to avoid altogether, and may be worth a closer look. The same comments apply for the **Single Eyeshadow** *($2.29)*, which has a small but decent selection of shades to choose from.

☺ **EYE AND BROW SHAPER: Eye Liner Pencils** *($0.99)* are strikingly similar (if not identical) to all of the other standard pencils in the cosmetics world, and work just as well. Don't let the price fool you; if you are used to using an eye pencil, these definitely work for lining the eye or filling in brows! Sharpening them is a pain but that's true for any non-twist-up pencil. **Jumbo Eye Pencil** *($2.29)* is a standard, thick pencil that applies easily and has a soft, powdery finish, so smudging is unlikely. If you prefer pencils and like a thicker line, this would be something to look into!

☺ **LIPSTICK AND LIP PENCIL: Liquid Lipstick** *($1.79)* is just a good, standard, emollient gloss. **Lip Tricks Mood Lipstick** *($1.59)* isn't much of a trick but it may take you back to a time when these were all the rage. It is just a light gloss with a hint of color. **Mega Colors Lipstick** *($1.59)* is more of a gloss than a lipstick, but would work just fine for a sheer, glossy look. **Mega Core Lipstick** *($1.59)* is virtually identical to the one above, only these have a clear "moisture core" meant to help with dry lips, only the ingredients for this aren't any different from those for the lipstick itself. **Mega Brites Lipstick** *($1.59)* is a very good, standard, creamy lipstick that has opaque coverage and a strong stain. Most of the colors are vivid, so they won't please everyone, but if you like bright shades on your lips these are an option. **Silk Finish Lipstick** *($.99)* is Wet 'n' Wild's standard lipstick; it's a sheer formula with a glossy finish and has plenty of shades to choose from. **Precious Metals Silk Finish Lipstick** *($1.49)* are identical to the Silk Finish reviewed above, only these all have a shiny, metallic finish and more eclectic colors. **Pretty Hot & Tempting Lips** *($1.49)* is the latest lipstick from Wet 'n' Wild, and is amazingly similar to the existing collection. These are slightly more "wet" looking and the colors are on the bold side, but that's about it. **Glassy Gloss Lip Gloss** *($1.69)* and **Mega Flavors Lip Gloss** *($1.99)* are both standard pot glosses with a sticky feel and a very shiny finish. Look no further if you've ever wondered what mango colada lip gloss tastes like. **Lip Crayon** *($2.59)* is a jumbo-sized lip pencil that serves up a creamy texture that has a sticky, iridescent finish. There is really no fashion reason to try these, but at this price, it may be logical enough to give it a try. **Lip Liner** *($0.99)* is similar to the Eye Pencil reviewed above and the same basic comments apply.

MASCARA: ☹ **Protein Mascara** *($1.59)* is pretty useless, building no length or thickness to speak of. Adding insult to injury, **MegaLash Mascara** *($2.29)* is an awful, sticky mess that clumps while you try in vain to build some modicum of length or thickness. **MegaLash Lengthening Mascara** *($1.99)* is a complete disappointment in all areas.

☺ **MegaWink Lash Curling Mascara** *($1.89)* is a decent mascara that adds a good amount of length but no thickness without clumping or smearing. It won't curl the lashes, but is worth considering for lengthening.

# *Yon-Ka Paris*

Yon-Ka Paris is a French line of cosmetics with a decidedly French accent, but that is where the élan of this pricey skin-care line starts and stops. The ads for Yon-Ka Paris declare that the company has a passion for the "world of plants ... that nourish and heal the body and soul and restore the beauty of skin and spirit." At these prices, that's the least you should expect. Adding to the allure is a description of the name Yon-Ka. "Yon is a river in China known as a place of eternal beauty and renewal, chosen to symbolize the purity of the products; Ka is Egyptian for vital energy, representing the life force that all botanicals possess." Wow! But that is incredibly overblown for some fairly standard products that contain some incredibly unnatural ingredients that range from propylene glycol to peg-33 castor oil, Vaseline, mineral oil, methylparaben, polyquaternium-11, diazolidinyl urea, TEA stearate, and on and on. Don't misunderstand, I don't think any of those ingredients are terrible or awful for skin, but Yon-Ka Paris says they are. It is just inexplicably ironic that Yon-Ka Paris makes it abundantly clear from its piles and piles of marketing information and training manuals that many of the ingredients in its own products are offensive to them.

I would love to challenge each and every outlandish claim made for these exceedingly standard formulations but there just isn't room—it would take volumes. Let me just say this: for a line boasting about passion and blending science with nature, there is very little science to be found. There are no sunscreens as part of the daily care routine, the products for oily or combination skin are destined to make matters worse, there is no disinfectant or effective AHA or BHA exfoliant, and the products for sensitive skin all contain sensitizing ingredients.

What is most shocking is the fact that the company states quite clearly in its brochure for sunscreens that its "Ultra Protection SPF 25 offers a solar block which totally disperses UVBs ... [while] allowing the tanning UVAs through." Clearly Yon-Ka Paris is in the dark about the fact that UVA rays cause skin cancer and are the primary source of wrinkles. Plus, there is almost no sun protection to speak of in any of its products. Why anyone would trust their skin to a company that would settle for this kind of pathetic, dangerous information is beyond me!

The moisturizers are good and the cleansers fairly run-of-the-mill, but many of the products contain irritating or sensitizing ingredients and, in comparison to many other lines that use a variety of water-binding agents and antioxidants and have well-formulated AHA and BHA exfoliants, these products just aren't that interesting or state of the art.

For more information about Yon-Ka Paris, call Eastern/Central (800) 533-6276 or Pacific/Mountain (800) 966-5255, or check out the Web site at www.yonka-paris.com.

☺ $$$ **Gel Nettoyant Cleansing Gel** (*$34 for 6.7 ounces*) is a very good, but very basic, water-soluble detergent-based cleanser for normal to oily skin. It does contain fragrance.

☹ $$$ **Lait Nettoyant Cleansing Milk** (*$34 for 6.6 ounces*) is as standard a wipe-off cleanser as it gets, and it can leave a greasy film on the skin. It is little more than expensive cold cream, but it is an option for someone with dry skin.

☹ **Nettoyant Creme, Non-Comedogenic, Wash Cream, for Very Sensitive Skin** (*$31 for 3.5 ounces*) contains peppermint and a few other potentially irritating ingredients. For very sensitive skin? What was this company thinking?

☹ **Gommage 303, Soft Clarifying Gel Peel with Botanical Extracts, for Normal to Oily Skin** (*$34 for 1.7 ounces*) contains way too many irritating ingredients, including lemon (the second ingredient), orange oil, lemon oil, lime oil, and lemon extract, to be good for any skin type.

☹ **Gommage 305, Soft & Clarifying Gel Peel with Botanical Extracts, for Dry or Sensitive Skin** (*$34 for 1.7 ounces*) is similar to the Gommage 303 above, only they left out most of the irritating ingredients except the lime oil. Why the company didn't know that would also be an irritant is anyone's guess.

☹ **Lotion, Non-Alcohol, Treated Lotion with Natural Essentials, for Normal or Oily Skin** (*$34 for 6.6 ounces*) contains several problematic ingredients for any skin type, including lime oil, nettle extract, and sodium lauryl sulfate.

☺ $$$ **Lotion, Alcohol Free Toner with Botanical Essential Oils, for Normal to Dry Skin** *($34 for 6.6 ounces)* includes fragrant oils that may smell nice, but they are all serious potential skin irritants. Other than that, this is just water, glycerin, and castor oil, with a sprinkling of coloring agents, which adds up to a complete waste of time for skin!

☺ $$$ **Lotion, Alcohol Free Toner with Botanical Essential Oils, for Normal to Oily Skin** *($34 for 6.6 ounces)* is almost identical to the Normal to Dry Skin version above and the same basic review applies.

☹ **Creme 11, Calming Treatment Cream for Visible Redness** *($43 for 1.4 ounces)* would have been a good, but extremely standard moisturizer for dry skin, but the arnica, yarrow, and nettle in here can cause skin irritation, which would only add redness to skin.

☺ $$$ **Creme 15, Purifying Treatment Cream with Botanical Extracts, for Problem Skin** *($40 for 1.7 ounces)* is almost identical to the Creme 11 above, which makes it a problem for problem skin. Actually the coltsfoot, sage, and birch, along with the fragrant oils, can all cause problems for any skin type.

☺ **Creme 28, Protective and Hydrating Cream with Botanical Essential Oils, for Dehydrated Skin** *($28 for 1.7 ounces)* would be a very good moisturizer for dry skin. It does contain retinol but only a very minute amount of the stuff.

☺ $$$ **Creme 83, Protective and Environmental Cream with Botanical Essential Oils** *($43 for 1.7 ounces)* is a good, though extremely standard moisturizer for dry skin. There is nothing in here that would protect the skin from the environment and there are far better-formulated moisturizers than this ho-hum version.

☺ $$$ **Creme 93, Protective and Balancing Cream with Botanical Essential Oils, for Combination Skin** *($43 for 1.7 ounces)* is almost identical to the Creme 83 above and the same basic review applies, except that contrary to what the label indicates it would absolutely not be appropriate for combination skin.

☺ $$$ **Creme PG, for Oily Skin** *($43 for 1.7 ounces)* is similar to the Creme 93 above and would be completely inappropriate for oily skin.

☺ **Creme PS, Protective and Nourishing Cream, for Dry Skin** *($43 for 3.52 ounces)* would be a good moisturizer for dry skin. This does contain a teeny amount of retinol.

☺ $$$ **Elastine Jour, Protective Age-Free Hydrating Cream, for All Skin Types** *($53 for 1.7 ounces)*. This is hardly appropriate for all skin types, and it won't stop one second of age, though it is a good, though very standard moisturizer for dry skin. Of course, without sunscreen, this is inappropriate for daytime.

☺ $$$ **Elastine Nuit, Age-Free Hydrating Cream, for All Skin Types** *($54 for 1.7 ounces)*. This good, but fairly standard moisturizer would be good for dry skin, but the inclusion of amniotic fluid is supposed to make you feel like your skin stands a chance of returning to the womb, and it can't.

☻ **Emulsion Pure, Purifying Emulsion with Botanical Essential Oils, for Blemishes** *($40 for 1.7 ounces).* The notion that there are essential oils that can help blemishes has no proof or substantiation. However, according to the American Academy of Dermatology and a recent article published in the *Journal of Cosmetic Dermatology,* fragrances (which is essentially what essential oils are) are potent potential irritants. Your face may smell nice, but with this product it will also run the risk of being red, irritated, and greasy.

☻ **Juvenil for Deep Acne** *($38 for 0.5 ounce)* is almost identical to the Emulsion Pure above and the same exact comments apply.

☻ **Fruitelia for Dry Sensitive Skin** *($60 for 1.7 ounces).* Even the brochure for this one states that it has a pH of 5.4, which isn't low enough for it to be an exfoliant (that calls for a pH of 3 to 4). The AHA content is disappointing anyway, with extracts of bilberry and lemon, which aren't AHAs.

☻ **Fruitelia for Normal to Oily Skin** *($60 for 1.7 ounces)* is similar to the Dry Sensitive Skin version above, and the same comments apply.

☻ **Nutri Contour, Eye & Lip Nourishing Protection Cream with Botanicals** *($39 for 0.5 ounce)* is an exceptionally boring moisturizer with standard thickeners and plant oils, though it also contains peppermint, which is a potent skin irritant particularly for the eye area.

☺ **$$$ Optimizer Cream** *($58 for 1.4 ounces)* is a good, though fairly uninteresting moisturizer for dry skin. It does contain a tiny amount of lactic acid (less than 1%), which isn't enough to do much of anything for the skin. The horsetail extract in here can be a skin irritant.

☺ **$$$ Optimizer Fluid** *($62 for 1 ounce)* is a very good, lightweight moisturizer for normal to dry skin. The horsetail extract in here can be a skin irritant.

☻ **Pamplemousse, Protective and Vitalizing Cream with Botanical Essential Oils, for Normal to Dry Skin** *($43 for 1.7 ounces)* contains grapefruit extract and lime oil, and that makes it a problem for dry skin. It does contain vitamin C, but the form is ascorbic acid, which is fine as a pH balancer but not as an antioxidant.

☻ **Pamplemousse, Protective and Vitalizing Cream with Botanical Essential Oils, for Normal to Oily Skin** *($43 for 1.7 ounces)* is almost identical to the Normal to Dry skin version above, and that means it can be irritating for all skin types. However, this does contain plant oils, which makes it an even bigger problem for oily skin types. Why does someone with oily skin need olive oil and pumpkin seed oil?

☹ **$$$ Phyto Contour, Eye Firming Cream with Rosemary Extracts, for Puffiness, Dark Circles** *($39 for 0.53 ounce).* The rosemary in here can be a skin irritant, which isn't great for puffy eyes, and the other ingredients just add up to a boring moisturizer for dry skin.

☻ **Alpha-Complex Deep Retexturing Night Gel** *($47 for 1 ounce)* does not contain any AHA ingredients so this cannot exfoliate skin, plus the grapefruit oil and other plant extracts here can be skin irritants.

☹ **Alpha-Contour, Anti-Wrinkles Eye and Lip Contour, Renewing Gel with Fruit Acids** *($39 for 0.88 ounce)*. The mint oil in here is a problem for all skin types, plus the extracts in here are not AHAs and do not have exfoliating properties you can rely on.

☹ **Dermol 1** *($38 for 0.5 ounce)* is more of a toner than anything else, but the inclusion of alcohol high up on the ingredient listing makes it a problem for all skin types.

☹ **Dermol 2** *($38 for 0.5 ounce)* is similar to the one above, and the same comments apply.

☹ **Dermol 3** *($38 for 0.5 ounce)* is similar to the one above, and the same comments apply.

☹ **3 Creme 410, Protective Sun Cream with Botanicals for Dark Skin** *($9.75 for 1.7 ounces)* doesn't have an SPF (required by the FDA for real sunscreens), so it's absolutely not recommended for any kind of exposure. The salesperson explained at length that this was an SPF 8 but that for legal reasons they couldn't list the SPF number. That is such garbage information I wanted to scream!

☹ **6 Creme 410, Protective Sun Cream with Botanicals, for Fair Skin** *($21.75 for 1.7 ounces)* is similar to the one above, and the same comments apply.

☹ **6 Creme 410 Teintee, Tinted Sun Cream with Botanicals, for Fair Skin** *($21.75 for 1.7 ounces)* is similar to the one above, and the same comments apply.

☹ **6 Lait Solaire, Protective Sun Tan Milk with Botanicals, for Fair Skin** *($21.75 for 5 ounces)* contains no sunscreen, and is unacceptable for outdoor use for any skin.

☺ **$$$ Ultra Protection, Age-Free Solar Block with AHAs and Botanicals, Water Resistant, SPF 25, UVA-UVB-IR** *($41 for 1 ounce)* is a part titanium dioxide–based sunscreen that contains no AHAs (the sugarcane extract this product contains is not the same as glycolic acid). It is a good, but standard moisturizing sunscreen for normal to dry skin. To suggest that there are far less expensive as well as far better formulated sunscreens than this one is an understatement.

☺ **Auto-Bronzant, Self-Tanning Lotion with AHAs and Botanicals, for Face and Body SPF 4** *($28.25 for 5 ounces)*, like all self tanners, contains dihydroxyacetone and would work as well as any. The claim about AHAs is strange, given that it doesn't contain any—while the SPF is useless.

☺ **Lait Apres Soleil, Soothing Hydrating After Sun Milk with Botanicals, for All Skin Types** *($33 for 5 ounces)*. I would imagine that after not using a sunscreen you would need something, but this standard moisturizer would only be OK for dry skin. For sunburn, you would be better off with pure aloe, but you would be far better off with appropriate sun protection, at least if you are interested in preventing skin cancer or wrinkles.

☺ **Masque 103, Purifying and Clarifying Clay Mask, for Normal to Oily Skin** *($38 for 3.52 ounces)*. This exceptionally standard clay mask is fine but not as effective as plain Philip's Milk of Magnesia.

☺ **Masque 105, Oxygenating and Clarifying Clay Mask, for Dry or Sensitive Skin** *($38 for 3.52 ounces)* is similar to the one above and the same basic review applies. The claim about supplying oxygen to the skin is impossible, because oxygen in skin-care products cannot permeate the skin, plus there is nothing in here that could deliver oxygen to the skin.

☹ $$$ **Halo 70, "Instant Glow" Vials with Natural Essential Oils, for All Skin Types** *($43 for 0.5 ounce)* is a burn, not for the skin, but for the claims, the cost, and the simplistic toner formulation. I should mention it does have a tint, but so what!

☹ $$$ **Phyto 52, Firming Treatment Cream with Rosemary Extracts, for All Skin Types** *($41 for 1.4 ounces)*. This standard moisturizer for dry skin won't firm anything, while the rosemary extract here is a potential skin irritant.

☹ $$$ **Phyto 54, Blending Treatment Cream for Visible Redness** *($43 for 1.4 ounces)* is almost identical to the Phyto 52 above, only with a different claim it can't deliver on.

☺ $$$ **Phyto 58, Rejuvenation Treatment Cream with Rosemary Extracts, for Normal to Dry Skin** *($50 for 1.4 ounces)* is a good moisturizer for dry skin, but it's completely incapable of creating any kind of rejuvenation.

☹ $$$ **Phyto 58, Rejuvenation Treatment Cream with Rosemary Extracts, for Normal to Oily Skin** *($50 for 1.4 ounces)* includes plant oils that are completely inappropriate for oily skin, and the lack of water-binding agents doesn't make this even an interesting option for someone with dry skin; plus rosemary can be a skin irritant.

☹ $$$ **Yon-Ka Serum** *($43 for 0.5 ounce)*. Skip the fragrance, which is a problem for the skin, and buy some pure corn oil and sunflower oil at the grocery store *(about $2 for 8 ounces)* and keep the change for yourself.

☹ $$$ **Mesonium 1** *($70 for 1 ounce)* is virtually identical to the Yon-Ka Serum above, and the same comments apply.

☹ $$$ **Mesonium 2** *($70 for 1 ounce)* is virtually identical to the Yon-Ka Serum above, and the same comments apply.

# Youngblood

What a great name for a cosmetics line! Youngblood suggests all kinds of images to women in search of beauty. Aside from the trendy name, this line's claim to fame is an assortment of loose powders called Youngblood. These supposedly revolutionary powders are promoted as an all-in-one product—foundation, concealer, and powder. The brochure states, "You'll be amazed at how lightweight and long lasting this powder is," plus it's "water resistant, [it] won't run, smear, or fade," it contains no "talc, fillers, perfumes, [and] dyes," and it isn't supposed to cause breakouts. The good news is that 50 percent of Youngblood's claims are valid: this is an amazing foundation that can double as concealer or loose powder. The bad news is that 50 percent of its claims are embellished and misleading, although that doesn't diminish the positives. Even better, they send out small sample packets of the powder in three or more shades, which makes this stuff incredibly easy to check out. (At least for those of you with normal to oily, combination, or normal skin. If your skin is even slightly dry, this powder will cause flaking, and if your skin is very oily, it can pool into the pores and look patchy.)

The brochure describes one of the ingredients, bismuth oxychloride, as a natural antiseptic that can be healing for problem skin. It can't. This earth mineral does have antiseptic properties, but it can also be a skin irritant, which doesn't make it all that healing. Also, the powders are supposed to give the skin "a translucent glow." The powder imparts a glow because it contains shiny, sparkly ingredients, including mica and iron oxides. If you have oily skin, you will not be happy with this much shine. However, these powders really do provide surprisingly even, smooth coverage; the colors are wonderfully neutral and easy to blend; they stay on incredibly well; and for most of the day they give the face a nice glow that only starts to look *too* shiny at the end of the day. Like most powder foundations, the Youngblood products did feel quite light, but they still provided completely opaque coverage and evened out most imperfections, especially when applied with a sponge instead of a brush.

If Youngblood piques your interest, you can call them at (888) YOUNGBLOOD or visit the Web site at www.ybskin.com.

## *Youngblood Skin Care*

☹ **Sudsing Cucumber Gel** *($16 for 6 ounces)* is a decent, water-soluble cleanser that uses standard detergent cleansing agents, which would make it an option for normal to oily skin except that the sodium lauryl sulfate, lemon, grapefruit, orange, lime, rosemary, mandarin, and citronella oils make this too potentially irritating for all skin types.

☹ **Papaya Enzyme Scrub** *($20 for 6 ounces)* lists one of the main cleansing agents as sodium C14-16 olefin sulfate, which makes this too potentially irritating and drying for all skin types.

☹ **Stimulating Toner** *($16 for 7 ounces)* contains several problematic irritating ingredients for all skin types, including witch hazel distillate, lemon, grapefruit, orange, lime, rosemary, mandarin, clary sage, geranium, and citronella oil. This is an irritation waiting to happen.

☺ **Nurturing Primrose Cream** *($30 for 2 ounces)* is a fairly standard moisturizer with plant oil, plant extracts, and fragrant oils. The primrose and hemp oil in here are good emollients but they aren't miracle oils for skin.

☺ $$$ **Nourishing Vitamin C Cream** (*$38 for 1 ounce*) does contain a minuscule amount of vitamin C, but even so the form is ascorbic acid and that is considered to be irritating and unstable. Other than that this is just OK for dry skin, but it would be far better with antioxidants and interesting water-binding agents. It does contain fragrance.

☹ **Oil Control Hydrating Fluid** (*$24 for 2 ounces*) lists the fifth ingredient as aluminum starch (octenylsuccinate), which is a decent, though potentially irritating absorbent. However, the rosemary, horsetail, pine, and lemon extracts in here can add to the irritation.

☺ $$$ **True Refine Rejuvenation Treatment** (*$36 for 1 ounce*) does contain about 4% AHA (glycolic acid) and about 1% BHA; however, the pH isn't low enough for these to be effective as exfoliants. Other than that, this is just a mediocre moisturizer.

☹ **Lyphazome, SPF 15 or 30** (*$18 for 4 ounces*) doesn't contain the UVA-protecting ingredients titanium dioxide, zinc oxide, or avobenzone, and is not recommended.

# *Youngblood Makeup*

☺ $$$ <u>FOUNDATION AND POWDER:</u> **Natural Mineral Foundation** (*$29.95*) is a talc-free, opaque loose powder that is billed as a foundation, concealer, and powder in one. It certainly offers enough coverage to function as a foundation, and it can be mixed with a moisturizer to create a regular foundation consistency, but this does have a drier texture, and used by itself it is best for normal skin. If your skin is even the slightest bit dry, this powder will cause flaking and if you're very oily it can pool in the pores and look patchy. With that said, this is incredibly easy to check out, as Youngblood willingly sends out samples of several shades on request. There are 14 colors to choose from, with options for very light and dark skins, and they are wonderfully neutral and easy to blend. Youngblood's claim that these powders give your skin a "glow" is true, because of the shiny minerals they contain. A word of caution: this product contains a fair amount of titanium dioxide, which explains why, as a loose powder, it can provide opaque coverage and stay in place so well. When I asked about the SPF rating, the salesperson explained that it wasn't rated ("It hasn't undergone the expensive testing required to give the SPF a number") but, she said, "it is comparable to an SPF 15." If this company doesn't want to spend the money necessary to rate this product, that's up to them, but making any unsupported statement about sun protection is disingenuous and irresponsible. If a product doesn't have an SPF rating, you can't know how much protection you're really getting.

☺ $$$ **Compact Foundation** (*$32.50*) is a talc-based pressed-powder foundation that goes against the trend of the other Youngblood powders that proclaim their talc-free status as some kind of benefit. There is no substantial evidence anywhere to suggest that using talc in face powders is harmful, but that's beside the point. This has a silky, soft texture and a smooth application that provides sheer to light coverage. The 11 shades are mostly neutral, but a few of them do cross the line into being a bit peach or orange for most skin tones.

☺ $$$ **Mineral Rice Setting Powder** *($17)* is talc-free and opts to use rice and cornstarch as its base. That can be problematic for those prone to breakouts due to the fact that the bacteria that contribute to breakouts feed off of these "natural" ingredients. However, this has a finely milled, light but very dry texture that provides very sheer coverage and comes in three good colors.

☹ <u>BLUSH:</u> **Crushed Mineral Blush** *($15.95)* is a shiny loose-powder blush that is messy to use and easy to apply unevenly. There really is no reason to try this, given the innumerable pressed-powder blushes available from almost every other line that are far easier to apply.

☹ <u>EYESHADOW:</u> **Crushed Mineral Eyeshadow** *($14)* is also in loose powder form and has the same application issues as the Mineral Blush above. There are 12 mostly pastel, ultra-shiny shades and a few labeled as matte that still have discernible shine, especially in daylight.

☺ <u>EYE AND BROW SHAPER:</u> **Eye Liner Pencil** *($10)* is a very standard pencil that glides smoothly and has a soft, dry finish, which means less smearing and smudging.

☹ <u>LIPSTICK AND LIP PENCIL:</u> The Youngblood **Lipsticks** *($14)* are creamy with a slightly too thick, waxy texture. It's nice that they're not greasy or too glossy but the application could certainly be smoother. By the way, Youngblood makes a big deal over the "natural minerals" used to create its lipstick colors, but you only have to take a cursory glance at the ingredient list to see they contain the same minerals and FD&C colorants found in thousands of other lipsticks. **Lip Pencil** *($12)* is just fine in terms of standard pencils, but you can find this same texture and finish in countless other pencils that sell for less, and many of them don't need to be sharpened.

☺ <u>BRUSHES:</u> Youngblood offers a small collection of mostly good **brushes** *($12 to $16.50)* that aren't the fullest or softest you may find, but are certainly affordable. The **Small** and **Large Kabuki Brushes** *($14 and $16.50)* are very full and are attached to a small base instead of a handle. This can be awkward to use and is not preferred to a standard, soft and full powder brush. The remaining brushes are worth a look if you happen upon a Youngblood display.

# Yves Rocher (Skin Care Only)

Like any other cosmetics line, Yves Rocher capitalizes on hyperbole and misleading information. Every gimmick in the book can be found in this vast assembly of products, from DNA and RNA in its A.D.N. line (as if you would want a cosmetic to affect your genetic structure), to yeast, a cornucopia of plants (of course, plants are always the answer for everything from acne to wrinkles), and vitamins.

Yves Rocher does have its good points. The products are not tested on animals, all of them have a 100 percent money-back guarantee, and there are some decent moisturizers to be found here (though the formulations are fairly dated, so you miss out on antioxidants or interesting water-binding agents). The company often has sales of its products and the prices aren't all that steep, although the sizes of the products are skimpy. You have to get past the extremely exaggerated claims and the really unnecessary diversity of the various lines to make a decision, and also avoid some really bad products for acne and some poorly formulated sunscreens. For more information, call (800) 321-9837 or (800) 321-3434, or visit the Web site at www.yvesrocherusa.com.

☺ **A.D.N. Revitalizing Resource Rinse-Off Cleansing Lotion, for Devitalized Skin** *($14 for 6.7 ounces)* is a fairly standard, mineral oil–based, wipe-off cleanser that can leave a greasy film on the skin, though it can be an option for someone with dry skin. It does contain fragrance.

☺ **A.D.N. Revitalizing Resource Refreshing Toner, Alcohol-Free, for Devitalized Skin** *($14 for 6.7 ounces)* is a very ordinary, irritant-free toner, but the fragrant plant water is more like applying eau de cologne to your face than a skin-care product.

☺ $$$ **A.D.N. Revitalizing Resource Age Defense Eye Contour Treatment, for Wrinkles and Puffiness** *($30 for 1 ounce)*. This very standard, overpriced moisturizer claims to have DNA and RNA that can somehow affect your skin; they can't, and it is insulting that the company suggests otherwise.

☺ **A.D.N. Revitalizing Resource Firming Intensive Night Cream, for Devitalized Skin** *($22 for 1.35 ounces)* is a good but extremely ordinary moisturizer for someone with normal to dry skin.

☺ **A.D.N. Revitalizing Resource Intensive Firming Serum, for Face and Throat** *($30 for 1.7 ounces)* is a good moisturizer for someone with normal to dry skin.

☹ **A.D.N. Revitalizing Resource Vital Defense Lotion, SPF 15 for Devitalized Skin** *($19 for 1.7 ounces)* doesn't contain the UVA-protecting ingredients avobenzone, zinc oxide, or titanium dioxide, and is not recommended.

☹ **A.D.N. Revitalizing Resource Vital Energizing Complex, for Devitalized Skin** *($24 for 1.35 ounces)* is supposed to contain fruit acids, a bogus name for AHAs. It doesn't contain any ingredients that can exfoliate the skin, it is just a good, though standard moisturizer for dry skin.

☺ **A.D.N. Revitalizing Resource Vital Moisture Day Cream, for Devitalized Skin** *($16 for 1.7 ounces)* is a good, but extremely standard, moisturizer for someone with dry skin, but because it lacks sunscreen, this "day" cream should only be used at night.

☺ $$$ A.D.N. Revitalizing Resource Energizing Mask, for Devitalized Skin ($16 for 1.7 ounces) is a good emollient mask for someone with dry skin.

☺ Bio-Calmille Gel Cleanser ($9.95 for 3.4 ounces) is a standard, detergent-based water-soluble cleanser that would be good for most skin types. It can be drying for someone with dry to sensitive skin. It does contain fragrance.

☹ Bio-Calmille Gentle Cleansing Lotion ($9.95 for 6.7 ounces) is a fairly standard, mineral oil–based cleanser with emollients that doesn't rinse off easily and can leave a greasy film behind on the skin. It can be an option for someone with dry skin. Any soothing benefit the Bio-Calmille products would have is reduced by the addition of fragrance in of all them.

☺ Bio-Calmille Eye Makeup Remover Gel ($9.95 for 3.4 ounces) is a standard, detergent-based eye-makeup remover. This one should work as well as any.

☺ Bio-Calmille Soothing Alcohol Free Toner ($9.95 for 6.7 ounces) is a very simple, ordinary, irritant-free toner. It would be OK for someone with normal to dry skin.

☺ Bio-Calmille Long-Lasting Day Cream ($11.95 for 1.7 ounces) is without sunscreen and should not be used during the day! At night this would be a good, though ordinary moisturizer for someone with dry skin. Urea in this amount can be an exfoliating agent.

☺ Bio-Calmille Soothing Night Cream ($15.95 for 1.7 ounces) is a good, though extremely ordinary moisturizer for someone with normal to dry skin.

☺ Bio-Calmille Relaxing Soothing Mask ($11.95 for 1.7 ounces) is a standard, mineral oil–based mask with thickening agents. It isn't particularly interesting but as a ho-hum moisturizer for dry skin it is just fine.

☹ Bionutritive Essential Cleansing Lotion ($9.95 for 6.7 ounces) is a fairly standard, mineral oil–based cleanser with emollients that can leave a greasy film behind on the skin, though it can be an option for someone with dry skin. It does contain fragrance.

☺ Bionutritive Essential Toning Lotion ($9.95 for 6.7 ounces). The plant extract is mugwort, which can be a skin irritant, and other than that this is just an OK toner for normal to dry skin.

☺ Bionutritive Enrichment Day Cream ($11.95 for 1.35 ounces) is without sunscreen and should not be used during the day! At night this would be a good though very ordinary moisturizer for someone with dry skin.

☺ Bionutritive Nourishing Night Cream ($17.95 for 1.35 ounces) is a good though ordinary moisturizer for someone with dry skin.

☹ Cel Defense Protective Foaming Cleanser ($10 for 5 ounces) is a standard, detergent-based cleanser that contains sodium lauryl sulfate somewhat high up on the ingredient list. That can be a skin irritant and drying for most skin types.

☹ **Cel Defense Age-Defying Toner** *($10 for 5 ounces)* is an alcohol-based toner and is absolutely not recommended.

☺ **Cel Defense Age-Defying Day Cream** *($17.50 for 1.35 ounces)* isn't much of a day cream (it has no sunscreen), but it is a good, though ordinary moisturizer for dry skin. The interesting ingredients are far at the end of the ingredient list and offer minimal to no benefit for skin.

☺ **Cel Defense Age-Defying Night Cream** *($19.50 for 1.35 ounces)* is similar to the Day Cream version above and the same comments apply.

☹ **Derma Controle Foaming Gel Cleanser** *($9.95 for 2.5 ounces)* contains a small amount of BHA (salicylic acid), which is completely wasted in a water-soluble cleanser because it would be rinsed down the drain before it could have an effect on the skin.

☹ **Derma Controle Normalizing Gel** *($11.95 for 2 ounces)* is yet another salicylic acid (BHA) product, this time in a gel, along with ingredients that could possibly cause breakouts, plus the pH of this product isn't low enough for the BHA to be effective as an exfoliant.

☹ **Derma Controle Purifying Lotion** *($9.95 for 4.2 ounces)* is an alcohol-based salicylic-acid toner. Alcohol only irritates the skin, causing dryness and redness that would be a problem for the skin in the long run.

☹ **Pro-Balance Skin-Balancing Cleanser** *($9.95 for 6.7 ounces)* is a fairly standard, oil-based cleanser with emollients that can leave a greasy film on the skin, which makes it completely inappropriate for someone with combination skin.

☹ **Pro-Balance Toner with Botanical Self Regulator** *($9.95 for 6.7 ounces)*. The oil part of this product will not make someone with combination skin happy.

☺ **Pro-Balance Day Cream with Botanical Self Regulator** *($11.95 for 1.7 ounces)* is without sunscreen and should not be used during the day! At night this would be a good moisturizer for someone with normal to slightly dry skin, but the oil would not be great for oily parts of the face.

☹ **Pro-Balance Fluid** *($13.95 for 1.7 ounces)*. Cornstarch can cause bacteria growth, increasing breakouts as well as irritation, and the plant oils just add grease to the skin. This product won't balance anything.

☹ **Pure Systeme Micro-Grain Gentle Cleansing Bar** *($15.95 for 4.4 ounces)* is a standard, tallow- and detergent-based bar cleanser. Tallow can cause breakouts and irritate the skin.

☹ **Pure Systeme Gentle Foaming Scrub** *($15.95 for 3.4 ounces)* is a standard, detergent-based scrub that uses synthetic particles (ground-up plastic) as the exfoliant. It's OK, but it does contain grapefruit and menthol, which can be irritating to the skin and won't do anything to reduce oil or breakouts.

☹ **Pure Systeme Gentle Skin Clarifier** *($16.95 for 6.7 ounces)* contains mostly water and alcohol. It won't control oil and can cause dryness and irritation.

☹ **Pure Systeme Oil-Free Balancing Gel, for Oily Skin** *($19.95 for 1.7 ounces)*. Alcohol and grapefruit extract are serious irritants, and one of the thickeners used in this gel can clog pores.

☹ **Pure Systeme Oil-Free Moisturizing Lotion** *($19.95 for 1.7 ounces)*. The grapefruit can be a skin irritant and can only hurt the skin—it provides no benefit for oily or acne-prone skin—and the absorbent in here, aluminum starch (octenylsuccinate), can also be an irritant.

☺ $$$ **Pure Systeme Oil-Free Absorbent Mask** *($14.95 for 2 ounces)* is a standard clay mask that can indeed help absorb oil. It does contain grapefruit, but hopefully not enough to cause problems for the skin.

☺ **Riche Creme Rinse-off Creme Cleanser, with 10 Botanical Oils** *($14 for 5 ounces)* is a fairly standard, mineral oil–based cleanser that can leave a greasy film behind on the skin, though it can be an option for someone with dry skin.

☺ **Riche Creme Alcohol-Free Toner, with Floral and Herbal Extracts** *($14 for 6.7 ounces)* contains several plant extracts that can be skin irritants (sage and rosemary) as well as plants that can be anti-irritants (mallow), which adds up to a waste. It's OK, but more of a waste of time for your skin.

☺ **Riche Creme Wrinkle Fighting Concentrate** *($26 for 1 ounce)*, as the name implies, is a very rich moisturizer. It won't change wrinkles but it is great for very dry skin.

☺ **Riche Creme Wrinkle Smoothing Day Cream, with 10 Botanical Oils** *($19 for 1.7 ounces)* would be a decent moisturizer for someone with dry skin but the interesting ingredients are barely present in this formula and have little to no benefit for skin. It also doesn't contain a sunscreen so this product should not be used during the day.

☺ **Riche Creme Wrinkle Smoothing Night Cream with 10 Botanical Oils** *($24 for 1.7 ounces)* does contain a lot of plant oils, lanolin, and emollients, but the first oil is mineral oil. This is a good but standard emollient moisturizer for someone with dry skin.

☺ $$$ **Riche Creme Wrinkle Smoothing Eye Cream, with Floral Extracts** *($24 for 0.5 ounce)* is an average moisturizer for dry skin.

☹ **Hydra Advance Solaire Intensive Moisture Sun Lotion SPF 8** *($13.95 for 5 ounces)* doesn't contain the UVA-protecting ingredients avobenzone, zinc oxide, or titanium dioxide, and is not recommended.

☹ **Hydra Advance Solaire Intensive Moisture Sun Lotion SPF 15** *($15.95 for 5 ounces)* doesn't contain the UVA-protecting ingredients avobenzone, zinc oxide, or titanium dioxide, and is not recommended.

☺ **Hydra Advance Solaire Moisture Replenishing Lotion After-Sun** *($11.95 for 5 ounces)* is a good emollient moisturizer for very dry skin.

☺ **Hydra Advance Solaire Moisturizing Self-Tanning Spray** *($15.95 for 4 ounces)*, like all self tanners, uses dihydroxyacetone to turn the skin brown; this one will work as well as any.

☺ **Hydra Advance Solaire Moisturizing Sun Block SPF 25** *($17.95 for 5 ounces)* is a good in-part titanium dioxide–based sunscreen offering UVA protection for someone with dry skin.

☹ **Hydra Advance Solaire Self-Tanning Face Cream SPF 10** *($11.95 for 1.35 ounces)* doesn't contain the UVA-protecting ingredients avobenzone, zinc oxide, or titanium dioxide, and is not recommended.

☹ **Response Nature Time Defense Daytime Protective Cream SPF 8** *($14 for 1.35 ounces)* doesn't contain avobenzone, zinc oxide, or titanium dioxide, and is not recommended.

☺ **Response Nature Time Defense Night Recovery Treatment** *($24 for 1.35 ounces)* is a very good emollient moisturizer for someone with dry skin. It does contain a tiny amount of vitamin A, as the name claims, but it won't help skin recover from anything.

☺ **Cap Soleil Sunless Self-Tanning Cream** *($11.95 for 3.5 ounces)*, like all self tanners, uses dihydroxyacetone to turn the skin brown. This one would work as well as any.

# Yves St. Laurent

While the Yves St. Laurent haute couture label is considered to be synonymous with international standards of beauty and glamour, the makeup sets no such comparative standards. In many ways this is the least impressive of all the French lines I've reviewed. The skin care is just OK but truly ordinary and lacking recent innovations in formulary standards; many of the foundation colors are a far cry from neutral, and virtually all of the eyeshadows and blushes are shiny. The only real positive is that the tester units at the Yves St. Laurent counters have improved and most of the products are easily accessible or require minimal assistance. For more information, call (800) 268-2499 or visit the Web site at www.beauty.com.

# Yves St. Laurent Skin Care

☹ **$$$ Demaquillant Douceur/Soothing Creme Cleanser** *($24 for 5 ounces)* is a standard, mineral oil–based cleanser that can leave a greasy film on the skin, though it can be an option for dry skin.

☹ **Gel Mousse Purete/Foaming Cleansing Gel** *($24 for 5 ounces)* is a standard, detergent-based water-soluble cleanser that rinses well and takes off all the makeup. The main detergent cleansing agent is sodium C14-16 olefin sulfate, which can be very drying and may cause skin irritation.

☺ $$$ **Lait Demaquillant Fraicheur/Instant Cleansing Milk** *($24 for 6.6 ounces)* is similar to the Soothing Creme Cleanser only in lotion form, and the same basic review applies.

☹ $$$ **Doux Demaquillant Pour Les Yeux/Gentle Eye Makeup and Lipstick Remover** *($22.50 for 2.5 ounces)* is just a synthetic emollient, slip agent, and preservatives. It will wipe off makeup, but it is just not worth the money.

☹ $$$ **Natural Action Exfoliator, Granule-Free, for All Skin Types** *($32 for 2.5 ounces)*. This waxy substance is rubbed over the skin and will help remove dead skin cells. Be careful, because the thickening agents in here can clog pores, and rubbing the skin isn't the best.

☹ **Tonique Soin Douceur/Extra-Gentle Tonic Alcohol-Free** *($24 for 6.6 ounces)* is mostly fragranced water, and several of the plant extracts can be skin irritants. It's about as do-nothing a skin-care product as I've ever seen.

☹ **Tonique Soin Fraicheur/Mild Clarifying Tonic** *($24 for 6.6 ounces)* is an alcohol-based toner that can be drying and irritating for all skin types.

☹ **Tonique Soin Purete/Oil-Control Tonic** *($24 for 6.6 ounces)* is a standard, alcohol-based toner that won't control oil, but will irritate the skin.

☺ $$$ **Hydratant Absolu/Absolute Hydration** *($57 for 1 ounce)*. There are some interesting water-binding agents at the end of the ingredient list, but that placement means they amount to little more than a dusting. This is a very standard, unimpressive moisturizer for someone with dry skin, and hardly worth the price.

☺ $$$ **Firm Effects Eye Complex** *($48 for 1 ounce)*. It's almost embarrassing how ordinary a moisturizing formula this is. The teeny amounts of yeast, soybean, and plankton extracts may have some tiny anti-irritant benefit, but in this ordinary group of ingredients, why bother?

☺ $$$ **Firm Effects Creme** *($65 for 1 ounce)*. Much like the Eye Complex above, this one has minuscule amounts of yeast, soybean, and plankton extracts that may have some tiny anti-irritant benefit, but in this ordinary, mundane, incredibly overpriced group of waxes and silicone they are all a complete waste of money.

☺ $$$ **Firm Effects Lotion** *($55 for 1 ounce)* is almost identical to the Firm Effects Creme above only in lotion form, but the same basic comments apply.

☺ $$$ **Firming Eye and Lip Creme** *($55 for 0.5 ounce)* is almost identical to the Firm Effects Creme above, only in lotion form, but the same basic comments apply. The only difference is the addition of a minuscule amount of cytochrome. Cytochrome is a protein found in blood cells that, with the aid of enzymes, serves a vital function in the transfer of energy within cells. There are three types of cytochromes, indicated by A, B, or C, with cytochrome C being the most stable. However, because cytochromes require a complex process that is triggered by a sequence of other components in order to be effective in their function of cellular respiration, they serve no function alone on skin.

☺ $$$ **Firm Effects Instant Lift Concentrate** *($70 for 1 ounces)* is almost identical to the Firm Effects Eye Complex above and the same basic comments apply. There is nothing in here that can lift skin even a fraction of a millimeter.

☺ $$$ **Soin Beaute Instantanee/Instant Firming Gel** *($60 for 1 ounce)* won't firm anything but it is a good lightweight moisturizer for dry skin.

☹ $$$ **Fruit Jeunesse/Firming Renewal Complex Glucohydroxy Acid** *($50 for 1.6 ounces)* is an OK 4% malic acid (AHA) product. However, malic acid is not considered the best option for AHAs—glycolic or lactic acid are considered better for penetration and reliable exfoliation. It's an option, but there are far better and less expensive AHA formulations than this one.

☹ **Hydra Fluide/Hydro-Light Day Lotion, SPF 15** *($50 for 1.3 ounces)* doesn't contain the UVA-protecting ingredients titanium dioxide, zinc oxide, or avobenzone, and is not recommended.

☺ $$$ **Intensive Nighttime Revitalizer, for Dry to Very Dry Skin** *($55 for 1 ounce)* is an exceptionally mundane moisturizer that isn't appropriate for very dry skin. It contains less than 1% AHA, which isn't enough to exfoliate skin. The minuscule amount of yeast in here has no benefit for skin.

☺ $$$ **Creme de Nuit Revitalisante/Nighttime Revitalizer, for Combination to Dry Skin** *($55 for 1 ounce)* is almost identical to the Intensive Nighttime Revitalizer for Very Dry Skin above, with a few minor differences. This is a good though fairly average moisturizer for dry skin, and definitely not worth the money.

☺ $$$ **Soin Lissant Immediat Contour de L'oeil/Smoothing Eye Contour Gel** *($45 for 0.5 ounce).* There are some other interesting water-binding ingredients here, but they come well after the preservatives, which makes them useless. Other than that, this is a good, though very ordinary, lightweight moisturizer for normal to slightly dry skin. The yeast and collagen in here are in such teeny amounts as to have no benefit for skin.

☺ $$$ **Precurseur Anti-Temps/Time Interceptor Fortifying Complex** *($65 for 1 ounce).* There are some other interesting water-binding agents here, but they come well after the preservatives, which makes them barely present and ineffective. This is an overpriced, fairly standard moisturizer for dry skin.

☺ $$$ **Prevention + /Time Prevention Day Creme** *($65 for 1.7 ounces)* is an overpriced, fairly standard moisturizer for dry skin.

☺ $$$ **Visible Energie Complete Day Creme for Dry Skin** *($50 for 1.7 ounces)* is a very ordinary moisturizer for normal to dry skin, but for the price you would expect more.

☺ $$$ **Visible Energie Complete Day Creme for Combination Skin** *($50 for 1.7 ounces)* contains several ingredients that could be problematic for combination skin. Aside from that, this is just a bunch of waxy thickening agents with a minuscule amount of water-binding agents.

☹ **Absolute Purifying Masque** *($35 for 2.5 ounces)* is a standard clay mask that contains orris root and zinc sulfate, both of which can be skin irritants, and that won't purify anything.

☺ **$$$ Masque Creme Hydro Actif/Hydro-Active Moisture Masque** *($35 for 1.6 ounces)* is an emollient, though completely ordinary moisturizer/mask for dry skin.

# Yves St. Laurent Makeup

**FOUNDATION:** ☺ **$$$ Teint Sur Mesure Creme Foundation** *($65)* is a two-part foundation that has a very smooth, light cream texture that dries to a natural, sheer finish. It comes with a pale-pink concealer color, and the notion is to use the concealer over any areas of the face you want to appear lighter—particularly the lines around the eyes, forehead, and mouth—or all over if you wish, before or after applying the foundation part. It's a standard technique that can be accomplished with any good concealer and foundation. In any event, this expensive way to do something quite basic would work well for someone with normal to dry skin. With only six colors it has a limited range of shades, of which Golden Honey and Light Amber can be too peach.

☺ **$$$ Teint Singulier Sheer Powder Creme Veil Foundation** *($38)* has a slippery texture that dries to a satin finish, providing sheer coverage that would work for someone with normal to dry skin. There are only six shades, with nothing for very light or darker skin tones, and #6, #8, and #9 can be too rose or too peach for most skins.

☺ **$$$ Premier Teint Long Lasting Radiant Primer** *($35)* is nothing more than sheer, shiny liquid that offers some strange colors and no coverage. For an artificial, tinted glow, it's fine, but the real question is, why bother?

☺ **$$$ Teint de Soie Line Smoothing Foundation** *($46)* is a moist foundation suitable for normal to dry skins seeking light to medium coverage and a soft, natural finish. Of the seven shades, most are too peach to look natural, but you may wish to consider (or test) #1, #2, #7, and #8.

☺ **$$$ Energie Teint Liquid Foundation SPF 12** *($46)* has a very good, avobenzone-based sunscreen for UVA protection, but SPF 15 would have been better. This one's creamy texture blends well and stays very moist on the skin, providing light to medium coverage. The seven shades are impressive compared to Yves St. Laurent's other choices, but there is nothing for very dark skin tones to consider. Only #3 and #6 are too peach for most skin tones. By the way, this comes in a pump bottle, which isn't the most economical way to use foundation, especially at this price.

☺ **$$$ Teint Matte Parfait Oil Free Foundation SPF 12** *($46.50)* comes with fancy marketing language that says this product contains microparticles that can capture sebum (oil). Those microparticles are just clay and magnesium—not the least bit fancy or unique. Other than that, this is a good, in-part titanium dioxide–based sunscreen foundation with a soft matte finish. This is best for someone with normal to slightly oily skin, but it won't hold back oil and stay in place like ColorStay Lite SPF 15 can. Of the six shades half are poor options, which is not great odds. The colors to avoid are #1, #5, and #6. This may not be available at all YSL counters, as the company seems indecisive about whether or not to keep it in wide distribution.

☺ $$$ **Teint Poudre Sur Mesure** *($50; $32.50 refills)* is a pressed-powder foundation that also features a tiny amount of a shiny highlighting powder. The powder is shiny as well, but it is subtle. The four shades are nice, but nothing special; many lines offer better alternatives for far less.

<u>CONCEALER:</u> ☺ $$$ **Radiant Touch** *($34)* is a pale-pink, slightly shiny concealer/highlighter that comes packaged in a pen with a brush tip. You click the bottom to "feed" concealer to the brush, and that can make it hard to control how much product comes out. As a highlighter it can work well and the texture is smooth, but it has limited use.

☹ **Concealer** *($27.50)* is a greasy mess and is also only available in one color.

<u>POWDER:</u> ☺ $$$ **Semi-Loose Powder** *($55)* comes in a cake form, but the container shaves off the top layer when you twist it, creating a loose powder. It's certainly less messy than conventional loose powder, but all of the colors are shiny and that eliminates the purpose of using a powder to dust down shine.

☺ $$$ **Silk Finish Pressed Powder** *($38.50)* comes in three very good colors and has a great, soft texture and smooth finish.

☹ **Soft Bronzing Powder** *($40)* is a standard, overly orange, and shiny bronzing powder that barely resembles a tanned appearance.

☹ <u>BLUSH:</u> **Variations Blush** *($36)* comes quad-style, with two matte and two intensely shiny colors, all subtle variations of the same shade. They go on sheer, but oh, that shine!

<u>EYESHADOW:</u> ☺ $$$ **Perfecting Eye Shadow** *($38)* are eyeshadow trios, each with a pale ivory base color and two shadow colors, one of which is iridescent. The only ones to seriously consider for a coordinated evening look are #3 and #5, which are almost matte.

☹ **Eyeshadow Powder Duo** *($36)* are too powdery and flaky for a smooth, even application, and all of the duos are ultra-shiny, with poor color combinations. **Perfecting Eyeshadow Duo Compact Kohl** *($38)* are identical to the Powder Duos above, except for the addition of a third color (deep brown or navy blue) for lining. The same comments apply to these. **Mono Eyeshadow** *($26)* supposedly are available in regular and pearly finishes, but the small assortment of colors are all shiny.

<u>EYE AND BROW SHAPER:</u> ☺ $$$ **Perfecting Eye Pencil** *($19.50)* is a dual-ended, standard pencil with one side being a light shade and the other a dark color. Both have a creamy texture that makes them prone to smudging.

☺ $$$ **Kohl Eye Pencil** *($16.50)* is also standard and creamy, but a bit more solid than the one above due to its soft powder finish. **Liquid Eyeliner** *($25)* has a decently workable brush that applies well, but all of the colors (except black) are shiny and easily smudge.

☹ **Eyebrow Pencil** *($20)* has a too-dry texture that is difficult to apply because it balls up on the skin as you draw it over the brow.

☺ $$$ **LIPSTICK AND LIP PENCIL:** **Rouge Pur Pure Lipstick** *($24.50)* offers dozens of shades in this fairly greasy lipstick with a good opaque finish. These are richly pigmented, which is nice, but they can easily bleed and feather into lines around the mouth. **Rouge Pur Matte Lipstick** *($24.50)* goes on moist and creamy and isn't matte in the least. The colors are vivid with a strong stain, which will aid in longer wear. **Rouge Singulier Lipstick** *($27.50)* is a very smooth, creamy lipstick whose long-lasting claims are easily refuted once you've tried this one on. **Rouge Pur Transparent Lipstick** *($24.50)* is an overpriced, extra-glossy lipstick with a bevy of frosted shades. **Lip Lacquer** *($22)* is an opaque, very shiny (and too sticky for comfort) gloss. **Intense Lip Colour** *($25)* is much nicer than the Lip Lacquer, although this price is ridiculous for standard, non-sticky lip gloss. **Lip Liner Pencil** *($18)* are standard pencils that are creamy and come in an attractive range of colors.

☺ $$$ **MASCARA:** **Mascara Moire** *($22.50)* applies relatively well, but may clump if you're not careful. Average length and some thickness are achieved, but this is by no means a must-have mascara. **Mascara Essentiel** *($22.50)* builds beautifully long, thick lashes and stays on well all day. There are now six shades, including blues and purples that do little to enhance the lashes.

☹ **BRUSHES:** Yves St. Laurent's **Brushes** *($20 to $30)* are an incomplete, poorly made collection that the salesperson did not even want to show me in spite of my insistence. I was told they are being eliminated, which from my perspective is a good idea.

# ZAPZYT

If the name of a product line was ever meant to tell a woman exactly what to expect, this one is it. Though the name is clear enough, don't expect much skin "clearing" from this assortment. The bar soap is too alkaline, which can be irritating and encourage the growth of bacteria, and the BHA products are in a pH that makes them relatively poor as exfoliants. The benzoyl peroxide gel is actually quite good, but it only comes in one strength and not all skin types can handle that. For more information about ZAPZYT, visit the Web site at www.zapzyt.com.

☹ **Cleansing Bar** *($3.29 for 3 ounces)* contains 3% sulfur, which is too irritating and problematic for most skin types. While sulfur can be a good disinfectant, there are far more effective and less corrosive options for skin. There is also well-documented research that points to a high pH as causing an increase in the presence of bacteria. With a pH of 8, this bar soap would definitely negate any positive effect from the disinfecting action of the sulfur.

☺ **10% Benzoyl Peroxide** *($4.99 for 1 ounce)* is a great option for treating acne. It contains no fragrance or any other irritating ingredient—well, except for the 10% benzoyl peroxide—but that is a good option for killing the bacteria that can cause blemishes. Keep in mind that 10% benzoyl peroxide is at the high end of the options available and is potentially quite drying and irritating. It should only be considered after lesser concentrations of 2.5% and 5% strengths have been tried.

☹ **Acne Wash Treatment** *($5.29 for 6.25 ounces)* is a standard, detergent-based cleanser that includes 2% salicylic acid (BHA). Its pH of 5 means the BHA isn't all that effective, and even if it were, in a cleanser it would quickly be rinsed down the drain, having minimal opportunity to get inside the pore where it needs to be to have the most impact.

☺ **Pore Treatment Gel** *($5.29 for 0.75 ounce)* is an option for a topical BHA (it contains 2% salicylic acid). This gel formula contains no other irritants and while the pH of 4 is on the high side for being effective as an exfoliant, it can still be helpful for some skin types.

# Zhen

Zhen (pronounced "Jen") is a line of skin-care and makeup products aimed at Asian women. Created by two Asian sisters who were frustrated at the lack of colors that suited their skin tones, this line boasts a "unique collection of yellow-toned foundations" appropriate for all skin types, but most specifically for Asian women. However, although I agree with the mission statement these sisters make, many of their foundations are not in the least bit yellow–based. In fact, I would call most of these glaringly pink, peach, or ash. Didn't the Yee sisters look at these colors in the daylight? Admittedly, many of the really poor colors have been discontinued since the last edition of this book, but there is still cause for concern, and overall there is nothing about this line that makes it better for Asian skin tones, or most other skin tones for that matter. Far better examples of appropriate yellow-based colors for Asians and others can be found in lines like Bobbi Brown, Clinique, M.A.C., and Maybelline, to name a few.

Zhen's brochure carries on with the Asian theme and is peppered throughout with "ancient Chinese secrets" that are nothing more than basic makeup tips such as powdering after applying foundation or using concealer to neutralize undereye circles. It also makes a big deal about its products not containing mineral oil, which, though greasy-feeling, is almost completely benign to the skin and actually a great ingredient for dry skin. Meanwhile, Zhen's skin-care products, touted as being developed for sensitive skin, contain a litany of irritating ingredients and plant extracts, such as lemon, clove, and witch hazel. These do nothing beneficial for the skin, except to cause irritation and redness. Those with sensitive skin would do well to avoid these skin-care products. Finally, none of the sunscreens offer the requisite UVA-protecting ingredients of titanium dioxide, zinc oxide, or avobenzone (though the sunscreens in the foundations do). For more information about Zhen, call (800) 457-8455 or visit the Web site at www.zhenbeauty.com.

# Zhen Skin Care

☹ **Cleanser for All Skin Types** (*$18 for 7 ounces*) contains way too many seriously irritating ingredients, including peppermint, clove, and cinnamon, and is not recommended.

☹ **Cleanser for Normal to Dry Skin** (*$18 for 8 ounces*) contains glycolic acid, which is a problem in a cleanser, but it also has other irritating ingredients that should not be put on the skin, particularly near the eyes, including lemon, arnica, lemongrass, orange, and pine.

☺ **Cleanser for Normal to Oily Skin** (*$18 for 8 ounces*) is a standard, detergent-based cleanser that can be an option for someone with normal to oily skin. There are a few irritating plant extracts in here but the amount is so small as to not be a problem for most skin types.

☹ **Papaya Face Scrub** (*$20 for 4 ounces*) contains several ingredients that are a problem for skin, including arnica, lemongrass, kiwi, and pine. Papaya itself is also a rather unstable enzyme that has minimal exfoliating properties, but especially minimal when it would just be rinsed off down the drain.

☹ **Toner for All Skin Types** (*$16.50 for 6 ounces*) contains peppermint, clove, and cinnamon, which are all too irritating, and that is absolutely not recommended for any skin type.

☹ **Toner for Normal to Oily Skin** (*$16.50 for 6 ounces*) has even more irritating ingredients than the one for All Skin Types above, and is not recommended for any skin type.

☹ **Toner for Normal to Dry Skin** (*$16.50 for 6 ounces*) doesn't contain as many irritants as the other two toners above, but it does contain lemon and orange, and that won't do for dry skin.

☹ **Moisturizer with SPF 15 for All Skin Types** (*$19.50 for 2 ounces*) doesn't contain the UVA-protecting ingredients avobenzone, zinc oxide, or titanium dioxide, and is not recommended.

☺ **$$$ Eye Creme** (*$22 for 0.5 ounce*) is an OK moisturizer for dry skin. It also has a tiny amount of glycolic acid, but not enough for it to be an exfoliant, nor is the pH of this one low enough for that purpose. The teeny amount of vitamins at the end of the ingredient listing are in such minute amounts as to have little benefit for skin.

☺ **Face Creme** *($25 for 1.25 ounces)* is a very good moisturizer for dry skin. The "respiratory enzyme" in here offers no benefit for skin, it will not help your skin breathe better. Please refer to the "Cosmetic Ingredient Dictionary" in the Appendix for more information about respiratory enzyme.

☻ **Eye Gel** *($22 for 0.75 ounce)*. The witch hazel in here can cause irritation; without that, this could have been a good lightweight moisturizer for normal to slightly dry skin.

☻ **Moisturizing Gel for Oily Skin** *($17.50 for 2 ounces)*. The witch hazel in here can cause irritation; without that, this could have been a good lightweight moisturizer for normal to slightly dry skin.

☻ **$$$ Papaya Mask** *($18 for 2 ounces)* is a good, but extremely standard clay mask that contains a handful of plant extracts, with some being anti-irritants and others being irritants. The teeny amount of papaya in here has no effect on skin.

☺ **Skin Lightening Cream** *($25 for 1 ounce)* is a very good hydroquinone-based skin-lightening product that can inhibit melanin production. This does contain sunscreen, but the SPF isn't stated and there are no UVA-protecting ingredients, so do not rely on this product for sun protection (which is also essential to prevent brown skin discolorations). It also contains magnesium ascorbyl phosphate, a form of vitamin C that can help inhibit melanin production, but it takes a 10% concentration to have that effect, and this product contains less than 0.1%.

# Zhen Makeup

**FOUNDATION:** ☹ **Matte Foundation** *($15.50)* is a decent matte foundation but the color selection of eight shades is lacking in range. Only Porcelain, Cream, and Sand are neutral enough to be considered true skin-tone colors. The rest are either too peach, yellow, or ash for most skin tones.

☹ **Light-Diffusing Foundation SPF 8** *($22.50)* is insufficient to rely on for daily sun-damage protection, even though the SPF contains in-part titanium dioxide. Even more bleak are the colors, which are mostly awful. You can consider Cream, Porcelain, or Sand, but why bother?

☹ **Foundation Stick with SPF 8** *($18)* has a creamy texture and a soft, opaque powder finish, but the eight shades are just not worth recommending. The colors lighten up a bit on the skin, but not enough to warrant trying the peach, rose, and ashy shades. The same SPF problems for the Light-Diffusing version above apply for this one too.

☺ **Dual Powder Foundation** *($20)* has a dry, matte finish and six colors that are mostly very good. Only Cashew and Honey are too peach or orange for most skin tones. This standard, talc-based powder foundation applies well and provides sheer to medium coverage.

☺ **Sheer Foundation with SPF 10** *($19.50)* has an in-part titanium dioxide–based sunscreen, though an SPF 15 is what is truly needed. It has a smooth, light texture that dries to a soft matte finish. This is an option for normal to slightly dry or slightly oily skin seeking light coverage, and the six shades present some good options. Cashew and Honey may be too peach for most skin tones. Be aware that you cannot rely on this foundation alone for sun protection.

☺ **Tinted Moisturizer SPF 15** *($18)* is very sheer and moist without being heavy, but of the two colors, only Beijing is an option. The SPF 15 comes without adequate UVA protection, making this a poor choice for daytime wear.

☺ **CONCEALER:** Zhen's tube **Concealer** *($10.50)* has a somewhat matte texture and smoothes on nicely without creasing. Unfortunately, it only comes in two colors, but if one of these works for you, it is worth a try, particularly if you have normal to oily skin.

**POWDER:** ☹ **Loose Powder** *($18)* and **Pressed Powder** *($20)* are both talc-based and have a sheer, light texture that feels great. The three shades for each are extremely yellow (Amber is almost a taxicab yellow!) and the Loose Powder has a subtle shine that kind of defeats the purpose of powder, doesn't it?

☺ **$$$ Mosaic Powder** *($25)* is simply a talc-based powder that is arranged in the compact as a multihued pattern of fragmented colors. When you place your brush over the colors it still comes out as one shade. These are nice to look at, but that is the only advantage they have over a single-hued pressed powder. Bronze Mosaic would make a suitable bronzing powder for light to medium skins.

☺ **BLUSH: Powder Blush** *($14.50)* comes in an attractive though small grouping of matte colors that are divided into Warm and Neutral groups. The Neutrals are really the Warm-toned shades, and those labeled as Warms are undeniably cool tones. But since when is fuchsia considered a warm color?

**EYESHADOW:** ☺ **Zodiac Eye Shadows** *($10)* have a soft texture that applies easily and sheer. The colors have been streamlined and are mostly neutral and matte, with a few shiny or blue exceptions. **Ying Yang Shadow Changer** *($10)* are duo eyeshadow sets that are pale, pastel, and iridescent. These are suggested in Zhen's brochure for an evening look, and I agree.

☺ **Sister Shadows** *($12)* feature six shades of softly shiny cream-to-powder eyeshadows named after each Yee sister. For some reason, Jane got stuck with the blue shade; the others, though shiny, are neutral.

☺ **EYE AND BROW SHAPER: Waterproof Eye Definer** *($11)* are standard eye pencils with a boring color selection; they work, but are no more waterproof than other pencils. **Liquid Eye Liner** *($11.50)* is a standard liquid liner that goes on smooth, and without peeling or chipping as the day goes by. The only shade is black, so this can look severe on anyone with fair skin. **Brow Pencil** *($9.50)* is a good but very basic brow pencil with a brush at one end to soften the color. **Brow Set** *($11)* is simply a clear gel (like hairspray) that will groom the brows. **Brow Duo** *($10)* offers a dark brown and charcoal matte powder color packaged together. This has a dry texture, but will work for the brows (or can be used wet as eyeliner). One question: what are blondes and redheads supposed to use? After all, this is supposed to be a line that suits all skin tones.

    <u>LIPSTICK AND LIP PENCIL:</u> ☺ **Cream Lipstick** *($10)* is a fairly creamy lipstick, bordering on greasy. **Matte Lipstick** *($10)* is an excellent matte lipstick with a smooth, non-drying finish. It stays on well and doesn't feather; too bad there are only six shades to choose from! **Moisture Lipstick** *($10)* is a good creamy lipstick with a creamy, not semi-matte, finish. This is as suitable for dry lips as any other creamy, emollient lipstick would be. **Lip Silks** *($10)* is a sheer, glossy lipstick that claims it protects lips from the sun but doesn't tell you how. **Lip Pencil** *($12)* is as standard as standard can get for a lip pencil.

    ☺ **Lip Primer** *($10)* and **Lip Base** *($10)* are two gimmicky lip products that claim to smooth the lips' creases and/or serve as a foundation base for the lips. Claims notwithstanding, these two products may keep lip color from changing but are largely unnecessary provided you have a good lipstick that doesn't feather and a matte concealer (if needed) to double up as a lip base.

    ☺ <u>MASCARA:</u> The **Mascara** *($12)* claims to be an extra-gentle formula for sensitive eyes, but that can't save this mascara's mediocrity. It tends not to smear, but doesn't do much else when it comes to length or thickness. **Lash Thickener** *($11)* is a thick-consistency lash primer that wouldn't be needed if Zhen's mascara performed better. If you're using a great mascara, that in and of itself is quite enough.

    ☺ <u>BRUSHES:</u> Zhen's **9-Piece Professional Brush Set** *($55)* is a good assortment of brushes that covers every inch of your face, including a very tiny and very good eyeliner brush, a great contour brush, large and small eyeshadow brushes, and more. At $55 for nine brushes, that averages out to just $6.10 per brush. The only brush that is a bit of a waste is the lip brush; it isn't retractable, which makes it a bit too large (as well as messy) to tote in your bag.

# Zia Natural Skin Care

    Zia Wesley Hosford is the founder of Zia Natural Skin Care, although, due to a falling out with her partners, the Zia line is no longer owned by Zia herself. However, the product philosophy remains the same and the "natural" bent is as hyped as ever. While there are plenty of plants in these products, there are synthetic ingredients here as well. Keep in mind that just because an ingredient has a natural source does not mean it's automatically better for the skin. Poison ivy is natural and you don't want that on your skin. There are lots of plants, particularly those with fragrant, volatile oils, that can cause skin irritation, and that's bad for skin. There are some very good products to consider in this line, but definitely those to stay away from, so choose carefully. For more information, call (800) 334-7546 or visit the Web site at www.ziacosmetics.com.

☺ **Natural Foundation SPF 8** *($14.95)* has an excellent titanium dioxide and zinc oxide sunscreen, but why they stopped at the SPF 8 is a mystery; 15 would've been much better for this smooth-textured foundation. This one offers light to medium coverage and a natural finish, but of ten shades, only four are worth considering: Alabaster and Moonstone (great for very light skins), and Sandstone and Mica.

☹ **Face Powder** *($14.95; $10.95 for refills)* is a talc-free pressed powder that has a very soft, silky texture and a satiny finish. The cornstarch in here can be problematic for those with breakout tendencies. This features six colors, best for light to medium skin tones. Avoid Pink Tourmaline (too ashy pink) and Bronze (too orange).

☹ **Absolutely Pure Aloe & Citrus Wash for All Skin Types** *($3.75 for 4 ounces)* definitely does contain citrus (it's actually the first ingredient), but just as orange juice can be drying and irritating to skin, this will have a similar impact. This one doesn't clean skin all that well and isn't the best for removing makeup.

☺ **Fresh Cleansing Gel, for Normal, Sensitive, Combination & Oily/Problem Skin Types** *($15.50 for 8 ounces)* is a mild, detergent-based cleanser that should work well for normal to dry skin. It does contain fragrance.

☹ **Moisturizing Cleanser, for Normal, Sensitive, Dry & Mature Skin Types** *($15.50 for 8 ounces)* is basically a wipe-off cleanser with thickening agents and plant oils. It can leave a greasy film on the skin, so it is only an option for someone with dry skin.

☹ **Fresh Papaya Enzyme Peel Non-Abrasive Exfoliant for All Skin Types** *($20.95 for 1.5 ounces)* contains papaya, which does contain papain, the enzyme that can exfoliate skin, but papaya extract has minimal papain present, which makes this a poor exfoliant, and even so the effective ingredient would just be rinsed down the drain before it had a chance to have an effect.

☹ **$$$ Balancing Elixir** *($16.95 for 4 ounces)* is supposed to be aromatherapy for the face. The plant extracts in here are all potential irritants, including lemon, grapefruit, lavender, and clary, which is disappointing, because the other ingredients make for a good toner. The teeny amount of tea tree extract in here is not enough to have any effect as a disinfectant.

☹ **$$$ Hydrating Elixir** *($16.95 for 4 ounces)* is almost identical to the Balancing version above only with different but equally problematic plant extracts.

☹ **$$$ Replenishing Elixir** *($16.95 for 4 ounces)* is almost identical to the Balancing version above only with different but equally problematic plant extracts.

☺ **Sea Tonic Aloe Toner for Normal, Sensitive, Combination & Oily/Problem Skin Types** *($14.75 for 8 ounces)* is similar to the Balancing version above only with different but equally problematic plant extracts.

☺ **Sea Tonic Rosewater & Aloe Toner for Normal, Dry & Mature Skin Types** *($14.75 for 8 ounces)* is similar to the Balancing version above only with different but equally problematic plant extracts.

☺ **Citrus Night Time Reversal Alpha Hydroxy Acid Creme for All Skin Types** *($25.95 for 1.5 ounces)* contains sugarcane extract, which is not related to glycolic acid (AHA) and the same is true for the citrus and milk solids (which are supposed to be associated with lactic acid). Putting milk or sugarcane on your skin doesn't give you the effectiveness of AHAs, because if it did you could just use them and forget this product altogether. Regardless, even if those were effective AHAs, the pH isn't high enough for them to be effective as exfoliants, so this is just an OK moisturizer for normal to dry skin, nothing more.

☹ **Ultimate Exfoliator** *($29.95 for 2 ounces)* contains lemon, lime, and citrus, which are too irritating for all skin types. Papaya is not a good exfoliant but it is a good irritant.

☺ **$$$ Essential Eye Gel** *($19.95 for 0.5 ounce)*. The plant extracts in here are a mix of irritants (ivy and witch hazel) and anti-irritants (seaweed and chamomile), which makes them all wasted. Other than that, this is a good lightweight moisturizer for normal to slightly dry skin.

☺ **Everyday Moisturizer, Fragrance Free for Normal, Sensitive, Combination & Dry Skin Types** *($18.95 for 2 ounces)* would be a very good moisturizer for someone with dry skin, but there are several ingredients in here that would be a definite problem for someone with combination skin. Fragrance-free is great, but why not make all the products fragrance-free given that it's clear this line recognizes fragrance is a problem for skin?

☺ **Herbal Moisture Gel Oil Free Moisturizer for Normal, Sensitive, Combination & Oily/Problem Skin Types** *($22.95 for 1.5 ounces)* is a very lightweight gel that contains an anti-irritant, thickeners, fragrance, and preservatives. This won't do much for skin, but if you have a touch of dry skin this could help soothe it.

☺ **Nourishing Creme Cellular Renewal for Normal, Dry & Mature Skin Types** *($12.75 for 1 ounce)* is a very good emollient moisturizer for dry skin, but it won't help cell renewal any more than any other emollient moisturizer. If you have sensitive skin, the fragrance in here, including lemon oil, can be irritating.

☺ **$$$ Ultimate "C" Serum** *($49.95 for 0.5 ounce)*. The plant extracts in here are a mix of irritants (horsetail) and anti-irritants (green tea), which is disappointing, because overall this is a very good moisturizer for normal to dry skin. The vitamin C in here is in such a minute amount it is inconsequential for skin, and the form used (ascorbic acid) is considered to be unstable and one of the more irritating forms of vitamin C.

☹ **$$$ Ultimate Eye Creme** *($29.95 for 0.5 ounce)*. The fragrance and witch hazel in here can be a problem for the eye area, which is a shame, because otherwise it contains very good moisturizing ingredients.

☺ **Ultimate Moisture** *($34.95 for 1.5 ounces)* is a very good moisturizer for normal to dry skin. The fragrant plant water in here can be a problem for some skin types.

☺ **$$$ Deep Moisture Repair Serum** *($29.95 for 0.3 ounce)* can't repair anything. However it is a good moisturizer for normal to slightly dry skin. The indication on the label that one of the ingredients is a "natural source of liposomes" is just bizarre; liposomes are not an ingredient but the way ingredients are delivered into the skin by a process in which the water and oil phase of the formulation are combined.

☺ **$$$ Seaweed Lift Serum** *($34.95 for 0.5 ounce)*. The apple juice is strange, but shouldn't be a problem for skin. This is still a good lightweight moisturizer for normal to slightly dry skin, even if it can't lift skin anywhere. The algae in here is a good anti-irritant, but that's about it.

☹ **Daily Moisture Sunscreen SPF 15** *($19.95 for 1.5 ounces)* does not contain the UVA-protecting ingredients titanium dioxide, zinc oxide, or avobenzone, and is not recommended.

☹ **Sunscreen SPF 15 Gel for the Face** *($15.95 for 1.8 ounces)* does not contain the UVA-protecting ingredients titanium dioxide, zinc oxide, or avobenzone, and is not recommended.

☹ **Sunscreen SPF 30 Gel for the Face** *($16.95 for 1.8 ounces)* does not contain the UVA-protecting ingredients titanium dioxide, zinc oxide, or avobenzone, and is not recommended.

☺ **Sans Sun Self Tanning Creme for All Skin Types** *($16.95 for 5 ounces)*, like all self-tanning products, uses dihydroxyacetone to turn the skin brown. This one would work as well as any.

☹ **15 Minute Face Lift for All Skin Types Especially Mature** *($19.95 for 4.4 ounces)* contains mostly cornstarch and egg white! If you want to believe that will lift your skin, whatever I have to say won't stop you.

☹ **Acne Treatment Mask for Combination & Oily/Problem Skin Types** *($19.95 for 5 ounces)* contains mostly alcohol, sulfur, and camphor. Any one of these would be enough to hurt blemish-prone skin, but together they can make skin red and irritated, and they have no benefit for skin.

☺ **Super Moisturizing Mask for Normal, Sensitive, Dry & Mature Skin Types** *($19.95 for 5 ounces)* is a good emollient moisturizer with lots of plant oils, lanolin, and thickeners. It would feel soothing for dry skin. It does contain fragrance, which is not appropriate for sensitive skin.

☺ $$$ **Ultimate Hydrating Mask** *($24.95 for 3 ounces)* is similar to the Super Moisturizing Mask above, only this one contains forms of algae that are good anti-irritants. However, they don't make this mask any more "ultimate" than the "super" one.

☺ $$$ **Eye Treatment Oil for All Skin Types** *($16.95 for 0.3 ounce)* would be a very good moisturizer for someone with dry skin, but there is nothing in here appropriate for normal to oily skin, despite the name.

The Reviews Z

# CHAPTER FOUR

# Baby's Skin-Care Products

When you are cleaning, softening, and soothing your child's skin, you also want to protect it and, of course, avoid applying anything that might cause problems for young, tender skin. Fortunately, there are some great products for this. But let me warn you about the baby products that can actually be anything but soothing or protecting for any skin type, but especially for a child's skin. My concern is that an alarming number of expensive baby products are being marketed to affluent consumers under the guise that they are better for young, delicate skin—when, for the most part, they aren't.

I know the baby sections in drugstores and at a growing number of cosmetic counters and health food stores have sweet, adorably packaged shampoos, moisturizers, cleansers, and sun products. Just from the packaging, you assume special care has been taken to use only ingredients that will be the most gentle to your baby's skin, but that assumption is sometimes not accurate. Think now about the wafting, appealing fragrances emanating from most all baby products and you are on the track of a major problem, one that makes me leery of using baby products for anyone's skin, let alone babies'! That delicious, recognizable aroma you could smell a mile away is nothing more than added fragrance, and can cause irritation. Moreover, baby products almost always have a pretty yellow or pink tint, which is contrived by coloring agents, another group of problematic skin-care ingredients for sensitive skin. If baby products were really gentler than what adults put on their skin, they would be fragrance free and contain no coloring agents. Sadly, only a few of those exist.

Cosmetics and hair-care companies know that mothers feel an impulsive emotional pull toward scents that trigger the image of their babies. That subconscious pull is difficult for a marketer to ignore, given the way women gravitate to the fragrance generated by other perfume-laden products. In other words, hair- and skin-care companies don't have much motivation to take these problematic ingredients out. That means you, the mother/consumer, as an advocate for your child, need to pay attention to this issue and choose fragrance-free and color-free products whenever you can!

When it comes to cleansing products, the group of ingredients considered the most gentle are called amphoteric surfactants (I generally use the term "detergent cleansing agent" for the more technical term "surfactant"). According to the *Cosmetic Science and Technology Series,* volume 17, *Hair and Hair Care,* amphoteric surfactants do not cleanse or foam as well as other surfactants; however, their one unique property is their very low potential for irritation. Amphoterics are so gentle that they can even reduce the irritation potential of other surfactants known for their sensitizing possibilities, such as sodium lauryl sulfate. According to *Hair and Hair Care,* a compilation of current hair-care research edited by Dale H. Johnson, "The skin irritancy of sodium lauryl sulfate in the presence of cocamidopropyl betaine [an amphoteric surfactant] is reduced substantially."

This explains why Johnson & Johnson's Baby Shampoo was such a phenomenal success when it launched in the 1960s. Johnson & Johnson's 1967 patent established the mild, nonirritating capacity for the amphoteric group of cleansing agents. As it turns out, the primary ingredient in Johnson & Johnson's baby shampoos is cocamidopropyl betaine, and that also explains why, when a mother tries to use baby shampoo on her own hair, it doesn't work very well. The amphoteric surfactants just can't clean like other surfactants can, and given the styling products and conditioners most adults use, it is essential to have a shampoo with good cleansing properties. Nowadays, most baby shampoos use a combination of cleansing agents to lower irritancy and improve cleansing, but they are still almost always more gentle than adult versions.

In general, a child's delicate skin would be better served by products that are fragrance- and color-free and that contain gentle cleansing agents. The basics for any child's skin are a gentle cleanser; a lightweight, soothing, nonirritating moisturizer (most of the fragrance-free versions are those packaged for adults, not children, like Cetaphil Moisturizer, Aquaphor, Eucerin, and Lubriderm, although they are excellent options for children); and a zinc oxide–based diaper-rash product (definitely fragrance-free—it hurts to put fragrance on red, rashy skin), and those at the drugstore are just fine for this. Then, a talc-free dusting powder—because you must never use talc on a baby's skin (see the Baby Powders section later in this chapter)—also, of course, fragrance free. Plain cornstarch is an excellent option for this; it is the primary ingredient in most talc-free baby powders, and plain cornstarch doesn't contain fragrance. (Cornstarch can be problematic for some sensitive skin types or in a pressed powder for an adult or teen struggling with breakouts.)

## Sun Care for the Little Ones

If you have babies or small children, the issue of sunscreen protection should absolutely be a primary concern. The delicacy of their skin is makes it even more sensitive to the sun's damaging energy. Whether or not you are diligent about using sunscreen for yourself, you must be diligent when it comes to the health of your children. It's easy to be attracted to the child-oriented products with pictures of cute babies on the label, but I have yet to see a formulation variance between products aimed at children and those for adults. Of greater concern to me is that I haven't seen many children's formulas that contains any amount of avobenzone, titanium dioxide, or zinc oxide. Sea & Ski for Kids SPF 30, Coppertone Water Babies SPF 45, and Coppertone Kids Colorblock SPF 40 all sound great for children, but not one offers appropriate protection from UVA damage to the skin when I reviewed them.

All sunscreen formulations that have an SPF are closely regulated by the FDA; the formulations don't differ in any way because of the age of the intended user. The only difference I've ever noted in baby products is the use of fragrance. Certain fragrances may make you think of little ones, but fragrance can be irritating for all skin types, and baby formulas tend to add more than most. **If you are looking for a less-irritating sunscreen for your kids, choose one that contains only pure titanium dioxide or zinc oxide as the active ingredient, which will definitely be less irritating than a product with other inorganic sunscreen agents.**

The following is an assortment of baby products available at drugstores, boutique cosmetics stores, and department store cosmetics counters, including general groupings for baby wipes, baby powders, and diaper ointments. You'll notice my ratings for baby products are more rigorous in regard to the fragrance issue. In defense of a baby's sensitive skin, there is no reason for a baby to put up with fragrance just because a mother thinks it smells better.

## Baby Magic Baby Care

What would really be magical is if these products didn't have such a noticeable scent to them.

☺ **Baby Bath, Original** (*$2.99 for 9 ounces*) is an exceptionally gentle cleanser with way too much fragrance.

☺ **Baby Bath with Aloe** (*$2.99 for 9 ounces*) is similar to the one above, only this one has a teeny amount of aloe.

☺ **Laugh and Splash Baby Bath** (*$3.49 for 15 ounces*) is virtually identical to the two above, and the same review applies.

☺ **Rich and Creamy Moisturizing Baby Bath, Original** (*$2.99 for 6.75 ounces*) is similar to those above, only this one has more thickening agents. It isn't in the least moisturizing for the skin.

☺ **Rich and Creamy Moisturizing Baby Bath with Aloe Vera** (*$2.99 for 6.75 ounces*) is similar to the one above, only with a tiny amount of aloe added.

☺ **Baby Lotion, Original** (*$2.99 for 9 ounces*) is a good moisturizer for dry skin, but the fragrance is overwhelming. Some skin types can be allergic to lanolin.

☺ **Baby Lotion with Aloe** *($2.99 for 9 ounces)* is similar to the one above only with a tiny amount of aloe added.

# Bobbi Brown Baby Essentials

All of the Bobbi Brown baby products have a distinctive fragrance, yet the ingredient listing doesn't include any. The fragrance isn't as bad as others but it is still unmistakably present.

☺ **Gentle Body Wash and Shampoo** *($18 for 6.7 ounces)* is a fairly gentle face and body wash using many of the ingredients mentioned above that make a shampoo gentle. It does contain fragrance, but it's not as bad as some.

☺ **Soothing Body Balm** *($22.50 for 8.5 ounces)* is a very good moisturizer for dry skin. It's good, but Eucerin Lite for half the price is just as good, and it's unscented.

☺ **Diaper Balm** *($14.50 for 2.5 ounces)* is a very good, emollient (although greasy) moisturizer for dry skin.

☹ **Massage Oil** *($16 for 4 ounces)*. Skip the fragrance-and-oil blend, and just use some pure soybean or almond oil from your pantry.

☹ **Silkening Powder** *($18 for 3.5 ounces)* is a pricey, talc-free powder that is highly fragranced and contains primarily cornstarch, oat flour, rice starch, preservatives, and fragrance. Plain cornstarch would work just as well without the fragrance and preservatives.

# Burt's Bees Baby Products

☹ **Buttermilk Soap** *($5 for 3.5 ounces)* is a standard (and overpriced) bar soap, and is too drying for most all skin types.

☺ **Buttermilk Bath** *($15 for 7.5 ounces)*. If there is a reason why a mother would want to soak her child in milk, I don't know it. OK, let's say there is a reason; in that case, this product is only nonfat dry milk, whole dry buttermilk, and fragrance. Forget the fragrance and just dump some nonfat dry milk in the bath. I'm not saying it's a good idea, but it's better than using this product.

☺ **Baby Bee Skin Creme** *($11 for 2 ounces)* is a good, extremely standard moisturizer for dry skin. The price is unwarranted for what you get.

☺ **Buttermilk Lotion** *($9 for 8 ounces)* contains mostly water, plant oils, glycerin, thickeners, vitamin E, aloe, buttermilk powder, thickeners, and fragrance.

☺ **Baby Bee Apricot Baby Oil** *($8 for 4 ounces)* pretty much contains what the name implies, so you can save a lot of money and take better care of your baby's skin by just using plain apricot oil and forgetting the fragrance in this product, but in this form it is still an option, though without fragrance would have been preferred.

☺ **Diaper Ointment** *($7 for 1.75 ounces)* contains mostly zinc oxide, plant oils, vitamin E, and plant extracts.

☹ **Dusting Powder** *($8 for 2.5 ounces)* contains mostly cornstarch, fragrance, and clay. Again, forget the fragrance and just use plain cornstarch from the grocery store.

☹ **Solid Perfume** *($7 for 0.3 ounce)*. I know there must be a reason why a mother would want to apply perfume to her child; I just can't think what it might be.

# Crabtree & Evelyn

☹ **Soap Collection** *($5 for 3 ounces)* is an assortment of standard, tallow-based bar soaps that can be drying and irritating for a baby's skin.

☹ **Baby Wash** *($10.50 for 8.5 ounces)* uses sodium lauryl sulfate as the cleansing agent and is not recommended.

☹ **Baby Shampoo** *($8.5 for 8.5 ounces)* is identical to the Baby Wash above, and the same comment applies.

☺ **Baby Lotion** *($10 for 8.5 ounces)* is a fairly emollient, though standard, moisturizer. It's good for dry skin but it would be better without the fragrance.

☺ **Cream for Baby** *($5 for 7 ounces)* is almost identical to the one above, only in cream form.

☺ **Baby Powder** *($8.5 for 3.5 ounces)* is mostly rice starch and cornstarch, with fragrance.

# Gerber Baby Products

If Gerber can sell baby food why not skin-care products? There are some options here, but also options to stay away from!

☺ **Baby Shampoo, Tear Free** *($3.79 for 15 ounces)* is a good, standard, detergent-based shampoo that would be gentle enough for your baby or you. It is not fragrance free.

☺ **Hair and Body Baby Wash** *($3.79 for 15 ounces)* is similar to the version above and the same comments apply.

☺ **Hair and Body Baby Wash, Calming Lavender** *($3.79 for 15 ounces)* is similar to the version above and the same comments apply. The lavender is not calming, although it can be a skin sensitizer. This version does contain fragrance and coloring agents.

☹ **Baby Vapor Bath** *($3.79 for 15 ounces)* contains menthol and eucalyptus, and as long as you only let your baby smell this stuff (though I would check with your pediatrician first) and you don't put any of it on baby's skin, it should be OK.

☹ **Baby Lotion, Hypoallergenic** *($3.79 for 15 ounces)* is hardly hypoallergenic, there are several problematic ingredients in here, including sodium hydroxide (rather high up on the ingredient listing), benzyl alcohol, and fragrance. There are better moisturizers for your baby, from Lubriderm to Cetaphil.

☺ **Baby Oil, Hypoallergenic** *($3.79 for 15 ounces)* is mostly mineral oil and fragrance. Why not skip the fragrance, which makes this hardly hypoallergenic; and just use plain mineral oil, which is great for dry skin for people of any age?

☺ **Baby Powder, Cornstarch with Aloe and Vitamin E** *($3.79 for 15 ounces)* contains 98% cornstarch, and the rest is mostly fragrance. The amount of aloe and vitamin E in here is just minute. For the money, and to avoid the sensitizing effect of fragrance, why not just use plain cornstarch from your kitchen cabinet?

☺ **Diaper Rash Lotion, Dimethicone** *($4.99 for 4 ounces)* would be soothing for any dry or rashy skin, and the lack of preservatives and fragrance is great.

☹ **Diaper Rash Ointment, Zinc Oxide** *($4.99 for 4 ounces)* contains menthol, which is extremely irritating and stinging for a sore baby bottom.

## Givenchy Baby Care

☺ **Delicate Bath Gel** *($20 for 8.4 ounces)* is an extremely standard, gentle cleanser that contains coloring agents and fragrance too.

☺ **Gentle Baby Lotion** *($18 for 8.4 ounces)* is a good, standard moisturizer. This one offers no benefit over the less-expensive ones I've mentioned above.

## Gymboree CradleGym Baby Care

☹ **Gentle Soap** *($3.50 for 3.65-ounce bar)* isn't gentle. It is a standard soap using detergent cleansing agents and fragrance.

☺ **Baby Shampoo** *($3.99 for 8 ounces)* is similar to other gentle baby shampoos. It would have been great if they had just left out the fragrance.

☺ **Moisturizing Lotion** *($4.49 for 8 ounces)* is a good moisturizer for dry skin, but Lubriderm or Eucerin Lite accomplish the exact same thing without fragrance.

☹ **Diaper Rash Cream** *($9.50 for 2 ounces)* is an emollient, 2% zinc-oxide cream. Even the thought of putting eucalyptus and tea tree oil on a baby's tender, irritated backside makes me want to scream.

## Johnson & Johnson Baby and Kids Products

☹ **Baby Bar** *($1.89 for 3-ounce bar)* is a standard bar cleanser that uses sodium cocoyl isethionate as the cleansing agent, which is fairly drying, plus the fragrance can just about knock you out.

☹ **Baby Bath** *($2.69 for 9 ounces)* almost reeks with fragrance. It is a gentle cleanser but that fragrance is an irritation or allergic reaction waiting to happen.

☺ **Head to Toe Baby Wash** *($2.69 for 9 ounces)* at least has a milder fragrance in comparison to the others in this line. This is a good, gentle cleanser using standard detergent cleansing agents.

☹ **Minnie Bath Bubbles** *($3.49 for 13.5 ounces)* is not only heavily fragranced but it isn't as gentle as most baby shampoos and cleansers.

☺ **Moisturizing Baby Bath with Aloe Vera and Vitamin E** *($3.69 for 15 ounces)* is far more gentle than those above, and if not for the fragrance, would be a great option.

⊗ **Ultra Sensitive Baby Cleansing Bar** *($2.29 for 3-ounce bar)* is a standard bar cleanser, but even with its minor fragrance (this product is one of the least fragrant I've reviewed), it still uses sodium cocoyl isethionate as the detergent cleansing agent, which makes it less gentle than other baby shampoos and cleansers.

☺ **Ultra Sensitive Baby Lotion** *($2.99 for 6.75 ounces)* is a good, but very basic, fragrance-free moisturizer.

☺ **Ultra Sensitive Baby Wash** *($2.49 for 6.75 ounces)* contains mostly water, detergent cleansing agents, thickeners, and preservatives.

☺ **Baby Cream, Soothes and Protects** *($3.73 for 4 ounces)* would be great for dry skin, but fragrance is the third ingredient in this product and that makes it a problem.

☺ **Baby Lotion** *($2.59 for 9 ounces)* is a highly fragrant, standard moisturizer for dry skin. There are far better moisturizers for a baby's skin than this one.

☺ **Baby Lotion with Aloe Vera and Vitamin E, Soothes and Nourishes Dry Skin** *($2.59 for 9 ounces)* is similar to the one above, and the same review applies. It does contain aloe and a tiny amount of vitamin E, which is OK but nothing special for a child's skin.

☺ **Baby Lotion with Daily UV Protection with SPF 15** *($3.59 for 4 ounces)* is a good, in-part titanium dioxide–based sunscreen in a lightweight, standard moisturizing lotion.

## Kiehl's Baby Care

☺ **Mild Gentle Shampoo for Babies** *($7.95 for 4 ounces)* is a standard detergent-based cleanser that is about as gentle as any including plant oils, and it contains no fragrance or coloring agents!

☺ **Baby Body Lotion** *($19.95 for 8 ounces)* is a nicely formulated, emollient moisturizer that is fragrance free and has no coloring agents.

☺ **Nourishing, Soothing Diaper Area Ointment** *($18.95 for 2 ounces)* is a fairly emollient ointment that would be very good for dry, irritated skin.

☺ **$$$ Diaper Rash Treatment Cream** *($26.50 for 6.2 ounces)* is similar to the one above and the same basic comments apply. There is no reason to spend this kind of money on a diaper rash product.

☺ **Baby Lip Balm** *($4.95 for 0.17 ounce)* is a very emollient lip balm with no fragrance or coloring agents; it contains mostly thickeners, plant oils, and preservative.

☺ **Sun Shield Sunblock with SPF 15** *($23.50 for 4 ounces)* is a very good, pure titanium dioxide–based sunscreen with no fragrance or coloring agents. What a shame it's so pricey, because this would be very good for a little one's skin.

## Little Forest Baby Care

☹ **Baby Soap** *($6.50 for 3.65 ounces)* is supposed to be pediatrician recommended, but that would only be because whoever it was didn't read the ingredient listing. This is soap, which can be drying, and the tea tree oil can be a skin irritant.

☹ **Baby Shampoo** *($8 for 4 ounces)* contains tea tree oil, eucalyptus oil, and grapefruit seed extract, and is absolutely not recommended.

☹ **Baby Oil** *($10 for 4 ounces)* contains tea tree oil, eucalyptus oil, and grapefruit seed extract, and is absolutely not recommended.

☹ **Baby Cream (for Diaper Rash)** *($10.59 for 2 ounces)*. This product made me want to cry when I thought some unsuspecting mother might use this on her baby's red, irritated skin not knowing it contains tea tree oil, eucalyptus oil, and grapefruit seed extract, and that they can be so terribly irritating even on skin that isn't abraded and raw.

☹ **Baby Powder** *($11.50 for 3 ounces)* contains tea tree oil, eucalyptus oil, and grapefruit seed extract, and is absolutely not recommended.

## Mustela Baby Products

☹ **Bain Mousse Bebe, Bubble Bath for Babies** *($9 for 6.8 ounces)* contains sodium lauryl sulfate and several other detergent cleansing agents that make it too irritating for all skin types, especially for a baby's skin.

☺ **Hydra Bebe Facial Hydrating Cream** *($9 for 1.4 ounces)* is a good, standard (albeit ordinary) moisturizer for dry skin.

## Origins Baby Care

While the Origins baby products end up being somewhat less fragrant than others, they are still far from fragrance-free.

☹ **Short Cake Baby Cleansing Bar** *($7.50 for 4.2-ounce bar)* contains several fragrant plant oils that be can irritating to skin, and the cleansing agents are not as gentle as those found in other baby products.

☹ **Bare Hug Baby Massage Cream** *($12.50 for 3.5 ounces)* would have been just a good, basic moisturizer containing thickeners and plant oils, but they included balsam, neroli, pine, and orange, and that's way too irritating for most babies' skin.

☹ **Love Me Tender Soothing Baby Lotion** *($13.50 for 6 ounces)* is similar to the one above except in lotion form. No baby needs cedarwood, geranium, cinnamon leaf, lavandin, patchouli, or styrax on its skin.

☺ **First Sun for Children Chemical Free SPF 15** *($14 for 3.5 ounces)* is a titanium dioxide–based sunscreen, and that part is great. However, it also contains many of the same fragrances that the other Origins baby products do.

☺ **Smooth Baby Baby Oil** *($11 for 8.5 ounces)* contains mostly soybean oil and fragrance. Skip the fragrance and just use some soybean oil from the grocery store.

☺ **Diaper Service Baby Bottom Balm** *($10 for 3.5 ounces)* is much like other baby balms at the drugstore, and contains castor oil, zinc oxide, plant oils, emollient, fragrance, and preservatives. The fragrance isn't necessary, so Johnson & Johnson Diaper Rash Ointment with 13% Zinc Oxide for half the cost is far better.

# Baby Wipe Products

☺ **Chubs Baby Wipe with Aloe** *($2.49 for 80 towelettes)* is a very gentle liquid cleanser soaked onto soft towelettes. It does contain fragrance, so forget this one and use the others that are fragrance-free.

☺ **Diaparene Baby Wash Cloths, Fragrance-Free** *($2.49 for 100 towelettes)* is almost identical to the Chubs above only without fragrance!

☺ **Huggies Baby Wipes Refills, Natural Care, Unscented** *($5.29 for 160 towelettes)* is almost identical to the Chubs above, only this one doesn't contain fragrance! Huggies does have a scented version, but why bother?

☹ **Kleenex Cottonelle Flushable Moist Wipes with Aloe** *($2.49 for 50 towelettes)*. The Kleenex brand name is recognizable but the formulation is problematic due to the inclusion of fragrance and propylene glycol. Propylene glycol is used in skin-care products to help other ingredients penetrate the skin better, and that is not necessary for a baby's skin.

☹ **Pampers Baby Fresh Tub, Original** *($3.19 for 84 towelettes)* is similar to the Kleenex brand above, and the same comments apply.

☺ **Pampers Baby Fresh Alcohol Free Wipe Refills, Unscented** *($5.99 for 168 towelettes)* is similar to the Kleenex brand above, minus the fragrance.

# Baby Powders

There is legislation pending that would require talc powders to carry a warning label as a result of studies indicating some cancer risks. While I feel strongly that the studies were not linked in any way to the talc used in makeup products for adults, I also feel that talc is something you would never want to use anywhere on your children.

☺ **Desitin Cornstarch Baby Powder** *($2.99 for 14 ounces)* is just fragranced cornstarch.

☹ **Caldesene Protecting Powder, Fresh Scent** *($3.79 for 5 ounces)* is a talc-based powder, and is not recommended.

☹ **Gold Bond Children's Medicated Baby Powder** *($3.99 for 4 ounces)* is a talc-based powder, and is not recommended.

☺ **Good Sense Baby Powder with Cornstarch** *($2.09 for 15 ounces)* definitely makes better sense than their talc version, but this one still contains fragrance and just plain cornstarch would be better.

☹ **Johnson & Johnson Baby Powder** *($3.69 for 22 ounces)* is a talc-based powder, and is not recommended.

☺ **Johnson & Johnson Corn Starch Baby Powder with Aloe Vera & Vitamin E** *($2.89 for 9 ounces)* is just fragranced cornstarch; the amount of aloe and vitamin E here is negligible.

☺ **Johnson & Johnson Medicated Baby Powder** *($2.29 for 9 ounces)* is fragranced cornstarch with zinc oxide. The fragrance doesn't add much benefit to the powder.

☺ **Suave Baby Care Powder with Cornstarch** *($2.29 for 15 ounces)* is fragranced cornstarch.

## Diaper Rash Ointments

☺ **A&D Diaper Rash Ointment** *($2.59 for 1.5 ounces)* is exceptionally emollient, containing mostly petrolatum, lanolin, cod liver oil, fragrance, mineral oil, and wax. It would be best if it didn't contain fragrance, but this is exceptionally moisturizing.

☺ **A&D Diaper Rash Ointment with 10% Zinc Oxide** *($5.49 for 4 ounces)* isn't as emollient as the one above and it also contains benzyl alcohol rather high up on the ingredient list. It's probably not a problem, but for a rash ointment I'd maybe think twice about this one.

☺ **A&D Original Ointment** *($4.29 for 4 ounces)* is just Vaseline with lanolin. That makes it very emollient and just fine for a moisturizer, and it's completely fragrance-free.

☹ **Balmex Diaper Rash Ointment** *($5.75 for 4 ounces)* uses balsam as one of the main ingredients, and that can be a skin irritant.

☹ **Boudreaux's Butt Paste** *($7.49 for 4 ounces)* has a great name, but the second ingredient is balsam, and that can be a skin irritant.

☺ **Desitin Zinc Oxide Ointment, 10% Zinc Oxide** *($5.29 for 4 ounces)* is a good, emollient, zinc oxide–based ointment with silicone, preservatives, mineral oil, Vaseline, and thickeners.

☹ **Desitin Diaper Rash Ointment, Hypoallergenic, Zinc Oxide (40%)** *($5.29 for 4 ounces)* is not hypoallergenic; it still contains fragrance.

☹ **Desitin Diaper Rash Ointment, Ultra Smooth Cream Formula** *($2.99 for 2 ounces)* is similar to the one above only in cream form.

☺ **Dr. Smith's Diaper Ointment** *($6.99 for 2 ounces)* is extremely emollient and doesn't contain fragrance! It contains mostly zinc oxide, Vaseline, lanolin, mineral oil, wax, plant oil, and preservative.

☺ **Johnson & Johnson Diaper Rash Ointment with 13% Zinc Oxide** *($3.99 for 2 ounces)* contains mostly zinc oxide, water, silicone, glycerin, Vaseline, lanolin, thickeners, and preservatives. Another fragrance-free, emollient ointment!

# CHAPTER FIVE

# Men's Skin-Care Products

Men generally don't read my books or newsletters. But I don't take that personally—men don't read fashion magazines either, even though the pages are filled with drop-dead gorgeous, scantily clad women. Men are about as comfortable dealing with skin care, hair care, or any subject related to beauty as they are with holding a woman's purse while she shops. The aversion to these topics determines in advance that most men aren't going to see this chapter, even though they should. That means I have to rely on you, my female readers, to share this section with the men in your lives. Men have faces too, and they definitely have skin-care needs, but you could never convince the vast majority of men to put even a fraction of the attention and energy into the issue that women do. One positive result of this lack of interest is that men don't waste their money on wrinkle creams or unnecessary products for their skin. While this monetary savings is significant, it probably means most men don't use sunscreen on a consistent basis and leave their skin at risk for cancer, not to mention wrinkles. On a less serious note it also means most men don't understand about staying away from irritating skin-care ingredients in their shave products, and end up with red, rashlike bumps and razor burn (which is really, more often than not, product burn).

What gives? Men definitely wrinkle as much as women (any notion suggesting otherwise is myth and a bias about how much better men look with wrinkles than women do). And don't they get dry skin, breakouts, ingrown hairs, and red, irritated spots from shaving? So why don't men seem to care as much as women do about taking care of their skin? Probably because toughing it out it is one of the last vestiges of legitimate machismo left to a man. In fact, the very marketing angles about gentleness, soothing, and antiwrinkling that sell skin-care products to women are the ones almost completely left off of men's products (the best men's products can use is that there are producs are good for "sensitive skin").

The morning shaving ritual is the most typical start to a man's day. Yet, if I may be so bold, it is also the first area where men make mistakes. Most shaving creams and preshave products contain irritating ingredients such as alcohol, menthol, mint, potassium or sodium hydroxide, and camphor. These skin irritants make the hair follicle and skin swell, forcing the hair up and away from the skin. While this does make the hair stand up to some extent, supposedly allowing for a closer shave, the irritation and resulting swelling cause some of the hair to be hidden by the swollen follicle and skin. So what might get the hair to rise to the occasion really doesn't make for a better shave, because the swollen skin prevents the razor from getting closer to the base of the hair. Additionally, after you shave, because some of the facial hair is hidden beneath swollen skin (which temporarily gives the impression of a close shave) the stubble will have a harder time navigating its way back out. If the hair begins to grow (which it does almost immediately) before the swelling is reduced, the likelihood of ingrown hairs is increased.

Moreover, a razor gliding over the face abrades the skin—granted, not all that much, but enough to cause havoc when an innocent-looking aftershave lotion with irritating ingredients is splashed over that broken skin. Think of splashing an aftershave on a cut or scrape on any other part of your body where you have an abrasion. Now, why would you want to do that to your face (other than the erroneous notion that this somehow protects the skin)? Basic skin-care rule number one for both men and women: if the skin-care product you're using repeatedly burns, irritates, tingles, causes the skin to become inflamed, or hurts, don't use it.

What should men use to take care of their skin when they shave? The list isn't all that different from the one that applies for women. To start with, all men's skin types need a gentle, water-soluble cleanser; a gentle shave product (foam, cream, or gel); followed by a gentle, nonirritating aftershave or shaving lotion (which for all intents and purposes is just a masculine name for a gentle toner). The same options follow for treating breakouts (disinfectant and BHA), sun care (SPF 15 with UVA protection), or dealing with dry skin (a good moisturizer). The one exception to selecting a parallel routine is that, for some skin types, it can prove to be too irritating for men to follow shaving with an AHA or BHA product.

On and off over the years I've heard people say that a man's skin doesn't age like woman's. It isn't true, at least not physiologically when it comes to wrinkles. There is some validity to the notion that in our society, wrinkles and other visible signs of aging—like a less-than-perfect physique or thinning hair—are more socially acceptable for men than for women. Age can make a man look distinguished, while a woman the same age can just seem over the hill. Men's clothing styles never reveal as much skin as do women's, nor are they as form-fitting. All that makes physical flaws far more obvious and thus less socially acceptable for women than for men.

But when it comes to sun exposure and genetic aging, men and women age in the exact same way, determined primarily by how much time they have spent in the sun without adequate sun protection (and for most of us, given how little we've known about sun protection over the years, that's likely to be a lot of time).

However, in terms of surface-cell turnover, men who shave have an advantage, because shaving removes the top layer of dead skin cells, improving cell turnover.

That's good, but it only accounts for a certain amount of surface smoothness over the shaved areas (encouraging cell turnover doesn't alter the way wrinkles are formed). And it doesn't help the areas of the face where men don't shave. It also doesn't mean that men have to pass by the advantages of using a retinoid—like Retin-A or Renova—or that they should omit using a reliable sunscreen. Men who shave on a daily basis are probably best off not using AHAs on the bearded area of the face. Shaving exfoliates the skin more than adequately in that area, and it isn't necessary to do more by using an AHA product. However, cell turnover is not stimulated in nonshaved areas. Using an AHA product over the nonshaved areas of the face, neck, or forehead along with a good sunscreen would be a good addition to a man's skin-care routine.

I thought some of you might find it interesting if I reviewed the lines that are supposedly designed to meet a man's special skin-care needs. You'll notice that many of these products seem to be designed with nothing but irritation in mind. The same way in which cosmetics companies believe women want wrinkle creams, they believe men need menthol, peppermint, or alcohol in their skin-care products to create a "strong smell—strong man" concept the consumer seems to want. Both notions may be what the consumer *wants*, but neither is what the skin actually *needs*.

## *American Crew for Men*

☹ **The Bar for Men** *($6.05 for 5.45-ounce bar)* is a standard bar cleanser that is quite similar to Dove, only with a more distinct fragrance. It can be drying and irritating for skin.

☹ **Scrub Total Body Wash** *($7.50 for 8.45 ounces)* uses TEA-lauryl sulfate as the main cleansing agent, which can be irritating and sensitizing for most skin types. Plus, to add insult to injury, this product also contains peppermint oil, for more unnecessary irritation.

☹ **Essential Shave Oil** *($10.95 for 1 ounce)* contains lots of plant oils, but the fragrant oils of clove and sandalwood, along with eucalyptus, peppermint, and menthol, make this way too irritating and sensitizing for all skin types.

☹ **Herbal Shave Cream** *($8.80 for 5.1 ounces)* would be a good, soaplike shave cream with mostly nonherbal ingredients, but the addition of clove, eucalyptus, peppermint, balm mint, and menthol makes it far too irritating to consider.

☹ **After Shave Moisturizer** *($8.80 for 5.1 ounces)* has the same problems as the Herbal Shave Cream above and should not be used.

## *Aqua Velva*

☹ **Classic Ice Blue Cooling After Shave** *($7.29 for 7 ounces)* lists the first ingredient as alcohol, and in addition it contains menthol! Ouch!

&#9785; **Ice Sport Cooling After Shave** *($4.29 for 3.5 ounces)* is almost identical to the Ice Blue and the same painful comments apply.

# *Aramis Lab Series*

&#9785; **Dual Action Face Soap** *($10 for 5.5 ounces)* is a standard bar soap, which is irritating enough, only this one adds camphor to the mix, assuring that it will be very irritating.

&#9786; **Lift Off! Power Wash** *($14 for 4.2 ounces)* is a standard, water-soluble cleanser that also contains papain, an enzyme meant to exfoliate skin. Papain is considered to be an unstable enzyme, so its effectiveness for the job wouldn't amount to much. In any case, in a cleanser it would just be rinsed down the drain.

&#9785; **Active Treatment Scrub** *($12.50 for 3.4 ounces)* contains alcohol and menthol, which makes it too irritating for all skin types.

&#9786; **Instant Moisture Complex** *($18.50 for 1.7 ounces)* is a good, extremely average moisturizer for normal to somewhat dry skin.

&#9786; **Lift Off! AHA Formula** *($37.50 for 3.4 ounces)* contains a minimal amount of AHA, though it does contain BHA (salicylic acid). That could work to exfoliate, except that the pH of this product is too high for the exfoliants to be effective.

&#9786; **Lift Off! Moisture Formula** *($37.50 for 3.4 ounces)* is supposed to exfoliate skin like the AHA Formula above, and this version does have slightly more AHA, but both its concentration and the product's pH are still not what's needed to make it an effective exfoliant. Other than that, this is just a good moisturizer for dry skin.

&#9786; **$$$ Eye Time Rescue Gel** *($23.50 for 0.5 ounce)* is a good, standard, lightweight moisturizer for normal to dry skin. It does contain a form of alkali aluminum silicate, which is found in deodorants or used as an absorbent, and it seems strange to find it in an eye product that is meant to moisturize.

&#9786; **U-Turn Age Defying Formula** *($28 for 1.7 ounces)* is quite similar to the Eye Time Rescue Gel above, only in lotion form, and the same basic comments apply. It won't change one wrinkle on anyone's skin.

&#9785; **Waterproof, Sweatproof Sun Protection Spray SPF 15** *($18 for 3.4 ounces)* contains no UVA-protecting ingredients and is not recommended.

&#9785; **Skin Clearing Lotion** *($10 for 3.4 ounces)* contains mostly alcohol and witch hazel, and that won't clear anything, although it will make skin red, irritated, and dry.

&#9785; **Electric Shave Solution** *($11 for 3.4 ounces)* has alcohol as its main ingredient, and that is a problem for skin.

&#9785; **Maximum Comfort Shave Cream** *($10.50 for 3.4 ounces)* includes eucalyptus and lemon, which make it far too potentially irritating to be considered "comforting."

☺ **Razor Burn Relief Plus** *($25 for 3.4 ounces)* is just a good, lightweight moisturizer for normal to dry skin. How thoughtful of Aramis to offer a product for razor-burn relief, given the number of products it sells that could make skin feel burnt!

☺ **Stop Shine Oil Control Formula** *($24.50 for 1.7 ounces)* won't stop oil—it's mostly a lightweight moisturizer similar to many in the Aramis line. It does contain BHA but the pH of the product makes it ineffective as an exfoliant. Besides, BHA doesn't absorb oil or affect oil production in any way. An effective BHA product can help improve the shape and size of the pore, thus improving the "natural" flow of oil and helping to prevent clogging. Besides, this moisturizer contains several emollients that would be problematic for oily skin.

☺ **Tri-Gel Extra Shave Formula** *($12 for 4.2 ounces)* does contain a few problematic plant extracts, but they are far enough down on the ingredient list to make this a potentially irritant-free shave gel. It is extremely standard and not worth the price.

## Aveda Men's Skin Care

☺ **After Shave Balm** *($13.50 for 1.7 ounces)* is a rather fragrant, though fairly nonirritating moisturizer for normal to dry skin.

☹ **Shave Cream** *($11 for 7.9 ounces)* contains peppermint extract, and that can be a problem for irritation.

## The Body Shop Skin Mechanics for Men

☹ **Menthol Shave Cream** *($6 for 3.5 ounces)* is a detergent-based shave cream with plant oils; it would work well for dry skin, but the menthol can be a problem for irritation and redness, especially over abraded skin.

☺ **Original Shave Cream** *($10 for 6 ounces)* is a standard shave cream indistinguishable from any of the Edge products reviewed below at one-third the price.

☹ **Face Scrub** *($10 for 3 ounces)* is more abrasive than most, using pumice for the scrub particles. Given that a man shaves on a regular basis, that is enough exfoliation for any face, and adding this product is completely unnecessary. It also contains menthol and alcohol—ouch!

☹ **After Shave Lotion** *($10 for 3.2 ounces)* would be a good emollient moisturizer for dry skin. The menthol is a problem for irritation and redness, and that isn't helpful for newly shaved skin.

☺ **After Shave Gel** *($10 for 3.4 ounces)* is more like putting aloe with fragrance and coloring agents on your skin, which isn't bad, but skip the unnecessary fragrance and dyes and just use plain aloe you get from a health food store.

☺ **Face Protector** *($10 for 3.4 ounces)* does not have an SPF (though it does contain sunscreen), so it can't be relied on for sun protection. Other than that, it is a good, standard moisturizer for dry skin.

## Callaway Golf by Nordstrom

☺ **Skin Fitness Face Moisturizer SPF 25** *($22.50 for 4 ounces)* is one in a line of sunscreens that all contain the sun-blocking ingredient avobenzone, and all have appropriate SPFs. The formulations are mostly for normal to dry skin. While these are worthwhile in terms of effectiveness, the drawback for all of them is the price—the cost isn't worth it, given that there are far less expensive avobenzone-based sunscreens. Plus, it is critical to remember that for any sunscreen to be effective (even if it has the right SPF number and UVA-protecting ingredients) it needs to be applied liberally. For this kind of money you may be reluctant to do that.

☺ **Sun Block Powder Dry Lotion SPF 15** *($17.50 for 4 ounces)* is similar to the one above only in a more matte formulation.

☺ **Sun Block Powder Dry Lotion SPF 20** *($17.50 for 4 ounces)* is similar to the one above and the same comments apply.

☺ **Sun Block All Over Oil-Free Spray SPF 15** *($17.50 for 4 ounces)*, like those above, contains avobenzone, and this one would work for normal to slightly oily or slightly dry skin.

☺ **Sun Block Quick Stick SPF 15** *($8.50 for 0.65 ounce)* is similar to those above only in a balm, and would work well for dry skin.

## Clinique Skin Supplies for Men

☹ **Face Soap Regular Strength** *($9.50 for 6-ounce bar)* is a standard bar soap, which makes it not all that different from Ivory and worth neither the price nor the dryness it can cause.

☹ **Scruffing Lotion 1¹/₂ for Sensitive Skin** *($9.50 for 6.7 ounces)* contains mostly alcohol, witch hazel, and menthol. There is no reason to use those ingredients on any skin type, but it is thoughtless to have them in a product for someone with sensitive skin.

☹ **Scruffing Lotion 2¹/₂ for Dry to Average Skin** *($9.50 for 6.7 ounces)* contains mostly alcohol and witch hazel, which makes it unnecessarily irritating for all skin types.

☹ **Scruffing Lotion 3¹/₂ for Oily Skin** *($9.50 for 6.7 ounces)* has the same problems as the 2¹/₂ version above and the same comments apply.

☹ **Scruffing Lotion 4¹/₂ for Very Oily Skin** *($9.50 for 6.7 ounces)* has the same problems as the 2¹/₂ version above and the same comments apply.

☹ **Face Scrub** *($13.50 for 3 ounces)* contains menthol, which makes it too irritating, especially in a scrub.

☺ M Lotion *($16.50 for 3.4 ounces)* is a good but standard moisturizer for dry to very dry skin.

☺ Turnaround Lotion *($24.50 for 1.7 ounces)* is a good basic moisturizer for normal to dry skin. It does contain BHA, but the product's pH is too high for it to be an effective exfoliant.

☹ Non-Streak Bronzer *(11.50 for 2 ounces)* is a very sheer, relatively tan-looking bronzer in a lightweight gel base. It can add a bit of color, but on very light skin it can have a slightly too-peach look.

☹ Creme Shave *($8 for 4 ounces)* would be a good shave cream but it contains menthol, and that can cause redness and irritation.

☺ M Shave Aloe Gel *($11 for 4.4 ounces)* is a good nonirritating shave gel, but it is also virtually identical to several versions from Gillette for far less money.

☹ Post Shave Healer *($13.50 for 2.5 ounces)* contains alcohol, witch hazel, and almond meal (a scrub), and none of those will help heal skin, though they will add to irritation and dryness.

## Colgate Shaving Care

☺ Aloe Shave Cream *($1.69 for 11 ounces)* is a standard shave cream with minimal risk of irritation. It does contain a small amount of sodium lauryl sulfate but probably not enough to be a problem for most all skin types.

☺ Regular Shave Cream *($1.69 for 11 ounces)* is almost identical to the Aloe Shave Cream above and the same comments apply.

☺ Sensitive Skin Shave Cream *($1.69 for 11 ounces)* is almost identical to the Aloe Shave Cream above, and the same comments apply.

## Crabtree & Evelyn for Men

☹ Nomad Soap *($18 for 1 bar)* contains eucalyptus, which makes it too irritating for all skin types (not to mention that this standard soap formulation can be drying and irritating in and of itself).

☹ Sandalwood Shaving Bowl *($15 for 3.2 ounces)* is more like shaving with soap than anything else. The cleansing agents in here can be drying for most skin types.

☺ Nomad Shave Gel *($10 for 4.2 ounces)* is a good basic shaving gel that would work well for all skin types, with minimal to no risk of irritation.

☹ Nomad Shave Cream *($10 for 3.5 ounces)* is indeed a good shave cream for normal to oily skin types, but it's not good for sensitive skin. The cleansing agents in here are rather drying and potentially irritating for sensitive skin, as well as for those with dry skin.

☺ **Shaving Cream** *($18.50 for 5.8 ounces)* is similar to the Nomad version above and the same comments apply.

# Edge ProGel

☺ **Extra Moisturizing Shave Gel** *($2.49 for 7 ounces)* is a good shave gel for most all skin types, with minimal to no risk of irritation or dryness.

☺ **Extra Protection from Nicks and Cuts** *($2.49 for 7 ounces)* is similar to the Extra Moisturizing version above and the same comments apply. There is nothing in this product to prevent cuts or nicks from shaving.

☹ **Extra Refreshing with Lime Splash** *($2.49 for 7 ounces)*. The lime in here is just fragrance, which can cause irritation.

☹ **Extra Soothing with Cooling Menthol** *($2.49 for 7 ounces)*. Menthol is indeed cooling but it is also irritating and can increase the risk of redness and breakouts from shaving.

☺ **Fragrance-Free for Irritated Skin and Razor Bumps** *($2.49 for 7 ounces)* is similar to the Extra Moisturizing version above, only this one includes triclosan, a topical disinfectant. That can be minimally helpful to prevent infection, but infection is rarely the reason the skin becomes irritated and bumpy after shaving.

☺ **Normal Skin Shave Gel** *($2.49 for 7 ounces)* is almost identical to the Extra Moisturizing version above and the same comments apply.

☺ **Sensitive Skin with Aloe Shave Gel** *($2.49 for 7 ounces)* is almost identical to the Extra Moisturizing version above and the same comments apply.

☺ **Skin Conditioning with Lanolin Shave Gel** *($2.49 for 7 ounces)* is almost identical to the Extra Moisturizing version above and the same comments apply.

☺ **Tough Beards with Beard Softeners Shave Gel** *($2.49 for 7 ounces)* is almost identical to the Extra Moisturizing version above and the same comments apply.

# Estee Lauder for Men

☺ **Skin Comfort Lotion** *($18.50 for 1.75 ounces)* is a good moisturizer for dry skin, regardless of gender!

☹ **Close-Shave Cream** *($10 for 3.4 ounces)* could have been a great shave cream—but it contains menthol, and on shaved, abraded skin, that can hurt.

☹ **After Shave** *($30 for 3.4 ounces)* is just alcohol and fragrance. Putting this on the face after shaving is irritation waiting to happen.

# Gillette

☺ **Gillette Series Shaving Cream Advanced Performance, Vitamin Enriched** *($2.52 for 9 ounces)* is a standard shave cream that would work well for most all skin types. It does contain a tiny amount of sodium lauryl sulfate but probably not enough to be a problem for even sensitive skin. It isn't vitamin "enriched" at all; the amount of vitamins in here is negligible.

☹ **Gillette Foamy, Lemon Lime** *($1.69 for 11 ounces)* is similar to the Vitamin Enriched above and the same basic comments apply. The lemon-lime fragrance can be a problem for sensitive skin types.

☺ **Gillette Foamy, Regular** *($1.69 for 11 ounces)* is similar to the Vitamin Enriched above and the same basic comments apply.

☺ **Gillette Foamy, Sensitive Skin** *($1.69 for 11 ounces)* is similar to the Vitamin Enriched above and the same basic comments apply.

☺ **Gillette Series Shaving Cream Advanced Performance** *($2.99 for 7 ounces)* is similar to the Vitamin Enriched above, only with more emollients and minus the sodium lauryl sulfate, making it better for slightly drier skin.

☺ **Gillette Series Shaving Gel Advanced Performance, Aloe Enriched** *($2.99 for 7 ounces)* is similar to the non-vitamin-enriched Advanced Performance version above, and the same comments apply.

☺ **Gillette Series Shaving Gel Advanced Performance, Extra Protection** *($2.99 for 7 ounces)* is similar to the non-vitamin-enriched Advanced Performance version above, and the same comments apply.

☺ **Gillette Series Shaving Gel Advanced Performance, Sensitive Skin** *($2.99 for 7 ounces)* is similar to the non-vitamin-enriched Advanced Performance version above, and the same comments apply.

☺ **Gillette Foamy, Aloe and Allantoin** *($1.69 for 11 ounces)* is similar to the non-vitamin-enriched Advanced Performance version above, and the same comments apply.

☺ **Gillette Foamy, Skin Conditioning** *($1.69 for 11 ounces)* is similar to the non-vitamin-enriched Advanced Performance version above, and the same comments apply.

☹ **Gillette Series After Shave Skin Conditioner Gel, Allantoin Enriched** *($3.19 for 3.25 ounces)*. The alcohol in here is too drying and irritating for all skin types.

☹ **Gillette Series After Shave Skin Conditioner Gel, Extra Moisturizing and Soothing** *($3.19 for 3.25 ounces)* is similar to the Allantoin Enriched version above, and the same warnings apply.

☹ **Gillette Series After Shave Skin Conditioner Gel, Sensitive Skin** *($3.19 for 3.25 ounces)* is similar to the Allantoin Enriched version above, and the same warnings apply.

☹ **Gillette Series After Shave Skin Conditioner Lotion, Alcohol Free** *($2.52 for 3.25 ounces)* is not much of a moisturizer and is actually a rather confused product. The second ingredient is aluminum starch (octenylsuccinate), an absorbing/thickening agent, which is good for absorbing oil, but it has no place in a "conditioner." The third ingredient is fragrance, and the next preservatives. That means the remaining ingredients are less than 0.1 percent of the content. This may be an option for oily skin but the remaining ingredients, though minor, are best for dry skin.

☹ **Gillette Series After Shave Skin Conditioner Lotion, Extra Moisturizing & Soothing** *($2.52 for 3.25 ounces)* is similar to the Alcohol Free version above, and the same comments apply.

☹ **Gillette Series After Shave Skin Conditioner Lotion, Sensitive Skin** *($2.52 for 3.25 ounces)* is similar to the Alcohol Free version above, and the same comments apply.

☹ **Gillette Series Non-Stinging After Shave Splash, Sensitive Skin** *($4.89 for 3.5 ounces)* contains menthol, which can irritate skin.

☹ **Gillette Series Non-Stinging After Shave Splash, Allantoin Enriched** *($4.89 for 3.5 ounces)* contains menthol, which can irritate skin.

☹ **Gillette Series Non-Stinging Moisturizing After Shave Splash** *($6.29 for 3.2 ounces)* contains menthol, which can irritate skin.

## *Kiehl's for Men*

☺ **Soothing, Nourishing Face Cream for Men, for Dry to Normal Skin Types** *($11.95 for 4 ounces)* is a standard shave cream that would work well for most skin types.

☺ **Close Shavers Squadron Ultimate Brushless Shave Cream, It's a "Goggle-Fogger" Formula, Blue Eagle with Aloe for Sensitive Skin** *($14.50 for 8 ounces)* has a great name for a standard shave cream that would work well for most all skin types.

☹ **Close Shavers Squadron Ultimate Brushless Shave Cream, It's a "Hair Raizer" Formula, White Eagle** *($14.50 for 8 ounces)* contains menthol and camphor, which are too irritating for all skin types.

☹ **Close Shavers Squadron Ultimate Brushless Shave Cream, "Take Off" Formula, Green Eagle** *($14.50 for 8 ounces)* contains peppermint oil—ouch!

☺ **The Ultimate Men's After Shave All Day Moisturizer** *($11.95 for 4 ounces)* is a good moisturizer for dry skin, but without sunscreen is also a serious problem for all-day use.

☹ **The Ultimate Men's After Shave All Day Moisturizer (Mentholated)** *($11.95 for 4 ounces)* contains menthol and camphor, which are too irritating for all skin types, but especially for newly shaved skin. This product does contain benzocaine, a very mild anesthetic. That wouldn't be necessary if men weren't using so many irritating products on their skin.

# Mary Kay for Men

☺ **Enriched Shave Cream for All Skin Types** *($5.50 for 6.75 ounces)* is a standard shave cream that would work well for most skin types.

☹ **Cleansing Bar for All Skin Types** *($8.50 for 5.5 ounces)* is a standard bar cleanser with all the drying, irritating problems that can accompany this kind of product.

☹ **Cooling Toner for All Skin Types** *($8.50 for 6 ounces)* contains alcohol, mint, and peppermint, making it an irritation waiting to happen.

☹ **Conditioner With Sunscreen SPF 8 for Dry and Normal Skin** *($13 for 3.5 ounces)* doesn't contain adequate UVA protection and, because it is only an SPF 8, is not recommended by me or the American Academy of Dermatology to meet the minimum sunscreen standard of SPF 15.

☹ **Oil Controller with Sunscreen SPF 8 for Combination and Oily Skin** *($13 for 3.5 ounces)* is similar to the one above and is absolutely not recommended.

☺ **Blemish Control Formula** *($8 for 2 ounces)* is a 10% benzoyl peroxide formula that also contains water, slip agent, and detergent cleansing agent. This is strong stuff and not the best over razor-abraded skin, at least not to start. However, for stubborn breakouts that don't respond to lesser concentrations of benzoyl peroxide, this one is an option to consider.

# Noxzema for Men

☺ **Medicated Shave Cream, Regular, Protective Formula** *($2.79 for 11 ounces)* is a good standard shave cream for most all skin types. There is nothing medicated in here. The active ingredient is a silicone, and that's just a good moisturizing ingredient.

☺ **Medicated Shave with Aloe and Lanolin, Dimethicone Skin Protectant Shave** *($2.79 for 11 ounces)* is similar to the one above and the same comments apply.

☺ **Medicated Shave for Sensitive Skin, Dimethicone Skin Protectant Shave** *($2.79 for 11 ounces)* is similar to the one above and the same comments apply.

# Old Spice

☺ **Moisturizing Shave Cream** *($2.49 for 11 ounces)* is a standard shave cream that would work well for most all skin types. It does contain a tiny amount of sodium lauryl sulfate but probably not enough to be a problem for even sensitive skin.

☹ **After Shave, Fresh** *($6.29 for 4 ounces)*. Keep this cologne of alcohol and fragrance off the face. If you want to smell like "old spice," put this anywhere but where you've just shaved.

☹ **After Shave Alcohol Free, Original** *($6.29 for 4 ounces)*. It's nice they left the alcohol out of this formulation but there is no reason to put this much fragrance on the face. It only adds to the risk of irritation.

☹ **After Shave Alcohol Free, Sensitive** *($6.29 for 4 ounces)* is similar to the Alcohol Free, Original above, and the same comments apply.

☹ **Soothing Gel After Shave & Moisturizer in One, Original** *($4.29 for 3.25 ounces)* contains too much alcohol to be used on the face.

## Phytomen by Phytomer

☺ **Softening Shaving Gel for Sensitive Skin** *($10.50 for 5 ounces)* is a good, extremely standard shave gel for most all skin types. It does contain a tiny amount of triclosan, a topical disinfectant, but that is in here more for preserving the product than for disinfecting the skin.

☺ **Soothing After Shave Balm with Hypericum** *($13.50 for 1.6 ounces)* is a good moisturizer for dry skin but absolutely nothing special, and the price is unwarranted for what you're getting. Hypericum is the herb St. John's wort, and it has no real benefit for skin. In fact, recent studies I've seen indicate that St. John's wort can be photosensitizing if taken or applied in quantity (though it does takes a lot to have that effect). Most likely, manufacturers are hoping that their products containing St. John's wort will convey to the consumer that they can have some kind of tranquilizing effect on skin. St. John's wort can't do that from the outside in.

☹ **Invigorating Body Splash** *($18 for 6.76 ounces)*. Alcohol and fragrance can be considered invigorating, but by most standards they are just irritating and drying.

## Ralph Lauren Polo Sport

☹ **Face and Body Soap** *($15 for 5.3 ounces)* is a standard bar based on lard and lye. That can dry and irritate the skin and clog pores.

☹ **Scrub Face Wash** *($12.50 for 2.5 ounces)* is a standard, detergent-based water-soluble scrub that uses synthetic particles as the abrasive. That would be OK, but this product also contains eucalyptus, peppermint, grapefruit, and menthol. The only thing I can think of is, ouch!

☹ **Lotion Sports Moisturizer** *($12.50 for 4.2 ounces)* could have been a decent though incredibly ordinary moisturizer, but for some inane, skin-irritating reason, this product also contains eucalyptus, mandarin, peppermint, and grapefruit.

☹ **After Shave** *($38 for 4.2 ounces)* contains fragrance and alcohol. Put this on the skin after a shave and you will be assured of having red dots and rashes most of the year.

☹ **Shave Comfort Gel** *($12.50 for 5.3 ounces)* would have been comforting except this product contains eucalyptus, mandarin, peppermint, and grapefruit. That isn't comforting, that's distressing.

☹ **Shave Fitness Skin Protecting Foam** *($12.50 for 5.3 ounces)* does foam, but the review for the Gel above applies here too.

☺ **Water Basics Post Shave Relief Balm** *($25 for 4.2 ounces)* is just a good emollient moisturizer with too much fragrance, but I imagine this balm would feel nice after using all the shave products above, given the list of irritating ingredients in them.

☹ **Face Fitness AHA Moisture Formula, SPF 8** *($25 for 4.2 ounces)* has an SPF 8; that's bad enough, but this product also doesn't contain avobenzone, zinc oxide, or titanium dioxide for UVA protection, and is not recommended.

☹ **Oil-Free Self-Tanning Spray SPF 8** *($15 for 3.5 ounces)* has the same review as the one above.

☹ **Sun Stick SPF 15** *($10 for 0.26 ounce)* has the same review as the one above.

☹ **Weatherproof Sun Block SPF 15** *($15 for 3.4 ounces)* has the same review as the one above.

☹ **Waterproof Sun Lotion SPF 8** *($15 for 3.4 ounces)* is a part titanium dioxide–based sunscreen, which gives some UVA protection, but the SPF 8 just doesn't cut it when SPF 15 is the minimum recommended, and so many other lines have great SPF 15s.

☹ **Weatherproof Sun Block SPF 8** *($15 for 3.4 ounces)* has the same review as the one above.

## Skin Bracer

☹ **Cooling Blue After Shave** *($3.69 for 3.5 ounces)* contains mostly alcohol. It also has menthol and is too irritating for all skin types.

☹ **Original After Shave** *($3.69 for 3.5 ounces)* contains mostly alcohol. It also has menthol and is too irritating for all skin types.

☹ **Pre-Electric Shave Lotion** *($5.29 for 5 ounces)* contains mostly alcohol. It also has menthol and is too irritating for all skin types.

☹ **Sport Talc After Shave** *($3.69 for 3.5 ounces)* contains mostly alcohol. It also has menthol and is too irritating for all skin types.

## Zirh Men's Skin Care

☹ **Clean Alpha Hydroxy Wash** *($12.50 for 8 ounces)* contains menthol, peppermint oil, and lemon oil, and is absolutely not recommended—plus the presence of AHA in a cleanser is wasted, because the ingredients get washed down the drain before they can have an effect.

☹ **Scrub, Aloe Facial Scrub** *($12.50 for 4 ounces)* uses sodium lauryl sulfate as the main cleansing agent, which is a problem for most skin types. The scrub particles are ground-up shells and can also be too abrasive for most skin types.

☹ **Protect Pycnogenol Clarifying Moisturizers SPF 8** *($22.50 for 4 ounces)* has an SPF of 8, far below the SPF 15 required by the American Academy of Dermatology; moreover, this product does not contain adequate UVA protection, and is not recommended.

☺ **$$$ Prevent Anti-Oxidant Nourishment from Grape Seed Extract** *($28.50 for 30 capsules).* If you want to believe that grape seed extract is the answer for skin and worth this absurd price, go for it, but there is no reason I can think of to consider this product.

☹ **Correct Pycnogenol Problem Solver** *($22.50 for 2 ounces)* contains several irritating plant extracts, including witch hazel, spearmint, cinnamon, and clove, as well as lemon oil. This won't correct skin problems but it could cause some.

# CHAPTER SIX

# The Best Products Summary

The product lists that follow summarize the individual reviews in Chapter Three. Be sure to read those more-detailed product evaluations before making any final decisions. I hope all of these recommendations will make you feel informed and confident when shopping for makeup and skin-care products or, at the very least, help you narrow down the field of choices.

I know my lists of suggestions can get quite long, and some women have complained that I should reduce the list to my absolute favorites, or to a top-ten list. I understand the frustration when looking at the number of products I do like, and although the field is even more narrowed with this edition than ever before, you still may wonder where to begin. I'm not quite sure how to get around the fact that the following products are all excellent formulations or perform beautifully; there really isn't a hierarchy. I wouldn't even suggest that someone start with my own products (Paula's Choice), as they are just some of the many products I find to be excellent. Most of you know I have a preference for superior formulations for the least amount of money, but this list simply concentrates on performance, regardless of cost.

In some ways this notion of narrowing down my list even further is a bit funny to me, because often I am criticized for hating the cosmetics industry and not liking anything that's out there. But then on the other hand, women complain that I like too many things and I should shrink my list down even further! Perhaps there is no way to please everyone. The best I can do is tell you what my extensive research and experience have found to be true, and then you the consumer can take it from there.

I should mention that one of the purposes of my newsletter, *Cosmetics Counter Update*, is to narrow the range of options, as it offers more detail and more explanation than I can provide in a compendium such as this book. In the "Dear Paula" section of my newsletter where readers write to me with their particular concerns and needs, I address those concerns and make specific recommendations depending on the individual situation and history. In this book, the goal is to bring more general information together all in one place, giving consumers enough room to find what works best for them among all the products with great, reliable formulations.

**First Beauty Note:** Most cosmetics companies recommend skin-care routines for specific skin types. It is my strong suggestion that you ignore their categories and the corresponding product names. A person with dry skin who follows the cosmetics companies' recommendations could end up using too many products that will overgrease the skin and cause buildup, making the skin look dull and possibly causing breakouts (particularly whiteheads). Someone with oily skin will most likely be sold products that contain strong irritants that can make oily and acned skin worse. **Please consider each product individually for its quality and value to your skin, instead of by its placement in a series of products, its promotional ads or brochures, or the sales pitches you are likely to hear.**

**Second Beauty Note:** Please keep in mind that a cosmetics company's name for a product does not always, if ever, correspond with my recommendations. Just because a product label says it "gets rid of wrinkles" or is recommended for sensitive skin, or says it is a firming or nourishing serum doesn't mean the formulation itself supports that label or claim. **The same is true for eye creams or throat creams. Despite what the cosmetics industry wants you to believe, those products can be used anywhere on the face, and what counts is what skin type they are good for.** Additionally, you will find many selections in the following list of recommended products with names that sound like they should be in the dry-skin group but that I have included in the oily-skin group, and vice versa. That's because what counts is how the product is formulated, not what the companies want you to believe about their products.

**Third Beauty Note:** Just as a reminder, I consider all moisturizers as being necessary only where the skin is dry. If you have oily skin, you do not need to use a moisturizer. Overusing moisturizer can hurt the skin's healing process and hinder cell turnover. As a result I provide no category for oily-skin moisturizers. Even when a product is labeled as being for someone with oily or combination skin, it is only meant to be used over dry areas and not over oily areas. If you have dry skin in areas where you are oily, then you either have a skin disorder such as rosacea, dermatitis, psoriasis, or seborrhea, or you are using skin-care products that are too drying and irritating for your skin. That doesn't require a moisturizer, but a change in how you are taking care of your skin, or an appointment with a dermatologist.

If you have oily skin but have dry areas under the eye or on the cheeks (and you are certain you have no skin disorders and are not using irritating skin-care products) then consider the moisturizers in the slightly dry or dry skin category below.

**The exception to this rule is sunscreens, which absolutely must be used all over, every day, 365 days a year!** To that end I do divide up my recommendations in skin-care categories. Unfortunately, there are very few options for women with oily skin. It is quite a search to find products that don't generate breakouts or feel greasy. Because of this I often recommend using a matte foundation with a good SPF and UVA protection, and then using a regular sunscreen on the rest of your body whenever it is exposed to the sun.

**Fourth Beauty Note:** The order for application for any given skin-care regime is described at length in my book *The Beauty Bible*. As a general rule, the following is a safe guideline, depending on the products your skin needs: **cleanser; scrub; eye-makeup remover** if needed—by using an eye-makeup remover after the cleanser to get the last traces of eye or face makeup off, you prevent the excessive pulling that can occur if that is the primary way you remove your makeup; **toner; AHA, BHA, topical disinfectant; topical retinoid** (retinoids cannot be used with benzoyl peroxide), **azelaic acid, Differin, MetroGel, or MetroCream; sunscreen** during the day; and at night a **moisturizer.** If you are using a **skin-lightening** product, it comes before the sunscreen or moisturizer. **Sunscreen is always the last item you apply during the day because you must never dilute a sunscreen.**

## *Best Cleansers*

The main criteria for this category, regardless of skin type, are that the cleanser be water-soluble, gentle, and able to thoroughly clean the skin without drying or leaving a greasy feel, and also contain no harsh, irritating, or sensitizing ingredients. I never recommend bar soap because the ingredients that keep bar soap in a bar form can clog pores, and the cleansing agents are almost always drying. I am not fond of cleansers that need to be wiped off or leave a film on the skin. The major reason for this is that the greasy residue can inhibit cell turnover and may encourage clogged pores. The other issue is that wiping off makeup tends to overpull skin, and that repetitive daily tugging can break down the skin's elasticity and promote wrinkles.

However, a major difference for this edition is that I am including a category for cleansers that need to be wiped off for those with dry to very dry skin. After a great deal of research and feedback from hundreds of women, it appears that it's a difficult task to create a water-soluble cleanser that removes makeup well and doesn't leave a greasy feel on the skin, but that someone with dry skin won't find drying. So, while I am not enthusiastic about using a wipe-off cleanser, for those women whose skin feels better with this type of product I have listed those that do the job well and gently.

One other exception about wiping off makeup has to do with the ultra-matte and stick foundations on the market. These foundations are just very difficult to simply wash off, no matter how strong the cleanser is. If you are wearing this type of foundation, the best option is to use a water-soluble cleanser along with a washcloth to be sure you are getting everything off at night. One reader of my newsletter suggested another alternative I'd like to pass along. She takes an eye-makeup remover and dabs it all over the face, without pulling. Then she splashes her face with water and then follows with a water-soluble cleanser. She says that works great without pulling and without using a washcloth (which she found too irritating). This process actually works well with some foundations and is worth a try.

One thing most cleansers have in common, regardless of price, are their ingredient listings. Within each category—normal to oily skin or normal to dry skin—the formulations are virtually identical. Spending a lot of money on cleansers does not in any way, shape, or form mean you are getting a better product.

For normal to oily/combination and/or blemish-prone skin types, the best water-soluble cleansers are: Adrien Arpel Oily Skin Sea Foam Gel Cleanser ($19 for 4 ounces) and Aromafleur Petal Daily Cleanser ($22.50 for 4.5 ounces); Alpha Hydrox Foaming Face Wash, for All Skin types ($5.57 for 6 ounces); Amway Clarifying Cleansing Gel for Normal to Oily Skin ($15.60 for 4.2 ounces); Ashley Skin Care pH Balancing Cleanser ($26 for 6 ounces); Aubrey Organics Green Tea Facial Cleansing Lotion ($7.25 for 4 ounces); Aveda All Sensitive Cleanser ($19 for 5.5 ounces) and Purifying Gel Cleanser ($18 for 5.5 ounces); Avon Anew Perfect Cleanser ($14 for 5.1 ounces) and Refraiche Me Cleansing Foam ($20 for 5 ounces); bare escentuals Tea Tree Foaming Cleanser Normal to Oily Skin ($18 for 5 ounces); Basis Comfortably Clean Face Wash ($4.09 for 6 ounces); BeautiControl Purifying Cleansing Gel ($12 for 8 ounces) and All Clear Skin Wash ($12 for 6 ounces); Beauty for All Seasons/Norma Virgin Makeup AlphaCeuticals Wash ($11.50 for 4 ounces); Bioelements Decongestant Cleanser ($18.50 for 6 ounces); BioMedic Purifying Cleanser ($25 for 6 ounces); Biore Cleansing Gel, Non-Foaming ($5.99 for 5 ounces) and Foaming Cleanser ($5.99 for 5 ounces); BioTherm Biosensitive Self-Foaming Gentle Cleanser ($19 for 5 ounces), BioPur Pure Cleansing Gel ($15 for 5 ounces), and Biosource Foaming Gel Cleanser ($15 for 5 ounces); Black Opal Oil Free Cleansing Gel ($4.51 for 6 ounces); Bobbi Brown Essentials Gentle Foaming Cleanser ($27 for 5 ounces); The Body Shop Balancing Cleansing Gel for Normal to Oily Skin ($9 for 6.76 ounces), Tea Tree Oil Facial Wash ($3 for 2 ounces), and Passion Fruit Cleansing Gel for Normal to Oily Skin ($8.15 for 8.4 ounces); CamoCare Camomile Light Foaming Cleanser ($9.95 for 4 ounces); Cellex-C Betaplex Gentle Foaming Cleanser ($23.20 for 3 ounces); Cetaphil Oily Skin Cleanser ($5.50 for 2 ounces); Chanel Aquamousse Foaming Cream Face Wash ($28.50 for 5 ounces), Gel Tendre Non-Foaming Makeup Remover Face and Eyes ($30 for 5 ounces), and Gel Purete Foaming Gel Face Wash ($30 for 5 ounces); Christian Dior Purifying Wash-Off Cleansing Foam ($22.50 for 6.8 ounces); Circle of Beauty Day Life Gentle Action Cleanse + Tone Foam, Combination Oily ($9.50 for 7 ounces) and Day Life Gentle Action Cleanse + Tone Foam, Oily ($9.50 for 7 ounces); Clairol Herbal Essences Foaming Face Wash Moisture-Balancing for Normal/Dry Skin ($4.99 for 6.8 ounces); Clarins Oil-Control Cleansing Gel Oily Skin with Breakout Tendencies ($18 for 4.4 ounces); Clean & Clear Sensitive Skin Foaming Facial Cleanser ($3.79 for 8 ounces), Foaming Facial Cleanser ($3.49 for 8 ounces), and Clean & Clear Oil Free Daily Pore Cleanser ($3.49 for 5.5 ounces); Clear LogiX Gentle Foaming Acne Cleanser *($5.99 for 6 ounces)*; <u>Clearasil</u> Daily Face Wash *($4.99 for 6.5 ounces)*; <u>DDF</u> Non-Drying Gentle Cleanser *($30 for 8.45 ounces)*, Sensitive Skin Cleansing Gel *($27.50 for 8.45 ounces)*, and Wash off Cleanser *($30 for 8.45 ounces)*; <u>Dermalogica</u> Special Cleansing Gel *($34 for 16 ounces)*; <u>DHC USA</u> Facial Wash for Oilier Skin *($18 for 6.7 ounces)*; <u>Dr. Mary Lupo</u> Gentle Purifying Cleanser *($22 for 7 ounces)*; <u>Ecco Bella</u> Purifying Cleanser for Normal to Oily Skin *($11.50 for 6.5 ounces)* and Soft and Soothing Cleanser for Normal to Dry Skin *($11.50 for 6.5 ounces)*; <u>Elizabeth Arden</u> Modern Skin Care 2-in-1 Cleanser *($17.50 for 4.2 ounces)*; <u>Epicuren</u> Herbal Cleanser *($48 for 4 ounces)*; <u>Estee Lauder</u> Perfectly Clean Foaming Gel Cleanser, Normal/Oily and Oily Skin *($16.50 for 4.2 ounces)*; <u>Eucerin</u> Gentle Hydrating Cleanser *($7.99 for 8 ounces)*; <u>Exuviance</u> Purifying Cleansing Gel *($18 for 8 ounces)*; <u>FACE Stockholm</u> Foaming Facial Cleanser Normal to Oily Skin *($12 for 4 ounces)*; <u>Fashion Fair</u> Botanical Cleansing Gel *($12 for 6.7 ounces)* and Gentle Facial Shampoo Mild for Dry Sensitive Skin *($10 for 2.1 ounces)*; <u>Flori Roberts</u> My Everything Foaming Gel Cleanser *($15 for 6 ounces)* and Optima Gel Cleanser Gold Oil-Free *($15 for 6 ounces)*; <u>Freeman Cosmetics</u> Blueberry & Lavender Facial Gel Cleanser *($2.85 for 6 ounces)* and Pineapple & Watermelon Alpha & Beta Hydroxy Skin Renewal Facial Wash *($3.29 for 8 ounces)*; <u>Garden Botanika</u> Skin Correcting Deep Cleansing Face Wash *($10 for 8 ounces)*, Citrus Cleansing Gel *($9 for 4 ounces)*, and Cucumber Cleansing Gel *($10 for 8 ounces)*; <u>Givenchy</u> Cleansing Foam *($22 for 4.2 ounces)* and Regulating Cleansing Gel, Purifying Care for Radiant Skin Combination and Oily Skins *($20 for 4.5 ounces)*; <u>Glymed</u> Plus Gentle Facial Wash *($29 for 8 ounces)*; <u>Hydron</u> Best Defense Antibacterial Facial Cleansing Gel *($9.97 for 4 ounces)*; <u>Iman</u> Liquid Assets Gentle Cleansing Lotion *($13 for 3 ounces)*; <u>Jafra</u> Cleansing Gel *($12.50 for 4.2 ounces)*, Purifying Gel Cleanser *($14 for 4.4 ounces)*, and Balancing Foam Cleanser *($14 for 4.2 ounces)*; <u>Jan Marini Skin Research</u> Bioglycolic BioClean Cleanser *($25 for 8 ounces)* and Jan Marini Skin Research C-Esta Cleansing Gel *($25 for 6 ounces)*; <u>Jane</u> ClenZing Gel, Gentle *($5.99 for 5 ounces)*; <u>Janet Sartin</u> Nourishing Cleanser *($25 for 6 ounces)*; <u>Jason Natural Cosmetics</u> Citrus 6-in-1 Facial Wash & Scrub with Ester-C *($7 for 4.5 ounces)*; <u>Jergens</u> Gentle Foaming Face Wash *($3.89 for 6 ounces)*; <u>Joan Rivers</u> Results Thoroughly Cleansing Facial Bath *($20 for 6.7 ounces)*; <u>Joey New York</u> Pure Pores Cleansing Gel with Vitamin C *($22 for 8 ounces)*; <u>La Mer</u> The Cleansing Gel *($65 for 6.7 ounces)*; <u>La Prairie</u> Foam Cleanser *($50 for 4 ounces)* and Essential Purifying Gel Cleanser *($50 for 7.3 ounces)*; <u>Lancome</u> Ablutia Fraicheur Purifying Foam Cleanser *($21.50 for 6.4 ounces)* and Clarifiance Oil-Free Gel Cleanser *($21.50 for 6.8 ounces)*; <u>Laura Mercier</u> One Step Cleanser *($35 for 8 ounces)*; <u>Le Mirador</u> Dual Action Facial Cleanser *($19 for 6 ounces)*; <u>Lorac</u> Oil Free Face Wash *($20 for 8 ounces)*; <u>L'Oreal</u> Hydra Fresh Deep Cleanser Foaming Gel for Normal to Oily Skin

*($4.99 for 6.5 ounces),* **Hydra Fresh Cleanser Foaming Cream for Normal to Dry Skin** *($4.99 for 6.5 ounces),* **Shine Control Foaming Face Wash with Pro-Vitamin B5** *($4.99 for 6.5 ounces),* and **RevitaClean Gentle Foaming Cleanser** *($7.29 for 6 ounces);* <u>M.A.C.</u> **Green Gel Cleanser** *($15 for 5 ounces);* <u>Marcelle</u> **Aquarelle Oil-Free Purifying Cleansing Gel for Oily Skin** *($11.95 for 170 ml),* **Cleansing Milk Combination Skin** *($11.25 for 240 ml),* **Cleansing Milk Oily Skin** *($11.25 for 240 ml),* **Gentle Foaming Wash All Skin Types** *($10.50 for 170 ml),* and **Hydractive Water Rinseable Cleansing Lotion for Dehydrated/Normal to Dry Skin** *($11.95 for 180 ml);* <u>Mario Badescu</u> **Seaweed Cleansing Lotion** *($15 for 8 ounces);* <u>Mary Kay</u> **Deep Cleanser Formula 3** *($10 for 6.5 ounces);* <u>M.D. Formulations</u> **Facial Cleanser Basic** *($16 for 8 ounces)* and **Sensitive Skin Cleanser** *($28 for 8 ounces);* <u>Merle Norman</u> **Luxiva Foaming Cleanser for Dry Skin** *($18 for 4 ounces);* <u>Models Prefer</u> **Skin Cleanser** *(5.1 ounces);* <u>Moisturel</u> **Sensitive Skin Cleanser** *($7.76 for 8.75 ounces);* <u>Murad</u> **AHA/BHA Exfoliating Cleanser, Deep Cleansing for All Skin Types** *($23 for 6 ounces),* **Moisture Rich Skin Cleanser** *($19.50 for 6 ounces),* **Refreshing Skin Cleanser** *($19.50 for 6 ounces),* and **Environmental Shield Facial Cleanser** *($30 for 6 ounces);* <u>Natura Bisse</u> **Sensitive Cleansing Cream for All Skin Types** *($27 for 7 ounces);* <u>Neutrogena</u> **Cleansing Wash for Skin Irritated by Drying Medications or Facial Peels** *($6.99 for 6 ounces),* **Fresh Foaming Cleanser Soap-Free Cleanser for Combination Skin** *($6 for 5.5 ounces),* and **Pore Refining Cleanser** *($7.99 for 6.7 ounces);* <u>Nicole Miller Skin Care</u> **Renew Foaming Facial Cleanser** *($24 for 4.2 ounces);* <u>Nivea Visage</u> **Foaming Facial Cleanser Deep-Cleansing Formula** *($5.49 for 6 ounces)* and **Vital Mild Foaming Cleanser, Provitamin B5** *($6.99 for 5 ounces);* <u>Noevir</u> **95 Herbal Facial Cleanser** *($30 for 3.5 ounces),* **105 Herbal Facial Cleanser** *($56 for 3.5 ounces),* **Clear Control Clean Wash** *($14 for 2.6 ounces),* **Herbal Skincare Line NHS Cleansing Foam** *($18 for 3.8 ounces),* and **Cleansing Crystals** *($25 for 2.4 ounces);* <u>Nu Skin USA</u> **Nu-Derm Gentle Cleanser** *($29 for 6.7 ounces);* <u>Obagi</u> **Nu-Derm Foaming Gel Cleanser** *($29 for 6.7 ounces)* <u>Olay</u> **Foaming Face Wash** *($3.87 for 6.78 ounces)* and **Age Defying Series Daily Renewal Cleanser** *($4.60 for 6.78 ounces);* <u>Orlane</u> **Wash-Off Cleansing Cream for All Skin Types** *($29 for 6.8 ounces);* <u>Osmotics</u> **Balancing Cleanser for Normal to Oily Skin** *($27 for 6 ounces),* **Calming Cleansing Milk for Sensitive Skin** *($27 for 6 ounces),* and **Hydrating Cleanser for Normal to Dry Skin** *($27 for 6 ounces);* <u>Paula's Choice</u> **One Step Face Cleanser for Normal to Oily/Combination Skin** *($10.95 for 8 ounces);* <u>Peter Thomas Roth</u> **Chamomile Cleansing Lotion** *($30 for 8 ounces),* **Gentle Cleansing Lotion** *($30 for 8 ounces),* **Foaming Face Wash** *($30 for 8 ounces),* **Extra Strength Cleansing Gel Oil-Free for Oily, Combination or Problem Skin** *($30 for 8 ounces),* **Sensitive Skin Cleansing Gel** *($30 for 8 ounces),* **Combination Skin Cleansing Gel** *($30 for 8 ounces),* **Glycolic Acid 3% Face Wash** *($30 for 8 ounces),* and **Beta Hydroxy Acid 2% Acne Wash**

($32 for 8 ounces); <u>philosophy</u> real purity cleanser ($15 for 6 ounces); <u>pHisoDerm</u> Daily Cleanser and Conditioner, for Normal to Oily Skin ($7.93 for 14 ounces), Daily Skin Cleanser and Conditioner, for Normal to Dry ($7.93 for 14 ounces), Daily Skin Cleanser and Conditioner, Sensitive Skin Formula, for Sensitive Skin ($7.93 for 14 ounces), and Gentle Skin Cleanser for Baby ($5.41 for 8 ounces); <u>Physicians Formula</u> Oil-Control Deep Pore Cleansing Gel for Normal to Oily Skin ($6.95 for 8 ounces); <u>Phytomer</u> Gentle Cleansing Cream ($27 for 5 ounces) and Purifying Cleansing Gel ($26 for 5 ounces); <u>Prescriptives</u> All Clean Fresh Foaming Cleanser ($19.50 for 6.7 ounces); <u>Principal Secret</u> Advanced Gentle 4-in-1 Cleanser ($24 for 6 ounces) and Gentle Deep Cleanser ($22 for 6 ounces); <u>Purpose</u> Gentle Cleansing Wash ($4.95 for 6 ounces); <u>reflect.com</u> Facial Cleanser, Foaming Cleanser ($17 for 6.7 ounces); <u>Rejuvenique</u> Purifying Cleanser ($18.50 for 4 ounces); <u>Sage Skin Care</u> Facial Shampoo, Facial Shampoo Extra Gentle, and Facial Shampoo Extra Strength ($30 for 8 ounces each); <u>Sea Breeze</u> Foaming Face Wash for Normal to Oily Skin ($3.78 for 6 ounces) and Foaming Face Wash for Sensitive Skin ($3.78 for 6 ounces); <u>Selleca Solution</u> Soothing Cleanser with Chamomile ($28, $19.50 for 6 ounces); <u>Shaklee</u> Purifying Cleansing Gel ($16.50 for 6 ounces); <u>Shiseido</u> Benefiance Creamy Cleansing Foam ($27 for 4.4 ounces), Vital Perfection Cleansing Foam ($22 for 4.5 ounces); <u>Shiseido</u> The Skin Care Gentle Cleansing Foam ($23.50 for 4.8 ounces); <u>SkinCeuticals</u> Simply Clean ($24 for 8 ounces); <u>SmashBox</u> Cleanser ($26 for 3.5 ounces); <u>St. Ives</u> Swiss Formula Peaches and Cream Renewal Wash ($3.34 for 12 ounces); <u>Suave</u> Balancing Facial Cleansing Gel ($2.75 for 8 ounces) and Foaming Face Wash ($2.75 for 8 ounces); <u>Tommy Hilfiger</u> Clean Scheme Gel Cleanser ($12 for 5 ounces); <u>Trish McEvoy</u> Essential Cleanser ($38 for 8 ounces); <u>Ultima II</u> CHR Double Action Gentle Cleanser for Dry Skin ($17.50 for 4.8 ounces), Vital Radiance Foaming Face Wash for Normal to Dry Skin ($17.50 for 5 ounces), and Vital Radiance Foaming Face Wash for Normal to Oily Skin ($17.50 for 5 ounces); <u>Vichy</u> Normaderm Express Cleansing Gel, for Acne Prone Skin ($9.99 for 150 ml) and Purete Thermale Hydra-Purifying Cleansing Gel ($14.95 for 125 ml); <u>Yon-Ka Paris</u> Gel Nettoyant Cleansing Gel ($34 for 6.7 ounces); <u>Yves Rocher</u> Bio-Calmille Gel Cleanser ($9.95 for 3.4 ounces); <u>Zhen</u> Cleanser for Normal to Oily Skin ($18 for 8 ounces); and <u>Zia Natural Skin Care</u> Fresh Cleansing Gel, for Normal, Sensitive, Combination & Oily/Problem Skin Types ($15.50 for 8 ounces).

For normal to dry and/or sensitive skin, the best cleansers are: <u>Signature Club A by Adrien Arpel</u> French Vanilla Meltdown, Cleansing Creme for Face & Eyes ($18 for 4 ounces) and Peaches & Cream Facial Cleanser ($32.50 in a set that includes 8-ounce cleanser, 8-ounce toner, and 9-ounce body cream); <u>Ahava</u> Advanced Deep Cleanser for All Skin Types ($20 for 2.5 ounces), Advanced Facial Cleansing Milk for Normal to Dry Skin ($20 for 2.5 ounces), and Advanced Facial Cleansing Milk for Oily Skin *($24 for 8.5 ounces)*; <u>Alexandra de Markoff</u> Balancing Cleanser *($28.50 for 6 ounces)* and Comfort Cleanser *($40 for 4 ounces)*; <u>Almay</u> Moisture Balance Cleansing Lotion for Normal/Combination Skin *($7.69 for 7.25 ounces)*, Moisture Renew Cleansing Cream for Dry Skin *($6.29 for 3.75 ounces)*, and Time-Off Age Smoothing Cleansing Lotion *($7.99 for 7.25 ounces)*; <u>Aloette</u> Aloepure Essential Cleansing Oil *($15.50 for 2 ounces)*; <u>Amway</u> Moisture Rich Cleansing Creme for Normal to Dry Skin *($15.60 for 4.2 ounces)* and Delicate Care Cleanser for Sensitive Skin Types *($15.60 for 4.2 ounces)*; <u>Aquanil</u> Aquanil Lotion *($6.99 for 8 ounces)*; <u>Arbonne</u> Bio-Matte Oil-Free Cleanser *($16 for 2 ounces)*, Cleansing Lotion *($14.50 for 3.25 ounces)*, and Cleansing Cream *($15.50 for 2 ounces)*; <u>Aveda</u> Purifying Cream Cleanser *($18 for 5.5 ounces)*; <u>Avon</u> Anew Ultra Force Hydrating Cleanser *($14 for 4 ounces)* and Naturally Almond Cleansing Milk *($20 for 5 ounces)*; <u>BeautiControl</u> Chamomile Balancing Cleansing Lotion for Combination Skin *($13.50 for 8 ounces)* and Mild Rosemary Cleansing Fluide for Dry Skin *($13.50 for 8 ounces)*; <u>Beauty Without Cruelty</u> Extra Gentle Facial Cleansing Milk Dry/Mature Skin Types *($7.49 for 8.5 ounces)* and Herbal Cream Facial Cleanser Normal/Dry Skin *($7.49 for 8.5 ounces)*; <u>BeneFit</u> All Types Skin Wash *($14 for 4 ounces)*; <u>Bioelements</u> Moisture Positive Cleanser *($18.50 for 6 ounces)*; <u>Biogime</u> Colloidal Cleanser *($15.95 for 6 ounces)*; <u>BioTherm</u> Biosensitive High Tolerance Fluid Cleansing Milk *($20 for 5 ounces)*, Biosource Express Cleansing Fluid *($20 for 8.5 ounces)*, Biosource Invigorating Cleansing Milk *($19 for 8.5 ounces)*, and Biosource Softening Cleansing Milk *($19 for 8.5 ounces)*; <u>The Body Shop</u> Cucumber Cleansing Milk for Normal to Dry Skin *($8.15 for 8.4 ounces)*, Foaming Cleansing Cream for Normal to Dry Skin *($9 for 6.7 ounces)*, Honey Cream Cleanser for Dry Skin *($9.70 for 3.5 ounces)*, Orchid Cleansing Milk for Normal to Dry Skin *($8.15 for 8.4 ounces)*, and Rich Cleansing Cream for Dry Skin *($9 for 6.7 ounces)*; <u>Burt's Bees</u> Farmer's Market Orange Essence Cleansing Creme *($9 for 4 ounces)*; <u>Calvin Klein</u> Balancing Milk Cleanser *($20 for 6 ounces)*; <u>CamoCare</u> Camomile Moisturizing Cleanser *($9.95 for 4 ounces)*; <u>Cetaphil</u> Gentle Skin Cleanser *($8.31 for 16 ounces)*; <u>Christian Dior</u> Softening Cleansing Milk for Face and Eyes *($22.50 for 6.8 ounces)* and Softening Wash-Off Cleansing Creme *($22.50 for 6.8 ounces)*; <u>Circle of Beauty</u> Day Life Gentle Action Cleanse + Tone Foam, Dry *($9.50 for 7 ounces)*, Day Life Gentle Action Cleanse + Tone Foam, Combination Dry *($9.50 for 7 ounces)*, Day Life Gentle Action Cleanse + Tone Foam, Dehydrated *($9.50 for 7 ounces)*, Come Clean Cleanser Dry Type 4 *($8.50 for 6 ounces)*, and Come Clean Cleanser Dehydrated Type 5 *($8.50 for 6 ounces)*; <u>Clarins</u> Extra-Comfort Cleansing Cream with Bio-Ecolia Very Dry or Sensitized Skin *($30 for 7 ounces)*; <u>Clinique</u> Water-Dissolve Cream Cleanser *($15.50 for 5 ounces)*; <u>Club Monaco</u> Face Lotion Wash *($14 for 6.7 ounces)* and Face Soothing Wash *($17 for 6.7 ounces)*; <u>Color Me Beautiful</u> Creamy Cleanser for Dry

Skin *($15.50 for 6 ounces)*; <u>Decleor Paris</u> Cleansing and Make-up Remover Cream *($26 for 8.4 ounces)*, Gentle Facial Cleanser *($24 for 5 ounces)*, Velvet Cleansing Milk *($24 for 8.4 ounces)*, and Whitening Cleanser *($33 for 8.4 ounces)*; <u>Dermalogica</u> Essential Cleansing Solution *($34 for 16 ounces)*; <u>DHC USA</u> Deep Cleansing Oil *($22 for 6.7 ounces)* and Mild Cleansing Cream for Drier Skin *($14 for 4.9 ounces)*; <u>eb5</u> Cleansing Formula *($15 for 6 ounces)*; <u>Elizabeth Arden</u> Millennium Hydrating Cleanser *($25.50 for 4.4 ounces)* and Visible Difference Deep Cleansing Lotion *($18.50 for 6.7 ounces)*; <u>Epicuren</u> Apricot Cream Cleanser *($31 for 4 ounces)*; <u>Erno Laszlo</u> Active pHelityl Oil Pre-Cleansing Oil for Dry to Slightly Oily Skin *($30 for 6.8 ounces)* and HydrapHel Cleansing Treatment Liquid Cleanser for Extremely Dry Skin *($25 for 4.3 ounces)*; <u>Estee Lauder</u> Perfectly Clean Foaming Lotion Cleanser, Normal/Dry and Dry Skin *($16.50 for 4.2 ounces)*, Tender Creme Cleanser *($26 for 8 ounces)*, and Soft Clean Rinse Off Cleanser *($16.50 for 6.7 ounces)*; <u>Exuviance by Neostrata</u> Gentle Cleansing Creme, Sensitive Formula *($18 for 8 ounces)*; <u>Fashion Fair</u> Cleansing Creme with Aloe Vera *($14.25 for 4 ounces)* and Deep Cleansing Lotion Balanced for All Skin Types *($15 for 8 ounces)*; <u>Forever Spring</u> Collagen Facial Cleanser *($14.25 for 4 ounces)*; <u>Garden Botanika</u> Chamomile Cleansing Milk *($8.50 for 8 ounces)*, English Violet Cleansing Milk *($8.50 for 8 ounces)*, and Linden Flower Cleansing Milk *($9.50 for 8 ounces)*; <u>Guerlain</u> Issima Foaming Milky Cleanser *($49 for 6.8 ounces)* and Issima Moisturizing Cleansing Milk *($32.50 for 6.8 ounces)*; <u>Hydron</u> Best Defense Gentle Cleansing Creme *($16.50 for 6 ounces)*; <u>Jafra</u> Cleansing Lotion for Dry to Normal Skin *($12.50 for 8.4 ounces)*, Replenishing Cream Cleanser *($14 for 4.4 ounces)*, Original Formula Cleansing Cream *($14 for 3 ounces)*, and Natural Fresh Face Rehydrating Cleanser *($9 for 8 ounces)*; <u>Karin Herzog Skin Care</u> Cleansing Milk *($30 for 7.05 ounces)* and Professional Cleansing Cream *($32 for 1.76 ounces)*; <u>Kiehl's</u> Gentle Foaming Facial Cleanser for Dry to Normal Skin Types *($13.50 for 8 ounces)*, Oil-Based Cleanser and Makeup Remover *($10.50 for 4 ounces)*, Ultra Moisturizing Cleansing Cream *($16.95 for 8 ounces)*, and Washable Cleansing Milk A Moisturizing Cleanser for Dry or Sensitive Skin *($13.50 for 8 ounces)*; <u>Kiss My Face</u> Gentle Face Cleanser for Normal to Dry *($10 for 4 ounces)*; <u>La Mer</u> The Cleansing Lotion *($65 for 6.7 ounces)*; <u>La Prairie</u> Purifying Creme Cleanser *($50 for 6.8 ounces)*; <u>L'Occitane</u> Cold Cream *($21 for 2.64 ounces)*, Extra Gentle Cleansing Milk *($16 for 8.4 ounces)*, and Very Mild Cleansing Lotion *($20 for 8.4 ounces)*; <u>L'Oreal</u> RevitaClean Cold Cream for Dry or Maturing Skin *($5.29 for 5 ounces)*; <u>M.A.C.</u> Cold Cream Cleanser *($15 for 4 ounces)* and Everyday Lotion Cleanser *($15 for 5 ounces)*; <u>Marcelle</u> Cleansing Cream *($7.98 for 240 ml)* and Cleansing Milk for Dry to Normal Skin *($11.25 for 240 ml)*; <u>Marilyn Miglin</u> Clean Tone *($25 for 4 ounces)*; <u>Mario Badescu</u> Cucumber Makeup Remover Cream *($10 for 4 ounces)* and Cleansing Milk with Carnation & Rice Oil *($10 for 4 ounces)*; <u>Mary</u>

Kay TimeWise 3-in-1 Cleanser ($18 for 4.5 ounces), Gentle Cleansing Cream Formula 1 ($10 for 6.5 ounces), and Creamy Cleanser Formula 2 ($10 for 6.5 ounces); Merle Norman Luxiva Collagen Cleanser ($18.50 for 6 ounces); Natura Bisse Dry Skin Milk Cleanser ($24 for 6.5 ounces); Neutrogena Extra Gentle Cleanser ($6.06 for 6.7 ounces) and Non-Drying Cleanser Lotion ($6 for 5.5 ounces); Nicole Miller Skin Care Renew Creamy Cleanser ($24 for 4.2 ounces); Noevir 95 Herbal Cleansing Massage Cream ($30 for 3.5 ounces), 105 Herbal Cleansing Massage Cream ($70 for 3.5 ounces), and Herbal Skincare Line NHS Deep Cleansing Cream ($18 for 3.5 ounces); Noxzema Sensitive Cleansing Cream ($3.67 for 10 ounces) and Sensitive Cleansing Lotion ($3.25 for 10.5 ounces); Nu Skin USA Cleansing Lotion ($10.50 for 4.2 ounces); Olay Facial Cleansing Lotion ($3.87 for 6.78 ounces) and Sensitive Skin Foaming Face Wash ($3.87 for 6.78 ounces); Orlane Gentle Cleansing Milk for Dry Sensitive Skins ($32 for 6.8 ounces); Parthena Sense & Sensibility Milk Orchid Cleanser ($19.50 for 8 ounces); Paula's Choice One Step Face Cleanser for Normal to Dry Skin ($10.95 for 8 ounces); Peter Thomas Roth Silky Cleansing Cream ($30 for 8 ounces); Pevonia Botanica Sevactive Cleanser ($19.75 for 6.8 ounces) and Botanica Lavandou Cleanser ($19.75 for 6.8 ounces); Physicians Formula Gentle Cleansing Lotion for Normal to Dry Skin ($7.25 for 8 ounces), Enriched Cleansing Concentrate for Dry to Very Dry Skin ($5.95 for 4 ounces), and Gentle Cleansing Cream for Dry to Very Dry Skin ($5.95 for 4 ounces); Phytomer Gentle Cleansing Milk ($25 for 6.8 ounces) and Neutralizing Cleanser ($34 for 6.8 ounces); Pond's Clear Cold Cream ($4.50 for 4 ounces) and Cleansing Lotion ($4.39 for 4 ounces); Prescriptives All Clean Rich Cream Cleanser ($19.50 for 6.7 ounces); reflect.com Facial Cleanser, Creamy Lotion Cleanser ($17 for 6.7 ounces); Remede Rinseable Cold Cream Deep Cleanser for All Skin Types ($32 for 6.8 ounces) and Dissolve ($22 for 3.4 ounces); Revlon Moon Drops Extra Gentle Cleansing Cream Water-Rinseable for Sensitive/Delicate ($5.99 for 4 ounces) and Moon Drops Replenishing Cleansing Lotion Water Rinseable for Normal to Dry ($5.99 for 8 ounces); Shaklee Hydrating Cleansing Lotion ($16.50 for 6 ounces); Shiseido Benefiance Creamy Cleansing Emulsion ($27 for 6.7 ounces), Pureness Cleansing Foam Oil-Control ($15 for 3.7 ounces), and Vital Perfection Cleansing Cream ($22 for 3.9 ounces); Shu Uemura Cleansing Beauty Oil Balancer ($40 for 8.4 ounces); Sisley Botanical Cleansing Milk with Hawthorn for Dry/Sensitive Skin ($65 for 8.4 ounces); SkinCeuticals Delicate Cleanser ($24 for 8 ounces); Sothys Paris Softening Skin Cleanser for Dry Skin ($26 for 6.7 ounces) and Comfort Soothing Skin Cleanser, Avocado Extract, for Sensitive Skins ($26 for 6.7 ounces); St. Ives Age-Defying Hydroxy Cleanser ($3.34 for 12 ounces) and Makeup Remover & Facial Cleanser ($2.32 for 7.5 ounces); Tommy Hilfiger Clean Break Daily Cleanser ($12 for 5 ounces); Ultima II CHR Cream Cleanser ($18.50 for 4 ounces); Vichy Purete Thermale Demaquillant Integral One-Step Cleanser for Face and Eyes 3-in-1 *($15.50 for 200 ml)*, Purete Thermale Dermo-Protective Cleansing Milk Dry Skin *($14.95 for 200 ml)*, and Purete Thermale Dermo-Protective Cleansing Milk Normal & Combination Skin *($14.95 for 200 ml)*; Yon-Ka Paris Lait Nettoyant Cleansing Milk *($34 for 6.6 ounces)*; and Yves Rocher A.D.N. Revitalizing Resource Rinse-Off Cleansing Lotion, for Devitalized Skin *($14 for 6.7 ounces)* and Lait Demaquillant Fraicheur/Instant Cleansing Milk *($24 for 6.6 ounces)*.

## Best Makeup Removers

It is definitely not best to wipe off eye makeup or face makeup, because pulling at the skin encourages sagging. However, water-resistant makeup, stubborn makeup, and ultra-matte foundations need more help in being removed than most gentle cleansers can provide, especially water-resistant eye makeup. Almost without exception all eye-makeup removers, regardless of price, are created equal. The formulations are so amazingly similar it is almost shocking. Regardless of the eye-makeup remover you choose, my strong recommendation is to get as much of your makeup off as possible by washing first with a water-soluble cleanser. Any traces of makeup left behind can then gently be removed with minimal pulling by using an eye-makeup remover. (Ultra-matte foundations can be removed with the aid of a washcloth and a water-soluble cleanser—but be gentle—and then you can go over those areas of the face with the eye-makeup remover too if you choose, or with a toner.) I prefer nonoily eye-makeup removers (meaning those with no plant oils or mineral oil) because they leave the least residue on the skin, but mineral oil and plant oils are best for dry skin or for removing waterproof makeup.

Best makeup removers that may leave a slight residue on skin (for dry skin or for removing waterproof makeup) are: Almay Moisturizing Eye Makeup Remover Lotion *($4.39 for 2 ounces)*, Moisturizing Eye Makeup Remover Pads *($3.29 for 35 pads)*, and Moisturizing Gentle Gel Eye Makeup Remover *($4.49 for 1.5 ounces)*; Awake Point Makeup Remover (Eye and Lip) *($25 for 2.1 ounces)*; BioTherm Biocils Waterproof Eye Make-up Remover *($18 for 4.2 ounces)*; Bobbi Brown Essentials Waterproof Eye Makeup Remover *($16.50 for 3.4 ounces)*; The Body Shop Soothing Eye Makeup Remover Gel *($9 for 3.38 ounces)*; Chanel Lait Tendre Gentle Makeup Remover Face and Eyes *($28.50 for 6.8 ounces)* and Demaquillant Yeux Intense Gentle Biphase Eye Makeup Remover *($22.50 for 3.4 ounces)*; Christian Dior Purifying Cleansing Gelee for Face and Eyes *($22.50 for 6.8 ounces)*; Clinique Extremely Gentle Eye Makeup Remover *($9.50 for 2 ounces)* and Take the Day Off Makeup Remover, for Lids, Lashes, and Lips *($14.50 for 4.2 ounces)*; Decleor Paris Cleansing Oil for the Face and Eyes *($31 for 8.4 ounces)*; Jafra Dual-Action Eye Makeup Remover *($9 for 2 ounces)*; La Prairie Cellular Eye Make-Up Remover

*($40 for 4.2 ounces);* Marcelle Creamy Eye Make-Up Remover *($6.99 for 50 ml),* Gentle Eye Make-up Remover—Sensitive Eyes *($9.98 for 120 ml),* and Eye Make-Up Remover Pads *($8.50 for 60 pads);* Mary Kay Oil-Free Eye Makeup Remover *($14 for 3.75 ounces);* Nu Skin USA Nu Color Eye Makeup Remover *($13.15 for 2 ounces);* Physicians Formula Eye Makeup Remover Lotion for Normal to Dry Skin *($4.50 for 2 ounces)* and Eye Makeup Remover Pads for All Skin Types *($4.75 for 60 pads);* Prescriptives Quick Remover for Face Makeup *($18.50 for 4.2 ounces);* Shiseido Vital Perfection Advanced Makeup Cleansing Gel *($23 for 4.2 ounces);* Sothys Paris Eye Make-Up Removing Lotion for All Skin Types *($25 for 6.7 ounces);* Ultima II Going Going Gone Makeup Remover *($13.50 for 4 ounces);* and Yves St. Laurent Doux Demaquillant Pour Les Yeux/Gentle Eye Makeup and Lipstick Remover *($22.50 for 2.5 ounces).*

Best makeup removers that leave no residue are: 5S Makeup Eraser *($9 for 2 ounces);* Ahava Eye Makeup Remover *($18 for 4 ounces);* Almay Non-Oily Eye Makeup Remover Lotion *($4.49 for 2 ounces),* Non-Oily Eye Makeup Remover Gel *($4.03 for 1.5 ounces),* and Non-Oily Eye Makeup Remover Pads *($2.80 for 35 pads);* Amway Eye & Lip Makeup Remover *($12.50 for 4 ounces);* Aveda Pure Gel Eye Makeup Remover *($15 for 3.7 ounces);* bare escentuals Eye Makeup Remover *($12 for 3 ounces);* Beauty Without Cruelty Extra Gentle Eye Makeup Remover *($5.89 4 ounces);* BeneFit Clean Sweep *($14 for 4 ounces);* BioTherm Biocils Soothing Eye Make-up Remover *($17 for 4.2 ounces);* Bobbi Brown Essentials Eye Makeup Remover *($16.50 for 4 ounces);* The Body Shop Chamomile Eye Make-up Remover *($10.95 for 8.4 ounces);* Calvin Klein Makeup Remover *($16 for 4 ounces);* Christian Dior Instant Eye Makeup Remover *($18.50 for 3.4 ounces);* Clarins Instant Eye Makeup Remover *($19 for 4.2 ounces);* Clinique Rinse-Off Eye Makeup Solvent *($12 for 4 ounces);* Club Monaco Eye Color Remover *($12 for 6.7 ounces);* Decleor Paris Cleansing Lotion for the Eyes *($18 for 4.2 ounces);* Dermalogica Soothing Eye Makeup Remover *($15 for 2 ounces);* DHC USA Oil-Free Makeup Remover *($15 for 3.3 ounces);* Erno Laszlo pHelitone Gentle Eye Makeup Remover *($18 for 3 ounces);* Estee Lauder Gentle Eye Makeup Remover *($13.50 for 3.4 ounces),* Lip and Eye Makeup Remover for Long Wear Formulas *($14.50 for 3.4 ounces),* and Take It Away Makeup Remover *($18 for 6.7 ounces);* Fashion Fair Eye Makeup Remover *($8.50 for 2 ounces);* Gale Hayman Total Eye Make-up & Facial Cleanser *($18.50 for 6.76 ounces);* Garden Botanika Gentle Eye Makeup Remover *($6 for 4 ounces);* Guerlain Issima Blue Voyage Ready to Go Cleanser *($27 for 0.8 ounce);* Hydron Best Defense Gentle Eye Make Up Remover *($17 for 4 ounces);* Janet Sartin Gentle Eye Makeup Remover *($17 for 4 ounces)* and Gentle Eye Makeup Remover Pads *($17 for 60 pads);* Jason Natural Cosmetics Quick Clean Eye Makeup Remover for All Skin Types, Oil Free *($7.49 for 75 pads);* Joey New York Extra Gentle Eye Makeup

Remover *($16 for 6 ounces)* and **Gentle Makeup Remover Pads** *($10 for 50 pads)*; L'Occitane Gentle Eye Makeup Remover *($15 for 5.1 ounces)*; Lorac Oil Free Makeup Remover *($15 for 4 ounces)* L'Oreal Refreshing Eye Makeup Remover *($4.99 for 4.2 ounces)*; M.A.C. Wipes *($12.50 for 45 sheets)*; Marcelle Eye Make-Up Remover Lotion Oil-Free *($8.50 for 120 ml)*; Merle Norman Luxiva Dual Action Eye Makeup Remover *($12.50 for 4 ounces)*; Murad Gentle Make-up Remover *($16.50 for 4.2 ounces)*; Natura Bisse Eye Make-up Remover Hypo-Allergenic Lotion *($23 for 3.3 ounces)*; Nicole Miller Skin Care Gentle Care Eye Makeup Remover *($15 for 4.6 ounces)*; Nivea Visage Eye Make-Up Remover *($4.99 for 2.5 ounces)*; Olay Daily Facials Cleansing Cloths, Normal to Oily *($6.99 for 30 cloths)*; Origins Well-Off Fast and Gentle Eye Makeup Remover *($11 for 3.4 ounces)*; Parthena Soothing Eye Makeup Remover *($16 for 4 ounces)*; philosophy change me make-up remover *($12 for 4 ounces)*; Physicians Formula Vital Lash Oil Free Eye Makeup Remover for Normal to Oily Skin *($4.50 for 2 ounces)*; Pond's Cleansing and Make-Up Remover Towelettes *($3.97 for 30 towelettes)*; Prescriptives Eye Makeup Remover *($15 for 4 ounces)*; reflect.com Facial Cleansing Cloths *($18.50 for 30 cloths)*; Revlon ColorStay Makeup Remover Pads *($5.47 for 80 pads)*; Selleca Solution Gentle Eye Makeup Remover *($25, $17.50 for 4 ounces)*; Serious Skin Care Eye Sweep *($15 for 2 ounces)*; Shaklee Eye Makeup Remover *($9.15 for 2 ounces)*; Stila H₂Off Cleansing Cloths *($25 for 40 cloths)*; Tova Cactine Eye Makeup Remover *($29 for 6.7 ounces)*; Trish McEvoy Eye Makeup Remover *($18.50 for 2 ounces)*; Ultima II Eye Makeup Remover for Sensitive Eyes *($12.50 for 3.6 ounces)*; Vichy Demaquillant Yeux Sensibles Eye Makeup Remover for Sensitive Eyes *($13.50 for 150 ml)*; Victoria Jackson Cosmetics Facial Cleanser and Eye Makeup Remover *($9.25, $13.50 for 4 ounces)*; and Yves Rocher Bio-Calmille Eye Makeup Remover Gel *($9.95 for 3.4 ounces)*.

## Best Toners

The essential criterion for any toner is that it be nonirritating, and I am pleased to say that the cosmetics industry has plenty of them to offer these days. But keep in mind that alcohol-free does not mean irritant-free. Unfortunately, many cosmetics lines stick other irritating ingredients, particularly irritating plant extracts, in their toners.

Toners and all the products that fall into this category (refining lotions, clarifying lotions, soothing tonics, stimulating lotions, fresheners, and astringents) are an extra cleansing step, and sometimes they can be soothing and slightly moisturizing. I evaluated these products strictly on how soothing or moisturizing and clean they felt on the face without drying the skin or leaving a greasy residue or irritating the skin. I expect a toner for normal to oily skin to leave the face soft and clean but not dry, and a toner for normal to dry skin to leave water-binding agents on the skin to help a moisturizer perform better. For oily skin, a good toner can be the only moisturizer that is needed.

There are excellent toners in all price ranges, but overall the formulations are amazingly redundant, with the primary components being water, glycerin, anti-irritants, water-binding agent, and fragrance. As a result of my being more critical of formulations in this edition, the list of good toners is far shorter than earlier editions of this book; however, even though a toner may have received only a neutral face doesn't mean it isn't still an option, it just didn't contain as many state-of-the-art water-binding agents or anti-irritants as those below. A toner is a great option for removing any last traces of makeup and, because of the soothing, soft feeling many irritant-free toners can provide, they can be beneficial for many skin types.

Note: If you have slightly dry skin, combination skin, or oily skin with dry areas, the toners listed for dry skin can be the only moisturizer your skin needs.

For normal to oily/combination skin, the best toners are: Beauty Without Cruelty Balancing Facial Toner for All Skin Types ($7.49 for 8.5 ounces); Black Opal Purifying Astringent ($3.99 for 6 ounces); CamoCare Camomile Stimulating Toner ($8.95 for 4 ounces); Chanel Lotion Tendre Soothing Toner ($28.50 for 6.8 ounces); Estee Lauder Verite Soothing Spray Toner ($22.50 for 6.7 ounces); Hydron Best Defense Botanical Toner ($14.50 for 6.5 ounces); Jason Natural Cosmetics Beta-Gold Rehydrating Freshener ($9 for 8 ounces); La Prairie Cellular Refining Lotion ($55 for 8.2 ounces); Neutrogena Alcohol-Free Toner ($6 for 8 ounces); Nivea Visage Alcohol Free Moisturizing Facial Toner ($5.49 for 6 ounces); Nu Skin USA NaPCA Moisture Mist ($19.80 for 8.4 ounces); Orlane Soothing Lotion Alcohol-Free for Dry or Sensitive Skin ($29 for 6.8 ounces); Osmotics Firming Tonic Facial Mist ($35 for 6.8 ounces); Paula's Choice Final Touch Toner for Normal to Oily/Combination Skin ($9.95 for 8 ounces); Pevonia Botanica Phyto-Aromatic Mist ($22.25 for 8.5 ounces); Physicians Formula Gentle Refreshing Toner for Dry to Very Dry Skin ($6.95 for 8 ounces); and Sea Breeze Alcohol-Free Toner ($3.99 for 10 ounces).

For normal to dry skin and/or sensitive skin, the best toners are: Signature Club A by Adrien Arpel Peaches & Cream Toner ($32.50 in a set that includes 8-ounce cleanser, 8-ounce toner, and 9-ounce body cream); Alexandra de Markoff Luxury Skin Toner, with Aloe Vera and Comfrey ($28.50 for 6 ounces) and Soothing Lotion Alcohol Free, for Dry or Sensitive Skins ($48 for 4 ounces); Aloette Aloepure Alcohol-Free Toner ($13.50 for 8 ounces); Amway Moisture Rich Toner for Normal to Dry Skin ($16.60 for 8.1 ounces); Aveda All Sensitive Toner ($18 for 5.5 ounces) and Skin Firming/Toning Agent ($18 for 5.5 ounces); The Body Shop Hydrating Freshener for Normal to Dry & Dry Skin ($8 for 6.76 ounces); Clarins Alcohol-Free

Toning Lotion for Dry to Normal Skin *($21 for 8.4 ounces)*; <u>Ecco Bella</u> Moisture-to-Go Spray On *($15.50 for 2 ounces)*; <u>Forever Spring</u> Ambrosia Skin Refresher *($14.50 for 4 ounces)*; <u>Givenchy</u> Gentle Toning Lotion *($28 for 6.7 ounces)*; <u>Jafra</u> Soothing Results Calming Toner for Sensitive Skin *($13 for 8.4 ounces)*; <u>La Mer</u> The Tonic *($60 for 6.7 ounces)*; <u>Marcelle</u> Hydractive Reviving Toner, Dehydrated and Normal to Dry Skin *($11.25 for 180 ml)*; <u>Paula's Choice</u> Final Touch Toner for Normal to Dry Skin *($9.95 for 8 ounces)*; <u>Revlon</u> Moon Drops Softening Toner Normal to Dry *($5.99 for 8 ounces)*; <u>Shiseido</u> Vital Perfection Balancing Softener *($30 for 5 ounces)*; <u>Shu Uemura</u> Refreshing Lotion *($35 for 8.4 ounces)*; and <u>Victoria Jackson Cosmetics</u> Toning Mist *($9.75, $14.50 for 4 ounces)*.

## *Best Topical Disinfectants*

For someone who struggles with blemishes, the toner step can be a topical disinfectant, which is essential to fight pimples (topical disinfectants do not have any impact on clogged pores or blackheads). I discuss this step at length in my book *The Beauty Bible* and to a lesser extent in Chapter Two of this book. All the recommendations below are for over-the-counter products that include benzoyl peroxide with no other irritating ingredients. A range of prescription-strength topical antibiotics are available from dermatologists. Alternative sources of topical disinfectants such as tea tree oil are an option; however, there were no formulations being sold that used enough tea tree oil for it to have effective disinfecting properties for skin.

<u>For blemish-prone skin for all skin types, the best topical disinfectants are:</u> <u>Avon</u> Clearskin 10% Benzoyl Peroxide Vanishing Cream *($3.99 for 0.75 ounce)*; <u>Clean & Clear</u> Persa-Gel 5, Regular Strength *($3.49 for 1 ounce)* and Persa-Gel 10, Maximum Strength *($3.49 for 1 ounce)*; <u>DDF</u> 2.5% Benzoyl Peroxide Gel *($13 for 2 ounces)* and Benzoyl Peroxide Gel 5% with Tea Tree Oil *($16.50 for 2 ounces)*; <u>Epicuren</u> Medicated Acne Gel *($49 for 4 ounces)*; <u>Glymed Plus</u> Serious Action Skin Medication No. 5 *($26.95 for 4 ounces)* and Serious Skin Medication No. 10 *($26.40 for 4 ounces)*; <u>Jan Marini Skin Research</u> Benzoyl Peroxide 2.5% *($25 for 4 ounces)*, Benzoyl Peroxide 5% *($25 for 4 ounces)*, and Benzoyl Peroxide 10% *($25 for 4 ounces)*; <u>Mary Kay</u> Acne Treatment Gel *($7 for 1.25 ounces)*; <u>M.D. Formulations</u> Benzoyl Peroxide 5% for Extremely Oily and Acne-Prone Skin *($25 for 4 ounces)* and Benzoyl Peroxide 10% for Extremely Oily and Acne-Prone Skin *($25 for 4 ounces)*; <u>Neutrogena</u> On-the-Spot Acne Treatment Tinted Formula 2.5% Benzoyl Peroxide *($6.75 for 0.75 ounce)* and On-the-Spot Acne Treatment Vanishing Formula 2.5% Benzoyl Peroxide *($6.75 for 0.75 ounce)*; <u>Oxy Balance</u> Oxy 10 Acne Medication Sensitive Skin Formula *($4.52 for 1 ounce)* and Oxy 10 Acne Medication Invisible Formula *($4.52 for 1 ounce)*; <u>Paula's Choice</u> Blemish Fighting Solution for All Skin Types *($12.95 for 4 ounces)* and Extra Strength Blemish Fighting Solu-

tion *($12.95 for 4 ounces)*; <u>Peter Thomas Roth</u> BPO Gel 2.5% *($20 for 3 ounces)*, BPO Gel 5% *($22 for 3 ounces)*, and BPO Gel 10% *($24 for 3 ounces)*; <u>ProActiv</u> Repairing Lotion *($22.95 for 2 ounces)*; <u>Sage Skin Care</u> Miracle Zit 2.5% *($20 for 4 ounces)*, Miracle Zit 5% *($20 for 4 ounces)*, Miracle Zit 10% *($20 for 4 ounces)*, Fix Zit 2.5% *($20 for 4 ounces)*, and Fix Zit 5% *($20 for 4 ounces)*; <u>Serious Skin Care</u> Clearz-It with 5% Benzoyl Peroxide *($19.95 for 4 ounces)* and Unplugged *($22 for 2 ounces)*; and <u>ZAPZYT</u> Benzoyl Peroxide *($4.99 for 1 ounce)*.

# Best Exfoliants
# (AHA, BHA, and Topical Scrubs)

Exfoliating the skin (getting rid of unwanted, dead, or built-up layers of sun-damaged skin cells and improving skin-cell turnover) can be beneficial for almost all skin types, and especially those with sun-damaged skin or a tendency toward breakouts or clogged pores, but even dry-skin types can benefit for many reasons. Despite the fact that most beauty experts, as well as dermatologists and plastic surgeons, agree that exfoliating the skin is a wonderful way to take care of both oily and dry skin, *how* to exfoliate is a bone of contention.

During most of the '70s and '80s, the only choices were topical, mechanical scrubs with ingredients such as honey and almond pits, cleansers with scrub particles, facial masks, and irritating toners. Most of these options took a toll on the face, and irritation or dry patches of skin with redness were typical problems. (Then and now my favorite recommendation for a topical scrub, as I've mentioned repeatedly throughout this book, is mixing Cetaphil Gentle Skin Cleanser with baking soda to create an effective, gentle, and inexpensive mechanical scrub. Other scrubs, with their detergent cleansing agents and wax bases, just can't compare and are far more expensive.)

Alpha hydroxy acids (AHAs) and salicylic acid (BHA) work by exfoliating the skin chemically instead of mechanically via abrasion. For many reasons, this can be less irritating and can create more even and smoother results, which is why facial scrubs have become less and less a part of most skin-care routines.

There is growing information that both overuse (using too many AHA or BHA products on the face) and the use of high concentrations of AHAs can be a problem for skin, and I concur with those concerns. Abundant research points to the fact that irritation and inflammation of any kind is bad for skin. Improper use, too frequent use, and use by those with sensitive skin are situations in which actual skin damage can occur. Even though many lines sell multiple products containing AHA or BHA, or high-concentration AHA products (over 10% has always been a concern of mine), using these together or too frequently can be too much for one face. The goal then is to use one effective AHA (10% concentration or less) *or* BHA (2% concentration or less) product, and only as needed—which may be twice a day, once a day, or once every other day, depending on your skin type.

The AHA and BHA products recommended below have formulations that meet the established criteria; they have a pH of 4 and below, with the appropriate concentrations of exfoliants.

If you decide to use an AHA or BHA product, particularly one from my list of recommendations, the question is, do you still need to use a physical scrub? The answer isn't all that easy, and you will have to judge that for yourself. Most women with normal to dry and/or sensitive skin should probably use only the AHA product and no other exfoliant (except maybe once in awhile). Someone with normal to oily skin should use a good BHA product and only use a mechanical scrub over breakouts once in awhile (say once or twice a week). Whatever you choose, always listen closely to your skin and remember that irritation is never the goal!

What about the products that contain both BHA and AHA, sometimes referred to as polyhydroxy acids? Because I feel strongly that AHAs are best for dry or sun-damaged skin and BHAs for blemish-prone or oily skin, I think mixed-acid products are unwise (I explain this at length in the introduction of this book).

**Note:** The lack of recommendations for scrubs is due to the fact that most scrubs are extremely abrasive, contain irritants, or have unnecessary waxy thickening agents that would be a problem for oily or blemish-prone skin types. Plus, what was true in the first edition of this book is still true today: I feel strongly that **Cetaphil Gentle Skin Cleanser** *($8.31 for 16 ounces)* mixed with baking soda, or just plain baking soda by itself, is the best topical scrub for any skin type.

**Second Note:** Because of my concern about higher concentrations of AHAs, I did not list those in this section. However, the only line that offers a significant selection of those is M.D. Formulations and its subdivision, M.D. Forte. If you are interested, please check out those sections in the book.

**Last Note:** If you have sensitive skin, it is more important to use an AHA, BHA, or scrub infrequently, though lower-concentration AHAs or BHA are an option.

**Okay, One More Note:** There are almost no AHA or BHA products that also contain an effective sunscreen. This is because, to be effective, it is crucial that AHA and BHA products have a low pH, while sunscreens need a pH that is higher to be effective (especially those with physical sunblocking agents of titanium dioxide and zinc oxide that protect against UVA radiation). Sunscreen ingredients prefer pH environments over 5 and AHAs and BHA need to be in a pH of 4 or less. While that may not seem significant, in terms of efficacy the difference between a pH of 4 and a pH of 5 is considerable. The only exception to this rule are **Exuviance by Neostrata's Essential Multi-Defense** sunscreens.

For normal to oily/combination and/or blemish-prone skin, the best scrubs are: Ashley Skin Care Gentle Exfoliating Polish *($32 for 6 ounces)*; BeautiControl Balancing Scrub for Combination Skin *($14 for 3 ounces)* and Renewing Scrub/Masque *($14 for 3 ounces)*; Beauty Without Cruelty Extra Gentle Facial Smoother *($7.49 for 4 ounces)*; Biore Mild Daily Cleansing Scrub *($4.94 for 5 ounces)*; The Body Shop Japanese Washing Grains for All Skin Types *($4.75 for 1.7 ounces)*, Peachy Clean Exfoliating Wash *($10 for 3.4 ounces)*, and Foaming Gel Scrub for Normal to Oily & Oily Skin *($12 for 3.7 ounces)*; Calvin Klein Micro-Exfoliator *($22 for 4 ounces)*; DDF Bergamot, Herbal, Strawberry, or Coconut Face and Body Polish *(each one is $22 for 8.45 ounces)*; Murad AHA/BHA Exfoliating Cleanser, Deep Cleansing for All Skin Types *($23 for 6 ounces)* and AHA/BHA Exfoliating Cleanser, Deep Cleansing for All Skin Types *($23 for 6 ounces)*; Principal Secret Gentle Deep Revitalizing Scrub *($22 for 4 ounces)*; reflect.com Facial Scrub *($16.50 for 5 ounces)*; and Sage Skin Care Corrective Grains Regular, Corrective Grains Extra Gentle, and Corrective Grains Extra Strength *(each one is $30 for 8 ounces)*.

For normal to dry and/or sensitive skin, the best scrubs are: Ahava Advanced Gentle Mud Exfoliator for All Skin Types *($24 for 3.4 ounces)*; Christian Dior Deep Radiance Exfoliating Creme *($25 for 2.4 ounces)*; Clarins Gentle Exfoliating Refiner for Face *($21 for 1.7 ounces)*; Clinique 7 Day Scrub Cream *($15 for 3.5 ounces)*, 7 Day Scrub Cream Rinse Off Formula *($14 for 3.4 ounces)*, and Gentle Exfoliator Rinse-Off Formula *($13.50 for 3 ounces)*; Club Monaco Face Mild Exfoliant *($15 for 3.3 ounces)*; Dr. Hauschka Skin Care Cleansing Cream *($15.95 for 1.7 ounces)*; Hydron Best Defense Micro-Exfoliating Creme *($16.75 for 3.6 ounces)*; Jafra Gentle Exfoliating Scrub for All Skin Types *($12.50 for 2.5 ounces)*; La Prairie Essential Exfoliator *($50 for 7 ounces)*; Lancome Exfoliance, Delicate Exfoliating Gel *($21 for 3.5 ounces)*; Physicians Formula Beauty Buffers Exfoliating Scrub All Skin Types *($5.95 for 2 ounces)*; Principal Secret Gentle Exfoliating Scrub *($20 for 4 ounces)*; and Remede Sweep *($36 for 2.7 ounces)*.

For all skin types, the best alpha hydroxy acid products (these can be worn under a moisturizer for someone with dry skin or alone for someone with normal to oily/combination and/or blemish-prone skin) are: Alpha Hydrox Extra Strength AHA Oil-Free Formula, 10% AHA Facial Treatment *($8.53 for 1.7 ounces)*; Amway Alpha Hydroxy Serum Plus *($40.20 for 1 ounce)*; BioMedic Phospholipid Gel *($30 for 2 ounces)*; Black Opal Skin Retexturizing Complex with Alpha-Hydroxy Acids *($9.95 for 1 ounce)*; Cellex-C Betaplex Line Smoother *($47.20 for 0.5 ounce)*; Dr. Mary Lupo AHA Renewel Gel I *($25 for 3.5 ounces)* and AHA Renewal Gel II *($25 for 3.5 ounces)*; Paula's Choice 8% Alpha Hydroxy Acid Solution *($12.95 for 4 ounces)*; Serious Skin Care Glycolic Renewal Gel *($20 for 4 ounces)*; Trish McEvoy Glycolic Lotion *($38 for 2 ounces)*; and Peter Thomas Roth Glycolic Acid 10%

Hydrating Gel *($45 for 2 ounces)* and AHA 12% Hydrating Ceramide Repair Gel *($45 for 2 ounces)*.

For normal to dry skin, the best alpha hydroxy acid products are: Alpha Hydrox AHA Creme, 8% AHA Facial Treatment for Normal Skin *($7.64 for 2 ounces)*, AHA Enhanced Creme, 10% AHA Facial Treatment, for Dry to Normal Skin *($8.41 for 2 ounces)*, AHA Lotion, 8% AHA Facial Treatment, for Dry Skin *($8.64 for 6 ounces)*, and AHA Sensitive Skin Creme, 5% AHA Facial Treatment *($7.64 for 2 ounces)*; Aqua Glycolic Face Cream Advanced Smoothing Therapy 10% Glycolic Compound *($11.29 for 2 ounces)*; Avon Stress Shield Serum *($12.50 for 1 ounce)*; BeautiControl Regeneration Extreme Repair for Dry and Damaged Skin *($30 for 4 ounces)*, Regeneration Gold *($55 for 1.8 ounces)*, and Regeneration Gold Eye Repair *($25 for 0.5 ounce)*; BioMedic Conditioning Cream *($27 for 2 ounces)* and Phospholipid Lotion *($30 for 2 ounces)*; Bobbi Brown Essentials Face Lotion *($38 for 2 ounces)*; Cellex-C Betaplex Smooth Skin Complex *($47.20 for 1 ounce)* and Betaplex Complexion Cream *($47.20 for 1 ounce)*; Color Me Beautiful Visible Results Glycolic Skin Conditioner for All Skin Types I *($18.50 for 1 ounce)*; DDF Glycolic Moisturizer 10% *($32.50 for 2 ounces)*; Dr. Mary Lupo AHA Renewal Lotion I *($25 for 3.5 ounces)* and AHA Renewal Lotion II *($25 for 3.5 ounces)*; Exuviance by Neostrata Hydrating Lift Eye Complex *($22.50 for 0.5 ounce)*; Glymed Plus Treatment Cream *($69.55 for 2 ounces)* and Derma Pigment Skin Brightener *($33.60 for 2 ounces)*; Hope Aesthetics Protective Eye Gel for All Skin Types *($40 for 0.5 ounce)* and Triplice Antioxidant Creme for Normal to Dry Skin *($50 for 2 ounces)*; Jan Marini Skin Care Bioglycolic Cream *($60 for 2 ounces)*, Bioglycolic Facial Lotion *($45 for 2 ounces)*, and Bioglycolic BioClear *($50 for 1 ounce)*; Janet Sartin Revitalizing Cream with Plant Extracts *($44 for 1.7 ounces)*, Revitalizing Lotion with Plant Extracts *($32 for 1 ounce)*, and Revitalizing Lotion Advance Strength with Plant Extracts *($35 for 1 ounce)*; Lac Hydrin Five Lotion *($10.99 for 8 ounces)* and Lac-Hydrin *($34.98 for 7.6 ounces)*; M.D. Formulations Facial Lotion with 12% Glycolic Compound *($55 for 2 ounces)*, Smoothing Complex with 10% Glycolic Compound *($35 for 0.5 ounce)*, and M.D. Forte Skin Rejuvenation Lotion I, 10% Glycolic Compound *($33.50 for 1 ounce)*; Murad Intensive Formula *($48 for 3.3 ounces)*; Neostrata Skin Smoothing Cream *($12.95 for 1.75 ounces)*, Skin Smoothing Lotion *($16.95 for 6.8 ounces)*, Polyhydroxy AHA Eye Cream *($22.95 for 0.5 ounce)*, Polyhydroxy AHA Ultra Moisturizing Face Cream *($22.95 for 1.75 ounces)*, and Sensitive Skin AHA Face Cream *($17.50 for 1.75 ounces)*; N.V. Perricone, M.D. Alpha Lipoic Acid Face Firming Activator with NTP Complex *($85 for 2 ounces)*; Osmotics Facial Renewal *($75 for 1.7 ounces)*; Peter Thomas Roth Glycolic Acid 5% Moisturizer *($40 for 2 ounces)* and Glycolic Acid 10% Moisturizer *($40 for 2 ounces)*; Pond's Clear Solutions Combination Skin Moisturizer *($5.69 for 4 ounces)*; and Principal Secret AHA Booster Complex *($45 for 1 ounce)*.

For all skin types, the best beta hydroxy acid products (these can be worn under a moisturizer for someone with dry skin or alone for someone with normal to oily/combination and/or blemish-prone skin) are: Estee Lauder Clear Difference Oil-Control Hydrator for Oily Normal/Oily and Blemish-Prone Skin *($27 for 1.7 ounces)*; Garden Botanika Skin Correcting Purifying Toning Lotion *($10 for 8 ounces)*; M.D. Formulations Vit-A-Plus Night Recovery Complex *($56.25 for 1 ounce)*; Neutrogena Deep Pore Treatment *($7 for 2 ounces)* and Clear Pore Treatment Nighttime Pore Clarifying Gel Salicylic Acid Acne Treatment *($6.75 for 2 ounces)*; Oxy Balance All Night Deep Pore Treatment *($4.84 for 2 ounces)*; Paula's Choice 2% Beta Hydroxy Acid Solution *($12.95 for 4 ounces)*; philosophy hope in a bottle oil-free moisturizer normal to oily skin *($30 for 2 ounces)*; Serious Skin Care Clarifying Treatment with 2% Salicylic Acid *($19.95 for 4 ounces)*; Ultima II Vital Radiance Skin Renewing Toner Normal to Dry Skin *($17.50 for 8 ounces)*; and ZAPZYT Pore Treatment Gel *($5.29 for 0.75 ounce)*.

For normal to dry and/or sensitive skin, the best beta hydroxy acid products are: Almay Time Off Revitalizer Daily Solution *($18 for 0.72 ounce)* and Time Off Daily Solution Pads *($18 for 112 pads)*; Avon Anew Perfecting Lotion for Problem Skin *($16 for 1.7 ounces)* and Mild Clarifying Lotion *($15.50 for 12 ounces)*; M.A.C. Oil Control Lotion *($22 for 1.7 ounces)*; Neutrogena Skin Clearing Moisturizer with 2% BHA *($11.99 for 1 ounce)*; and Paula's Choice 1% Beta Hydroxy Acid Solution *($12.95 for 4 ounces)*.

# *Best Moisturizers*

One huge departure from the last edition of this book is that I am not listing individual best moisturizers for normal to dry skin, but only for normal to slightly dry skin (meaning extremely lightweight gel, serum, or lotion formulations). For best moisturizers for normal to dry skin (and for those who prefer a more emollient feel on their skin), I am only listing the names of companies that have the best selection available. Even with my new strict criteria for what makes a great moisturizer for normal to dry skin, there are still over 500 moisturizers that got a happy face rating, which makes for an almost endless, unusable listing. Almost without exception, every line has its share of great moisturizers; you really can't make a mistake (other than believing the questionable claims and wasting your money). Even those products with neutral face ratings will work wonderfully to reduce dry skin, though they may not be state-of-the-art. In fact, it is almost impossible to buy a bad moisturizer. I wish there was a way to narrow this down for you but there just isn't. The redundancy is an issue created by the cosmetics industry and there isn't just a "best" but, rather, lots and lots of good ones to consider.

My strong recommendation is to consider one of the lines listed below that have many good moisturizers available and then look up that line's review and read over the moisturizers it sells and see which ones may be suitable for what you're looking for.

I included a listing of the best moisturizers for normal to slightly dry skin because there are far fewer products meeting these criteria (a lightweight formulation with minimal chance of clogging pores), and because finding them is rather difficult, at least in comparison to the scads of moisturizers for normal to dry skin.

Because many of you are curious about products containing retinol (vitamin A), I have listed those that contain relatively reliable concentrations (though exactly what is reliable is unknown) and that are packaged to keep the product stable.

I did not create a list of vitamin C products. It is an understatement to say that there is no consensus on which is the best form of vitamin C, much less how much of it to use to receive whatever the unproven, hyped results are supposed to produce. In the vitamin C wars, lines like Jan Marini Skin Care, N.V. Perricone, M.D., Peter Thomas Roth, and SkinCeuticals, among others, all claim to have THE best form and the correct amount of vitamin C. Who to believe is up to you. The research says not to believe any of it (at least not beyond the belief than vitamin C can increase the effectiveness of a sunscreen for UVB damage and that it's a good antioxidant—which is fine, but not better than other antioxidants).

Please keep in mind that products claiming that they are antiaging, antiwrinkling, lifting, firming, repairing or rejuvenating; can give the skin oxygen; or contain any number of miracle ingredients are telling fairy tales (except for sunscreens). What isn't a fantasy is the fact that there are a lot of great moisturizers to be found that can help soothe the skin and eliminate dryness (at least while you wear them—the effect is gone once you wash you face), and help make wrinkles look less pronounced—but stop using the product, whatever the exotic name, promise, or claim, and the wrinkles are back in short order. The most frustrating aspect of the moisturizer craze is the belief that using moisturizers can somehow slow down or stop the wrinkling process, so that a lot of women end up using moisturizers who shouldn't be, with the result being that many women are overmoisturizing, and that can hurt the skin's healing process.

Regardless of what they are called on the label—wrinkle creams, day creams, replenishers, liposome creams, eye creams, throat creams, lotions, serums, gels, and nourishing creams—all these concoctions and combinations do the same thing—moisturize the skin—and, for the most part, they do an excellent job. What is offensive is that many of these formulations don't warrant the outlandish claims, ridiculous prices, or your belief that you've finally found the fountain of youth (because a new antiwrinkle product launch is just a month or so down the road, and yet we're still wrinkling!).

Please note: There are no products that can change dark circling under the eye (unless the dark circling is caused by sun damage, which requires a well-formulated skin-lightening product).

When it comes to day moisturizers versus night moisturizers, the only difference should be whether or not the day moisturizer contains a sunscreen (most sunscreen formulations have a moisturizing base).

The moisturizer you use on your face will always work around your eyes and throat, on your chest, or wherever. Try to disregard the scare tactics at the cosmetics counters and the brochures that carry on about special formulations designed exclusively for the eye, throat, or chest area. These claims are not substantiated by the ingredients in the products, which are identical to products supposedly designed just for the face.

Women with oily skin should not get sucked into believing that all skin types, even oily-skin types, require a moisturizer to prevent the skin from wrinkling or to combat surface dehydration. Unless we are talking about a UVA-protecting sunscreen with an SPF of 15, or dealing with isolated areas of dryness, someone with oily skin should not being using a moisturizer. Remember that the words "oil-free" don't mean a product won't feel slick, greasy, or oily on the skin. Many ingredients that don't sound like "oil" have a very slick, oily texture. The product recommendations for oilier skin types refer to lighter-weight, less-emollient formulas, but they should still be used onlyover dry areas of the face.

Please Remember: The only reason to use a moisturizer is if you have dry skin; if you don't have dry skin, it is not helpful for your skin. For those areas of your face that have dryness, you can use one of the toners listed above or one of the moisturizers for normal to dry skin below; if you are only looking for an extremely lightweight moisturizer, the section below for normal to slightly dry skin is what you want to check.

The companies that have the largest choices well-formulated moisturizers for normal to dry skin (please keep in mind that every line has great moisturizers—these are the companies that have the best selection for a variety of skin types and preferences) are: Amway; Arbonne; Aveda; Avon; Awake; BeautiControl; Beauty Without Cruelty; BioMedic; BioTherm; Cellex-C; Chanel; Christian Dior; Circle of Beauty; Clarins; Clinique; DDF; Decleor Paris; Dermalogica; DHC USA; Diane Young; Dr. Hauschka Skin Care; Elizabeth Arden; Epicuren; Erno Laszlo; Estee Lauder; Forever Spring; Garden Botanika; Glymed Plus; Hydron; Jafra; Jan Marini Skin Care; Jason Natural Cosmetics; Kiss My Face; La Prairie; L'Oreal; Marcelle; Marilyn Miglin; Mary Kay; Nicole Miller Skin Care; Nu Skin USA; N.V. Perricone, M.D.;Origins; Orlane; Osmotics; Parthena; Paula's Choice; Peter Thomas Roth; Pevonia; philosophy; Prescriptives; RoC; Sothys Paris; St. Ives; Tova; Vichy; Yon-Ka Paris; and Zia Natural Skin Care.

The best lightweight moisturizers for normal to slightly dry or combination skin are: Ashley Skin Care Hyaluronic Serum *($48 for 1.01 ounces)* and Dermaceutical Eye Lift *($40 for 1.01 ounces)*; Aveda Firming Fluid *($32 for 1 ounce)* and Oil-Free Hydraderm *($26 for 5 ounces)*; Avon Anew Eye Force Vertical Lifting Complex *($18 for 0.5 ounce)*; Awake Hydro Plus *($40 for 1.4 ounces)*, Nano Essence AX Dry Skin *($60 for 0.8 ounce)*, and Skin Renovation *($95 for 1 ounce)*; bare escentuals Habit Skin Care Bare Aloe Vera *($8 for 2 ounces)*; BeautiControl Microderm Oxygenating Firming Gel *($29.50 for 2 ounces)*; Beauty for All Seasons/Norma Virgin Makeup Chamomile Calming Eye Gel *($10.50 for 0.5 ounces)*; Beauty Without Cruelty Green Tea Nourishing Eye Gel *($14.49 for 1 ounce)*; Bioelements Jet Travel, Moisture Boost for Low Humidity *($31.50 for 1 ounce)*, Stress Solution *($31.50 for 1 ounce)*, Urban Detox *($31.50 for 1 ounce)*, and Oxygen Cocktail Natural Defense Against Visible Skin Aging *($31.50 for 1 ounce)*; BioMedic High Density Gel *($26 for 2 ounces)*; BioTherm Aquasource Oligo-Thermal Moisturizing Gel for Dry Skin *($29 for 1.7 ounces)*, Aquasource Oligo-Thermal Moisturizing Gel for Normal Skin *($29 for 1.7 ounces)*, and Symbiose Daily Aging Treatment Liposome Gel *($45 for 1.7 ounces)*; Bobbi Brown Essentials Revitalizing Eye Gel *($32.50 for 0.5 ounce)*; The Body Shop Hydrating Moisture Lotion for Normal to Dry Skin *($16 for 3.38 ounces)* and Tea Tree Oil Moisturizing Gel, for Oily or Blemished Skin *($13.50 for 8.4 ounces)*; Calvin Klein Oil Control Hydrator *($30 for 1.7 ounces)*; Cellex-C Hydra 5 B-Complex Moisture Enhancing Gel for All Skin Types *($55 for 1 ounce)* and Salicea Gel for All Skin Types *($45 for 1 ounce)*; Chanel HydraMax Balanced Hydrating Gel *($40 for 1.7 ounces)*; Clarins Extra Firming Concentrate *($52.50 for 1 ounce)*; Color Me Beautiful Eye Lift Firming Gel *($18.50 for 0.5 ounce)*; Coppertone Aloe Aftersun Gel *($4.49 for 16 oz)*, Cool Beads! Aftersun Aloe Gel, Light, Summertime Fragrance *($5.49 for 16 ounces)*, Cool Beads! Aftersun Moisturizer with Vitamins A + E *($4.99 for 12 ounces)*, Cool Gel Aloe Aftersun *($5.49 for 16 ounces)*, and Gold After Sun Cool Gel, with Vitamin E & Aloe *($5.29 for 12 ounces)*; DDF Soothing Eye Gel *($35 for 1 ounce)* and Erase Eye Gel *($37.50 for 0.5 ounce)*; Decleor Paris Instant Beauty Booster for All Skin Types *($42 for 1.69 ounces)*; Dermalogica Intensive Moisture Concentrate *($45 for 1 ounce)* and Specific Skin Concentrate *($45 for 1 ounce)*; DHC USA Soothing Lotion for Drier Skin *($12 for 6 ounces)*, AntioxC *($32 for 1.4 ounces)*, and Oil-Free Hydrator for Oilier Skin *($22 for 3.3 ounces)*; Diane Young Years Younger Serum *($45.50 for 1 ounce)*; Elizabeth Arden Ceramide Advanced Time Complex Capsules *($55 for 0.97 ounce, includes 60 capsules)*; Hydron Oil Balancing Serum *($19.75 for 0.45 ounce)* and Best Defense Line Smoothing Complex *($37.75 for 0.5 ounce)*; Iman Time Control Renewal Complex *($29.50 for 1 ounce)*; Jafra Elasticity Recovery Hydrogel *($35 for 1 ounce)*; Jason Natural Cosmetics Oil Free NaPCA Naturally Lite Moisturizing Creme *($7.50* *for 4 ounces);* <u>L'Occitane</u> Firming Serum *($20 for 0.5 ounce);* <u>Marcelle</u> Hydractive Eye Contour Gel *($11.95 for 15 ml);* <u>M.D. Formulations</u> Moisture Defense Anti-oxidant Hydrating Serum *($42 for 1 ounce);* <u>Models Prefer</u> Skin Serum *(1 ounce);* <u>Natura Bisse</u> Sensitive Concentrate Calming Concentrate for All Sensitive Skin Types *($120 for 6 ampoules totaling 1.2 ounces)* and Sensitive Eye Gel Calming Gel for the Eyes *($52 for 0.8 ounce);* <u>Neutrogena</u> Combination Skin Moisture Oil-Free *($9.50 for 4 ounces);* <u>Nicole Miller Skin Care</u> Delicate Repair Eye Gel *($32 for 0.5 ounce)* and Multi-Action Vitamin Complex *($40 for 1 ounce);* <u>Noevir</u> Eye Treatment Gel *($65 for 0.52 ounce);* <u>Nu Skin USA</u> Celltrex Skin Hydrating Fluid *($26.75 for 0.5 ounce),* Enhancer Skin Conditioning Gel *($29.15 for 2.5 ounces),* HPX Hydrating Gel *($49.95 for 1.5 ounces),* and NaPCA Moisturizer *($19.80 for 2.5 ounces);* <u>Origins</u> Line Chaser Stop Sign for Lines *($25 for 0.5 ounce);* <u>Orlane</u> Normalane Foam Cleansing Gel for Mixed and Oily Skins *($25 for 4.2 ounces);* <u>Paula's Choice</u> Completely Non-Greasy Moisturizing Lotion *($12.95 for 4 ounces);* <u>Peter Thomas Roth</u> Environmental Repair Hydrating Gel *($35 for 2 ounces);* <u>Pevonia</u> Eye Gel *($29.75 for 0.7 ounce);* <u>Pond's</u> Revitalizing Eye Capsules *($10.99 for 20 capsules totaling 0.26 ounce)* and Skin Smoothing Capsules *($10.99 for 26 capsules);* <u>Prescriptives</u> Super Line Preventor *($45 for 1 ounce);* <u>Principal Secret</u> Eye Relief *($30 for 0.5 ounce);* <u>reflect.com</u> Facial Moisturizer for Combination or Blemish Prone Skin *($29.50 for 1 ounce);* <u>Remede</u> Resistance Anti-Oxidant Firming Complex *($65 for 1 ounce);* <u>RoC</u> Hydra+ Light Mat Cream *($12.17 for 1.35 ounces);* <u>Serious Skin Care</u> A Force Vitamin A Serum *($25 for 1 ounce)* and Refirm Firming Eye Gel *($16.50 for 0.5 ounce);* <u>SkinCeuticals</u> Eye Gel *($42 for 0.5 ounce)* and Intense Line Defense *($50 for 1 ounce);* <u>Sothys Paris</u> Soothing Skin Lotion, with Allantoin Extract, for Sensitive Skin *($26 for 6.7 ounces);* <u>Trish McEvoy</u> Oil-Controlling Gel *($28 for 2 ounces)* and Moisture Gel (Oil-Free) *($19 for 1 ounce);* <u>Ultima II</u> Vital Radiance Skin Renewing Night Serum *($25 for 0.95 ounce);* <u>Vichy</u> Optalia Restructuring Eye Gel *($28.50 for 15 ml)* and Heliocalm Calming Reparative Gel for Face and Body *($15.50 for 100 ml);* <u>Victoria Jackson Cosmetics</u> Eye Repair Gel *($12.50, $19.50 for 0.5 ounce);* <u>Yves St. Laurent</u> Soin Beaute Instantanee/Instant Firming Gel *($60 for 1 ounce);* and <u>Zia Natural Skin Care</u> Essential Eye Gel *($19.95 for 0.5 ounce),* Herbal Moisture Gel Oil Free Moisturizer for Normal, Sensitive, Combination & Oily/Problem Skin Types *($22.95 for 1.5 ounces),* Deep Moisture Repair Serum *($29.95 for 0.3 ounce),* and Seaweed Lift Serum *($34.95 for 0.5 ounce).*

<u>Best products containing retinol:</u> <u>Alpha Hydrox</u> Retinol Night ResQ Anti-Wrinkle Firming Complex *($11.99 for 1.05 ounces);* <u>Avon</u> Anew Retinol Recovery Complex P.M. Treatment *($17.50 for 1 ounce);* <u>BeautiControl</u> Regeneration Retinol PM *($35 for 1 ounce);* <u>BioMedic</u> Microencapsulated Retinol Cream 15, 30, or 60 *(15: $30 for 1.05 ounces; 30: $32 for 1.05 ounces; 60: $35 for 1.05 ounces);* <u>Circle</u>

of Beauty Night Life Oxygen-Retinol Repair Cream, Oily *($15 for 2 ounces)*, Night Life Oxygen-Retinol Repair Cream, Dry *($15 for 2 ounces)*, Night Life Oxygen-Retinol Repair Cream, Combination Dry *($15 for 2 ounces)*, Night Life Oxygen-Retinol Repair Cream, Dehydrated *($15 for 2 ounces)*, and Night Life Oxygen-Retinol Repair Cream, Combination Oily *($15 for 2 ounces)*; Color Me Beautiful Retinol PM Capsules, Cellular Recovery Complex *($22.50 for 30 capsules)*; Erno Laszlo Retinol Reparative Therapy *($85 for 1 ounce)*; Jan Marini Skin Care Factor-A Cream *($45 for 1 ounce)* and Factor-A Lotion *($40 for 1 ounce)*; Lancome ReSurface *($52.50 for 1 ounce)*; L'Oreal Line Eraser Pure Retinol Concentrate *($12.49 for 1 ounce)*; Neutrogena Healthy Skin Anti-Wrinkle Cream with Retinol *($12.49 for 1.4 ounces)*; Nu Skin USA Ideal Eyes Vitamins C & A Eye Refining Creme *($40 for 0.5 ounce)*; N.V. Perricone, M.D. Alpha Lipoic Acid Evening Facial Emollient with NTP Complex and Retinol *($80 for 2 ounces)*; philosophy help me *($45 for 1.05 ounces)*; Prescriptives Px Retinol LSW *($50 for 1 ounce)*; RoC Retinol Actif Pur Anti-Wrinkle Treatment, for Night *($15.99 for 1.01 ounces)* and Retinol Actif Pur-Eye Contour Cream *($15.99 for 0.51 ounce)*; Sothys Paris Retinol-15 Night Cream, Time Interceptor Line *($48 for 1 ounce)* and Retinol-30 *($48 for 1 ounce)*; and St. Ives Vitamin A Anti-Wrinkle Serum *($6.99 for 14 0.16-ounce capsules)* and Multi Vitamin Retinol Anti-Wrinkle Cream *($10.99 for 0.5 ounce)*.

## *Best Sunscreens*

I've discussed at length why sunscreens are essential for skin care day in and day out, 365 days a year (they are the only true antiwrinkle products), why UVA-protecting ingredients (either avobenzone, zinc oxide, or titanium dioxide) are so crucial, and why an SPF number should be 15 or greater, because these are the only real options for preventing wrinkles or skin damage.

The only thing left to reiterate is why the lists below are so disproportionate, with vastly more sunscreens for normal to dry skin than for normal to oily. The answer is not reassuring, at least not to those with oily skin or skin prone to breakouts. Sunscreen agents work better in an emollient emulsion than in a matte base or liquid. When a lightweight liquid is available, often the base includes alcohol, and that is just hard on skin due to irritation. Plus, the UVA-protecting ingredients of zinc oxide and titanium dioxide can clog pores! As I mentioned before, from the chin up, someone with oily skin may prefer using a foundation with a good SPF and from the neck down any other good sunscreen formulation. This is one area of skin care that is difficult for someone with oily skin, and it takes experimentation to find what works well for you.

All of the following sunscreens have an SPF 15 or greater and contain either avobenzone, titanium dioxide, or zinc oxide as one or more of the *active* ingredients (finding them someplace else on the ingredient list does not count toward sun protection).

Please note that avobenzone may be listed on an ingredient label as Parsol 1789 or butyl methoxydibenzoylmethane.

For normal to oily/combination skin, the best sunscreens (but keep in mind that foundations with sunscreens work great for oily and combination skin types) are: Signature Club A by Adrien Arpel Flower Acid Wrinkle Remedy Day Face Creme with Sunscreen SPF 20 *(sold in a set, 2 ounces)*; Avon Skin So Soft Kids Sunblock SPF 40 *($9 for 4.2 ounces)*, Sun So-Soft Kids Sunblock SPF 40 *($9 for 4.2 ounces)*, Sun So-Soft Moisturizing Suncare Plus SPF 15 *($9 for 4.2 ounces)*, and Sun So-Soft Moisturizing Suncare Plus SPF 30 *($9 for 4.2 ounces)*; Calvin Klein Protective Moisture Lotion SPF 15 *($30 for 1.7 ounces)*; Chanel Rectifiance Day Lift Refining Oil-Free Lotion SPF 15 *($50 for 1.7 ounces)* and Fluide Multi-Protection Daily Protection Lotion SPF 25 *($25 for 1 ounce)*; Christian Dior UV 30 Ultra UV Face Coat *($31 for 1 ounce)*; Club Monaco Face Day Protection Fluid SPF 15 *($19 for 1.7 ounces)*; Coppertone Shade UVA Guard Sunblock Lotion with Parsol 1789 SPF 30 *($6.99 for 4 ounces)*; Dr. Mary Lupo Full Spectrum Sunscreen UVA/UVB SPF 27 *($17.50 for 3 ounces)*; Glymed Plus Photo-Age Environmental Protection Gel SPF 20 *($47.25 for 7 ounces)*; Lancome SPF 15 Face and Body Lotion with Pure Vitamin E *($21 for 5 ounces)*, SPF 25 Face and Body Lotion with Pure Vitamin E *($21 for 5 ounces)*, and SPF 15 Water-Light Spray *($21 for 5 ounces)*; Marcelle Protective Block No Chemical Sunscreen Spray SPF 15 *($12.95 for 120 ml)*; Neutrogena Pore Refining Cream SPF 15 *($13.99 for 1 ounce)* and UVA/UVB Sunblock SPF 45 *($7.99 for 4 ounces)*; Paula's Choice Essential Non-Greasy Sunscreen SPF 15 *($11.95 for 6 ounces)* and All Day Cover Non-Greasy Sunscreen SPF 30+ with Antioxidants Waterproof *($11.95 for 6 ounces)*; ProActiv Oil Free Moisture with SPF 15 *($25 for 1.7 ounces)*; Sage Skin Care SPF 25 Sunblock *($21 for 4 ounces)*; and Shiseido Gentle Sun Block Cream SPF 22 *($20 for 3.8 ounces)* and Ultra Light Sun Block Lotion SPF 30 *($25 for 3.3 ounces)*.

For normal to dry, extra dry, and/or sensitive skin, the best sunscreens are: Almay Time-Off Lasting Moisture SPF 25 *($14.99 for 3.8 ounces)*; Aveda Daily Light Guard SPF 15 *($16.50 for 5 ounces)*; Avon Anew Day Force Vertical Lifting Force SPF 15 *($20 for 1 ounce)*, Luminosity Skin Brightener SPF 15 *($20 for 1.7 ounces)*, Anew Perfect Eye Care Cream SPF 15 *($13.50 for 0.53 ounce)*, and Sun-So-Soft SPF 25 Sunscreen Stick *($7.50 for 0.42 ounce)*; Bain de Soleil UV Sense SPF 50 *($9.89 for 3.12 ounces)*, Bebe Block SPF 50 *($9.89 for 3.12 ounces)*, All Day Extended Protection Sunscreen SPF 30 *($9.19 for 4 ounces)*, All Day Extended Protection Sunblock SPF 15 *($6.99 for 4 ounces)*, All Day Waterproof Sunblock

SPF 15 *($9.19 for 4 ounces)*, **Gentle Block Sunblock** SPF 30 *($8.99 for 4 ounces)*, **Mademoiselle Sunblock** SPF 15 *($6.99 for 4 ounces)*, and **Kids Sunblock** SPF 30 *($8.99 for 4 ounces)*; <u>Basis</u> **Face the Day Lotion** SPF 15 *($6.55 for 4 ounces)* and **One Step Face Cream** SPF 15 *($6.55 for 1.5 ounces)*; <u>Beauty for All Seasons/Norma Virgin Makeup</u> **Moisturessence** SPF 18 *($20 for 4 ounces)* and **SPF 15 Daily Facial Lotion, Benefits All Skin Types** *($9.49 for 4 ounces)*; <u>Bioelements</u> **Sun Diffusing Protector** SPF 15 *($29.50 for 6 ounces)* and **Sun Protector** SPF 15 *($17.95 for 4 ounces)*; <u>BioMedic</u> **Facial Shield** SPF 20 *($30 for 2 ounces)* and **Pigment Shield** SPF 18 *($30 for 2 ounces)*; <u>Bobbi Brown Essentials</u> SPF 15 **Face Lotion** *($38 for 1.7 ounces)*; <u>The Body Shop</u> **Vitamin C Protective Daywear Moisturizer with SPF 15** *($12 for 2.5 ounces)* and **Facial Sun Stick** SPF 30 *($6.50 for 0.6 ounce)*; <u>Calvin Klein</u> **Protective Moisture Cream** SPF 15 *($30 for 1.7 ounces)*; <u>Cetaphil</u> **Daily Facial Moisturizer** SPF 15 *($7.99 for 4 ounces)*; <u>Chanel</u> **Rectifiance Day Lift Refining Cream** SPF 15 *($60 for 1.7 ounces)* and **Rectifiance Day Lift Refining Lotion** SPF 15 *($50 for 1.7 ounces)*; <u>Clarins</u> **Extra-Firming Day Lotion** SPF 15 *($57.50 for 1.7 ounces)* and **Hydration-Plus Moisture Lotion** SPF 15 for All Skin Types *($30 for 1.7 ounces)*; <u>Clinique</u> **Weather Everything** SPF 15 *($37.50 for 1.7 ounces)*, **City Block** SPF 15 *($13.50 for 1.4 ounces)*, and **Super City Block** SPF 25 Oil-Free Daily Face Protector *($14.50 for 1.4 ounces)*; <u>Darphin</u> **Ecran Soleil** SPF 30 *($50 for 1.7 ounces)*, **Soleil Filtrant** SPF 25 *($48 for 5 ounces)*, and **Vital Protection Day Fluid** SPF 15 *($75 for 1 ounce)*; <u>DDF</u> **Organic Sunblock** SPF 30 *($21 for 4 ounces)*; <u>Dermalogica</u> **Total Eye Care** SPF 15 *($33 for 0.75 ounce)*; <u>DHC USA</u> **Dual Defense** SPF 25 *($24 for 3.5 ounces)*; <u>Dr. Hauschka Skin Care</u> **Sunscreen Lotion** SPF 15 *($15.95 for 3.4 ounces)*, **Sunscreen Lotion** SPF 20 *($17.95 for 3.4 ounces)*, and **Sunscreen Cream for Children** SPF 22 *($19.95 for 3.4 ounces)*; <u>Dr. Mary Lupo</u> **Daily Age Management Oil Free Moisturizer** SPF 15 *($23 for 2 ounces)*; <u>Ecco Bella</u> **Skin Survival Day Cream** SPF 15 *($21.50 for 2 ounces)*; <u>Epicuren</u> **Zinc Oxide Sunblock Sunscreen** SPF 20 *($58 for 4 ounces)*; <u>Estee Lauder</u> **New Resilience Lift** SPF 15 Face and Throat Cream *($45 for 1 ounce)*, **New Resilience Lift** SPF 15 Face and Throat Lotion *($45 for 1 ounce)*, **Day Wear Super Anti-Oxidant Complex** SPF 15 *($37.50 for 1.7 ounces)*, **Sun Block for Face** SPF 15 *($18.50 for 1.7 ounces)*, and **Sun Block for Face** SPF 30 *($19.50 for 1.7 ounces)*; <u>Eucerin</u> **Advanced Sun Defense** SPF 15 *($7.99 for 6 ounces)* and **Facial Moisturizing Lotion,** SPF 25 *($8 for 4 ounces)*; <u>Jafra</u> **Advanced Time Protector Daily Defense Cream,** SPF 15 *($38 for 1.7 ounces)*; <u>Jan Marini Skin Care</u> **Bioglycolic Facial Lotion** SPF 15 *($45 for 2 ounces)*; <u>Janet Sartin</u> SPF 15 **Sunblock Face Cream with Plant Extracts** *($39 for 1.85 ounces)*, **Sunblock** SPF 15 Waterproof **Lotion with Plant Extracts** *($18 for 4 ounces)*, and **Sunblock** SPF 25 Waterproof **Lotion with Plant Extracts** *($18 for 4 ounces)*; <u>Jason Natural Cosmetics</u> SPF 16 **Sun Block** *($9 for 4 ounces)*, SPF 26 **Total Sun Block** *($9.50 for 4 ounces)*, SPF 36 **Family**

Sun Block *($10.50 for 4 ounces)*, SPF 40 Active Sun Block *($10.75 for 4 ounces)*, SPF 46 Kids Sun Block *($11 for 4 ounces)*, SPF 20 Natural Lip Protection on a String *($5 for 0.16 ounce)*, and SPF 26 Sun Block Sport Stick *($8 for 0.75 ounce)*; Joey New York Green Tea with Multivitamins SPF-30 *($20 for 1 ounce)*; Kiehl's Sun Shield Sunblock with SPF 15 *($23.50 for 8 ounces)*; Kiss My Face Oat Protein Sunblock SPF 18 *($9 for 4 ounces)* and Oat Protein Sunblock SPF 30 *($10 for 4 ounces)*; La Prairie Age Management Stimulus Complex SPF 25 *($150 for 1 ounce)*, Cellular Brightening System Day Emulsion with SPF 15 *($125 for 1 ounce)*, Cellular Defense Shield Eye Cream, SPF 15 *($100 for 0.5 ounce)*, Cellular Time Release Moisture Lotion SPF 15 *($125 for 1.7 ounces)*, Cellular Purifying Systeme Hydrating Fluid SPF 15 *($100 for 1.7 ounces)*, Suisse De-Sensitizing Systeme Barrier Shield SPF 15 *($100 for 1 ounce)*, Soleil Suisse Cellular Anti-Wrinkle Sun Cream SPF 30 *($100 for 1.7 ounces)*, and Soleil Suisse Cellular Anti Wrinkle Sun Block SPF 50 *($125 for 1.7 ounces)*; Lancome High Protection SPF 30 Face Creme with Pure Vitamin E *($23 for 1.7 ounces)*, UV Expert SPF 15 Sunscreen, Daily UVA/UVB Protection Water-Lite Fluide *($30 for 1 ounce)*, and Soleil Expert Sun Care SPF 30 High Protection Sun Stick *($19.50 for 0.26 ounce)*; Laura Mercier Mega Moisturizer Cream with SPF 15 *($38 for 2 ounces)* and Moisturizer Cream with SPF 15 *($38 for 2 ounces)*; Le Mirador Triple Action Revitalizing Moisturizer SPF 15 *($21.71 for 2 ounces)* and Formula Sunscreen Protection SPF 15 *($14.50 for 6 ounces)*; Marcelle Moisture Cream Eye with Gingko Biloba SPF 15 *($12.50 for 15 ml)*, Multi-Defense Cream Daily Moisturizer SPF 15 *($15.25 for 60 ml)*, Protective Block No Chemical Sunscreen Cream SPF 25 *($12.95 for 50 ml)*, and Protective Block No Chemical Sunscreen Lotion SPF 25 *($12.95 for 120 ml)*; Mario Badescu Oil Free Moisturizer SPF 17 *($20 for 2 ounces)* and Aloe Moisturizer SPF 15 *($35 for 4 ounces)*; Mary Kay Day Solutions SPF 15 *($30 for 1 ounce)*; M.D. Formulations Total Daily Protector SPF 15 *($15 for 2.5 ounces)*, Total Protector 30 *($20 for 2.5 ounces)*, M.D. Forte Total Daily Protector SPF 15 *($12.50 for 2.5 ounces)*, and M.D. Forte Sun Protector 30 *($18 for 2.5 ounces)*; Merle Norman Luxiva Preventage Firming Defense Creme for Oily and Normal/Combination Skin Types SPF 15 *($36 for 2 ounces)*, Luxiva Preventage Firming Defense Creme for Dry Skin SPF 15 *($36 for 2 ounces)*, Luxiva Preventage Firming Eye Crème SPF 15 *($19.50 for 0.5 ounce)*, and Luxiva Changing Skin Treatment SPF 15 *($42 for 1 ounce)*; Murad Environmental Shield Essential Day Moisture SPF 15 *($40 for 1.4 ounces)*, Daily Defense Oil Free Sunblock SPF 15 (Light Tint) *($16.50 for 4.2 ounces)*, Daily Defense Hydrating Sunscreen SPF 15 *($16.50 for 4.2 ounces)*, and Waterproof Sunblock SPF 30 Face and Body *($19 for 4.2 ounces)*; Neutrogena Sensitive Skin UVA/UVB Block SPF 17 *($8.99 for 4 ounces)* and Sensitive Skin UVA/UVB Block SPF 30 *($8.99 for 4 ounces)*; Nu Skin USA Sunright 28 Ultimate Sunscreen Protection *($17.45 for 3.4 ounces)*; Nu Skin 180 UV Block Hydrator SPF 18 *1 ounce)*; <u>Dr. Obagi</u> Nu-Derm Sunblock SPF 25 *($37 for 2 ounces)*; <u>Olay</u> Complete UV Protective Moisture Lotion SPF 15 (Fragrance and Fragrance Free) *($6.59 for 4 ounces)* and Complete UV Protective Moisture Cream SPF 15 (Fragrance and Fragrance Free) *($6.59 for 4 ounces)*; <u>Ombrelle</u> Sunscreen Lotion SPF 15 *($10 for 4 ounces)*, Sunscreen Lotion SPF 30 *($10 for 4 ounces)*, and Kids Spray SPF 28 *($8.69 for 4 ounces)*; <u>Origins</u> Let the Sunshine SPF 14 *($13.50 for 5 ounces)* and Silent Treatment Instant UV Face Protector SPF 15 *($15 for 1.7 ounces)*; <u>Orlane</u> Creme Solaire Total Block Sun Cream for the Face 30+ UVA 11 *($30 for 1.7 ounces)*; <u>Osmotics</u> Protection Extreme Total Body SPF 15 *($30 for 4.25 ounces)* and Protection Extreme Total Body SPF 25 *($32 for 4.25 ounces)*; <u>Paula's Choice</u> Essential Moisturizing Sunscreen SPF 15 *($11.95 for 6 ounces)*, Essential Pure Block Sunscreen SPF 15 *($12.95 for 6 ounces)*, and All Day Cover Moisturizing Sunscreen SPF 30+ with Antioxidants Waterproof *($11.95 for 6 ounces)*; <u>Peter Thomas Roth</u> Daily Defense Moisture Cream SPF 20 *($25 for 4 ounces)*, Oil-Free Sunblock SPF 20 *($25 for 4 ounces)*, Oil-Free Sunblock SPF 30 *($25 for 4 ounces)*, Water Resistant Sunblock SPF 20 *($25 for 4 ounces)*, Water Resistant Sunblock SPF 30 *($25 for 4 ounces)*, Max Sheer All-Day Moisture Defense Lotion SPF 30 *($37 for 1.7 ounces)*, Titanium Dioxide Sunblock SPF 15 *($25 for 4 ounces)*, Titanium Dioxide Sunblock SPF 30 *($6.26 for 1 ounce)*, and Ultra Lite Oil-Free Sunblock SPF 30 with Parsol 1789 *($25 for 4 ounces)*; <u>Pevonia</u> Sunblock Dry to Sensitive Skin, SPF 15 *($28.25 for 2.5 ounces)*, Sunblock Combination to Oily Skin, SPF 15 *($28.25 for 2.5 ounces)*, and Sunblock Body Milk, SPF 15 *($29.25 for 5 ounces)*; <u>Physicians Formula</u> Sun Shield Sensitive Skin Formula Chemical Free Sunscreen SPF 25 *($8.50 for 4 ounces)*, Sun Shield for Faces Sensitive Skin Formula SPF 15 for All Skin Types *($8 for 2 ounces)*, Vital Defense Sun Stick for Faces SPF 30 for All Skin Types *($6.95 for 0.55 ounce)*, and Vital Defense Oil Free Lotion with SPF 15 for Normal to Oily Skin *($8 for 6 ounces)*; <u>Pond's</u> Nourishing Moisture Lotion with SPF 15 *($5.99 for 2.5 ounces)*; <u>Prescriptives</u> Px Insulation Anti-Oxidant Vitamin Cream with SPF 15 *($40 for 1.7 ounces)* and Any Wear SPF 15 *($19.50 for 1 ounce)*; <u>Principal Secret</u> Sun Block SPF 20 *($17 for 4 ounces)*; <u>Purpose</u> Dual Treatment Moisturizer with SPF 15 Protection *($7.89 for 4 ounces)*; <u>reflect.com</u> Facial Moisturizer UV Facial Cream SPF 15 *($25 for 1.7 ounces)* and Facial Moisturizer UV Facial Lotion SPF 15 *($19.50 for 6.7 ounces)*; <u>RoC</u> ChronoBlock Active Preventive Daily Moisturizing Cream SPF 15 *($16.99 for 1.35 ounces)*; <u>Shiseido</u> Sun Block Face Cream SPF 35 *($22 for 1.7 ounces)*, Sun Block Stick SPF 35 *($18 for 0.31 ounce)*, Translucent Sun Block Stick SPF 30 *($20 for 0.31 ounce)*, and The Skin Care Day Protective Moisturizer SPF 15 *($30 for 1.4 ounces)*; <u>Sisley</u> Botanical Sun Block SPF 20 *($100 for 1.5 ounces)*; <u>SkinCeuticals</u> Daily Sun Defense SPF 20 *($28 for 3 ounces)*, and Ultimate UV Defense SPF 30

*($34 for 3 ounces)*, **Ultimate UV Defense SPF 45** *($34 for 3 ounces)*; <u>Sothys Paris</u> **SPF 25 Sunblock** *($23 for 2.5 ounces)*; <u>Trish McEvoy</u> **Protective Shield Moisturizer SPF 15** *($38 for 2 ounces)* and **Sport Cream SPF 30** *($19 for 4 ounces)*; <u>Ultima II</u> **Glowtion Skin Brightening Moisture Cream SPF 15** *($21.50 for 2 ounces)*, **Glowtion Skin Brightening Moisturizer SPF 25** *($21.50 for 2 ounces)*, and **Under-It-All Makeup Perfector SPF 25** *($13.50 for 1.25 ounces)*; <u>Vichy</u> **Capital Soleil Protective Gel-Cream SPF 15** *($15.50 for 120 ml)*, **Capital Soleil Protective Lotion SPF 15** *($15.50 for 120 ml)*, **Capital Soleil Sunblock Cream for the Face SPF 25** *($15.50 for 50 ml)*, **Capital Soleil Sunblock Lotion SPF 25** *($15.50 for 120 ml)*, **Capital Soleil Total Sunblock Lotion SPF 30** *($15.50 for 120 ml)*, **Capital Soleil Total Sunblock Cream SPF 45** *($15.50 for 50 ml)*, **Capital Soleil Total Sunblock Cream SPF 60** *($19.50 for 50 ml)*, **Capital Soleil Sunblock Lotion for Children SPF 25** *($15.50 for 120 ml)*, **Capital Soleil Sunblock Lotion for Children SPF 35** *($19.50 for 120 ml)*, and **Capital Soleil Sunblock Stick SPF 25** *($9 for 3 ml tube)*; <u>Yon-Ka Paris</u> **Ultra Protection, Age-Free Solar Block with AHAs and Botanicals, Water Resistant, SPF 25, UVA-UVB-IR** *($41 for 1 ounce)*; and <u>Yves Rocher</u> **Hydra Advance Solaire Moisturizing Sun Block SPF 25** *($17.95 for 5 ounces)*.

    <u>For normal to dry, sensitive skin the best tinted sunscreens are:</u> <u>Aveda</u> **Moisture Plus Tint SPF 15** *($25)*; <u>Bobbi Brown Essentials</u> **SPF 15 Tinted Moisturizer** *($35)*; and <u>Peter Thomas Roth</u> **Tinted Protective Day Cream SPF 30** *($40 for 2.3 ounces)*.

    <u>The best foundations with sunscreen for normal to dry, sensitive skin:</u> See the section below for Best Foundations. Those products with adequate UVA protection as an SPF 15 have an asterisk.

    <u>The best foundations with sunscreen for someone with oily/combination and/or blemish-prone skin:</u> See the section below for Best Foundations. Those products with adequate UVA protection as an SPF 15 have an asterisk.

    <u>The best lip products with sunscreen:</u> <u>Cover Girl</u> **Triple Lipstick SPF 15** *($5.89)*; <u>Nu Skin USA</u> **Sunright Lip Balm 15** *($5.65 for 0.25 ounce)*; <u>Olay</u> **Color Moist Lipstick SPF 15** *($8.89)*; <u>Paula's Choice</u> **Total Protection Lip Care SPF 15** *($6.95 for 0.5 ounce)*; <u>Pevonia</u> **Botanica Sunblock Eye & Lip, SPF 15** *($17.25 for 0.5 ounce)*; and <u>Prescriptives</u> **Lavish Lipstick SPF 15** *($16)*.

# Best Facial Masks

    Although I am rarely a woman of few words, I'm not one to get too excited about facial masks. First, I feel quite comfortable stating that there are not many exciting, interesting, or particularly helpful facial masks to choose from. Many facial masks use clay as their main ingredient and then add thickening agents, water-binding agents, or plants (so you think you're getting something special), which isn't necessarily bad for skin, but isn't necessarily helpful either. What is most disturbing are the number of facial masks that add a host of irritating ingredients to the mix so the skin tingles and you feel that is doing something for the face—but all it's doing is causing damage. There are also an array of masks that use a plasticizing agent that is then pulled or peeled off the skin. These do impart a temporary soft feeling on the skin by pulling off a layer of skin, but that is hardly beneficial or lasting. Facial masks can be a pampering interval for women, but for good skin care, what you do daily is vastly more important than what you do once a week or once a month.

For normal to oily/combination and/or blemish-prone skin, the best masks are: Alpha Hydrox Purifying Clay Masque 4% AHA Facial Masque, for Normal to Oily Skin *($8.35 for 4 ounces)*; Amway Deep Cleansing Masque *($16.15 for 3.3 ounces)*; Arbonne Mild Masque *($17 for 5 ounces)*; Beauty Without Cruelty Purifying Facial Mask *($8.49 for 4 ounces)*; BeneFit Shrink Wrap Mask, For Combo/Oily Skin *($26 for 2 ounces)*; The Body Shop Honey & Oatmeal Scrub Mask for Dry Skin *($11.25 for 2.4 ounces)*; CamoCare Revitalizing Mask *($13.39 for 2 ounces)*; Circle of Beauty Pore Purge Clay Mask *($10.50 for 8 ounces)*; DDF Detoxification Mask *($22.50 for 2 ounces)*; Dermalogica Skin Refining Masque *($27.50 for 2.5 ounces)*; Estee Lauder So Clean Deep Pore Mask *($19.50 for 3.4 ounces)*; Freeman Cosmetics Avocado & Oatmeal Mineral Mud Mask *($2.85 for 6 ounces)*; Garden Botanika Skin Correcting Activated Charcoal Mask *($10 for 3.4 ounces)* and Desert Mud Mask *($7.50 for 2 ounces)*; Janet Sartin Skin Clarifying Mask with Green Tea *($25 for 1.7 ounces)*; Jason Natural Cosmetics Meditation Masque, Anti-Stress Aromatherapy, Soothing, and Refreshing Masque *($7.50 for 4 ounces)*; La Mer Refining Facial *($75 for 3.4 ounces)*; Murad Purifying Clay Masque *($22.50 for 2.25 ounces)*; Nu Skin USA Clay Pack *($13.60 for 2.5 ounces)*; Orlane B21 Oligo Vit-a-Min Vitalizing Masque *($32.50 for 1.7 ounces)*; Paula's Choice Oil-Absorbing Facial Mask Oily/Combination Skin *($9.95 for 6 ounces)*; philosophy stuck in the mud *($18 for 2 ounces)*; reflect.com Facial Mask for Combination Skin *($24 for 5 ounces)*; Vichy Purifying Thermal Mask *($19.95 for 50 ml)*; Yon-Ka Paris Masque 103, Purifying and Clarifying Clay Mask, for Normal to Oily Skin *($38 for 3.52 ounces)* and Masque 105, Oxygenating and Clarifying Clay Mask, for Dry or Sensitive Skin *($38 for 3.52 ounces)*.

For normal to dry and/or sensitive skin, the best masks are: Bioelements Restorative Clay Active Treatment Mask *($21.50 for 2.5 ounces)*; Biogime Refining Sea Mud *($36.95 for 5.5 ounces)*; The Body Shop Passion Flower Massage Mask *($11 for 3.5 ounces)*; Chanel Masque Lift Express *($32.50 for 2.6 ounces)* and Masque Force Hydratante *($28.50 for 2.6 ounces)*; Clarins Gentle Soothing Mask *($30 for 1.7 ounces)* and Extra Firming Facial Mask *($40 for 2.7 ounces)*; Clinique Skin Calming Moisture Mask *($18.50 for 3.4 ounces)*; Decleor Paris Timecare Mask *($34 for 1.69 ounces)*, Contour Mask for Eyes and Lips All Skin Types *($31 for 1 ounce)*, and

Moisturizing Creamy Face Mask for All Skin Types *($32 for 1.69 ounces)*; Dermalogica Intensive Moisture Masque *($32.50 for 2 ounces)* and MultiVitamin Power Recovery Masque *($35 for 2.5 ounces)*; Diane Young Moisture Lift Eye Mask *($29.75 for Age Eraser Eye Kit)*; Dr. Hauschka Moisturizing Mask *($33.95 for 1.1 ounces)*; Origins Drink Up 10 Minute Moisture Mask *($17.50 for 3.4 ounces)*; Estee Lauder So Moist Hydrating Mask *($19.50 for 3.4 ounces)*, Stress Relief Eye Mask *($27.50 for ten 0.4-ounce packets)*, and Triple Creme Hydrating Mask *($27.50 for 2.5 ounces)*; FACE Stockholm Sage and Aloe Mask All Skin Types *($18 for 2 ounces)*; Jafra Refreshing Moisture Mask for Dry and Dry to Normal Skin *($12.50 for 2.5 ounces)* and Soothing Results Cooling Yogurt and Honey Mask, for Sensitive Skin *($12.50 for 2.6 ounces)*; Janet Sartin Triple Performance Moisture Mask with Kalaya Oil *($25 for 1.7 ounces)*; La Prairie Cellular Moisture Mask *($65 for 1 ounce)*; Le Mirador Firming Eye Mask with Honey *($16 for 1 ounce)*; Marcelle Gentle Purifying Mask *($10.95 for 50 ml)*; Nicole Miller Skin Care Cellular Delivery Hydrating Mask *($24 for 4.2 ounces)*; Osmotics Facial Refining Masque *($30 for 2 ounces)*; Pevonia Lavandou Mask *($30.75 for 1.7 ounces)*; Phytomer Gentle Mask for Sensitive Skin *($31 for 1.7 ounces)*; Sothys Paris Beauty Mask for Normal to Combination Skin *($31 for 1.7 ounces)*; Sage Skin Care Gelloid Moisturizer and Masque *($40 for 4 ounces)*; Shiseido Benefiance Firming Massage Mask *($37 for 1.9 ounces)*; Shu Uemura Balancing Mask *($33 for 2.2 ounces)*; Tova Cactine Moisture Masque *($29.50 for 4 ounces)*; University Medical Skin Care Face Lift Deep Wrinkle Mask *($19.99 for 3.4 ounces)*; Yves Rocher A.D.N. Revitalizing Resource Energizing Mask, for Devitalized Skin *($16 for 1.7 ounces)*; Zia Natural Skin Care Super Moisturizing Mask for Normal, Sensitive, Dry & Mature Skin Types *($19.95 for 5 ounces)* and Ultimate Hydrating Mask *($24.95 for 3 ounces)*.

# Best Skin-Lightening Products

Only a small group of products fit into this category of effective skin-lightening treatments. The preponderance of evidence indicates that the best ingredient for effectively inhibiting melanin production is hydroquinone. Over-the-counter hydroquinone products are available in strengths of 1% to 2%, and higher concentrations are available from dermatologists and plastic surgeons. Some formulations include kojic acid, magnesium ascorbyl palmitate, mulberry extract, bilberry extract, and arbutin as alternatives. While all of those have been shown to inhibit melanin production to one degree or another, very few products contain enough of them to have an effect.

There are a handful of lines that do contain some amount of magnesium ascorbyl palmitate, a stable derivative of ascorbic acid (vitamin C). When used in a 10% concentration in a cream, magnesium ascorbyl palmitate was shown to inhibit melanin production. It has also been shown to have a protective effect against inflammation caused by UVB sun exposure. If you are curious to see if those products may be of help, please see the section under Best Moisturizers for products that contain a substantial amount of vitamin C.

Keep in mind that no skin-lightening product will work if an effective sunscreen is not used on a daily basis.

<u>For all skin types the best skin-lightening products are:</u> <u>Alpha Hydrox</u> Fade Cream *($8.99 for 3.5 ounces)*; <u>Avon</u> Banishing Cream Skin Lightening Treatment *($8.50 for 2.5 ounces)*; <u>Bioelements</u> Pigment Discourager *($18.50 for 0.5 ounce)*; <u>Black Opal</u> Advanced Dual Phase Fade Creme with Sunscreen *($11.95 for 1.75 ounces)* and Advanced Dual Complex Fade Gel *($11.95 for 0.75 ounce)*; <u>DDF</u> Fade Gel 4 *($42.50 for 1 ounce)* and Holistic Skin Lightener *($37.50 for 2 ounces)*; <u>Fashion Fair</u> Vantex Skin Bleaching Creme with Sunscreens *($14 for 2 ounces)*; <u>Givenchy</u> Whitening Concentrate *($48 for 1 ounce)*; <u>Glymed Plus</u> Derma Pigment Bleaching Fluid *($33.60 for 2 ounces)*; <u>Jan Marini Skin Research</u> Bioglycolic Even Tone Pigment Lightening Gel *($35 for 2 ounces)*; <u>M.D. Formulations</u> Skin Bleaching Gel with 2% Hydroquinone in a Base Containing 10% Glycolic Compound *($30 for 1.5 ounces)*; <u>Dr. Obagi</u> Nu-Derm Blender *($48 for 2 ounces)*; <u>Parthena</u> Skin Lightening Cream *($24.50 for 1 ounce)*; <u>Paula's Choice</u> Remarkable Skin Lightening Lotion for All Skin Types *($12.95 for 4 ounces)*; <u>Peter Thomas Roth</u> Potent Botanical Skin Brightening Gel Complex *($45 for 2 ounces)*, Potent Botanical Skin Brightening Lotion Complex *($45 for 2 ounces)*, Potent Skin Lightening Gel Complex *($50 for 2 ounces)*, Potent Skin Lightening Lotion Complex *($50 for 2 ounces)*, and Ultra Gentle Skin Lightening Gel Complex *($50 for 2 ounces)*; <u>Pevonia</u> Skin Care Radiance Lightening Gel *($33.75 for 1 ounce)*; <u>philosophy</u> when lightening strikes *($45 for 4 ounces)*; <u>Serious Skin Care</u> Lighten Up Skin Lightener *($15 for 2 ounces)*; <u>University Medical Skin Care</u> Face Lift Ultra Skin Lightener *($19.99 for 2 ounces)*; and <u>Zhen</u> Skin Lightening Cream *($25 for 1 ounce)*.

# *Best Self Tanners*

Because all self tanners use the exact same ingredient, dihydroxyacetone, to turn the skin brown, there is no way to differentiate one from another: they all perform essentially the same. Where self tanners do differ is in the amount of dihydroxyacetone they contain; however, there is no way for me to determine how much is actually in each product. Even if I could find out how much dihydroxyacetone was in a given formula, the way the skin can interact with the amount of the active ingredient varies so widely that there isn't any reliable way of telling how much is too much or too little, and whether that's either a positive or a negative thing. It all depends on your skin and, even more primarily, on your application technique. For more personal evaluations please visit the **Web site** at **www.sunless.com**; it is both an entertaining and informative look at dozens of self tanners.

# Best Foundations

Perhaps no area of makeup is more treacherous and just plain hard to get exactly right than finding the perfect foundation. The problems are many, but the most difficult to overcome are hopes for flawless-looking skin, perfect color choice, and silky-smooth texture that doesn't look too dry or too oily. Women want a foundation that fits like a second, secret skin but still provides coverage and camouflage, erases wrinkles, hides blemishes, and reflects a radiant look. That is no short order! Foundations have their limitations, and some women find that hard to accept and keep looking endlessly for the right one. For instance, some women make a personal quest of finding an oil-free foundation that will last into the evening. If you have oily skin, that just isn't possible without intermittent touch-ups during the day. Plus, selecting oil as the only nefarious ingredient is irrationally narrow. There are lots of ingredients that aren't an oil or oily but that are still notorious for clogging pores. Light-reflecting or "diffusing" foundations promise to diminish the appearance of wrinkles, and those claims are equally bogus. All it takes is one application to check out how impossible that is to achieve with a foundation. Indeed, there are lots of great foundations, but only some (certainly not all) of your high hopes can be fulfilled.

Choosing the right foundation color is not only time-consuming, it is exceedingly frustrating. **The only way to discover what fits is to apply the foundation on your skin, perhaps two different colors on either side of your face, and then to check it in the daylight. If the color isn't an exact match, you have to go back in and try again.**

The last hurdle is finding a pleasing texture, one that feels soft and silky but doesn't streak, cake, or look thick, and that takes experimentation too. Now tell me that isn't a challenge!

If you can splurge on only one product, foundation is it. This is the one area where spending a little bit more is the best option, not because expensive means better, but because it's just way too risky to buy a foundation you can't try on first.

<u>Beauty Note:</u> I feel strongly that pressed powder–style foundations are best for normal to slightly dry or slightly oily skin. Because these are a unique group of products to use as a foundation, and involve personal preference more than skin type, I've included them in a separate category. Also, most stick or cream-to-powder foundations are best for those with normal to slightly dry or slightly oily skin. The ingredients that keep those types of foundations in the their cream or stick form can be problematic for oily or blemish-prone skin and the powder part of these can be too drying for dry skin.

*Very Important Note: The foundations listed below with SPF do not necessarily have UVA-protecting ingredients. The foundations with effective sun protection (meaning they contain UVA-protecting ingredients and an SPF 15 or greater) have an asterisk before the product name.

For very oily skin, the best foundations are: Almay Amazing Lasting Sheer Makeup SPF 12 ($10.49); BeautiControl Color Freeze Liquid Makeup SPF 12 ($19.50); Black Opal True Color Liquid Foundation Oil Free ($6.99); The Body Shop Oil-Free Liquid Foundation SPF 8 ($12.50); Clarins Oil-Free Ultra Matte Foundation ($31); Clinique SuperFit Makeup ($18.50) and Stay-True Makeup Oil-Free Formula ($15.50); Fashion Fair Oil-Free Liquid ($17.50); Lancome Maquicontrole ($32.50) and Tient Idole ($32.50); Maybelline Great Wear Makeup ($6.39); Revlon *ColorStay Lite Makeup SPF 15 ($12.59); and SmashBox Studio Matte Oil-Free Foundation SPF 15 ($28) and Anti-Shine Foundation ($26).

For normal to oily/combination skin, the best foundations are: Avon Clear Finish Oil Free Foundation Anti Acne Treatment ($5.25); Amway Absolute Oil Control Foundation SPF 15 ($24.25); Awake Oil Free Foundation ($32); Biotherm Aqua Teint Mat Fluid Makeup ($19); Black Opal True Color Maximum Coverage Foundation ($8.39); Bobbi Brown Essentials Oil-Free Foundation ($35); Chanel Teint Lift Eclat SPF 8 ($50); Circle of Beauty Skin Image Soft Matte Makeup SPF 8 ($11.50) and On and On Flawless Cover Makeup ($11.50); Clinique Stay-True Makeup Oil-Free Formula ($15.50); Corn Silk Zero Shine Powder Makeup ($7.23); Cover Girl *Fresh Look Makeup Oil-Free SPF 15 for Combination to Oily Skin ($7.79) and CG Smoothers All Day Hydrating Makeup ($7.29); Elizabeth Arden Flawless Finish Mousse Makeup ($28) and Flawless Finish Complete Control Matte Makeup SPF 10 ($28); Erno Laszlo *Multi-pHase Oil Free Foundation SPF 15 ($30); Estee Lauder Enlighten Skin-Enhancing Makeup with SPF 10 ($27.50); FACE Stockholm Matte Foundation ($21); Flori Roberts Maximum Matte Souffle Oil-Free Makeup ($20); Iman Second to None Oil-Free Makeup SPF 8 ($16.50); Lancome Photogenic Makeup SPF 15 ($32.50); Laura Mercier Oil-Free Foundation ($38); M.A.C. Hyper Real Foundation ($24) and Studio Finish Matte Foundation SPF 8 ($19.50); Mary Kay Day Radiance Formula III Oil-Free for Oily and Combination Skin ($11); Maybelline Shine Free Oil Control Makeup ($3.99); NARS Oil Free Foundation ($30); Neutrogena Healthy Skin Liquid Makeup SPF 20 ($9.99); Olay All Day Moisture Foundation ($9.99); Origins Original Skin Some, More, and Most Coverage ($14.50 each); Paula Dorf Cosmetics Moisture Foundation Oil-Free ($34); Prescriptives Virtual Skin Oil Free SPF 10 ($30), 100% Oil Free Makeup SPF 15($30), and Invisible Finish Foundation SPF 15 ($29); Shiseido *Benefiance Enriched Revitalizing Foundation SPF 15 ($40); Shu Uemura *UV Liquid Foundation SPF 21 ($30); Tommy Hilfiger Set It Up

Oil-Free Foundation SPF 15 *($15)*; <u>Victoria's Secret Cosmetics</u> Liquid Lingerie Oil-Free Makeup SPF 10 *($17.50)*; <u>Vincent Longo</u> Water Canvas *($40)*; and <u>Zhen</u> Sheer Foundation with SPF 10 *($19.50)*.

For normal to dry skin, the best foundations are: <u>Alexandra de Markoff</u> Countess Isserlyn Matte Makeup *($47.50)*; <u>Amway</u> *Self-Defining Sheer Foundation SPF 15 *($22.45)*; <u>Aveda</u> Base Plus Balance *($20.50)* and *Moisture Plus Tint SPF 15 *($25)*; <u>Bath & Body Works</u> Fresh Face Liquid Makeup SPF 15 *($10)*; <u>BioTherm</u> Naturel Perfection Foundation with Fruit Extracts *($19)*; <u>Bobbi Brown</u> Essentials Moisturizing Foundation *($35)* and Essentials Fresh Glow Cream Foundation *($35)*; <u>The Body Shop</u> Everyday Foundation *($10)* and Skin Treat Foundation SPF 8 *($15)*; <u>Calvin Klein</u> *Sheer Foundation with SPF 20; <u>Cargo</u> Liquid Foundation *($22)*; <u>Circle of Beauty</u> Skin Image Dewy Moist Makeup SPF 8 *($11.50)*; <u>Clarins</u> Matte Finish Foundation *($31)*; <u>Clinique</u> *Almost Makeup SPF 15 *($16.50)*, Balanced Makeup Base *($14.50)*, and Soft Finish Makeup *($18.50)*; <u>Club Monaco</u> Oil-Free Foundation *($19)*; <u>Color Me Beautiful</u> Liquid Foundation *($16)*; <u>Cover Girl</u> CG Smoothers Tinted Moisturizer *($7.29)* and Continuous Wear Makeup *($7.39)*; <u>Darphin</u> Teint de Rose Foundation *($45)*; <u>Elizabeth Arden</u> Flawless Finish Hydro-Light Foundation SPF 10 *($30)* and Flawless Finish Smartwear Makeup SPF 15 *($28)*; <u>Erno Laszlo</u> Multi-pHase Light Diffusing Foundation SPF 15 *($30)*; <u>Estee Lauder</u> Lucidity Light-Diffusing Makeup SPF 8 *($27.50)* and Futurist Age-Resisting Makeup SPF 15 *($32.50)*; <u>FACE Stockholm</u> Liquid Foundation *($21)*; <u>Fashion Fair</u> Liquid Sheer Foundation *($12.50)*; <u>Jane</u> True to You Sheer Finish Foundation *($2.99)*; <u>La Prairie</u> *Cellular Treatment Foundation Satin SPF 15 *($60)* and *Cellular Treatment Creme Finish SPF 15 *($70)*; <u>Lancome</u> Photogenic Makeup SPF 15 *($32.50)*, MaquiLibre SPF 15 *($32.50)*, Maquivelours *($32.50)*, and Teint Optim' Age SPF 15 *($32.50)*; <u>Laura Mercier</u> Moisturizing Foundation *($38)*; <u>Lorac</u> Translucent Cream Makeup *($35)*; <u>L'Oreal</u> Visible Lift Line Minimizing Makeup SPF 12 *($12.29)*; <u>M.A.C.</u> Studio Finish Satin Foundation SPF 8 *($19.50)*, EPT Day Emulsion *($24)*, and *Sheer Coverage Foundation SPF 15 *($19)*; <u>Mary Kay</u> Day Radiance Formula II for Normal to Dry Skin SPF 8 *($11)*; <u>Maybelline</u> True Illusion Makeup SPF 10 *($6.39)*; <u>NARS</u> Balanced Foundation *($37)*; <u>Olay</u> *Complete Radiance Foundation SPF 15 *($13.99)*; <u>Prescriptives</u> Virtual Skin Oil Free SPF 10 *($30)*, Makeup + *($30)*, Custom Blend Foundation Oil Free *($55)*, and Custom Blend Foundation Moisturizing Formula *($55)*; <u>Revlon</u> Age Defying Makeup with SPF 10 *($11.98)* and *Age Defying All Day Lifting Foundation SPF 20 *($13.89)*; <u>Shiseido</u> Fluid Foundation *($30)*; <u>Shu Uemura</u> Foundation Fluide S SPF 8 *($26)* and Foundation Fluid N SPF 8 *($26)*; <u>Sisley</u> Transmat *($68)*; <u>SmashBox</u> Liquid Foundation *($28)*; <u>Sonia Kashuk</u> Perfecting Liquid Foundation *($9.99)*; <u>Stila</u> Complete Coverage *($40)* and Oil-Free Liquid Makeup *($30)*; <u>Tommy Hilfiger</u>

Set It Up Oil-Free Foundation SPF 15 *($15)*; Trucco Pro Coverage Opaque Foundation SPF 8 *($20.75)*; Ultima II *Beautiful Nutrient Nourishing Makeup SPF 15 *($21.50)* and Glowtion Skin Brightening Makeup *($17.50)*; Vincent Longo Water Canvas *($40)* and Dew Finish Liquid Canvas *($30)*; Yves St. Laurent Energie Teint Liquid Foundation SPF 12 *($46)*; and Zia Natural Skin Care Natural Foundation SPF 8 *($14.95)*.

For any skin type, the best sheer foundations (please note that some of these are repeated from the listings above for normal to dry skin) are: Almay Amazing Lasting Sheer Makeup SPF 12 *($10.49)*; Amway Self-Defining Sheer Foundation SPF 15 *($22.45)*; Awake Oil Free Foundation *($32)*; Bath & Body Works Fresh Face Liquid Makeup SPF 15 *($10)*; Bobbi Brown Essentials *SPF 15 Tinted Moisturizer *($35)*; Calvin Klein *Sheer Foundation with SPF 20 *($29)*; Dermalogica Treatment Foundation *($29)*; Elizabeth Arden Flawless Finish Mousse Makeup *($28)*; Jane True to You Sheer Finish Foundation *($2.99)*; M.A.C. EPT Day Emulsion *($24)*; NARS Gel Fraicheur *($30)*; Shiseido Vital Perfection Tinted Moisturizer SPF 10 *($26)*; Trish McEvoy Natural Tint Foundation Oil-Free *($35)*; and Zhen Sheer Foundation with SPF 10 *($19.50)*.

For extra dry skin, the best foundations are: Alexandra de Markoff Countess Isserlyn Creme Makeup *($47.50)*; Avon Face Lift Moisture Firm Foundation *($9)*; Chanel Teint Extreme Lumiere with Non-Chemical SPF 8 *($50)*; Circle of Beauty Advanced Formula Anti-Aging Makeup SPF 15 *($13.50)*; Clinique Soft Finish Makeup *($18.50)*; M.A.C. Sheer Coverage Foundation SPF 15 *($19)*; Mary Kay Day Radiance Formula I Foundation for Dry Skin SPF 8 *($11 for refill, $8 for compact)*; and NARS Balanced Foundation *($37)*.

For maximum coverage regardless of skin type, the best foundations are: Estee Lauder *Maximum Coverage with Non-Chemical SPF 15 *($25)*; and Dermablend Foundations *($14.50 to $23)*.

Best pressed-powder foundations (generally best for normal to slightly dry or slightly oily skin and best used as powder, not foundation) are: Amway Versatile Matte Pressed Powder Foundation *($18.20)*; Anna Sui Makeup Compact Powdery Foundation *($25 for powder, $8.50 for compact)*; Aveda Dual Base Minus Oil *($19.50 without compact, $30 with)*; Awake Fine Finish Foundation *($38 with compact, $28 refill, $4 for sponge)*; BeautiControl Perfecting Wet/Dry Finish Foundation *($20.50)*; BeneFit Sheer Genius *($26)*; The Body Shop All-in-One Face Base *($15; refills $11)*; Chanel Double Perfection Makeup SPF 8 *($42)*; Chantecaille Compact Makeup *($45)*; Christian Dior Teint Dior Poudre Foundation *($42.50; refills $29.50)*; Clarins Ultra Smooth Compact Foundation SPF 15 *($31)* and Compact Powder Foundation *($29.50)*; Clinique Super Powder Double Face Powder Foundation *($15.50)*; Color Me Beautiful Perfection Microfine Powder Foundation *($20)*;

Elizabeth Arden Flawless Finish Dual Perfection Makeup *($28)*; Erno Laszlo Multi-pHase Dual Option Foundation SPF 8 *($32)*; Estee Lauder Compact Finish Double Performance Makeup *($27.50)*; FACE Stockholm Powder Foundation *($24)*; Garden Botanika Natural Color Powder Plus *($12.50)*; Jane Iredale *Purepressed Base SPF 17 *($32.50)* and Global Shades *($32.50)*; La Prairie Cellular Treatment Powder Finish SPF 10 *($60)*; Lancome Dual Finish *($30)*; M.A.C. StudioFix Powder Plus Foundation *($21)*; Olay *Complete Radiance Compact Foundation SPF 15 *($13.99)*; Orlane Compact Cake Foundation, Dual Effect *($42.50)*; Paula's Select Soft Pressed Powder *($9.95)*; Shiseido Dual Compact Powdery Foundation *($30)* and *Sun Block Compact SPF 32 *($25)*; Shu Uemura *UV Powder Foundation SPF 26 *($30)*; SmashBox Wet/Dry Foundation *($32)*; Stila Illuminating Powder Foundation *($22 for powder, $20 for compact)*; T. Le Clerc Powder Compact Foundation *($45)*; Trish McEvoy Dual Powder *($28)*; Trucco Prepair Duo Powder Foundation *($21.50)*; Urban Decay Surreal Skin Makeup 4 in 1 Powder *($25)*; Youngblood Natural Mineral Cosmetics Compact Foundation *($32.50)*; and Zhen Dual Powder Foundation *($20)*.

Best cream-to-powder or liquid-to-powder foundations (generally best for normal to slightly dry or slightly oily skin) are: Awake *Hydro-Touch Foundation SPF 18 *($40 with compact; $30 for refills)*; Chantecaille Real Skin Foundation *($47)*; Christian Dior Teint Glace *($35)*; Clinique *City Base Compact Foundation SPF 15 *($20)*; Color Me Beautiful *Illusion Age Defying Foundation SPF 15 *($20)*; Iman Second to None Cream to Powder Foundation SPF 8 *($18.50)*; Jane Lightweight Liquid Powder *($2.38)*; L'Oreal Feel Naturale Compact Light Softening One Step Makeup *($12.29)*; Marcelle Dual Cream Powder Makeup *($11.95)*; Mary Kay Cream-to-Powder Foundation *($11 for refill, $8 for compact)*; Maybelline True Illusion Liquid to Powder Makeup SPF 10 *($5.99)*; Prescriptives *Photochrome Compact Makeup SPF 15 *($35)*; Revlon *Age Defying Makeup and Concealer SPF 20 *($13.89)*, *ColorStay Compact Makeup SPF 25 Nonchemical *($13.89)*, and *New Complexion One Step Makeup SPF 15 *($12.59)*; Shu Uemura *UV Cream Foundation SPF 31 *($30)*; Trish McEvoy Cream Powder Makeup *($40)*; and Ultima II Beautiful Nutrient Nourishing Compact Makeup SPF 12 *($23.50)*.

Best stick foundations (generally best for normal to slightly dry or slightly oily skin) are: Almay One Coat Light and Easy Makeup *($12.49)*; Aveda Cooling Calming Cover Sheer Face Tint *($18)*; Avon Hydra Finish Stick Foundation SPF 8 *($9)*; Bath & Body Works Fast Fix Makeup SPF 10 *($12)*; BeneFit PlaySticks *($30)*; Chantecaille New Stick SPF 8 *($38)*; Clarins Smartstick *($31)*; Clinique *City Stick SPF 15 *($20)*; Cover Girl Clean Makeup Sheer Stick Foundation *($7.49)*; Estee Lauder *Minute Makeup SPF 15 *($27.50)*; Lancome Stick Express Teint Idole Foundation *($32.50)*; Laura Mercier Foundation Stick to Go *($35)*; L'Oreal

Quick Stick Foundation *($11.49);* <u>Maybelline</u> *3 in 1 Express Makeup SPF 15 *($7.44);* <u>Olay</u> All Day Moisture Stick Foundation *($13.59);* <u>Prescriptives</u> *Matchstick Foundation SPF 15 *($35);* <u>Revlon</u> *ColorStay Stick Makeup SPF 15 *($13.89);* <u>Shiseido</u> Stick Foundation *($30);* <u>SmashBox</u> Foundation Stick *($28);* and <u>Trish McEvoy</u> Foundation Stick *($38).*

<u>Best cosmetic lines with foundations for very light skin tones are:</u> Alexandra de Markoff; Anna Sui Makeup; Avon; Awake; Chanel; Circle of Beauty; Corn Silk; Cover Girl; Elizabeth Arden; Erno Laszlo; Estee Lauder; Lancome; Laura Mercier; M.A.C.; NARS; Prescriptives; Revlon; Shu Uemura; SmashBox; Stila; Trish McEvoy; Victoria's Secret Cosmetics; Vincent Longo; and Zia.

<u>Best cosmetic lines with foundations for darker skin tones are:</u> Black Opal; Bobbi Brown Essentials; Circle of Beauty; Clinique; Cover Girl; Iman; M.A.C.; Mary Kay; Maybelline; NARS; Prescriptives; Tommy Hilfiger; Trish McEvoy; and Victoria's Secret Cosmetics.

# *Best Concealers*

Finding a good under-eye concealer is a task that has become a great deal easier since the last edition of this book. A concealer shouldn't be too dry or too creamy, should definitely not crease into the lines under the eye (this requirement cannot be ignored, particularly by those of us with an increasing number of under-eye lines), and should provide good, even coverage. I found some great concealers in all price categories. I also found a lot of concealers that are still too thick, too greasy, too peach, too pink, too dark, or too expensive. Here are the great ones.

<u>The best concealers for all skin types are:</u> <u>Almay</u> Amazing Lasting Concealer *($6.69),* Cover-Up Stick *($5.79),* Extra Moisturizing Undereye Cover Cream *($5.73),* Time-Off Age Smoothing Concealer *($6.69),* and Sensitive Care Concealer *($6.69);* <u>Aveda</u> Conceal Plus Protect *($13.50);* <u>Awake</u> Concealer *($18);* <u>Bath & Body Works</u> Imperfection Correction Creme *($7);* <u>Black Opal</u> Flawless Concealer *($3.89);* <u>The Body Shop</u> Liquid Concealer *($8.50);* <u>Calvin Klein</u> Concealer *($18);* <u>Chanel</u> Quick Cover *($32.50);* <u>Clinique</u> Quick Corrector *($10.50)* and Soft Conceal Corrector *($11.50);* <u>Club Monaco</u> Concealer *($11);* <u>Corn Silk</u> Liquid Powder Concealer *($4.29);* <u>Cover Girl</u> Invisible Concealer *($3.99);* <u>Estee Lauder</u> Smoothing Creme Concealer SPF 8 *($16)* and Double Wear Concealer SPF 10 *($16.50);* <u>Jafra</u> White Souffle Highlighter *($9);* <u>Lancome</u> Effacernes *($19.50)* and Maquicomplet *($19.50);* <u>L'Oreal</u> Feel Naturale Concealer *($7.49),* Hydra Perfecte Concealer SPF 12 *($6.39),* and Visible Lift Line Minimizing Concealer *($9.69);* <u>M.A.C.</u> Concealer SPF 15 *($11.50);* <u>Maybelline</u> Great Wear Concealer *($4.69)* and Undetectable Creme Concealer *($4.99);* <u>Paula's Select</u> No Slip Concealer *($6.95);* <u>Prescriptives</u> Camouflage Cream *($15);* <u>Principal Secret</u> Perfect Concealer SPF 8 *($15);* <u>Tommy Hilfiger</u>

Fixer Upper Concealer *($10)*; <u>Ultima II</u> WonderWear Concealer SPF 6 *($14.50)*; and <u>Zhen</u> Concealer *($10.50)*.

# *Best Powders*

While there is little variation among powder formulations, I can't muster much enthusiasm for the finishing powders available at the drugstore. Not that many of these aren't superior products, but more often than not there is no way to test the color. In regard to drugstore finishing powders, I made my suggestions based on what I think are the safest choices for the products with the best texture, but if you are inexperienced or haven't had luck finding the best color, trying on a powder is generally the best way to make a decision.

**Note:** The recommendations for skin type that follow are more interchangeable than you might think. Choosing a powder truly has more to do with your preference (what kind of finish you like), how much of the product you use, and what kind of foundation you wear.

<u>The best finishing powders (both loose and pressed) for all skin types (except very dry skin) are:</u> <u>Almay</u> Moisture Balance Pressed Powder for Normal to Combination Skin *($6.06)*, Moisture Balance Oil Control Oil Blotting Powder for Oily Skin *($7.19)*, Time Off Age Smoothing Pressed Powder *($9.19)*, Clear Complexion Light and Perfect Pressed Powder *($8.59)*, and Skin Stays Clean Powder *($10.98)*; <u>Amway</u> Loose Powder *($17.50)*; <u>Arbonne</u> Translucent Pressed Powder *($16)*; <u>Aveda</u> Pressed Powder Plus Antioxidants *($17.50 without compact, $29 with)* and Pure Finish Loose Powder Plus Antioxidants *($18)*; <u>Avon</u> Translucent Loose Powder *($8)* and Translucent Pressed Powder *($8)*; <u>bare escentuals</u> bareMinerals mineral veil *($18)* and pressed mineral veil *($18)*; <u>Bath & Body Works</u> Once Over Pressed Powder *($11.50)*; <u>BeautiControl</u> Loose Perfecting Powder *($10.50)* and Oil-Free Translucent Pressed Powder *($11.50)*; <u>Beauty for All Seasons/Norma Virgin Makeup</u> Line-Diffusing MicroPowder *($17.50)*; <u>BeneFit</u> Powder Tint *($22)*; <u>Black Opal</u> Oil Absorbing Pressed Powder *($6.99)* and Color Fusion Pressed Powder *($9.89)*; <u>Calvin Klein</u> Pressed Powder *($27)* and Loose Powder *($32)*; <u>Cargo</u> Pressed Powder *($22)*; <u>Chanel</u> Perfecting Pressed Powder *($38.50)* and Luxury Compact *($100)*; <u>Christian Dior</u> Poudre Diorlight Loose Powder *($42.50)*, Diorlight Pressed Powder *($35)*, and Poudre Plus Fine Loose Powder *($42.50)*; <u>Clinique</u> Blended Face Powder & Brush *($15.50)* and Stay Matte Sheer Pressed Powder Oil-Free *($15.50)*; <u>Club Monaco</u> Loose Powder *($19)* and Pressed Powder *($19)*; <u>Color Me Beautiful</u> Translucent Loose Powder *($13.50)*; <u>Cover Girl</u> CG Smoothers Fresh Look Pressed Powder Combination to Oily Skin *($5.59)*, CG Smoothers Fresh Look Pressed Powder Normal to Dry Skin *($5.59)*, and Clean Pressed Powder Normal Skin *($3.99 in regular or fragrance-free)*; <u>Erno Laszlo</u> Controlling Face Powder Loose *($28)*, Duo-

pHase Face Powder Loose *($28)*, Controlling Face Powder Pressed *($25)*, and Duo-pHase Pressed Powder *($25)*; <u>Estee Lauder</u> Enlighten Skin Enhancing Powder *($20)*, Double-Matte Oil-Free Loose Powder *($18.50)*, and Double-Matte Oil-Free Pressed Powder *($20)*; <u>FACE Stockholm</u> Loose Powder *($18)*; <u>Gale Hayman of Beverly Hills</u> Semi-Translucent Face Powder *($17)*; <u>Garden Botanika</u> Pressed Powder *($8.50)*; <u>Guerlain</u> Compact Powder for the Face *($50)*; <u>Iman</u> Luxury Loose Powder *($17.50)* and Luxury Pressed Powder *($18)*; <u>Janet Sartin</u> Dual Performance Compact Powder *($24)* and Face Powder Loose *($21)*; <u>Laura Mercier</u> Loose Setting Powder *($30)* and Pressed Setting Powder *($28)*; <u>Lancome</u> Poudre Blanc Neige *($28.50)*; <u>Lorac</u> Loose Powder *($28)* and Perfect Powder *($32 with compact, $24 refill)*; <u>L'Oreal</u> Visible Lift Line Minimizing Powder *($12.29)*; <u>M.A.C.</u> Studio Finish Face Powder *($17)*, Professional Face Powder *($22)*, Pressed Powder Compact *($18.50)*, and Blot Powder *($14.50)*; <u>Mary Kay</u> Powder Perfect Loose Powder *($12.50)* and Powder Perfect Pressed Powder *($7.50)*; <u>NARS</u> Pressed Powder *($24)* and Loose Powder *($30)*; <u>Neutrogena</u> Fresh Finish Loose Powder *($11.75)*, Fresh Finish Pressed Powder *($11.75)* and SPF 30 Pressed Powder *($14.29)*; <u>Olay</u> Pressed Powder *($9.99)*; <u>Origins</u> Original Skin Loose Powder *($17)* and Original Skin Pressed Powder *($17.50)*; <u>Paula's Select</u> Soft Pressed Powder *($9.95)*; <u>Paula Dorf Cosmetics</u> Pressed Powder *($25)*; <u>Prescriptives</u> Virtual Skin Pressed Powder *($23)*; <u>Revlon</u> New Complexion Powder Normal to Oily Skin *($11.49)*, Age Defying Smoothing Powder *($12.59)*, and Age Defying Pressed Loose Powder *($11.98)*; <u>Rimmel</u> Light Finish Compact Powder *($3.97)*; <u>R Pro</u> Pressed Powder *($7.99)* and Loose Powder *($8.99)*; <u>Shu Uemura</u> Face Powder *($25)*; <u>Sonia Kashuk</u> Dual Coverage Powder Foundation *($9.99)*, Bare Minimum Pressed Powder *($7.99)*, and Barely There Loose Powder *($7.99)*; <u>Stila</u> Loose Powder *($27)* and Pressed Powder *($32)*; <u>Tommy Hilfiger</u> Powder Up Pressed Powder *($15)*; <u>Trish McEvoy</u> Loose Powder *($20)* and All Over Face Powder*($28)*; <u>Trucco</u> Touch Up Pressed Powder *($15.50)* and Final Touch Loose Powder *($13.75)*; <u>Vincent Longo</u> Loose Powder *($30)*; <u>Wet 'n' Wild</u> Pressed Powder *($2.49)*; and <u>Zhen</u> Mosaic Powder *($25)*.

<u>The best finishing powders (both loose and pressed) for dry skin are:</u> <u>Alexandra de Markoff</u> Countess Isserlyn Loose Powdermist *($40)* and Countess Isserlyn Pressed Powdermist *($35)*; <u>Almay</u> Luxury Finish Loose Powder *($9.19)*; <u>Awake</u> Loose Powder *($28)*; <u>The Body Shop</u> Translucent Loose Powder *($10)* and Pressed Face Powder *($10)*; <u>Cargo</u> Loose Powder *($22)*; <u>Christian Dior</u> Poudre Plus Fine Pressed Powder *($35)*; <u>Clinique</u> Soft Finish Pressed Powder *($15.50)*; <u>Estee Lauder</u> Lucidity Translucent Loose Powder *($26)* and Lucidity Translucent Pressed Powder *($20)*; <u>Jafra</u> Translucent Face Powder *($12)* and Pressed Powder *($12)*; <u>Lorac</u> Translucent Touch Up Powder *($32)*; <u>Orlane</u> Translucent Powder *($35)*; <u>Prescriptives</u> Magic Liquid Powder *($30)*; <u>Rimmel</u> Stay Matte Pressed Powder *($2.97)*; <u>Shiseido</u> Natu-

ral Pressed Powder *($23.50)* and Rich Matte Film *($29)*; SmashBox Loose Powder *($28)* and Pressed Powder *($24)*; and Victoria's Secret Cosmetics Powdered Silk Finishing Powder *($15)*.

The best bronzing products are: Black Opal Color Fusion Bronzer *($9.49)*; Bobbi Brown Essentials Bronzing Stick *($28)* and Bronzing Powder *($26)*; The Body Shop Tinted Bronzing Powder *($11)* and Multi-Swirl Bronzer *($16.50)*; Bonne Bell Gel Bronze Face and Body Bronzer *($3.49)*, Cream Bronze Face Bronze *($3.49)*, and Powder Bronze *($3.49)*; Clinique Quick Bronze Tinted Self Tanner *($14.50 for 1.7 ounces)*; Club Monaco Bronzers *($21)*; FACE Stockholm Bronzer *($18)*; Models Prefer Makeup Bronzer with Spiral Brush and Bag *($27.50)*; Origins Sunny Disposition Liquid Bronzer *($15)* and Sunny Disposition Powder Bronzer *($17.50)*; Orlane Translucent Powder *($35)*; Revlon New Complexion Bronzing Powder *($11.59)*; and Wet 'n' Wild Bronzer *($2.79)*.

# Best Blushes

Blush is probably one of the easiest cosmetics to get right because it is hard to buy a bad blush. Not that there aren't some real losers out there, but there are far more winners. The problem with blush is usually application, and that is where good brushes come into play. Using the proper brushes is essential for getting blushes to go on correctly.

Blushes received high marks if most of the colors were matte; had a soft, nongrainy texture; blended on smoothly; did not fade or dissipate with time; and came in a good selection of colors. There are plenty that qualify, so don't spend a lot of money on blush unless you need to test the color first. Many drugstore blushes are of a superior quality and provide the same results as those at the department store.

The best powder blushes are from the following companies: Almay; Arbonne; Aveda; Awake; Bath & Body Works; BeautiControl; Black Opal; Bobbi Brown Essentials; The Body Shop; Calvin Klein; Cargo; Chanel; Chantecaille; Christian Dior; Circle of Beauty; Clarins; Clinique; Club Monaco; Color Me Beautiful; Cover Girl, Ecco Bella; Elizabeth Arden; Estee Lauder; FACE Stockholm; Fashion Fair; Garden Botanika; Guerlain; Iman; Jafra; Jane; Jane Iredale; Janet Sartin; Lancome; Lorac; L'Oreal; M.A.C.; Marcelle; Max Factor; Maybelline; Merle Norman; NARS; Neutrogena; Origins; Paula's Select; Paula Dorf Cosmetics; philosophy; Prescriptives; Prestige Cosmetics; Profaces; Revlon; Sears T.I.M.E.; Shiseido; Shu Uemura; Sisley; Sonia Kashuk; Tommy Hilfiger; Trish McEvoy; Ultima II; Victoria Jackson Cosmetics; Victoria's Secret Cosmetics; Vincent Longo; Wet 'n' Wild; and Zhen.

The best traditional cream blushes are: Alexandra de Markoff Outlasting Cream Blush *($31.50)*; Clarins Multi-Blush *($20)*; M.A.C. Cream Color Base *($14)*; Marcelle Cream Blusher *($9.25)*; Merle Norman Luxiva Creme Blush *($13.50)*; and Sonia Kashuk Beautifying Blush Cream *($7.99)*.

The best cream-to-powder or stick blushes are: Bobbi Brown Essentials Cream Blush Stick ($25); Cargo ColorTube ($24); Chanel Face Brights ($35); Estee Lauder Minute Blush Creme Stick For Cheeks ($25); Jane Sweet Cheeks Instant Blush ($2.99); Lancome Pommette ($24) and Couleur Flash Blush Stick ($27.50); Laura Mercier Cheek Color Stick To Go ($25); L'Oreal Quick Stick Face and Body Blush ($12.29); Paula Dorf Cheek Color Creme ($17); Prescriptives Mystick Swivel Stick Cream Blush ($25); Revlon Age Defying Cheek Color ($11.98); Trish McEvoy Lip & Cheek Pencils ($18.50) and Cream Blush Sticks ($32); Ultima II Nourishing Blush Stick ($17); Vincent Longo Creme Blush ($16); and Wet 'n' Wild Twist-Up Blush Stick ($1.99).

The best gel or gel-stick blushes are: Aveda Cooling Calming Cover Sheer Face Tint ($18); BeneFit BeneTint ($26); Cover Girl CG Smoothers Cheek Glaze ($5.99); L'Oreal Translucide Luminous Gel Blush ($9.25); NARS Color Wash ($24); Origins Pinch Your Cheeks ($10); and philosophy the supernaturals cheek, lip tint and lip lacquer ($15).

# Best Eyeshadows

By now many of you know my opinions about shiny as well as blue, green, or any brightly colored eyeshadow. It still is my goal to find the best matte shades available, and I am thrilled to say that the cosmetics industry does deliver (though the recent resurgence of shine has made finding these somewhat more difficult). However, there are more than enough matte shades available in all price ranges. You can shop both the drugstores and cosmetics counters and find wonderful textures and colors. You still have lots of shiny products to wade through—or to choose, if that's your preference.

The best eyeshadows can be found in the following lines: Arbonne; Aveda; Black Opal; Bobbi Brown Essentials; Clarins; Club Monaco; Elizabeth Arden; Estee Lauder; FACE Stockholm; Garden Botanika; Iman; Jane; Jane Iredale; Lancome; Laura Mercier; Lorac; M.A.C.; Origins; Paula's Select; Paula Dorf Cosmetics; philosophy; Physicians Formula; Prescriptives; Prestige Cosmetics; Principal Secret; Profaces; Rimmel; Shu Uemura; Sonia Kashuk; Stila; Tommy Hilfiger; Trish McEvoy; Ultima II; and Zhen.

# Best Eye and Brow Shapers

Some cosmetics companies sell two different eye pencils, one for the brow and the other for lining the eye. Other cosmetics companies are more straightforward and sell only one that does both jobs. That is the practical and honest approach. There is usually little to no difference between eye and brow pencils; the contrasts mainly involve color choice. When there is a difference, the brow pencil often has a drier consistency. That can make drawing on a brow difficult, though it does tend to look less greasy, so what you choose is a matter of personal preference and experimentation.

An eye pencil with a dry texture makes it difficult to line the eyelid after you've applied your eyeshadows; if the pencil is on the greasy side, it will line the lid more easily, but it is also more likely to smear under the lower lashes in a very short time. **I have always preferred (and still do) to line the eyes with regular eyeshadow powder and a small, thin eyeliner brush.** I usually line my lower lashes with a soft brown eyeshadow and my eyelid with a black or dark brown eyeshadow. You can also wet the brush and apply the eyeshadow as you would a liquid liner in a more vivid line. In fact, even when I line my eyes with a pencil, I go over it with an eyeshadow to make sure it has a better chance of staying all day. The difference in the look and in how long it lasts, compared with using a pencil alone, is amazing—particularly if you have oily or combination skin. If, however, the technique of lining your eyes with an eyeshadow and a tiny brush isn't for you and you prefer pencils, there are still many good ones. You can shop the more expensive lines, but it is a waste of money, because, regardless of the price, almost all the pencils I tested in all price ranges had more similarities than differences.

Eyebrow pencil has long been (and it still is) the standard method for making eyebrows appear thicker or more defined, but greasy pencils look overly made-up and dry ones are not that easy to apply and can still look thick and heavy. It is my strong recommendation that you fill in the brow with a powder, either an eyeshadow or a specific eyebrow powder.

Several companies sell colored eyebrow gels as a way to fill, lift, and define the brow. There are also a few companies that make a clear brow gel that isn't much different from using hairspray on a toothbrush and brushing it through the brow. For the most part, the natural-colored brow gels are great. I strongly recommend them as another way to make eyebrows look fuller but not artificial. If you can learn how to use the eyebrow gels, they can be a great alternative to pencils.

I did not list every brow or eye pencil because every line has its share of extremely standard but very good pencils, so there is no "best" due to their overwhelming equality. However, be aware that liquid liners, brow powders, and brow gels do differ.

<u>The best liquid or cake eye liners are:</u> <u>Alexandra de Markoff</u> Professional Secrets Liquid Eyeliner *($19)*; <u>Almay</u> I-Liner *($6.69)*; <u>Amway</u> Fine Liner *($13.45)*; <u>Chanel</u> Eyelines *($45)* and **Double Effect Eye Pencil** *($23.50)*; <u>Christian Dior</u> Diorliner *($30)*; <u>Cover Girl</u> Liquid Pencil Felt Tip Eyeliner *($5.29)*; <u>FACE Stockholm</u> Cake Eyeliner *($11)*; <u>Givenchy</u> Perfect Liquid Eyeliner *($24)*; <u>Jane</u> Express Lines Liquid to Powder Liner *($2.99)*; <u>Lip Ink</u> Eye Liner *($15)* and Brow Liner *($15)*; <u>Lord & Berry</u> Ink Well *($3.99)* and Liquid Liner *($4.99)*; <u>M.A.C.</u>

Creme Liner *($11)* and Liquid Liner *($15)*; <u>Prestige</u> Cosmetics Liquid Eyeliner *($4.49)*; <u>R Pro</u> Liquid Eyeliner *($4.99)*; <u>Revlon</u> Wet/Dry Eyeliner *($6.49)*; <u>Tommy Hilfiger</u> Retroliner Liquid Eyeliner *($10)*; and <u>Yves St. Laurent</u> Liquid Eyeliner *($25)*.

<u>The best eyebrow powders and pencils with a powder finish (but also refer to the list of matte eyeshadows as definite options for brow powders) are:</u> <u>Beauty for All Seasons/Norma Virgin Makeup</u> Natural Brow *($10.50)*; <u>The Body Shop</u> Eyebrow Powder Makeup *($8)*; <u>Chanel</u> Sculpting Brow Pencil *($25.50)*; <u>Clinique</u> Brow Shaper *($13.50)*; <u>FACE Stockholm</u> Brow Shadow *($16)*; <u>Hard Candy</u> Training Brow Compact *($28)*; <u>Lancome</u> Brow Artiste *($28)*; <u>Maybelline</u> Ultra-Brow Brush-On Brow Color *($3.39)*; <u>Merle Norman</u> Only Natural Brow Powder *($11)*; <u>Paula Dorf Cosmetics</u> Brow Duet *($20)*; <u>Revlon</u> Softstroke Powderliner *($6.79)*; Revlon ColorStay Brow Color *($8.19)*; <u>Stila</u> Brow Filler *($15)*; <u>Trucco</u> Hi-Brow Trio *($28)*; and <u>Zhen</u> Brow Duo *($10)*.

<u>The best brow gels are:</u> <u>Beauty for All Seasons/Norma Virgin Makeup</u> Controla Brow *($10.50)*; <u>Chanel</u> Brow Shaper *($28.50)*; <u>Christian Dior</u> Brow Gel *($16)*; <u>FACE Stockholm</u> Brow Fix *($12)*; <u>Garden Botanika</u> Brow Gel *($7.50)*; <u>Jane</u> Brow Beaters Tinted Brow Groomer *($2.99)*; <u>Lancome</u> Modele Sourcils Brow Groomer *($17.50)*; <u>M.A.C.</u> Brow Set *($11)*; <u>Merle Norman</u> Tinted Brow Sealer *($11)*; <u>Origins</u> Just Browsing *($12)* and Brow Fix *($12)*; <u>Paula Dorf</u> Perfect Brow *($12)*; <u>Paula's Select</u> Brow/Hair Tint *($7.95)*; <u>Revlon</u> ColorStay Brow Color *($8.19)*; <u>Trucco</u> Brow Shaper *($11)*; and <u>Zhen</u> Brow Set *($11)*.

## *Best Lipsticks and Lip Pencils*

Suffice it to say is that there are no bad lipsticks, there are no all-day lipsticks, and most lipsticks are truly great—it just depends on your color and texture preferences. There are a handful of products with decent to very good stains that have surprising staying power, but those still do not look or feel like lipstick. Almost without exception the greasier or glossier the lipstick, the less likely it is to last, and the more matte the lipstick, the longer it is likely to stick around, although if it is too matte it may be too drying. If you don't have a problem with dry lips and you want to try a matte look, mattes and ultra-mattes are certainly an option. It is very difficult to make lipstick suggestions. There are great discussions on the Web about the best lipstick and lip pencil, but this is one area where preference plays a bigger role than any other issue (and women change their impressions and selections all the time).

If you do want to use a lip gloss or a sheer glossy lipstick during the day, it would be best if the lipstick contained a good SPF with UVA protection.

All the lines in this book have great lipsticks, lip glosses, and lip pencils available that differ only in terms of color and slight texture variations. For the most part they all work great, with differences reflected only in terms of your personal preference rather than performance. Instead of listing every product or product line—which is virtually every company—I am only including a list of specialty lipstick products that are relatively unique. Just keep in mind that price has nothing to do with how well a lipstick performs.

The best matte lipsticks are: FACE Stockholm Matte Lipstick ($15); M.A.C. Mattes ($13.50); Paula's Select Soft Matte Lipstick ($6.95); and Zhen Matte Lipstick ($10).

The best ultra-matte lipsticks are: Almay Amazing Lasting Lip Color ($8.49); Clinique Superlast Cream Lipstick ($13.50); Jafra Always Color Stay-On Lipstick ($9.50); L'Oreal Colour Endure Stay On Lip Colour ($9.19); Maybelline Great Wear Budgeproof Lip Color ($4.74); reflect.com Long Lasting Lipstick ($12); and Shu Uemura Powder Lipstick Rouge ($27).

The best lipstains are: Lip Ink ($15) and Stila Lip Rouge ($26).

The best lip exfoliants to prevent chapped lips are: Adrien Arpel Freeze-Dried Protein Lip Peel and Salve ($39.50 for 1 ounce of peel and 0.25 ounce of salve); BeautiControl Lip Apeel ($16 for 1.25 ounces); and Paula's Choice Exfoliating Lip Treatment ($7.95 for 0.5 ounce).

## Best Mascaras

I am still surprised by how many good mascaras there are at both drugstores and department stores. In fact, I think they've improved all around. And excellent mascaras can be found in all price ranges. Obviously, it is foolish to buy the most expensive mascara when reasonably priced ones are equally good. Given that this is one product you can't readily test at the counters, try a few of the inexpensive ones I suggest and see what works for you. It really is the most sensible and beautiful decision.

The best mascaras are: Almay One Coat Mascara Lengthening ($6.69), One Coat Mascara Thickening ($6.69), Longest Lashes Mascara ($6.23), and The Insider ($6.85); Amway Smudgeproof Mascara 200 ($14.50); Anna Sui Makeup Mascara ($19); Awake Volumizing Mascara ($15); Bobbi Brown Essentials Defining Mascara ($16) and Thickening Mascara ($16); Chanel Instant Lash Mascara ($20), Sculpting Mascara Extreme Length ($20), and Extreme Length Fine Lashes ($20); Christian Dior Diorcil ($19), Fascination ($19), and Diorific ($22); Clarins Lengthening Mascara ($17); Clinique Naturally Glossy Mascara ($11), Full Potential Mascara ($11), and Supermascara ($11); Color Me Beautiful Lush Lash ($9.50); Cover Girl Super Thick Lash ($4.69) and Natural Lash Darkener ($4.69); Elizabeth Arden Defining Mascara ($16.50) and Natural Volume Mascara ($16.50); Erno Laszlo Multi-pHase Mascara ($19); Estee Lauder More Than Mascara ($16.50), Individualist Lash Building Mascara ($16.50), Futurist Mascara ($16.50), and Lash

Luxe *($25)*; <u>Givenchy</u> Makeup Mascara *($19)*; <u>Jane</u> Flashes Ultra-Rich Mascara *($2.99)*; <u>La Prairie</u> Cellular Treatment Intensified Mascara *($25)*; <u>Lancome</u> Definicils *($19)*, Immencils *($19)*, Intencils *($19)*, and Extencils *($19)*; <u>Lorac</u> Lashes *($17)*; <u>L'Oreal</u> Lash Out Extending Mascara *($6.69)*, Le Grand Curl *($7.39)*, and Voluminous Mascara *($6.69, straight or curved brush)*; <u>M.A.C.</u> Mascara S *($12)*, Mascara N *($12)*, and Mascara X *($12)*; <u>Max Factor</u> 2000 Calorie Mascara *($5.79)*, S-T-R-E-T-C-H Mascara *($5.79)*, and Lash Enhancer No. 1 Mascara *($5.79)*; <u>Maybelline</u> Illegal Lengths Mascara *($4.29)*, Volum' Express Mascara *($3.29; regular or curved brush)*, and Full N' Soft Mascara *($6.39)*; <u>Olay</u> Beauty Mascara *($5.99)*; <u>Origins</u> Fringe Benefits Mascara *($12)*; <u>Paula's Select</u> Lush Mascara *($6.95)* and Epic Lengths Mascara *($6.95)*; <u>Paula Dorf Cosmetics</u> Mascara *($14)*; <u>Physicians Formula</u> Eyebrightener Mascara *($4.84)*; <u>Revlon</u> Lashfull Mascara *($6.79)*, Everylash Mascara *($6.69)*, and ColorStay Extra Thick Lashes Mascara *($6.99)*; <u>Rimmel</u> Extra Super Lash Mascara *($1.97)* and Exaggerate Mascara *($3.97)*; <u>Shu Uemura</u> Mascara Basic *($27)*; <u>SmashBox</u> Mascara *($14)*; <u>Sonia Kashuk</u> Lashify Mascara *($5.99)*; <u>T. Le Clerc</u> Mascara *($19)*; <u>Tommy Hilfiger</u> Big Deal Volumizing Lash Color *($10)*; <u>Tony & Tina</u> Herbal Eye Mascara *($18)*; <u>Trish McEvoy</u> Mascara *($16)*; <u>Ultima II</u> WonderWear Mascara *($13)* and LashFinder Mascara *($11)*; <u>Victoria Jackson Cosmetics</u> Dual Black Mascara *($8.50; $13.95)* and Mascara *($14.95)*; <u>Wet 'n' Wild</u> MegaWink Lash Curling Mascara *($1.89)*; and <u>Yves St. Laurent</u> Mascara Moire *($22.50)*.

<u>The best waterproof mascaras are:</u> <u>Bobbi Brown Essentials</u> Lash Lustre Waterproof Mascara *($16)*; <u>Chanel</u> Extreme Wear Waterproof Mascara *($20)*; <u>Clinique</u> Gentle Waterproof Mascara *($11.50)*; <u>Cover Girl</u> Professional Waterproof Mascara *($2.61)*; <u>Elizabeth Arden</u> Two-Brush Mascara Regular & Waterproof *($16.50)*; <u>Lancome</u> Aquacils *($19)* and Eternicils *($19)*; <u>L'Oreal</u> Voluminous Waterproof Mascara *($6.69)* and Le Grand Curl Waterproof Mascara *($7.39)*; <u>Max Factor</u> 2000 Calorie Aqualash Mascara *($5.79)*; <u>Maybelline</u> Volum' Express Waterproof Mascara *($3.29)*, Illegal Lengths Waterproof Mascara *($4.29)*, Great Lash Waterproof Mascara *($2.19)*, and Full N' Soft Waterproof Mascara *($3.99)*; <u>Merle Norman</u> Waterproof Mascara *($12.50)*; <u>Revlon</u> ColorStay Waterproof Mascara *($6.99)*; <u>Shiseido</u> Waterproof Mascara *($18)*; and <u>Vincent Longo</u> Waterproof Mascara *($16)*.

## Best Brushes

More than ever before, professional-sized brushes are available in all price ranges. Keep in mind that the texture of the brush is more important than the source of the bristles. While many cosmetics companies love bragging about the type of animal hair used, you are not buying a mink coat. What counts is softness and firmness, no matter where it comes from.

<u>The best assortments of brushes are from the following companies:</u> Aveda;

bare escentuals; Bath & Body Works; BeneFit; Bobbi Brown Essentials; Cargo; Chanel; Club Monaco; Elizabeth Arden; FACE Stockholm; Garden Botanika; Jane Iredale; J.C. Penney Professionals; La Prairie; Laura Mercier; Lorac; M.A.C.; Mary Kay; Mojave Magic; NARS; Origins; Paula's Select; Paula Dorf Cosmetics; Prescriptives; Prestige Cosmetics; Profaces; R Pro; Sephora; Shu Uemura; Sisley; Sonia Kashuk; Stila; Tony & Tina; Trish McEvoy; Trucco; Urban Decay; Victoria's Secret Cosmetics; and Zhen.

## *Best Specialty Products*

This is a list of miscellaneous products that have interesting effects that just don't fit in the above categories. For more details please refer to Chapter Three for the reviews for these products.

Christian Dior Highlights for Hair *($19.50)*

Lancome Touche Optim' Age *($22.50 for 0.52 ounce)*

M.A.C. Matte Creme Matifiance *($16.50)*

MetroGel, MetroLotion, and MetroCream *(prescription only)*

philosophy the coloring book *($160)*

Prescriptives Magic Invisible Line Smoother *($35 for 0.5 ounce)*

Rejuveness *($39.50 to $295, depending on the size ordered)*

Trish McEvoy Face Planners *($35 to $45 for the case; $12 to $14 for the pages)*

# Appendix

## *Cosmetic Ingredient Dictionary*

Almost all of my comments regarding the efficacy of the plant extracts used in products throughout this edition and in the following list were based on information listed in the Information Resource section at the end of this book.

**Note.** Repeatedly in the literature regarding research or studies for plant extracts, you will find the constant reminder that efficacy is dependent on the part of the plant being used (stems, for example, may have very different contents and benefits than the leaf), the time of year plants are collected, the type of extraction or preservation methods used, and the amount of the extract applied. The cosmetics industry has no standards for any of these concerns.

Another frequent reminder found in trustworthy sources is that much of the information about plant extracts, when it pertains to their use and efficacy, is anecdotal, meaning without substantiation, proof, or information about interaction with other substances.

When valid studies and research do exist for various plant extracts, it is important to realize that all of the comments regarding efficacy are the outcome of research that examined a pure concentrate or a pure tincture (a plant substance in an alcohol solution). There are few studies for any plant extracts with respect to their use when mixed into a cosmetic at fractional amounts.

<u>All of the following comments relate to external application only. Oral, systemic benefits for the plant extracts or vitamins listed can be very different from those for topical application. For oral, systemic benefits, please refer to www.drweil.com or the Web sites listed below.</u>

Cosmetic formulations are very hard to understand by just reading listings of ingredients. Although ingredient listings impart a great deal of information, having some knowledge about formulary standards is also crucial. I have spent years working with cosmetic formulators and reading the research about how products are formulated and how the actual substances (in myriad combinations) are created. My strong suggestion is to use this dictionary to help you understand the significance of an ingredient in terms of a product's claims and potential for irritation.

For a specific condition, like clogged pores, the actual formulation preference and potential for helping the problem is very hard to discern from an interpretation of a formula. Your best approach for determining a product's chance of causing breakouts is how thick it is and how emollient (rich) it feels. The thicker a product, the more likely that the thickening/emollient ingredients it contains could find their way into a pore and cause problems. The lighter in weight a product is (as long as it doesn't contain irritating ingredients), the far less likely it is to cause problems.

*Acacia senegal.* An herb that can have anti-inflammatory properties but is primarily a thickening agent. *See* **gums.**

**acetic acid.** An acid found in vinegar, some fruits, and human sweat. It can be a potent skin irritant and drying to skin, though it also has disinfecting properties.

**acetone.** A strong solvent that removes nail polish.

**acetyl glucosamine.** An amino acid sugar and the primary constituent of **mucopolysaccharides** and **hyaluronic acid.** It is an agent that has good water-binding properties for skin. In large concentrations it can be effective for wound healing. There is research (*Cellular-Molecular-Life-Science*, 1997 Feb; 53(2): 131–40) showing that chitins (chitosan—which is comprised of acetyl glucosamine) can help wound healing in a complex process. That is a few generations removed from the tiny amount of acetyl glucosamine being used in cosmetics, and wrinkles are not related to wounds.

**acetyl glyceryl ricinoleate.** *See* **glyceryl esters.**

**acetylated castor oil.** *See* **glyceryl esters.**

**acetylated hydrogenated cottonseed glyceride.** *See* **glyceryl esters.**

**acetylated lanolin.** An emollient derived from lanolin. Considered to be less of an allergen than pure lanolin.

**acetylated palm kernel glycerides.** *See* **glyceryl esters.**

*Achillea millefolium.* *See* **yarrow extract.**

**acid.** Anything with a pH lower than 7—above 7 is alkaline. Water has a pH of 7. Skin has an average pH of 5.5.

**acrylates.** *See* **film former.**

**acrylates/C10-30 alkyl acrylate crosspolymer.** *See* **film former.**

**active ingredients.** The part of an ingredient label regulated by the FDA. The amount and exact function of each active ingredient is controlled and must be approved by the FDA. Active ingredients include such substances as sunscreen ingredients, skin lightening agents, and benzoyl peroxide.

*Aesculus hippocastanum.* *See* **horse chestnut.**

**agar.** *See* **algae.**

**age spot.** There is no such thing as an "age spot." The skin can develop brown patches for many reasons, but the small characteristic ones on the hands, arms, and face are caused by sun damage. These are possibly indications of precancerous conditions and should be watched carefully for changes.

**AHAs.** Ingredients extracted from various plant sources or milk. However, 99% of the AHAs used in cosmetics are synthetically derived. In low concentrations (less than 3%) these work as water-binding agents. At over 4% and in a pH of 3 to 4, these can exfoliate skin cells by breaking down the substance in skin that holds skin cells together. The most effective and well-researched AHAs are glycolic acid and lactic acid. Malic acid, citric acid, and tartaric acid may also be effective but are considered less stable and less skin friendly. AHAs may irritate mucous membranes and cause irritation. *See also* **BHA**.

**ahnfeltia extract**. *See* **sea kelp**.

**albumin**. Found in egg white and can leave a film over skin.

*Alchemilla vulgaris*. Constricts skin which can cause irritation.

**alcloxa**. More technically known as aluminum chlorhydroxy allantoinate. It has constricting properties that can be irritating for skin.

**alcohol**. Organic compounds that have a vast range of forms and uses in cosmetics. In some benign forms they are glycols used as humectants and help deliver ingredients into skin. When fats and oils (*see* **fatty acids**) are chemically reduced, they become a group of less-dense alcohols called **fatty alcohols** that can have emollient properties or become detergent cleansing agents. When alcohols have low molecular weights they can be drying and irritating. The alcohols to be concerned about in skin-care products are ethanol, denatured alcohol, ethyl alcohol, methanol, benzyl alcohol, isopropyl, and SD alcohol. These can be extremely drying and irritating to skin.

**alfalfa extract**. Can be an antioxidant in skin-care products.

**algae**. Very simple chlorophyll-containing organisms with more than 20,000 different known species. A variety of algae are used in cosmetics as thickening agents, water-binding agents, and antioxidants.

**algin**. Brown algae. *See* **algae**.

**alginic acid**. Obtained by treating dry seaweed with acid to create a very thick, gelatin-like substance. It is used as a thickening agent in cosmetics.

**aliphatic hydrocarbon**. A hydrocarbon contained in natural gas and mineral oils. It is a synthetic fluid with varying properties that range from solvent to slip agent. *See* **solvent** and **slip agents**.

**alkaline**. Anything with a pH higher than 7—above 7 is alkaline. Water has a pH of 7. Skin has an average pH of 5.5.

**alkyloamides**. Identified on skin-care labels as **DEA** and **MEA**. These are used primarily for their foaming ability in shampoos, but they can also be used as thickening or binding agents. Because alkyloamides contain a free amine that can combine with specific types of preservatives in cosmetics, there is concern that they may form carcinogens.

**allantoin**. A by-product of uric acid extracted from urea and considered an effective anti-irritant.

**all-trans-retinoic acid.** *See* **Retin-A.**

**almond oil PEG-6 esters.** *See* **glyceryl esters.**

**almond oil.** An oil extracted from the seeds of almonds and used as an emollient.

*Aloe barbadensis. See* **aloe vera.**

**aloe extract.** *See* **aloe vera.**

**aloe juice.** *See* **aloe vera.**

**aloe vera.** Has been shown to have anti-irritant and soothing properties; however, aloe is an unstable ingredient and these benefits are best obtained from the fresh plant or a refrigerated pure-aloe product stored in a tightly capped dark glass bottle.

**alpha bisabolol.** *See* **bisabolol.**

**alpha hydroxy acid.** *See* **AHAs.**

**alpha lipoic acid.** An enzyme that applied topically on skin can be a very good antioxidant.

*Althaea rosea. See* **mallow.**

**althea extract.** *See* **mallow.**

**alumina.** Aluminum oxide, used as an abrasive, thickening agent, and absorbent in cosmetics.

**aluminum chlorohydrate.** A salt used in antiperspirant preparations. It can be extremely irritating on abraded skin.

**aluminum magnesium silicate.** *See* **kaolin.**

**aluminum silicate.** *See* **kaolin.**

**aluminum starch (octenylsuccinate).** A powdery thickening agent and absorbent that can be a skin irritant and cause contact dermatitis.

**amino acids.** Proteins are comprised of amino acids. In skin-care products, these types of ingredients, of which there are many, work as water-binding agents. *See also* **protein.**

**aminobutyric acid.** An amino acid that has water-binding properties for skin and may be an anti-inflammatory. It supposedly also increases growth hormone when taken orally, but the only support for this is a single obscure study that was conducted more than two decades ago in fewer than 20 subjects, and the results have yet to be replicated by other scientists.

**aminomethyl propanediol.** Used to adjust pH in cosmetics.

**ammonium chloride.** An alkaline salt used as a pH balancer in skin-care products; it is not used in concentrations that would be problematic for skin.

**ammonium laureth sulfate.** Can be derived from coconut; it is used primarily as a detergent cleansing agent and is considered to be gentle and effective.

**ammonium lauryl sulfate** Can be derived from coconut; it is used primarily as a detergent cleansing agent and is considered to be gentle and effective.

**amodimethicone.** *See* **silicone.**

**amyris oil.** *See* **sandalwood.**

**andiroba oil.** Extracted from the Brazilian mahogany tree; it has anti-inflammatory properties.

**angelica:** A potential skin irritant, though it can have antibacterial properties on skin.

**anise.** Can have antibacterial properties, but its fragrant component makes this a potential skin irritant.

**annato extract.** A natural plant colorant derived from the flesh surrounding the seed of *Bixa orellana,* a shrub native to South America, producing yellow-orange tones.

*Anthyllis vulneraria.* A member of the legume family; can impart fragrance, and may also constrict the skin, which can cause irritation.

**antibacterial.** Any ingredient that destroys or inhibits the growth of bacteria, particularly in the case of those causing blemishes.

**anti-inflammatory.** Any ingredient that reduces certain signs of inflammation, such as swelling, tenderness, fever, and pain.

**antioxidant.** Any ingredient that can reduce the harmful effects of oxygen, sunlight, or other sources of free-radical cellular damage. However, there is no evidence that antioxidants can prevent wrinkling; their primary effect on skin seems to be their ability to reduce inflammation and irritation. Antioxidants include many plant extracts, vitamins, and synthetic ingredients.

**aorta extract.** Obtained from hearts of animals. It is supposed to have rejuvenating properties for skin, but this has never been proven in research of any kind. Much like any part of a human or animal body, the heart tissue is a source of proteins, amino acids, and other water-binding agents for skin.

**apple cider vinegar.** *See* **vinegar.**

**apricot kernel oil.** An emollient plant oil pressed from the seeds of apricots, and similar to other nonvolatile plant oils.

**apricot kernel.** A seed that, especially when finely ground, is a natural exfoliant.

**arachidic acid.** Derived from peanut oil and used as an emollient and thickening agent in cosmetics.

**arachidonic acid.** Produced from phospholipids and fatty acids. There is research pointing to it being potentially unsafe when used topically, though more research is needed to decide this conclusively.

**arachidyl alcohol.** A waxy substance used as a thickening agent and emollient in cosmetics.

**arachidyl propionate.** A waxy substance used as a thickening agent and emollient in cosmetics.

*Arachis hypogaea extract.* Commonly known as the peanut. It can have emollient and anti-inflammatory properties for skin.

**arbutin.** A naturally occurring form of **hydroquinone**, which can suppress melanin production, though this has only been shown in vitro.

*Arctium lappa. See* **burdock root.**

**arginine.** An **amino acid** effective as a water-binding agent.

**arnica extract.** It is repeatedly stated in all of the herbal journals mentioned in the Appendix that arnica should not be applied to unbroken skin. *The PDR Family Guide to Natural Medicines & Healing Therapies* says: "Repeated contact with cosmetics containing arnica can cause itching, blisters, ulcers, and dead skin." It can increase blood flow to areas where it is applied.

**arrowroot.** A thickening agent; it has no known benefit for skin.

*Artemesia vulgaris. See* **mugwort extract.**

**artichoke extract.** Contains tannins that can constrict skin and cause irritation with repeated application.

*Ascophyllum nodosum.* A form of seaweed. *See* **algae.**

**ascorbic acid.** A form of vitamin C considered to be unstable in solution and that can also cause skin irritation.

**ascorbyl palmitate.** A form of vitamin C and considered a good antioxidant.

**asparagine.** An **amino acid.**

*Asparagopsis armata extract.* A form of seaweed. *See* **algae.**

**aspartic acid.** An **amino acid.**

*Avena sativa.* The oat plant; oat extract can have some anti-irritant properties. *See also* **oatmeal.**

**avobenzone.** Sunscreen ingredient that can protect against the entire range of UVA rays.

**avocado oil.** An emollient oil similar to other nonvolatile plant oils.

**awapuhi.** A plant from the ginger family; it can be a skin irritant.

**azelaic acid.** The active ingredient in a prescription drug called Azelex, and some over-the-counter products. It is often prescribed for acne due to its exfoliating and disinfecting properties and also for skin lightening. It is derived from *Pityrosporum ovale,* a form of yeast. It is considered a weak skin-lightening agent, though it can compare to **hydroquinone** when combined with high concentrations of glycolic acid.

**azuki beans.** Used as abrasives in scrub products.

**azulene.** A chamomile extract used primarily as a coloring agent in cosmetics.

**babassu oil.** A plant oil that can have emollient properties for skin.

*Bacillus subtilis.* A bacterium that is used as a fungicide on plants and has some medical benefits when taken orally, though there is no known benefit when applied to skin.

**balm mint extract.** A fragrant plant that poses some risk of irritation. It also has some reported antibacterial and antifungal properties. Claims that it can help heal wounds are not substantiated.

**barium sulfate.** An earth mineral used as a whitening agent in cosmetics. It can be a skin irritant.

**bay leaf oil.** Considered a potent skin irritant and should never be applied directly to skin.

**bearberry extract.** Has antibacterial properties for skin. It also contains **arbutin**. Arbutin can inhibit melanin production, though this has only been shown in vitro. However, the amounts of bearberry extract used in skin-care products are unlikely to affect skin or melanin.

**bee pollen.** Can be a good antioxidant, but there is no reported value for topical application.

**beeswax.** A substance made by bees to build the walls of their hives. It is a thickening agent and has some emollient properties.

**behenic acid.** A **fatty acid** used as a thickening agent and **surfactant**.

**behenyl alcohol.** A thickening agent used in cosmetics. It is not related to irritating forms of alcohol.

**bentonite.** A claylike material used as an absorbent in cosmetics. It can be drying and irritating to skin.

**benzoic acid.** A preservative used in skin-care products; it is considered to be less irritating than other forms of preservatives.

**benzoin extract.** A balsam resin that has some disinfecting and fragrant properties, and may be a skin irritant.

**benzophenones.** Used in cosmetics as sunscreen agents to protect mostly from UVB radiation.

**benzothonium chloride.** Used as a preservative in cosmetics. It is generally considered to be less irritating than other forms of preservatives.

**benzoyl peroxide.** An antibacterial agent primarily effective for killing the bacteria that cause blemishes. It can be drying or sensitizing for some skin types.

**benzyl alcohol.** *See* **alcohol**.

**bergamot.** A volatile oil extracted from the bergamot orange. It can have antibacterial properties, but is used primarily for fragrance and can be a skin irritant. *See* **volatile oils**.

**beta glucan.** Can be derived from **yeast**. It is a polysaccharide, meaning a sugar (such as starch and cellulose), and considered a good water-binding agent and antioxidant.

**beta hydroxy acid.** *See* **salicylic acid**.

**beta-carotene.** A potentially good antioxidant, although recent research published in the *Journal of the American Medical Association* has called this into question.

*Betula alba.* *See* **birch bark**.

**BHA.** The abbreviation for butylated hydroxyanisole, a synthetic, potent antioxidant. BHA in this form should not be confused with beta hydroxy acid (**salicylic**

**acid**), an exfoliant. Salicylic acid is abbreviated as BHA but it would never be shown that way on an ingredient list.

**BHT.** Butylated hydroxytoluene, a synthetic, potent antioxidant.

**bifida ferment lysate.** A bacteria found in the digestive system. It has no known effect on skin.

**bilberry extract.** Can dilate blood vessels and potentially may cause surfaced capillaries to appear more noticeable. Some naturopathic medicine claims that when taken internally bilberry is supposed to strengthen capillary walls to prevent leakage, but this is not supported by research.

**bioflavinoids.** *See* flavonoids.

**biotin.** Part of the B-complex vitamins. It has no reported topical benefit for skin.

**birch bark.** Comes from the plant *Betula alba,* also called white birch. It can have astringent properties, which makes it a potential irritant for skin.

**birch leaf extract.** *See* birch bark.

**bisabolol.** Can be derived synthetically or extracted from chamomile. It is an anti-irritant.

**bis-diglyceryl polyacyladipate-1.** *See* glyceryl esters.

**bis-diglyceryl polyacyladipate-2.** *See* glyceryl esters.

**black currant oil.** *See* gamma linoleic acid.

**black pepper oil.** Can cause inflammation and irritation to skin.

**bladderwrack extract.** Has a tightening, drying effect on skin and can be a skin irritant.

**bloodroot.** Is a potent skin irritant.

**bloodwort.** *See* yarrow extract.

*Bora cocos. See Poria cocos.*

**borage extract.** Can have anti-irritant, anti-inflammatory properties.

**borage oil.** Can have anti-irritant properties. *See* gamma linoleic acid.

**borates.** According to *A Consumer's Dictionary of Cosmetic Ingredients,* 5th edition, boric acid is still being used despite warnings about toxicity and severe irritation.

**boric acid.** According to *A Consumer's Dictionary of Cosmetic Ingredients,* 5th edition, boric acid is still being used despite warnings about toxicity from the American Medical Association.

**boron nitride.** An earth mineral that has antibacterial properties. It can also be a skin irritant.

*Boswellia carterii. See* frankincense extract.

**boxwood extract.** Can have constricting properties, which makes it a skin irritant.

**brewer's yeast.** A good antioxidant but can be a skin irritant.

**broad spectrum.** Meant to refer to a sunscreen's ability to protect the skin from both UVA and UVB rays from the sun. This term is not regulated by the FDA, so a cosmetic can make this claim when the product does not actually provide adequate broad-spectrum protection.

**bromelain.** An enzyme found in pineapple. Like all enzymes (papain and other proteases), bromelain breaks down the connecting structure that holds surface skin cells together, which creates exfoliation but can also cause irritation.

**bronopol.** A preservative used in minuscule amounts in cosmetics to prevent contamination.

*Bupleurum falcatum* **extract.** Can have anti-inflammatory properties.

**burdock root.** Has been shown to have antibacterial and anti-inflammatory benefits and is also a good antioxidant.

**butcher's broom extract.** Has anti-inflammatory properties.

**butcher's broom.** Can have anti-inflammatory properties for skin.

**butyl acetate.** A solvent used in nail polish and many other products.

**butylene glycol.** *See* **propylene glycol**.

**butyl methoxydibenzoymethane.** *See* **avobenzone**.

**butylparaben.** *See* **parabens**.

*Buxus sempervirens.* *See* **boxwood extract**.

**C10-18 triglycerides.** *See* **glyceryl esters**.

**C12-15 alkyl benzoate.** Used as an emollient and thickening agent in cosmetics.

**C12-18 acid triglyceride.** *See* **glyceryl esters**.

**C18-36 acid triglyceride.** *See* **glyceryl esters**.

**cabbage rose extract.** A highly fragrant substance that can be a skin irritant.

**caffeine.** A substance with a high tannin content, which constricts skin and can cause irritation. When consumed in coffee, caffeine can be a strong diuretic, but there is no evidence that this effect can take place when caffeine is applied to skin (so it would not have the effect of "flushing" away fluid in tissues around the eyes that can accumulate as you sleep).

**calcium carbonate.** Chalk; is used as an absorbent in cosmetics.

**calcium silicate.** *See* **silicate**.

**calendula extract.** Commonly known as marigolds; it has been shown to have antibacterial properties, but can be a skin irritant.

*Calophyllum tacamahaca.* A plant oil that has emollient and anti-irritant properties.

*Camellia sinensis.* *See* **green tea**.

**camphor.** Can cause skin irritation and dermatitis with repeated use.

**cananga extract.** A fragrance used in cosmetics; it can be a skin irritant, much like ylang-ylang.

*Cananga odorata.* *See* **ylang-ylang**.

**candelilla wax.** Derived from candelilla plants; used as a thickening agent and emollient to give products such as lipsticks or stick foundations their form.

**caprylic/capric triglyceride.** Derived from coconut, and considered to be good emollient and thickening agents in cosmetics.

**capsicum oleoresin.** A fatty resin derived from capsicum. It can be a skin irritant and should not be applied to abraded skin. *See* **capsicum**.

**capsicum.** Describes plants in the pepper family; substances derived from peppers can cause allergic reactions and skin irritation. Should not be applied to abraded skin.

**caramel.** A natural coloring agent.

**carbomers.** Thickening agents used primarily to create gel-like formulations.

**carbopol.** *See* **carbomer**.

**cardamom.** A plant from the ginger family, used as fragrance in cosmetics. It can be a skin irritant and sensitizer.

**carmine.** Natural red color that comes from the dried female cochineal beetle. It is sometimes used to color lip gloss, lipsticks, and other cosmetics.

**carnauba wax.** A vegetable wax that has as a hard, firm texture, and is used in cosmetics as a substantial thickening agent.

**carnitine.** A carboxylic acid that may be erroneously labeled an amino acid (which it is not); it has been claimed to have miraculous properties (unsubstantiated) for enhancing the metabolization of fat when taken orally; however, there is no known benefit for skin when applied topically.

**carnosic acid.** Extracted from **rosemary** and considered to be a potent antioxidant.

**carnosol acid.** *See* **carnosic acid**.

**carrageenan.** A seaweed gum used in cosmetics as a thickening agent with water-binding properties.

**carrot oil.** An emollient plant oil similar to other nonvolatile plant oils.

**casein.** A substance derived from milk protein that has some water-binding properties for skin.

**castor oil.** A vegetable oil derived from the castor bean. It is used in cosmetics as an emollient, though its unique property is that when dry it forms a solid film that can have water-binding properties. It is rarely associated with skin irritation or allergic reactions but its feel on skin can be slightly sticky.

**catalase.** An enzyme that decomposes hydrogen peroxide into water and oxygen.

*Caulerpa taxifolia* **extract.** *See* **algae**.

**cedarwood.** A fragrant plant extract that can be a skin irritant.

**celandine.** An extract from the plant also known as *Chelidonium majus* that has antiviral properties.

**cellulose.** The main fiber component of plants. It is used in cosmetics as a thickening agent and to bind other ingredients together.

*Centaurea cyanus*. *See* **cornflower**.

*Centella asiatica*. An herb that may appear on labels as asiatic acid, hydrocotyl, or gotu kola. Has some antibacterial properties, but can also constrict skin and may be a sensitizer and skin irritant.

*Cera alba*. Beeswax, used as a thickening agent in cosmetics.

ceramides. Naturally occurring skin lipids (fats). When used in skin-care products, they are good water-binding agents.

ceresin. Derived from clay, it is a waxy ingredient used as a thickening agent in cosmetics. It can be sensitizing for some skin types.

ceteareth-20. A **fatty alcohol** that is used to thicken cosmetics and keep ingredients mixed together and stable.

cetearyl alcohol. A **fatty alcohol** used as an emollient, emulsifier, thickener, and carrying agent for other ingredients. Can be derived naturally, as in coconut fatty alcohol, or synthetically.

cetyl alcohol. A **fatty alcohol** used as an emollient, emulsifier, thickener, and carrying agent for other ingredients. Can be derived naturally, as in coconut fatty alcohol, or synthetically. It is not an irritant and unrelated to SD alcohol or ethyl alcohol.

chamomile. An herb that has been shown to have anti-irritant and soothing properties.

charcoal. Baked wood that is mainly carbon. One teaspoonful of Activated Charcoal USP has a surface area of more than 10,000 square feet, which gives charcoal unique absorption properties. It also can disinfect wounds.

chaulmoogra oil. Taken internally it was once the treatment for leprosy worldwide. Topically it is an emollient that can also cause skin irritation.

chitosan. A dietary fiber derived from chitin. Chitin is a type of polysaccharide that comes from the shells of shellfish, which means it has good water-binding properties on skin.

chlorella. *See* **algae**.

cholesterol. A phospholipid (a type of human or animal fat) used in cosmetics as a stabilizer, an emollient, and a water-binding agent.

choline. One of the B-complex vitamins that may be an antioxidant but probably has no effect on skin.

*Chondrus crispus*. A form of red seaweed. *See* **carrageenan**.

chrysanthemum extract. Can have anti-inflammatory benefit for skin.

*Chrysanthemum parthenium* extract. *See* **feverfew extract**.

cinnamomum. *See* **cinnamon**.

cinnamon. Can be a skin irritant.

citric acid. Derived from citrus and used primarily to adjust the pH of products to prevent them from being too alkaline.

*Citrullus colocynthis*. Bitter apple; is considered to be a skin irritant.

clary oil. Used as fragrance, and can be a skin irritant or sensitizer.

clay. *See* **bentonite** and **kaolin**.

*Clematis vitalba* extract. A plant extract with no known benefit to skin; it may be a skin sensitizer.

clove oil. A potent skin irritant when used repeatedly.

clover blossom. Contains **eugenol**, which can be a skin sensitizer and cause photosensitivity.

clover leaf oil. *See* clover blossom.

cobalt gluconate. An element found in trace amounts in tissues of the body. While cobalt plays a vital role in the formation of some body systems, there is no evidence it serves any purpose topically on skin, though it may be an antioxidant.

cocamide DEA and MEA. *See* alkyloamides.

cocamide DEA. *See* DEA.

cocamidopropyl betaine. Considered to be one of the more gentle surfactants (*see* surfactant) used in skin-care products.

cocamidopropyl hydroxysultaine. A mild **surfactant**.

cocoa butter. An oil extracted from cocoa beans used as an emollient similar to the properties of all nonfragrant plant oils.

cocoglycerides. *See* glyceryl esters.

coconut oil. Has degreasing properties, which is why detergent cleansing agents are frequently derived from coconut oil.

*Codium tomentosum* extract. *See* algae.

coenzyme Q10. Can be an antioxidant in skin-care products.

*Coleus barbatus*. A member of the mint family; can be a skin irritant.

collagen. The major component of skin that gives it structure. Sun damage causes collagen in skin to deteriorate. Collagen can be derived from both plant and animal sources and is used in cosmetics as a good water-binding agent. Collagen in cosmetics, regardless of the source, has never been shown to have an effect on the collagen in skin.

colloidal oatmeal. *See* oatmeal.

colloidal silver. Refers to ground-up silver suspended in solution. *See* silver.

colostrum. The clear/cloudy "pre-milk" that female mammals secrete prior to producing milk. Colostrum contains immunoglobulins (disease resistance factors). While there is a small body of evidence indicating that adult consumption of colostrum may have disease-fighting potential, this is hardly substantiated and there is no known benefit when colostrum is applied topically to skin.

coltsfoot. According to *The PDR Family Guide to Natural Medicines & Healing Therapies*, coltsfoot has potential carcinogenic activity from its pyrrolizidine alkaloid content and is not recommended for repeated use.

comfrey extract. A plant source of allantoin, which gives this extract anti-irritant and anti-inflammatory properties.

**coneflower.** *See* **echinacea.**

**copper gluconate.** A mineral found in trace amounts in tissues of the body. While copper plays a vital role in the formation of many body systems, there is no evidence it serves any purpose topically on skin, though it may be a good antioxidant.

**copper peptides.** Substances that have a positive effect in wound healing, but despite claims, that does not translate to having an effect on wrinkles, as wrinkles are not wounds.

*Corallina officinalis* **extract.** *See* **algae.**

**coriander.** Also known as cilantro; is used as a fragrant component and can be a potential skin irritant. It may also have some antibacterial and antifungal properties, but this has not been established for skin.

**corn glycerides.** *See* **glyceryl esters.**

**corn oil.** An emollient oil with similar properties to other nonvolatile plant oils.

**cornflower.** A plant source of a blue dye used in skin-care products, though there is minimal evidence it may have antibacterial properties.

**cornstarch.** A starch obtained from corn and used as an absorbent; it can cause contact dermatitis, drying of skin, and can cause breakouts.

*Cornus* **extract.** *See* **dogwood.**

*Crataegus monogina* **extract.** From hawthorn plants; can have antibacterial properties. *See* **hawthorn extract.**

**crataegus.** *See* **hawthorn extract.**

**cucumber extract.** May have some anti-inflammatory properties but there is no real proof of this and the only notation seems to be anecdotal.

**cyanocobalamin.** Vitamin B12; has no known benefit when used topically on skin.

*Cyanotis arachnoidea.* A form of **guar gum.**

**cyclamen aldehyde.** A synthetic fragrant component in products; it can be a skin irritant.

**cyclomethicone.** A silicone with a drier finish than dimethicone.

*Cymbopogon martini.* *See* **geranium.**

*Cynara scolymus.* *See* **artichoke extract.**

**cysteine.** An **amino acid.**

**cytochrome.** A protein found in blood cells that, with the aid of enzymes, serves a vital function in the transfer of energy within cells. There are three types of cytochromes, indicated by A, B, or C, with cytochrome C being the most stable. However, because cytochromes require a complex process that is triggered by a sequence of other components in order to be effective in their function of cellular respiration, it serves no function alone on skin.

**D&C.** According to the FDA, D&C is an identification that indicates a coloring agent has been approved as safe in drug and cosmetics products but not in food.

**dandelion.** Can be particularly sensitizing for some atopic skin types but may also be irritating in general. It can also have water-binding and moisturizing properties.

**dandelion extract.** May have some anti-inflammatory properties, but this information is anecdotal and not supported by research.

**DEA.** A foaming agent in shampoos that can form nitrosamines.

**dead nettle extract.** When taken orally it can be of help for benign prostatic hyperplasia. Topically it has astringent properties and can be a skin irritant with repeated use.

**decyl glucoside.** Used as a gentle detergent cleansing agent.

**deionized/demineralized water.** Filtered water used in cosmetics. All water used in cosmetic formulations goes through this process to remove components that could interfere with a product's stability and performance.

***Delesseria sanguinea* extract.** *See* **algae**.

**denatured alcohol.** *See* **alcohol**.

**detergent cleansing agents.** *See* **surfactant**.

**dextran.** A polysaccharide that has water-binding properties for skin. *See also* **polysaccharide**.

**dextrin.** *See* **glycogen**.

**DHA.** *See* **dihydroxyacetone**.

**DHEA.** According to *HealthNews*, a newsletter from the publishers of *The New England Journal of Medicine*, though there is a small body of research showing that oral intake of DHEA may be helpful, for many reasons it may have more risks than positives. It is, most likely, a potent "steroid hormone called dehydroepiandrosterone, a chemical cousin of testosterone and estrogen ... Since DHEA is converted into testosterone, some women who take it grow body or facial hair and, if they are under age 50 or so, can stop menstruating. DHEA has also been shown to decrease levels of HDL ('good') cholesterol in women, and could increase the risk of heart disease." There is no research showing any positive or negative effects when it is used topically on skin.

**diatomaceous earth.** A light-colored porous rock composed of skeletons of minute sea creatures called diatoms, used typically as an abrasive material in scrub products.

**diazolidinyl urea.** A formaldehyde-releasing **preservative**.

**diethanolamine.** *See* **DEA**.

***Digenea simplex* extract.** *See* **algae**.

**dihydroxyacetone.** Reacts with amino acids found in the top layers of skin to create a shade of brown that takes place within two to six hours and builds color depth with every reapplication.

**dimethicone copolyol.** *See* **silicone**.

dimethicone. *See* silicone.

dipotassium glycyrrhizinate. *See* licorice extract.

disodium diglyceryl phosphate. *See* glyceryl esters.

disodium glyceryl phosphate. *See* glyceryl esters.

disodium lauraminopropionate. A mild surfactant (*see* surfactant).

disodium laureth sulfosuccinate. A mild surfactant.

DMDM hydantoin. Used with hydantoin to form a preservative. It slowly releases formaldehyde to give bactericidal properties to lotions.

DNA. The abbreviation for deoxyribonucleic acid, found in all cells. It is the primary component of genes—and genes are the way cells transmit hereditary characteristics. DNA is the basis for all genetic structure; its components include adenine (A), guanine (G), thymine (T), and cytosine (C). It is the mapping of these substances that is revealing the genetic code of human traits. The notion that putting DNA, RNA, or any of their components on skin can affect your own genetic structure is absolutely *not* possible.

dog rose. *See* rose hips.

dogwood. Can be an anti-irritant and anti-inflammatory on skin.

*Dong quai.* An herbal substance that was found to be no better than a placebo in treating hot flashes.

dulse. *See* algae.

*Durvillea antartica. See* seaweed.

echinacea. There are several types of echinacea but only *Echinacea purpurea* and *Echinacea pallida* have been shown to have effectiveness. These may have antibacterial and anti-inflammatory properties on skin.

ecosapentanoic acid. Derived from salmon oil; it is a good emollient for skin.

EDTA. The abbreviation for ethylenediaminetetraacetic acid. It is a stabilizer used in cosmetics to prevent ingredients in a given formula from binding with trace elements that can exist in water and other ingredients; the technical term for this function is a chelating agent.

egg yolk. Egg yolk is mostly water and lipids (fats), especially cholesterol, which makes it a good emollient and water-binding agent for skin.

*Elaeis guineesis.* Palm oil, which has emollient properties for skin, the same as any nonvolatile plant oil.

elastin. The major component of skin that gives it flexibility. Sun damage causes elastin in skin to deteriorate. Elastin can be derived from both plant and animal sources and is used in cosmetics as a good water-binding agent. Elastin in cosmetics has never been shown to affect the elastin in skin.

elderberry. May have anti-inflammatory properties on skin, though the evidence for this is mostly anecdotal.

**elecampane.** Can be very irritating to the skin and can trigger allergic reactions.

**emollients.** Substances that prevent water loss and have a softening and soothing effect on the skin. They can be natural, like almond oil, or manufactured, like mineral oil.

**emu oil.** An oil extracted from a large bird native to New Zealand. It is a good emollient and water-binding agent and has anti-inflammatory properties. It is not a miracle for the skin.

*Enteromorpha compressa* **extract.** An extract from a form of green algae. *See* **algae.**

**enzyme.** A biological catalyst that allows reactions between substances to take place.

*Ephedra sinica* **extract.** An extract from a Chinese herb also known as Ma huang; it has a high tannin and volatile oil content, which means it can be a skin irritant.

*Epilobium angustifolium* **extract.** Commonly known as fireweed. Can have anti-irritant properties for skin.

*Equisetum arvense. See* **horsetail extract.**

**ergocalciferol.** The technical name for vitamin D. *See* **vitamin D.**

**ergothioneine.** An amino acid with strong antioxidant properties; it is effective as a water-binding agent.

**erythritol.** A naturally occurring sugar found in plants and animal. Like all sugars, it has water-binding properties.

**erythrulose.** A substance chemically similar to the self-tanning agent **dihydroxyacetone.** Depending on your skin color, there can be a difference in the color effect for erythrulose. However, dihydroxyacetone completely changes the color of skin within two to six hours, while erythrulose needs about two to three days for the skin to show a color change.

**esculin.** A glycoside compound obtained from the horse chestnut tree. It is a good water-binding agent.

**essential oils.** *See* **volatile oils.**

**ethanol.** *See* **alcohol.**

**ethyl acetate.** A compound made from acetic acid and ethyl alcohol, that is used as a solvent in nail polish and nail-polish removers. May irritate skin.

**ethyl alcohol.** *See* **alcohol.**

**ethylene glycol.** *See* **propylene glycol.**

**ethylparaben.** *See* **parabens.**

**etidronic acid.** *See* **alcohol.**

**eucalyptus extract.** Can have antibacterial properties on the skin. It can also be a potent skin irritant, particularly on abraded skin.

**eucalyptus oil.** *See* **eucalyptus extract.**

*Eugenia caryophyllus. See* **clove oil.**

**eugenol.** *See* **clove oil** and **methyleugenol.**

*Euglena gracilis. See* **algae.**

*Euphrasia officinalis. See* eyebright.

evening primrose oil. Can have anti-inflammatory and emollient benefits for skin.

ext. D&C. According to the FDA, when Ext. D&C is followed by a color, it means the color is certified as safe for use only in drugs and cosmetics when used externally and not around the eyes or mouth. It is not safe for foods.

eyebright. A plant, and though the name sounds like it would be beneficial for the eye area, no known external benefit is attributed to this plant extract. The information for this plant on skin is strictly anecdotal.

*Fagus sylvatica* extract. Beech tree extract has no known benefit for skin. It can be used as a fragrant extract. (*See* volatile oils.)

farnesol. Extracted from plants and used in cosmetics primarily for fragrance. There is research demonstrating farnesol's effect in reducing pancreatic cancer in mice, but there is no evidence that this translates to a positive effect on skin.

farnesyl acetate. *See* farnesol.

fatty acids. Typically found in plant and animal lipids (fat), such as glycerides, sterols, and phospholipids. These are used in cosmetics as emollients, thickening agents, and when mixed with glycerin, cleansing agents.

fatty alcohols. Made from fatty acids (*see* fatty acids), and in cosmetics are thickening agents and emollients.

FD&C. According to the FDA, when FD&C is followed by a color, it is certified as safe for use in food, drugs, and cosmetics.

fennel extract. An extract from the fennel plant that can be a skin irritant.

fennel oil. A volatile, fragrant oil that can cause skin irritation and sensitivity.

*Ferula galbaniflua. See* galbanum.

feverfew extract. Can have anti-inflammatory benefit for skin.

fibronectin. A plasma protein. As is true for all proteins, regardless of their origin, it is a good water-binding agent for skin.

*Filipendula rubra. See* meadowsweet.

film former. Include ingredients such as PVP and acrylates that are used in hairstyling products to hold hair in place. When used in very small amounts in skin-care products, they can leave a smooth feel on skin and are good water-binding agents. They can be skin sensitizers for some individuals.

fir needle oil. A volatile, fragrant oil that can cause skin irritation and sensitivity.

flavonoids. Phenolic compounds found in plants, particularly broccoli, that are known to have potent antioxidant properties. Topically on skin, phenolic compounds can cause skin irritation.

floralozone. One of a number of synthetic fragrant components.

folic acid. Part of the B-vitamin complex; when taken orally, is considered a good antioxidant. That benefit has not been demonstrated on skin.

**fragrance.** A blend of either volatile, fragrant plant oils or synthetically derived oils that impart aroma and odor to products. *See* **volatile oils**.

**frankincense extract.** A fragrant component used in skin-care products that can be a skin irritant.

**free-radical damage.** Damage caused by reactive, volatile molecules. The damage is responsible for many human and nonhuman reactions, ranging from paint hardening to wrinkles and degenerative disease. The primary causes of free-radical damage are air and sunlight, but it can also triggered by cigarette smoke, herbicides, pesticides, pollution, and solvents. Antioxidants are a way to reduce and potentially neutralize the rampage of free-radical damage.

**fruit acids.** *See* **sugarcane extract**.

*Fu ling.* *See* **Poria cocos extract**.

*Fucus serratus* **extract.** *See* **algae**.

**galbanum.** A fragrant substance that, because of its resin and volatile oil content, can be extremely irritating and sensitizing on abraded skin.

**gamma linolenic acid.** Also known as GLA, a **fatty acid** used in cosmetics as an emollient and antioxidant. GLA is considered to promote healthy skin growth and is an anti-inflammatory agent. Good sources of GLA are black currant oil or seeds, evening primrose oil, and borage oil.

*Gan jiang.* *See* **ginger**.

**gelatin.** A protein obtained from plants or animals and that is used in cosmetics as a thickening agent.

*Gelidiela acerosa* **extract.** A type of algae. *See* **algae**.

**gentian extract.** A strongly bitter-tasting plant; it can have irritating and inflammatory properties.

**geranium oil.** A fragrant oil that can be a skin sensitizer or irritant.

**germanium.** According to Dr. Andrew Weil's Web site, "[There is] an FDA import ban aimed at germanium, a trace element used in the production of computer chips, which sometimes is identified as vitamin O. The FDA noted that consumption of germanium has caused kidney injury and death when used chronically by humans, even at dosages suggested on product labels. It has banned germanium imports intended for human consumption on the grounds that these products are either poisonous and deleterious to health or unapproved new drugs."

**ginger oil.** *See* **ginger**.

**ginger.** Can be a potent skin irritant.

*Gingko biloba.* An herb used in cosmetics for its anti-inflammatory, antioxidant, and anti-irritant properties.

**ginseng.** There is no evidence that any of the several kinds of ginseng can improve the appearance of the skin or that ginseng has any benefit topically.

**GLA.** *See* **gamma linolenic acid.**

**glucose oxidase.** An enzyme that has antibacterial and water-binding properties when used on skin.

**glucose tyrosinate.** *See* **tyrosine.**

**glutamic acid.** Is derived from wheat gluten and is an **amino acid** that can have water-binding properties for skin.

**glutamine.** An **amino acid.**

**glycereth-6 laurate.** *See* **glyceryl esters.**

**glycereth-17 cocoate.** *See* **glyceryl esters.**

**glycereth-20 stearate.** *See* **glyceryl esters.**

**glycereth-26 phosphate.** *See* **glyceryl esters.**

**glycerin.** A viscous fluid derived either synthetically or from plants. It is an emollient, a slip agent, and a humectant (*see* **water-binding agent**) and can keep water in skin. Myths about glycerin taking water out of the skin are inaccurate and do this great skin-care ingredient a disservice.

**glycerine.** *See* **glycerin.**

**glycerol.** *See* **glycerin.**

**glyceryl cocoate.** *See* **glyceryl esters.**

**glyceryl dipalmitate.** *See* **glyceryl esters.**

**glyceryl distearate.** *See* **glyceryl esters.**

**glyceryl esters.** A vast group of ingredients that are a mixture of **fatty acids** such as glycerides or **glycerin** mixed with other nonvolatile alcohols. These fats and oils are used in cosmetics as emollients and lubricants as well as binding and thickening agents.

**glyceryl glycyrrhetinate.** *See* **glyceryl esters.**

**glyceryl hydroxystearate.** *See* **glyceryl esters.**

**glyceryl isopalmitate.** *See* **glyceryl esters.**

**glyceryl isostearate.** *See* **glyceryl esters.**

**glyceryl palmitate.** *See* **glyceryl esters.**

**glyceryl ricinoleate.** *See* **glyceryl esters.**

**glyceryl stearate.** *See* **glyceryl esters.**

*Glycine soja.* Soybean oil, which has emollient properties for skin the same as any nonvolatile plant oil.

**glycine.** An **amino acid.**

**glycogen.** A common polysaccharide; it has water-binding properties for skin. *See* **polysaccharide.**

**glycolic acid.** *See* **AHAs.**

**glycolipids.** A fat effective as a **water-binding agent**.

**glycoproteins.** Used as water-binding agents.

**glycosaminoglycans.** A component of skin tissue that is used in skin-care products as a good water-binding agent.

**glycyrrhetic acid.** *See* **licorice extract.**

*Glycyrrhiza glabra.* The licorice plant. *See* **licorice extract.**

**goldenseal.** May have antibacterial or antiviral properties when taken orally, but there is no evidence that effect occurs when applied topically on skin. It can be a skin irritant.

**gotu kola.** *See Centella asiatica.*

**grape seed extract.** Has antioxidant properties.

**grape seed oil.** An emollient oil that also has good antioxidant properties. *See also* **linoleic acid.**

**grapefruit oil.** Can have antibacterial properties but can also be a potent skin irritant, especially on abraded skin.

**green tea.** An antioxidant that also has anti-irritant properties.

**guaiac wood.** Used as a fragrant extract in cosmetics and is a potent skin irritant.

*Guaiacum officinale.* *See* **guaiac wood.**

**guanine.** *See* **DNA.**

**guar gum.** A plant-derived thickening agent.

**guarana.** Guarana contains two and a half times more caffeine (*see* **caffeine**) than coffee. It can have constricting properties on skin and can therefore be a skin irritant.

**guava extract.** A fruit extract that can have constricting properties on skin, which makes it a potential skin irritant when used regularly.

**gums.** Substances that have water-binding properties but are primarily used as thickening agents in cosmetics. Some gums have a sticky feel and are used as film-forming agents in hairsprays, while others can constrict skin and have irritancy potential. Natural thickeners such as acacia, tragacanth, and locust bean are types of gums.

*Hamamelis virginiana.* *See* **witch hazel.**

**hamamelitannin.** The **tannin** concentration found in **witch hazel.** It can be a skin irritant.

*Haslea ostrearia.* Also known as blue algae. It is an extract that in pure concentrations can have antiviral properties on skin. *See also* **algae.**

**hawthorn extract.** Can have antibacterial properties, but may also dilate capillaries, making surfaced capillaries occur or look worse.

**hayflower extract.** A plant extract that, due to its constricting effect on skin, can be an irritant. There is no research supporting the claim it can regenerate skin cells.

**hedione.** A synthetic fragrant component in products that can be a skin irritant.

**helianthus oil.** *See* **sunflower oil.**

**helichrysum.** A plant family that includes strawflower. These plant extracts can have antibacterial properties for skin.

**hematin.** The iron-containing portion of blood. It has no known benefit for skin.

**hemp seed oil.** A fatty acid and an emollient. Other claims about healing skin are not substantiated.

**heptamethylnonane.** *See* **isohexadecane.**

**hesperidin.** A bioflavinoid that has antioxidant and water-binding properties for skin. It is also called "vitamin P," though it is not a vitamin and there is no such thing as vitamin P.

**hexylene glycol.** *See* **propylene glycol.**

**himanthalia.** *See* **algae.**

**histidine.** An **amino acid** that is effective as a water-binding agent.

**Hoelen.** *See* ***Poria cocos* extract.**

**honey.** Has antibacterial and preservative properties and can also function as a water-binding agent.

**honeysuckle.** A fragrant plant extract that can be a skin irritant but may also have anti-swelling properties.

**hops.** An aromatic plant that has astringent properties, which means it can be a skin irritant with repeated use.

**horse chestnut.** May have anti-inflammatory properties for skin, but it can also stimulate circulation, which can be a problem for those with surfaced capillaries. Orally it has been shown to reduce edema in the lower leg.

**horse-elder.** *See* **elecampane.**

**horseradish.** Can irritate skin and should never be applied to abraded skin.

**horsetail extract.** Can have skin-constricting properties, but it is a skin irritant and should not be used repeatedly on skin.

**humectant.** *See* **water-binding agent.**

**hyaluronic acid.** A component of skin tissue that is used in skin-care products as a good water-binding agent.

***Hydnocarpus anthelmintica.*** *See* **chaulmoogra oil.**

***Hydrastis canadenis.*** *See* **goldenseal.**

**hydrocortisone.** A hormone from the adrenal gland that can be synthetically derived. It has potent anti-inflammatory properties for skin, but prolonged use can destroy collagen in the skin.

**hydrocotyl extract.** *See* ***Centella asiatica.***

**hydrogenated castor oil hydroxystearate.** *See* **glyceryl esters.**

**hydrogenated coco-glycerides.** *See* **glyceryl esters.**

**hydrogenated lecithin.** *See* **lecithin.**

**hydrogenated palm glyceride.** *See* **glyceryl esters.**

**hydrolyzed reticulin.** Reticulin are fibers found in skin and thought to be part of a systematic network that surrounds collagen fibers and assists in holding them together. There is no evidence that when reticulin is applied externally to skin it can have any effect on collagen whatsoever. Hydrolyzed alters the form of the reticulin so it can be mixed into a skin-care product.

**hydrolyzed silk.** *See* **silk.**

**hydroquinone.** A substance that can reduce the intensity of freckles, melasma, and general brown patching by inhibiting melanin production. For continued and increased effectiveness it must be used for a longer term. Sun exposure should be avoided because it reverses the effect of hydroquinone by increasing melanin production. Occasionally, at higher concentrations, persons with a darker skin type will experience increased pigmentation, but this is rare. It can cause mild skin irritation and the possibility of an allergic reaction.

**hydroxylated lecithin.** *See* **lecithin.**

**hypericum extract.** Has no reported benefit for skin. It is taken orally for depression.

*Hypnea musciformis* **extract.** *See* **algae.**

**hyssop.** A fragrant plant extract with no known benefit for skin; it may be a mild skin irritant.

**illicium.** *See* **anise.**

**imidazolidinyl urea.** A commonly used cosmetic preservative (*see* **preservative**) that can cause contact dermatitis.

**Inositol.** Is not a vitamin (though it is sometimes mistaken for a B vitamin). It is a major component of **lecithin** and may have water-binding properties for skin.

*Inula helenium.* *See* **elecampane.**

**Irish moss extract.** *See* **algae.**

**iron oxides.** Compounds of iron that are used as colorings in some cosmetics. Also known as jewelers' rouge, and in crude form as rust.

**isocetyl salicylate.** *See* **sodium salicylate.**

*Isodonis japonicus* **extract.** A fragrant plant extract that contains terpenes (*see* **volatile oils**). It can be a skin irritant.

*Isodonis trichocarpus* **extract.** A fragrant plant extract that contains terpenes (*see* **volatile oils**). It can be a skin irritant.

**isohexadecane.** Used as a detergent cleansing agent, emulsifier, and thickening agent in cosmetics.

**isoleucine.** An amino acid.

**isopropyl alcohol.** *See* **alcohol.**

**isopropyl lanolate.** Used in cosmetics as a thickening agent and emollient.

**isopropyl myristate.** A substance known to cause clogged pores. According to *A Consumer's Dictionary of Cosmetic Ingredients,* 5th edition, this ingredient is associated with an increase in the risk of **nitrosamine** absorption.

**isopropyl palmitate.** Used in cosmetics as a thickening agent and emollient and, as is true for any emollient or thickening agent, can potentially clog pores, depending on the amount used in the product.

**ivy extract.** Can be a skin irritant due to its stimulant and astringent (skin-constricting) properties.

**Japan wax.** A vegetable wax obtained from sumac berries. It is used as a thickening agent and emollient in cosmetics.

**Japanese dandelion.** Can have anti-irritant properties.

**jasmine oil.** A fragrant oil, often used as a source of perfume, that can be a skin irritant or sensitizer. The oil is considered antidepressant and relaxing, and is used externally to soothe dry or sensitive skin.

**jojoba oil.** An emollient oil similar to all nonvolatile plant oils.

**jonquil extract.** A fragrant plant extract with a strong risk of skin irritation.

*Ju hua. See* **chrysanthemum extract.**

**juniper berry.** May have antibacterial properties but can be a skin irritant.

*Juniperus communis. See* **juniper berry.**

**kaolin.** A natural claylike mineral (silicate of aluminum) that is used in cosmetics for its absorbent properties.

**kava extract.** An extract from the plant *Piper methysticum* that has analgesic properties, which makes it an anti-inflammatory and anti-irritant for skin.

**kawa extract.** *See* **kava extract.**

**kelp.** May have anti-inflammatory properties for skin.

*Kigelia africana* **extract.** An extract from an African plant commonly known as Sausage Tree. The African lore about this extract is that it can firm breast tissue, but there is no supporting research for this myth.

**kiwi extract.** Used as a fragrance in cosmetics.

*Ko ken. See* **kudzu root.**

**kojic acid.** An extract of fungi (mushrooms) that has some reported value for preventing melanin production, though it is not as effective as **hydroquinone**. Kojic acid is considered to be more irritating than hydroquinone though kojic acid does have antioxidant properties.

**kola nut.** Can have anti-inflammatory properties; the major active ingredient of the nut is **caffeine**.

*Krameria triandra.* Commonly known as rhatany; it has a high tannin content and skin constricting properties, making it a significant skin irritant.

**kudzu.** An herb with no known benefit for skin. When taken internally it can dilate capillaries. If this effect is repeated on the skin it can be a problem for creating surfaced capillaries.

**lactates.** Natural or synthetic ingredients used in cosmetics as emollients, thickening agents, and lubricants.

**lactic acid.** An alpha hydroxy acid (*see* **AHAs**) extracted from milk, though most forms used in cosmetics are synthetic. It exfoliates cells on the surface of skin by breaking down the material that holds skin cells together. It may irritate mucous membranes and cause irritation.

**lactobacillus ferment.** A beneficial bacteria that is used to brew beer. It has no known benefit for skin.

**lactoferrin.** A protein usually derived from milk (particularly breast milk); it can also be found in saliva. It can have antiviral, antibacterial, and anti-inflammatory effect on skin.

**lactoperoxidase.** An enzyme derived from milk that has antibacterial properties for skin.

**lady's mantle extract.** *See* ***Alchemilla vulgaris***.

**lady's thistle extract.** Can have anti-inflammatory properties.

**laminaria.** *See* **algin**.

***Lamium album.*** *See* **dead nettle extract**.

**lanolin alcohol.** An emollient derived from lanolin; it is considered to be less of an allergen than pure lanolin.

**lanolin.** Derived from the sebaceous glands of sheep. It is considered to be very emollient for dry skin but can be a skin allergen for some.

**lappa extract.** *See* **burdock root**.

**L-ascorbic acid.** Considered to be a good antioxidant and anti-inflammatory agent, but claims about its eliminating or preventing wrinkles are not substantiated.

**lauramphocarboxyglycinate.** A mild surfactant (*see* **surfactant**).

**laureths.** Substances that in various combinations create a wide range of mild detergent cleansing agents called surfactants (*see* **surfactant**).

**lauryl alcohol.** *See* **surfactant**.

**lavender oil.** A fragrant oil that can be a skin irritant and a **photosensitizer**.

**lecithin.** A **phospholipid** (a type of human or animal fat) used in cosmetics as a stabilizer, surfactant, and water-binding agent.

**lemon balm.** *See* **balm mint**.

**lemon oil.** Can be a skin irritant, especially on abraded skin.

**lemon.** A potent skin sensitizer and irritant. Though it can have antibacterial properties, the irritation can hurt the skin's immune response.

**lemongrass extract.** Can be irritating and sensitizing for skin but may have antibacterial properties.

***Lentinus edodes*** **extract.** An extract from the shiitake mushroom that has antimicrobial and antibacterial properties. Shiitake mushrooms have a long history of use in Japan to prevent certain cancers and tumors; however, there is no information about their effect on skin.

**lettuce extract.** Can have anti-inflammatory properties for skin.

leucine. An amino acid.

licorice extract. Contains corticosteroids and has anti-inflammatory properties.

licorice root. *See* licorice extract.

lime oil. *See* lemon oil.

*Limnanthes alba*. *See* meadowfoam.

linalool. A fragrant component of plants that can be can a skin irritant or sensitizer.

linden flower extract. When taken internally it can increase perspiration and may have cardiotoxic effects. Topically, it has been shown to have skin-constricting properties that can prove to be irritating for skin.

linoleic acid. A fatty acid used as an emollient and thickening agent in cosmetics.

linolenic acid. *See* gamma linoleic acid.

linseed oil. *See* gamma linoleic acid.

lipids. A wide range of ingredients found in plants and skin that includes fatty acids, sebum, and fats. In skin-care products, these are emollients and thickening agents.

liposomes. A delivery system (not an ingredient) capable of holding other ingredients and releasing them once the liposome is absorbed into the skin. The research first establishing liposomes as a worthwhile delivery system has not held up over time.

*Litsea cubeba*. *See* lemongrass.

locust bean. *See* gums.

*Lonicera japonica*. *See* honeysuckle.

lupin oil. An extract of *Lupinus albus*, a legume, in oil form; it has emollient properties.

lupine. *See* lupin oil.

*Lupinus albus* extract. *See* lupin oil.

lysine. An amino acid.

macadamia nut oil. An emollient oil similar to all nonvolatile plant oils.

*Macrocystis pyrifera*. *See* algin.

magnesium aluminum silicate. A powdery, dry-feeling white solid that can be used as a thickening agent and powder in cosmetics.

magnesium ascorbyl palmitate. A stable derivative of ascorbic acid. When used in a cream with a 10% concentration, magnesium ascorbyl palmitate was shown to inhibit melanin production. It has also been shown to have a protective effect against inflammation caused by UVB sun exposure. It is considered to be a good antioxidant and anti-inflammatory agent, but claims about its eliminating or preventing wrinkles are not substantiated.

magnesium ascorbyl phosphate. *See* magnesium ascorbyl palmitate.

magnesium hydroxide. The active ingredient in milk of magnesia. It is an absorbent and has antibacterial properties for skin.

magnesium laureth sulfate. A mild detergent cleansing agent.

magnesium oleth sulfate. A mild detergent cleansing agent.

**magnesium stearate.** Used as a thickening agent in cosmetics.

**magnesium.** An earth mineral that has strong absorbent properties and some disinfecting properties.

**malic acid.** *See* **AHAs.**

**mallow.** Can be used as a thickening agent in cosmetics and may have anti-inflammatory properties.

**malvacae extract.** There are 1,000 species of malvacea, found in tropical and temperate regions the world over. There is no information about the effect any of these have for skin.

**mandarin orange.** A volatile oil used as a fragrance that can be a skin irritant.

**manganese gluconate.** A mineral found in trace amounts in tissues of the body. While manganese plays a vital role in the formation of many body systems, there is no evidence it serves any purpose topically on skin, though it may be an antioxidant.

**mannan.** A **polysaccharide** that is a good water-binding agent and film-forming agent.

**marigold.** *See* **calendula extract.**

**matricaria oil.** *See* **chamomile extract.**

**MEA.** *See* **alkyloamides.**

**meadowsweet.** Can have anti-inflammatory properties and benefit for skin.

*Melaleuca alternifolia.* *See* **tea tree oil.**

*Melia azadirachta.* *See* **neem extract.**

**melibiose.** A saccharide that can have good water-binding properties. *See* **mucopolysaccharide.**

*Melissa officinalis.* *See* **balm mint.**

*Mentha arvensis.* *See* **mint.**

*Mentha piperita.* *See* **peppermint.**

*Mentha spicata.* *See* **spearmint.**

**menthol.** Is derived from peppermint, and can have the same irritating effect on skin.

**menthyl lactate.** *See* **menthol.**

**methanol.** *See* **alcohol.**

**methionine.** An amino acid.

**methylchloroisothiazolinone.** A preservative that should be used only in rinse-off products as it can be too irritating when left on skin.

**methyldihydrojasmonate.** Synthetic fragrant components.

**methyleugenol.** A natural constituent of such plant oils as rose, basil, blackberry, cinnamon, and anise. According to the November 9, 1998, issue of *The Rose Sheet* (an insider cosmetics-industry newsletter), the National Toxicology Program Board of Scientific Counselors concluded that "methyleugenol, a component of a number of essential oils, has shown clear evidence of carcinogenic activity in male and female rats and mice." The study is an animal model and so it may or may not relate to humans.

**methylisothiazolinone.** A preservative that should be used only in rinse-off products as it can be too irritating when left on skin.

**methylparaben.** *See* parabens.

**methylsilanol mannuronate.** *See* silicone.

**methylsilanol PEG-7 glyceryl cocoate.** *See* glyceryl esters.

**mica.** An earth mineral used to give products sparkle and shine.

**micrococcus lysate.** An enzyme derived from bacteria. It can break down foods and is present in the human body. It has no known benefit in skin care.

**milk protein.** *See* proteins.

**mimosa.** A volatile oil used as a fragrance that can be a skin irritant.

**mineral oil.** A clear, odorless oil derived from petroleum that is widely used in cosmetics because it rarely causes allergic reactions and can't become a solid and clog pores. Despite mineral oil's association to petroleum and the hype that it is bad for skin, keep in mind that petroleum is a natural ingredient derived from the earth and that once it becomes mineral oil, it has no resemblance to the original petroleum.

**mink oil.** Considered to be similar to human sebum and therefore an effective emollient. The miraculous claims made for this ingredient are not proven, and in moisturizers it is not preferable to or more effective than plant oils.

**mint.** Can be a skin irritant and cause contact dermatitis.

**mixed fruit acids.** *See* sugarcane extract.

**mixed fruit extracts.** *See* sugarcane extract.

**montmorillonite.** *See* bentonite.

**mucopolysaccharide.** A natural component of skin that is used in skin-care products as a good water-binding agent.

**mugwort extract.** Can have antibacterial properties but can also be a skin irritant.

**mulberry extract.** Has some value in preventing melanin production though there is only one study demonstrating this. However, the pure concentration was minimally effective when compared to **hydroquinone** and **kojic acid.**

**myristates.** Generally forms of **fatty acids** used in cosmetics as thickening agents and emollients. As is true for any emollient, these can potentially clog pores, depending on the amount used in the product.

**myristic acid.** A detergent cleansing agent that also creates foam and can be drying.

**myristyl myristate.** Used in cosmetics as a thickening agent and emollient.

**N-acetyl-L tyrosine.** *See* tyrosine.

**NaPCA (sodium PCA).** *See* sodium PCA.

**neem extract.** A plant extract that has antibacterial properties.

**neopentanate.** Used in cosmetics as a thickening agent and emollient.

**neopentyl glycol dicaprylate/dicaprate.** Used as an emollient and thickening agent.

**neroli oil.** A fragrant plant oil; it can be a skin irritant or sensitizer.

**nettle extract.** Depending on the plant parts used for the extract, it can be a skin irritant. However, this is primarily found in fresh plants. It can have an antibacterial effect on skin.

**niacinamide.** Vitamin B3. There are a handful of studies demonstrating that when a 4% concentration of niacinamide is applied topically in gel form, it can have similar effects to the topical prescription drug clindamycin. However, this research is primarily from the company that makes this product (Papulex, 4% Niacinamide), and it can still cause dryness and inflammation. Some existing animal studies and in vitro studies on human fibroblasts (cells that produce connective tissue such as collagen) have demonstrated that niacinamide may have an effect on skin tumors. However, there is no research for niacinamide in relation to wrinkles or anything else having to do with sun-damaged skin.

**niaouli oil.** Extracted from a plant variety of **melaleuca**; has similar properties as a possible topical disinfectant.

**nitrosamines.** Can be formed in cosmetics when amines (DEA, MEA, or TEA) are combined with a formaldehyde-releasing preservative (bronopol or quaternium-15, among others). Nitrosamines are known for their carcinogenic properties. There is controversy as to whether or not this poses a real problem for skin given the fractional concentrations used and the question of whether or not nitrosamines can even penetrate skin.

**nonacnegenic.** A term meant to indicate a product will not clog pores and cause breakouts. This term is not regulated by the FDA or any organization, so a cosmetic company can make this claim regardless of proof or substantiation of any kind.

**noncomedogenic.** A term meant to indicate a product will not clog pores. This term is not regulated by the FDA or any organization, so a cosmetic company can make this claim regardless of proof or substantiation of any kind.

**nonoxynols.** Used as mild surfactants. *See* **surfactant.**

**nylon-12.** A powder substance that is used as an absorbent and thickening agent.

**oak root extract.** May have antibacterial properties on skin but can also be a skin irritant.

**oatmeal.** Has absorptive, soothing, and anti-inflammatory properties.

**octocrylene.** A sunscreen agent that protects from the UVB range of sunlight.

**octyl methoxycinnamate.** A sunscreen agent used to protect primarily from the sun's UVB rays.

**octyl palmitate.** Used in cosmetics as a thickening agent and emollient.

**octyl salicylate.** A sunscreen agent used to protect primarily from the sun's UVB rays.

**octyl stearate.** Used in cosmetics as a thickening agent and emollient.

**o-cymen-5-ol.** A preservative.

**oleic acid.** A mild surfactant. *See* **surfactant.**

**oleic/linoleic triglyceride.** *See* **glyceryl esters.**

**oleths.** Mild surfactants. *See* **surfactant.**

**olibanum extract.** *See* **frankincense extract.**

**olive oil PEG-6 esters.** *See* **glyceryl esters.**

**olive oil.** An emollient plant oil similar to all nonvolatile plant oils.

*Opuntia ficus-indica* **extract.** An extract from the Indian fig or prickly pear cactus. Orally there is some evidence it can alleviate prostate inflammation. For skin it can have some emollient properties.

**orange (bitter).** Can have antibacterial benefit on skin but, due to the fragrant component, it can also be a skin irritant.

**orange (sweet).** Can have antibacterial benefit on skin but, due to the fragrant component, it can also be a skin irritant.

**orange blossom.** A fragrant extract that can also be a skin irritant.

**orange flower extract.** Can be a skin irritant and sensitizer.

**orchid.** A fragrant extract that can be a skin irritant.

*Origanum majorana.* The herb marjoram. Its fragrant component is used in cosmetics and can be a skin irritant.

**orris root.** Causes frequent allergic or sensitizing skin reactions.

**osmanthus.** A fragrant plant used in perfumes that can also be a skin irritant.

**oxybenzone.** A sunscreen agent that protects primarily from the sun's UVB rays.

**ozokerite.** A mineral that is used as a thickening agent in cosmetics, especially for lipsticks and stick foundations.

*P. elisabethae.* The "*P.*" is short for *Pseudopterogorgia. See* **sea whip extract.**

**PABA.** *See* **para-aminobenzoic acid.**

**padimate O.** A sunscreen agent that protects primarily from the sun's UVB rays.

*Paeonia suffruticosa* **extract.** *See* **peony extract.**

**palm glyceride.** *See* **glyceryl esters.**

**palmarosa oil.** *See* **geranium.**

**palmitates.** Generally, forms of **fatty acids** used in cosmetics as thickening agents and emollients. As is true for any emollient, they can potentially clog pores, depending on the amount used in the product.

**palmitic acid.** A detergent cleansing agent that also creates foam and can be drying.

*Panax schinseng. See* **ginseng.**

**panthenol.** A substance derived from the vitamin B-complex. It has a thick, syrupy texture with humectant properties. It is also used as an emollient.

**papain.** *See* **bromelain.**

**papaya extract.** A source of papain (*see* **bromelain**) that can have exfoliating properties on skin. However, papaya extract is not the same thing as papain any more than wood is the same as paper. Papaya can be a skin irritant.

**para-aminobenzoic acid (PABA).** A sunscreen ingredient rarely used because of strong possible allergic reactions.

**parabens. Preservatives** used in cosmetics to prevent bacterial and fungal growth in products. The amounts used are so small they are considered safe unless a person has specific allergies to this type of ingredient.

**paraffin.** A waxy petroleum-based substance. Used as a thickener for cosmetics.

**paraffinum liquidum.** *See* **mineral oil**.

**Parsol 1789.** *See* **avobenzone**.

**patchouli.** A fragrant oil from mint. It contains **eugenol** and can be a skin sensitizer and irritant.

*Paullinia cupana.* *See* **guarana**.

**pawpaw extract.** *See* **papaya**.

**pea extract.** May have some antioxidant benefit for skin.

**peanut oil.** An emollient plant oil similar to all nonvolatile plant oils.

**pectin.** A natural substance found in plants, especially apples, and used in cosmetics as an emulsifier and thickening agent.

**PEG compounds.** PEG stands for polyethylene glycol. Various forms of PEGs are mixed with fatty acids and fatty alcohols to create a variety of substances that have diverse functions in cosmetics, including surfactants, binding agents (to keep ingredients blended), stabilizers, and emollients.

**PEG-80 sorbitan laurate.** A mild surfactant (*see* **surfactant**).

*Pelargonium graveolens* **oil.** *See* **geranium oil**.

**pellitory.** An herb that can have antibacterial properties for skin, though it can also constrict skin tissue and be an irritant; it also has potential for causing contact dermatitis.

**peony extract.** There is no research demonstrating this to have any effectiveness for skin.

**peppermint (oil or extract).** Can have an irritating, sensitizing effect on skin.

**perfluoropolymethylisopropyl ether.** A film-forming agent.

*Perilla ocymoides* **oil.** Derived from the seeds of the *Perilla ocymoides* plant and used to make varnishes, printing ink, and paints; in cosmetics it is used as a fragrance additive. It can be a skin irritant.

*Persea gratissima.* *See* **avocado oil**.

**petitgrain mandarin.** *See* **mandarin orange**.

**petrolatum.** Vaseline is petrolatum. *See also* **mineral oil**.

*Phellodendron amurense* **extract.** An extract of the Amur Corktree; it can have anti-inflammatory benefits.

**phenoxyethanol**. A formaldehyde-releasing **preservative**.

**phenyl trimethicone**. A **silicone** with a drier finish than dimethicone.

**phenylalanine**. An **amino acid**.

**phospholipids**. *See* **water-binding agent** and **glyceryl esters**.

**photosensitizer**. Ingredients that can cause the skin to have an irritated or inflammed reaction when exposed to sunlight.

**phytic acid**. A natural plant antioxidant.

**phytonadione**. *See* **vitamin K**.

*Pimpinella anisum*. *See* **anise**.

**pine needle extract**. *See* **pine oil**.

**pine oil**. Can be a skin irritant and should never be used on abraded or chafed skin.

**pineapple extract**. Contains the enzyme **bromelain**, which can break down the connecting layers between skin cells to exfoliate skin. However, bromelain is a more effective source of exfoliation without the other irritating properties of the pineapple.

*Piper nigrum*. *See* **black pepper**.

**placenta protein**. *See* **placenta** and **protein**. Protein works the same on skin regardless of the source. It is just a good water-binding agent.

**placenta**. Obtained from the afterbirth of animals. It is supposed to have rejuvenating properties for skin, but this claim has never been proven in research of any kind. Much like any part of a human or animal body, the placenta is a source of proteins, amino acids, and other water-binding agents for skin. It cannot make skin act young just because the source is young.

**placental extract**. *See* **placenta**.

**plasticizing agents**. Ingredients that place a thin layer of plastic over the skin; typically these are used in facial masks so they can be peeled off the skin. *See* **film former**.

*Pogostemon cablin*. *See* **patchouli**.

**poloxamers**. *See* **surfactant**.

**polyethylene glycol**. Polyethylene is the most typical form of plastic used in the world. It is flexible and has a smooth, waxy feel. When ground up, the small particles are used in scrubs as a gentle abrasive. When mixed with glycol, it becomes a viscous liquid that in pure concentrated form is antifreeze. In the minuscule amounts used in cosmetics, it helps keep products stable and performs functions similar to **glycerin**. Because polyethylene glycol can penetrate skin, it is also a vehicle that helps deliver other ingredients deeper into the skin. It is even used internally in medical procedures to flush and clean the intestinal tract.

**polyethylene**. *See* **polyethylene glycol**.

**polyglucuronic acid**. *See* **film former**.

**polyglyceryl methacrylate**. *See* **film former**.

**polyglyceryl-2 caprate**. *See* **glyceryl esters**.

**polyquaterniums.** A group of thickening agents with very distinct properties that are compatible to skin and hair. Polyquats have an affinity for the surface of skin and leave a soft, pleasant film on the skin.

**polysaccharide.** A natural component of skin that can be a good water-binding agent and antioxidant for skin.

**polysorbates. Fatty acids** that are used as emollients and thickening agents in cosmetics.

**polyvinyl alcohol.** *See* **plasticizing agents.**

**polyvinylpyrrolidone.** Usually listed on ingredient labels as PVP or PVP copolymer. It is one of the primary ingredients used in hairstyling products to hold hair in place. Used in minuscule amounts in skin-care products, it places an imperceptible film over the skin that is considered to be water-binding and that helps give the appearance of firmer skin. It can be a skin sensitizer for some individuals. *See also* **film former.**

**pomegranate extract.** Contains ellagic acid, and is considered to be effective as an anticarcinogen when taken orally. Its role in skin care is as an antioxidant.

*Poria cocos* **extract.** Derived from a mushroom with antiviral and antibacterial properties. Also known as Hoelen and Fu ling.

*Porphyridium cruentum.* A type of red algae. *See* **algae.**

**potassium hydroxide.** Also known as potash lye, and is a highly alkaline ingredient used to modulate the pH of a product. It is also used as a cleansing agent in some cleansers.

**potassium myristate.** A detergent cleansing agent that is a constituent of soap that can be drying and sensitizing for some skin types.

**potassium thiocyanate.** A salt that can be a potent skin irritant and can also have antibacterial properties for skin.

**potassium.** An earth mineral that has strong absorbent properties and some disinfecting properties but can also be a potent skin irritant.

**pregnenolone acetate.** A precursor to other hormones; it can affect levels of progesterone and estrogen in the body when taken orally. When applied to skin it may work as a water-binding agent. There is no information if absorption through skin is possible.

**preservatives.** Substances used in cosmetics to prevent bacterial and microbial contamination of products. While there is definitely a risk of irritation from these types of ingredients, the risk to skin and eyes from using a contaminated product is considered by many scientists to be even greater.

*Primula veris* **extract.** Derived from primrose or cowslip plants. It has no known benefit for skin.

**progesterone.** Because the issue of using USP progesterone is so complicated, please refer to the section in this book on "Battling Hormones" for more information.

*See also* **wild yams** in this glossary.

**prolamine extract.** A protein that has water-binding and antioxidant properties.

**proline.** An **amino acid**.

**propolis.** A brownish, resinous material that is collected by bees and is then used in the formation of the hive. It has antibacterial and anti-inflammatory properties for skin. The belief that this is a miracle skin-care ingredient is myth and not based on any research or data.

**propylene glycol.** A clear, colorless, slightly syrupy liquid that is an aliphatic alcohol compound (that means it is derived chemically from the alcohols—*see* **alcohol**). All the glycols help enhance the effectiveness and penetration of active or other ingredients in a formula, and have water-binding and moisturizing properties. Despite a lot of misleading information in the cosmetics industry, the glycols are safe as used in cosmetics. According to the U.S. Department of Health and Human Services' Public Health Service's Agency for Toxic Substances and Disease Registry, "Studies also have not shown these chemicals [propylene or the other glycols as used in cosmetics] to be carcinogens."

**propylparaben.** *See* **parabens**.

**protein.** A fundamental component of human and plant life. In skin-care products, proteins act as emollients and water-binding agents. They cannot affect, change, or rebuild the structure of skin. Whether the protein is derived from an animal or a plant, the skin can't tell the difference.

*Prunus armeniaca.* Apricot extract.

*Pueraria lobata.* *See* **kudzu**.

**pullulan.** Produced by black yeast. It is a glucan gum that contains **polysaccharides**, which makes it a good water-binding agent, thickening agent, and antioxidant.

**purified water.** *See* **deionized water**.

**PVP.** *See* **polyvinylpyrrolidone**.

**PVP copolymer.** *See* **polyvinylpyrrolidone**.

**pyridoxine hydrochloride.** Vitamin B6; can have antibacterial and antioxidant benefits for skin when applied topically.

*Pyrus cydonia.* *See* **quince seed**.

*Pyrus malus.* A species of apple; the pectin derived from it is used as a thickener in cosmetics; as an extract, it is used for its acidic quality.

**quaternium-15.** A formaldehyde-releasing **preservative** used in cosmetics. It can be a skin sensitizer, as can all preservatives.

**quercus.** *See* **oak root extract**.

**quillaja extract.** Is extracted from Chilean soap bark tree. It contains a good amount of saponins, which have some cleansing, antimicrobial, and water-binding properties for skin. *See* **saponins**.

**quince seed.** Used as a thickening agent in cosmetics, but this also has skin-constricting properties and can cause skin irritation.

**raspberry extract.** Can be a skin irritant or sensitizer with no known benefit for skin.

**red algae.** *See* algae.

**red clover flowers.** *See* **clover flower.**

**red raspberry extract.** Can be a skin irritant or sensitizer with no known benefit for skin.

*Rehmannia glutinosa.* A Chinese herb known as Di huang that has no known benefit for skin.

**Renova.** *See* **Retin-A.**

**resorcinol.** Considered an effective, though overly irritating topical disinfectant. It is rarely used any longer for treating blemishes.

**respiratory enzyme.** Enzymes that interact with several other biological and physiological processes for the activation and use of oxygen in the body. There is no evidence that any respiratory enzyme can do anything topically for skin.

**Retin-A.** The active ingredient in Retin-A and Renova is tretinoin (technically, all-trans retinoic acid). This is the acid form of vitamin A. There is a great deal of research establishing tretinoin as being effective in improving abnormal cell production often caused by sun damage. Tretinoin is a valid method of addressing wrinkles and overall making an improvement in cell production. Applying tretinoin doesn't produce miraculous results, but the positive outcome in terms of skin health is indisputable. *However*, irritation from using tretinoin on the skin is highly possible and a major drawback of this prescription drug.

**retinoic acid.** The active ingredient in **Retin-A** and Renova.

**retinol.** The technical name for (preformed) vitamin A (vitamin A is created in the body from beta-carotene). Cosmetics companies from Estee Lauder to Neutrogena, Avon, and others all have their assortment of products containing retinol or retinyl palmitate, and their claims mirror those made for **Retin-A** and Renova. But can cosmetics containing retinol or retinyl palmitate perform like tretinoin? The answer is, maybe but probably not. Retinol must become all-trans retinoic acid to work like tretinoin, and that process requires a series of steps and changes. The notion that the skin can perform this action with retinol is unproven and considered by many to be unlikely. It is even more improbable for this to happen with the ingredient retinyl palmitate. Retinyl palmitate is an ester of vitamin A. An ester is a compound several generations removed from the original form. This means that while retinol has to go through several steps to become all-trans retinoic acid in the skin, retinyl palmitate has to go through even more of a change. Because retinol is such an unstable ingredient, its packaging is of vital concern. Any container that allows sunlight and air exposure means the retinol will not be stable for very long if at all after opening.

retinyl palmitate. *See* retinol.

rhatany. *See* krameria extract.

*Rhus succedanea. See* Japan wax.

rice bran oil. An emollient oil similar to other nonvolatile plant oils.

rice starch. An absorbent substance used in place of talc. It can cause allergic reactions and as a food derivative (as opposed to a mineral derivative like talc), it can generate bacteria growth in the pore.

ricinoleate. Used in cosmetics as a thickening agent and emollient.

*Ricinus communis. See* castor oil.

RNA. *See* DNA.

*Rosa canina. See* rose hips.

*Rosa centifola. See* cabbage rose extract and rose flower.

*Rosa roxburghii* extract. An extract from the chestnut rose; it can be a source of antioxidants for skin, and does not impart fragrance.

rose flower. A highly fragrant substance that can be a skin irritant.

rose hips oil. A good emollient oil that has antioxidant properties.

rose hips. A source of vitamin C. May have some antioxidant benefit for skin.

rose oil. A fragrant, volatile oil that can be a skin irritant and sensitizer.

rosemary extract. Can have some antioxidant benefit for skin but can also be a skin sensitizer.

rosemary oil. Can have some antioxidant benefit for skin but may also be a skin sensitizer and irritant due to its constricting properties on skin.

*Rosmarinus officinalis. See* rosemary extract.

royal jelly. A milky white, thick substance secreted by worker bees that has been shown to have some antibacterial and emollient benefit on skin. The myriad other claims for stopping wrinkles and healing acne are all anecdotal with no researched substantiation.

*Rubus idaeus. See* red raspberry extract.

*Ruscus aculeatus. See* butcher's broom extract.

rutin. A bioflavinoid that is extracted from various plants and used as an antioxidant and emollient.

saccharames. *See* yeast.

saccharide isomerate. A good water-binding agent and emollient for skin.

saccharides. *See* mucopolysaccharides.

*Saccharum officinarum.* Sugarcane plant. Glycolic acid is derived from sugarcan. However, sugarcane extract does not have the same exfoliating properties as glycolic acid. *See* AHAs.

safflower oil. An emollient plant oil similar to all nonvolatile plant oils.

sage extract. Can be a potent antioxidant, but it also contains camphor and phenolic compounds and can be a skin irritant. It can also have antibacterial properties for skin.

**salicylic acid.** The active ingredient in aspirin. It is used in cosmetics as an exfoliant, and is the only source of beta hydroxy acid (BHA). As an exfoliant, in concentrations of 8% to 12%, it is effective in wart-remover medications. In concentrations of 0.5% to 2% it is far more gentle, and, much like AHAs (*see* **AHAs**), can exfoliate the surface of skin. BHA also has the ability to penetrate into the pore (AHAs do not), and can exfoliate inside the pore as well; it is thus considered effective for reducing clogged pores and breakouts. Because BHA is related to aspirin (both are salicylates), it retains some of aspirin's anti-inflammatory properties. In this regard BHA is anecdotally considered a good option for those with rosacea.

*Sambucus nigra.* *See* **elderberry.**

**sandalwood oil.** A fragrant oil that causes skin irritation or allergic reactions.

*Sang zhi.* Derived from twigs of the mulberry tree and has some effect on reducing swelling.

**sanguinaria.** *See* **bloodroot.**

*Santalum album.* *See* **sandalwood.**

*Saponaria officinalis* extract. *See* **soapwort.**

**saponin.** A group of plant constituents known as glycosides that have a distinctive foaming, soapy characteristic. As a glycoside, a saponin can have water-binding properties for skin. There is some evidence that saponins can have antimicrobial benefit for skin.

*Sargassum filipendula* extract. *See* **algae.**

**saturated fat.** A type of fat usually of animal origin. Chemically, when fatty-acid chains can't accommodate any more hydrogen atoms, they are saturated.

**sausurrea.** A volatile oil and fragrant component used in cosmetics; it can be a skin irritant. It is known to cause contact dermatitis.

**saw palmetto.** An herb that may have an anti-inflammatory influence on the skin. Saw palmetto's primary reputation is about reducing the presence of the male hormone dihydrotestosterone and it could thereby reduce hair loss, which has not been proven. There is some anecdotal information that it can have estrogenic effects, but that is unlikely, and is highly improbable when applied topically.

*Saxifraga sarmentosa* extract. *See* **strawberry begonia.** Has no known benefit for skin.

**sclareolide.** Extracted from **sage** and used as a fragrant component in cosmetics.

**sclerotium gum.** Used as a thickening agent.

**scullcap extract.** A herbal extract that has antibacterial and anti-inflammatory properties for skin.

*Scutellaria baicalensis* extract. *See* **scullcap extract.**

**SD alcohol.** *See* **alcohol.**

**sea whip extract.** An extract from a form of coral reef creature, known for its anti-inflammatory properties. Harvesting part of the ocean's coral reef system is of serious ecological concern.

**seaweed.** A group of sea plants with a gelatin-like consistency. Seaweed has antioxidant properties but other claims and benefits are not proven. *See* **algae.**

**sebaceous glands.** Glands in the skin that open into hair follicles and from which sebum is secreted.

**sebacic acid.** Used as a pH adjuster.

**selenium.** A mineral considered to be a potent antioxidant.

**sericin.** *See* **silk.**

**serine.** An **amino acid** effective as a water-binding agent.

**serum protein.** *See* **protein.**

**sesame oil.** An emollient oil similar to other nonvolatile plant oils.

**sesquioleate.** Used in cosmetics as a thickening agent and emollient.

**Shao-yao.** *See* **peony root.**

**shea butter.** An emollient plant lipid that is used as a rich emollient in cosmetics.

*Sigesbeckia orientalis.* A Chinese herb also known as St. Paul's wort. It has anti-inflammatory properties.

**silica.** A mineral found abundantly in sandstone, clay, and granite, as well as parts of plants and animals. It is the principal ingredient of glass. In cosmetics it is used as an absorbent powder and thickening agent.

**silicate.** An inorganic salt that has potent absorbing and thickening properties.

**silicone.** A substance derived from silica (sand is a silica). The unique fluid properties of silicone give it a great deal of slip and in its various forms it can feel like silk on the skin, impart emolliency, and be a water-binding agent that holds up well, even when skin becomes wet.

**silk.** As used in cosmetics it is a protein with good water-binding and moisturizing properties, just the same as any other protein. Whether the protein is derived from animals or plants, the skin can't tell the difference.

**silver.** A metal that in cosmetics can have disinfecting properties; however, prolonged contact can turn skin grayish-blue and can be irritating to skin.

**slip agents.** A term used to describe a range of ingredients that help other ingredients spread over the skin, as well as help ingredients to penetrate into the skin. Slip agents also have humectant properties. Slip agents include propylene glycol, butylene glycol, polysorbates, and glycerin, to name a few. They are as basic to the world of skin care as water.

**slippery elm bark.** Can be an anti-irritant and anti-inflammatory.

**soap.** A bar-type cleanser. Its composition is specifically controlled by the FDA. In order for a product to be called a soap it must contain lye and fat. It can be drying and irritating to skin.

**soapwort.** A plant extract with detergent cleansing properties.

**sodium ascorbate.** *See* **ascorbic acid.**

**sodium bisulfite.** Used in acid permanent waves to alter the shape of hair. It is less damaging than alkaline permanent waves but it is also limited as to how much change it can affect in hair. It can be a skin irritant.

**sodium borate.** Considered a potent skin irritant, especially if used on abraded skin.

**sodium C14-16 olefin sulfate.** Can be derived from coconut. It is used primarily as a detergent cleansing agent but is considered to be potentially drying and irritating for skin.

**sodium carbonate.** An absorbent salt used in cosmetics that can also be a skin irritant.

**sodium chloride.** Common table salt. It is used primarily as a binding agent in skin-care products and occasionally as an abrasive in scrub products.

**sodium cocoyl isethionate.** Derived from coconut and is a somewhat mild detergent cleansing agent (*see* **surfactant**).

**sodium hyaluronate.** *See* **hyaluronic acid.**

**sodium hydroxide.** The scientific name for lye. It is a highly alkaline ingredient used to modulate the pH of a product. It is also used as a cleansing agent in some cleansers.

**sodium laureth sulfate.** Can be derived from coconut; it is used primarily as a detergent cleansing agent. It is considered to be gentle and effective.

**sodium laureth-13 carboxylate.** *See* **surfactant.**

**sodium lauryl sulfate.** Can be derived from coconut; it is used primarily as a detergent cleansing agent. There is a great deal of misinformation about this ingredient. It is not toxic or dangerous for skin. However, it is considered to be a potent irritant, and is the standard irritancy substance used (meaning it is assumed it will net an irritated reaction) to measure and compare the irritancy potential of other ingredients.

**sodium metabisulfite.** A reducing agent that alters the structure of hair. It can also be used as a preservative in formulations, and can be a skin irritant.

**sodium methyl taurate.** A mild surfactant (*see* **surfactant**).

**sodium PCA.** A natural component of skin that is also a very good water-binding agent.

**sodium salicylate.** The salt form of salicylic acid (BHA). When it is no longer an acid, salicylic acid no longer has exfoliating properties.

**sodium silicate.** A highly alkaline and potentially irritating antiseptic and mineral used in cosmetics.

sodium sulfite. A reducing agent that alters the structure of hair. It can also be used as a preservative in cosmetic formulations, and can be a skin irritant.

sodium thioglycolate. *See* thioglycolates.

sodium trideceth sulfate. *See* surfactant.

*Solanum lycopersicum. See* tomato extract.

soluble fish collagen. *See* collagen.

sorbitan stearate. Used to thicken and stabilize cosmetic formulations.

sorbitol. Can be derived synthetically or from natural sources. It is a humectant, thickening agent, and slip agent. It is similar to glycerin.

soybean extract. An antioxidant and soothing agent for skin. However, the estrogenic effects it can have when taken orally are not duplicated when the extract is applied topically to skin.

soybean oil. An emollient oil similar to all nonvolatile plant oils.

spearmint oil. A fragrant, volatile oil that can cause skin irritation and allergic reactions.

spikenard. A plant that has antibacterial properties for skin.

*Spiraea ulmaria. See* meadowsweet.

spirulina. *See* algae.

squalane. *See* squalene.

squalene. An oil derived from shark liver or from plants and sebum. It is considered a good emollient for skin.

St. John's wort. *See* hypericum extract.

star anise. *See* anise.

stearalkonium chloride. An antistatic ingredient used in hair-care products to control flyaways and aid in combability.

stearates. *See* stearic acid.

stearic acid. A fatty acid (*see* fatty acids) used as an emollient and to help keep other ingredients intact in a formulation (*see* thickening agent).

stearyl alcohol. A fatty alcohol (*see* fatty alcohols) used as an emollient and to help keep the other ingredients intact in a formulation.

strawberry begonia. A plant that as no known benefit for skin.

strawberry leaves. Can be a skin irritant and skin sensitizer, with no known benefit for skin.

sugarcane extract. Ingredients like sugarcane extract, fruit extracts, mixed fruit extracts, and milk solids claim an association with AHAs, but they are not the same thing nor do they have the same effect on skin. While glycolic acid (*see* AHAs) is indeed derived from sugarcane, assuming that sugarcane will net you the same result as glycolic acid would be like assuming you could write on a tree the way you can on paper. Even though paper is derived from wood, that still doesn't mean you can use wood the same way you can paper. The pure form does not have the same effect as the derived effective ingredient. The same is true for lactic acid derived from milk. If milk were as acid as lactic acid (*see* **AHAs**) you would not be able to drink it without serious complications. There is a vast difference between the extracted, pure ingredient versus the original form it may have come from.

**sulfur.** A mild antibacterial agent that can be a potent skin irritant and sensitizer. Sulfur also has a high pH, and that can encourage the growth of bacteria on skin.

**sumac.** A plant that can be a skin irritant.

**sunflower oil.** An emollient plant oil similar to all nonvolatile plant oils.

**surfactant.** Surfactant is an acronym for <u>Surface</u> <u>Active</u> <u>Agent</u>. These agents degrease and emulsify oils and fats and suspend soil, allowing them to be washed away. I refer to these substances throughout my writing as detergent cleansing agents. They are used in all forms of cleansers and are, for the most part, considered to be gentle and effective for most skin types. They can be sensitizing for some.

**sutilain.** *See Bacillus subtilis.*

**sweet almond oil.** *See* **almond oil.**

**tangerine oil.** A fragrant, volatile oil that can be a skin irritant.

**tannin.** Can be extracted from a number of plant sources ranging from tea to sumac. It has constricting properties on skin, which may help with wound healing, but can be a skin irritant when applied repeatedly to skin.

*Taraktogenos kurzii. See* **chaulmoogra oil.**

*Taraxacum officinale. See* **dandelion.**

*Taraxacum platycarpum. See* **Japanese dandelion.**

**tartaric acid.** *See* **AHAs.**

**tea tree oil.** Also known as **melaleuca.** According to the *Healthnotes Review of Complementary and Integrative Medicine,* "[5% tea tree oil and 2.5% benzoyl peroxide] were effective in reducing the number of inflamed lesions [blemishes] throughout the trial, with a significantly better result for benzoyl peroxide when compared to the tea tree oil. Skin oiliness was lessened significantly in the benzoyl peroxide group versus the tea tree oil group." There are presently no skin-care products that contain more than 1% of tea tree oil and most contain less.

**TEA.** *See* **triethanolamine.**

**TEA-lauryl sulfate.** *See* **sodium lauryl sulfate.**

*Terminalia sericea.* A plant extract with a high incidence of irritation or contact dermatitis.

**tetrasodium EDTA.** A water softener; this substance is a bonding agent that links with minerals to prevent them from causing microbial growth.

*Thea sinensis* extract. *See* **green tea.**

**thickening agents.** Substances that can have a soft to hard waxlike texture or a creamy, emollient feel, and can be great lubricants. There are literally thousands of ingredients in this category that give every lotion, cream, lipstick, foundation, mascara, and so on its distinctive feel and form.

**thioglycolates.** Compounds used in permanent waves and depilatories either to alter the structure of hair or to dissolve it. These are potent skin irritants.

**thiotaurine.** A good antioxidant.

**threonine.** An **amino acid** that is effective as a water-binding agent.

*Thuja occidentalis* **extract.** Also known as extract of red or yellow cedar. It has antibacterial properties on skin but it also has constricting properties and can be a skin irritant.

**thyme extract.** From the thyme plant; has no established benefit for skin though it may have antibacterial properties and can cause inflammation.

**thymus extract.** *See* **thymus hydrolysate.**

**thymus hydrolysate.** A form of animal thymus derived by acid, enzyme, or other method of hydrolysis. It can have water-binding properties for skin but has no other special or unique benefit.

*Thymus vulgaris.* *See* **thyme extract.**

**Tian men dong.** A Chinese herbal asparagus extract; it has no known benefit for skin.

*Tilia cordata.* *See* **linden flower extract.**

**tissue respiratory factor (TSP).** A protein present on the surfaces of cells. As an extract in skin-care products it may offer some water-binding benefits, but there is no evidence it has any other function on skin.

**titanium dioxide.** An inert earth mineral used as a thickening, whitening, lubricating, and sunscreen ingredient in cosmetics. It protects from UVA and UVB radiation and is considered to have no risk of skin irritation.

**tocopherol acetate.** *See* **vitamin E.**

**tocopheryl lineolate.** *See* **vitamin E.**

**toluene.** A solvent used in nail polishes; it is considered toxic with repeated use.

**tomato extract.** May have some water-binding properties, but without specifics about what part of the plant the extract comes from, there is no way to know whether it may also be irritating for skin.

**tormentil extract.** From the plant *Potentilla erecta*, a tuber that is used for its reddish dye content.

**tragacanth.** A natural **gum** used as a thickener in cosmetics.

**tranexamic acid.** When used orally is an antihemophilic medicine; topically it is an anti-inflammatory agent.

**tretinoin.** The active ingredient in the prescription medication **Retin-A** and Renova.

**triacetin.** *See* **glyceryl esters.**

**tribenzoin.** *See* **glyceryl esters.**

**triclosan.** A disinfectant primarily used in products claiming to kill germs on the hands. There is little evidence that these products are helpful for reducing bacterial or viral infections.

tridecyl salicylate. The salt form of salicylic acid (BHA). When it is no longer an acid, salicylic acid no longer has exfoliating properties.

tridecyl stearate. Used in cosmetics as a thickening agent and emollient.

tridecyl trimellitate. Used in cosmetics as a thickening agent and emollient.

triethanolamine. Used in cosmetics as a pH balancer. Like all amines, it has the potential for creating nitrosamines. There is controversy as to whether or not this poses a real problem for skin, given the fractional concentrations used in cosmetics and the theory that nitrosamines can't penetrate skin.

Trifolium pratense. See clover blossom.

triglyceride. See glyceryl esters.

trilaurin. Used as an emollient and thickening agent in cosmetics.

trioctanoin. An emollient and thickening agent used in cosmetics.

tristearin. Used as an emollient and thickening agent in cosmetics.

Triticum vulgare. See wheat germ oil.

tuberose. See orchid.

turmeric. A natural food coloring.

Tussilago farfara. See coltsfoot.

tyrosine. In skin, tyrosine is an amino acid that initiates the production of melanin (melanin is the component of skin that gives it "color"). According to information on the FDA's Web site, tyrosine's "use is based on the assumption that it penetrates the skin, increases the tyrosine content of the melanocytes, and thus enhances melanin formation. This effect has not been documented in the scientific literature. In fact, an animal study reported a few years ago demonstrated that ingestion or topical application of tyrosine has no effect on melanogenesis [the creation of melanin]."

ubiquinone. See coenzyme Q10.

Ulva lactuca extract. An extract from the plant known as sea lettuce. It has some water-binding and antioxidant properties for skin.

umbilical extract. Much like any part of any human or animal body, the umbilical cord is a source of proteins, amino acids, and other water-binding agents for skin. It cannot make skin act young just because the source is young.

urea. A component of urine, though synthetic versions are used in cosmetics. Urea has good water-binding and exfoliating properties for skin.

Uva ursi extract. See bearberry.

VA/crotonates copolymer. See VA/crotonates.

VA/crotonates. A type of film-forming agent.

Vaccinium myrtillus. See bilberry extract.

valerian. An herb that has no known benefit for skin.

**valine**. An **amino acid**.

**verbena**. A fragrant extract that can be a skin irritant.

**vetiver oil**. A fragrant component in skin-care products that can also be a skin sensitizer.

**vinegar**. Consists of **acetic acid** and water. The alcoholic liquor used to ferment the acetic acid (such as apple cider or wine) determines the color and flavor. It does have mild disinfecting and antifungal properties, but according to a study in *Infection Control and Hospital Epidemiology*, January 2000, commercial disinfectants are far more able to kill germs and bacteria than vinegar. Vinegar can be a skin irritant.

**vitamin A**. Considered a good antioxidant. Claims that it can perform like the active ingredient in Renova are not substantiated.

**vitamin C**. Considered a good antioxidant. Claims that it can prevent or eliminate wrinkling are not proven.

**vitamin D**. Provides no known benefit for skin though it may have antioxidant benefits.

**vitamin E**. Considered one of the more stable and reliable antioxidants used in cosmetics, but may be an allergen for some people. There is no evidence that it can help heal scars, and because of skin sensitivity, it can actually impede the healing process for some.

**vitamin K**. The primary claims for the use of vitamin K cosmetics are to reduce the appearance of dark circles under the eyes and reduce the appearance of surface capillaries. Yet there is no independent research showing vitamin K to be effective for any aspect of skin care. The study quoted for this proof was done by the patent holder and the company selling vitamin K products.

**volatile oils**. Volatile fluids derived primarily from plants used in cosmetics primarily as fragrant additives. These components most often include a mix of alcohols, ketones, phenols, linalool, borneol, terpenes, camphor, pinene, acids, ethers, aldehydes, and sulfur, which all have extremely irritating and sensitizing effects on skin.

**walnut extract**. A coloring agent in cosmetics.

**walnut oil**. An emollient, nonvolatile plant oil.

**walnut-shell powder**. An abrasive used in scrub products.

**water-binding agent**. A wide range of ingredients that help skin retain water. Glycerin is one of the more typical and effective water-binding agents used in cosmetics. One group of water-binding agents can mimic the skin's actual structure and can be of benefit in a formulation; these include ceramide, lecithin, glycerin, polysaccharides, hyaluronic acid, sodium hyaluronate, mucopolysaccharides, sodium PCA, collagen, elastin, proteins, amino acids, cholesterol, glucose, sucrose, fructose, glycogen, phospholipids, glycosphingolipids, and glycosaminoglycans. No single one of these is preferred over the other, as none of them can change the actual structure of skin.

**watercress extract**. A source of mustard oil, which can be a skin irritant. It can have antibacterial properties for skin.

**wheat germ glycerides.** *See* **glyceryl esters.**

**wheat germ oil.** An emollient plant oil similar to all nonvolatile plant oils.

**wheat protein.** *See* **protein.**

**white oak bark extract.** *See* **oak root extract.**

**wild yam extract.** Does not contain progesterone or anything else that would act like progesterone. According to *The PDR Family Guide to Natural Medicines & Healing Therapies* and the *American Journal of Obstetrics and Gynecology*, volume 18, 1999, wild yam is used in the production of artificial [synthetic] progesterone in the laboratory, but it will not yield the hormone in the absence of a chemical conversion process that the body can't supply on its own.

**willow bark.** Contains salicin, a substance that when taken orally is converted by the digestion process to **salicylic acid** (beta hydroxy acid). The process of converting willow bark to salicylic acid requires the presence of enzymes to turn the salicin into salicylic acid. The digestive conversion process that turns salicin into saligenin, and then into salicylic acid, is complicated. Further, salicin, much like salicylic acid, is stable only under acidic conditions. The likelihood that willow bark in the tiny amount used in cosmetics can mimic the effectiveness of salicylic acid is at best problematic, and in all likelihood impossible. However, willow bark may indeed have some anti-inflammatory benefits for skin because, in this form, it appears to retain more of its aspirin-like composition.

**wintergreen oil.** A very irritating and skin-sensitizing ingredient.

**witch hazel.** Though witch hazel can have minimal anti-inflammatory properties in its pure form, according to the *Consumer's Dictionary of Cosmetic Ingredients,* fifth edition, "Witch hazel can have an ethanol [alcohol] content of 70 to 80 percent. Witch hazel water … contains 15% ethanol." The alcohol content can be an irritant. Witch hazel also has a high tannin content that can also be irritating when it is used repeatedly on skin, though when used for initial swelling from burns it can reduce inflammation.

**Wu wei zi.** Also know as *Schisandra chinensis,* this is an herb that can have a constricting effect and can be a skin irritant.

**xanthan gum.** Used as a thickening agent.

**Xi xin.** *See* **ginger extract.**

**ximenia oil.** Plum oil; can have emollient properties.

**xylitol.** *See* **sorbitol.**

**yarrow extract.** A plant extract that can be a skin irritant due to its constricting effect on skin.

**yeast.** A group of fungi that ferment sugars. Yeast is a source of **betaglucan**, which is considered a good antioxidant.

**ylang-ylang.** A fragrant, volatile oil (*see* **volatile oils**) that can also be a skin irritant.

**yucca extract.** A plant extract that can have anti-inflammatory benefits.

**zinc gluconate.** A combination of zinc with a form of glucose (a sugar) that is commonly used in cold lozenges for its antiviral effects. There is no other known benefit topically for skin. *See also* **zinc.**

**zinc.** Studies in the 1970s linked zinc to having a positive effect on acne, but those studies were never duplicated or considered to have any real significance for skin. Taken orally, zinc may have effects for wound healing and other health benefits, but this is not experienced topically. It can be a skin irritant.

**zinc oxide.** An inert earth mineral used as a thickening, whitening, lubricating, and sunscreen ingredient in cosmetics. One manufacturer of zinc oxide has heavily promoted this ingredient as being the only option for broad-spectrum sun protection. This has not been proven out from other independent research. Along with titanium dioxide, it is considered to have no risk of skin irritation, though both of these minerals can clog pores.

**zinc sulfate.** Results from the interaction of zinc with sulfuric acid. *See* **zinc.**

# Animal Testing and Cosmetics

For more information please refer to NAVS's book *Personal Care for People Who Care*, now in its tenth edition, or visit the Web site at www.navs.org.

**Companies that do not use animal testing on their finished products:**

Acne-Statin
Adrien Arpel
Alexandra de Markoff
Almay
Aloette
Alpha Max
Amway
Arbonne
Aubrey Organics
Aveda
Avon
bare escentuals and
  bareMinerals
Bath & Body Works
Beauty for All Seasons/
  Norma Virgin Makeup
Beauty Without Cruelty
Bioelements
Biogime
BioMedic
BioTherm
Black Opal
Blistex
Bobbi Brown
The Body Shop
Bonne Bell
Burt's Bees
CamoCare
Cellex-C
Chanel
Clarins
Clear LogiX
Clinique
Color Me Beautiful
Decleor Paris
Dermablend
Dr. Hauschka Skin Care

eb5
Ecco Bella
Estee Lauder
Exuviance by Neostrata
Fashion Fair
Flori Roberts
Forever Spring
Freeman Cosmetics
Guinot
Iman
Jafra
Jane
Janet Sartin
Jason Natural Cosmetics
Kiehl's
L'Oreal
La Mer
La Prairie
Lancome
Lord & Berry
M.A.C.
Marilyn Miglin
Mario Badescu
Mary Kay
Maybelline
Merle Norman
Moisturel
Murad
Neutrogena
Nivea Visage and
  Nivea Vital
Noevir
Nu Skin USA
Obagi
Origins
Orlane
Paula's Choice and
  Paula's Select
philosophy

Prescriptives
PropapH
R Pro
Rachel Perry
Ralph Lauren Polo Sport
Rejuveness
Revlon
Serious Skin Care
Shaklee
Shu Uemura
Smash Box
St. Ives
TheraCel
Tommy Hilfiger
Tova
Trish McEvoy
Ultima II
Victoria's Secret Cosmetics
Wet 'n' Wild
Yves Rocher
Zhen
Zia Natural Skin Care

**Companies that continue to use animal testing:**

5S
Aapri
Aveeno
Bain de Soleil
Calvin Klein
Cetaphil (Galderma)
Clairol
Clean & Clear
Clearasil
Coppertone
Coty
Cover Girl
Dove
Elizabeth Arden
Erno Laszlo

Johnson & Johnson
Lac Hydrin
  (Bristol-Myers Squibb)
Lubriderm
Max Factor
Noxzema
Olay
Oxy Balance
Pond's
Purpose
RoC
Sea Breeze
Shiseido
Suave
Vaseline Intensive Care

**Companies with unknown animal-testing status:**

Ahava
Alpha Hydrox
Anna Sui Makeup
Aqua Glycolic
Ashley Skin Care
Awake
Basis
BeautiControl
BeneFit
Cargo
Chantecaille
Christian Dior
Circle of Beauty
Clinac
Club Monaco
Corn Silk
Darphin
DDF
Dermalogica
DHC USA
Diane Young
Dr. Mary Lupo
English Ideas
Epicuren
Eucerin
Exact
FACE Stockholm

Fashion Fair
Gale Hayman of
  Beverly Hills
Givenchy
Glymed Plus
Guerlain
Hard Candy
Hope Aesthetics
Hydron
IGIA
J.C. Penney Professionals
Jan Marini
Jane Iredale
Janet Sartin
Jergens
Joan Rivers Results
Karin Herzog Skin Care
Kinerase
Kiss My Face
Laura Mercier
Le Mirador
Lip Ink
Liz Earle Naturally Active
  Skin Care
L'Occitane
Lorac
Lush
M.D. Formulations and
  M.D. Forte
Marcelle
Mederma
Models Prefer
Mojave Magic
Moisturel
NARS
Natura Bisse
Nature's Cure
Neostrata
Nicole Miller Skin Care
N.V. Perricone, M.D.
Ombrelle
Osmotics
Pan Oxyl
Parthena
Paula Dorf Cosmetics

Peter Thomas Roth
Pevonia
pHisoDerm
Physicians Formula
Phytomer
Prestige Cosmetics
Principal Secret
ProActiv
Reflect.com
Rejuvenique
Remede
Renew Skin Care Formula
Ré Vive
Rimmel
Sage Skin Care
Sears Studio Makeup and
  Sears T.I.M.E.
Selleca Solution
Sephora
Sisley
SkinCeuticals
Sonia Kashuk
Sothys Paris
Stila
Stridex
Sudden Youth
Three Custom Color
T. Le Clerc
Tony & Tina
Vichy
Victoria Jackson Cosmetics
Vincent Longo
University Medical
  Skin Care
Urban Decay
Yves St. Laurent
Yon-Ka Paris
Youngblood
ZAPZYT

# Research Sources for This Edition

*Botanicals: A Phytocosmetic Desk Reference*
D'Amelio
CRC Press, 1999
2000 Corporate Boulevard NW
Boca Raton, FL 33431

*The Chemistry and Manufacture of Cosmetics*
Allured Publishing Corp.
362 S. Schmale Road
Carol Stream, IL 60188-2787
Tel: (630) 653-2155

*Concise Science Dictionary of Cosmetics Ingredients, 3rd Edition*
Oxford University Press, 1996
Great Clarendon Street
Oxford, England OX2 6DP

*A Consumer's Dictionary of Cosmetic Ingredients, 5th Edition*
Winter
Three Rivers Press, 1999
201 East 50th Street
New York, NY 10022

*Cosmeceuticals, Active Skin Treatment*
Allured Publishing Corp.
362 S. Schmale Road
Carol Stream, IL 60188-2787
Tel: (630) 653-2155

Cosmetic Dermatology *(journal)*
Quadrant HealthCom Inc.
26 Main Street
Chatham NJ, 07928-2402
Tel: (973) 701-8900

Cosmetic, Toiletry, and Fragrance Association (CTFA)
1101 17th Street N.W., Suite 300
Washington, DC 20036-4702
Tel: (202) 331-1770

*Cosmetic, Toiletry, and Fragrance Association (CTFA) Scientific/Regulatory Reference Guide, 1997 Edition*
Cosmetic Ingredient Review Board
1101 17th Street N.W., Suite 300
Washington, DC 20036-4702
Tel: (202) 331-1770

*Cosmetics & Toiletries* (magazine)
Allured Publishing Corp.
362 S. Schmale Road
Carol Stream, IL 60188-2787
Tel: (630) 653-2155

*Drug & Cosmetics Industry (DCI)* (magazine)
Advanstar Communications
P.O. Box 5045
Pittsfield, MA 01203-9683
Tel: (888) 527-7008

*Encyclopedia of Common Natural Ingredients, 2nd edition*
by Albert Y. Leung and Steven Foster
John Wiley & Sons, Inc.
605 Third Avenue
New York, NY 10158-0012
Tel: (212) 850-6000

*F-D-C Reports*—The Rose Sheet *(newsletter)*
5500 Friendship Blvd., Suite One
Chevy Chase, MD 20815-7278
Tel: (800) 844-8974

*The Food and Drug Law Journal*
1000 Vermont Ave. N.W., Suite 200
Washington, DC 20005-4903
Tel: (202) 371-1420

*Healthnotes Review of Complementary and Integrative Medicine*
Healthnotes Inc.
1505 SE Gideon Street, Suite 200
Portland, OR 97202

*Household & Personal Products Industry (HAPPI)* (magazine)
Rodman Publishing
17 South Franklin Turnpike
Ramsey, NJ 07446
Tel: (201) 825-2552

*The Journal of the American Medical Association*
Subscriber Services Center
P.O. Box 10945
Chicago, IL 60610
Fax: (312) 464-5831

*The New England Journal of Medicine*
Massachusetts Medical Society
10 Shattuck Street
Boston, MA 02115-6094
Tel: (617) 734-9800

*The PDR Family Guide to Natural Medicines & Healing Therapies*
Ballantine Publishing, 1999
201 East 50th Street
New York, NY 10022

*Personal Care for People Who Care*,
9th edition
National Anti-Vivisection Society
53 W. Jackson Blvd.
Chicago, IL 60604
Tel: (800) 888-6287

*Personal Care Formulas*
Allured Publishing Corp.
362 S. Schmale Road
Carol Stream, IL 60188
Tel: (630) 653-2155

*http://BoDD.cf.ac.uk/ BoDDHomePage.html*
(Botanical Dermatology Database)

*http://metalab.unc.edu/herbmed/eclectic/ kings/main.html*
(King's American Dispensatory)

*http://onhealth.com/alternative/resource/ herbs/*
(Onhealth with WebMd Herbal Index)

*www.AAD.org*
(on-line information from the American Academy of Dermatology)

*www.botanical.com/*
(Aromatic and Medicinal Plants Index)

*www.egregore.com/Misc/herbindx.htm*
(Medicinal Herbs On Line)

*www.FDA.gov*
(Web site for the U.S. Food and Drug Administration)

*www.hcrc.org*
(Health Care Reality Check—Science-based Information on Alternative and Complementary Medicine)

*www.healthlink.com.au/nat_lib/index.htm*
(Health Link OnLine Resources)

*www.herb.com*
(Global Botanical Exchange)

*www.herbalgram.org*
(American Botanical Council Online)

*www.hort.purdue.edu/newcrop/med-aro/ toc.html*
(Aromatic and Medicinal Plants Index)

*www.lancet.com*
(medical journal on-line)

*www.matrix.ucdavis.edu/DO/desk/ desk.html*
(Dermatology Online Journal)

*www.Medscape.com*
(medical journal on-line)

www.ncbi.nlm.nih.gov/pubmed
(Web site for the National Library of Medicine)

*www.thorne.com/altmedrev/index.html*
(Alternative Medicine Review)

*www.vitamins.com/encyclopedia/Index*
(Herbal Encyclopedia)